Nutrition and Diagnosis-Related Care

FIFTH EDITION

Sylvia Escott-Stump, MA, RD, LDN

Dietetic Programs Director
East Carolina University
Greenville, North Carolina
and
Consulting Dietitian
Nutritional Balance
Winterville, North Carolina

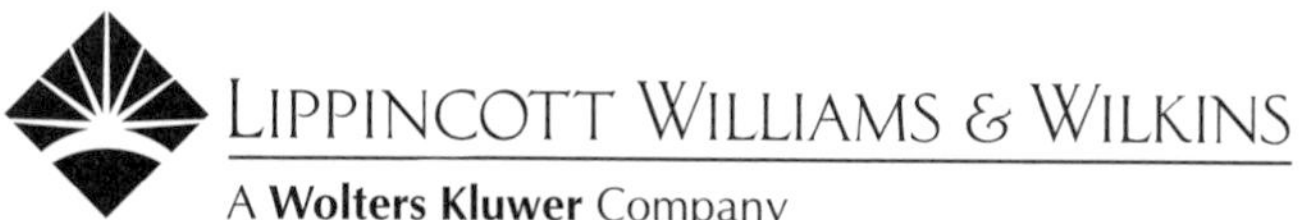

Philadelphia • Baltimore • New York • London
Buenos Aires • Hong Kong • Sydney • Tokyo

Editor: David Troy
Managing Editor: Matt Hauber
Marketing Manager: Paul Jarecha
Production Editor: Christina Remsberg
Compositor: Peirce Graphic Services
Printer: Courier

351 West Camden Street
Baltimore, Maryland 21201-2436 USA

530 Walnut Street
Philadelphia, PA 19106

Printed in the United States of America

First Edition, 1985
Second Edition, 1988
Third Edition, 1992
Fourth Edition, 1997

Library of Congress Cataloging-in-Publication Data

Escott-Stump, Sylvia.
Nutrition and diagnosis-related care / Sylvia Escott-Stump.—5th ed.
p. ; cm.
Includes bibliographical references and index.
ISBN 0-7817-3760-5
1. Diet therapy—Handbooks, manuals, etc. 2. Nutrition—Handbooks, manuals, etc. I. Title.
[DNLM: 1. Diet Therapy—Handbooks. 2. Nutrition—Handbooks. WB 39 E74n 2002]
RM217.2 .E83 2002
615.8'54—dc21

2002069452

The publishers have made every effort to trace the copyright holders for borrowed material. If they have inadvertently overlooked any, they will be pleased to make the necessary arrangements at the first opportunity.

To purchase additional copies of this book, call our customer service department at **(800) 638–3030** or fax orders to **(301) 824–7390.** International customers should call **(301) 714–2324.**

Visit Lippincott Williams & Wilkins on the Internet: http://www.LWW.com. Lippincott Williams & Wilkins customer service representatives are available from 8:30 am to 6:00 pm, EST.

05
3 4 5 6 7 8 9 10

Diagnosis-Related Care

FIFTH EDITION

FOREWORD

This book is a valuable resource for registered dietitians, dietetic students, and other healthcare professionals involved or interested in medical nutrition therapy (MNT). Given the increasing time demands confronting healthcare professionals, efficient time management is essential for delivering high quality patient care. The ever-changing healthcare environment necessitates that registered dietitians efficiently and effectively maintain their high level of practice skills. Maintaining and growing practice skills in a time-effective manner are essential to provide maximum time for patient-care activities. This book "fits the bill" as a key resource for prioritizing patient care and appropriately planning a nutrition treatment course. The guidance provided by *Nutrition and Diagnosis-Related Care* will be of immense value in charting the clinical course for each patient. It will be of great value for both routine and familiar cases and especially valuable in dealing with clinical conditions that the practitioner does not routinely treat.

Notable features of the book include an extensive array of clinical conditions that are dealt with routinely in dietetic practice including normal nutrition situations such as pregnancy and lactation. This book presents an extensive compilation of nutrition-care information in a most succinct way. An impressive attribute is that the germane information required by dietitians is presented in a single resource. This greatly simplifies the development of nutrition-care plans for patients. Thus, this book provides dietetic practitioners with superb guidance they can use to maintain outstanding practice skills. This book is a resource that can help achieve excellence in dietetic practice.

Penny Kris-Etherton PhD, RD
Pennsylvania State University

Karen Kubena, PhD, RD
Texas A & M

PREFACE

Healthcare professionals must identify all elements of patient care capable of affecting nutritional status and outcomes. With limitations on length of hospital stay, the registered dietitian must provide nutritional care in a practical, efficient, timely, and effective manner in any setting. Various environments provide unique and special considerations for the nutrition counselor. The astute dietitian is sensitive to the patient/client's current status in the continuum of care and adapts the nutritional care plan accordingly. The most important element is communication between staff of different facilities to save time in screenings and assessments. Data and summary reports should be shared from one practitioner to the next, regardless of setting. Confidential, computerized medical records enable the dietetic practitioner to maintain current updates for all patients in a readily accessible format.

Nutrition and Diagnosis-Related Care was developed to supplement other texts and references used by practitioners, instructors, interns, and students to quickly assimilate and implement medical nutrition therapy (MNT) for numerous disorders. This manual can be used to help write protocols, to establish priorities in nutritional care, to demonstrate therapies at lower cost than certain medications and total parenteral nutrition (TPN), and to categorize disorders in which nutritional input can reduce costs by lessening complications, further morbidity, mortality, and lengthy hospital stays. Adequate nutritional intervention often results in financial savings for the patient, the family, and the healthcare system.

The fifth edition was written to include the latest guidance in medical nutrition therapy. Each section of the book was thoroughly reviewed by leading practitioners in the field. New diagnostic terminology is used. In addition, the format of the book has been updated to improve navigation of the text and allow easier and quicker retrieval of information. The new Dietary Reference Intakes have been used, but at the time of printing, the macronutrient tables were not yet available. To find the new data, access the search at the Institute of Medicine site (http://wwwsearch.nationalacademies.org/)

Appendix C provides more Case Studies in a concept map format. A Nutritional Acuity Level Ranking for dietitian services is included for most conditions; it is the summary consensus from a survey of over 50 sites that includes clinical nutrition managers, clinical experts, and practitioners. This acuity ranking may be used to identify or to negotiate nutrition staffing patterns, to identify patients at moderate to high nutritional risk, and to plan adequate follow-up services from one site to another (see Appendix D for a summary table.)

Herbal and botanical interventions are compiled in a new Appendix E. This information is critical for dietitians to know because of the use and interest by the public and medical community. Side effects are often unknown except through anecdotal evidence. Where evidence from clinical trials is mentioned, information is included.

Nutrition care plans and goals must be created individually for each patient. The reader is encouraged to maintain current educational knowledge and skills in order to revise local nutritional guidelines as new evidence suggests. Evidence-based practice and use of this manual as a tool serve as the stimulus for improving medical nutrition therapy in all settings.

ASSUMPTIONS ABOUT THE READER

For this text, the following assumptions have been made:

1. The reader has an adequate background in nutritional sciences, physiology and pathophysiology, medical terminology, biochemistry, and interpretation of laboratory data to understand the abbreviations, objectives, and interventions.
2. An individualized drug history review is required for all patients; only a few commonly used medications are listed in this manual. Herbs and botanicals and dietary supplements are included because they are often used without prior consultation with a dietitian or a physician; they may have side effects as well as perceived or real benefits.
3. The Patient Education section assumes that the reader will acquire or provide appropriate diet information sheets and tools. Other tips are available from this guide to prepare the patient for independent functioning. The nutrition counselor will share all relevant information based on the Nutritional and Dietary Recommendations section, as deemed appropriate, with the patient or significant other(s).
4. Shortened lengths of stay have forced healthcare practitioners to prioritize nutritional care during hospital stays. Dietitians have found additional roles in ambulatory centers, extended care facilities, subacute or rehabilitative centers, private practices, and home care. The "seamless" flow from one site to another affords the possibility of lifelong patient connections, which are now a reality with appropriate tracking and follow-up.
5. The Profile section lists tests, disease markers, and common biochemical evaluations used by either the physician or the dietitian for the condition. Fewer laboratory tests are available in nonhospital settings for monitoring nutritional status. The major assessment tools (such as weight changes) remain essential. Physical changes and signs of malnutrition are as important for assessment purposes and should be identified whenever possible.
6. A current diet manual or diet therapy text should be used to acquire complete lists of diet modifications since lists are not included with this book. Use of standard Medical Nutrition Therapy guidelines from The American Dietetic Association is also highly recommended to provide predictable services over multiple visits.
7. Except when specifically noted for children, medical nutrition therapy plans are for adults over the age of 18.
8. Vitamin and mineral supplements in large doses may cause food–drug interactions. They are needed in cases of a documented or likely deficiency. Otherwise, plan meals and nourishments carefully to avoid the need for supplements.

Athletes, women, elderly individuals, and vegetarians tend to take vitamin and mineral supplements more often than other individuals.

9. Much evidence points to the benefits of whole foods to acquire known and unknown phytochemicals and substances as yet unidentified. Healthy persons should obtain nutrients from food, not pills. Single-dose nutrients cannot halt the progression of acute or chronic illness. Where listed in this text, single nutrients are suggested as the focus of dietary meal planning. If necessary, a balanced multiple vitamin–mineral supplement may be warranted.

10. In general, the rules include use of a well-balanced, varied diet with the USDA Food Guide Pyramid as the basis for dietary plans. The many ethnic, vegetarian, children's, geriatric, and diabetes food pyramids are excellent tools for menu planning and design.

11. Ethics, cultural sensitivity, and a concern for patient rights should be considered and practiced at all times. When available, the wishes and advanced directives of the patient are to be followed.

12. Interesting and varied websites have been included for the reader to use to acquire additional insights into various diseases, conditions, and nutritional interventions. This list is not comprehensive and was current at the time of printing.

ACKNOWLEDGMENT

Thanks to Brooke Sikes, MS, RD, and Nawakish Ali Kahn, MD who helped with edits for this edition, and to the reviewers of the section content, who made valuable suggestions for changes.

Sylvia Escott-Stump, MA, RD, LDN

REVIEWERS

SECTION 1

Pregnancy and Lactation
Cathy Fagen, PhD, RD
Long Beach Memorial Medical Center, Long Beach, CA

Infant, Childhood, and Adolescent Nutrition
Barbara Gaffield, MS, RD (Now retired)
Division of Developmental and Behavioral Pediatrics, Children's Hospital of Oakland, Oakland, CA

Cristine Trahms, MS, RD, FADA
PKU and Biochemical Genetics Program;
Head, Nutrition Center on Human Development and Disabilities,
University of Washington, Seattle, WA

Sports Nutrition
Jackie Berning, PhD, RD
University of Colorado, Colorado Springs, CO

Adult and Geriatric Nutrition
Nancy Harris, MS, RD, FADA
Lecturer, East Carolina University, Greenville, NC

SECTION 2

Cultural Foods, Food Allergies, and Food Safety
Robert Earl, MPH, RD
National Association of Food Processors, Washington, DC

SECTION 3

Special Pediatric Disorders
Leila Beker, PhD, RD, LD
Director, Bionutrition Research Core; General Clinical Research Center
George Washington University, Children's National Medical Center, Washington, DC

Dianne Frazier, PhD, MPH
Associate Professor of Pediatrics
University of North Carolina Medical Center
Division of Genetics and Metabolism
Chapel Hill, NC

SECTION 4

Neurological and Psychiatric Disorders
Kathrynne Holden, MS, RD
Consultant, National Parkinson's Foundation

Charlie Kresho, RD, Physician's Assistant
East Carolina University, Greenville, NC

SECTION 5

Pulmonary Disorders
John Lamberson, MS, RD
Albemarle Hospital, Elizabeth City, NC

SECTION 6

Cardiovascular Disorders
Sonja Connor, MS, RD, LD
Research Associate Professor
Department of Medicine, Oregon Health & Science University, Portland, OR

Debra Krummel, PhD, RD
Assistant Professor, Community Medicine
West Virginia University, Morgantown, WV

SECTION 7

Gastrointestinal Disorders
Peter Beyer, MS, RD
University of Kansas Medical Center, Kansas City, KS

SECTION 8

Hepatic, Pancreatic, and Biliary Disorders
Jeannette Hasse, PhD, RD, LD, FADA, CNSD
Transplant Nutrition Specialist, Transplantation Services
Baylor University Medical Center, Dallas, TX

SECTION 9

Endocrine Disorders
Joan Heins, MS, RD
School of Medicine, Washington University, St. Louis, MO

SECTION 10

Weight Control and Malnutrition
Kathy Kolasa, PhD, RD
Section Head, School of Medicine, East Carolina University, Greenville, NC

Kimberly Shovelin, MPH, RD
East Carolina University, Greenville, NC

SECTION 11

Musculoskeletal, Arthritic, and Collagen Disorders
Sarah Morgan, MD, RD, FADA, FACP
University of Alabama at Birmingham, Birmingham, AL

SECTION 12

Hematology: Anemias and Blood Disorders
Carol Mitchell, PhD, RD, LDN
Professor, University of Memphis, Memphis, TN

SECTION 13

Cancer
Abby Bloch, PhD, RD
Consultant, New York, NY

Barbara Eldridge, RD
Clinical Research Associate
St. Alphonsus Cancer Treatment Center, Boise, ID

SECTION 14

Surgical Disorders
Walter Pories, MD
Department of Surgery, School of Medicine, East Carolina University, Greenville, NC

Marion Winkler, MS, RD, LDN, CNSD
School of Medicine, Brown University, Providence, RI

SECTION 15

AIDS and HIV
Laura McNally, MPH, RD, FADA
DHHS, Health Resources and Services Administration, Washington, DC

Hypermetabolic, Infectious, Traumatic, and Febrile Conditions
Marion Winkler, MS, RD, LDN, CNSD
School of Medicine, Brown University, Providence, RI

SECTION 16

Renal Disorders
Jessie Pavlinac, MS, RD, CS, LD
Clinical Nutrition Manager, Oregon Health & Science University, Portland, OR

SECTION 17

Enteral and Parenteral Nutrition
Marion Winkler, MS, RD, LDN, CNSD
School of Medicine, Brown University, Providence, RI

APPENDIX A

Nutritional Review
Margie Gallagher, PhD, RD
Professor, Department of Nutrition and Hospitality Management
East Carolina University, Greenville, NC

APPENDIX B

Dietetic Process, Forms and Counseling Tips
Cynthia Brylinsky, MS, RD
Geisinger Health System, Danville, PA

Esther Myers, PhD, RD, FADA
The American Dietetic Association, Chicago, IL

APPENDIX C

Multiple Condition Case Studies
Candyce Roberts, MS, RD

APPENDIX D

Nutritional Acuity Ranking for Dietitian Services
Esther Myers, PhD, RD, FADA
The American Dietetic Association, Chicago, IL

APPENDIX E

Complementary Nutrition—Herbals and Botanicals
Esther Myers, PhD, RD, FADA
The American Dietetic Association, Chicago, IL

COMMON ABBREVIATIONS

AA amino acid
abd abdomen, abdominal
ABW average body weight
ACE angiotensin-converting enzyme
ACTH adrenocorticotropic hormone
ADA American Dietetic Association
Alb albumin
alk phos alkaline phosphatase
ALT alanine aminotransferase
amts amounts
ARF acute renal failure
ASHD atherosclerotic heart disease
AST aspartate aminotransaminase
ATP adenosine triphosphate
BCAAs branched-chain amino acids
BEE basal energy expenditure
BF breast-feeding, breast-feeder
BMR basal metabolic rate
BP blood pressure
BS blood sugar
BSA body surface area
BUN blood urea nitrogen
BW body weight
bx biopsy
C cup(s)
C coffee
CA cancer
Ca++ calcium
CABG coronary artery bypass grafting
CBC complete blood count
CF cystic fibrosis
CHD cardiac heart disease
CHF congestive heart failure
CHI creatinine-height index
CHO carbohydrate
chol cholesterol
circum circumference
Cl, Cl− chloride
CNS central nervous system
CO_2 carbon dioxide
CPK creatine phosphokinase
CPR cardiopulmonary resuscitation
CrCl creatine clearance
CRP C-reactive protein
CT computed tomography
Cu copper
CVA cerebrovascular accident
DAT diet as tolerated
dec decreased
decaf decaffeinated
def deficiency
DJD degenerative joint disease
dL deciliter
DM diabetes mellitus
DNA deoxyribonucleic acid
DOB date of birth
DRI dietary reference intake
DV daily value
dx diagnosis
D5W 5% dextrose solution in water
EAA essential amino acid
ECG, EKG electrocardiogram
EEG electroencephalogram
EFAs essential fatty acids
elec electrolytes
elim eliminate, elimination
EN enteral nutrition
ESRD end-stage renal disease
ETOH ethanol/ethyl alcohol
Fe, Fe++ iron
F & V fruits and vegetables
FSH follicle-stimulating hormone
FTT failure to thrive
FUO fever of unknown origin
G, g gram(s)
GA gestational age
GBD gallbladder disease
GE gastroenteritis
gest gestational
GFR glomerular filtration rate
GI gastrointestinal
gluc glucose
GN glomerular nephritis
GTT glucose tolerance test
H & H hemoglobin and hematocrit
HBV high biologic value
HBW healthy body weight
HCl hydrochloric acid
Hct hematocrit
HDL high-density lipoprotein
HbA1c hemoglobin A1c test (glucose)
HLP hyperlipoproteinemia or hyperlipidemia
HPN, HTN hypertension
ht height
Hx history
I infant
I & O intake and output
IBD inflammatory bowel disease
IBS irritable bowel syndrome
IBW ideal body weight
IDDM insulin-dependent diabetes mellitus
IEM inborn error of metabolism
IU international units
IUD intrauterine device
IV intravenous
jc juice
K, K+ potassium
kcal food kilocalories
kg kilogram(s)
L liter(s)
lb pound(s)
LBM lean body mass
LBV low biological value
LBW low birth weight

LCT	long-chain triglycerides
LDH	lactic acid dehydrogenase
LDL	low-density lipoproteins
LE	lupus erythematosus
LGA	large for gestational age
LH	luteinizing hormone
LI	large intestine
lytes	electrolytes
M	milk
MAC	midarm circumference
MAMC	midarm muscle circumference
MAO	monoamine oxidase
MBF	meat-base formula
MCH	mean cell hemoglobin
MCT	medium-chain triglycerides
MCV	mean cell volume
MI	myocardial infarction
Mg, Mg++	magnesium
mg	milligram(s)
μg	micrograms
mm	millimeter(s)
MODS	multiple organ dysfunction syndrome
MSG	monosodium glutamate
MUFA	monounsaturated fatty acids
N&V	nausea and vomiting
N	nitrogen
Na+	sodium
NCEP	National Cholesterol Education Program
NEC	necrotizing enterocolitis
NG	nasogastric
NIDDM	non-insulin-dependent diabetes mellitus
NP	nonprotein (as in NP calories)
NPO	nil per os (nothing by mouth)
NSI	Nutrition Screening Initiative
O_2	oxygen
OCs	oral contraceptives
OJ	orange juice
OT	occupational therapist
oz	ounce(s)
P	phosphorus
PCM	protein-calorie malnutrition
pCO_2	partial pressure of carbon dioxide
PG	pregnant, pregnancy
PKU	phenylketonuria
PN	parenteral nutrition
pO_2	partial pressure of oxygen
prn	pro re nata (as needed)
prot	protein
PT	pro-time or physical therapy
PTH	parathormone
PTT	prothrombin time
PUFA(s)	polyunsaturated fatty acid(s)
PVD	peripheral vascular disease
RAST	radioallergosorbent test
RBC	red blood cell count
RDAs	recommended dietary allowances
RDS	respiratory distress syndrome
REE	resting energy expenditure
RQ	respiratory quotient
Rx	treatment
SFA	saturated fatty acids
SGA	small for gestational age
SI	small intestine
SIADH	syndrome of inappropriate antidiuretic hormone
SIDS	sudden infant death syndrome
SOB	shortness of breath
Sub	substitute
Sx	symptoms
"t"	teaspoon(s)
T	tablespoon
TB	tuberculosis
TF	tube feeding; tube fed
TIBC	total iron-binding capacity
TLC	total lymphocyte count
TPN	total parenteral nutrition
TG	triglycerides
TSF	triceps skinfold
UA	uric acid
UTI	urinary tract infection(s)
UUN	urinary urea nitrogen
VMA	vanillylmandelic acid
VO_2 max	maximum oxygen intake
WBC	white blood cell count
WNL	within normal limits
Zn	zinc

TABLES

FIGURES

TABLE OF CONTENTS

ALPHABETICAL LIST OF TOPICS

SECTION 1

NORMAL LIFE-CYCLE CONDITIONS

CHIEF ASSESSMENT FACTORS

- EDUCATIONAL BACKGROUND, SOCIO-ECONOMIC STATUS
- GENERAL STATE OF HEALTH, RECENT SURGERY/HOSPITALIZATIONS, WEIGHT HISTORY, PERCENTAGE OF BODY MASS INDEX (BMI) OR IDEAL BODY WEIGHT (IBW) OR HEALTHY BODY WEIGHT (HBW) FOR HEIGHT, LOSS OF LEAN BODY MASS (LBM), PREVIOUS WEIGHT CURVE, FATIGUE, WEAKNESS, CACHEXIA
- CHILLS, SWEATING, TREMORS, ANOREXIA, NAUSEA, DIARRHEA, VOMITING, BLOOD PRESSURE, TEMPERATURE, PULSE
- HAIR OR NAIL CHANGES, SKIN RASHES, ITCHING, LESIONS, TURGOR, PETECHIAE, PALLOR
- HEADACHE, SEIZURES, OTITIS MEDIA, GLAUCOMA, CATARACTS, GLASSES, BLURRING OF VISION, SINUSITIS, ALTERED SENSE OF SMELL, NASAL OBSTRUCTION
- DENTURES, LOOSE OR MISSING TEETH, CARIES, BLEEDING GUMS, ORAL HYGIENE, TASTE ALTERATIONS, DYSPHAGIA
- CHEST PAIN, DYSPNEA, WHEEZING, COUGH, HEMOPTYSIS, VENTILATOR SUPPORT, BLOOD GASES
- ELECTROLYTE BALANCE, HYPERTENSION, CYANOSIS, EDEMA, ASCITES, CARDIAC OUTPUT
- ANEMIAS, HEART RATE, ARRHYTHMIAS, BLOOD LOSS
- APPETITE, JAUNDICE, CONSTIPATION, INDIGESTION, ULCERS, HEMORRHOIDS, MELENA, STOOL CHARACTERISTICS, SPECIAL DIETS
- SKINFOLDS, VISCERAL PROTEINS, BASAL ENERGY EXPENDITURE (BEE), WEIGHT CHANGES, NITROGEN BALANCE
- VITAMIN/MINERAL INTAKE, NUTRITIONAL SUPPORT, BLOOD GLUCOSE, DIETARY PATTERNS AND TYPICAL INTAKE , ALCOHOL INTAKE

- MEDICATIONS, SIDE EFFECTS, FOOD–DRUG INTERACTIONS, THERAPIES, EFFECTS ON NUTRITIONAL STATUS, USE OF HERBS/BOTANICALS/SUPPLEMENTS, USE OF OVER-THE-COUNTER MEDICATIONS
- HEMATURIA, FLUID REQUIREMENTS, SPECIFIC GRAVITY, URINARY TRACT INFECTIONS
- HORMONE BALANCE, GOITER, GLUCOSE INTOLERANCE, CELLULAR IMMUNITY
- ALLERGY, SENSITIVITY, INTOLERANCES
- PAIN, ARTHRITIS, NUMBNESS, AMPUTATIONS, RANGE OF MOTION, MUSCULAR STRENGTH
- CONVULSIONS, ALTERED SPEECH, PARALYSIS, GAIT, ANXIETY, MEMORY LOSS, SLEEP PATTERNS, DEPRESSION, SUBSTANCE ABUSE, MOTIVATION

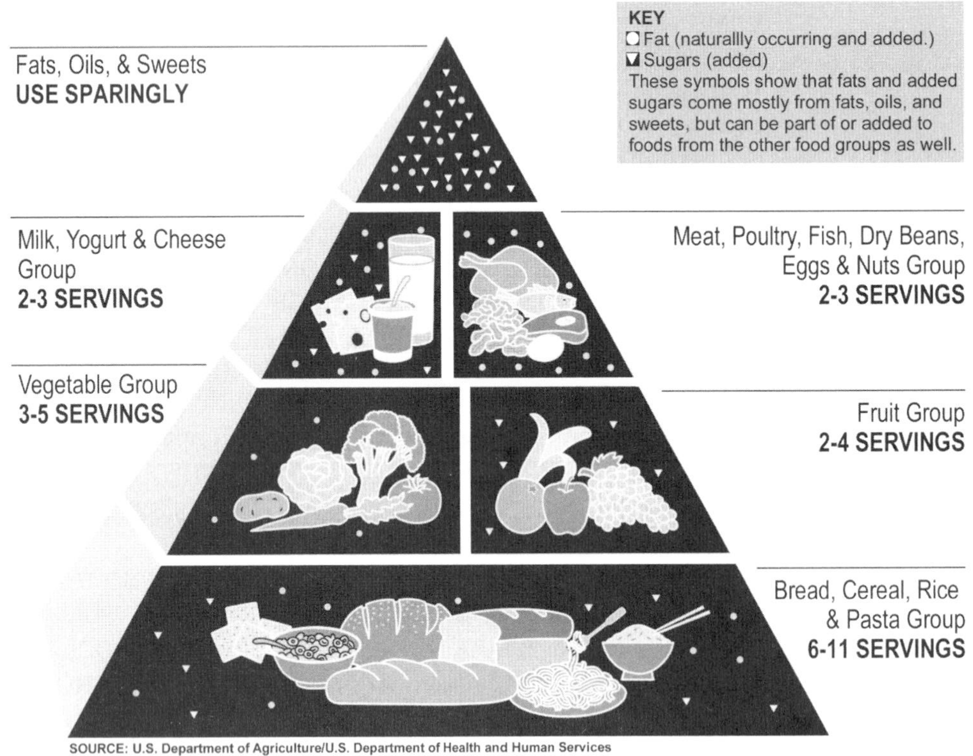

Food Guide Pyramid Resources:

- Resources for educators—http://www.nal.usda.gov/fnic/Fpyr/guide.pdf
- Ethnic and regional practices for diabetes– http://www.eatright.org/catalog/diabetes/html
- New Americans project— http://www.monarch.gsu.edu/nutrition/download/htm

TEN GREAT PUBLIC HEALTH ACHIEVEMENTS IN THE UNITED STATES, 1900–1999

Development of vaccines
Increased motor vehicle safety
Safer workplaces
Control of infectious diseases
Decline in deaths from coronary artery disease and stroke
Safer and healthier foods
Healthier mothers and babies
Better family planning
Fluoridation of drinking water
Recognition of tobacco as a health hazard

Source: Morbidity and Mortality Weekly Report, June 1999

TABLE 1–1 Dietary Guidelines

Dietary Guidelines for Americans (Dietary Guidelines Advisory Committee, U.S. Department of Health and Human Service, 2000)

Aim for fitness:	Aim for a healthy weight.
	Be physically active each day.
Build a healthy base:	Let the Pyramid guide your food choices.
	Choose a variety of grains daily, especially whole grains.
	Choose a variety of fruits and vegetables daily.
	Keep food safe to eat.
Choose sensibly:	Choose a diet that is low in saturated fat and cholesterol and moderate in total fat.
	Choose beverages and foods to moderate your intake of sugars.
	Choose and prepare foods with less salt.
	If you drink alcoholic beverages, do so in moderation.

Chinese Dietary Guidelines and Food Guide Pagoda (Ge and McNutt, 2000):

Eat a variety of foods with cereals as the staple.
Consume plenty of vegetables, fruits, and tubers.
Consume milk, beans, or dairy and bean products every day.
Consume appropriate amounts of fish, poultry, eggs, and lean meat.
Reduce fatty meat and animal fat in your diet.
Balance food intake with physical activity to maintain a healthy body weight.
Choose a light diet that is also low in salt.
If you drink alcoholic beverages, do so in limited amounts.
Avoid unsanitary and spoiled foods.

PREGNANCY

NUTRITIONAL ACUITY RANKING: LEVEL 1 (UNCOMPLICATED); LEVEL 3 (HIGH RISK PREGNANCY)

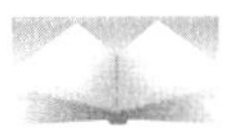

DEFINITIONS AND BACKGROUND

Pregnancy is an anabolic state, which affects maternal tissues using hormones synthesized to support successful pregnancy. Progesterone induces fat deposition to insulate the baby, supports energy reserves, and relaxes smooth muscle, which will cause a decrease in intestinal motility for greater nutrient absorption. Estrogen increases tremendously during pregnancy for growth promotion, uterine function, and water retention.

Tissue growth in pregnancy= breast, 0.5 kg; placenta, 0.6 kg; fetus, 3–3.5 kg; amniotic fluid, 1 kg; uterus, 1 kg; increase in blood volume, 1.5 kg; and extracellular fluid, 1.5 kg. Adequate weight gain is needed to ensure optimal fetal outcome. During late pregnancy (PG) and lactation, energy expenditure and respiratory quotient (RQ) increase; the latter confirms the preferential use of glucose by the fetus and mammary gland (Butte et al., 1999.)

Greater maternal weight before pregnancy increases the risk of late fetal death, although it protects against the delivery of a small for gestational age (SGA) infant. Obesity is associated with increased risk of macrosomia and perinatal mortality; underweight is associated with SGA or preterm deliveries (Cnattingius et al., 1998.)

Recent research (Godfrey and Barker, 2000) suggests that several of the major diseases of later life, including cardiac heart disease (CHD), hypertension (HPN), and type 2 diabetes, originate in impaired intrauterine growth and development. These diseases may be consequences of programming, whereby a stimulus or insult at a critical, sensitive time has permanent effects on structure, physiology, and metabolism. People who are small or disproportionate (thin or short) at birth may have high rates of CHD, high BP, high cholesterol concentrations, and abnormal glucose-insulin metabolism, independent of length of gestation. CHD may be related to growth restriction rather than to premature birth, which suggests the importance of fetal adaptations when maternal-placental nutrient supply fails to match fetal nutrient needs. In addition, high serum total cholesterol levels during pregnancy induce changes in the fetal aorta that increase the child's long-term susceptibility to fatty-streak formation and subsequent atherosclerotic heart disease (ASHD) (Napoli et al., 1999.) Approximately 35% of major cardiac defects may be prevented by maternal use of multivitamins during the peri-conceptual period (Botto et al., 2000.)

Bulimia nervosa during pregnancy can lead to miscarriage, inappropriate weight gain (excessive or inadequate), complicated delivery, low birth weight, prematurity, infant malformation, low Apgar scores, and other problems; it must be identified and carefully addressed (Morrill and Nickols-Richardson, 2001.)

Nutritional deficits are also serious in pregnancy. Planned pregnancies usually have the most favorable outcomes. Continuous dietary monitoring of pregnant women and pregnant teens is essential, especially for calcium, magnesium, zinc, iron, fiber, folate, and vitamins D and E (Giddens et al., 2000.) Table 1–2 lists risk assessments and indicators of potentially poor maternal or fetal outcomes. The American Dietetic Association suggests three visits for medical nutrition therapy in high-risk pregnancy http://www.knowledgelinc.com/ada/mntguides/.

OBJECTIVES

- Meet increased needs for fetus and tissues. Prevent hypoglycemia and ketosis.
- Provide additional nutrients and calories (net cost of pregnancy: 80,000 kcal). Studies indicate needs vary from 20,000–80,000 kcal. Women carrying more than one fetus must add extra kilocalories to support multiple births. Energy deficit may contribute to low infant birth weight.
- Provide adequate amino acids to meet fetal and placental growth. Approximately 950 g of protein are synthesized for fetus and placenta. Low protein intake may lead to a reduced infant head circumference.
- Provide adequate weight gain during course of pregnancy. Underweight women (BMI under 18.5) should gain 28–40 lb. Normal weight women (BMI 19–24.9)

TABLE 1–2 Prenatal Risk Assessments and Indicators of Potentially Poor Outcomes

Prepregnancy

- ✦ Adolescence (poor eating habits, greater needs).
- ✦ History of three or more pregnancies in past 2 years, especially miscarriages.
- ✦ History of poor obstetrical/fetal performance.
- ✦ Overweight and obesity, which can cause a higher risk for gestational diabetes, preeclampsia, eclampsia, C-section, and/or delivery of infant with macrosomia (Baeten et al., 2001).

Prepregnancy or During Pregnancy

- ✦ Economic deprivation.
- ✦ Food faddist; smoker; user of drugs/alcohol; practice of pica with related iron or zinc deficiencies; anorexia nervosa or bulimia.
- ✦ Modified diet for chronic systemic diseases.
- ✦ Prepartum weight of less than 85% or more than 120% of IBW (may reflect inability to attain proper weight or poor dietary habits).
- ✦ Deficient Hgb (less than 11 g) or hematocrit (Hct) (less than 33%).
- ✦ Any weight loss during PG or gain of less than 2 lb/month in the last two trimesters; dehydration; hyperemesis.
- ✦ Risk of toxemia (2-lb weight gain per week or more).
- ✦ Poorly managed vegetarian diet.
- ✦ Poor nutrient or energy intakes over the course of the pregnancy – assess intakes over the duration.
- ✦ Poor intake of magnesium, zinc, calcium, and other key nutrients.

should gain 25–30 lb total. Overweight women (BMI 25–29.9) should gain 15–25 lb. Obese women (BMI over 30) should gain under 15 lb. For twins, 35–45 lb is recommended; for triplets, overall gain of 50 lb (Brown and Carlson, 2000).

- Encourage proper rate of gain: 2–4 lb first trimester, 10–11 lb second trimester, 12–13 lb third trimester. More weight should be gained if patient is below IBW before pregnancy; this is especially true for young women. Overweight women should gain ⅔ lb per week.
- Promote development of an adequate fetal immune system (during first trimester).
- Prevent or correct deficiencies of iron or folic acid, common in 50–75% of pregnancies. Folate deficiency may cause miscarriage and neural tube defects; iron deficiency may cause low infant birth weight and premature birth. A woman with a history of spontaneous abortion in her immediate prior pregnancy may be at increased risk for a pregnancy affected by a neural tube defect; short interpregnancy interval increases this risk (Todoroff and Shaw, 2000). In addition, neural tube defects, stillbirth, and clubfoot may be related to elevated homocysteine levels (Vollset et al., 2000).
- Avoid or treat other complications, such as pregnancy-induced hypertension, nausea and vomiting of pregnancy (NVP) or morning sickness, hyperemesis gravidarum, and gestational diabetes. See appropriate entries.
- Vitamin A deficiency is strongly associated with depressed immune system and higher morbidity and mortality due to infectious diseases such as measles, diarrhea, and respiratory infections. Vitamin A deficiency is often related to mother to infant HIV transmission (Azais-Braesco and Pascal, 2000). On the other hand, avoid excesses of vitamin A; doses of 10,000–30,000 IU/day can cause birth defects (Miller et al, 1998).
- Calcium is important, but supplementation during PG does not necessarily prevent preeclampsia (Morris et al., 2001). In the Calcium for Preeclampsia Prevention study, 4,314 women were followed during pregnancy and 7.6% had preeclampsia and 17% had pregnancy-associated hypertension; high body mass index and race were more commonly related to these conditions than any of the 23 nutrients that were also studied.
- Avoid vitamin D deficiency, which may lead to a low infant birth weight.
- Supply sufficient iodine to prevent cretinism with mental and physical retardation.
- Provide zinc to prevent congenital malformations.
- Only extremely high serum levels of paraxanthine (a caffeine metabolite) are associated with spontaneous abortion (Klebanoff et al., 1999). Therefore, moderate caffeine intake is unlikely to cause an increased risk of miscarriage. Limit intake to two cups daily.
- Avoid alcohol. Mothers who drink relatively high levels of alcohol around the time of conception increase the risk of orofacial clefts in their offspring (Shaw and Lammer, 1999).
- Maintain adequate gestational duration and avoid preterm delivery.
- Develop or improve good eating habits to prevent or delay onset of chronic health problems postnatally.

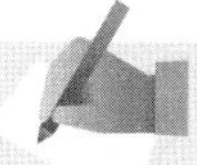

DIETARY AND NUTRITIONAL RECOMMENDATIONS

- Include in diet: 1 g protein/kg body weight daily (or 10–15 g in excess of recommended dietary allowances [RDA] for age). Young teens: 11–14 years (1.7 g/kg); 15–18 years (1.5 g/kg); over 19 years of age (1.7 g/kg); high risk (2 g/kg).
- Calories: first trimester, add 50–150 kcal/day. In second and third trimesters, add 200–300 kcal/day. May add more or less calories depending on activity. Evaluate teens individually according to age and prepregnancy weight, for an average of 36–40 kcal/kg/day, 15% protein, 55% carbohydrate (CHO), and 30% fat (American Diabetes Association, 1994).
- Adequate weight gain can also be estimated from BMI: BMI<20, gain 28–40 lb; BMI=20–25, gain 25–35 lb; BMI=26–29, gain 16–25 lb.
- The diet should include 200 kg extra folacin, 27 mg ferrous iron (diet + supplemental), and 5 mg increase in intake of zinc (from meats).
- The RDA for calcium in pregnancy is 1,000 mg for women over age 19; 1,300 mg for women under age 19.
- Encourage use of vitamin C with iron-rich foods or an iron sulfate supplement. Supplemental vitamins C and E may help prevent preeclampsia (Chappell et al., 1999).
- Use adequate vitamins A and D. Avoid hypervitaminosis, which may lead to fetal damage. Monitor use of diet and supplements carefully.
- Be sure to use iodized salt but avoid excess.
- Desired pattern of food intake: 3 cups milk group (calcium, protein); 7 oz meat or protein substitute (protein, iron, zinc); 5 fruits and vegetables, including citrus (vitamin C) and rich sources of vitamin A and folacin; 7 servings of grains and breads, three of which are whole grain or enriched breads/substitutes (iron, calories); 3 servings of fat.
- Omit alcohol. Reduce caffeine intake to the equivalent of two cups of coffee; this includes intake from colas, chocolate, and tea.
- Use cereal grains, nuts, green vegetables, and seafood for extra magnesium. Magnesium seems to play a role in preventing or correcting high blood pressure in susceptible women (Dawson et al., 2000).
- Essential fatty acids from fats, such as safflower oil, should equal 1–2% of daily calories. Fish and seafood (e.g., tuna, mackerel, salmon) should be encouraged for omega-3 fatty acids several times weekly, if no related allergy exists.
- Extra B6 and copper will be needed. These are readily obtained from a planned diet.
- Vegan vegetarians will need a B12 supplement and perhaps zinc, calcium, and vitamin D.
- In cases of severe gastrointestinal problems, as in women with inflammatory bowel disease (IBD), pancreatitis, or anorexia nervosa, total parenteral nutrition (TPN) may be needed. Adequate lipids (10–20% of calories) are needed for the fetus, as well as protein and CHO. Check blood sugar regularly. Be sure to use adequate fluid (2–3 L for some). Complications of TPN in pregnancy may include bacteremia, decreased renal function with preexisting disease,

neonatal hypoglycemia, and possible subclavian vein thrombosis.

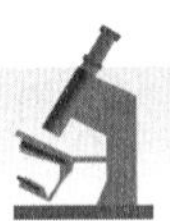

PROFILE

Clinical/History

- Gravida (number of pregnancies)
- Para (number of births)
- Abortus (number of abortions)
- Hx births with neural tube defects
- Use of alcohol
- Smoking habits and drug use
- Nausea (frequency, duration, impact on intake)
- Vomiting (frequency, duration, impact on intake)
- Blood pressure (BP)
- Height
- Prepregnancy weight (% standard)
- Weight grid or prenatal BMI (19.8–20.0)
- Present weight for gestational age
- Desired weight at term

Lab Work

- Hemoglobin and hematocrit (H & H) (goal higher than 11.0 and 33%)
- Serum Fe
- Urea N
- Glucose (gluc) (by 24–28 weeks)
- Ca++, Mg++
- Albumin (alb) or prealbumin (if needed)
- Transferrin
- Ceruloplasmin
- T3, T4
- Blood urea nitrogen (BUN)
- Creat
- Cholesterol (chol) (inc.)
- Alkaline phosphatase (alk phos) (inc.)
- Total iron-binding capacity (TIBC) (inc. in late PG)

Common Drugs Used and Potential Side Effects

- After the fourth month, encourage use of a basic vitamin-mineral supplement between meals (with liquids other than milk, coffee, or tea) for better utilization. Supplements vary greatly; read labels carefully. Iron is the only nutrient that cannot be met from diet alone (30 mg needed after the first trimester).
- Avoid taking iron supplements with antacids. Bedtime is a good time to take an iron supplement.
- Avoid taking isotretinoin (Accutane) or 13-cis retinoic acid for acne; they have been linked to birth defects.
- Avoid excesses of vitamin A, especially in the first trimester. Be wary of 10,000 IU of vitamin A or more; birth defects may result.
- Insulin may be needed with consistently high blood glucose levels over 120 mg/dL; monitor overfeeding.
- Anti-NVP agents may include ondansetron (Zofran), cyclizine (Marezine), buclizine (Bucladin-S), metoclopramide (Reglan), meclizine (Antivert), prochlorperazine (Compazine), promethazine (Phenergan), or antihistamines such as Benadryl. Side effects vary but may include sedation, dizziness, changes in blood pressure, and/or tachycardia (Erick and Bunnell, 2000). Diclectin and Bendectin (doxylamine with vitamin B6) are only available in Canada at this time; they are safe for the fetus.
- Discuss the relevance of tolerable upper intake levels (ULs) from the latest dietary reference intakes of the National Academy of Sciences. These levels were set to protect individuals from receiving too much of any nutrient from diet and dietary supplements.

Herbs, Botanicals and Supplements

- Pregnant women should not use herbs and botanical supplements without checking with their physician first. Women who are using such supplements should stop immediately when they discover they are pregnant.
- Pregnant women should not take kava, chasteberry, dong quai, Asian ginseng, licorice root, and Saw Palmetto.

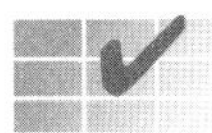

PATIENT EDUCATION

✓ Describe an adequate pattern and rate of weight gain in pregnancy. Explain the rationale for such gain. Individualize according to goals (e.g., short women at lower range

Nutrient	*Recommendation for Ages 18 or under*	*Recommendation for Ages 19–30*	*Recommendation for Ages 31–50*
Calories:	1st tri = +50–150 kcal/d; 2nd–3rd tri = +200–300 kcal/d	1st tri = +50–150 kcal/d; 2nd–3rd tri = +200–300 kcal/d	1st tri = +50–150 kcal/d; 2nd–3rd tri = +200–300 kcal/d
Protein:	60 g/d	60 g/d	60 g/d
Calcium:	1,300 mg/d	1,000 mg/d	1,000 mg/d
Iron:	27 mg/d	27 mg/d	27 mg/d
Folate	600 μg/d	600 μg/d	600 μg/d
Phosphorus:	1,250 mg/d	700 mg/d	700 mg/d
Vitamin A:	750 μg	770 μg	770 mg/d
Vitamin C:	80 mg/d	85 mg/d	85 mg/d
Thiamin:	1.4 mg/d	1.4 mg/d	1.4 mg/d
Riboflavin:	1.4 mg/d	1.4 mg/d	1.4 mg/d
Niacin:	18 mg/d	18 mg/d	18 mg/d

of gain). Excess equals more than 6.5 lb gained monthly after 20 weeks. Inadequate intake equals less than 2 lb gained monthly after the first trimester.

- ✔ Explain to the patient what to do for NVP (morning sickness); share available handouts. Try lemonade and potato chips rather than just than ginger ale and saltines; minimize offensive odors (Erick and Bunnell, 2000). Avoid large meals and spicy and high-fat foods if not tolerated. Eat dry crackers before rising in the morning. If necessary, drink fluids between meals rather than with meals. Multivitamin mineral supplements may also trigger NVP. It may be helpful to try a different brand. Rehydration may be essential. NVP often abates by 17 weeks of pregnancy.
- ✔ Encourage adequate calcium intake. Discuss what to do for milk allergy/intolerance and lactose intolerance, suggesting alternative foods and ways to include calcium.
- ✔ Discourage faddist behavior, low-nutrient-density foods, and the habit of skipping breakfast. Discuss ketosis from low glucose levels and its effect on the fetus, e.g., brain development.
- ✔ Encourage stress reduction, which has an effect on nitrogen and calcium. Encourage pleasant mealtimes and a healthy appetite.
- ✔ Encourage breast-feeding (except for women who are HIV-positive). Explain reasons for doing so, e.g., immunological benefits, bonding, and weight stabilization.
- ✔ For excessive weight gain, the goal should be to restore eating patterns to match a normal growth curve. Severe calorie restriction should be avoided, and at least 150 g of CHO will be needed.
- ✔ Discuss fluoride and iodine intake from water, table salt, and related sources (e.g., seafood). A balance of both nutrients is needed, but excesses are to be avoided.
- ✔ Discuss effects of marijuana (e.g., decreased birth weight, congenital malformations), cocaine, alcohol, and other drugs, as needed. Discourage smoking because of the effect on the fetus.
- ✔ Limit intake of aspartame-sweetened foods to 3–4 servings per day (Carroll, 1990). Other sweeteners should be used in moderation.
- ✔ Eligible women should be referred to participate in the WIC Program to decrease low birth weight. Many barriers hinder low-income women's participation in nutrition education programs. Women cite problems with relocation, conflicting activities, negative feelings about nutrition education, and lack of transportation or child care as major problems (Damron, 1999).
- ✔ Postpartum concerns should be discussed, including physical activity, breast-feeding, anemia, and control of hyperglycemia.
- ✔ For constipation, extra fluid is recommended (2–3 quarts). Extra fiber and activity are needed. Avoid use of laxatives.
- ✔ For swelling of ankles, hands, and legs, become more physically active; avoid excessive salt at the table but do not restrict salt severely.
- ✔ For heartburn, eat smaller meals more frequently, eat slowly, and cut down on spicy or high-fat foods. Avoid antacids unless approved by the physician.
- ✔ For hyperemesis gravidarum (intractable vomiting), hospitalization with tube feeding may be needed (Gulley et al., 1993). When eating orally, liquids taken between meals, extra B complex and vitamin C, and limited fat may be beneficial. Hyperemesis affects 20% of pregnancies. Electrolyte imbalances must be avoided. Metoclopramide (Reglan) may help some women.
- ✔ Pica prevalence is sometimes identified among women enrolled in WIC and is associated with ice, freezer frost, baking soda, baking powder, cornstarch, laundry starch, baby powder, clay, or dirt (Rainville 1998). Pica practices are associated with significantly lower hemoglobin levels at delivery; counselors must be aware. Food cravings and aversions usually subside after pregnancy.
- ✔ Avoid soft cheeses such as feta, Brie or Camembert, Roquefort, and Mexican soft cheese; they may have been contaminated with Listeria, which can cause fetal death or premature labor. If they are used, cook until boiling first.
- ✔ Avoid raw eggs, raw fish, and raw and undercooked meats because of potential food-borne illnesses.
- ✔ Pregnant women should not eat shark, swordfish, king mackerel, and tilefish. These long-lived larger fish contain the highest levels of methyl mercury that may harm an unborn baby's developing nervous system. These women should select a variety of other kinds of fish, i.e., shellfish, canned fish, smaller ocean fish, or farm-raised fish. They can safely eat 12 oz of cooked fish per week, with a typical serving size being 3–6 oz. Keep fish and shellfish refrigerated or frozen until ready to use.

For More Information

- ✦ American College of Nurse-Midwives (ACNM)
  818 Connecticut Avenue, NW, Ste. 900
  Washington DC 20006
  888-MIDWIFE
  http://www.midwife.org
- ✦ American Dietetic Association
  High Risk Pregnancy protocol
  http://www.eatright.org
- ✦ Healthy Mothers, Healthy Babies National Coalition
  121 N. Washington St., Suite 300
  Alexandria, VA 22314
  703-836-6110
  http://www.hmhb.org/
- ✦ National Association of Childbearing Centers
  3123 Gottschall Road
  Perkiomenville, PA 18074
- ✦ National Center for Education in Maternal-Child Health
  http://www.ncemch.org/
- ✦ National Foundation-March of Dimes
  1275 Mamaroneck Ave.
  White Plains, NY 10605
  888-MODIMES
  http://www.noah.cuny.edu/providers/mod.html
- ✦ WIC Program—Supplemental Food Programs Division
  Food and Nutrition Service--USDA
  3101 Park Center Drive
  Alexandria, VA 22302
  703-305-2746
  http://www.fns.usda.gov/wic/

LACTATION

NUTRITIONAL ACUITY RANKING: LEVEL 1 (NOT FORMALLY RANKED)

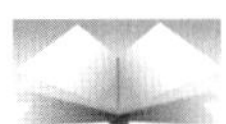

DEFINITIONS AND BACKGROUND

Breastfeeding (BF) should be supported and encouraged because of its immunological, physiological, economic, social, and hygienic effects on mother and infant. Broad-based efforts are needed to break the many barriers to breastfeeding (American Dietetic Association, 2001). Because maternal intake and breastfeeding practices vary over the duration of lactation, assess regularly and determine whether or not the infant needs supplemented foods or nutrients. It is an anabolic state requiring extra energy.

Composition of breast milk varies over time. Colostrum contains mainly immunological factors (days 1–4); then there is a short transition (days 5–9). The function of breast milk secreted between days 9 and 28 is primarily nutritional. Breast milk is balanced in its functions of immunity and nutrition between days 28 and 84 (Montagne et al., 2000).

Infants digest and absorb human milk better than other forms of milk. It has more polyunsaturated fatty acid (PUFA) (DHA and arachidonic acid for normal cognitive and visual development) and carnitine for mitochondrial oxidation of these long-chain fatty acids. It also has less sodium and a proper protein ratio. Breast milk has 1.5 times as much lactose as cow's milk; consequently, protein is absorbed better. The whey:casein ratio of 80:20 is more desirable than that of many formulas. In comparison, cow's milk has twice as much protein and ash. Breast milk yields 1 mg iron/L with a 49% absorption rate. Cholesterol content is 15–23 mg/dL regardless of maternal intake. The composition of breast milk also changes to meet the baby's changing needs, i.e., the fat content decreases over time.

Food allergies are less frequent in infants who are exclusively breastfed. Breast milk has more antibodies than cow's milk formulas and more than 45 bioactive factors such as digestive enzymes, hormones, immune factors, and growth factors. The promotion of nearly universal breastfeeding has played an important role in improving child health by providing optimum nutrition and protection against common childhood infections and by promoting child spacing (Weinberg, 2000).

Infants receive beneficial nucleotides from human milk, which tends to protect against diarrhea (Carver, 1999), respiratory illnesses, ear infections, and allergies (Wright et al., 2001). Bacterial flora of breastfed infants are generally *Lactobacillus,* not *Escherichia coli,* like those of formula-fed infants. Formula-fed infants have more illnesses and cost the healthcare system more money than BF infants; this difference averages between $331–475 per never-breastfed infant during the first year of life (Ball and Wright, 1999).

Unfortunately, breastfeeding is responsible for much of the increasing burden of worldwide pediatric human immunodeficiency virus (HIV) infection. In developing nations, where adequate sanitary replacement feeding is not available, the decision to withhold breastfeeding so as to decrease HIV transmission may lead to increased rates of child morbidity and mortality from diarrheal and respiratory diseases and malnutrition (Weinberg, 2000). Women must be fully informed about the risks of breastfeeding transmission of HIV and the expense and availability of obtaining formula. If an uninterrupted access to a nutritionally adequate breast milk substitute that can be safely prepared is ensured (as in industrialized countries), HIV-infected women should be counseled not to breastfeed their infants (Weinberg, 2000). The infant should not be breastfed if the mother uses alcohol or illicit drugs or is receiving chemotherapy. Breastfeeding should also be avoided if the infant has galactosemia.

Women should be encouraged to breastfeed as long as they can until the child is 1 year of age, when weaning should be complete; in developing countries, this timing may be by age 2. Mothers should not deprive themselves, however. The volume of milk decreases in a poorly nourished mother. New mothers who are breastfeeding should try not to lose weight rapidly during this time.

The long-term effects of breastfeeding an infant include possibly lower incidence of type 2 diabetes, Crohn's disease, lymphoma, allergies, and neurologic disabilities. The intake of several minerals found in milk has been demonstrated to have an inverse relationship with blood pressure; peptides formed during the digestion of milk proteins have also been demonstrated to have a blood pressure lowering effect, which may play a protective role later in life (Groziak and Miller, 2000). Breast milk consumption is associated with lower later blood pressure in children born prematurely. Evidence suggests programming of a cardiovascular risk factor by early diet and further supports the long-term beneficial effects of breast milk (Singhal et al., 2001).

Better cognitive development in the infant is also a benefit. Even after adjustment for key cofactors, breastfeeding is associated with significantly higher cognitive development than with formula feeding; the enhancement remains until about age 15 (Anderson et al., 1999). Breastfed infants are often more mature, secure, and assertive and tend to score higher on developmental tests. Healthy People 2010 includes a goal of increasing to 75% the proportion of mothers who breastfeed upon discharge from the hospital, and 50% still breastfeeding at 6 months of age.

A minimum of $3.6 billion would be saved if breastfeeding were increased from current levels (64% in-hospital, 29% at 6 months) to those recommended by the U.S. Surgeon General (75 and 50%); this figure underestimates total savings because it represents cost savings from the treatment of only three childhood illnesses: otitis media, gastroenteritis, and necrotizing enterocolitis (Weimer, 2001). Breastfeeding may also reduce the risk of breast and ovarian cancers and may protect bone mineral density in the mother (American Dietetic Association, 1997).

Hospital practices tend to influence the duration of breastfeeding. Giving infants formula in the hospital, giving mothers discharge packs of formula, removing the infant from the mother's room for more than 60% of their time in the hospital, and not putting the infant to the breast within the first few hours of life seem to negatively affect the duration of lactation (Wright et al., 1996). The nutrition counselor should support the mother as much as possible to continue breastfeeding for 1 year and longer for developing countries. See Table 1–3 for common problems.

OBJECTIVES

- Normalize body composition gradually so that the mother returns to ideal weight.
- Breast milk can meet nutrient needs during the first 6 months with possible exception of vitamin D and iron in certain populations (Dewey, 2001).
- Provide for adequate lactation (usual secretion, 750–800 mL/day). Human milk provides 67 calories/dL. Good calorie intake does impact milk production, mainly in undernourished women.
- Have the mother continue breastfeeding beyond several months. The ideal time for the mother to discontinue lactation is when the infant is 1-year-old. WHO recommends breastfeeding for up to 2 years in developing countries.
- Decrease nutritional risks (e.g., use of alcohol, etc.) while mother is breastfeeding. Alcohol intake inhibits letdown reflex (oxytocin).
- Promote adequate infant growth and development, including bone mineralization. Lactation doubles normal daily loss of calcium for the mother. The decrease in bone mineral density (BMD) during lactation and subsequent increase in BMD after weaning are negatively influenced by parity; bone loss may be decreased by a high ratio of dietary calcium to protein (Krebs et al., 1997).
- Discourage excessive use of stimulants, including caffeine from coffee (limit to 2 cups daily) and from tea, colas, and chocolate.
- Promote gradual weight loss even in obese women; poor lactation performance may be associated with obesity (Hilson et al., 1997). In overweight women who are exclusively breastfeeding, weight loss of .5 kg per week between 4–14 weeks after delivery does not affect the growth of their infants (Lovelady et al., 2000).

TABLE 1–3 Common Problems During Breastfeeding and Reasons Why Women Discontinue Breastfeeding

Engorgement: The best way to prevent engorgement is to begin breastfeeding as soon as possible after birth followed by nursing regularly throughout the day. Rapid filling of the breasts and blocked mammary ducts may cause a painful engorgement. Frequent nursing, breast massage, or warm shower before feedings, use of cold packs shortly after nursing, wearing a firm bra that is not too tight, and avoiding the use of nipple shields can help alleviate this condition.

Jaundice: Breast milk jaundice occurs in about 1% of the population of breastfeeding newborns, caused by the presence of a substance that alters liver function and may cause red cell hemolysis. Mothers should be encouraged to breastfeed 10–12 times per day to correct elevated serum bilirubin levels.

Mastitis: Breast infection causes fever, chills, redness, flu-like symptoms, and breast sensitivity. A clogged mammary duct, maternal anemia, stress, or an infection carried from the baby may cause mastitis. The primary goal is emptying the infected breast; frequent nursing is encouraged. The physician should be notified so that antibiotics or pain relievers are often prescribed. Application of heat to the breast, drinking plenty of fluids, and adequate rest are useful measures for treatment.

Nipple Confusion: Infants who are breastfed may refuse to take a bottle as the weaning of breastfeeding occurs. If the mother plans to feed formula from a bottle at any time during the first year of life, have her offer a bottle during the first 2–4 weeks of life and then offer one bottle per week thereafter to decrease the incidence of nipple confusion. The bottle feedings can be given using expressed breast milk.

Inadequate Milk Supply: Poor milk supply can be a cause of failure to thrive in breastfeeding infants. Maternal causes of poor milk supply are hypothyroidism, excessive antihistamine use, smoking, oral contraceptive use, excessive caffeine intake (over 2 cups of coffee and caffeinated sodas), illness, poor diet, decreased fluid intake, infrequent nursing, or fatigue. Correction of any of these causes may improve milk supply.

Sore Nipples: Frequent, short nursing, repositioning the infant at the breast, applying cold packs or heat to breasts, avoiding irritating soaps or lotions on nipples, air-drying nipples after nursing, exposing nipples to direct sunlight or 60 watt bulb for 15 minutes several times per day, applying vitamin E squeezed from capsules or ointment such as vitamins A and D or pure lanolin cream to nipples, and avoiding the use of nipple shields may help ease the pain. Occasionally, sore nipples are caused by *Candida albicans;* the breasts may not appear to have a fungal infection, but cultures of nipple surfaces will be positive for *Candida albicans*.

Reasons Why Women Discontinue Lactation

Hospital practices that do not support breastfeeding (Wright et al., 1996); physician apathy or misinformation
Acute infections in the mother
Mother's return to work
Mother's inability to provide 50% of the infant's needs
Mother's chronic illness (e.g., tuberculosis, severe anemia, chronic fevers, cardiovascular or renal disease)
Infant's inability to nurse due to weakness
Infant's inability to nurse adequately because of oral anomalies
Lack of information and support
Inadequate preparation
Lack of part-time jobs, flexible scheduling, and convenient day-care for mothers who must work

Nutrient	*Recommendation for Ages 18 yrs or under*	*Recommendation for Ages 19–30 yrs*	*Recommendation for Ages 31–50 yrs*
Calories:	1st 6 mos = +500 kcal/d; 2nd 6 mos= +400 kcal/d	1st 6 mos = +500 kcal/d; 2nd 6 mos = +400 kcal/d	1st tri = +500 kcal/d; 2nd 6 mos= +400 kcal/d
Protein:	65 g/d	65 g/d	65 g/d
Calcium:	1,300 mg/d	1,000 mg/d	1,000 mg/d
Iron:	10 mg/d	9 mg/d	9 mg/d
Folate	500 μg/d	500 μg/d	500 μg/d
Phosphorus:	1,250 mg/d	700 mg/d	700 mg/d
Vitamin A:	1,200 μg	1,300 μg	1,300 mg/d
Vitamin C:	115 mg/d	120 mg/d	120 mg/d
Thiamin:	1.4 mg/d	1.4 mg/d	1.4 mg/d
Riboflavin:	1.6 mg/d	1.6 mg/d	1.6 mg/d
Niacin:	17 mg/d	17 mg/d	17 mg/d

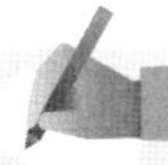

DIETARY AND NUTRITIONAL RECOMMENDATIONS

- In the first 6 months, increase the mother's caloric intake to +500 over RDA for age. In the next 6 months, use +400 over RDA for age. Recommendations may vary because individuals vary in prepregnancy weights, activity levels, and rates of weight gain (Fagan, 2000).
- Consider the special needs of adolescents or women older than 35 years of age. Energy and nutrient requirements will change accordingly.
- Increase the mother's intake of protein by 15 g (or approximately 65 g for average age). Encourage intake of sources of high biologic value (HBV) protein.
- Encourage intake of usual sources of vitamins and minerals. Intake of calcium should be 1,000–1,300 mg a day. Increases of B complex (thiamine and vitamin B6), and of vitamins A and C should be included in the diet. Supplementation may be needed for women with poor dietary intakes or chronic illnesses.
- Adequate vitamin D will be needed if maternal intake is poor or if infant receives little sunshine exposure. Dark-skinned, breastfed infants should be given vitamin D supplements to prevent nutritional rickets (Kreiter et al., 2000).
- Levels of both iron and copper decrease with progression of lactation; there is no evident need for supplementation in the first 6 months of lactation (Dorea, 2000).
- Increase intake of fluids.
- Forbid the use of alcohol unless permitted by physician.
- Beyond 3 months of lactation, the mother should increase her caloric intake if her weight loss has been excessive.
- Women who follow vegan diets may need zinc, calcium, vitamin D, or vitamin B12 supplementation. These diets also may be low in carnitine.
- If a tube feeds breast milk, fat losses can occur. Standard pediatric formula may be needed instead.

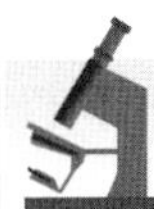

PROFILE

Clinical/History

BP
Smoking
Height
Current weight
Weight history
Prepregnancy weight
Date of birth (DOB) for infant
Goal for return to usual body weight

Lab Work

Gluc
Alb
H & H, Serum Fe
Alk phos
Physical therapy (PT)
Chol
Trig
Ca++
Serum phosphorus

Common Drugs Used and Potential Side Effects

- Alcohol, smoking, and many drugs are transmitted through breast milk to infants. Their use should be discouraged, unless permitted by a physician. Cigarette smoking also reduces the amount of milk produced. Moderate amounts of caffeine are acceptable (the recommendation is equivalent to no more than 2 cups of coffee).
- Cimetidine, lithium, cyclosporine, ergotamine, and other drugs may be contraindicated.
- Be careful about hypervitaminosis A and D. Read supplement labels carefully.
- Parlodel (bromocriptine mesylate) inhibits secretion of prolactin (decreases lactation) and is used for this purpose for women who do not wish to breastfeed. Constipation or anorexia may result.
- Drugs that may be used during breastfeeding: acetaminophen, some antibiotics and antihistamines, codeine, decongestants, insulin, quinine, ibuprofen, and thyroid medications.

- Discuss the relevance of tolerable upper intake levels (ULs) from the latest dietary reference intakes of the National Academy of Sciences. These levels were set to protect individuals from receiving too much of any nutrient from diet and dietary supplements.

Herbs, Botanicals and Supplements

- Herbs and botanical supplements should not be used without discussing with the physician. In general, these supplements have not been proven to be safe for breastfeeding mothers and their infants.
- Fenugreek, anise, fennel, garlic, and Echinacea have been suggested but have not been studied in this population for side effects.
- Lactating women should not take kava, chaste berry, dong quai, Asian ginseng, licorice root, and saw palmetto.

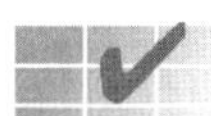

PATIENT EDUCATION

✓ Explain the composition of breast milk and the benefits of breastfeeding. Show the mother how to care for her nipples. Discuss how stools of breastfed babies differ from formula-fed infants (more loose, etc.).

✓ Women who are at risk for delayed onset of lactation need additional support during first week postpartum; frequent nursing should be recommended (Chapman and Perez-Escamilla, 1999).

✓ Explain the meaning of a balanced diet. Encourage the mother to normalize weight after delivery, but while the mother is nursing, she should not be placed on a weight loss program (Dewey et al., 1993). Other than postpartum diuresis, average loss is 0.67 kg/month.

✓ Guidance for lactating women should stress food sources of nutrients likely to be limited in their diets: calcium, zinc, folate, and vitamins E, D, and B6 (Mackey et al., 1998).

✓ Explain the requirements of infant nutrition after the infant has been weaned. Refer to the WIC program, if available, for eligible children.

✓ If necessary, omit chocolate, gas-forming foods, and highly seasoned foods. Amounts of food antigens in breast milk may be controlled by modifying the maternal diet (Fukushima et al., 1997).

✓ Moderate exercise seems to have no adverse effects on breastfeeding among healthy mothers (McCrory, 2001).

✓ Infant feeding methods do not alter the rate of postpartum weight loss (but total weight gained during pregnancy does). Mothers should not attempt rapid losses during the breastfeeding period; they should try to maintain their postpartum weight during lactation. Weight loss should not be initiated until breastfeeding is discontinued, with no more than 1 lb/week.

✓ Human milk can be stored safely for 24 hours at 15°C, for 4 hours at 25°C, but not at 38°C because bacterial growth and lipolysis are rapid at room temperature (Hamosh et al., 1996). Milk to be used within 48 hours can be refrigerated; for longer days, try freezing (up to 6 months) immediately.

✓ Lactating women are at high risk of energy and nutrient inadequacies, especially in low-income communities. Strategies to ensure adequate intakes must be planned (Doran and Evers, 1997).

✓ Nursing mothers should not eat shark, swordfish, king mackerel, and tilefish. These long-lived larger fish contain the highest levels of methyl mercury, which may harm a baby's developing nervous system. These women should select a variety of other kinds of fish, e.g., shellfish, canned fish, smaller ocean fish, or farm-raised fish. They can safely eat 12 ounces of cooked fish per week, with a typical serving size being 3–6 oz. They should avoid raw fish to reduce the risk of viral and bacterial illness.

For More Information

✦ Breastfeeding Promotion Committee
Healthy Mothers, Healthy Babies National Coalition
121 M. Washington St., Suite 300
Alexandria, VA 22314
703-836-6110
http://www.hmhb.org/

✦ Center for Breastfeeding Information
La Leche International
847-519-7730
http://www.lalecheleague.org/

✦ Lactation Institute and Breastfeeding Clinic
16430 Ventura Blvd., Suite 303
Eucino, CA 91436
818-995-1913
http://www.lactationinstitute.org/

✦ International Lactation Consultant Association
4101 Lake Boone Trail, Suite 201
Raleigh, NC 27607
http://www.ika.org/

INFANT, NORMAL (0–6 MONTHS)

NUTRITIONAL ACUITY RANKING: LEVEL 1

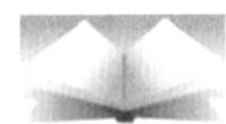

DEFINITIONS AND BACKGROUND

The average birth weight of an infant ranges between 5.5 and 10 lb; the average is approximately 7–7.5 lb. Normal gestation is 40 weeks. For assessment of an infant, monitoring growth is the best way to evaluate intake. For infants who are ill, special techniques (doubly labeled water studies or test weighing) may be used for determining intakes of breast milk. Mixed feedings of formula, breast milk, and foods complicate the process in older infants, and eating patterns vary from one month to the next because appetite regulates growth.

Healthy, full-term infants lose some weight in the first days after birth but tend to regain it within approximately 1 week (Fagan, 2000). Infants often double their birth weight within 4–6 months and triple it within 1 year (Fagan, 2000). Head circumference increases about 40% during the first year, and brain weight should almost double. Infants are composed of approximately 75–80% water, compared with adults, who are composed of 60–65% water. Infants may become dehydrated easily, especially in hot weather or after bouts of diarrhea.

Infants are born with a 4- to 6-month supply of iron if maternal stores were adequate during gestation and if the mother was not anemic during pregnancy. Infants of vegan mothers may require zinc, calcium, and vitamin B12 supplementation. Some research suggests that infants who are at risk for sudden infant death syndrome (SIDS) have low levels of magnesium in their bloodstreams, which may contribute to an inability to lift the neck muscles from a prone position (Caddell, 2001). A bigger problem is vitamin D intake during infancy and the risk of rickets, which is becoming more common. Over-supplementation should be avoided in all cases. High blood pressure in adults may be linked to maternal nutrition; studies are being conducted in this area (Rosebloom et al., 2001).

Breastfeeding takes longer than cup or bottle feeding, but has the most benefits and is the preferred method. When breastfeeding is not possible or not desired, formula feeding is used.

For formula feedings in infants with oral or developmental problems, administration times, amounts ingested, and physiologic stability of infants are similar when newborn infants are fed using a bottle or a cup. If using a cup, use a small plastic medicine cup and stroke the lower lip to stimulate rooting (Howard et al., 1999). Section 3 describes conditions where alternative feeding methods may be needed.

The Committee on Nutrition of the American Academy of Pediatrics supports the following practices during infancy (American Academy of Pediatrics, 1998):

- Exclusive breastfeeding for the first 6 months. Supplement with vitamin D from birth and iron supplementation as ferrous sulfate drops or iron-fortified cereal after 4 months of age. Fluoride supplementation may be required after 6 months of age depending on the fluoride content of the city water. Feeding of iron-fortified commercial infant formula for the first year as an alternative to breastfeeding.
- Delaying the use of whole cow milk until after one year of age. Early introduction of whole cow milk protein during infancy may contribute to iron-deficiency anemia by increasing gastrointestinal blood loss. Whole cow milk has an increased renal solute load compared to infant formulas.
- Reduced fat milks should be delayed until after the second year of life. Adequate fat intake is important for the developing brain and milk is usually the primary source of fat for infants and toddlers.
- Delaying the introduction of semi-solid foods until 4–6 months of age or until the infant demonstrates signs of developmental readiness, such as head control and ability to sit with support.

OBJECTIVES

- Promote normal growth and development: assess sleeping, eating, and attentiveness habits. Compare infant's growth to the chart of normal growth patterns. Weight for length (height) is the most meaningful measurement. Use updated CDC growth charts and monitor growth trends, not a singular value. Malnutrition results in decreased weight, then height, then head circumference (if chronic.)
- Overcome any nutritional risk factors or complications, such as otitis media or dehydration.
- Evaluate use and discourage early introduction of solids and cow's milk.
- Encourage the mother to use breast milk as the infant's main source of nutrition for the first 6 months, introducing solids and juices slowly beginning at approximately 4 months of age.
- If the infant is breastfed, assess the mother's prepregnancy nutritional status and risk factors, weight gain pattern, food allergies, and medical history (such as toxemia, chronic illnesses, or anemia). Discuss any current conditions that may affect lactation (e.g., smoking, use of alcohol, family history of allergies.)
- If the infant is formula-fed, the mother should learn about nursing-bottle caries syndrome prevention and about potential overfeeding problems. Overnutrition is associated with subsequent fatness (Martorelli et al., 2001).
- Promote growth and development through adequate fatty acid intake—linoleic acid n-6 and linolenic n-3 (Agostoni, 1994).
- Soy diets are known to induce goiter because they increase thyroxine requirements; soy contains a mildly goitrogenic factor (Chorazy et al., 1995). Effects of soy formulas on the thyroid must be monitored in infants with hypothyroidism. Iodine has been added to most infant formulas; check labels.

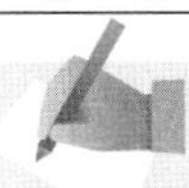

DIETARY AND NUTRITIONAL RECOMMENDATIONS

- Fluid requirements may include the following: 60–80 mL/kg water in newborns; 80–100 mL/kg by 3 days of age; 125–150 mL/kg up to 6 months of age. Assess individual needs according to status.
- Calorie needs are estimated by RDA to decrease from 115–105 kcal/kg between birth and 6 months. This can be obtained in about 28–32 oz human milk or infant formula.
- Protein requirement is generally 2.2 g/kg, or about 13 g/day. Sick infants may need a higher ratio. Use nutrient recommendation chart (below.)
- If infant is breastfed, discourage mother from use of drugs and alcohol; keep caffeine intake limited to the equivalent of 2 cups of coffee per day. Teach parents about use of diluted fruit juice (perhaps apple) at 4 months of age. Breastfed infants may require 200 IU vitamin D, 0.01 mg of fluoride; and sometimes iron supplements (at about 3 months of age). Mothers of infants predisposed to allergies should avoid fish, cow's milk, and nuts. Do not introduce cow's milk before 12 months of age.
- Formula-fed infants: type of formula—milk-based, soy, etc. Check list of significant ingredients and amount used for 24 hours. No calorie-containing formula should be given in the crib—only water. Sweetened beverages should not be used between meals or at bedtime. Be careful in warming bottles: folacin and vitamin C may be destroyed. Iron-fortified formula is often used after 2–3 months (American Academy of Pediatrics, Committee on Nutrition, 1999).
- The inhibitory effect of calcium and phosphorus on iron absorption is not clinically important in infants fed iron-fortified formulas (Dalton et al., 1997). No fluoride supplement is needed unless the water supply provides less than 0.3 ppm. Discourage use of evaporated milk formula, which is low in vitamin C and high in protein, sodium, and potassium; it is not for use with infants.
- Standard formulas have a 60:40 whey:casein ratio, which is desirable in a formula; they provide 20 kcal/oz. Breast milk yields an 80:20 whey:casein ratio and approximately the same calories. Standard formulas include Enfamil, Similac, Gerber Formula, Good Start, and others.
- Special formulas are available for special needs—ProSobee, Carnation Alsoy, or Isomil for cow's milk allergies; soy formulas are fortified with zinc and iron. Alimentum, Portagen, or Pregestimil are available for malabsorption and inclusion of medium-chain triglycerides (MCT); Nutramigen, Alimentum, or Pregestimil for other complex gastrointestinal (GI) problems. Nutramigen may also be used for allergies to both soy and cow's milk protein. Contact nutritional formula companies for updated information.
- Soy formulas now include carnitine, which generally is available in breast milk.
- At 4–6 months, introduce plain (not mixed, sweetened, or spiced) strained or pureed baby cereals, then nonallergenic vegetables (such as carrots or green beans), and then fruits. Start with 1–2 teaspoons and progress as appetite indicates. Try a single new item for 7+ days to detect any signs of food allergy. The intake of solids should not decrease breast milk or formula intake to less than 32 oz daily. Avoid giving too much juice (Dewey, 2001); 4–6 oz daily is sufficient.
- Ensure that the RDAs are being met for all other nutrients for each stage of growth. Vitamin D fortification in milk may be unpredictable, for example, and signs of any problem should be noted. When in doubt, a multi-vitamin mineral supplement is advisable (Dewey, 2001).
- For tube-fed infants, PediaSure, Kindercal, Nutren Junior, and Resource Just for Kids are specifically for pediatrics. If an elemental diet is needed for severe protein intolerance or cow's milk allergy, Pediatric Vivonex, Neocate One Plus, and Elecare may be useful. Monitor carefully for hydration; don't modify nutrients because of changing osmolality. Breast milk has an osmolality of 285 mOsm/kg; formulas vary from 150–380 mOsm/kg. Formulas with over 400 mOsm/kg can cause diarrhea or vomiting. Formula should contain 10–20% protein, 30–40% fat, 40–60% CHO. Fat should not be excessive so that the infant does not experience ketosis.
- Minimal enteral feeding (MEF) favors secretion of gastrointestinal hormones in sick premature infants. Early MEF seems to be preferable to late feeding since it allows a faster secretion related to volume of the formula; MEF does not increase abdominal complications (Ordaz-Jimenez et al., 1998). See Low Birth Weight entry in Section 3.
- For special conditions, TPN may be used. 1–2% essential fatty acids (EFAs) may be necessary to prevent signs of deficiency, such as inadequate wound healing, growth, immunocompetence, and platelet formation. Linoleic and linolenic acids seem to be required.

Nutrient	*Recommendation for Infants Ages 0–6 mos*
Calories	115–105 kcal/kg
Protein	13 g/d
Calcium	210 mg/d
Iron	0.27 mg/d
Folate	65 μg/d
Phosphorus	100 mg/d
Vitamin A	400 μg
Vitamin C	40 mg/d
Thiamin	.2 mg/d
Riboflavin	.3 mg/d
Niacin	2 mg/d

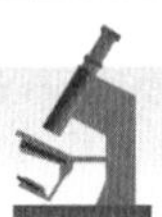

PROFILE

Clinical/History		
Birth weight Gestational age Length Percentile weight/ length (goal between 5th and 95th)	Head circumference Apgar scores Sucking reflex Prematurity Physical handicaps Mother's prenatal history Appetite Hydration status; intake and output (I & O)	**Lab Work** Alb Serum Fe Gluc H & H (after 3 months)

Herbs, Botanicals and Supplements

- Infants and children may be even more susceptible to some of the adverse effects and toxicity of these products because of differences in physiology, immature metabolic enzyme systems, and dose per body weight (Tomassoni and Simone, 2001). Herbs and botanical supplements should not be used without discussing with the physician. In general, these types of supplements have not been proven to be safe for infants (Gardinier and Kemper, 2000).
- Discuss the relevance of tolerable upper intake levels (ULs) from the latest dietary reference intakes of the National Academy of Sciences. These levels were set to protect adults from receiving too much of any nutrient from diet and dietary supplements; infants are especially at risk for toxicities.

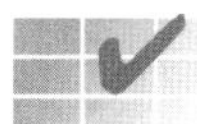

PATIENT EDUCATION

- ✓ Explain the proper timing and sequence of feeding (Sullivan and Birch, 1994). Discuss successful feeding as trusting and responding to cues from the infant about timing, pace, and eating capacity.
- ✓ Explain growth patterns, e.g., an infant who is 4–6 months of age should double his or her birth weight. Discuss problems related to inadequate growth, e.g., for children with atopic dermatitis, the method of feeding does not seem to affect growth rate; other factors may be involved by ages 6–12 months (Agostoni et al., 2000).
- ✓ Emphasize the importance of adequate bonding.
- ✓ Explain the proper care of infant's teeth, including risks of nursing-bottle caries syndrome.
- ✓ Explain the proper timing and sequence of solid food introduction. Avoid use of stringy foods or foods like peanut butter that are hard to swallow. Hard candies, grapes, and similar foods may increase the risk of aspiration.
- ✓ Discuss the rationale for delaying introduction of cow's milk (risks for allergy, gastrointestinal bleeding).
- ✓ Discuss why fluid intake is essential, and explain that infant needs are much greater than for adults, according to weight.
- ✓ If the infant is breastfed, discuss the normalcy of 4–6 soft stools each day. Compare the normal stool with symptoms of diarrhea.
- ✓ For special feeding problems, see Table 1–4

For More Information

- American Academy of Pediatrics http://www.aap.org/
- Clinical Practice Guidelines (constipation, gastroenteritis, etc.) http://www.aap.org/policy/paramtoc.html

TABLE 1–4 Special Problems in Infant Feeding*

Spitting up or Reflux. If there is no weight loss concern, just offer encouragement that the problem will resolve in a few months. Positioning is an important consideration during feeding. Feed more slowly and burp often. Use feeding volumes and a schedule that is set. Avoid exposure to second-hand smoke. Offer parental reassurance.

Regurgitation. Position the infant in an upright, 40–60 degree position after feeding for approximately 30 minutes; have the doctor rule out other problems. Use smaller, more frequent feedings to avoid overfeeding. Thickening of formula with a small amount of cereal has been recommended; now there are prethickened formulas available if the doctor thinks it is necessary.

Diarrhea. Replace fluids and electrolytes (e.g., Pedialyte) as directed by the doctor. After an extended period of time, have the doctor rule out allergy. Monitor weight loss and fluid intake carefully.

Pale, oily stools. Check for fat malabsorption. Use an MCT-containing formula if necessary.

Constipation. The doctor will make a careful assessment and may suggest adding 1 t of a carbohydrate source to 4 oz of water or formula, one to two times daily. Avoid use of honey and corn syrup to prevent infant botulism.

Colic. Check for hunger, food allergy, incorrect formula temperature, stress, or other underlying problems. Give small, frequent feedings and parental encouragement. Colic is equally common in breastfed or formula-fed infants. If breastfed, continue to breastfeed. Rarely, removal of cow's milk products from the mother's diet is useful. If formula-fed, expensive elemental formulas should be discontinued if symptoms do not improve. Curved bottles allow infants to be fed while they are held upright (Juszczyk Balon, 1997). Collapsable bags decrease swallowing of air. Infants should be burped regularly during feedings.

Allergy. Primary prevention through a hypoallergenic diet may reduce the prevalence of food allergy, eczema, and urticaria (Arshad, 2001). Breastfeeding should be recommended for all children. Introduce new foods at the appropriate age and singly; try for at least 7 days before introducing any new foods. Discuss any symptoms with the doctor immediately. Avoid cow's milk strictly, and delay introduction of egg, nuts, wheat, and fish (Arshad, 2001).

*See also: ADA Pediatric Manual of Clinical Dietetics and the ADA/DDPD Children with Special Health Care Needs: a Community Nutrition Pocket Guide.

- Growth Charts
  http://www.cdc.gov/growthcharts
- Mead Johnson (products for infants)
  http://meadjohnson.com/products/index.html
- National Perinatal Association
  http://www.nationalperinatal.org/
- Ross Laboratories (products for infants)
  http://rosslabs.com
- Sudden Infant Death Syndrome
  IDS Hotline: 800–221-SIDS

INFANT, NORMAL (6–12 MONTHS)

NUTRITIONAL ACUITY RANKING: LEVEL 1

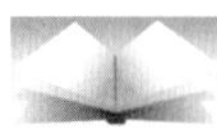

DEFINITIONS AND BACKGROUND

Infants older than 6 months of age are beginning the developmental stages that will lead to walking and talking. Many of the same principles associated with infant feeding during the first 6 months will continue with the greater use of solids. The growth pattern of breastfed and formula-fed infants differs in the first 12 months of life. The new CDC growth charts were developed with a larger proportion of breastfed infants. Growth indices in breastfed groups, high at birth and closer than expected to the reference at 12 months, may reflect differences in genetic factors, intrauterine conditions, or both (Agostoni et al., 2000). Overall, infant feeding mode (i.e., breastfeeding or formula) is associated with differences in body composition in early infancy, which do not persist into the second year of life (Butte et al., 2000).

Timing of the introduction of complementary foods (solids) is an important consideration. Early introduction is considered to be at 3–4-months-old, late introduction at 6-months-old. A recent study monitored the effect of introduction of complementary foods on iron and zinc status among formula-fed infants at 12, 24, and 36-months-old; iron and zinc status were not influenced by timing of the introduction of complementary foods (Kattelmann et al., 2001).

Introduction of cow's milk at 12-months-old brings new problems and risks related to essential fatty acid deficiency if low-fat or skim milks are used. It seems that long-chain fatty acids are useful in normal growth and development of infants and young children. It is not necessary to alter the diets of young children to prevent heart disease or to lower cholesterol, etc.

While the relationship between the type of feeding and one's later intelligence may relate to social environment rather than to nutritional qualities of milk received (Gale and Martyn, 1996), recent studies confirm the effects of fatty acids on later intelligence. Breastfed and formula-fed infants maintain a characteristic serum cholesterol ester fatty acid pattern after age 7 months even after they begin to receive solid food; breastfed infants have significantly higher levels of arachidonic acid and docosahexaenoic acid (Salo et al., 1997); they tend to have better cognitive development.

Growth and development at this stage are affected by underlying or acute illnesses, nutritional intake, and related factors. Children with severe atopic dermatitis, for example, will suffer a progressive impairment in growth irrespective of the early type of feeding. The severity of disease may be an independent factor negatively influencing growth (Agostoni, 2000).

OBJECTIVES

- Continue to promote normal growth and development during this second stage of very rapid growth. Use updated CDC growth charts. Monitor trends in growth, not a singular value.
- Prevent significant weight losses from illness or inadequate feeding. Malnutrition results in decreased weight, then height, then head circumference.
- Avoid dehydration.
- Prevent or correct such complications as diarrhea, constipation, and otitis media. Otitis media is more common in bottle-fed infants.
- Introduce new solids, at appropriate periods of time, singly. Support feeding skills development—new tastes at 4–6 months (fortified rice cereal); sitting at 6–7 months (vegetables, fruits); pincer grasp at 8–9 months (protein foods and finger foods); reaching for food at 10–12 months (soft table foods, encourage self-feeding.)
- Begin to encourage greater physical activity; prepare for walking by ensuring adequate calorie intake.
- Continue to emphasize the role of good nutrition in the development of healthy teeth.
- Delay allergenic foods until 12 months of age (e.g., citrus, egg white, cow's milk, corn). Be wary of peanut and nut butters because they are often highly allergenic.
- Use of follow-up formulas with higher percentage of kilocalories from protein and CHO and less from fat have questionable benefits at this time.
- Prevent nutrient deficiencies upon weaning, e.g., zinc.

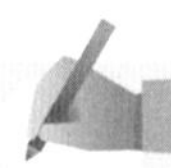

DIETARY AND NUTRITIONAL RECOMMENDATIONS

- Fluid requirements may include approximately 125–150 mL/kg up to 1-year-old. Fluid needs may decline slightly during this stage.
- For energy needs, the RDA suggests 90–100 kcal/kg body weight. See nutrient recommendations chart. Monitor according to the CDC growth charts and identify problems early.
- Continue to provide breast milk or iron-fortified formula

Nutrient	*Recommendation for Infants Ages 6 mos–1 yr*
Calories	850 kcal/d
Protein	14 g/d
Calcium	270 mg/d
Iron	11 mg/d
Folate	80 μg/d
Phosphorus	275 mg/d
Vitamin A	500 μg
Vitamin C	50 mg/d
Thiamin	0.3 mg/d
Riboflavin	0.4 mg/d
Niacin	4 mg/d

during this stage. Avoid use of excessively sweetened beverages. The use of special milk substitutes is not necessary unless there is an allergy to soy protein or cow's milk.

- Protein requirement for a 6-month-old infant is generally 1.56 g/kg, changing as the infant grows. This equals about 14 g/day. By 12 months, the need is only 1.14 g/kg. See nutrient recommendations chart.
- Introduce more solids as indicated: egg yolk at 8–9-months-old; meat and cottage cheese at 9–10-months-old; and finger foods at 10–12-months-old, e.g., peeled and cooked fruit, dry toast, vegetable bits, and zwieback or arrowroot crackers. Toddler or junior foods may be used, but selection of those items that are single foods rather than mixed dishes may be more appropriate (e.g., some mixed dishes are primarily starch and not meat). Read labels carefully.
- Avoid raw vegetables and fruits (other than ripe banana or soft peeled apple). Beware of foods that may cause choking (e.g., hot dogs, popcorn, nuts, grapes, seeds).
- As tolerated, introduce coarsely ground table foods at 10–12-months-old.
- Introduce cow's milk at 12-months-old, ensuring that intake does not go above 1 quart daily to prevent anemia. Use whole milk.
- Whole egg may be offered at 12-months-old, using caution because of allergy to the egg whites.
- Begin to offer fluids by cup at approximately 9–12-months-old; weaning often occurs by about 1 year of age. Avoid sweetened beverages at this age whenever possible.
- Spicy foods often are not liked or not tolerated. Taste buds are very acute at this stage. This is also affected by culture and the seasoning of foods that are introduced.
- Continue use of approximately 6 T of iron-fortified baby cereal after 12 months of age to ensure adequate intake. Adult cereals often are inappropriate for infants and children younger than 4. Approximately 10 mg of iron is required. WIC-approved cereals are iron fortified.
- Children who require tube feeding require specialty care. If the infant needs a tube feeding (for poor weight gain, low volitional intake, 5th percentile or lower for weight for height and age, slow and prolonged feeding times over 4–6 hours because of oral/motor problems), a standard isotonic tube feeding formula that provides 30 kcal/oz, intact proteins may be used. If necessary, lactose-free and gluten-free formulas are available. Added fiber and a mix of long-chain and medium-chain fatty acids may be useful. Osmolality of 260–650 mOsm/kg is common; monitor tolerances regularly. Be sure to use sufficient water. The infant may tolerate bolus feedings in the day and continuous feedings at night.

Herbs, Botanicals and Supplements

- Infants and children may be even more susceptible to some of the adverse effects and toxicity of these products because of differences in physiology, immature metabolic enzyme systems, and dose per body weight (Tomassoni and Simone, 2001). Herbs and botanical supplements should not be used without discussing with the physician. In general, these types of supplements have not been proven to be safe for infants (Gardinier and Kemper, 2000).
- Discuss the relevance of tolerable upper intake levels (ULs) from the latest dietary reference intakes of the National Academy of Sciences. These levels were set to protect adults from receiving too much of any nutrient from diet and dietary supplements; infants are especially at risk for toxicities.

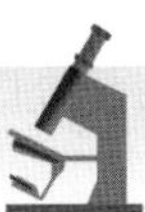

PROFILE

Clinical/History		
Length	Head circumference	Persistent vomiting
Current weight	Developmental stage	Diarrhea
Birth length/weight	Hydration status	**Lab Work**
Percentile weight/length	Tooth development	Gluc
Age in months	Physical handicaps	Serum Fe
	Appetite	Alb
	I & O	pCO2, pO2
		H & H

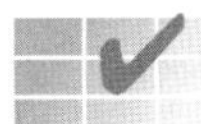

PATIENT EDUCATION

- Discuss adequate weight pattern: infants generally double or triple birth weight by 12-months-old; body length increases by about 55%; head circumference by about 40%, and brain weight doubles.
- Discuss overfeeding, iron intake, fluid intake, and other nutritional factors related to normal growth and development.
- When brushing teeth, be careful not to use a large amount of fluoridated toothpaste. A very small amount suffices.
- Discuss role of fat-soluble vitamins and their presence in whole milk. Discuss also the role of essential fatty acids in normal growth and development of the nervous system.
- Bottled waters are not a substitute for formula. Hyponatremia may result.
- Fluoridated water is recommended; check the community status. Be wary of use of fluoride supplements when the water is fluoridated and the infant receives adequate water from this source. Note that well water is not fluoridated and that supplementation may be needed in this case.
- Lead poisoning should be monitored in growing children, especially in older homes or buildings where there are day-care centers. Toddlers may eat lead-based paint that is chipping away from walls. Lead replaces calcium in the bone; deposition may be seen in x-rays of the knee, ankle, or wrist. Lead also depletes iron. When using tap water, let the water run 2 minutes to clear pipes prior to making formula or offering water to drink.

- ✓ For planning vegan diets in infancy, breast milk should be the sole food with soy-based formula as an alternative; breastfed vegan infants may need supplements of vitamin B12, zinc, and vitamin D (Reed, Mangels, and Messina, 2001). Protein sources for older infants may include tofu and dried beans.

For More Information

- Feeding Kids Newsletter
  http://www.nutritionforkids.com/Feeding_Kids.htm
- Growth Charts
  http://www.cdc.gov/growthcharts
- Kids Health
  http://www.kidshealth.org/
- USDA/ARS Children's Nutrition Research Center
  1100 Bates Street, Houston, Texas 77030 Phone: 713-798–7971
  http://www.bcm.tmc.edu/cnrc/

Manufacturers:

- Beech Nut
  800-523-6633
  http://www.babycenter.com/solidfoods/product.html
- Gerber
  1–800-4-gerber
  http://www.gerber.com/
- Heinz
  1–800-USA-BABY
  http://www.heinzbaby.com/

CHILDHOOD

NUTRITIONAL ACUITY RANKING: LEVEL 1

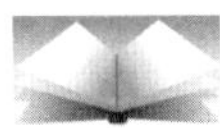

DEFINITIONS AND BACKGROUND

Goals of development (Erikson, 1963): toddler (1–3-years-old)—autonomy; preschooler (4–6-years-old)—initiative; school age (6–12-years-old)—industry. Children are not "little adults" and should be treated differently, even nutritionally. A surrogate is usually required to discuss nutritional intakes; the ability to recall is often limited in children in relation to vocabulary, literacy level, and attention span. Even under the best conditions (i.e., reporting within 90 minutes after eating school lunch), children have difficulty reporting what they have eaten; accuracy decreases markedly the longer the time span after eating (Baxter and Domel, 1997). Observation by an adult is often needed to assess accurate intakes.

Growth during this stage involves changes in appetite, physical activity, and frequency of illnesses. The CDC growth charts provide a guideline for monitoring successful growth as it relates to weight, height, and age. Body mass index (BMI) calculations are now available for use with children and calculations may be used to identify underweight, potential stunting, or obesity in children. Prevalence for low height for age (stunting) and low weight for age (wasting) seems to be higher among children from persistently poor families than from the general population (Miller and Korenman, 1994).

During the early years of life, eating occurs primarily as a result of hunger and satiety cues. Evidence suggests that by the time children are 3- or 4-years-old, eating is no longer driven by real hunger but is influenced by a variety of environmental factors, including presentation of larger portions (Rolls et al., 2000). Girls with mothers who are dieting have more ideas about dieting than those with moms who do not diet (Abramaovitz and Birch, 2000). Restricting young girls' access to palatable foods may promote the intake of restricted foods and may generate negative feelings about their consumption (Orlet, Fisher, and Birch, 2000).

Children from underserved, ethnically diverse population groups tend to have increased risk for obesity, increased serum lipids, and dietary consumption patterns that do not meet suggested dietary guidelines (Bronner, 1996). Intake of dairy products, fruits, and vegetables tends to be significantly lower in the black population (Lindquist et al., 2000). Children are becoming more overweight and less active; type 2 diabetes usually affects those over age 45, but more children are given a diagnosis of maturity-onset diabetes in youth (MODY) (Trissler, 1999). There have been numerous recent reports of case series of type 2 diabetes mellitus (DM) in American Indian, African American, Hispanic, Asian American, and white children from North America. Prevalence and incidence estimates vary depending on the age and ethnicity of the population, but it is estimated that type 2 DM represents 8–45% of patients with DM currently diagnosed in large U.S. pediatric centers; however, this is likely to be an underestimation (Fagot-Campagna, 2000). Allow overweight children to grow into their weights rather than restricting energy intakes. For more information, see Childhood Obesity in Section 3.

Almost 23% of children under the age of 18 in the U.S. live in poverty; some may be exposed to lead poisoning, and iron deficiency anemia is the biggest risk. Even mild undernutrition affects brain growth and function (Pollitt, 1995). Food assistance programs should be used whenever possible. It is also essential that school-aged children have adequate meals to eliminate transient hunger, which tends to interfere with classroom performance. Attention is easily diverted at this age; total intake may vary. Scheduling of lunch after recess results in greater intake of all foods and calories (Getlinger et al., 1996).

Misconceptions must be corrected, such as "good foods/bad foods" or "foods that are good for you taste bad." Dietary fat restriction may compromise growth and should not be implemented. There is no proof of long-term safety and efficacy for restricting fat in the diets of children. Lower content of calcium, zinc, Mg++, phosphorus, vitamins E and B12, thiamin, niacin, and riboflavin intakes must be considered (Olson, 2000).

Adequate calcium is essential during growth, especially during rapid bone growth and mineralization during puberty. Current mean dietary intakes are below desired levels; children may need encouragement to increase their intakes of skim and low-fat dairy products and may need information about calcium supplements (American Academy of Pediatrics, 1999; Stallings, 1997). Dietary calcium needs of children who take medications that alter bone metabolism is uncertain; provide at least RDA levels for calcium and for vitamin D. Rickets is becoming more common in children (Carvalho et al., 2000).

Recent estimates suggest that malnutrition (measured as poor anthropometric status) is associated with about 50% of all deaths among children. The strongest relationship to malnutrition is observed for diarrhea and acute respiratory infection, and also some evidence for a potentially increased risk for death from malaria or from measles (Rice et al., 2000). Infectious diseases of childhood may be related to poor nutrition, especially a lack of vitamin C (Seaton and Devereux, 2000). Children who are prone to repetitive illness may benefit from a basic multiple vitamin–mineral supplement in addition to a carefully planned diet.

OBJECTIVES

- Assess growth patterns, feeding skills, dietary intake, activity patterns, inherited factors, and intellectual development. Promote adequate growth and development patterns such as increased independence at 12–18 months (stop bottle, begin eating with a spoon), growth slowdown from 18 months–2 years (less interest in food; begin eating with utensils), calorie intake varies from 2–3 years (control exerted), brain growth triples by age 6.

- Monitor long-term drug therapies and related side effects (e.g., use of anticonvulsants and the effects on folate, growth, etc.).
- Assess nutritional deficiencies, especially iron. If possible, detect and correct pica (eating nonfood items or any one food to the exclusion of others—even ice chips). Prevent "milk anemia" that may originate from drinking too much milk with meals and not consuming enough iron-rich meats, grains, and vegetables.
- Avoid food deprivation, which may decrease ability to concentrate, cause growth failure or anemia, aggravate stunting, and lead to easy fatigue.
- Evaluate status of the child's dental health. Prevent dental decay.
- Promote adequate response to immunizations.
- Promote adequate intake of calcium, fiber, and zinc—nutrients that are often poorly consumed by young children.
- Help reduce onset of chronic diseases later in life (e.g., high blood pressure, cardiovascular diseases, diabetes) by prudent menu planning and meal intakes. Risk for nutritional inadequacy does not appear to be higher among children who eat moderate-fat versus higher-fat diets. Higher-fat diets are not necessarily more protective against nutritional inadequacy (Ballew et al., 2000).
- Encourage physical activity and aerobic fitness.
- Avoid mislabeling children as "fat," which may aggravate an eating disorder later.
- Children should be treated respectfully. Initiate conversation with the child personally rather than only talking with parents or caregivers. As with any counseling relationship, a personalized conversation elicits the most effective response.
- The school and community have equal responsibility for achieving integrity of school food service. Nutrition integrity is a guaranteed level of performance that all foods available contribute to the overall RDA for children and contribute to lifelong healthy eating habits (American Dietetic Association, 2000).
- To promote proper growth, especially for stature, parents and caretakers should limit fruit juice and sweetened beverage intake to 12 fl oz per day (Dennison et al., 1999; Skinner et al., 1999). Excesses of products that contain sorbitol may also cause diarrhea.
- Emphasize food variety to reduce fear of new foods (neophobia), which may reduce nutritional status (Falciglia et al., 2000).

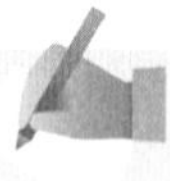

DIETARY AND NUTRITIONAL RECOMMENDATIONS

- See charts for energy requirements and protein. Calorie needs are approximately 100 kcal/kg at the onset of childhood, gradually decreasing to 55 kcal/kg by the teen years.
- Provide fat as 30–35% total kcal. After 2 years of age, replace some high-fat foods with lower-fat foods; use low-fat techniques for preparation of meals; and use less added fat from foods, e.g., use jelly on bread instead of butter (Sigman-Grant, 1993). Use of 10% kcal as saturated fatty acids and less than 300 mg of cholesterol are beneficial guidelines from the National Cholesterol Education Program (NCEP).
- Offer calcium as indicated in nutrient charts to increase mineral density. Yogurt, plain or chocolate milk, calcium-fortified juices, and cheeses are generally well accepted by children.
- Phosphorus intake should be similar to calcium intakes.
- Encourage exposure to sunlight and monitor dietary intake of vitamin D. Adequate folate, magnesium, selenium, and vitamin E are important to obtain from dietary sources.
- Day-care meals given for a 4- to 8-hour stay should provide for one-third to one-half of daily needs. School lunch programs generally provide one-third of daily needs. Meals at home should be planned carefully to make up the differences.
- Give 50–60 mL/kg fluid daily. Milk, fruit and vegetable juices, and water should be the basic fluids offered.
- To increase fiber in the diet, use the "age +5 rule" (Williams, 1995). From 8 g/day at 3-years-old to 25 g/day by 20-years-old is suggested. Fiber from fruits, vegetables, grains, and legumes may help to prevent or correct constipation.
- Include a variety of foods in proper portions for age.
- Suggested pattern of food intake: preschool children—milk and dairy products, 3/4 cup four times daily; meat and meat substitutes, 1/4 cup twice daily; fruits and vegetables, 4 oz four times daily—check for sufficient intake of vitamins A and C; 4–6 servings of bread or substitute daily.
- Suggested pattern of food intake: school age children—milk and dairy products, 3/4–1 cup four times daily; meat and meat substitutes, 1/3–1/2 cup twice daily; fruit and vegetables, 4–6 oz four times daily—check for sufficient intake of vitamins A and C; six or more servings of bread or substitute daily.

Nutrient	*Recommendation for Ages 1–3 yrs*	*Recommendation for Ages 4–8 yrs*
Calories:	1,300 kcal/d	1,800 kcal/d
Protein:	16 g/d	24 g/d
Calcium:	500 mg/d	800 mg/day
Iron:	7 mg/d	10 mg/d
Folate	150 μg/d	200 μg/d
Phosphorus:	460 mg/d	500 mg/d
Vitamin A:	300 μg	400 μg
Vitamin C:	15 mg/d	25 mg/d
Thiamin:	0.5 mg/d	0.6 mg/d
Riboflavin:	0.5 mg/d	0.6 mg/d
Niacin:	6 mg/d	8 mg/d

Common Drugs Used and Potential Side Effects

- Nutritional supplements should be taken only when prescribed by a physician, although over-the-counter use is common. Avoid serving cereals to children that fulfill the adult RDAs for vitamins and minerals (e.g., Total cereal.)

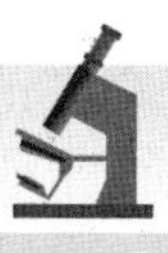

PROFILE

Clinical/History	Hydration (I & O)	Lab Work
Age Weight Height Growth percentile for age Dental status Physical handicaps Appetite	Triceps skinfold (TSF) Midarm muscle circumference (MAMC), midarm circumference (MAC)	Alb Trig Transferrin H & H, Serum Fe Chol Gluc Alk phos Ca++

- Anticonvulsants may cause problems with the child's growth and normal body functions. Diet should be adjusted carefully.
- Corticosteroids may cause growth stunting if given over an extended time in large doses.
- Poly-Vi-Fluor contains fluoride; use caution in areas where water is fluoridated. Too much can cause fluorosis.
- Tofranil may be used for some cases of bedwetting. Dry mouth may result.

Herbs, Botanicals and Supplements

- Herbs and botanical supplements should not be used without discussing with the physician. These supplements have not been proven to be safe for children.
- Discuss the relevance of tolerable upper intake levels (ULs) from the latest dietary reference intakes of the National Academy of Sciences. These levels were set to protect individuals from receiving too much of any nutrient from diet and dietary supplements; children are more prone to toxicity than adults.

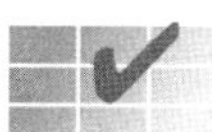

PATIENT EDUCATION

- ✔ Explain the appropriate diet for children. The diet should contain sufficient protein of approximately 50% high-biologic-value sources.
- ✔ Encourage parents to use finger foods for toddlers. Older children need nutritious snacks. Iron-rich desserts may also be used on occasion. Cheese cubes are good snacks for the teeth.
- ✔ Encourage a relaxed atmosphere at mealtime. There should be no pressure to eat, hurry, or finish meals.
- ✔ Explain to parents that bribery or rewards for eating should never be used. Rewards can actually decrease acceptance.
- ✔ Remind parents that children have food jags and that they also prefer single foods.
- ✔ Encourage parents to avoid sweetened beverages and empty-calorie foods.
- ✔ Teach the parents about food intake and dietary practices that affect learning and problems.
- ✔ With toddlers, continued use of iron-fortified cereal can be beneficial. Include juices that are naturally high in vitamin C.
- ✔ Children should be allowed to vary in their food acceptance, choices, and intakes, just as adults.
- ✔ Children who have chronic illnesses fare better if parents give them responsibilities, such as meal planning and taking their own medications. Tasks should be age-appropriate. Section 3 addresses pediatric illnesses in greater detail.
- ✔ A proper emotional atmosphere is important to children, especially at mealtimes.
- ✔ Parents must be careful about "control" issues around meals or foods; disordered eating may result in later years. Treatment of childhood obesity by targeting the parents as the sole agents for change may have the added benefit of improving the eating patterns and activity levels of the parents (Golan et al., 1999).
- ✔ Children tend to prefer sweets and must be helped to choose balanced meals (Story and Brown, 1987). Many children have low intakes of fruits, vegetables, and vitamin C. Children with desirable vitamin C intakes tend to have more healthful diets, drink more milk, and eat more vegetables than their peers (Hampl et al., 1999).
- ✔ Despite all current knowledge, many children still do not eat breakfast each day. Monitor and discuss the importance regarding abilities to concentrate, learn, and retain new information.
- ✔ Too much television watching with low energy expenditure has been indicated as a problem for children who become overweight (Gortmaker et al., 1996). The dramatic increase in childhood obesity is related to many things, including decreased physical activity and fitness levels and minimal physical education in schools (Lucas, 2001).
- ✔ It is essential that school-aged children have adequate meals to eliminate transient hunger, which interferes with classroom performance. Attention is easily diverted at a young age; total intake may vary. Scheduling of lunch after recess results in greater intake of all foods and calories (Getlinger et al., 1996).
- ✔ The food guide pyramid and 5-A-Day recommendations provide guidelines for food selection, beginning in childhood. Knowledge and training are needed to improve food consumption patterns as children consume foods away from home and as they take on greater responsibility for meal preparation and food selection (Melnick et al., 1998).
- ✔ Vegan children should be encouraged to consume adequate sources of vitamin B12, riboflavin, zinc, calcium, and vitamin D, if sun exposure is not adequate (Messina and Reed Mangels, 2001).
- ✔ Special considerations for children are found in Table 1–5. Attention deficit disorder is described in Table 1–6.

For More Information

- ✦ Alliance for Food and Fiber
  http://www.foodsafetyalliance.org/

Table 1–5 Special Considerations for Children

Measles and Blindness in Children (Gilbert and Foster, 2001): The major causes of blindness in children vary widely from region to region in the world. In high-income countries, lesions of the optic nerve and higher visual pathways predominate; retinopathy from prematurity is an important cause in middle-income countries; corneal scarring from measles, vitamin A deficiency, harmful traditional eye remedies, and ophthalmia neonatorum are the major causes in low-income countries. Other causes in all nations include cataract, congenital abnormalities, and hereditary retinal dystrophies. In almost half of the children who are blind today, the underlying cause could have been prevented, or the eye condition treated to preserve or restore sight. In the United States, as many as 15 million individuals may lack humoral immunity against measles (Hutchins et al., 2001). Control of blindness in children is a priority within the World Health Organization's VISION 2020 program; strategies are region specific, based on activities to prevent blindness in the community. Measles immunization, health education, control of vitamin A deficiency, and provision of eye care facilities for conditions that require specialist management are part of this plan.

Lead Poisoning: Lead is a confirmed neurotoxicant. Data show an inverse relationship between blood lead concentration and scores on four measures of cognitive functioning: arithmetic scores, reading scores, nonverbal reasoning, and short-term memory; deficits occur at blood lead concentrations lower than 5 mg/dL (Lanphear et al., 2000). Although past public health efforts have reduced lead exposure significantly, lead poisoning remains the most common environmental health problem affecting American children. Lead exposure occurs through ingestion of lead-contaminated household dust and soil in older housing containing lead-based paint; exposure can be increased with housing deterioration or renovation (Campbell and Osterhoudt, 2000). Bottled water is not guaranteed as a safe alternative. Lead replaces calcium in the bone; deposition may be seen in x-rays of the knee, ankle, or wrist. Anemia may also occur. Nutritional interventions involve provision of regular meals with adequate amounts of calcium and iron and supplementation for iron deficiency. Lead chelation should complement environmental, nutritional, and educational interventions, when indicated. Educational efforts address parental awareness of lead exposure pathways, hygiene, and housekeeping measures to prevent ingestion of dust and soil. Use drinking water from the cold tap, not hot water tap. Blood lead screening is often recommended universally at ages 1 and 2. For more information, visit the website http://www.cdc.gov/nceh/lead/lead.htm.

TABLE 1–6 Attention Deficit Hyperactivity Disorder (ADHD)

Attention deficit hyperactivity disorder (ADHD) is a set of symptoms. Children with ADHD need positive interactions, especially correlated with their attention deficits. Decreased appetite may occur. Stimulants like methylphenidate (Ritalin) or dextroamphetamine (Dexedrine) may cause anorexia, growth stunting, nausea, stomach pain, and weight loss. EFA deficiency is being researched, along with many other possibilities.

PET scan comparisons between the brain of a normal child and the brain of an ADHD child show a significant difference between the two. Because glucose is the brain's main energy source, it can give researchers a sense of the activity level of the brain according to these scan reports. Scientists have found that particular brain regions, which inhibit impulses and control attention, actually use less glucose in the brain of an ADHD child, meaning the areas are less active than normal. This decreased activity in the brain leads to inattention in the person's behavior.

Researchers believe the inactivity in the brains of ADHD children is associated with neurotransmitters that lack the ability to send complete chemical messages across synapses. Often, activity levels mostly affect the attention, concentration, planning, and organization areas of the brain, which is why glucose could be a link to ADHD. Furthermore, ADHD children who are given medication to correct the chemical instability in their brains show more normal PET scans than ADHD children not on the medication. Researchers continue to look into the possible effects of drug use, toxemia, and other complications seen during pregnancies as causes of ADHD. After birth, such things as meningitis, seizures, and even lead toxicity are being questioned. There are no concrete explanations for ADHD, but hopefully, further improvements in technology will aid in discovering the true secret to this baffling disorder. http://www.nimh.nih.gov/publicat/adhd.cfm#adhd14

- American Academy of Pediatrics
  http://www.aap.org/
- American School Foodservice Association
  700 S. Washington St., Suite 300
  Alexandria, VA 22314
  http://www.asfsa.org/
- Attention Deficit Disorders
  1–800-487–2282
- Beech Nut
  http://www.babycenter.com/solidfoods/product.html
- Bright Futures
  http://www.brightfutures.org
- Children's Nutrition Research Center – Baylor University
  http://www.bcm.tmc.edu/cnrc/
- Gerber
  http://www.gerber.com/
- Growth Charts
  http://www.cdc.gov/growthcharts
- Healthy School Meals
  http://schoolmeals.nal.usda.gov:8001/
- Heinz
  http://www.heinzbaby.com/
- Mead Johnson (products for infants)
  http://meadjohnson.com/products/index.html
- National Perinatal Association
  http://www.nationalperinatal.org/
- Ross Laboratories (products for infants)
  http://rosslabs.com
- School Foodservice Association
  http://www.asfsa.org/
- USDA Child Nutrition Home Page
  http://www.fns.usda.gov/cnd/Default.htm

ADOLESCENCE

NUTRITIONAL ACUITY RANKING: LEVEL 1

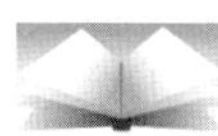

DEFINITIONS AND BACKGROUND

Tanner staging indicates physiological growth better than chronological age. According to Erickson's psychological stages of development (1963), teens (12–18-years-old) are working on "identity." For cognitive development, the concrete, "here and now," lasts from ages 11–14 in girls and from ages 13–15 in males. Early abstract thinking and daydreams are common among 15- to 17-year-old females and 16- to 19-year-old males. True abstract thinking and idealism occurs for young women aged 18–25 but not for males until 20–26 years of age.

Teens require increased nutrients to provide for the accelerated growth that takes place; nutritional deficiencies in adolescence can lead to loss of height, osteoporosis, and delayed sexual maturation (Herbold and Frates, 2000). When the teen years begin, the adolescent has achieved 80–85% of final height, 53% of final weight, and 52% of final skeletal mass. Teens may almost double their weight and can add 15–20% in height. With longer life expectancy than in past decades, half of the girls and one-third of the boys today can expect to live to 85 years of age.

Intakes change often during teen years, especially during growth spurts and varying stages of physical maturation. Sociocultural influences are known to affect adolescent eating patterns and behaviors, i.e., some teens reject a meat-based diet to become vegetarians, others take up dieting to lose weight and may subsequently develop an eating disorder (Herbold and Frates, 2000). Meal skipping, snacks at odd hours, laxative or diuretic use, fasting, bulimia, self-induced vomiting, and sports requirements are issues that should be addressed in a nutritional assessment. Dietary recalls are challenging. More than 60% of the incidence of obesity in children and teens may be related to excessive time spent watching television, i.e., 5 or more hours compared with 2 or fewer hours in those not overweight (Gortmaker et al., 1996).

RDAs divide teens by preteen ages 9–13 and teen years from 14–18. The growth spurt of girls occurs at 9-½–13-½ years of age; menarche generally is at 12-½ years. For boys, the growth spurt occurs during the ages of 11-¾–14-½. Sexual maturation occurs at ages 10–12 for girls and at ages 12–14 for boys. The increase in percent of total body fat in girls is 1.5–2 times that of boys at this time. Boys have greater increases in lean body mass (muscle) and greater increases in height before epiphyseal closure of long bones occurs. Most skeletal growth is completed by 19 years of age. Girls have more total body fat and less total body water than boys.

Dietary intake and body size influence age at menarche and growth patterns in teen girls. Puberty comes early for some girls because of a gene (CYP1B1) that speeds up the body's breakdown of androgens. Age at menarche is also inversely related to percentage of energy intake from dietary protein at ages 3–5, fat intake at ages 1–2; and percentage of energy from animal protein at ages 6–8 influences age of peak growth (Berkey et al., 2000). These factors may have implications for later development of diseases whose risks are associated with adolescent growth, including breast cancer and heart disease.

OBJECTIVES

- Modify diet to meet the needs of an ongoing or potential growth spurt.
- Prevent or correct nutritional anemias.
- Evaluate the patient's weight status. Offer appropriate guidance.
- Provide adequate energy for growth and development.
- Protein intake should be 45–60 g/day for boys, 44–46 g/day for girls.
- Evaluate use of fad diets, skipping meals, unusual eating patterns, or tendency toward eating disorders. If problems are noted, seek immediate assistance. Family therapy may be beneficial, especially at 10–11 years of age (Flodmark, 1993).
- Prevent future tendency toward osteoporosis. During short periods of inadequate calcium intake, girls absorb calcium more efficiently and lose less in their urine; bone resorption is increased during low calcium intake (O'Brien et al., 1996).
- Introduce food changes one at a time; reassure patient regarding nutrition and fast foods.
- Determine girl's sexual maturity (menarche, etc.), and whether oral contraceptives or intrauterine devices are being used. Growth spurt and onset of menstruation are associated with depletion of iron (Ilich-Ernst et al., 1998). Alter diet accordingly to provide sufficient vitamins and minerals.
- Encourage healthy food choices according to the factors of greatest interest to teens (taste and appearance). Health, calories, and price are not viewed as essential at this stage (Stewart and Tinsley, 1995).
- Vegetarians should be encouraged to consume adequate sources of vitamin B12, riboflavin, zinc, iron, calcium, protein, and energy for growth. Cobalamin deficiency, in the absence of hematologic signs, may lead to impaired cognitive performance in adolescents (Louwman et al., 2000). Vegan children tend to have higher intakes of fiber and lower intakes of saturated fatty acids and cholesterol than omnivore children; they may need to increase intake of omega-3 fatty acids (Messina and Reed Mangels, 2001).
- Girls may have total cholesterol concentration greater than 5.2 mmol/L; boys have a higher mean fitness score than girls (Anding et al., 1996). Some of this may be related to differences in male and female hormones.

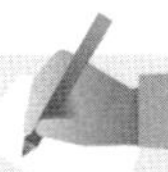

DIETARY RECOMMENDATIONS

- The food pyramid: 4 cups of milk or equivalent source of calcium; 2–3 servings of meat or equivalent; 6–12 servings from the bread group; 2–4 servings of fruit or juices; 3–5 servings from vegetable group.

- Adequate zinc for growth and sexual maturation; iodized salt.
- Calcium is needed for bone growth; iron is needed for menstrual losses in girls; vitamins D and A are essential.
- For calorie needs, see nutrient recommendation charts. Snacks should be planned as healthy inclusions in the diet.
- Debut age of drinking (alcohol) is important. If drinking begins before age 15, there is twice the risk of substance abuse and four times the risk of dependence.
- Diet for athletes: an acceptable diet for the athlete would be a normal diet for age, sex, and level of activity, plus adequate intake of carbohydrates and fluids. Avoid excesses of protein and inadequate replacement of electrolytes (see Sports Nutrition).

PROFILE

Clinical/History		Lab Work
Age	Tanner ratings of sexual maturation	H & H, Serum Fe
Height	Hydration status (I & O)	Gluc
Weight	Physical activity level	Alk phos
Weight/height percentile	Athletics	Retinol-binding protein (RBP)
BMI or Ideal/Healthy body weight IBW/HBW	Physical handicaps	Chol
Recent changes (height, weight)	Disordered eating patterns	Trig
	GI complaints	Alb
		Ca++, serum phosphorus
		Mg++

Common Drugs Used and Potential Side Effects

- Vitamin–mineral supplements are not needed, except for pregnant teens or teens whose diets are generally inadequate (such as those following an unplanned vegetarian pattern or restricted energy plans). The majority of American teens do not use supplements; those who do use them tend to eat a more nutrient-dense diet than those who do not. Vitamins A and E, calcium and zinc tend to be low regardless of use of supplements among all teens (Stang, 2000). In addition, excesses of these nutrients are not recommended and may lead to toxic levels of vitamins A and D, if taken indiscriminately.
- Discuss the relevance of tolerable upper intake levels (ULs) from the latest dietary reference intakes of the National Academy of Sciences. These levels were set to protect individuals from receiving too much of any nutrient from diet and dietary supplements.
- Monitor use of nonprescription medications (such as aspirin, cold remedies, etc.) and use of marijuana, alcohol, and illegal drugs. Side effects may include poor oral dietary intakes of several nutrients. Smoking cigarettes tends to decrease serum levels of vitamin C.
- For *Teenage Girls:* contraceptive steroids decrease serum levels of vitamins C, B6, B12, and folic acid and increase serum levels of vitamin A, copper, and lipids. Adjust diets accordingly. Users of intrauterine devices should increase their intake of iron and vitamin C to counteract increased menstrual losses.

Herbs, Botanicals and Supplements

- Herbs and botanical supplements should not be used without discussing with the physician. In general, these supplements have not been proven to be safe for adolescents.

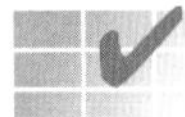

PATIENT EDUCATION

- ✓ Explain the food pyramid and the rationale behind the concept.
- ✓ Explain the relation of diet to the needs of the adolescent athlete, and its influence on skin, weight control, and general appearance. Educate the patient regarding acceptable snacks.

Nutrient	*Recommendation for Ages 9–13 yrs*	*Recommendation for Males 14–18 yrs*	*Recommendation for Females 14–18 yrs*
Calories:	2,000 kcal/d	2,500 kcal/d	2,200 kcal/d
Protein:	1 g/kg per day	0.9 g/kg per day	.08 g/kg/day
Calcium:	1,300 mg/day	1,300 mg/d	1,300 mg/d
Iron:	8 mg/d	12 mg/d	15 mg/d
Folate:	300 μg/d	400 μg/d	300 μg/d
Phosphorus:	1,250 mg/d	1,250 mg/d	1,250 mg/d
Vitamin A:	600 μg	1000 μg	800 μg
Vitamin C:	45 mg/d	45 mg/d	45 mg/d
Thiamin:	0.9 mg/d	0.9 mg/d	0.9 mg/d
Riboflavin:	0.9 mg/d	0.9 mg/d	0.9 mg/d
Niacin:	12 mg/d	12 mg/d	12 mg/d

- ✔ Help the family recognize the adolescent's need for independence. This may include choosing meals and snack items.
- ✔ Emphasize dental health and oral hygiene in relation to diet.
- ✔ Diets of teens are often low in vitamins A and C, folate, and iron. Discuss the concept of nutrient density; food comparison charts are useful. Encourage 5 servings of fruits and vegetables daily.
- ✔ Discuss the role of heroes and peer pressure. Boys generally want larger biceps, shoulders, chest, and forearms. Girls often want smaller hips, waistlines, and thighs and larger bust lines.
- ✔ Emphasize the importance of not skipping meals, especially breakfast. Discourage obsessions with dieting and weight.
- ✔ Discuss calcium; half of adolescent girls consume inadequate amounts. Low-fat dairy products should be used in amounts of 3–4 servings daily.
- ✔ Cigarette smoking and the use of alcohol or other drugs should be presented for their effects on various nutrients.
- ✔ Teens respond well to discussions that respect their independence.
- ✔ Encourage family meals, but discuss nourishing options for meals eaten away from home ("portable foods," etc.).
- ✔ A wide variety of foods should be consumed—vitamin A: chicken liver, cantaloupe, mango, spinach, and apricots, vitamin C: citrus fruits and juices, broccoli, spinach, melon, and strawberries, calcium: low-fat milk, yogurt, broccoli, cheddar cheese, shakes made with low-fat milk, and skim-milk cheeses, iron: liver, rice, whole milk, raisins, baked potatoes, and corn, vitamin B6: white meats, bananas, potatoes, and egg yolks, folacin: wheat germ, spinach, asparagus, and strawberries, zinc: apples, chicken, peanut butter, tuna, rice, and whole milk.
- ✔ Table 1–7 discusses special needs of the pregnant teenager.

For More Information

- ✦ Academy of Eating Disorders
  http://www.acadeatdis.org/
- ✦ Attention Deficit Hyperactivity Disorder
  http://www.nimh.nih.gov/publicat/adhd.cfm#adhd14
- ✦ Bright Futures—Adolescence
  http://www.brightfutures.org/adolescence/adtoc.htm
- ✦ National Coalition on Adolescent Health
  http://www.ama-assn.org/

TABLE 1–7 Special Considerations for Adolescent Pregnancy

- ✦ 95% of pregnant teens are keeping their babies (Trissler, 1999). Low birth weight (LBW) and prematurity are common. Increased weight in the last trimester is helpful in lessening LBW.
- ✦ Fetuses grow more slowly in 10- to 16-year-olds. Check gynecologic age (chronological age less age of menarche) to determine future potential growth of the mother.
- ✦ The diet for the pregnant adolescent should provide for optimal fetal growth and maintain an optimal nutritional status during and after gestation.
- ✦ By the end of the pregnancy, the mother's desired weight gain should be between 25 and 35 lb.
- ✦ For teen pregnancy, add the desired increments for calories for the RDA for same-age nonpregnant teens, or monitor the weight gain pattern to assess the adequacy of the present diet.
- ✦ Protein requirement is 1.5–1.7 g/kg body weight.
- ✦ Problem nutrients include calcium (1,300 mg under age 18), zinc (need 13 mg), iron (need 27 mg), vitamin A (need 750 μg), and vitamin C (need 80 mg/day).
- ✦ The physician should prescribe prenatal vitamins.
- ✦ Diet may include 5 cups of milk, 3 servings of meat, 4 servings of fruits/vegetables, and 4 servings of breads/cereals. Three snacks daily will be needed; discourage skipping of meals.
- ✦ Cravings are common, especially for chocolate, fruit, fast foods, pickles, and ice cream. Watch for aversions to meat, eggs, and pizza.
- ✦ Note that the dietitian may be seen as another authoritarian figure rather than as a friend; encourage the teen to see herself as having a key role in providing good nutritional support for her new family.
- ✦ Encourage enrolling in organized programs such as WIC where an individualized nutrition risk profile is developed for each pregnant teen, and a specific nutrition rehabilitation program is effective. Positive outcomes are noted in birth weight, rates of low or very low birth weight, preterm delivery, maternal morbidity, and perinatal morbidity/mortality (Dubois et al., 1997).
- ✦ Women who conceive during or shortly after adolescence are likely to enter pregnancy with low or absent iron stores. Iron deficiency anemia (IDA) during pregnancy is associated with significant morbidity for mothers and infants; supplementation during adolescence is a strategy to improve iron balance in pregnant teens (Lynch, 2000).
- ✦ Pregnant teens are more likely to smoke, to deliver preterm infants, and to have their infants die in the first year than mothers in any other age group (Trissler, 1999). Counseling methods must consider that they are still teens.

SPORTS NUTRITION

NUTRITIONAL ACUITY RANKING: LEVEL 2

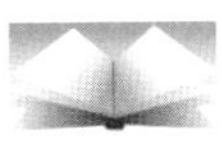

DEFINITIONS AND BACKGROUND

During high physical activity, energy and protein intakes must be met to maintain body weight, replenish glycogen stores, and provide adequate protein for building and repairing tissues (American Dietetic Association, 2000). Sports training does not appear to affect growth, maturation, or nutritional status during puberty (Fogelholm et al., 2000). Female children and adolescents who participate regularly in sports may develop certain medical conditions, including disordered eating, menstrual dysfunction, and decreased bone mineral density; pediatricians play an important role in monitoring the health of young female athletes (American Academy of Pediatrics. Committee on Sports Medicine and Fitness, 2000).

Many athletes are involved in running, jogging, weight lifting, or wrestling (active sports) when they seek nutritional guidance. Weight control guidance, disordered eating patterns, and wellness guidance are most common. Often, only a few athletes who seek help from a nutritionist have a true clinical concern, as for diabetes, Crohn's disease, or irritable bowel syndrome.

The primary fuel for athletic events using less than 50% VO2max (or aerobic capacity) is fat. Muscle glycogen and blood glucose supply half of the energy for aerobic exercise during a moderate (at or below 60% of VO2max or aerobic capacity) workout and nearly all the energy during a hard (above 80% of aerobic capacity) workout. In short-duration events of more than 70% VO2max (as in events like swimming or sprint running), glycogen is the key fuel. In long-duration events or activities of more than 70% VO2max (such as long-distance running, cycling, or swimming), muscle glycogen can be depleted in 100–120 minutes; maintaining a high carbohydrate daily diet while training for adequate glycogen replenishment is necessary in these cases.

CHO ingestion during prolonged exercise and CHO loading before exercise can have different effects on fuel substrate kinetics. CHO loading before exercise reduces the relative contribution of plasma glucose to total CHO oxidation; CHO ingestion during exercise may spare liver and muscle glycogen, cause reductions in gluconeogenesis, and delay onset of hypoglycemia (Bosch et al., 1996). Elite athletes metabolize CHO more effectively than nonathletes but nutritional factors still affect glycemic control in well-trained athletes (Tegelman et al., 1996).

Performance in endurance events is dependent upon maximal aerobic power as sustained by the availability of substrates (carbohydrates and fats). Protein has the role of maintaining and repairing muscle mass and tissues; a sufficient but not excessive intake is important. Excessive protein intakes may cause dehydration. In a study of gymnasts, it was found that they had a lower weekly calorie intake but a higher intake from dietary protein than the nonathletes. Gymnasts are often at risk of malnutrition, which when compounded with intense physical exercise, could lead to immunosuppression in these athletes (Lopez-Varela et al., 2000).

Fatigue is associated with reduced muscle glycogen; increasing muscle glycogen or blood glucose prolongs performance, while increasing fat and decreasing CHO decreases performance. This has led to an emphasis on CHO intake in athletes in endurance sports, which quite often leads to low caloric intake (Pendergast et al., 2000). Trained individuals have higher levels of fat oxidative capacity, which spares glycogen during endurance sports. Use of isocaloric high-fat diets (42–55%) maintains adequate CHO levels compared to diets composed of low fat intake (10–15%). Endurance runners who eat a low-fat diet may not consume enough energy, EFAs and some minerals, especially zinc; these inadequate intakes may compromise their performance (Horvath et al., 2000). Pendergast suggests consideration of a diet comprising 20% protein, 30% CHO, and 30% fat with the remaining 20% of the calories distributed between CHO and fat based on the intensity and duration of the sport.

Athletes should be well hydrated before the start of exercise and should drink enough fluid during and after exercise to balance fluid losses. Consumption of sport drinks containing carbohydrates and electrolytes during exercise will provide fuel for the muscles, help maintain blood glucose and the thirst mechanism, and decrease the risk of dehydration or hyponatremia (American Dietetic Association, 2000).

OBJECTIVES

- Promote healthy, safe eating habits and activities that can be continued throughout life. Aerobic activity is especially beneficial, as is resistance (weight) training.
- Correct faddist beliefs, erroneous trends, meal skipping, and other unhealthy eating behaviors.
- Promote improved performance.
- Enhance overall health and fitness. Evaluate body fatness and counsel accordingly (see Table 1–8).
- Help prevent injuries, dehydration, overhydration, and hyponatremia.
- Prevent or correct amenorrhea, which may result from poor energy and fat intake. Monitor or correct eating disorders, such as bulimia or anorexia nervosa. Female athletes are under intense pressure to have a low percentage of body fat for performance, which may result in a vulnerable athlete resorting to disordered eating, developing amenorrhea, and suffering the consequences of osteoporosis, the "female athlete triad" (Sanborn et al., 2000). Prevention efforts require a de-emphasis of a low percentage of body fat and an adequate emphasis on good nutrition. The consequences of lost bone mineral density can be devastating for the female athlete; premature osteoporotic fractures can occur, and lost bone min-

eral density may never be regained (Hobart and Smucker, 2000). The female athlete triad is a serious syndrome that requires a multidisciplinary approach.

- Meet extra calorie requirements created by a higher BMR for metabolically active muscle mass.
- Maintain healthy body weight.

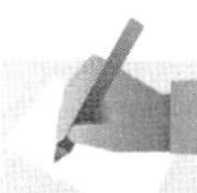

DIETARY AND NUTRITIONAL RECOMMENDATIONS

- For active individuals, use a normal diet for age and sex with special attention to calorie needs for the specific activity and frequency. 50–60% CHO is generally a good target.
- Protein requirements should be calculated by age and sex with a slightly higher requirement (e.g., 1.2–1.7 g/kg) in strenuous or endurance sports activity; 1 g/kg for mild and moderate activities, including strength activities. Avoid excesses of protein, but be aware of the role that an adequate protein/calorie ratio plays in preventing amenorrhea and in maintaining an adequate iron status. It is important to avoid running out of glycogen, when protein would be used for energy.
- Extra riboflavin may be needed to meet muscle demands. Inclusion of dairy foods should be sufficient for all except the most strenuous activities.
- Fluid replacement may be essential with a calculation of 1 mL/kcal used for an average. Do not dilute sports drinks, because they have been formulated to have between 6 and 8% CHO along with an appropriate amount of electrolytes.
- Electrolytes must be carefully monitored and replaced. Newer sports drinks on the market contain glucose polymers with lower osmolality than sugared drinks or fruit juice. Gatorade and other recently formulated sports drinks products are acceptable.
- Because athletes train almost daily, glucose loading is not recommended for endurance activities. Athletes training hard for several hours per day should consume 1.5 g of CHO per kg within 30 minutes postexercise followed by an additional 1.5 g of CHO per kg 2 hours later for glycogen synthesis. Based on time spent training, most athletes should consume 6–10 g of CHO per kg of body weight on a daily basis (Berning, 2000). In addition, complex CHO in the form of starch can help with glycogen storage; popular choices include bagels, fruit, or cereal approximately 2 hours before an event.
- Avoid fads, such as omission of meat from the diet. Heme iron is important, and meat is also a good source of zinc. Dried beans and enriched cereals are also good suggestions for iron.
- Ensure adequate calcium intake for women (i.e., 1–1.5 g/day) to prevent osteoporosis and to reduce muscle cramping and stress fractures. Weight-bearing exercises, such as walking and running in moderation, tend to be beneficial for bone mineral density accumulation.
- Maintain total fat intake at a level determined by age, medical status, and type of performance and endurance required.
- Prevent meal skipping. Breakfast is especially important in maintaining homeostasis. Small meals or frequent small snacks are useful for some individuals.
- There is some evidence that antioxidant foods may be useful for correcting "oxidative stress." Supplemental sources are not recommended in lieu of foods rich in these substances (Clarkson, 1995). Table 1–13 is a useful reference.

TABLE 1–8 Body Fat Standards

Clinical obesity	26%+ in men, 29%+ in women
*Reference levels	14% newborn (3.4 kg BW)
	13% 10-year-old boy (31 kg BW)
	19% 10-year-old girl (32 kg BW)
	15% adult man (72 kg BW)
	28% adult female (58 kg BW)
Athletes	12–15% men, 20–25% women
Top athletes	7–10% men, 12–18% women
Essential for life	5% men, 11% women

*From: Shils M, et al. *Modern nutrition in health and disease*. 9th ed. Philadelphia: Lippincott Williams & Wilkins, 1999:799.

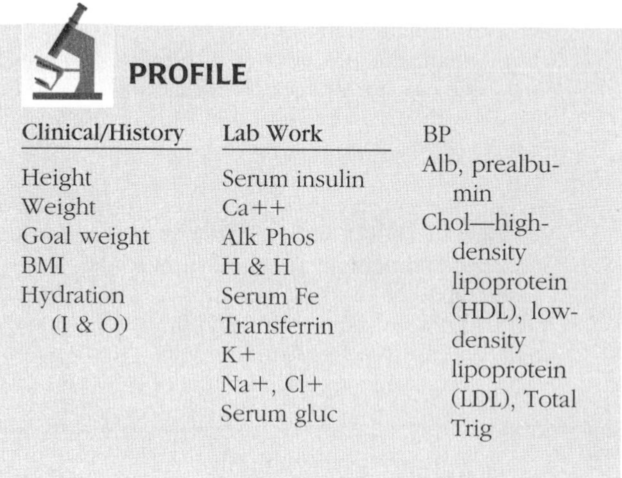

PROFILE

Clinical/History	Lab Work	
Height	Serum insulin	BP
Weight	Ca++	Alb, prealbumin
Goal weight	Alk Phos	Chol—high-density lipoprotein (HDL), low-density lipoprotein (LDL), Total
BMI	H & H	Trig
Hydration (I & O)	Serum Fe	
	Transferrin	
	K+	
	Na+, Cl+	
	Serum gluc	

Common Drugs Used and Potential Side Effects

- Steroids may affect numerous nutritional parameters. Take a careful drug history and discuss all side effects as appropriate.
- Salt tablets should be discouraged; water intake is generally the requirement during athletic events.
- Discuss the fact that excessive use of vitamin–mineral supplements can lead to toxicity, especially for vitamins A and D.
- If an athlete is in a sport that requires drug testing, check first before using any drug with the U.S. Olympic Committee or the NCAA. Androstenedione and anabolic steroids do promote muscle mass enhancement but are not allowed.

- Hormone replacement therapy should be considered early to prevent the loss of bone density (Hobart and Smucker, 2000).
- Discuss the relevance of tolerable upper intake levels (ULs) from the latest dietary reference intakes of the National Academy of Sciences. These levels were set to protect individuals from receiving too much of any nutrient from diet and dietary supplements.

Herbs, Botanicals and Supplements

- Herbs and botanical supplements should not be used without discussing with the physician, especially for underlying medical conditions.
- Ergogenic aids are expensive and not necessary; use with caution only. A well-balanced diet will suffice for most athletic events (American Dietetic Association, 2000).
- Creatine supplementation increases the capacity of skeletal muscle to perform work during periods of alternating intensity exercises, possibly because of increased aerobic phosphorylation and flux through the creatine kinase system (Rico-Sanz, Mendez Marco, 2000). Creatine supplements have a slight beneficial effect with strength training (Becque et al., 2000).
- L-tryptophan, the precursor to serotonin, has sometimes been used to enhance performance. It should not be used with MAO inhibitors, antidepressants, or serotonin receptor antagonists. It can exaggerate conditions of psychosis.
- Zinc supplements are sometimes taken to enhance performance. It should not be taken with immunosuppressants, fluoroquinolones, and tetracycline.
- Ginseng may be used for performance enhancement. It should not be taken with warfarin, insulin, oral hypoglycemics, CNS stimulants, caffeine, steroids, hormones, antipsychotics, aspirin, or antiplatelet drugs.

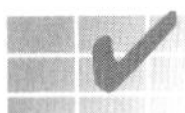

PATIENT EDUCATION

- ✓ Dispel such myths as "milk is for children only," "meat is bad for you," "carbohydrates are fattening," and "dieting is the key to fluid control." Discuss appropriate alternatives.
- ✓ If the client is an adult child of alcoholic parents, he or she may need help in reducing such traits as perfectionism, compulsive or controlling behaviors, or the need for attention. Many athletes are driven by such traits and can cope more effectively with personalized counseling; refer to the appropriate health provider as needed.
- ✓ For weight control problems, address not only body weight but also family genetics and body type. Body fatness is another key issue; see Table 1–4. Parenting styles, socioeconomic issues, and environmental cues also play important roles in managing weight.
- ✓ Pre-event diets should be eaten up to an hour before the activity (Berning, 2000). Complex carbohydrates should be consumed, using less fat and protein because of their effect on digestive processes. The meal may contain 300–1,000 calories with 60–70% from carbohydrates. After an event, recovery carbohydrate intake is suggested.
- ✓ Discuss how to obtain a high-calorie, high-complex carbohydrate diet with attention to the individual's preferences. In vigorous training programs, 3,000–6,000 kcal may be needed, especially for ultramarathons.
- ✓ Water is necessary to avoid dehydration. Drink fluids before, during, and after exercising. Weigh before and after events. Drink 1–2 cups of cool fluids 2 hours before the event, 4–8 oz immediately after the event, 8–16 oz after exercise, 8 oz of fluid between meals, and 8 oz of fluid with meals; replacement drinks should contain 80–120 mg sodium per 8 oz (Berning, 2000). Alcoholic beverages do nothing to promote performance and may negatively affect neurologic and cardiac systems. Caffeine promotes mild physical endurance and alertness but is limited in competitive sports.
- ✓ There is no such thing as "quick energy." The habit of eating candy before a game can cause an insulin overshoot, leading to hypoglycemia. A balanced diet is more practical.
- ✓ Although female athletes with subclinical eating disorders tend to have dietary intakes of energy, protein, CHO, and certain micronutrients below RDA and Dietary reference intakes (DRI) levels; micronutrient status appears relatively unaffected, probably due to use of supplements (Beals and Manore, 1998). Instituting an appropriate diet and moderating the frequency of exercise may result in the natural return of menses (Hobart and Smucker, 2000).
- ✓ Blacks may have lower resting metabolic rates (RMRs), total daily expenditures, and physical activity energy expenditures than do whites. If these findings are confirmed, interventions designed to decrease energy intake and to increase physical activity targeted to blacks may become especially important to reduce the high obesity rates and associated metabolic disorders (Gannon et al., 2000).

For More Information

- American College of Sports Medicine
  401 W. Michigan St.
  Indianapolis, IN 46202-3233
  http://www.acsm.org/
- American Council on Exercise
  http://acefitness.org
- American Alliance for Health, Physical Education, Recreation and Dance
  http://www.aahperd.org
- American Dietetic Association
  Sports and Cardiovascular Nutritionists
  http://www.nutrifit.com
- President's Council on Physical Fitness and Sports
  http://www.surgeongeneral.gov/ophs/pcpfs.htm
- US Olympic Committee
  http://www.olympic-usa.org/
- Women's Sports Foundation
  http://www.womenssportsfoundation.org/

ADULTHOOD

NUTRITIONAL ACUITY RANKING: LEVEL 1 (NOT RANKED)

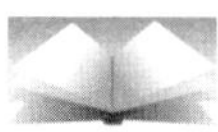

DEFINITIONS AND BACKGROUND

The period of young adulthood is 18–40-years-old when careers are a priority. The period of middle adulthood is 40–65-years-old, and family is the primary focus. It is important to alter poor dietary habits, to review family history, and to assess the potential role of genetic counseling regarding chronic disease. Eventually, gene therapy could provide a cure for diseases such as cystic fibrosis; the mutant gene in a germ cell is replaced with a single copy of the normal gene (Tolstoi et al., 1999).

Americans are eating less fat but not necessarily fewer calories, and nutrient density has not necessarily improved (Fishman, 1996). Zinc, pyridoxine, and iron intakes often are low in diets designed to meet the Dietary Guidelines for Americans (Dollahite, 1995).

Composite sensory experience of taste, olfaction, and trigeminal sensation is what is perceived as flavor (Duffy, 1996). Both genetics and conditioning influence preferences; taste seems to be innate and responses to odors, conditioned. The influence of genetic variation in taste on food intake depends on how perceptible sweet, fat, or bitter components are in foods and beverages as well as the value of sensory factors versus other factors (e.g., health, convenience) on personal dietary choices (Duffy and Bartoshuk, 2000). Female super-tasters of bitterness may avoid high fat or sweet foods because these oral sensations are too intense and thus less pleasant. Super-tasters may taste more bitterness in vegetables but still enjoy eating them because of healthfulness and because condiments can be used to block bitterness (Duffy and Bartoshuk, 2000).

Dietary patterns characterized by omission of food groups are associated with mortality in both men and women, according to National Health and Nutrition Survey (NHANES) data (Kant et al., 1993). Men who maintain or improve their physical fitness are less likely to die from cardiovascular disease than men who are not physically fit (Blair et al., 1995). The same is likely to be true for women. Healthy People 2010 proposes many ideal changes in health and nutritional behaviors to improve quality of life and to increase longevity. Community programs designed to change behavior are challenged when the costs of new behavior are high and when the personal benefits are intangible (Rangan et al., 1996). Peer pressure and moral persuasion may help promote long-term changes in behavior by adults (Rangan et al., 1996).

Nutrition is involved in the 10 leading causes of death in women. Osteoporosis and extremes in body weight are approaching epidemic proportions (American Dietetic Association, 1999); osteoporosis affects 20 million women. Women have 66% more doctor visits than men and are hospitalized 15% more often; they account for 75% of long-term care (LTC) stays (Finn, 1997). Heart disease is the number one disabler and killer of women in the U.S., whereas cancer is the leading cause of premature death. When adults are hospitalized, declines occur in nutritional status with higher hospital charges (about $15,000 more) and more complications are likely (Braunschweig et al., 2000.) Table 1–9 lists some considerations for women.

OBJECTIVES

- Maintain quality of nutrition while compensating for energy needs lower than during growth.
- Prevent obesity resulting from a sedentary lifestyle where relevant. Highly sedentary people lose 20–24% of overall muscle mass and strength. Every adult should accumulate 30 minutes or more of moderate intensity physical activity on most days of the week (Pate et al., 1995). Also useful are: strength training (resistance or weight training with 8–12 repetitions), isotonics, and aerobics (20 minutes of walking, jogging, swimming, or bicycling).
- Prevent or delay the onset of medical conditions, e.g., hypertension, osteoporosis, cardiovascular disease, renal disorders, and oncologic conditions. Treat problems as they occur.
- Promote adequate bone mass density, which peaks at 25–30 years of age.
- Improve nutrient density of meals, especially those eaten away from home. The average American eats 3–4 meals away from home each week.
- Iron deficiency affects approximately one-half of all women. Correct through diet as far as possible. Avoid excesses, especially in men.
- Identify problems with food insecurity and its relationship to available foods and consumption patterns; fruit and vegetable intakes decrease when incomes are decreased (Kendall et al., 1996).

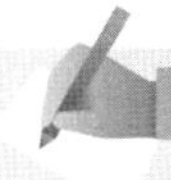

DIETARY AND NUTRITIONAL RECOMMENDATIONS

- Ensure intake from the food pyramid: 2–3 servings of milk, 2–3 servings of meat or substitute, 3–5 servings of vegetables, 2–4 servings of fruits, and 6–12 bread group servings. Fats, oils, sugars, and sweets are to be controlled as needed to increase or decrease caloric intake. Be aware that foods from the fats/sweets/alcohol group often replace nutrient-dense foods in the American diet, often up to 33% of kcal (Kant and Schtzkin, 1994).
- Follow the Dietary Guidelines (see Table 1–1).
- Modify diet as needed for special medical conditions. P:M:S fat ratio should be 1:1:1.
- Calorie needs: females, 35 kcal/kg IBW; males, 40 kcal/kg IBW—vary by sedentary or active status. In addition, after 23 years of age only underweight individuals need to gain weight. See nutritional recommendation charts.
- For most healthy adults, 0.8–1 g of protein/kg will suffice.

TABLE 1–9 Special Nutrition-Related Concerns of Women

Premenstrual Syndrome (PMS): PMS symptoms include edema, hypoglycemia, migraines, hypothyroidism, and slightly elevated prolactin levels. A low-fat vegetarian diet is associated with increased serum sex-hormone binding globulin concentration and reductions in body weight, dysmenorrhea duration and intensity, and premenstrual symptom duration; symptom effects might be mediated by dietary influences on estrogen activity (Barnard et al., 2000). Women may want to omit alcohol and excesses of caffeine or chocolate from their diets 7–14 days before menstruation, if they suffer from PMS or anxiety. A balanced diet with adequate protein, calcium, magnesium, manganese, and vitamin B6 should be consumed. Calcium has been found to be of benefit in PMS sufferers; limited evidence suggests that Vitamin E and CHO supplements may be useful; vitamin B6 has had conflicting results (Bendich, 2000). A daily magnesium supplement reduces symptoms associated with PMS in the second cycle of administration with less weight gain, swelling of extremities, breast tenderness, and abdominal bloating (Walker et al., 1998). Herbals have no supporting data in PMS; black cohosh may cause hypotension, vomiting, headache, dizziness, GI distress, and limb pain. Six small meals may be better tolerated. The doctor may recommend a general multivitamin/mineral capsule. For some, spironolactone by prescription may be helpful. PMS Hotline: (800) 222-4767.

Fibrocystic Breast Conditions: Fibrocystic breast conditions, formerly considered benign breast or fibrocystic breast disease, actually affect about half of all women and present with breast nodularity, swelling, and pain (Horner and Lampe, 2000). Excessive estrogen or sensitivity is the dominant theory. Randomized controlled studies have failed to support nutrition interventions commonly recommended. For instance, decreased sodium or fluid and caffeine, and increased use of primrose oil and herbal teas have been promoted. Adequate intakes of vitamins A, C, E, and B6, iodine, omega-3 fatty acids, and selenium have been suggested. Overall, use of a low-fat (15–20% kcals), adequate fiber diet (30 g/day) and soy isoflavones seem to be most useful (Horner and Lampe, 2000).

Infertility and Spontaneous Abortions: High caffeine intakes (over 500 mg daily) may delay conception in fertile women (Bolumar et al., 1997). Weight loss in obese infertile women results in improvement in reproductive outcomes for all forms of fertility treatment (Clark et al., 1998). Five cups or more of regular coffee each day seemed to be related to spontaneous abortions at twice the normal risk (Klebanoff et al., 1999). A normal female has body fat levels that are suitable for normal reproduction; avoid having either too much or too little body fat.

Menopause: Needs during menopause change because of declining levels of estrogens and other hormones and because of cessation of menstrual periods (decreasing need for extra iron, etc.). Exogenous estrogens may be a concern in the development of adenoma of the endometrium. Postmenopausal osteoporosis may lead to bone fractures. Encourage regular physical examinations. Exercise, calcium or Calcitriol, and hormonal therapy are being reviewed for their roles in preventing fractures. Women need less iron at this time. Vitamins C and E and soy may be useful to lessen hot flashes and vaginal dryness, although not yet proven. Black cohosh, used by some women for menopausal symptoms, may cause hypotension, vomiting, headache, dizziness, GI distress, and limb pain. Some studies now suggest that Alzheimer's disease may be related to low levels of estrogen; this condition tends to be common for postmenopausal women.

Osteoporosis: Women of all ages must carefully select diets that provide sufficient calcium and vitamin D. Excesses of protein should be avoided. Weight-bearing activity is generally useful, whereas excessive heavy exercises may lead to osteoporotic fractures; walking is considered the best activity for lifelong bone health. Estrogen loss in the decades after menopause or ovarian removal contributes to accelerated bone loss and osteoporosis (Writing Group for the PEPI Trial, 1996). Hormone replacement therapy is useful for many women for increasing bone mineral density. Fosamax, calcium bone replacement, and other options are also now available (see Section 11).

Use fish, poultry, and nonmeat entrees (e.g., dry beans, peas, nuts) regularly instead of just meat-centered meals.

- A careful sodium to potassium balance (ratio of 1:1) should be maintained, along with adequate levels of calcium and magnesium.
- Adequate vitamins A, C, and E and selenium foods should be consumed for their antioxidant properties. Foods rather than supplements are recommended because of the yet unknown properties that may be beneficial.
- Phytochemicals are now recognized for their potential effect on prevention of chronic disorders. Soybeans, fruits, and vegetables seem to yield the greatest risk reductions. Soy protein, as in tofu and meat extenders, may reduce serum cholesterol and possibly reduce risks of prostate and breast cancers (Messina and Erdman, 1995). See Table 13–2.
- Women of childbearing age should include foods rich in folic acid, now available through fortification of grains, to

Nutrient	*Recommendation for Males 19–30 yrs*	*Recommendation for Males 31–50 yrs*	*Recommendation for Males 51–70 yrs*
Calories:	2,900 kcal/d	2,900 kcal/d	2,300 kcal/d
Protein:	58 g/d	63 g/d	63 g/d
Calcium:	1,000 mg/d	1,000 mg/d	1,200 mg/d
Iron:	8 mg/d	8 mg/d	8 mg/d
Folate:	400 μg/d	400 μg/d	400 μg/d
Phosphorus:	700 mg/d	700 mg/d	700 mg/d
Vitamin A:	900 μg	900 μg	900 μg
Vitamin C:	90 mg/d	90 mg/d	90 mg/d
Thiamin:	1.2 mg/d	1.2 mg/d	1.2 mg/d
Riboflavin:	1.3 mg/d	1.3 mg/d	1.3 mg/d
Niacin:	16 mg/d	16 mg/d	16 mg/d

Nutrient	*Recommendation for Females 19–30 yrs*	*Recommendation for Females 31–50 yrs*	*Recommendation for Females 51–70 yrs*
Calories:	2,200 kcal/d	2,200 kcal/d	1,900 kcal/d
Protein:	46 g/d	50 g/d	50 g/d
Calcium:	1,000 mg/d	1,000 mg/d	1,200 mg/d
Iron:	18 mg/d	18 mg/d	8 mg/d
Folate:	400 μg/d	400 μg/d	400 μg/d
Phosphorus:	700 mg/d	700 mg/d	700 mg/d
Vitamin A:	700 μg	700 μg	700 μg
Vitamin C:	75 mg/d	75 mg/d	75 mg/d
Thiamin:	1.1 mg/d	1.1 mg/d	1.1 mg/d
Riboflavin:	1.1 mg/d	1.1 mg/d	1.1 mg/d
Niacin:	14 mg/d	14 mg/d	14 mg/d

prevent neural tube defects. Men may need to eat more folic-acid-rich foods to lower serum homocysteine levels; high levels are a cardiac risk factor. Cold cereals, cooked pinto and navy beans, asparagus, and spinach, as well as orange juice, should be planned into the diet regularly to increase folic acid intake.

Common Drugs Used and Potential Side Effects

For Women of Childbearing Years

- Contraceptive steroids decrease serum levels of vitamins B6, B12, folic acid, and vitamin C and increase serum levels of vitamin A, copper, and lipids. Adjust diet accordingly. Nausea or vomiting may occur secondary to dietary adjustment. Limit use of caffeine to the equivalent of 2 cups of regular coffee per day.
- Users of intrauterine devices should increase their intake of iron and vitamin C to counteract increased menstrual losses.

PROFILE

Clinical/History	Lab Work	
BP	Alb, prealbumin	H & H, Serum Fe
Height	BUN, Creat	Gluc
Weight—current	Na+, K+	Chol—HDL/LDL, Total
Weight—usual	Mg++	Trig
BMI or IBW/HBW	Ca++	Serum homocysteine
Recent weight changes		Serum folic acid
Body fat analysis		Serum B12
Smoking		
Alcohol use		

For Menopausal Women

- Low doses of Megace (megestrol acetate) may be used to decrease hot flashes in postmenopausal women

TABLE 1–10 5-A-Day For Better Health

Eat at least one vitamin A-rich fruit or vegetable such as apricots, cantaloupe, carrots, sweet potatoes, spinach, collards, or broccoli each day.
Eat at least one vitamin C-rich fruit or vegetable such as oranges, strawberries, green peppers, or tomatoes each day.
Eat at least one high-fiber fruit or vegetable such as apples, grapefruit, broccoli, or cauliflower each day.
Eat blueberries often; they have been highly rated for their antioxidant properties (anthocyanins).
Eat cabbage family vegetables such as cauliflower, broccoli, Brussels sprouts, and cabbage several times every week.

Tips for eating more fruits and vegetables

Add fruit to cereal or plain yogurt.
Use fruit juice instead of water when preparing cakes and muffins.
Drink 100% fruit juice instead of soda.
Snack on dried fruits, such as dried apricots, peaches, raisins, or "craisins."
Eat a piece of fruit for a morning snack; choose a grapefruit or an orange for an afternoon snack.
Choose the darkest green or red leaf lettuce greens for salads; add carrots, red cabbage, and spinach.
Add more vegetables to soups and stews; add tomato juice to soups and stews for more vitamins A and C.
Choose pizza with extra green pepper, onion, broccoli, and tomatoes.
Munch on raw vegetables with a low fat dip for an afternoon snack.
When eating out, choose a side dish of vegetables.
Fill up most of the plate with vegetables at lunch or dinner.
Choose fortified foods and beverages such as juice with added calcium.

who cannot take estrogen. Megace can cause increased appetite, edema, and sodium retention.
- Raloxifene (Evistal) is a designer estrogen that protects bones while reducing breast cancer risk. It may cause hot flashes.
- Alendronate (Fosamax) may be used to maintain bone density without breast cancer risk.

For Men—Infertility, Erection Dysfunction
- Adequate supplementation with vitamin C (1 g/day) has helped some couples overcome problems with infertility. Otherwise, excessive supplemental vitamin C use may lead to high serum levels and sometimes a delayed insulin response to a high glucose load (Johnston and Yen, 1994).
- Viagra (sildenafil) has been widely used to treat erectile dysfunction (ED), but it is not without potential health risks (Mulhall, 2000). Studies and clinical trials of similar drugs are underway.

For Men—Baldness
- Use of Rogaine (minoxidil) to treat baldness may cause diarrhea, altered blood pressure, nausea, vomiting, and weight gain; it is a vasodilator. A low-sodium, low-calorie diet may be needed.

For Men—Prostate Problems
- Proscar and other medications are used with some relief. Monitor blood pressure and other side effects. No nutritional side effects are noted.
- There is some evidence that saw palmetto may be useful (see below).
- Discuss the relevance of tolerable upper intake levels (ULs) from the latest dietary reference intakes of the National Academy of Sciences. These levels were set to protect individuals from receiving too much of any nutrient from diet and dietary supplements.

Herbs, Botanicals and Supplements

- Herbs and botanical supplements should not be used without discussing with the physician, especially for underlying medical conditions. For infertility: cauliflower, ginseng, spinach, ginger, guava, and sunflower have been proposed, but there are no studies that confirm effectiveness. For endometriosis: soybean, peanut, flax, and alfalfa have been suggested; no studies confirm any effects. For impotence: no studies confirm usefulness of fava bean, anise, gingko, yohimbe, and cardamom. For motion sickness: ginger and raspberry have anecdotal recommendations only. For insomnia: lemon balm, lavender, camomile, and hops have been suggested. For menopause: alfalfa, licorice, and red clover have been suggested but have not been studied for efficacy.
- Black cohosh may cause hypotension, vomiting, headache, dizziness, GI distress, and limb pain.
- Chaste berry may be used for premenopausal symptoms, dysmenorrhea, or menopause but should not be taken with hormone replacement therapy or oral contraceptives.
- Dong Quai is Chinese women's tonic for menstrual cramps and other symptoms; it should not be taken with warfarin, aspirin, or ticlopidine. It has coumadin-like substances.
- Evening primrose oil can be taken for menopausal symptoms. Avoid use with antiseizure medications, antiepileptics, chlorpromazine, fluphenazine, and mesoridazine.
- Brewer's Yeast should not be taken with MAO inhibitors such as Nardil, Parnate.
- Saw palmetto is useful for prostate health but should not be taken with oral contraceptives, estrogens, or anabolic steroids.
- Echinacea may be used as an immune system stimulant. It should not be taken with steroids, cyclosporine, or immunosuppressants.
- Ginseng may be used for stress adaptation, performance enhancement, impotence, or as a digestive aid. It should not be taken with warfarin, insulin, oral hypoglycemics, CNS stimulants, caffeine, steroids, hormones, antipsychotics, aspirin, or antiplatelet drugs. A double-blind study showed that it does not enhance psychologic well being (Cardinal and Hermann-J. Engels, 2001).
- Kava is sometimes used as a sleep aid but should not be taken with sedatives, alcohol, antipsychotics, or other CNS depressants.
- L-tryptophan, the precursor to serotonin, has sometimes been used to promote sleep or to correct depression. It should not be used with MAO inhibitors, antidepressants, or serotonin receptor antagonists. It can exaggerate conditions of psychosis.
- Melatonin has been used as a sleep aid or a jet lag adjuster but should not be used with CNS depressants such as alcohol, barbiturates, corticosteroids, or immunosuppressants.
- Valerian may be used as an antianxiety drug or sleep aid. Benzodiazepines, sedatives, alcohol, and other CNS depressants should not be used at the same time because of the risk of additional sedation.
- Zinc supplements are sometimes taken to prevent viral illness, enhance performance, and correct male infertility. They should not be taken with immunosuppressants, fluoroquinolones, and tetracycline.

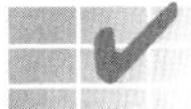

PATIENT EDUCATION

- ✓ Explain the benefits of weight management and exercise for the adult.
- ✓ Describe the effects of the "business lunch" with alcohol on nutritional status. Daily alcohol intake may equal 300 kcal or more. Discourage intake of more than two alcoholic drinks per day for men and one for women.
- ✓ Discuss food choices when eating away from home. For jet lag, adjust meal times to match new time zone, which may help the liver adjust more readily.
- ✓ Help plan a diet in accordance with individual lifestyle. Nutrient density, food cost, and portion sizes should be explained. About 75% of Americans believe there is too much conflicting information about diet (Hogbin and Hess, 1999). Some of this confusion is related to the difference between a "serving" and a "portion."
- ✓ Discuss calcium alternatives for people who exclude milk products.

- ✓ Discuss fiber, nonmeat vegetarian meals, cooking methods for nutrient preservation, and phytochemicals. Functional foods may reduce the risk of coronary heart disease, cancers, hypertension, and osteoporosis (Klotzbach-Shimomura, 2001). Nutrition messages that lead to increased consumption of dietary fiber need to be strengthened; good taste and convenience are critical components (Auld et al., 2000).
- ✓ Determine psychological readiness to change and the individual's stage (Prochaska, 1996)—precontemplation, contemplation, preparation, action, maintenance, or termination. Partnerships with patients, developing understanding of the patient's experience, starting where the patient is, and concentrating on small changes for success are keys (Glover and Jocelyn, 1998).
- ✓ Peer education seems to be effective in increasing fruit and vegetable intakes in adults with low socioeconomic status (Butler et al., 2000).
- ✓ Safe food handling and sanitation techniques are important to discuss.
- ✓ Most adults do not know how to use the food label and the Daily Values (DV) (%) but are able to moderate fat intake using labels (Levy et al., 2000). Label reading may be a marker for other dietary behaviors that predict healthful food choices and should therefore be discussed. See Table 1–11.
- ✓ The American Council on Science and Health (ACSH) ranked consumer magazines as sources of reliable nutrition information. Parents, Cooking Light, and Good Housekeeping ranked the highest for excellence.

TABLE 1–11 Labeling Terms and Authorized Health Claims

% Fat Free = food must be a low-fat or fat-free food to include this value
Free = food contains 0% of the indicated nutrient
Good Source = contains 10–19% of the daily value (DV) for a nutrient
High = contains 20% or more DV for a nutrient
Lean = food (meat) is no more than 10% fat by weight, not calories; contains 10 g fat or less and 95 mg cholesterol or less (Extra lean = 5% fat by weight)
Less = food contains 25% less than original food
Light/Lite = food contains fewer calories or 50% less fat than original food OR description of color (if indicated as such on the label)
Low = low fat as 3 g or less; low sodium as 140 mg or less; very low sodium as 35 mg or less; low cholesterol as 20 mg or less; low calorie as 40 calories or less
More = food contains 110% or more DV than original food
Reduced = product has been altered to contain 25% less of a nutrient or the usual calories of that food
Reduced Cholesterol = the food contains 75% or less of the cholesterol found in the original product

Authorized Health Claims

The Food and Drug Administration has authorized certain health claims for use in food labeling:

Calcium and Osteoporosis: Typical Foods: Low-fat and skim milks, yogurts, tofu, calcium-fortified citrus drinks, and some calcium supplements. Requirements: Food or supplement must be "high" in calcium and must not contain more phosphorus than calcium. Claims must cite other risk factors; state the need for regular exercise and a healthful diet; explain that adequate calcium early in life helps reduce fracture risk later by increasing as much as genetically possible a person's peak bone mass; and indicate that those at greatest risk of developing osteoporosis later in life are white and Asian teenage and young adult women, who are in their bone-forming years. Claims for products with more than 400 mg of calcium per day must state that a daily intake over 2,000 mg offers no added known benefit to bone health.

Sodium and Hypertension: Typical Foods: Unsalted tuna, salmon, fruits and vegetables, low-fat milks, low-fat yogurts, cottage cheeses, sherbets, ice milk, cereal, flour, and pastas (not egg pastas). Requirements: Foods must meet criteria for "low sodium." Claims must use "sodium" and "high blood pressure" in discussing the nutrient-disease link.

Dietary Fat and Cancer: Typical Foods: Fruits, vegetables, reduced-fat milk products, cereals, pastas, flours, and sherbets. Requirements: Foods must meet criteria for "low fat." Fish and game meats must meet criteria for "extra lean." Claims may not mention specific types of fats and must use "total fat" or "fat" and "some types of cancer" or "some cancers" in discussing the nutrient-disease link.

Dietary Saturated Fat and Cholesterol and Risk of Coronary Heart Disease: Typical Foods: Fruits, vegetables, skim and low-fat milks, cereals, whole-grain products, and pastas (not egg pastas). Requirements: Foods must meet criteria for "low saturated fat," "low cholesterol," and "low fat." Fish and game meats must meet criteria for "extra lean." Claims must use "saturated fat and cholesterol" and "coronary heart disease" or "heart disease" in discussing the nutrient-disease link.

Fiber-Containing Grain Products, Fruits, and Vegetables and Cancer: Typical Foods: Whole-grain breads and cereals, fruits, and vegetables. Requirements: Foods must meet criteria for "low fat" and, without fortification, be a "good source" of dietary fiber. Claims must not specify types of fiber and must use "fiber," "dietary fiber," or "total dietary fiber" and "some types of cancer" or "some cancers" in discussing the nutrient-disease link.

Fruits, Vegetables, and Grain Products That Contain Fiber, Particularly Soluble Fiber, and Risk of Coronary Heart Disease: Typical Foods: Fruits, vegetables, and whole-grain breads and cereals. Requirements: Foods must meet criteria for "low saturated fat," "low fat," and "low cholesterol." They must contain, without fortification, at least 0.6 g of soluble fiber per reference amount, and the soluble fiber content must be listed. Claims must use "fiber," "dietary fiber," "some types of dietary fiber," "some dietary fibers," or "some fibers" and "coronary heart disease" or "heart disease" in discussing the nutrient-disease link. The term "soluble fiber" may be added.

(continued)

TABLE 1–11 Labeling Terms and Authorized Health Claims (*Continued*)

Fruits and Vegetables and Cancer: Typical Foods: Fruits and vegetables. Requirements: Foods must meet criteria for "low fat" and, without forti-fication, be a "good source" of fiber, vitamin A, or vitamin C. Claims must characterize fruits and vegetables as foods that are low in fat and may contain dietary fiber, vitamin A, or vitamin C; characterize the food itself as a "good source" of one or more of these nutrients, which must be listed; refrain from specifying types of fatty acids; and use "total fat" or "fat," "some types of cancer" or "some cancers," and "fiber," "dietary fiber," or "total dietary fiber" in discussing the nutrient-disease link.

Folate and Neural Tube Birth Defects: Typical Foods: Enriched cereal grain products, some legumes (dried beans), peas, fresh leafy green vegetables, oranges, grapefruit, many berries, some dietary supplements, and fortified breakfast cereals. Requirements: Foods must meet or exceed criteria for "good source" of folate—that is, at least 40 μg of folic acid per serving (at least 10% of the DV). A serving of food cannot contain more than 100% of the DV for vitamins A and D because of their potential risk to fetuses. Claims must use "folate," "folic acid," or "folacin" and "neural tube defects," "birth defects spina bifida or anencephaly," "birth defects of the brain or spinal cord anencephaly or spina bifida," "spina bifida and anencephaly, birth defects of the brain or spinal cord," "birth defects of the brain and spinal cord," or "brain or spinal cord birth defects" in discussing the nutrient-disease link. Folic acid content must be listed on the Nutrition Facts panel.

Dietary Sugar Alcohol and Dental Caries (cavities): Typical Foods: Sugarless candy and gum. Requirements: Foods must meet the criteria for "sugar free." The sugar alcohol must be xylitol, sorbitol, mannitol, maltitol, isomalt, lactitol, hydrogenated starch hydrolysates, hydrogenated glucose syrups, erythritol, or a combination of these. When the food contains a fermentable carbohydrate, such as sugar or flour, the food must not lower plaque pH in the mouth below 5.7 while it is being eaten or up to 30 minutes afterwards. Claims must use "sugar alcohol," "sugar alcohols," or the name(s) of the sugar alcohol present and "dental caries" or "tooth decay" in discussing the nutrient-disease link. Claims must state that the sugar alcohol present "does not promote," "may reduce the risk of," "is useful in not promoting," or "is expressly for not promoting" dental caries.

Dietary Soluble Fiber, such as that found in Whole Oats and Psyllium Seed Husk, and Coronary Heart Disease: Typical Foods: Oatmeal cookies, muffins, breads, and other foods made with rolled oats, oat bran, or whole oat flour; hot and cold breakfast cereals containing whole oats or psyllium seed husk; and dietary supplements containing psyllium seed husk. Requirements: Foods must meet criteria for "low saturated fat," "low cholesterol," and "low fat." Foods that contain whole oats must contain at least 0.75 g of soluble fiber per serving. Foods that contain psyllium seed husk must contain at least 1.7 g of soluble fiber per serving. Claim must specify the daily dietary intake of the soluble fiber source necessary to reduce the risk of heart disease and the contribution one serving of the product makes toward that intake level. Soluble fiber content must be stated in the nutrition label. Claims must use "soluble fiber" qualified by the name of the eligible source of soluble fiber and "heart disease" or "coronary heart disease" in discussing the nutrient-disease link. Because of the potential hazard of choking, foods containing dry or incompletely hydrated psyllium seed husk must carry a label statement telling consumers to drink adequate amounts of fluid, unless the manufacturer shows that a viscous adhesive mass is not formed when the food is exposed to fluid.

For More Information

- American Association of Family and Consumer Sciences
  1555 King St., Alexandria, VA 22314
  703-706-4600
  http://www.aafcs.org/
- American Public Health Association
  http://www.apha.org/
- Association for Worksite Health Promotion
  http://www.awhp.org/
- Centers for Disease Control & Prevention
  http://www.cdc.gov/
- Food & Drug Administration
  http://www.fda.gov/
- Food Guide Pyramid—USDA
  http://www.nal.usda.gov/fnic/Fpyr/pyramid.html
- Foundation for Better Health Care
  http://fbhc.org/modules/menopause.cfm
- Health Statistics
  http://www.cdc.gov/nchs/fastats/Default.htm
- International Food Information Council
  http://ificinfo.health.org/
- National Women's Health Resource Center
  http://www.4woman.org/
- Recipes: www.intelihealth.com; www.deliciousdecisions.org; www.cookinglight.com; www.mealsforyou.com; www.allrecipes.com
- Shape Up America
  http://www.shapeup.org/
- Women's Health Initiative
  http://www.nhlbi.nih.gov/whi/index.html

GERIATRIC NUTRITION

NUTRITIONAL ACUITY RANKING: LEVEL 2–3

The Nutrition Screening Initiative (NSI) reports that 24% of elderly individuals are at high nutritional risk; 38% are at moderate risk (see Table 1–12).

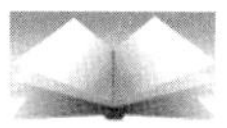

DEFINITIONS AND BACKGROUND

Aging involves a progression of physiological changes with cell loss and organ decline; decreased glomerular filtration rate (GFR) and creatinine-height index (CHI), constipation, decreased glucose tolerance, and lowered cell-mediated immunity can occur. Need for calories related to basal metabolism can decrease as much as 10% for ages 50–70 and by 20–25% thereafter. After 70 years of age, body weight declines; physical activity can prevent unnecessary losses in lean body mass. Nutritional assessment challenges include limited recall, hearing and vision losses, changes in attention span, and variations in dietary intake from day to day.

Although the term "life span" describes the maximal potential for humans (estimated to be between 120–140 years), life expectancy is the mean length of life projected for a population at a given age (Harris, 2000). Nutritional well-being is an integral part of successful aging; aging need not imply disability (American Dietetic Association, 1996).

Individuals older than 65 years of age currently comprise 13% of the United States population. Only 4–5% of elderly individuals are in nursing homes, the others live in the community (often alone). Approximately 48% of medical and 50% of surgical hospital admissions have malnutrition as a complication, especially among the elderly. Although the stress response to surgery (decrease in albumin and transferrin) is not affected by age, serum protein levels return to normal more slowly in older individuals (Puskarich-May et al., 1996). This factor must be considered for all older patients undergoing surgery.

TABLE 1–12 Nutrition Screening Initiative (NSI) DETERMINE Checklist

The NSI is targeted for identification of elderly individuals who are at nutritional risk. The following are warning signs for malnutrition that should be addressed (Nutrition Screening Initiative, 1994).

D = Disease (illness affects nutritional intake)
E = Eating poorly, especially fewer than two meals daily
T = Tooth loss, mouth pain, chewing difficulty
E = Economic hardship (too few dollars to buy food)
R = Reduced social contact; eating meals alone
M = Multiple medicines (three or more prescribed or over-the-counter medications)
I = Involuntary weight loss or gain (10 lb in 6 months)
N = Needs assistance with self-care (shopping, cooking, eating)
E = Elderly years (older than 80 years of age), with increasing frailty

Reprinted with permission by the Nutrition Screening Initiative, a project of the American Academy of Family Physicians, The American Dietetic Association and the National Council on the Aging, Inc., and funded in part by a grant from Ross Products Division, Abbott Laboratories Inc.

The term "frail elderly" refers to individuals with low lean body mass, often far below the desired range for their height. Undernutrition may be associated with dysphagia, slow eating, low protein intake, anorexia (often from depression), tube feeding, and age (Keller, 1993). Malnutrition is a frequent condition and is likely to affect health status and life expectancy among the elderly.

Unexpected weight loss is a pathologic condition, recently categorized in one of three ways—sarcopenia, wasting and cachexia according to criteria of nutritional intake, and functional abilities and age-related body composition modifications. The relationship to frailty, failure to thrive, and homeostatic balance failure syndrome must be identified. With the latter term, it is widely represented in the late stages of malnutrition that often evolves in multiple organ system failure and lastly in death (Vetta et al., 1999).

Two-thirds of persons age 75 are edentulous. Decreased salivation and absorption, as well as declining taste and smell, are also common. BMR declines 2% with each decade of life; LBM declines 6% with each decade and generally is replaced by fat.

The oldest age attained by humans seems to be 114 years. Energy deprivation or control may play a part in increasing longevity, although being too thin is risky to the immune system of elderly individuals. In general, weight loss in elderly individuals is not desirable because it usually is difficult for them to recover lost weight (Roberts, 1994; Wallace et al., 1995).

In long-term care facilities, 20–50% of residents are likely to be undernourished. Protein-energy undernutrition may contribute to pressure ulcers, immune dysfunction, infections, hip fractures, anemia, muscle weakness, fatigue, edema, cognitive changes, and mortality. Weight loss, depression, dehydration, and feeding problems are the easiest clues to monitor; serum albumin levels below 3.5 are also important to correct. Where possible, include activity and exercise to help stimulate an improved appetite. Use of Megace may help improve poor nutritional intake over a 3-month period (Yeh et al., 2000).

Older adults seem to need more vitamin B6 to maintain glucose tolerance and functional immunity (Blumberg, 1994). Almost 90% of older persons with low serum levels of vitamin B12 show evidence of tissue deficiency as well (Metz et al., 1996). Increased intakes of vitamins B12 and E, folic acid, and zinc also may be needed to counteract changes in hydrochloric acid and decreased intakes. Multivitamin supplementation in healthy older persons can enhance hypersensitivity skin test responses (Bogden et al., 1994). New RDAs for the "oldest old" individuals may be necessary at some point.

Precipitously declining cholesterol appears to be a marker for mortality and may help explain the low cholesterol–mortality association in older nursing home patients (Grant et al., 1996). Other prospective studies also report higher nonatherosclerotic disease rates in people with low serum total cholesterol, below 150 mg/dL. Higher cholesterol may be a marker for other protective substances such as fat-soluble antioxidants, may result in enhanced delivery of lipids to cells during the immune response or tissue repair, or may enhance defense against endotoxins and viruses (Jacobs and Iribarren, 2000). Low cholesterol might mark poor nutrition, as in depression; more research is needed to elucidate any biologic basis for these relationships, especially among the elderly.

In the Cardiovascular Health Study, 5,888 participants age 65 years and older were followed for several years (Burke et al., 2001). Data from this study suggest that a number of modifiable behavioral factors (physical activity, smoking, and obesity) and cardiovascular risk factors (diabetes, HDL cholesterol, and blood pressure) are associated with maintenance of good health in older adults.

OBJECTIVES

- Provide proper nutrition for weight control, healthy appetite, and prevention of acute illness or complications of chronic diseases (e.g., osteoporosis, fractures, anemias, obesity, diabetes, heart disease, and cancers).
- Correct existing nutritional deficiencies. Malnutrition may be caused by poverty, ignorance, depression, chronic disease, poor dietary intake, polypharmacy, and mental or physical disability. Avoid restrictive diets unless absolutely necessary (Buckler, 1994). Malnourished elderly patients receiving oral supplemental beverages gain more fat-free mass and make more protein compared to those not receiving any supplements (Bos et al., 2000).
- Determine baseline functional level and evaluate changes over time.
- Provide foods of proper consistency by status of dentition. Dentures increase bitter and sour taste sensations. In addition, elderly individuals have fewer taste buds, especially for sweets and salt. More sweet flavorings and salty foods (or equivalent seasoning) may be required to satisfy the appetite.
- Evaluate for laxative, enema, or alcohol abuse. Recommend suitable alternatives and interventions.
- Provide a diet of correct texture that excludes hard, sticky foods that are difficult to chew and swallow.
- Choose an appropriate regimen: "if the gut works, use it." Maintain weight through oral diet or tube feeding. However, for individuals who are unable to regain significant lost weight, TPN may be required.
- Investigate all major shifts in body weight. Ensure adequate hydration. Diminishing thirst mechanisms and incontinence play a part in dehydration, a common reason for hospital admissions (Chernoff, 1994; Warren et al., 1994; Weinberg, 1995).
- Assess the environment. (i.e., Who shops? Who cooks? How are finances handled? How many meals are eaten away from home?)
- Encourage physical activity, especially resistance training, to maintain metabolically active tissue and to correct mild constipation.
- Correct "the dwindles," which is similar to "failure to thrive" in infants and children (Verdery, 1995; Kimball and Williams-Burgess, 1995). Evaluate family and social support. Depression, use of many medications, underlying medical illnesses, and other factors should be addressed.

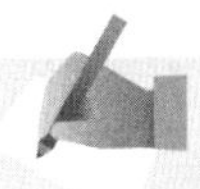

DIETARY AND NUTRITIONAL RECOMMENDATIONS

- Ensure intake of the food pyramid: 3–4 servings of milk, dairy products, or calcium substitute, 2–3 servings of meat or substitute, 3–5 servings of vegetables, 2–4 servings of fruits, and 6–12 bread-group servings. Fats, oils, sugars, and sweets are to be controlled to increase or decrease caloric intake, as appropriate for the individual.
- Diet should provide adequate intake of protein: 1 g/kg body weight (Campbell, 1994). This may mean 63 g for men and 50 g for women. Consider liver and renal impairments and decrease as needed. Increase for pressure ulcers, cancers, and other conditions requiring a high protein intake.
- Consume 1,200 mg of calcium (from milk and yogurt when possible). Include the B vitamins, 10 mg of iron, and 12–15 mg of zinc. Follow RDAs for other nutrients according to the patient's age and sex.
- Calories: 25–35 kcal/kg. The average 75-year-old female needs 1,900 kcal; males need 2,100 kcal if ambulatory. Fewer calories are needed for nonambulatory persons. Nutritional supplements may be useful for elderly nursing home residents who have lost weight; improvements in albumin, total lymphocyte count (TLC), cholesterol, and hemoglobin often result (Johnson et al., 1993).
- If patient has cardiovascular disease, encourage lower intake of saturated fat and use a no-added-salt diet. Liberalize where possible to keep intake at a sufficient level. Extra vitamin E may be useful from nuts, some vegetable oils, and more fruits and vegetables.
- The consistency of the food should be altered (i.e., ground, strained, or chopped) as required. Try to maintain whole textures as often as possible to enhance the food's appeal and to increase mastication with saliva.
- Adequate fiber and fluid intakes are necessary. Prudent increases in fiber (e.g., from prunes and bran) can reduce laxative abuse. Dehydration is a common cause of confusion.
- Adequate amounts of vitamins C and D, folic acid, and iron are needed; these nutrients frequently are deficient in the diets of elderly individuals.

Nutrient	*Recommendation for Males over 70 yrs*	*Recommendation for Females over 70 yrs*
Calories:	2,100 kcal/d	1,900 kcal/d
Protein:	63 g/d	50 g/d
Calcium:	1,200 mg/d	1,200 mg/d
Iron:	8 mg/d	8 mg/d
Folate:	400 μg/d	400 μg/d
Phosphorus:	700 mg/d	700 mg/d
Vitamin A:	900 μg	700 μg
Vitamin C:	90 mg/d	75 mg/d
Thiamin:	1.2 mg/d	1.1 mg/d
Riboflavin:	1.3 mg/d	1.1 mg/d
Niacin:	16 mg/d	14 mg/d

- When taste and olfactory sensations are weak, the diet should provide adequate intake of zinc, folate, and vitamins A and B12. Season with herbs and spices; add butter-flavored seasonings, garlic, maple or vanilla extract, and cheese or bacon-flavored seasonings. Consider all possible taste enhancers.
- About 10–30% of people over the age of 50 may have protein-bound vitamin B12 malabsorption; these people need to consume a majority of their RDA from synthetic forms rather than from food form (Ho et al., 1999).
- Increased thiamine may be needed because of decreased metabolic efficiency. Men are especially susceptible.
- Reduce intake of excessive sugar; poor glucose tolerance and insulin resistance are common after 65 years of age.
- If early satiety is a problem, having the main meal at noon may help.
- Encourage socialization at mealtimes. Individuals tend to eat more when they are in a group setting.
- Offer substitutes for major foods not consumed. Consult the dietitian if intake is chronically poor.

PROFILE

Clinical/History		
Age	Skin condition and pressure ulcers	TLC
Height (actual)	Urinary incontinence	Ca++
Weight, current	Hx surgery, radiation, chemotherapy	Urinary N
Weight, usual	Mini-Mental State Examination	Na+, K+
BMI or IBW/HBW	Incontinence, indwelling catheter	H & H, Serum Fe
Recent weight changes	Clinical signs of malnutrition	Serum B12, methylmalonic acid
Temp (hypothermia is more common)	Hydration status, I & O	Serum folate
BP		Serum homocysteine
Dentition	**Lab Work**	Chol, Trig
Eyesight	Transferrin	Alb (may be deceptively high in dehydration)
Hearing		Prealbumin
Difficulty in chewing		Gluc
Dysphagia		TSF, MAC, MAMC
Constipation, bowel habits		BUN, Creat

Common Drugs Used and Potential Side Effects

- Many drugs affect the nutritional status of the patient. A thorough drug history is needed. Polypharmacy is common in elderly individuals.
- Use of mineral oil as a laxative should be discouraged because it decreases absorption of fat-soluble vitamins and calcium.
- Evidence exists that a long-term, high-carbohydrate, low-protein diet may be undesirable with drug therapies of many types. Drug metabolism is slowed down, which is a potentially dangerous occurrence.
- Drug metabolism and detoxification require adequate methionine, vitamins A, C, and E, choline, folacin, selenium, other sulfur amino acids, and vitamin B12.
- Sulfonamides decrease levels of vitamin K and the B complex.
- Diuretics can decrease serum levels of potassium, magnesium, calcium, and zinc.
- Cimetidine (Tagamet) can decrease vitamin B12 levels.
- Aspirin decreases serum folate, vitamin C, and iron.
- Estrogens (Premarin) may cause nausea, vomiting, and weight changes.
- Long-term diuretic therapy is one central pharmacologic therapy of heart insufficiency and HPN. Diuretics not only lead to an increased urinary excretion of electrolytes but also of water-soluble vitamins. Thiamin deficiency is a real risk; a low dose thiamin supplement may be useful to prevent a subclinical beri-beri in older subjects on diuretics (Suter et al., 2000).
- Megestrol acetate improves appetite and well-being after 12 weeks of treatment in older adults, who have cachexia (Yeh et al., 2000).
- Discuss the relevance of tolerable upper intake levels (ULs) from the latest dietary reference intakes of the National Academy of Sciences. These levels were set to protect individuals from receiving too much of any nutrient from diet and dietary supplements.

Herbs, Botanicals and Supplements

- Herbs and botanical supplements should not be used without discussing with the physician, especially for underlying medical conditions.
- Gingko biloba has been studied for its beneficial effects on memory. While some studies have demonstrated some effectiveness for treatment of age-related memory loss or dementia, others have not (van Dongen et al., 2000).
- Age-associated increase in prostaglandin E2 production contributes to the decline in T-cell mediated function with age. Black currant seed oil rich in both gamma and alpha linoleic acids has a moderate immune-enhancing effect related to its ability to reduce production of PGE2 (Wu et al., 1999).
- Echinacea may be used as an immune system stimulant. It should not be taken with steroids, cyclosporine, or immunosuppressants.
- Kava is sometimes used as a sleep aid. Kava should not be taken with sedatives, alcohol, antipsychotics, or other CNS depressants.
- Ginseng may be used for stress adaptation, performance enhancement, impotence, or as a digestive aid. It should not be taken with warfarin, insulin, oral hypoglycemics,

CNS stimulants, caffeine, steroids, hormones, antipsychotics, aspirin, or antiplatelet drugs.

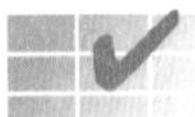

PATIENT EDUCATION

- ✔ Emphasize the need to consume adequate amounts of calcium, vitamin D, folic acid, vitamins A and E, and iron.
- ✔ Be aware of income limitations when planning a menu—less expensive protein sources may be necessary. Discuss shopping and meal preparation tips.
- ✔ Prevent excessive use of caffeine (e.g., coffee, colas, and tea), which may prevent intake of other desirable juices and beverages. Three 6–9 oz cups of coffee per day poses no specific health risk; monitor effects of anxiety, medications, etc.
- ✔ Ensure that the diet uses sources of fluid and fiber to alleviate constipation. Discuss exercises such as walking and resistance training.
- ✔ Determine whether the patient is using alcohol because multiple deficiencies may result, especially thiamine, B12, folacin, and zinc. Make appropriate referrals.
- ✔ Encourage participation in Meals-on-Wheels, food stamps, or congregate feeding programs.
- ✔ Ensure adequate fluid intake where permitted.
- ✔ Encourage exercise as prescribed (e.g., strength conditioning).
- ✔ Discuss adding herbs and spices to foods. Flavorful foods may release endorphins, which help boost the immune system (Duffy, 1995).
- ✔ Because depression affects 20–40% of older Americans but is not a normal part of aging, and because it causes a lot of weight loss in nursing homes and in the community, it must be identified and treated (Ryan and Shea, 1996). Tables 1–13, 1–14, and 1–15 can be used to determine weight and stature among the elderly.
- ✔ Hypothermia is common in the elderly (i.e., body temperature of 95 degrees or lower). Fatigue, weakness, poor coordination, lethargy, slurred speech, and drowsiness can occur. Give hot beverages and place in a warm bed. When body temperature reaches 90 degrees, the individual is likely to die.
- ✔ A key list of important nutrients in fruits and vegetables is provided in Table 1–16. Top choices include: papaya, kiwifruit, cantaloupe, mango, apricot, broccoli, spinach, tomato, sweet potato, and collards.
- ✔ Restorative dining may require specialized attention from a dietitian. The American Dietetic Association suggests 3 visits for medical nutrition therapy in restorative dining procedures (http://www.knowledgelinc.com/ada/mntguides/).
- ✔ For patients with a history of, current status of, or risk for dehydration, The American Dietetic Association suggests 2 medical nutrition therapy visits (http://www.knowledgelinc.com/ada/mntguides/).

For More Information

- ✦ Administration on Aging
  http://www.aoa.dhhs.gov/
- ✦ Aging Well–New York State
  http://agingwell.state.ny.us/index.html
- ✦ American Association of Retired Persons (AARP)
  http://www.aarp.org/
- ✦ American Dietetic Association
  Restorative Dining and Dehydration/Fluid Maintenance protocols
  http://www.eatright.org
- ✦ American Federation for Aging Research
  http://www.afar.org/

TABLE 1–13 Weight Table for Men Aged 70 and Over

Height Inches	*Ages 70–74*	*Ages 75–79*	*Ages 80–84*	*Ages 85–89*	*Ages 90–94*	*Ages Over 94*
5′1″ (61)	128–156	125–153	123–151	120–145	118–142	113–139
5′2″ (62)	130–158	127–155	125–153	122–148	119–143	114–140
5′3″ (63)	131–161	129–157	127–155	122–150	120–146	115–141
5′4″ (64)	134–164	131–161	129–157	124–152	122–148	116–142
5′5″ (65)	136–166	134–164	130–160	127–155	125–153	117–143
5′6″ (66)	139–169	137–167	133–163	130–158	128–156	120–146
5′7″ (67)	140–172	140–170	136–166	132–162	130–160	122–150
5′8″ (68)	143–175	142–174	139–169	135–165	133–163	126–154
5′9″ (69)	147–179	146–178	142–174	139–169	137–167	130–158
5′10″ (70)	150–184	148–182	146–178	143–175	140–172	134–164
5′11″ (71)	155–189	152–186	149–183	148–180	144–176	139–169
6′0″ (72)	159–195	156–190	154–188	153–187	148–182	143–173
6′1″ (73)	164–200	160–196	158–192	157–189	156–187	155–177
6′2″ (74)	169–205	165–201	163–197	162–190	160–188	158–181

Source: Adapted from *Journal of the American Medical Association*, Vol. 177, p. 658, with permission of American Medical Association, Copyright 1960. American Medical Association.

TABLE 1–14 Weight Table for Women Aged 70 and Over

Height Inches	*Ages 70–74*	*Ages 75–79*	*Ages 80–84*	*Ages 85–89*	*Ages 90–94*	*Ages Over 94*
4′7″ (55)	117–143	106–132	107–132	94–113	86–108	85–107
4′8″ (56)	118–144	108–134	108–133	95–114	88–110	87–109
4′9″ (57)	119–145	110–136	109–134	96–115	90–112	89–110
4′10″ (58)	120–146	112–138	111–135	97–118	94–115	93–114
4′11″ (59)	121–147	114–140	112–136	100–122	99–121	98–120
5′0″ (60)	122–148	116–142	113–139	106–130	102–124	101–123
5′1″ (61)	123–151	118–144	115–141	109–133	104–128	103–129
5′2″ (62)	125–153	121–147	118–144	112–136	108–132	107–131
5′3″ (63)	127–155	123–151	121–147	115–141	112–136	107–131
5′4″ (64)	130–158	126–154	123–151	119–145	115–141	108–132
5′5″ (65)	132–162	130–158	126–154	122–150	120–146	112–136
5′6″ (66)	136–166	132–162	128–157	126–154	124–152	116–142
5′7″ (67)	140–170	136–166	131–161	130–158	128–156	120–146
5′8″ (68)	143–175	140–170	137–164	134–162	131–160	124–150
5′9″ (69)	148–180	144–176				

Source: Adapted from *Journal of the American Medical Association,* Vol. 177, p. 658, with permission of American Medical Association, Copyright 1960. American Medical Association.

- American Geriatrics Society
  http://www.americangeriatrics.org/
- American Society on Aging
  833 Market Street, Suite 511
  San Francisco, CA 94103-1824
  415-974-9600
  http://www.asaging.org/ASA_Home_New5.cfm
- The Gerontological Society of America
  1030 15th Street NW Suite 250
  Washington DC 20005
  202-842-1275
  http://www.geron.org/
- Meals on Wheels
  1414 Prince St., Suite 202
  Alexandria, VA 22314
  703-548-5558
  http://www.mealsonwheelsassn.org/
- Medicare Information
  http://www.medicare.gov/
- National Aging Information Center
  330 Independence Ave., SW--Room 4656
  Washington, DC 20201
  202-619-7501
  http://www.aoa.dhhs.gov/naic/
- National Association of Nutrition and Aging Services Programs
  http://www.nanasp.org/
- National Council on Aging (NCOA)
  http://www.ncoa.org/
- National Institute on Aging (NIA)
  31 Center Dr., MSC 2292--Building 31, Room 5C27
  Bethesda, MD 20892
  http://www.nih.gov/nia/
- National Policy and Resource Center on Nutrition and Aging
  http://www.fiu.edu/~nutreldr
- Nutrition Screening Initiative (NSI)
  1010 Wisconsin Ave. NW, Suite 800
  Washington, DC 20007
  http://home.aafp.org/nsi/index.html
- USC Leonard Davis School of Gerontology
  http://www.usc.edu/dept/gero/nutrition/

TABLE 1–15 Formula for Calculating Stature Using Knee Height

Stature for men = 64.19 − (0.04 × age) + (2.02 × knee height)
Stature for women = 84.88 − (0.24 × age) + (1.83 × knee height)

Source: Reprinted with permission of Ross Laboratories, Columbus, Ohio, from *Nutritional Assessment of the Elderly through Anthropometry* by W.C. Chumlea, © 1984 Ross Laboratories.

TABLE 1–16 Key Nutrients in Fruits and Vegetables

FRUITS	*Vitamin A >500 IU*	*Vitamin C >6 mg*	*Folate >.04 mg*	*Potassium >350 mg*	*Dietary Fiber >2 g*
Apple, with skin (1 medium)		X			X
Apricot, dried (3)	X	X		X	X
Banana (1 medium)		X		X	X
Blackberries (1/2 cup)					X
Blueberries (1 cup)		X			X
Cantaloupe (1 cup)	X	X		X	
Grapefruit (1/2 medium)		X			
Grapefruit juice (3/4 cup)		X		X	
Grapes (1/2 cup)		X			
Honeydew melon (1 cup)		X		X	X
Kiwifruit (2 medium)		X	X	X	X
Mango (1 medium)	X	X			X
Nectarine (1 medium)	X	X			X
Orange (1 medium)		X	X		X
Orange juice (3/4 cup)		X	X	X	
Papaya (1 medium)	X	X	X	X	X
Peach, with skin (1 medium)	X	X			X
Pear, with skin (1 medium)		X			X
Pineapple (2, 3/4 slices)		X			X
Plum, with skin (2 medium)		X			X
Prunes (4) (Dried Plums)	X				X
Raspberries (1 cup)		X			X
Strawberries (1/2 cup)		X			X
Watermelon (1 cup)	X	X			
VEGETABLES					
Artichokes (1 medium)					X
Asparagus (5 spears)		X	X		X
Beans, kidney (1/2 cup)			X	X	X
Beans, lima (1/2 cup)			X	X	X
Black-eyed peas (1/2 cup)			X		X
Bok choy (1 cup cooked)		X			
Broccoli (1/2 cup)	X	X	X		X
Brussels sprouts (1/2 cup)		X			
Carrots (1 medium)	X	X			X
Cauliflower (1 cup)		X	X		X
Collards (1/2 cup)	X	X	X		X
Corn (1 cup)		X	X	X	X
Green beans (1/2 cup)		X			X
Green pepper (1 medium)	X	X			X
Kale (1/2 cup)	X	X			X
Lentils (1/2 cup)			X	X	X
Peas, green (1/2 cup)		X	X		X
Peas, split (1/2 cup)			X	X	X
Potato (1 medium)		X		X	
Potato, with skin (1 medium)		X		X	X
Romaine lettuce (6 leaves)	X	X	X		
Spinach, cooked (1/2 cup)	X	X	X	X	X
Squash, winter (1/2 cup)	X	X		X	X
Sweet potato (1 medium)	X	X		X	X
Tomato (1 medium)	X	X		X	
Turnip greens (1/2 cup)	X	X	X		

X indicates that the item provides 10% or more of the DV in the serving size specified or at least 2 grams of dietary fiber.
Used by permission from: SUPERMARKET SAVVY (tm) newsletter, Linda McDonald Associates Inc., www.supermarketsavvy.com.

REFERENCES

Pregnancy—Cited References

American Dietetic Association. Position of The American Dietetic Association: nutrition care for pregnant adolescents. *J Am Diet Assoc.* 1994;94:450.

Azais-Braesco V, Pascal G. Vitamin A in pregnancy: requirements and safety limits. *Am J Clin Nutri.* 2000;71:1325S.

Baeten JM, et al. Pregnancy complications and outcomes along overweight and obese nulliparous women. *Am J Public Health.* 2001;91:436.

Botto LD, et al. Occurrence of congenital heart defects in relation to maternal multivitamin use. *Am J Epid.* 2000;151:878.

Brown JE, Carlson M. Nutrition and multifetal pregnancy. *J Am Diet Assoc.* 2000;100:343.

Butte NF, et al. Adjustments in energy expenditure and substrate utilization during late pregnancy and lactation. *Am J Clin Nutri.* 1999;69:299.

Carroll P. Safe ingestion of aspartame during pregnancy. *Clin Nutri.* 1990;5:1.

Chappell LC, et al. Effect of antioxidants on the occurrence of preeclampsia in women at increased risk: a randomized trial. *Lancet.* 1999;354:810.

Cnattingius S, et al. Prepregnancy weight and the risk of adverse pregnancy outcomes. *N Engl J Med.* 1998;338:147.

Damron D, et al. Factors associated with attendance in a voluntary nutrition education program. *Am J Health Promotion.* 1999;149:268.

Dawson EB, et al. Blood cell lead, calcium, and magnesium levels associated with pregnancy-induced hypertension and preeclampsia. *Biol Trace Elem Res.* 2000;74:107.

Dubois S, et al. Ability of the Higgins Nutrition Intervention Program to improve adolescent pregnancy outcome. *J Am Diet Assoc.* 1997;97:871.

Erick M, Bunnell MK. Nausea and vomiting of pregnancy: manifestations and current interventions. *Female Patient.* 2000;25:59.

Giddens JB, et al. Pregnant adolescent and adult women have similarly low intakes of selected nutrients. *J Am Diet Assoc.* 2000;100: 1334.

Godfrey KM, Barker DJ. Fetal nutrition and adult disease. *Am J Clin Nutri.* 2000;71S:1344.

Gulley R, et al. Treatment of hyperemesis gravidarum with nasogastric feeding. *Nutri Clin Pract.* 1993;8:33.

Klebanoff MA, et al. Maternal serum paraxanthine, a caffeine metabolite, and the risk of spontaneous abortion. *N Engl J Med.* 1999;341:1639.

Miller RK, et al. Periconceptional vitamin A use: how much is teratogenic? *Repro Toxicol.* 1998;12:75.

Morrill ES, Nickols-Richardson HM. Bulimia nervosa during pregnancy: a review. *J Am Diet Assoc.* 2001;101:448.

Morris CD, et al. Nutrient intake and hypertensive disorders of pregnancy: evidence from a large prospective cohort. *Am J Obstet Gynecol.* 2001;184:643.

Napoli C, et al. Influence of maternal hypercholesterolemia during pregnancy on progression of early atherosclerotic lesions in childhood: Fate of Early Lesions in Children (FELIC) study. *Lancet.* 1999;354:1234.

Rainville A. Pica practices of pregnant women are associated with lower maternal hemoglobin level at delivery. *J Am Diet Assoc.* 1998;98:293.

Shaw GM, Lammer EJ. Maternal periconceptional alcohol consumption and risk for orofacial clefts. *J Pediatr.* 1999;134:298.

Todoroff K, Shaw GM. Prior spontaneous abortion, prior elective termination, interpregnancy interval, and risk of neural tube defects. *Am J Epid.* 2000;151:505.

Vollset SE, et al. Plasma total homocysteine level and complications and outcomes of pregnancy. *Am J Clin Nutri.* April 2000;71:962.

Pregnancy—Suggested Readings

Badart-Smook A, et al. Fetal growth is associated positively with maternal intake of riboflavin and negatively with maternal intake of linoleic acid. *J Am Diet Assoc.* 1997;97:867.

Bailey LB. New standard for dietary folate intake in pregnant women. *Am J Clin Nutri.* 2000;71S:1304.

Broussard CN, Richter JE. Nausea and vomiting of pregnancy. *Gastroenterology Clin North Am.* 1998;27:123.

Erick M. Nutrition via jejunostomy feeding in refractory hyperemesis gravidarum: a case report. *J Am Diet Assoc.* 1997;10:1154.

Hardy DS. A multiethnic study of the predictors of macrosomia. *Diab Educator.* 1999;25:925.

Kiely M, et al. Low molecular weight plasma antioxidants and lipid peroxidation in maternal and cord blood. *Euro J Clin Nutri.* 1999;53:861.

Kramer-LeBlanc C, et al. Review of the Nutritional Status of WIC Participants. Center for Nutrition Policy and Promotion, USDA, Sept 1999.

Lenders C, et al. Gestational age and infant size at birth are associated with dietary sugar intake among pregnant adolescents. *J Nutri.* 1997;127:1113.

Neggers Y, et al. Plasma and erythrocyte zinc concentrations and their relationship to dietary zinc intake and zinc supplementation during pregnancy in low-income, African-American women. *J Am Diet Assoc.* 1997;97:1296.

Owen A, Owen G. Twenty years of WIC: a review of some effects of the program. *J Am Diet Assoc.* 1997;97:777.

Scholl TO, et al. Use of multivitamin/mineral prenatal supplements: influence on the outcome of pregnancy. *Am J Epid.* 1997;146:134.

Scholl TO, Johnson WG. Folic acid: influence on the outcome of pregnancy. *Am J Clin Nutri.* 2000;71:1295.

Shaw G, et al. Risk of neural tube defect-affected pregnancies among obese women. *J Am Med Assoc.* 1996;275:1093.

Siega-Riz A, et al. Maternal underweight status and inadequate rate of weight gain during the third trimester of pregnancy increases the risk of preterm delivery. *J Nutri.* 1996;126:146.

Stanure M, et al. High hemoglobin and hematocrit levels and pregnancy outcomes. *Top Clin Nutri.* 1999;14:25.

Stoler JM, et al. The prenatal detection of significant alcohol exposure with maternal blood markers. *J Pediatr.* 1998;133:346.

Strychar IM, et al. Psychosocial and lifestyle factors associated with insufficient and excessive maternal weight gain during pregnancy. *J Am Diet Assoc.* 2000;00:353.

Tepper BJ, Seldner AC. Sweet taste and intake of sweet foods in normal pregnancy complicated by gestational diabetes mellitus. *Am J Clin Nutri*. 1999;70:277.

Werler M, et al. Multivitamin supplementation and risk of birth defects. *Am J Epid*. 1999;150:675.

Widga AC, Lewis NM. Defined, in-home prenatal nutrition intervention for low-income women. *J Am Diet Assoc*. 1999;99:1058.

Worthington-Roberts B. The role of maternal nutrition in the prevention of birth defects. *J Am Diet Assoc*. 1997;97:S184.

Lactation—Cited References

American Dietetic Association. Position of The American Dietetic Association: breaking the barriers to breastfeeding. *J Am Diet Assoc*. 2001;101:1213.

Anderson JW, Johnstone BM, and Remley DT. Breastfeeding and cognitive development: a meta-analysis. *Am J Clin Nutri*. 1999;70:525.

Ball TM, Wright AL. Healthcare costs of formula-feeding in the first year of life. *Pediatrics* 1999;103(S):870.

Carver JD. Dietary nucleotides: effects on the immune and gastrointestinal systems. *Acta Pediatr Suppl*. 1999;88:83.

Chapman D, Perez-Escamilla R. Identification of risk factors for delayed onset of lactation. *J Am Diet Assoc*. 1999;99:450.

Dewey KG. Nutrition, growth, and complementary feeding of the breastfed infant. *Pediatr Clin North Am*. 2001;48:87.

Dewey KG, et al. Maternal weight-loss patterns during prolonged lactation. *Am J Clin Nutri*. 1993;58:162.

Doran L, Evers S. Energy and nutrient inadequacies in the diets of low-income women who breastfeed. *J Am Diet Assoc*. 1997;97:1283.

Dorea JG. Iron and copper in human milk. *Nutrition*. 2000;16:209.

Fagan K. Nutrition during pregnancy and lactation. In: Mahan K, Escott-Stump S, eds. *Krause's food, nutrition and diet therapy*. 10th ed. Philadelphia: WB Saunders, 2000.

Fukushima Y, et al. Consumption of cow milk and egg by lactating women and the presence of B-lactoglobulin and ovalbumin in breast milk. *Am J Clin Nutri*. 1997;65:30.

Groziak SM, Miller GD. Natural bioactive substances in milk and colostrum: effects on the arterial blood pressure system. *Br J Nutri*. 2000;84:119S.

Hamosh M, et al. Breastfeeding and the working mother: effect of time and temperature of short-term storage on proteolysis, lipolysis, and bacterial growth in milk. *Pediatrics*. 1996;97:492.

Hilson J, et al. Maternal obesity and breastfeeding success in a rural population of white women. *Am J Clin Nutri*. 1997;66:1371.

Krebs N, et al. Bone mineral density changes during lactation: maternal, dietary, and biochemical correlates. *Am J Clin Nutri*. 1997;65:1738.

Kreiter SR, et al. Nutritional rickets in African American, breastfed infants. *J Pediatr*. 2000;137:153.

Lovelady CA, et al. The effect of weight loss in overweight, lactating women on the growth of their infants. *N Engl J Med*. 2000;342:449.

Mackey A, et al. Self-selected diets of lactating women often fail to meet dietary recommendations. *J Am Diet Assoc*. 1998;98:297.

McCrory MA. Does dieting during lactation put infant growth at risk? *Nutri Rev*. 2001;59:18.

Montagne PM, et al. Dynamics of the main immunologically and nutritionally available proteins of human milk during lactation. *J Food Composition and Anal*. 2000;13:127.

Ordaz-Jimenez MR, et al. Gastrointestinal hormones during minimal enteral feeding of sick premature infants. *Rev Invest Clin*. 1998;50:37.

Singhal A, et al. Early nutrition in preterm infants and later blood pressure: two cohorts after randomized trials. *Lancet*. 2001;357:413.

Weimer J. The economic benefits of breastfeeding: a review and analysis. ERS Food Assistance and Nutrition Research Report No. 13, March 2001.

Weinberg GA. The dilemma of postnatal mother-to-child transmission of HIV: to breastfeed or not? *Birth*. 2000;27:199.

Wright AL, et al. Changing hospital practices to increase the duration of breastfeeding. *Pediatrics*. 1996;97:669.

Wright AL, et al. Factors influencing the relation of infant feeding to asthma and recurrent wheeze in childhood. *Thorax*. 2001;56:192.

Lactation—Suggested Readings

Bakker EC, et al. Early nutrition, essential fatty acid status, and visual acuity of term infants at 7 months of age. *Euro Clin J Nutri*. 1999;53:872.

Beshgetoor D, et al. Attitudes toward breastfeeding among WIC employees in San Diego County. *J Am Diet Assoc*. 1999;99:86.

Bruin NC, et al. Energy utilization and growth in breastfed and formula-fed infants measured prospectively during the first year of life. *Am J Clin Nutri*. 1998;67:885.

Dorea JG. Magnesium in human milk. *J Am Col Nutri*. 2000;19:210.

Fly AD, et al. Major mineral concentrations in human milk do not change after maximal exercise testing. *Am J Clin Nutri*. 1998;68:345.

Innis SM, King DJ. Trans fatty acids in human milk are inversely associated with concentrations of essential allo-cis n-6 and n-3 fatty acids and determine trans, but not n-6 and n-3 fatty acids in plasma lipids of breastfed infants. *Am J Clin Nutri*. 1999;70:383.

Janney C, et al. Lactation and weight retention. *Am J Clin Nutri*. 1997;66:1116.

Kalkwarf HJ and Harrast SD. Effects of calcium supplementation and lactation on iron status. *Am J Clin Nutri*. 1998;67:1244.

Murtaugh M. Optimal breastfeeding duration. *J Am Diet Assoc*. 1997;97:1252.

Orlet-Fisher J, et al. Breastfeeding through the first year predicts maternal control in feeding and subsequent toddler energy intakes. *J Am Diet Assoc*. 2000;100:641.

Raisler J, et al. Breastfeeding and infant illness: a dose-response relationship? *Am J Public Health*. 1999;89:25.

Sharma M and Petosa R. Impact of expectant fathers in breastfeeding decisions. *J Am Diet Assoc*. 1997;97:1311.

Wright AL, et al. Increasing breastfeeding rates to reduce infant illness at the community level. *Pediatrics* 1998;101:837.

Zimmer JP, et al. Postpartum maternal blood helper T (CD3+CD4+) and cytotoxic (CD3+CD8+) cells: correlation with iron status, parity, supplement use, and lactation status. *Am J Clin Nutri*. 1998;67:897.

Infant, Normal (0–6 Months)—Cited References

Agostoni C, et al. Effects of diet on the lipid and fatty acid status of full-term infants at 4 months. *J Am Col Nutri*. 1994;13:658.

Agostoni C, et al. Growth pattern of breastfed and nonbreastfed infants with atopic dermatitis in the first year of life. *Pediatrics*. 2000;106:73E.

American Academy of Pediatrics' Committee on Nutrition. Iron fortification of infant formulas. *Pediatrics*. 1999;104:119.

American Academy of Pediatrics' Committee on Nutrition. *Pediatric Nutrition Handbook*. 4th edition. Elk Grove, Ill: American Academy of Pediatrics, 1998.

American Academy of Pediatrics' Committee on Nutrition. Soy protein-based formulas: recommendations for use in infant feeding. *Pediatrics.* 1998;101:148.

Arshad SH. Food allergen avoidance in primary prevention of food allergy. *Allergy.* 2001;67:113S.

Caddell JL. Magnesium deficiency promotes muscle weakness, contributing to the risk of sudden infant death (SIDS) in infants sleeping prone. *Magnes Res.* 2001;14:39.

Chorazy P, et al. Persistent hypothyroidism in an infant receiving a soy formula: case report and review of the literature. *Pediatrics* 1995;96:148.

Dalton M, et al. Calcium and phosphorus supplementation of iron-fortified infant formula. *J Am Diet Assoc.* 1997;97:921.

Forsyth J, et al. Relation between early introduction of solid food to infants and their weight and illnesses during the first two years of life. *BMJ.* 1993;306:1572.

Gardiner P, Kemper KJ. Herbs in Pediatric and adolescent medicine. *Pediatrics in Review.* 2000;21:44.

Howard CR, et al. Physiologic stability of newborns during cup and bottle-feeding. *Pediatrics.* 1999;104:1204.

Juszczyk-Balon A. Management of infantile colic. *Am Fam Phys.* 1997;55:235.

Martorelli R, et al. Early nutrition and later adiposity. *J Nutri.* 2001;131:874S.

Rosebloom TJ, et al. Maternal nutrition during gestation and blood pressure in later life. *J Hypertens.* 2001;19:29.

Sullivan S, Birch L. Infant dietary experience and acceptance of solid foods. *Pediatrics.* 1994;93:271.

Tomassoni AJ, Simone K. Herbal medicines for children: an illusion of safety? *Curr Opin Pediatr.* 2001;13:162.

Trahms C. Nutrition in infancy. In: Mahan K, Escott-Stump S, eds. *Krause's food, nutrition, and diet therapy.* 10th ed. Philadelphia: WB Saunders, 2000.

Infant, Normal (0–6 Months)—Suggested Readings

American Dietetic Association. *Pediatric Manual of Clinical Dietetics.* Chicago, IL: The American Dietetic Association, 1998.

Coutsoudis A, et al. The effects of vitamin A supplementation on the morbidity of children born to HIV-infected women. *Am J Public Health.* 1995;85:1076.

Drewnowski A, Rock C. The influence of genetic taste markers and food acceptance. *Am J Clin Nutri.* 1995;62:506.

Graham G, et al. Protein requirements of infants and children: growth during recovery from malnutrition. *Pediatrics.* 1996;97:499.

Lonnerdal B. Genetic engineering: opportunities and challenges in infant nutrition. Proceedings of a symposium held in Palm Beach, Florida, Dec 1994. *Am J Clin Nutri.* 1996;63:621S.

Mennella J. A cross-cultural perspective: infant feeding. *Nutrition Today.* 1997;32(4):144.

Schwartz J, et al. Does WIC participation improve breastfeeding practices? *Am J Public Health.* 1995;85:729.

Infant, Normal (6–12 Months)—Cited References

Agostoni C, et al. Growth pattern of breastfed and nonbreastfed infants with atopic dermatitis in the first year of life. *Pediatrics.* 2000;106:73E.

Agostoni C, et al. Growth patterns of breastfed and formula-fed infants in the first 12 months of life: an Italian study. *Arch Dis Child.* 1999;81:395.

Butte NF, et al. Infant feeding mode affects early growth and body composition. *Pediatrics.* 2000;106:1355.

Gale C, Martyn C. Breastfeeding, dummy use and adult intelligence. *Lancet.* 1996;347:1072.

Gardiner P, Kemper KJ. Herbs in pediatric and adolescent medicine. *Pediatrics in Review.* 2000;21:44.

Kattelmann KK, et al. Effect of timing of introduction of complementary foods on iron and zinc status of formula-fed infants at 12, 24, and 36 months of age. *J Am Diet Assoc.* 2001;101:443.

Reed-Mangels A, Messina V. Considerations in planning vegan diets: infants. *J Am Diet Assoc.* 2001;101:670.

Salo P, et al. Milk type during mixed feeding: contribution to serum cholesterol ester fatty acids in late infancy. *J Peds.* 1997;130:110.

Tomassoni AJ, Simone K. Herbal medicines for children: an illusion of safety? *Curr Opin Pediatr.* 2001;13:162.

Childhood—Cited References

Abramovitz BA, Birch LL. Five-year-old girls' ideas about dieting are predicted by their mothers' dieting. *JAMA.* October 2000;100:1157.

American Academy of Pediatrics' Committee on Nutrition. Calcium requirements of infants, children, and adolescents. *Pediatrics.* 1999;104:1152.

American Dietetic Association. Position of The American Dietetic Association: local support for nutrition integrity in schools. *J Am Diet Assoc.* 2000;100:108.

Ballew C, et al. Nutrient intakes and dietary patterns of young children by dietary fat intakes. *J Pediatr.* 2000;136:181.

Baxter S, Domel, et al. Impact of gender, ethnicity, meal component, and time interval between eating and reporting on accuracy of fourth-graders' self-reports of school lunch. *J Am Diet Assoc.* 1997;97:1293.

Bronner Y. Nutritional status outcomes for children: ethnic, cultural, and environmental contexts. *J Am Diet Assoc.* 1996;96:891.

Carvalho NF, et al. Severe nutritional deficiencies in toddlers resulting from health food milk alternatives. Rickets is increasingly common in children. *Pediatrics.* 2001;107:46E.

Dennison BA, et al. Children's growth parameters vary by type of fruit juice consumed. *J Am Col Nutri.* 1999;18:346.

DuRant R, et al. The relationship among television watching, physical activity, and body composition of young children. *Pediatrics.* 1994;94:449.

Erikson E. *Childhood and society.* 2nd ed. New York: WW Norton & Company, 1963.

Fagot-Campagna A. Emergence of type 2 diabetes mellitus in children: epidemiological evidence. *J Pediatr Endocrinol Metab.* 2000;13:1395S.

Falciglia GA, et al. Food neophobia in childhood affects dietary variety. *J Am Diet Assoc.* 2000;100:1474.

Getlinger MJ, et al. Food waste is reduced when elementary school lunch children have recess before lunch. *J Am Diet Assoc.* 1996;96:906.

Gilbert C, Foster A. Childhood blindness in the context of VISION 2020—the right to sight. *Bull World Health Organ.* 2001;79:227.

Golan M, et al. Impact of treatment for childhood obesity on parental risk factors for cardiovascular disease. *Prevent Med.* 1999;29:519.

Gortmaker S, et al. Television viewing as a cause of increasing obesity among children in the United States, 1986–1990. *Arch Pediatr Adolesc Med.* 1996;150:356.

Hampl JS, et al. Intakes of vitamin C, vegetables, and fruits: which schoolchildren are at risk? *J Am Col Nutri.* 1999;18:582.

Hutchins SS, et al. National serologic survey of measles immunity among persons 6 years of age or older, 1988–1994. *Med Gen Med.* 2001;24:E5.

Lanphear BP, et al. Cognitive deficits associated with blood lead concentrations <10 mg/dL in US children and adolescents. *Public Health Rep.* 2000;115:521.

Lindquist CH, et al. Role of dietary factors in ethnic differences in early risk of cardiovascular disease and type 2 diabetes. *Am J Clin Nutri.* 2000;71:725.

Lucas B. Ensuring healthy and well-nourished children. *J Am Diet Assoc.* 2001;101:628.

Melnick T, et al. Food consumption patterns of elementary schoolchildren in New York City. *J Am Diet Assoc.* 1998;98:159.

Messina V, Reed-Mangels A. Considerations in planning vegan diets: children. *J Am Diet Assoc.* 2001;101:661.

Miller J, Korenman S. Poverty and children's nutritional status. *Am J Epidemiol.* 1994;140:233.

Olson R. Is it wise to restrict fat in the diets of children? *J Am Diet Assoc.* 2000;100:28.

Orlet-Fisher J, Birch LL. Parents' restrictive feeding practices are associated with young girls' negative self-evaluation of eating. *J Am Diet Assoc.* 2000;100:1341.

Pollitt E. The relationship between undernutrition and behavioral development in children. *J Nutri.* 1995;125(8):2211.

Rice AL, et al. Malnutrition as an underlying cause of childhood deaths associated with infectious diseases in developing countries. *Bull World Health Organ.* 2000;78:1207.

Rolls B, Engell D, Birch LL. Serving portion size influences 5-year-old but not 3-year old children's food intakes. *J Am Diet Assoc.* 2000;100:232.

Seaton A, Devereux G. Diet, infection, and wheezy illness: lessons from adults. *Pediatr Allergy Immunol.* 2000;13:37.

Sigman-Grant M, et al. Dietary approaches for reducing fat intake of preschool-age children. *Pediatrics.* 1993;91:955.

Skinner JD, et al. Fruit juice intake is not related to children's growth. *Pediatrics.* 1999;103:58.

Stallings V. Calcium and bone health in children: a review. *Am J Therapeutics.* 1997;4:259.

Story M, Brown J. Do young children instinctively know what to eat? The studies of Clara Brown revisited. *N Engl J Med.* 1987;316:103.

Trissler RJ. Type 2 diabetes on the rise in children: is the American lifestyle coming home to roost? *J Am Diet Assoc.* 1999;99:1354.

Williams C. Importance of dietary fiber in childhood. *J Am Diet Assoc.* 1995;95:1140.

Childhood—Suggested Readings

American Dietetic Association. Position of The American Dietetic Association: nutrition standards for child-care programs. *J Am Diet Assoc.* 1999;99:981.

American Dietetic Association. Position of The American Dietetic Association: dietary guidance for healthy children aged 2–11 years. *J Am Diet Assoc.* 1999;99:93.

Ames SK, et al. Effects of high compared with low calcium intake on calcium absorption and incorporation of iron by red blood cells in small children. *Am J Clin Nutri.* 1999;70:44.

Bonjour JP, et al. Calcium-enriched foods and bone mass growth in prepubertal girls: a randomized, double-blind, placebo-controlled trial. *J Clin Invest.* 1997;99:1287.

Carruth BR, et al. The phenomenon of "picky eater": a behavioral marker in eating patterns of toddlers. *J Am Col Nutri.* 1998;17:180.

Cutting TM, et al. Like mother, like daughter: familial patterns of overweight are mediated by mothers' dietary disinhibition. *Am J Clin Nutri.* 1999;69:608.

Dwyer J. Should dietary fat recommendations for children be changed? *J Am Diet Assoc.* 2000;100:36.

Evers C. Empower children to develop healthful eating habits. *J Am Diet Assoc.* 1997;97: S116.

Falorni A, et al. Using obese-specific charts of height and height velocity for assessment of growth in obese children and adolescents during weight excess reductions. *Euro J Clin Nutri.* 1999;53:181.

Friedman BJ, Hurd-Crixell SL. Nutrient intake of children eating school breakfast. *J Am Diet Assoc.* 1999;99:219.

Gunnell DJ, et al. Childhood obesity and adult cardiovascular mortality. *Am J Clin Nutri.* 1998;67:1111.

Himes JH, Story M. Obesity in childhood and adolescence: assessment, prevention and treatment. Papers emanating from a conference held in Minneapolis, Minnesota, May 1997. *Int J Obesity and Related Metabolic Disorders.* 1999;23:1.

Hopman E, et al. Eating habits of young children with Down syndrome in the Netherlands: adequate nutrient intakes but delayed introduction of solid food. *J Am Diet Assoc.* 1998;98:7.

Krebs NF, Johnson SL. Guidelines for healthy children: promoting eating, moving, and common sense. *J Am Diet Assoc.* 2000;100:37.

Leslie J, et al. Development and implementation of a school-based nutrition and fitness promotion program for ethnically diverse middle-school girls. *J Am Diet Assoc.* 1999;99:967.

Lytle LA. In defense of a low-fat diet for healthy children. *J Am Diet Assoc.* 2000;100:39.

Lucas B. Nutrition in childhood. In: Mahan K, Escott-Stump S, eds. *Krause's food, nutrition, and diet therapy.* 10th ed. Philadelphia: WB Saunders, 2000.

Nickerson HJ, et al. Treatment of iron deficiency anemia and associated protein-losing enteropathy in children. *J Pediatr Hematol Oncol.* 2000;22:50.

Pietrobelli A, et al. Body mass index as a measure of adiposity among children and adolescents. *J Pediatr.* 1998;132:204.

Reimers T, et al. Maternal acceptability of a dietary intervention designed to lower children's intake of saturated fat and cholesterol: the Dietary Intervention Study in Children (DISC). *J Am Diet Assoc.* 1998;98:31.

Robertson SM, et al. Factors related to adiposity among children aged 3–7 years. *J Am Diet Assoc.* 1999;99:938.

Satter E. A moderate view on fat restriction for young children. *J Am Diet Assoc.* 2000;100:32.

Sentongo TA, et al. Resting energy expenditure and prediction equations in young children with failure to thrive. *J Pediatrics.* 2000;136:345.

Sicherer SH, et al. Use assessment of self-administered epinephrine among food-allergic children and pediatricians. *Pediatrics.* 2000; 105:359.

Skinner JD, et al. Longitudinal study of nutrient and food intakes of white preschool children aged 24–60 months. *J Am Diet Assoc.* 1999;99:1514.

Spencer T. Growth deficits in children with attention deficit hyperactivity disorder. *Pediatrics.* 1998;102:501.

Stanek K, et al. Lead consumption of 18- to 36-month-old children as determined from duplicate diet collections: nutrient intakes, blood lead levels, and effects on growth. *J Am Diet Assoc.* 1998;98:155.

Tanner J, et al. Tanner-Whitehouse bone age reference values for North American children. *J Peds.* 1997;131:34.

Baer M, Harris A. Pediatric nutrition assessment: identifying children at risk. *J Am Diet Assoc.* 1997;97:S107.

Tershakovec AM, et al. Age-related changes in cardiovascular disease risk factors of hypercholesterolemic children. *J Pediatr.* 1998;132:414.

Tershakovec AM, et al. Insurance reimbursement for the treatment of obesity in children. *J Pediatrics.* 1999;134:573.

Van Horn L. Primary prevention of cardiovascular disease starts in childhood. *J Am Diet Assoc.* 2000;100:41.

Wildley MB, et al. Fat and sugar levels are high in snacks purchased from student stores in middle schools. *J Am Diet Assoc.* 2000;100: 319.

Will SM, et al. The effects of a high-protein, low-fat, ketogenic diet on adolescents with morbid obesity: body composition, blood chemistries, and sleep abnormalities. *Pediatrics.* 1998;101:61.

Young RJ, et al. Increasing oral fluids in chronic constipation in children. *Gastroenterol Nurs.* 1998;21:156.

Adolescence—Cited References

Anding J, et al. Blood lipids, cardiovascular fitness, obesity, and blood pressure: the presence of potential coronary heart disease risk factors in adolescents. *J Am Diet Assoc.* 1996;96:238.

Berkey CS, et al. Relation of childhood diet and body size to menarche and adolescent growth in girls. *Am J Epid.* 2000;152:446.

Flodmark C, et al. Prevention of progression to severe obesity in a group of obese school children treated with family therapy. *Pediatrics.* 1993;91:880.

Gortmaker S, et al. Television viewing as a cause of increasing obesity among children in the United States, 1986–1990. *Arch Pediatr Adolesc Med.* 1996;150:356.

Herbold NH, Frates SE. Update of nutrition guidelines for the teen: trends and concerns. *Curr Opin Pediatr.* 2000;12:303.

Ilich-Ernst JZ, et al. Iron status, menarche, and calcium supplementation in adolescent girls. *Am J Clin Nutri.* 1998;68:880.

Louwman MW, et al. Signs of impaired cognitive function in adolescents with marginal cobalamin status. *Am J Clin Nutri.* 2000;72:762.

Lynch SR. The potential impact of iron supplementation during adolescence on iron status in pregnancy. *J Nutri.* 2000;130(S):448.

Messina V, Reed-Mangels A. Considerations in planning vegan diets: children. *J Am Diet Assoc.* 2001;101:661.

O'Brien K, et al. Increased efficiency of calcium absorption during short periods of inadequate calcium intake in girls. *Am J Clin Nutri.* 1996;63:579.

Stang J, et al. Relationships between vitamin and mineral supplement use, dietary intake, and dietary adequacy among adolescents. *J Am Diet Assoc.* 2000;100:905.

Stewart B, Tinsley A. Importance of food choice influences for working young adults. *J Am Diet Assoc.* 1995;95:227.

Adolescence—Suggested Readings

DeBourdeauhuij I, Van Oost P. Family members' influence on decision making about food: differences in perception and relationship with healthy eating. *Am J Health Promotion.* 1998;13:73.

Harnack L, et al. Soft drink consumption among U.S. children and adolescents: nutritional consequences. *J Am Diet Assoc.* 1999;9:436.

Neumark-Sztainer D, et al. Lessons learned about adolescent nutrition from the Minnesota Adolescent Health survey. *J Am Diet Assoc.* 1998;98:1449.

Neumark-Sztainer D, et al. Factors influencing food choices of adolescents: findings from focus-group discussions with adolescents. *J Am Diet Assoc.* 1999;99:929.

Popkin BM, JR Udry. Adolescent obesity increases significantly in second and third generation U.S. immigrants: the National Longitudinal Study of Adolescent Health. *J Nutri.* 1998;128:701.

Rickert V, ed. *Adolescent nutrition assessment and management.* New York: Chapman & Hall, 1996.

Spear B. Nutrition in adolescence. In: Mahan K, Escott-Stump S. *Krause's food, nutrition and diet therapy.* 10th ed. Philadelphia: WB Saunders, 2000.

Story M, et al. Dieting status and its relationship to eating and physical activity behaviors in a representative sample of U.S. adolescents. *J Am Diet Assoc.* 1998;98:10.

Story M, et al. Availability of foods in high schools: is there cause for concern? *J Am Diet Assoc.* 1996;96:123.

Trissler RJ. The child within: a guide to nutrition counseling for pregnant teens. *J Am Diet Assoc.* 1999;99:916.

Vaisman N, et al. Weight perception of adolescent dancing school students. *Arch Pediatr Adolesc Med.* 1996;150:187.

Sports Nutrition—Cited References

American Academy of Pediatrics' Committee on Sports Medicine and Fitness. Medical concerns in the female athlete. *Pediatrics.* 2000;106:610.

American Dietetic Association. Position of the American Dietetic Association and the Canadian Dietetic Association: nutrition for physical fitness and performance for adults. *J Am Diet Assoc.* 2000;100:1543.

American Dietetic Association. Timely statement of The American Dietetic Association: nutrition guidance for child athletes in organized sports. *J Am Diet Assoc.* 1996;96:610.

American College of Sports Medicine, The American Dietetic Association, International Food Information Council. For a healthful lifestyle: promoting cooperation among nutrition professional and physical activity professionals. *J Am Diet Assoc.* 1999;99:994.

Becque MD, et al. Effects of oral creatine supplementation on muscular strength and body composition. *Med Sci Sport Ex.* 2000;32:654.

Berning J. Nutrition in athletic performance. In: Mahan K, Escott-Stump S, eds. *Krause's food, nutrition, and diet therapy.* 10th ed. Philadelphia: WB Saunders, 2000.

Bosch A, et al. Fuel substrate kinetics of carbohydrate loading differs from that of carbohydrate ingestion during prolonged exercise. *Metabolism.* 1996;45:415.

Clarkson P. Antioxidants and physical performance. *Crit Rev Food Sci Nutri.* 1995;35(1&2):131.

Fogelholm M, et al. Growth, dietary intake, and trace element status in pubescent athletes and school children. *Med Sci Sport Ex.* 2000;32:738.

Gannon B, et al. Do African Americans have lower energy expenditure than Caucasians? *Int J Obesity & Related Metabolic Disorders.* 2000;24:4.

Hobart JA, Smucker DR. The female athlete triad. *Am Fam Physician.* 2000;61:3357.

Lopez-Varela S, et al. Nutritional status of young female elite gymnasts. *Int J Vitam Nutri Res*. 2000;70:185.

Pendergast DR, et al. A perspective on fat intake in athletes. *J Am Col Nutri*. 2000;19:345.

Rico-Sanz J, Marco MT. Creatine enhances oxygen uptake and performance during alternating intensity exercise. *Med Sci Sport Ex*. 2000;32:379.

Sanborn CF, et al. Disordered eating and the female athlete triad. *Clin Sports Med*. 2000;19:199.

Tegelman R, et al. Influence of a diet regimen on glucose homeostasis and serum lipid levels in male elite athletes. *Metabolism*. 1996;45:435.

Sports Nutrition—Suggested Readings

Aschenbach W, et al. Effect of oral sodium loading on high-intensity arm ergometry in college wrestlers. *Med Sci Sport Ex*. 2000;32:669.

Beals K, Manore M. Nutritional status of female athletes with subclinical eating disorders. *J Am Diet Assoc*. 1998;98:419.

Bourique S, et al. Twelve weeks of endurance exercise training does not affect iron status measures in women. *J Am Diet Assoc*. 1997;97:1116.

Bryner RW, et al. Effects of resistance vs aerobic training combined with an 800 calorie liquid diet on lean body mass and resting metabolic rate. *J Am Col Nutri*. 1999;18:115.

Campbell WW, et al. Effects of an omnivorous diet compared with a lacto-ovovegetarian diet on resistance training induced changes in body composition and skeletal muscle in older men. *Am J Clin Nutri*. 1999;70:1032.

Cullinen K, Caldwell M. Weight training increases fat-free mass and strength in untrained young women. *J Am Diet Assoc*. 1998;98:414.

Dale KS, Landers DM. Weight control in wrestling: eating disorders or disordered eating? *Med Sci Sport Ex*. 1999;31:1382.

Deutz RC, et al. Relationship between energy deficits and body composition in elite female gymnasts and runners. *Med Sci Sport Ex*. 2000;32:659.

Ebbeling CB, Rodriguez NR. Effects of exercise combined with diet therapy on protein utilization in obese children. *Med Sci Sport Ex*. 1999;31:378.

Gill JMR, Hardman AE. Postprandial lipemia: effects of exercise and restriction of energy intake compared. *Am J Clin Nutri*. 2000;71:465.

Horvath PJ, et al. The effects of varying dietary fat on the nutrient intake in male and female runners. *J Am Col Nutri*. 2000;19:42.

Hunter GR, et al. Racial differences in energy expenditure and aerobic fitness in premenopausal women. *Am J Clin Nutri*. 2000;71:500.

King N, et al. Effects of exercise on appetite control: implications for energy balance. *Med Sci Sport Ex*. 1997;29:1076.

Klausen B, et al. Increased intensity of a single exercise bout stimulates subsequent fat intake. *Int J Obesity & Related Metabolic Disorders*. 1999;23:1282.

Leddy J, et al. Effect of a high- or a low-fat diet on cardiovascular risk factors in male and female runners. *Med Sci Sport Ex*. 1997;29:17.

Murgatroyd PR, et al. Effects of inactivity and diet composition on human energy balance. *Int J Obesity & Related Metabolic Disorders*. 1999;23:1269.

Nujika I, et al. Creatine supplementation and sprint performance in soccer players. *Med Sci Sport Ex*. 2000;32:518.

Okano G, et al. Effect of elevated blood FFA levels on endurance performance after a single fat meal ingestion. *Med Sci Sport Ex*. 1998;30:763.

Plunkett BT, Hopkins WG. Investigation of the side pain "stitch" induced by running after fluid ingestion. *Med Sci Sport Ex*. 1999;31:1169.

Rosenbloom C, ed. *Sports nutrition: a guide for the professional working with active people*. 3rd ed. Chicago: Sports and Cardiovascular Nutrition and the American Dietetic Association, 2000.

Ryan M. Sports drinks: research asks for reevaluation of current recommendations. *J Am Diet Assoc*. 1997;97:S197.

Schabort EJ, et al. The effect of a pre-exercise meal on time to fatigue during prolonged cycling exercise. *Med Sci Sport Ex*. 1999;31:464.

Volek J, et al. Performance and muscle fiber adaptations to creatine supplementation and heavy resistance training. *Med Sci Sport Ex*. 1999;31:1147.

Volek J, et al. Creatine supplementation enhances muscular performance during high-intensity resistance exercise. *J Am Diet Assoc*. 1997;97:765.

Wagner DR. Hyper-hydrating with glycerol: implications for athletic performance. *J Am Diet Assoc*. 1999;99:207.

Wee SL, et al. Influence of high and low glycemic index meals on endurance running capacity. *Med Sci Sport Ex*. 1999;31:393.

Youngstedt SD, et al. Acute exercise reduces caffeine-induced angiogenesis. *Med Sci Sport Ex*. 1998;30:740.

Adulthood—Cited References

American Dietetic Association. Position of the American Dietetic Association and Dietitians of Canada: women's health and nutrition. *J Am Diet Assoc*. 1999;99:738.

Auld GW, et al. Reported adoption of dietary fat and fiber recommendations among consumers. *J Am Diet Assoc*. 2000;100:52.

Barnard ND, et al. Diet and sex-hormone binding globulin, dysmenorrhea, and premenstrual symptoms. *Ob Gynecol*. 2000;95:245.

Bendich A. The potential for dietary supplements to reduce premenstrual syndrome (PMS) symptoms. *J Am Col Nutri*. 2000;19:3.

Blair S, et al. Changes in physical fitness and all-cause mortality. *J Am Med Assoc*. 1995;273:1093.

Bolumar F, et al. Caffeine intake and delayed conception: a European multicenter study on infertility and subfecundity. *Am J Epid*. 1997;145:324.

Braunschweig C, et al. Impact of declines in nutritional status on outcomes in adult patients hospitalized for more than 7 days. *J Am Diet Assoc*. 2000,100:1316.

Butler DB, et al. Randomized trial testing the effect of peer education at increasing fruit and vegetable intake. *J Nat'l Cancer Inst*. 2000;91:1491.

Cardinal BJ, Hermann-Engels J. Ginseng does not enhance psychological well-being in healthy young adults: results of a double-blind, placebo-controlled, randomized clinical trial. *J Am Diet Assoc*. 2001;101:655.

Clark AM, et al. Weight loss in obese infertile women results in improvement in reproductive outcomes for all forms of fertility treatment. *Hum Repro*. 1998;13:1505.

Dollahite J, et al. Problems encountered in meeting the recommended dietary allowances for menus designed according to the Dietary Guidelines for Americans. *J Am Diet Assoc*. 1995;95:341.

Duffy V. The flavor of food? It's all in your head! *J Am Diet Assoc*. 1996;96:655.

Finn S. Women in the new world order: where old values command new respect. *J Am Diet Assoc*. 1997;97:475.

Fishman P. Healthy people 2000: what progress toward better nutrition? *Geriatrics*. 1996;51:38.

Ge K, McNutt K. How the Chinese link dietary advice to their national plan of action for nutrition. *J Am Diet Assoc*. 2000;100:885.

Fahm E, Jocelyn J. Changing behaviors to optimize women's health: a multidisciplinary seminar. *J Am Diet Assoc*. 1998;98:818.

Hogbin M, Hess MA. Public confusion over food portions and servings. *J Am Diet Assoc*. 1999;99:1209.

Horner NK, Lampe JW. Potential mechanisms of diet therapy for fibrocystic breast conditions show inadequate evidence of effectiveness. *J Am Diet Assoc*. 2000;100:1368.

Johnston C, Yen MF. Megadose of vitamin C delays insulin response to a glucose challenge in normoglycemic adults. *Am J Clin Nutri*. 1994;60:735.

Kant A, et al. Dietary diversity and subsequent mortality in the first NHANES epidemiological follow-up study. *Am J Clin Nutri*. 1993;57:434.

Kant A, Schtzkin A. Consumption of energy-dense, nutrient-poor foods by the US population: effect on nutrient profiles. *J Am Col Nutri*. 1994;13:285.

Kendall A, et al. Relationship of hunger and food insecurity to food availability and consumption. *J Am Diet Assoc*. 1996;96:1019.

Klebanoff MA, et al. Maternal serum paraxanthine, a caffeine metabolite, and the risk of spontaneous abortion. *N Engl J Med*. 1999;341:1639.

Klotzbach-Shimomura. Functional foods: the role of physiologically active compounds in relation to disease. *Top Clin Nutri*. 2001;16:68.

Levy L, et al. How well do consumers understand percentage daily value on food labels? *Am J Health Promotion*. 2000;14:157.

Lussner-Cacon S, et al. Plasma total homocysteine in healthy subjects: sex-specific relation with biological traits. *Am J Clin Nutri*. 1996;64:587.

Messina M, Erdman J. First international symposium on the role of soy in preventing and treating chronic disease. *J Nutri*. 1995;125(3):567.

Mulhall JP. Current concepts in erectile dysfunction. *Am J Manag Care*. 2000;6:S625.

Palmer D, Abusabha R. The fifth edition of the Dietary Guidelines for Americans: lessons learned along the way. *J Am Diet Assoc*. 2001;101:631.

Pate R, et al. Physical activity and public health: a recommendation from the Centers for Disease Control and Prevention and the American College of Sports Medicine. *J Am Med Assoc*. 1995;273:402.

Prochaska J. "Just do it" isn't enough: change comes in stages. *Tufts U Diet & Nutrition Newsletter*. 1996;14(7):4.

Rangan V, et al. Do better at doing good. *Harvard Bus Rev*. 1996;74:42.

Rock C, et al. Nutritional characteristics, eating pathology, and hormonal status in young women. *Am J Clin Nutri*. 1996;64:566.

Tolstoi LG, et al. Human Genome Project and cystic fibrosis—a symbiotic relationship. *J Am Diet Assoc*. 1999;99:1421.

Walker AF, et al. Magnesium supplementation alleviates premenstrual symptoms of fluid retention. *J Women's Health*. 1998;7:1157.

Writing Group for the PEPI Trial. Effects of hormone therapy on bone mineral density: results from the postmenopausal estrogen/progestin interventions (PEPI) trial. *J Am Med Assoc*. 1996;276:1389.

Adulthood—Suggested Readings

American Dietetic Association. Position of the American Dietetic Association: food and water safety. *J Am Diet Assoc*. 1997;97:184.

American Dietetic Association. Position of the American Dietetic Association: food fortification and dietary supplements. *J Am Diet Assoc*. 2001;101:115.

American Dietetic Association. Position of the American Dietetic Association: food irradiation. *J Am Diet Assoc*. 2000;100:246.

American Dietetic Association. Position of the American Dietetic Association: functional foods. *J Am Diet Assoc*. 1999;99:1278.

American Dietetic Association. Position of the American Dietetic Association: food and nutrition misinformation. *J Am Diet Assoc*. 2002;102:260.

American Dietetic Association. Position of the American Dietetic Association: the role of nutrition in health promotion and disease prevention. *J Am Diet Assoc*. 1998;98:205.

Barrocas A. Complementary and alternative medicine: friend, foe or OWA? *J Am Diet Assoc*. 1997;97:1373.

Bayerl CT. Nutrition in the community. In: Mahan K, Escott-Stump S, eds. *Krause's food, nutrition, and diet therapy*. 10th ed. Philadelphia: WB Saunders, 2000.

Brown J, et al. Predictors of red cell folate level in women attempting pregnancy. *J Am Med Assoc*. 1997;277:548.

Carlton DJ, et al. Design, development, and formative evaluation of "Put Nutrition into Practice," a multi-media nutrition education program for adults. *J Am Diet Assoc*. 2000;100:555.

Devine CM, et al. Life-course events and experiences: association with fruit and vegetable consumption in three ethnic groups. *J Am Diet Assoc*. 1999;99:309.

DiSogra L, Glanz K. The 5-A-Day virtual classroom: an on-line strategy to promote healthful eating. *J Am Diet Assoc*. 2000;100:349.

Dodd, J. Incorporating genetics into dietary guidance. *Food Technology*. 1997;51:80.

Duffy VB, Bartoshuk LM. Food acceptance and genetic variation in taste. *J Am Diet Assoc*. 2000;100:647.

Earl R, Borra S. Dietary planning. In: Mahan K, Escott-Stump S, eds. *Krause's food, nutrition, and diet therapy*. 10th ed. Philadelphia: WB Saunders, 2000.

Clemens L, et al. The effect of eating out on quality of diet in premenopausal women. *J Am Diet Assoc*. 1999;99:442.

Frankenfield D, et al. The Harris-Benedict studies of human basal metabolism: history and limitations. *J Am Diet Assoc*. 1998;98:439.

Greene G, et al. Dietary applications of the Stages of Change Model. *J Am Diet Assoc*. 1999;99:673.

Hahn NI. Are phytoestrogens nature's cure for what ails us? A look at the research. *J Am Diet Assoc*. 1998;98:9.

Haines PS, et al. The Diet Quality Index revised: a measurement instrument for populations. *J Am Diet Assoc*. 1999;99:697.

Harnack L, et al. Guess who's cooking? The role of men in meal planning, shopping, and preparation in U.S. families. *J Am Diet Assoc*. 1998;98:995.

Kant AK, et al. A prospective study of diet quality and mortality in women. *J Am Med Assoc*. 2000;283:2109.

King S, Gibney M. Dietary advice to reduce fat intake is more successful when it does not restrict habitual eating patterns. *J Am Diet Assoc*. 1999;99:685.

Kloeblen AS. Folate knowledge, intake from fortified grain products, and periconceptual supplementation patterns of a sample of low-income pregnant women according to the Health Belief Model. *J Am Diet Assoc*. 1999;99:33.

Kristal A, et al. How can stages of change be best used in dietary interventions? *J Am Diet Assoc*. 1999;99:679.

Lee CD, et al. Cardiorespiratory fitness, body composition and all-cause and cardiovascular disease mortality in men. *Am J Clin Nutri*. 1999;69:373.

Leitzmann MF, et al. A prospective study of coffee consumption and the risk of symptomatic gallstone disease in men. *J Am Med Assoc*. 1999;281:2106.

Lindberg R. Active living: on the road with the 10,000 Steps program. *J Am Diet Assoc*. 2000;100:878.

Ma J, et al. Antioxidant intakes and smoking status: data from the Continuing Survey of Food Intakes by Individuals 1994–1996. *Am J Clin Nutri*. 2000;71:774.

Mathai K. Nutrition in adulthood. In: Mahan K, Escott-Stump S, eds. *Krause's food, nutrition, and diet therapy*. 10th ed. Philadelphia: WB Saunders, 2000.

Moore-Kenner M, et al. Primary care providers need a variety of nutrition and wellness patient education materials. *J Am Diet Assoc*. 1999;99:462.

Nitzke S, et al. Stages of change for reducing fat and increasing fiber among dietitians and adults with a diet-related chronic disease. *J Am Diet Assoc*. 1999;99:728.

Ounpuu S, et al. Defining stage of change for lower-fat eating. *J Am Diet Assoc*. 2000;100:674.

Patterson RE, et al. The genetic revolution: change and challenge for the dietetics profession. *J Am Diet Assoc*. 1999;99:1412.

Peterson S, et al. Impact of adopting lower-fat food choices on energy and nutrient intake of American adults. *J Am Diet Assoc*. 1999;99:177.

Raikkonen K, et al. Anger, hostility, and visceral adipose tissue in healthy, postmenopausal women. *Metabolism: Clin & Experi*. 1999;48:1146.

Singer A, et al. Improvements are needed in hospital diets to meet dietary guidelines for health promotion and disease prevention. *J Am Diet Assoc*. 1998;98:639.

Sloan A. Food industry forecast: consumer trends to 2020 and beyond. *Food Technology*. 1998;52:37.

Suter PM, et al. Diuretic use: a risk for subclinical thiamine deficiency in elderly patients. *J Nutri Health Ageing*. 2000;4:69.

Tai M, et al. Thermic effect of food during each phase of the menstrual cycle. *Am J Clin Nutri*. 1997;66:1110.

Viteri FE, et al. Long-term weekly iron supplementation improves and sustains nonpregnant women's iron status as well or better than currently recommended short-term daily iron supplementation. *J Nutri*. 1999;129:2013.

Weinsier RL, et al. Energy expenditure and free-living physical activity in black and white women: comparison before and after weight loss. *Am J Clin Nutri*. 2000;71:1138.

Geriatric Nutrition—Cited References

American Dietetic Association. Position of The American Dietetic Association: nutrition, aging and the continuum of care. *J Am Diet Assoc*. 1996;96:1048.

Blumberg J. Nutrient requirements of the healthy elderly—should there be specific RDAs? *Nutri Rev*. 1994;52(8):S15.

Bogden J, et al. Daily micronutrient supplements enhance delayed hypersensitivity skin test responses in older people. *Am J Clin Nutri*. 1994;60:437.

Bos C, et al. Short-term protein and energy supplementation activates nitrogen kinetics and accretion in poorly nourished elderly subjects. *Am J Clin Nutri*. 2000;71:1129.

Buckler D, et al. The use of dietary restrictions in malnourished nursing home patients. *J Am Geriatr Soc*. 1994;42:1100.

Burke GL, et al. Factors associated with healthy aging: the cardiovascular health study. *J Am Geriatr Soc*. 2001;49:254.

Campbell W, et al. Increased protein requirements in elderly people: new data and retrospective reassessments. *J Clin Nutri*. 1994;60:501.

Chernoff R. Thirst and fluid requirements. *Nutri Rev*. 1994;52(8):S3.

Duffy V, et al. Olfactory dysfunction and related nutritional risk in free-living, elderly women. *J Am Diet Assoc*. 1995;95:879.

Grant M, et al. Declining cholesterol and mortality in a sample of older nursing home residents. *J Am Geriatr Soc*. 1996;44:31.

Harris N. Nutrition in aging. In: Mahan LK, Escott-Stump S. *Krause's food, nutrition, and diet therapy*. 10th ed. Philadelphia: WB Saunders, 2000.

Ho C, et al. Practitioners' guide to meeting the vitamin B12 Recommended Dietary Allowance for people aged 51 and older. *J Am Diet Assoc*. 1999;99:725.

Jacobs DR, Iribarren C. Invited commentary: low cholesterol and non-atherosclerotic disease risk: a persistently perplexing question. *Am J Epidemiol*. 2000;151:748.

Johnson L, et al. Oral nutritional supplement use in elderly nursing home patients. *J Am Geriatr Soc*. 1993;41:947.

Keller H. Malnutrition in institutionalized elderly: how and why? *J Am Geriatr Soc*. 1993;41:1212.

Kimball M, Williams-Burgess C. Failure to thrive: the silent epidemic of the elderly. *Arch Psychiatr Nurs*. 1995;IX:99.

Metz J, et al. The significance of subnormal serum B12 concentration in older people: a case control study. *J Am Geriatr Soc*. 1996;44:1355.

Puskarich-May C, et al. The change in serum protein concentration in response to the stress of total joint surgery: a comparison of older versus younger patients. *J Am Geriatr Soc*. 1996;44:555.

Roberts S, et al. Control of food intake in older men. *J Am Med Assoc*. 1994;272:1601.

Ryan C, Shea M. Recognizing depression in older adults: the role of the dietitian. *J Am Diet Assoc*. 1996;96:1042.

Wallace J, et al. Involuntary weight loss in older outpatients: incidence and clinical significance. *J Am Geriatr Soc*. 1995;43:329.

Warren W, et al. The burden and outcomes associated with dehydration among U.S. elderly. *Am J Public Health*. 1994;84:1265.

Weinberg A, et al. Dehydration: evaluation and management in older adults. *J Am Med Assoc*. 1995;274:1552.

Wu D, et al. Effect of dietary supplementation with black currant seed oil on the immune response of healthy elderly subjects. *Am J Clin Nutri*. 1999;70:536.

Van Dongen MC, et al. The efficacy of gingko for elderly people with dementia and age-associated memory impairment: new results of a randomized clinical trial. *J Am Geriatr Soc*. 2000;48:1183.

Verdery R. Failure to thrive in the elderly. *Clin Geriatr Med*. 1995;11(4):653.

Vetta F, et al. The impact of malnutrition on the quality of life in the elderly. *Clin Nutri*. 1999;18:259.

Yeh SS, et al. Improvement in quality of life measures and stimulation of weight gain after treatment with megestrol acetate oral suspension in geriatric cachexia: results of a double-blind, placebo-controlled study. *J Am Geriatr Soc*. 2000;48:485.

Geriatric Nutrition—Suggested Readings

American Dietetic Association. Position of The American Dietetic Association: liberalized diets for older adults in long-term care. *J Am Diet Assoc*. 1998;98:201.

American Dietetic Association. Position of The American Dietetic Association: nutrition, aging, and the continuum of care. *J Am Diet Assoc.* 2000;100:580.

Bernard M, et al. Common health problems among minority elders. *J Am Diet Assoc.* 1997;97:771.

Blaum C, et al. Validity of the minimum data set for assessing nutritional status in nursing home residents. *Am J Clin Nutri.* 1997;66: 787.

Chandra R. Graying of the immune system: can nutrient supplements improve immunity in the elderly? *J Am Med Assoc.* 1997;97:1398.

Chidester J, Spangler A. Fluid intake in the institutionalized elderly. *J Am Diet Assoc.* 1997;97:23.

Chumlea W, et al. Stature prediction equations for elderly non-Hispanic white, non-Hispanic black, and Mexican-American persons developed from NHANES III data. *J Am Diet Assoc.* 1998;98:137.

Coakley EH, et al. Lower levels of physical functioning are associated with higher body weight among middle-aged and older women. *Int J Obes Rel Metab Disord.* 1998;22:958.

Covinsky KE, et al. The relationship between clinical assessments of nutritional status and adverse outcomes in older hospitalized medical patients. *J Am Geriatr Soc.* 1999;47:532.

Cummings DE, Meriam GR. Age-related changes in growth hormone secretion: should the somatopause be treated? *Semin Repro Endocrinol.* 1999;17:311.

DiPietro L, et al. Excess abdominal adiposity remains correlated with altered lipid concentrations in healthy older women. *Int J Obes Rel Metab Disord.* 1999;23:432.

Duffy V, et al. Olfactory dysfunction and related nutritional risk in free-living, elderly women. *J Am Diet Assoc.* 1995;95:879.

Evans J, et al. Relation of colonic transit to functional bowel disease in older people: a population-based study. *J Am Geriatr Soc.* 1998;46:83.

Evans W. Nutrition, exercise, and healthy aging. *J Am Diet Assoc.* 1997;97:632.

Kuzmarskei M, Kuzmarski RJ, Najjar M. Descriptive anthropometric reference data for older Americans. *J Am Diet Assoc.* 2000;100:59.

Fortes C, et al. The effect of zinc and vitamin A supplementation on immune response in an older person. *J Am Geriatr Soc.* 1998;46:19.

French SA, et al. Prospective study of intentionality of weight loss and mortality in older women: the Iowa Women's Health Study. *Am J Epid.* 1999;149:504.

Garry PJ, et al. Effects of iron intake on iron stores in elderly men and women: longitudinal and cross-sectional results. *J Am Col Nutri.* 2000;19:262.

Harari D, et al. Bowel habit in relation to age and gender: findings from the National Health Interview Survey and clinical implications. *Arch Int Med.* 1996;156:315.

Heuser M, Adler W. Immunological aspects of aging and malnutrition. *Clin Geriatr Med.* 1997;13(4):697.

Holben DH, et al. Fluid intake compared with established standards and symptoms of dehydration among elderly residents of a long-term care facility. *J Am Diet Assoc.* 1999;99:1447.

Houston DK, et al. Age-related hearing loss, vitamin B12, and folate in elderly persons. *Am J Clin Nutri.* 1999;69:564.

Hurley R, et al. Comparative evaluation of body composition in medically stable elderly. *J Am Diet Assoc.* 1997;97:1105.

Jacobs DR, et al. Is whole grain intake associated with reduced total and cause-specific death rates in older women? The Iowa Women's Health Study. *Am J Public Health.* 1999;89:322.

Jensen G, Rogers J. Obesity in older persons. *J Am Diet Assoc.* 1998;98:1308.

Kalmijn S, et al. The association of body weight and anthropometry with mortality in elderly men: the Honolulu Heart Program. *Int J Obes Rel Metab Disord.* 1999;23:395.

Katz I, DiFilippo S. Neuropsychiatric aspects of failure to thrive in late life. *Clin Geriatr Med.* 1997;13(4):623.

Kerschner H, Pegues J. Productive aging: a quality of life agenda. *J Am Diet Assoc.* 1998;98:1445.

Klein G, et al. Nutrition and health for older persons in rural America: a managed care model. *J Am Diet Assoc.* 1997;97:885.

Landi F, et al. Body mass index and mortality among older people living in the community. *J Am Geriatrics Soc.* 1999;47:1072.

Langlois J, et al. Weight change between age 50 years and old age is associated with risk of hip fracture in white women aged 67 years and older. *Arch Int Med.* 1996;156:989.

LaRue A, et al. Nutritional status and cognitive functioning in a normally aging sample: a 6-year reassessment. *Am J Clin Nutri.* 1997;65:20.

LeBoff MS, et al. Occult vitamin D deficiency in postmenopausal U.S. women with acute hip fracture. *J Am Med Assoc.* 1999;281:1505.

Losonczy K, et al. Vitamin E and vitamin C supplement use and risk of all-cause mortality in older persons. The Established Populations for Epidemiologic Studies of the Elderly. *Am J Clin Nutri.* 1996;64:190.

Metz J, et al. The significance of subnormal serum B12 concentration in older people: a case control study. *J Am Geriatr Soc.* 1996;44:1355.

Meydani M. Dietary antioxidants modulation of aging and immune-endothelial cell interaction. *Mech Ageing Dev.* 1999;111:123.

Meydani S, et al. Vitamin E supplementation and in vivo immune response in healthy elderly subjects: a randomized controlled trial. *J Am Med Assoc.* 1997;277:1380.

Moore AA, et al. Drinking habits among older persons: findings from the NHANES I Epidemiologic Study (1982–1984). *J Am Geriatr Soc.* 1999;47:412.

Morley J. Anorexia of aging: physiologic and pathologic. *Am J Clin Nutri.* 1997;66:760.

Mouton CP, et al. Health Screening in older women. *Am Fam Physician.* 1999;59:1835.

Mouton CP. Special health considerations in African-American elders. *Am Fam Phys.* 1997;55:1243.

Nilsson K, et al. The plasma homocysteine concentration is better than that of serum methylmalonic acid as a marker for sociopsychological performance in a psychogeriatric population. *Clin Chem.* 2000;46:691.

Obisesan T, et al. Moderate wine consumption is associated with decreased odds of developing age-related macular degeneration in NHANES-1. *J Am Geriatr Soc.* 1998;46:1.

Perrig W, et al. The relation between antioxidants and memory performance in the old and very old. *J Am Ger Soc.* 1997;45:718.

Philip KA, Greenwood CE. Nutrient contribution of infant cereals used as fluid thickening agents in diets fed to the elderly. *J Am Diet Assoc.* 2000;100:549.

Porter C, et al. Dynamics of nutrition care among nursing home residents who are eating poorly. *J Am Diet Assoc.* 1999;99:1444.

Quill TE, Byock IR. Responding to intractable terminal suffering: the role of terminal sedation and voluntary refusal of food and fluids. *Annals of Internal Medicine.* 2000;132:408.

Reuben DB, et al. The predictive value of combined hypoalbuminemia and hypocholesterolemia in high functioning community-dwelling older persons. MacArthur Studies of Successful Aging. *J Am Geriatr Soc.* 1999;47:402.

Riggs K, et al. Relations of vitamin B12, vitamin B6, folate, and homocysteine to cognitive performance in the Normative Aging Study. *Am J Clin Nutri.* 1996;63:306.

Ritchie C, et al. Nutritional status of urban homebound older adults. *Am J Clin Nutr.* 1997;66:815.

Russell RM, et al. Modified Food Guide Pyramid for people over 70 years of age. *J Nutr.* 1999;129:751.

Sayhoun N, et al. Nutrition Screening Initiative checklist may be a better awareness/educational tool than a screening one. *J Am Diet Assoc.* 1997;97:760.

Shoaf LR, Bishirjian KO, Schlenker ED. The Gerontological Nutritionists Standards of professional practice for dietetics professionals working with older adults. *J Am Diet Assoc.* 1999;99:863.

Stabler S, et al. Vitamin B12 deficiency in the elderly: current dilemmas. *Am J Clin Nutr.* 1997;66:741.

Stein MS, et al. Falls relate to vitamin D and parathyroid hormone in an Australian nursing home and hostel. *J Am Geriatrics Soc.* 1999;47:1195.

Stevens J, et al. The effect of age on the association between body-mass index and mortality. *N Engl J Med.* 1998;338:1.

Suleiman S, et al. Effect of calcium intake and physical activity level on bone mass and turnover in healthy, white postmenopausal women. *Am J Clin Nutr.* 1997;66:937.

Sullivan DH, et al. Protein-energy under utilization among elderly hospitalized patients: a prospective study. *J Am Med Assoc.* 1999;281:2013.

Sullivan DH, Walls RC. Protein-energy undernutrition and the risk of mortality within 6 years of hospital discharge. *J Am Col Nutr.* 1998;17:571.

Sullivan D, et al. Nightly enteral nutrition support of elderly hip fracture patients: a phase 1 trial. *J Am Col Nutr.* 1998;17:136.

Sullivan D, Lipschitz D. Evaluating and treating nutritional problems in older patients. *Clin Geriatr Med.* 1997;13(4):753.

Taaffe D, et al. Accuracy of equations to predict basal metabolic rate in older women. *J Am Diet Assoc.* 1995;95:1387.

Thun M, et al. Alcohol consumption and mortality among middle-aged and elderly U.S. adults. *N Engl J Med.* 1997;337:1705.

Toth MJ, Poehlman ET. Energetic adaptation to chronic disease in the elderly. *Nutr Rev.* 2000;58:61.

Tripp F. The use of dietary supplements in the elderly: current issues and recommendations. *J Am Diet Assoc.* 1997;97:S181.

Turic A, et al. Nutrition supplementation enables elderly residents of long-term care facilities to meet or exceed RDAs without displacing energy or nutrient intakes from meals. *J Am Diet Assoc.* 1998;98:1457.

Wallace J, Schwartz R. Involuntary weight loss in elderly outpatients: recognition, etiologies, and treatment. *Clin Geriatr Med.* 1997;13 (4):717.

Wang S, et al. Longitudinal weight changes, length of survival, and energy requirements of long-term care residents with dementia. *J Am Geriatr Soc.* 1997;45:1189.

Warsama J, et al. Dietary antioxidants and cognitive function in a population-based sample of older persons: the Rotterdam Study. *Am J Epid.* 1996;144:275.

Weinberg A, et al. Dehydration: evaluation and management in older adults. *J Am Med Assoc.* 1995;274:1552.

Weir DG, Scott JM. Brain function in the elderly: role of vitamin B12 and folate. *Br Med Bull.* 1999;55:669.

Wellman N, et al. Elder insecurities: poverty, hunger, and malnutrition. *J Am Diet Assoc.* 1997;97:S120.

Wilkinson T, et al. The response to treatment of subclinical thiamine deficiency in the elderly. *Am J Clin Nutr.* 1997;66:925.

Williamson DF. Prospective study of intentional weight loss and mortality in overweight white men aged 40–64 years. *Am J Epid.* 1999;149:491.

Yeh SS, et al. Improvement in quality-of-life measures and stimulation of weight gain after treatment with megestrol acetate oral suspension in geriatric cachexia: results of a double blind, placebo controlled study. *J Am Geriatr Soc.* 2000;48:485.

SECTION 2

Dietary Practices and Miscellaneous Conditions

CHIEF ASSESSMENT FACTORS

- CULTURAL PATTERNS
- USE OF HERBAL AND BOTANICAL PRODUCTS
- RELIGIOUS PREFERENCES, KOSHER DIETS, MUSLIM PRACTICES
- VEGETARIAN DIETS
- MOUTH: DENTAL PROBLEMS, PERIODONTAL DISEASES, DENTURES (ILL-FITTING), MISSING OR LOOSE TEETH, CARIES, DENTAL CARE, INCREASED SALIVATION, DRYNESS, LESIONS
- PROBLEMS WITH SELF-FEEDING
- VISION: CATARACTS, VISUAL FIELD CHANGES, DIPLOPIA, GLAUCOMA, BLINDNESS
- SKIN: TEXTURE OR COLOR CHANGES, DRYNESS, ECCHYMOSES, LESIONS, MASSES, PETECHIAE, PRESSURE ULCERS
- SIGNS OF VITAMIN DEFICIENCIES
- FOOD ALLERGIES OR INTOLERANCES
- HEAD/FACE: MIGRAINE HEADACHES, PAIN, PAST TRAUMA, SYNCOPE, UNUSUAL OR FREQUENT HEADACHES
- EARS: PROBLEMS, VERTIGO, DISCHARGE, INFECTIONS, TINNITUS
- FOOD-BORNE ILLNESSES

For More Information

- American Dietetic Association–Nutrition Education for the Public
  http://www.dietetics.com/nepdpg/
- Center for Disease Control–Index for consumer questions
  http://www.cdc.gov/health/diseases.htm
- Federal Consumer Information Center
  http://www.pueblo.gsa.gov/food.htm
- Federal Trade Commission
  http://www.ftc.gov/
- Health Finder
  http://www.healthfinder.gov/
- Health Fraud and Quackery
  http://www.quackwatch.com/
- Health Statistics
  http://www.cdc.gov/nchswww/
- Healthy People 2010
  http://web.health.gov/healthypeople/
- Physicians' Desk Reference for Consumers
  http://consumer.pdr.net/consumer/index.htm
- Public Med-line
  http://www.ncbi.nlm.nih.gov/PubMed/
- Tufts University Nutrition Navigator
  http://search.tufts.edu/custom/navigator/
- USDA
  Food Composition tables–http://www.nal.usda.gov/fnic/pubs/bibs/gen/2001fdcomp.html
  Nutrient Data Tables–http://www.nal.usda.gov/fnic/foodcomp/
  Herb and Supplement Resource List–http://www.nal.usda.gov/fnic/pubs/bibs/gen/dietsupp.html

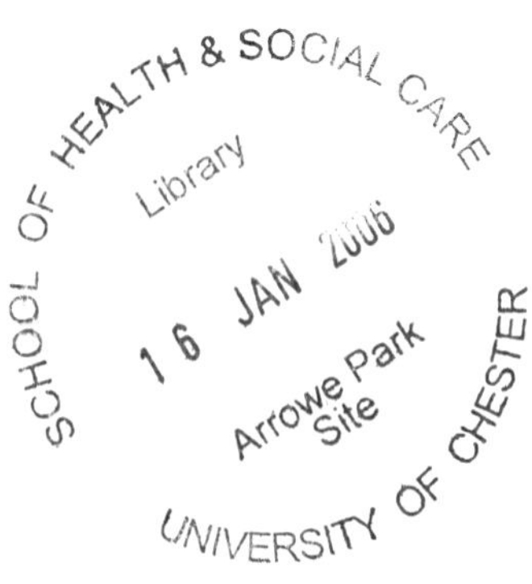

CULTURAL FOOD PATTERNS AND INTEGRATIVE MEDICINE

NUTRITIONAL ACUITY RANKING: LEVEL 2 (ADAPTATIONS, ADVISEMENT)

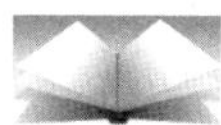

DEFINITIONS AND BACKGROUND

Varied dietary intakes by age, culture, gender, and years in the United States are known and accepted (Kim et al., 2000.) Assessment of a patient's cultural food preferences is essential to determine adequacy of nutritional intake. Nutrition planning for immigrant and minority patients will be more effective if tailored to the level of dietary acculturation; the ability to accurately assess dietary acculturation is an important component of nutrition education, interventions, and counseling in these populations (Satia et al., 2001).

In addition to planning for individual patients, effective prevention initiatives require use of available findings about individual cultures. Reinforcement of positive traditional dietary habits, adaptation of healthy Western food items, and development of strategies that will effectively correct likely deficiencies in diet are important intervention goals (Kim et al., 2000). Dietetics practitioners can use the information presented here to study nutrition-related chronic diseases in public health planning and in nutrition education efforts directed toward ethnic-specific groups (Bermudez et al., 2000).

Integrative medicine incorporates herbal and botanical products that are used for preventive or medicinal purposes. Different cultures apply different herbs and practices, some of which are traditionally known as folk medicine. There is currently much research in this area.

OBJECTIVES

- Become aware of one's own cultural values; avoid imposing them on others. For example, the desire to be thin is more common among Caucasians than other races.
- Assess values, attitudes, beliefs, practices, and rituals of the patient/client before attempting to discuss any lifestyle changes. Observe and interact appropriately.
- Provide individualization for cultural patterns that differ from the standard in the region. Do not assume that each person fits a typical pattern but be prepared to understand the differences from the "typical American" diet.
- Determine which habits, if any, are detrimental for healthy lifestyles. In addition, review any patterns or food intakes that aggravate existing or predisposing chronic or acute conditions for each person. Build on healthy practices.
- Correct the diet for deficits, such as calcium and riboflavin, in dietary patterns in which dairy products or milk are excluded or not tolerated.
- Offer suggestions for changes in food preparation (e.g., reducing fat or salt use) rather than changing foods themselves.
- Understand and interpret customs, festive occasions, fasting, ceremonial activities, and offer reasonable suggestions.
- Functional foods, including whole foods and fortified, enriched, or enhanced foods have a potentially beneficial effect on health when consumed as part of a varied diet on a regular basis at effective levels (American Dietetic Association, Functional foods, 1999). Each culture may have foods that have special attributes.

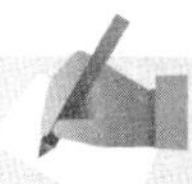

DIETARY PATTERNS

- Chinese and Traditional Asian patterns. Diet may be low in calcium and riboflavin because milk often is not tolerated or consumed. Encourage use of tofu, green vegetables, and fish containing small bones. Diet may be high in sodium if monosodium glutamate (MSG) and soy sauces are used. The traditional Chinese diet is 80% grains, legumes, and vegetables (Earl and Borra, 2000). Stir-frying, deep fat frying, and steaming are common cookery methods. Pork is the preferred meat. "Hot" and "cold" foods may be used during pregnancy or illness; these terms do not refer to food temperatures. Korean Americans tend to have a greater intake of carbohydrates and vitamins A and C and a lower intake of total fat, cholesterol, and saturated fat (Kim et al. 2000). See Figure 2–1.
- Hmong (Southeast Asian) patterns. Milk is seldom used, often related to lactose intolerance, and calcium may be a problem. Fish, chicken, and pork are common entrees. Rice may be eaten at nearly every meal. A highly salted fish sauce is used. Snacking is rare in the family diet. Anemia may result from parasite infestation because many individuals have been refugees (Earl and Borra, 2000). Like Chinese patterns, hot–cold patterns are sometimes observed (American Dietetic Association, Hmong, 1999). A website is available for Vietnamese foods at http://monarch.gsu.edu/nutrition/Vietnamese1.htm. Figure 2–1 is also useful for a pattern.
- Hispanic (Mexican and Latin American) patterns. Whole milk may be used rarely, but cheese is a common additive to meals. Fruits and vegetables may be viewed as luxuries, but chili peppers, mangos, and avocados are common. The main starch is corn or flour tortilla. The diet may be high in sugar and saturated fat (lard). A common main dish is beans with rice. Hot and cold foods are concepts commonly found. Salsa or sofrito seasonings are used frequently. Rice is the major contributor of energy among the elderly; more acculturated Hispanic elders consume fewer ethnic foods and more foods related to the non-Hispanic-white eating patterns than those less acculturated (Bermudez et al., 2000). Obesity and type 2 diabetes may be problems in this population; snacking is more common with higher levels of acculturation. See Figure 2–2.

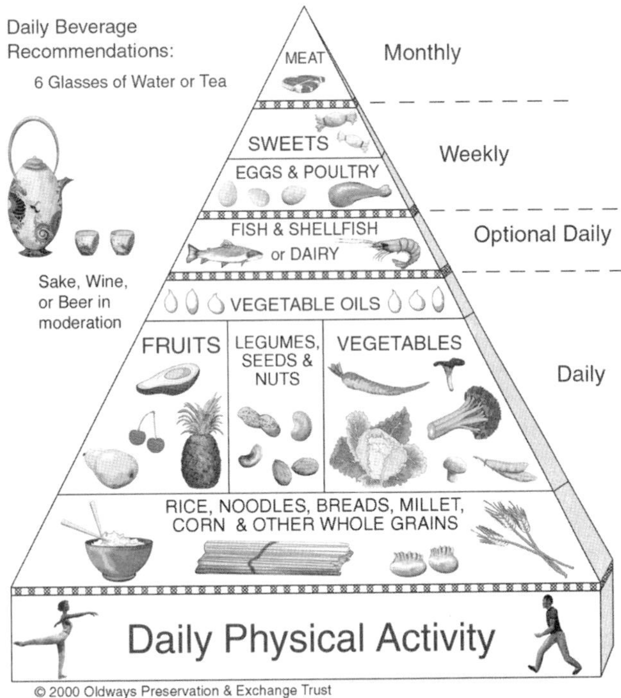

Figure 2–1 Traditional Asian Diet Pyramid. (Reprinted with permission of Oldways Preservation and Exchange Trust.)

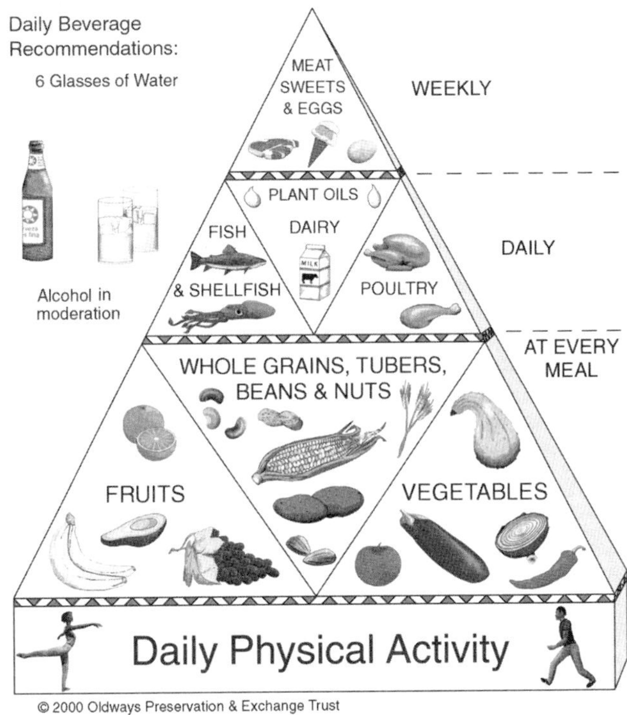

Figure 2–2 Traditional Latin Diet Pyramid. (Reprinted with permission of Oldways Preservation and Exchange Trust.)

- Southern/Soul/Cajun patterns. Milk often is not tolerated or consumed. Broccoli, greens, and evaporated milk often constitute the calcium source. Pork, ham, black-eyed peas, beans, and nuts are typical protein sources. Rice, cornbread, and hominy grits make up the starches, in addition to bread. High-sodium salt pork and bacon are used as seasonings. Low-potassium intakes are common. Problems may include obesity, hypertension, diabetes, heart disease, and end-stage renal disease. Insufficient exercise may relate to obesity.
- Mediterranean patterns. Some research suggests that this dietary pattern has advantages for reducing cardiac disease and cancers. Vegetable fat such as olive oil; fish, poultry, and eggs rather than beef; breads, fruits, and vegetables in abundance, and lots of beans/legumes, yogurt, and cheeses make up this pattern. Exercise and wine are also mainstays. The patterns reflect the habits of populations of Italy, Crete, and Greece. A recent study showed that the Mediterranean model is restricted to older people and to rural areas, whereas urbanized young people depart from it (Scali et al., 2001). See Figure 2–3.
- Indian/Pakistani patterns. (American Dietetic Association, Ethnic and . . ., 1996). Indian immigrants are about 83% Hindu, whereas Pakistani immigrants are mostly Muslims. Vegetarianism is the primary practice among Indians, deriving from religious beliefs in which the cow is sacred. Lentils and legumes are a primary source of protein; in some families, eggs, fish, shrimp, and milk are consumed. Sattvic foods are believed to create a healthy life; these include milk products (except cheese made from rennet), rice, wheat, and legumes. Rajasic foods are believed to contribute to aggression; these include meats, eggs, and rich or very salty foods. Tamasic foods are believed to contribute to slothfulness or dullness; these include garlic, pickled foods, stale or rotten foods, and alcohol used for pleasure or to excess. Lack of portion control may be a factor in diabetes, which is common in this population. Combination foods include Biryani (grain, meat), Samosas (grain, vegetable, meat, fat), Kheer "rice pudding" (grain, milk), and Curry (meat, vegetable). Not all Muslims are vegetarian. A Hindi food pyramid is available at http://monarch.gsu.edu/nutrition/hindi1.htm. An Arabic food pyramid (primarily Muslim) is available at http://monarch.gsu.edu/nutrition/arabic1.htm.
- Native American patterns (American Indian and Alaskan Native). Food has great religious and social significance and is commonly part of many celebrations (Earl and Borra, 2000). Fried foods, fried bread, corn, mutton, and goat are foods frequently used by American Indians, whereas seafood and game are more common among Alaskan natives. Obesity and type 2 diabetes are very common in these populations. See the following website

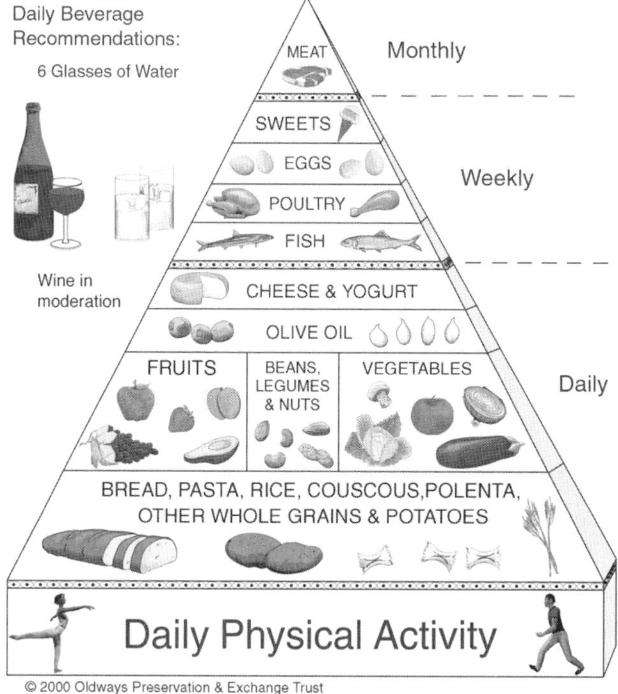

Figure 2–3 Mediterranean Diet Pyramid. (Reprinted with permission of Oldways Preservation and Exchange Trust.)

for more information about Native American foods: http://www.aaip.com/tradmed/tradmedfoodguide.html.

Herbs, Botanicals and Supplements

- Many cultures use herbs and botanicals as part of their meal patterns, rituals, and celebrations. Identify those that are used and monitor for potential side effects. HerbMedR, an interactive, electronic herbal database, provides hyperlinked access to the scientific data including clinical trials and efficacy. The National Center for Complementary and Alternative Medicine is also one of many reliable resources.
- Green tea has thermogenic properties and promotes fat oxidation; these properties are not explained by caffeine alone. It may be related to the sympathetic nervous system's activation of thermogenesis, fat oxidation, or both (Dulloo et al., 1999). Green tea is popular in several cultures.

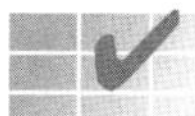

PATIENT EDUCATION

- ✓ Demonstrate respect for the beliefs, values, and practices of the patient and family members.
- ✓ Alternative solutions to dietary patterns must be gently offered. There is no "one right way" for dietary patterns.
- ✓ Understanding background, health problems, statistics, social issues, and disease patterns is useful when providing multicultural education.
- ✓ Build relationships through sensitivity and communication.
- ✓ Remove assumptions and stereotypes. Cultures are ever changing, growing, and dynamic.
- ✓ Family beliefs and behaviors may sabotage a client's efforts; be aware and be helpful.
- ✓ Development of an intuitive counseling style may be beneficial (Curry, 2000).
- ✓ Offer tips on food selection, preparation, and storage within a cultural context. Identify resources, ethnic stores, and agencies that may be useful (Harris-David and Haughton, 2000).

For More Information

- American Botanical Council
  http://www.herbalgram.org/
- Alternative Medicine Foundation
  HerbMed®–interactive, electronic herbal database
  http://www.herbmed.org/
- CAM on PubMed—searchable database
  http://www.nlm.nih.gov/nccam/camonpubmed.html
- Cultural Food Pyramids
  http://www.semda.org/info/
- Ethnic Foods
  http://www.eatethnic.com/
- Food and Nutrition Information Center
  Agricultural Research Service, USDA
  National Agricultural Library
  10301 Baltimore Avenue, Room 304
  Beltsville, MD 20705-2351
  301-504-5719
  Fax: 301-504-6409
  http://www.nal.usda.gov/fnic/
- Nutrition Education/Food Pyramids for various cultures
  http://monarch.gsu.edu/nutrition/download.htm
- National Center for Alternative and Complementary Medicine
  http://nccam.nih.gov/
- Oldways Cultural Food Pyramids
  http://www.oldwayspt.org/index.htm
- USDA Food Pyramid–Ethnic and Cultural versions
  http://www.nal.usda.gov/fnic/Fpyr/pyramid.html

VEGETARIANISM

NUTRITIONAL ACUITY RANKING: LEVEL 2 (ADVISEMENT ON PLANNING)

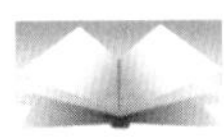

DEFINITIONS AND BACKGROUND

Vegetarian diets are basically plant based, with fruits, vegetables, legumes, seeds, and nuts (American Dietetic Association, Vegetarian, 1997). There are three major categories of vegetarianism: vegan, a very strict vegetarian food pattern ("pure" vegetarianism); lacto, a vegetarian food pattern using milk; and lacto-ovo, a vegetarian food pattern using milk and eggs. Conscious combining of complementary protein sources does not appear to be necessary (American Dietetic Association, Vegetarian, 1997).

In review of dietary intakes from the Continuing Survey of Food Intake by Individuals (CSFII) 1994–1996, diet quality was evaluated (Kennedy et al., 2001). Diets that were high in carbohydrates and low to moderate in fat tended to be lower in energy; lowest energy intakes and BMIs were found among those on a vegetarian diet.

Vegetarian diets can be healthful when carefully planned and monitored; they can improve obesity, constipation, coronary heart disease, diabetes, hypertension, and diverticular disease. They also may reduce the incidence of breast cancer, colon cancer, and gallstones. Vegetarians tend to have less appendicitis, hiatal hernia, irritable bowel syndrome, hemorrhoids, and varicose veins. The National Cancer Institute recommends intake of 25–35 g of fiber per day; vegetarian diets can easily provide this level.

Vegetarians usually consume less fat and generally have more favorable lipid levels (Bederova et al., 2000) and lower intakes of cholesterol, LDL-cholesterol, atherogenic index, and saturated fatty acids. Vegetarian diets usually provide higher levels of HDL-cholesterol, polyunsaturated fatty acids, and vitamins E and C. Vegetarians tend to have significantly higher levels of all antioxidant vitamins as a result of a higher consumption of vegetables, fruits, plants, fat, and sprouts (Bederova et al., 2000).

Potential Complications of a Vegetarian Diet (http://www.oldwayspt.org/html/p_veg7.htm): **Iron-deficient Anemia.** Females should be sure to obtain an adequate amount of absorbable iron. The iron in dairy, eggs, and plant foods is largely nonheme, of which only about 2–20% is absorbed. **Vitamin B12 deficiency.** An individual following a vegan diet should use supplements to obtain this vitamin. **Vitamin D deficiency or Rickets.** The human body can synthesize Vitamin D from sunlight, but this is only possible when the sun reaches a certain intensity level. For many people who live in North America, this means that for a few months of the year they will have to seek other sources of Vitamin D because the sun is not intense enough. Milk is generally fortified with Vitamin D, but for vegans who do not consume dairy products, supplements are necessary. **Bulky diets.** In some circumstances, this regimen can restrict energy intake in the first few years of life. This is also true for adults who consume large amounts of fiber to the extent that many other nutrients are not able to be absorbed in the small intestine. **Omega-3** polyunsaturated fatty acids and essential amino acids **methionine** and **lysine** are found in significantly lower amounts in vegetarian diets. **Calcium** absorption may be inhibited in vegetarians as a consequence of the presence of phytates in plant foods; vegetarian nutrition represents a risk for pregnant women, children, and adolescents if the values of iron and calcium are not carefully planned.

OBJECTIVES

- Encourage use of a wide variety of foods in adequate quantity and balance of amino acids to achieve a balance of amino acids during the day (see Table 2–1).
- Provide nutritionally adequate menus with sufficient calories for weight maintenance/idealization. Discourage excessive use of sweets.
- Monitor fiber intake, because excesses interfere with absorption of calcium, zinc, and iron.
- Monitor the diet carefully if the patient is a pregnant woman or lactating mother. In addition, monitor elderly persons following a vegetarian diet.
- Infants and children on vegan diets should be monitored closely to ensure adequate energy intake and mineral and vitamin intakes. High-fiber diets may replace calories and cause some stunting or other growth deficits.
- Prevent or correct anemia.

TABLE 2–1 Complementary Protein Relationships (American Dietetic Association, 1997.)

Different food combinations provide essential amino acids that produce higher quality proteins. Plant sources of protein can provide adequate amounts of essential amino acids; using a variety of plant foods is key, and energy needs should be met. Research suggests that complementary proteins do not need to be consumed at the same time and that consumption of various sources of amino acids over the course of the day should ensure adequate nitrogen retention and use in healthy persons (Young and Pellett, 1994). Although vegetarian diets are lower in total protein and a vegetarian's protein needs may be somewhat elevated because of the lower quality of some plant proteins, protein intake in both lacto-ovo-vegetarians and vegans appears to be adequate (Messina and Messina, 1996).

Be aware of the limiting amino acids in typical protein foods: wheat (lysine), rice (lysine and threonine); corn (lysine and tryptophan); beans (methionine); and chick-peas (methionine). Varying choices will be useful, e.g., serving grains and milk: bread and milk, rice and cheese, or pasta and cheese; serving grains and legumes: rice and beans, bread and beans, or corn and beans; serving seeds and legumes: garbanzos and sesame seeds (as in dips) and beans (as in roasted snacks); serve vegetables with nuts, dairy products, rice, sunflower seeds, or wheat germ.

The Traditional Healthy
Vegetarian Diet Pyramid

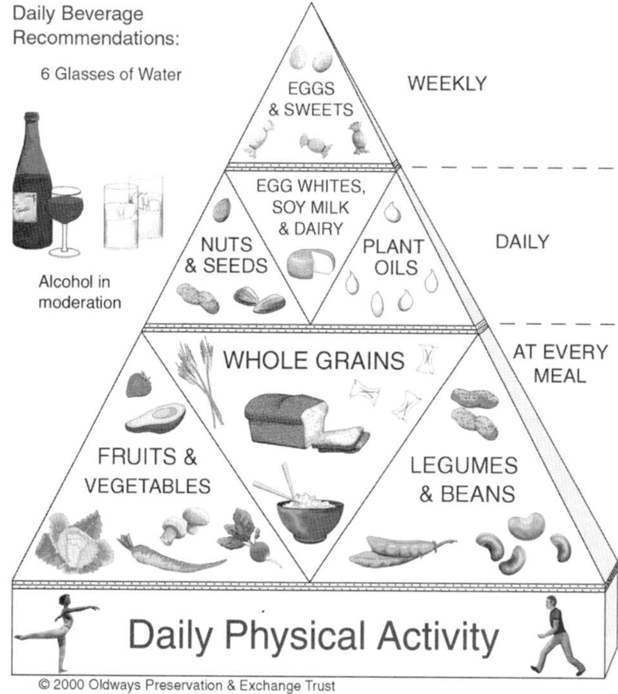

Figure 2–4 Vegetarian Pyramid. (Reprinted with permission of Oldways Preservation and Exchange Trust.)

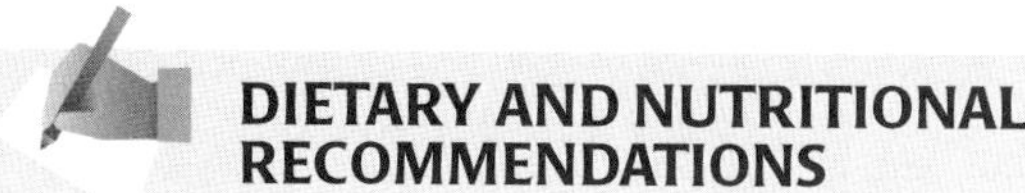

DIETARY AND NUTRITIONAL RECOMMENDATIONS

American Dietetic Association recommends consultation with a registered dietitian or other qualified nutrition professional, especially during periods of growth, breastfeeding, pregnancy, or recovery from illness.

- For a balanced diet, minimize intake of less nutritious foods such as sweets and fatty foods. Choose whole or unrefined grain products instead of refined products. Choose a variety of nuts, seeds, legumes, fruits, and vegetables, including good sources of vitamin C to improve iron absorption. Choose low-fat or nonfat varieties of dairy products, if they are included in the diet. Follow the vegetarian pyramid. See Figure 2–4.
  6–12 servings from the bread group
  2–3 servings of legumes, nuts or seeds, or eggs (if used)
  2–3 servings from the dairy group (if used); tofu, yogurt, or fortified soy milk may be substituted
  4^{+} servings of vegetables
  3^{+} servings of fruits
  2–3 servings of fats and oils, including olives and avocado
- Followers of a lacto-vegetarian diet should be monitored for deficiencies in iron, phosphorus, potassium, B complex, and protein. **Iron** is in legumes, tofu, green leafy vegetables, dried fruit, whole grains, and iron-fortified cereals and breads, especially whole-wheat. (Absorption is improved by vitamin C found in citrus fruits and juices, tomatoes, strawberries, broccoli, peppers, dark green leafy vegetables, and potatoes with skins). **Protein** is in tofu and other soy-based products, legumes, seeds, nuts, grains, and vegetables
- Followers of a vegan diet should be monitored for deficiencies in calcium, iron, iodine, vitamin B12, vitamin D, protein, riboflavin, and zinc. For **calcium,** calcium-processed tofu and calcium-fortified soy milk provide sources for vegans. **Zinc** is in whole grains (especially the germ and bran), whole-wheat bread, legumes, nuts, and tofu. **Vitamin B12** can be found in fortified soy beverages and cereals. **Vitamin D** can be found in sunshine or in fortified soy beverages.
- Use iodized salt, if seafood and other sources are not consumed, to prevent **iodine** deficiency.
- Suggest dark leafy greens for calcium, riboflavin, and iron. Avoid excessive intake of oxalates from spinach, rhubarb, kale, and chard.
- Ensure adequate calorie intake since vegetarian diets tend to be lower in calories than typical American patterns.
- Vegan diets for infants can be nutritious and support adequate growth if planned carefully, according to the following guidelines by Mangels and Messina (2001): Use breast milk for the first 4–6 months, with soy-based infant formula as an alternative. Breastfed vegan infants may need vitamin B12 supplements if maternal diet is inadequate; older infants may need zinc supplements and good sources of iron, vitamins D, and B12. Commercial soy milk should not be the major beverage until after age 1. Timing of solid food introduction is similar to that recommended for nonvegetarians. Tofu, dried beans, and meat analogs are introduced as protein sources around 7–8 months.
- For children and teenagers, ensure adequate intakes of calories, vitamin D, calcium, iron, and zinc; sufficient calories are important.
- Take iron and folate (folic acid) supplements during pregnancy. In addition, for vegans: Use properly fortified food sources of vitamin B12, such as fortified soy beverages or cereals, or take a supplement.
- If sunlight exposure is inadequate, take a vitamin D supplement during pregnancy or while breastfeeding.

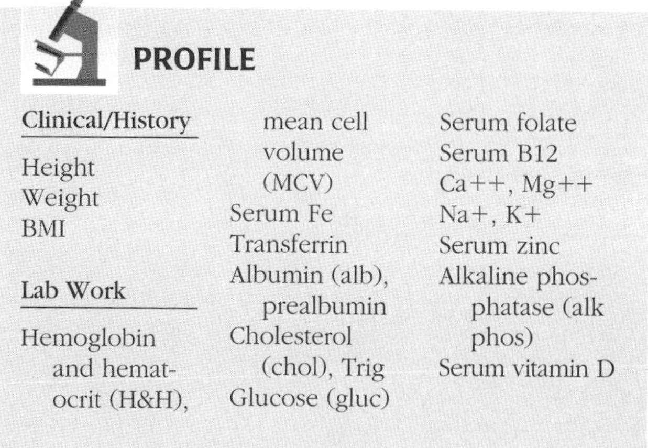

PROFILE

Clinical/History		
Height	mean cell volume (MCV)	Serum folate
Weight	Serum Fe	Serum B12
BMI	Transferrin	Ca++, Mg++
Lab Work	Albumin (alb), prealbumin	Na+, K+
Hemoglobin and hematocrit (H&H),	Cholesterol (chol), Trig	Serum zinc
	Glucose (gluc)	Alkaline phosphatase (alk phos)
		Serum vitamin D

Herbs, Botanicals and Supplements

- Many cultures use herbs and botanicals as part of their meal patterns, rituals, and celebrations. Identify those that are used and monitor side effects.
- Counsel about use of herbal teas, especially regarding toxic substances.

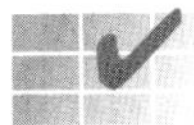

PATIENT EDUCATION

- ✔ Explain patterns of food intake that provide complementary amino acids. Whole grains, legumes, seeds, nuts, and vegetables contain sufficient essential and nonessential amino acids if taken in the right combinations.
- ✔ Emphasize the importance of a balanced diet.
- ✔ Describe the role vegetarian diets play in lowering serum cholesterol, triglycerides, and glucose.
- ✔ Counsel about appropriate products for infants and children (e.g., fortified soy formula). Protein may be the biggest problem. Soy milk also should be fortified with calcium and vitamin B12.
- ✔ Unless otherwise advised by a doctor, those taking dietary supplements should limit the dose to 100% of the Daily Reference Intakes (Recommended Daily Allowances.)

For More Information

- North American Vegetarian Society
  http://www.navs-online.org/
- Seventh-Day Adventist Dietetic Association
  PO Box 75
  Loma Linda, CA 92354
  (909) 793-8918
  http://www.adventist.org/
- World Guide to Vegetarianism
  http://www.veg.org/veg/
- Vegetarian Cuisine
  http://vegweb.com/
- Vegetarian Network Victoria
  http://www.vnv.org.au/
- Vegetarian Resource Group
  PO Box 1463
  Baltimore, MD 21203
  (410) 366-8343
  http://www.vrg.org/
- Vegetarian Society of the United Kingdom
  http://www.vegsoc.org/

JEWISH OR KOSHER DIETARY PRACTICES

NUTRITIONAL ACUITY RANKING: LEVEL 2 (ADVISEMENT/PLANNING)

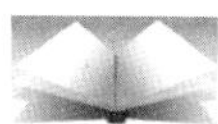

DEFINITIONS AND BACKGROUND

The term "kosher" applies to foods "fit, proper, and in accordance with the Kashruth" (Jewish dietary laws). Products labeled with "K," "U," or "pareve" are foods made without milk or meat or their derivatives. A kosher diet forbids all foods that are not in accordance with Mosaic law.

When a pregnant woman wishes to honor her religious beliefs by keeping kosher, attention to separating milk and meat and serving only kosher foods must be part of the planning process. The same is true for other individuals with medical conditions.

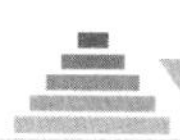

OBJECTIVES

- Observe dietary practices as followed by the kosher laws of Judaism: meats are limited to cud-chewing animals with cloven hooves (cows, sheep). Pork (including ham and all pork products), shellfish, and scavenger fish are forbidden.
- Separate utensils are to be used for preparation and eating and especially for separating meat and milk foods.
- Remember that the kosher diet tends to be high in cholesterol, saturated fats, and sodium.
- Reduce lactose and sodium in sensitive individuals.

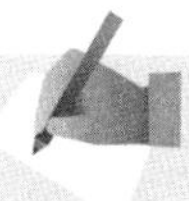

DIETARY AND NUTRITIONAL RECOMMENDATIONS

Meat and dairy dishes are eaten separately. Separate dishes and cooking utensils are used in a strict kosher kitchen.

- Meat. No pork, ham, bacon, pork products, rabbit, shellfish, or eel may be eaten. Eggs are pareve (neutral) foods.
- Dairy. Milk may be consumed before a meal, but once meat is eaten, 3–6 hours must pass before dairy products can be consumed.
- Kosher products must be used. On food labels, "U" or "K" denotes a kosher food. "Pareve" indicates that the food is neutral.
- Fruits, vegetables, and grains can be used, except that breads made with milk products are forbidden with meat meals.
- Leavened (raised) bread is forbidden during Passover. Matzoh bread or crackers may be used. Haroset and fried matzoh are traditional Passover foods. Seder plates and other items appropriate for the Seder dinner are important additions to the menu at this time.
- Omit lactose if necessary; provide other sources of calcium and riboflavin.
- Frozen kosher meals may be available in some areas.
- Common food choices include matzoh ball soup, chicken soup with kreplach, gefilte fish with beet horseradish, cheese blintz with sour cream, flanken tzimmes, chopped liver, noodle Kugel, and kishka.
- Fasting is common during Rosh Hashanah and Yom Kippur.
- Hanukkah may require use of special breads such as challah bread, latkes, and sour cream.

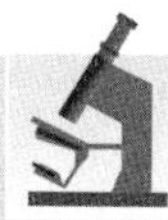

PROFILE

Clinical/History	Blood pressure (BP)	Serum Na+
Height		K+
Weight	**Lab Work**	Ca++
BMI		Mg++
Recent weight changes	Gluc	Alk phos
	Chol, Trig	H&H
		Serum Fe

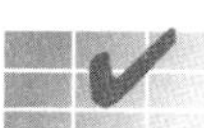

PATIENT EDUCATION

- Show the patient how to limit foods high in cholesterol/fat, if weight and elevated lipid levels are a problem.
- Discuss sodium and obesity in relationship to hypertension, as appropriate. Recommend other herbs, spices, and cooking methods.
- Low-fat cheeses should be substituted for high-fat cheeses such as cream cheese.
- Note that food labels with "U" are kosher.
- Discuss holiday preferences and alternatives where needed.
- Foods labeled "pareve" could present a problem for individuals with milk allergy because of trace contamination from airborne dust in a food processing plant (Hubbard-Wilson, 2000).

For More Information

- Hebrew Food Pyramid
  http://monarch.gsu.edu/nutrition/hebrew1.htm
- Union for Traditional Judaism
  http://www.utj.org/
  (800) 843-8825

MUSLIM DIETARY PRACTICES

NUTRITIONAL ACUITY RANKING: LEVEL 2 (ADVISEMENT/PLANNING)

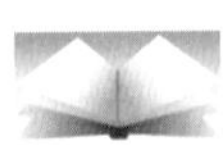

DEFINITIONS AND BACKGROUND

Islam is an Arabic word that means submission, surrender, and obedience; it also means peace, as it is derived from the word "SALAM," peace. As a religion, Islam stands for complete submission and obedience to God. Followers of the Islamic faith are known as Muslims. Muslims promote the concept of eating to live, not living to eat; they advise not eating to capacity and always sharing food (Earl and Borra, 2000). The flesh of animals must be slaughtered according to Islamic law or *halal*. Muslims may use kosher meats for this reason. Improper slaughtering is identified as *haram*.

OBJECTIVES

- Monitor dietary patterns, which include fasting 3 days a month. Pregnant and breastfeeding mothers need not fast but must make up fasting days later (Earl and Borra, 2000).
- During Ramadan, fasting occurs from dawn to sundown and eating occurs only before dawn and after sunset.

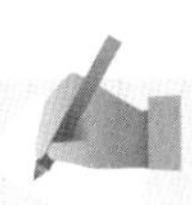

DIETARY AND NUTRITIONAL RECOMMENDATIONS

- Pork and pork products are forbidden, including gelatin.
- Alcohol is not used, even in vanilla extract and other preparations.
- Foods such as dates, seafood, honey, sweets, yogurt, milk (goat's milk also), meat, and olive or vegetable oils are encouraged. Beef, chicken, and lamb are commonly used. Couscous, pita bread, rice, millet, and bulgur are used.
- Typical combination foods include: falafel (meat, fat), hummus (meat, fat), kibbeh (meat, grain, fat), tabouli (vegetable, grain, fat), baba ghannouj (vegetable, fat), pilaf (grain, fat), stuffed grape leaves (meat, grain, fat), and shawarma (meat, grain, fat).

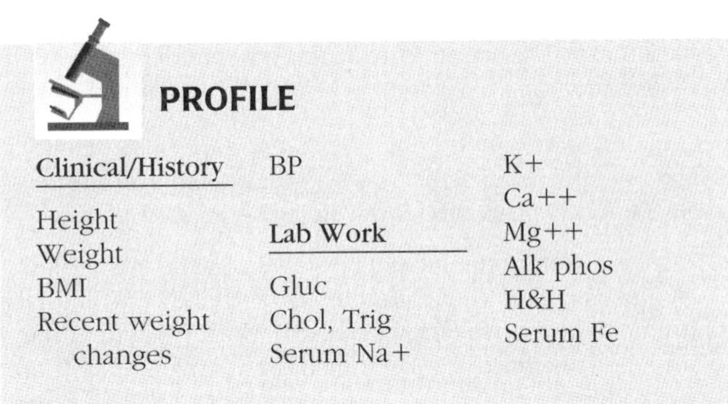

PROFILE

Clinical/History		
Height	BP	K+
Weight	**Lab Work**	Ca++
BMI	Gluc	Mg++
Recent weight changes	Chol, Trig	Alk phos
	Serum Na+	H&H
		Serum Fe

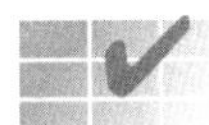

PATIENT EDUCATION

- ✔ No specific medical conditions have been identified in the Muslim population.
- ✔ Fasting is not recommended for persons who have diabetes, cancer, or HIV-AIDS. Discuss menu planning for religious occasions.

DENTAL DIFFICULTIES AND ORAL DISORDERS

NUTRITIONAL ACUITY RANKING: LEVEL 2

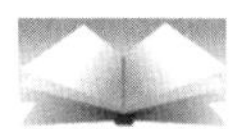

DEFINITIONS AND BACKGROUND

Cell turnover is rapid in the tongue and oral mucosa; therefore, the oral cavity is one of the first areas that signs of systemic disease appears. Health professionals should monitor changes in the oral/dental health of a patient. Assessment of the teeth should include missing, loose teeth; presence of dentures and whether they fit well; and presence of rampant tooth decay. Tooth loss can prevent proper bite and may lessen the ability to chew foods properly. About 40% of Americans lack fluoridated water, an effective safeguard against dental cavities. Those who are poor or have no dental insurance are also at risk for cavities.

In dental caries, a chronic infectious disease leads to progressive destruction of tooth substances from interactions between bacteria and organic tooth compounds. *Streptococcus mutans* and *Lactobacillus* are common culprits; acid forms 20 seconds–30 minutes after contact. Erosion of tooth enamel may occur in patients who chronically consume acidic beverages and/or keep such beverages or foods in the mouth for a period of time (e.g., sucking lemons, chewing vitamin C tablets, chewing lemon hard candies).

Some dental problems are age-specific. Infants should be monitored for the nursing-bottle caries syndrome; dental decay often occurs during the growth spurts of adolescents; and elderly patients should be monitored for changes in eating habits and use of an inadequate diet, as well as caries. Keep in mind also that poor oral hygiene can increase the likelihood of gingival abnormalities in scorbutic conditions.

Fracture of the lower jaw (mandible) is a common injury. Treatment involves intermaxillary fixation (wiring). Patients with wired jaws face a whole new lifestyle for up to 6 weeks following maxillofacial surgery. Patients will learn ways to care for their bodies, to eat their meals, and to communicate at this time. Proper presurgical patient education is essential

With tongue disorders, mastication of food may be affected. The ability to push mashed food with the tongue and anterior hard palate will be affected.

Other oral problems may cause pain, problems with chewing, dysphagia, mouth dryness, or infection including aphthous stomatitis, cheilosis, oral cancer, lichen planus, herpes simplex I, candidiasis, thrush, or xerostomia. Today, treatment and prevention of leukoplakias are improving; the importance of candidosis has become evident (Scully, 2000). Many of these conditions occur because of altered immunity and debility, as in cancer or HIV/AIDS. Proper nutrition is essential.

Table 2–2 provides a list of the key nutrients needed for healthy oral mucosa and teeth. Plasma ascorbate and plasma retinol are significantly associated with dental status (Sheiham et al., 2001).

TABLE 2–2 Nutrients Needed for Proper Oral Tissue Synthesis and Dental Care

- Vitamin A: Necessary for epithelial tissue and enamel. Beta-carotene may play a role in oral cancer prevention.
- Vitamin C: Enables connective tissue cells to elaborate intercellular substances. Deficiency can lead to easy bleeding or swelling of gums and gingivitis. Forms collagen. Helps to heal wounds and bleeding gums.
- Vitamin K: Aids with calcium absorption in bone; adequate blood clotting; helps healing.
- Calcium, phosphorus, vitamin D: Necessary for dentin and bony tissue synthesis. Poor mineralization occurs with deficiency. Maintains jawbone sufficiency.
- Magnesium: Helps in bone development. Enhances use of vitamin C. Deficiency may lead to calcium resorption.
- Fluoride: Reduces susceptibility of teeth to caries formation (American Dietetic Association, 2000). Drinking water should contain 1 ppm. Toothpaste, mouth rinses, and topical treatments also help.
- B-complex vitamins: Deficiencies show a bright scarlet tongue and stomatitis in niacin deficiency; magenta tongue, cheilosis, and angular stomatitis in ariboflavinosis; smooth tongue in vitamin B12 deficiency.
- Protein: Needed for healthy tissue growth and maintenance.
- Folacin: Needed for a healthy blood supply.
- Iron: Helps produce red blood cells; promotes resistance to disease; improves health of the teeth, skin, and bones
- Copper: Aids in bone formation and healing.
- Zinc: Regulates the inflammatory process; aids in wound healing. Deficiencies can lead to poor healing, susceptibility to infection, and loss of taste.

OBJECTIVES

Edentulism

- Provide proper consistency to allow the patient to eat.
- Monitor for deficiencies in fiber and vitamins A and C if whole grains; fruits and vegetables are not consumed (Touger-Decker, 2000).

Broken or Wired Jaw

- Provide adequate nourishment to allow healing while reducing jaw movement.
- Decrease fever, nausea, and vomiting.
- Prevent excess weight loss (usually 10%).
- Maintain a patent airway.

Mouth Ulcers or Pain

- Lessen mouth soreness to increase dietary intake; some mouth sprays may be available to lessen pain while eating.

- Promote healing for a return to normal eating patterns.
- Prevent weight loss or other consequences.

Tongue Disorders
- Provide adequate nourishment despite acute or chronic disability.

Dental Caries
- Alter dietary habits; deprive bacteria of substrate; reduce acid; keep pH at 7.0.
- Maintain frequent fluoride contact with tooth surfaces as directed by a dental professional.

Baby Bottle Tooth Decay (BBTD)
- BBTD is a preventable dental disease. It affects over 50% of Native Indian/Alaska Native (NI/NA) children (Bruerd and Jones, 1996).
- Enamel erodes and tooth surface is permanently damaged.
- Education is the biggest factor.

Tube Feeding
- Children on tube feedings often have dental problems; therefore, these children should receive more dental care than those fed orally (Dyment and Casas, 1999).
- Adults will require special attention to oral hygiene and mouth care while on tube feedings.

Xerostomia
- Dry mouth is more permanent with radiation therapy than with other causes such as diabetes or autoimmune disorders (Garg and Malo, 1997).
- Artificial saliva agents may be useful for some, but not all patients find relief.
- Good oral hygiene may prevent dental decay.

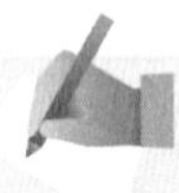

DIETARY AND NUTRITIONAL RECOMMENDATIONS

Edentulism
- A chopped, ground, strained, or pureed diet should be followed as required. Use the least restricted diet and progress as tolerated.
- Identify potential solutions such as obtaining new dentures, repairing current dentures, etc.

Broken or Wired Jaw
- A diet of pureed and strained foods, as well as liquids of high protein/calorie content is necessary.
- Adequate amounts of vitamin C should be taken to aid healing.
- Monitor food temperatures carefully.
- Six to eight meals are needed.
- Follow meals with salt-water rinse.
- Products such as TwoCal HN, Ensure Plus, and Sustacal HC may be useful.
- Double-strength milk may also be used to keep protein intake high.

Mouth Ulcers or Pain
- Foods low in acid and spices should be taken (e.g., citrus juices are not allowed).
- Supplement the diet with vitamin C, protein, and calories to speed the rate of healing.
- Small, frequent meals and oral supplements may be beneficial to prevent weight loss.
- Moist foods and blenderized foods with additional liquid are helpful.
- Soft, cold foods such as canned fruits, ice cream, popsicles, yogurt, cottage cheese, or cold pasta dishes may be used.
- Use of a straw may be helpful.
- Cut or grind meats or vegetables.
- Extra butter, mild sauces, and gravies may be needed.
- Follow meals by brushing teeth to reduce caries.

Tongue Disorders
- If the patient is unable to chew, tube feeding is necessary.
- Liquids may be added to the diet as tolerated. Some foods are tolerated if liquefied and blenderized.

Dental Caries
- Decrease sucrose and cooked or sticky starches, as well as the frequency of snacking and duration of exposure time. *Streptococcus mutans* is a common bacterial culprit; others include *Lactobacillus casein* or *Streptococcus sanguis* (Touger-Decker, 2000).
- Use a balanced diet, eating sweets or starches with meals.
- Fluoride exposure should be adequate, including from water supplies.
- The sequence of eating foods, the combination of foods, the form of foods and beverages consumed, and nutrient composition of foods/beverages must be evaluated and altered accordingly (Touger-Decker, 2000).

Baby Bottle Tooth Decay

The American Academy of Pediatric Dentistry has developed the following guidelines for preventing baby bottle tooth decay (http://www.cdc.gov/ncidod/hip/abc/facts02.htm)
- Don't allow a child to fall asleep with a bottle containing milk, formula, fruit juices, or other sweet liquids. Never let a child walk with a bottle in his/her mouth.
- Comfort a child who wants a bottle between regular feedings or during naps with a bottle filled with cool water.
- Always make sure a child's pacifier is clean and never dip a pacifier in a sweet liquid.
- Introduce children to a cup as they approach 1 year of age. Children should stop drinking from a bottle soon after their first birthday.
- Notify the parent of any unusual red or swollen areas in a child's mouth or any dark spot on a child's tooth so that the parent can consult the child's dentist.
- Never put an infant or child to bed with a bottle that is filled with sugar-containing beverages, including fruit juice or Kool-aid. Good oral hygiene is needed. Wean children by age 2 years.

Tube Feeding
- Good oral hygiene and mouth care will be needed, even if a patient is not fed by mouth. Tube feeding should include all key nutrients to meet patient needs. See Section 17.

Xerostomia
- Moisten foods.
- Avoid too many added spices.
- Avoid excessively chewy foods like steak, crumbly foods

like crackers or cake, dry foods like chips, or sticky foods such as peanut butter (Touger-Decker, 2000).

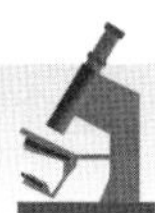

PROFILE

Clinical/History		Lab Work (continued)
Height Weight BMI Recent weight changes Mouth or tongue lacerations Caries Missing or loose teeth Taste alterations	Sore or bleeding gums Dentures, especially poorly fitting **Lab Work** Alb, prealbumin Ca++ Mg++ Alk Phos H&H	Serum Fe Phosphorus Triceps skinfold (TSF), midarm muscle circumference (MAMC), midarm circumference (MAC) for wired jaw X-rays (such as mandible)

Common Drugs Used and Potential Side Effects

- Luride is a fluoride supplement for children to strengthen teeth against tooth decay. Avoid use with calcium or dairy products because it may form a nonabsorbable product.
- For patients with cancer, various therapies affect the mouth and gums. Monitor closely.
- Oral side effects of drugs are adverse effects that interfere with client function and increase risks for infection, pain, and possible tooth loss (Spolarich, 2000).

Herbs, Botanicals and Supplements

- Herbs and botanicals may be used; identify and monitor side effects.
- Counsel about use of herbal teas, especially regarding toxic substances.

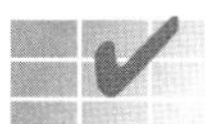

PATIENT EDUCATION

- ✓ If needed, blended foods and/or tube feedings should be prepared. Sometimes, a bulb syringe may be useful.
- ✓ Provide the patient with creative ideas for the seasoning and flavoring of foods. Discuss acceptable restaurant options.
- ✓ Ensure that fluoride is provided in some way by the diet and water supply.
- ✓ Encourage good habits in oral hygiene and diet: detergent foods (e.g., raw fruits and vegetables) should be recommended rather than sticky or impactant foods (e.g., soft cookies, bread, sticky sweets, dried fruits, etc.). Cariogenic foods include dried fruits, candy, cookies, pies, cakes, ice cream, canned fruit, soft drinks, fruit drinks, lemonade, gelatin desserts, snack crackers, pretzels or chips, and muffins. Cariostatic foods should be encouraged, such as cheese, raw fruits and vegetables, peanuts, and cocoa.
- ✓ Read milk labels to ensure vitamin D fortification.
- ✓ Use cheese after meals or sugary snacks to normalize pH.
- ✓ Most dental researchers consider fluoride and dental sealants to be highly effective caries prevention measures; in contrast, WIC nutritionists consider oral hygiene to be most important (Faine and Oberg, 1995).

For More Information

- ✦ American Dental Association
  211 East Chicago Avenue
  Chicago, IL 60611
  (312) 440-2658
  http://www.ada.org/
- ✦ American Academy of Dental Schools
  1619 Massachusetts Avenue NW
  Washington, DC 20036
  (202) 667-9433
- ✦ Academy of General Dentistry
  http://www.agd.org/
- ✦ American Academy of Pediatric Dentistry
  http://www.aapd.org/
- ✦ American Academy of Periodontology
  http://www.perio.org/
- ✦ American Dental Association
  Statement on Fluoridation of Water
  http://www.ada.org/prof/prac/issues/statements/fluoride2.html
- ✦ Dentistry online
  http://www.floss.com/dental_nutrition.htm
- ✦ International Association for Disability and Oral Health
  http://www.iadh.org/
- ✦ National Children's Dental Health Association
  (800) 947-4746
  http://www.ada.org/consumer/ncdhm/nc-menu.html
- ✦ National Institute of Dental and Craniofacial Research (NIDCR)
  Bldg. 31, Room 2C35
  31 Center Drive, MSC 2290
  Bethesda, MD 20892-2290
  301-496-4261
- ✦ National Oral Health Information Clearinghouse
  1 NOHIC Way
  Bethesda, MD 20892-3500
  301-402-7364
  http://www.nohic.nidcr.nih.gov
- ✦ Oral Health America
  http://www.oralhealthamerica.org/
- ✦ Special Care in Dentistry
  http://www.foscod.org/

SELF-FEEDING PROBLEMS

NUTRITIONAL ACUITY RANKING: LEVEL 2–3 (VARIES BY SEVERITY)

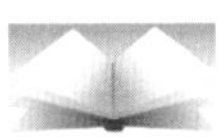

DEFINITIONS AND BACKGROUND

Four areas of concern in management of self-feeding as part of the activities of daily living are blindness, coordination problems, chewing problems, and dysphagia. Where appropriate, these factors are also mentioned in relation to specific disorders in other sections.

OBJECTIVES

- Promote independence in self-feeding, when possible.
- Address all nutritional deficiencies and complications individually.
- Promote overall wellness and health.
- Increase interest in eating.
- Prevent malnutrition and weight loss.
- Decrease instances in which constipation, anorexia, or other problems affect nutritional status.
- Increase pleasure associated with mealtimes.
- Educate the caregiver about adaptive equipment, utensils, and special food modifications.

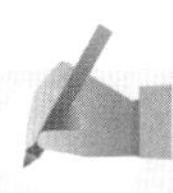

DIETARY AND NUTRITIONAL RECOMMENDATIONS

Blindness

- Provide special plate guards, utensils, double handles, and compartmentalized plates with foods placed in similar locations at each meal. Explain placement of foods. Open packets if needed.
- Work with occupational therapist (OT) or family to practice kitchen safety and to determine ability to have independence at mealtimes.
- Create a feeling of usefulness by delegating appropriate tasks related to mealtime, such as drying dishes and assisting with simple meal tasks that are safe for the individual.
- The individual may benefit from companionship during meals, especially if any problems occur or if anything else is needed.
- Use straws for beverages, if there are no problems with dysphagia.

Coordination Problems

- Self-feeding requires the ability to suck, to sit with head and neck balanced, to bring hand to mouth, to grasp cup and utensil, to drink from a cup, to take food from a spoon, to bite, to chew, and to swallow.
- Each person should be assessed individually to determine which, if any, aspects of coordination have been affected by his or her condition. Adjust self-feeding accordingly.
- Use of clothing protectors may be useful for maintaining dignity.
- Assist with feeding if needed. Adjust table or chair height; use adaptive feeding equipment as needed (such as weighted utensils, large-handled cups, larger or smaller silverware than standard.)

Chewing Problems

- Decrease texture in foods as necessary (e.g., use a mechanical soft, pureed, or liquid diet as needed). Season as desired for individual taste. Try to progress in textures if possible because chewing is important for saliva production and proper digestion of foods.
- Liquid or blenderized foods may be beneficial. If needed, use a tube feeding.
- For some persons, a straw may be helpful; for others, it is not. Speech therapists may be helpful in assessment of this ability.
- Protein foods such as tofu, cottage cheese, peanut butter, eggs, cheese, and milk products can be used when meats or nuts cannot be chewed.
- Edentulousness without dentures may contribute to deterioration in the systemic health of the elderly. Dentures should fit well and be adjusted or replaced as needed, such as after weight loss.

Dysphagia

- Dysphagia has been recognized as a variable that increases hospital length-of-stay (LOS) and influences patient outcome. In young children, it can seriously affect physical and intellectual development (Perlman, 1999). Airway protection and adequacy of nutrient intake must be considered. Fiberoptic endoscopic evaluation of swallowing (FEES) may identify patients who are at high risk for pulmonary aspiration due to swallowing dysfunction after prolonged intubation. Based on the results of FEES, dietary recommendations can be made to decrease the incidence of aspiration after prolonged intubation (Ajemian et al., 2001). Some institutions offer up to 4 levels of dysphagia diets. More information is in Section 7 (gastrointestinal disorders).

Herbs, Botanicals and Supplements

- Herbs and botanicals may be used; identify and monitor side effects. For <u>glaucoma:</u> oregano, jaborandi, bilberry, kaffir potato, and pansy have been recommended but have not been confirmed as effective. For <u>cataract:</u> bilberry, rosemary, carrot, catnip, Brazil nut, and capers have been recommended but have not been studied for efficacy.
- Counsel about use of herbal teas, especially regarding toxic substances.

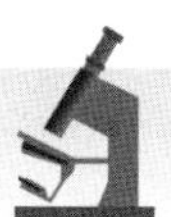

PROFILE

Clinical/History		Lab Work
Height Weight BMI Recent weight changes Mouth or tongue lacerations Missing or loose teeth Sore or bleeding gums	Dentures, especially poorly fitting Blindness or vision problems Dysphagia Chewing problems Coordination problems	Alb, prealbumin Ca++ Mg++ Alk Phos H&H Serum Fe Phosphorus TSF, MAMC, MAC for wired jaw X-rays (such as mandible)

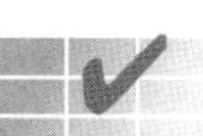

PATIENT EDUCATION

- ✓ Discuss the importance of various therapies and medications for recovery.
- ✓ Discuss the role of nutrition in health, weight control, and recovery or repair processes.
- ✓ Provide instruction regarding simplified meal planning and preparation.
- ✓ Refer to agencies such as Meals-on-Wheels, etc.
- ✓ For dysphagia: moisten foods with appropriate gravies, sauces, milk, and other liquids. Discuss which foods may cause aspiration. Foods served at hot or cold temperatures trigger the swallowing reflex more effectively than foods served at room temperature. See section 7.
- ✓ For healthy eyes, nutrition plays an essential role. See Table 2–3 for a description of this role.

For More Information

- ✦ American Association of Ophthalmology
  http://www.eyenet.org/
- ✦ American Council for the Blind
  (800) 424-8666
  http://www.acb.org/
- ✦ Age-Related Macular Degeneration Alliance
  http://www.amdalliance.org/
- ✦ American Dietetic Association
  Restorative Dining protocol
  http://www.eatright.org
- ✦ National Eye Institute, NIH
  http://www.nei.nih.gov/
- ✦ Prevent Blindness America
  (800) 331-2020

TABLE 2–3 Key Nutrients in Ophthalmology

In proper eye health, key nutrients include vitamins A (for healthy cornea and conjunctiva), B6 (for healthy conjunctiva), and C (for healthy conjunctiva and vitreous humor), zinc (for healthy retina and optic nerve), riboflavin (for corneal vascularization), vitamin B12 (for retina and nerve fibers), and thiamine (for normal retinal and optic nerve functioning). Niacin is also important.

According to the National Eye Institute, age-related macular degeneration (ARMD, or AMD) and cataract are the leading causes of visual impairment and blindness in the United States. Both diseases increase dramatically after age 60. Although excellent treatments for cataract are available, there are no equivalent treatments for ARMD.

ARMD is a vascular condition that damages the retina; diets high in saturated fat may also promote higher risk (Cho et al., 2001). High intakes of linoleic acid and trans-fatty acids significantly raise ARMD risk, while high intakes of omega-3 fatty acids and fish are protective (Cho et al., 2001). Eating fish just once a week and cutting back on saturated fatty acids may helpful in reducing age-related macular degeneration (Smith et al., 2000). Abdominal obesity has also been implicated. Further studies are warranted.

Studies suggest that some types of blindness and ARMD can be prevented by proper intake of antioxidants, especially carotenoids (Eye Disease Case-Control Study, 1993). Lutein and zeaxanthin, found mostly in green leafy vegetables (e.g., kale, collards, spinach), are the carotenoids most associated with reduced risk of macular degeneration (Seddon et al., 1994). The Eye Institute tested large doses of zinc oxide (80 mg), vitamin C (500 mg), vitamin E (400 IU), and beta-carotene (15 mg) given with copper to prevent anemia with some promising results. However, it is too early to support these large doses for the general population because of potential side effects, including use of beta-carotene supplements by smokers (Age-Related Eye Disease Research Group, 2001).

For cataracts, long-term vitamin C supplement use may prevent or delay early age-related lens opacities (Jacques et al., 1997). In addition, a low-sodium diet may be protective against development of cataracts (Cummings et al., 2000).

PERIODONTAL DISEASE

NUTRITIONAL ACUITY RANKING: LEVEL 2

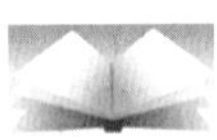

DEFINITIONS AND BACKGROUND

Periodontal disease is a painless, chronic inflammatory disease generally caused by dental plaque and microbial flora. A poor diet and inadequate dental hygiene can also cause destruction of the jawbone. Periodontal disease is evident approximately 10 years before osteoporosis; it most commonly manifests as pyorrhea alveolaris. In the United States, periodontal disease affects 75% of the population. At risk in particular are pregnant women, diabetics, alcoholics, smokers, and persons on certain medications. Abnormal blood glucose levels may be found in some patients with periodontal disease (Katz, 2001). Usually, dental caries and periodontal disease are not present in the same patients because the microbial flora differs.

Tissues that support teeth in the jaws are collectively known as the periodontium (gums, alveolar bone, periodontal membrane). Any abnormality that leads to a visible change or loss of integrity of any component of the supporting tissue is listed as a periodontal disease. Periodontitis involves a gross breakdown of supporting tissues with progressive loosening and loss of teeth; it is a major cause of tooth loss in adults. Periodontoclasia involves destruction of tissues around the teeth.

Gingivitis involves minor inflammatory change; it may be acute or chronic, local or generalized. Vitamin C deficiency has been implicated. Acute necrotizing ulcerative gingivitis (Vincent's disease or trench mouth) is an acute ulceration affecting marginal gingiva with inflamed or necrotic interdental papillae. The onset is abrupt and painful with slight fever, malaise, excess salivation, and fetid breath. It can be caused by systemic disease. A bland diet may be useful.

There have been advances in evidence-based periodontology over the past decade: adjunctive antimicrobial therapy, regenerative periodontal surgery, periodontal plastic surgery, bone regeneration surgery and implant treatment, and advanced soft tissue management at implant sites (Tonetti, 2000).

OBJECTIVES

- Reduce inflammation.
- Promote healing.
- Correct poor nutritional habits that can lead to chronic subclinical nutritional deficiencies in levels of vitamin C, amino acids, riboflavin, folacin, vitamin A, zinc, and calcium.
- Prevent further decline in status of bones and gums.
- Protect the jawbone with adequate calcium.

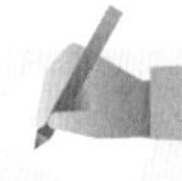

DIETARY AND NUTRITIONAL RECOMMENDATIONS

- Ensure adequate intake of calcium, protein, and phosphorus.
- Vitamin D-fortified milk should be used.
- Ensure adequate intake of vitamin C, fluoride, vitamin A, and zinc.
- Use high detergent foods (firm, fresh fruits and raw vegetables).
- If needed, a plan should be designed to control timing and frequency of meals and snacks to reduce exposure of susceptible gum tissue and teeth to the acids that form plaque.

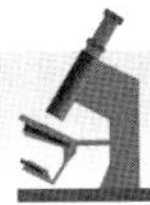

PROFILE

Clinical/History		Lab Work
Height Weight BMI Gums—color, friability Oral examination for	tooth mobility, calculus Presence of dental caries Missing teeth Mouth sores Overall nutritional status	Serum ascorbic acid Serum Fe Alb, prealbumin H&H

Common Drugs Used and Potential Side Effects

- Oral contraceptives may lower serum levels of folate and vitamin C, thereby jeopardizing gingival health.
- Sodium bicarbonate may be used as a mouthwash. Patients with high blood pressure should not swallow this wash.
- Peridex is an oral rinse to control bleeding gums. Taste changes may occur with its use.

Herbs, Botanicals and Supplements

- Herbs and botanicals may be used; identify and monitor side effects. For gingivitis: bloodroot, Echinacea, purslane, camomile, licorice, and sage have been recommended but not confirmed for efficacy.
- Counsel about use of herbal teas, especially regarding toxic substances.
- A Connective Tissue Nutrient Formula that contains vitamins A, C, and D, glucosamine sulfate, magnesium, oligoproanthocyanindins, copper, zinc, manganese, boron, silicon, and calcium is prescribed to enhance the integrity of key connective tissue elements and improve their resistance to degradation. Naturopathic physicians prescribe Panax ginseng, Withania som-

nifera, and Eleutherococcus senticosus to reverse the impact of bacterial and psychosocial stressors. A clinical trial is being designed to study the effects of these therapies (http://www.clinicaltrials.gov/).

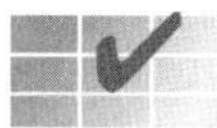

PATIENT EDUCATION

- ✓ Encourage a proper diet, especially a correct calcium:phosphorus ratio and recommended dietary allowances (RDAs) for age.
- ✓ Recommend meticulous oral hygiene and regular dental examinations to maintain dental hygiene.
- ✓ Encourage pregnant women and persons with diabetes, cancer, HIV/AIDS, or leukemia to pay special attention to oral hygiene.

For More Information

- ✦ American Academy of Periodontology
  Suite 924, 211 East Chicago Avenue
  Chicago, IL 60611

TEMPOROMANDIBULAR JOINT DYSFUNCTION

NUTRITIONAL ACUITY RANKING: LEVEL 1

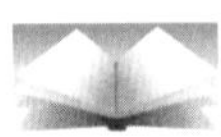

DEFINITIONS AND BACKGROUND

Temporomandibular joint (TMJ) disorders result from local or systemic causes, such as rheumatoid or osteoarthritis and connective tissue disorders. The TMJ is a diarthrodial joint with moving elements (mandible) and fixed elements (temporal bone). With this dysfunction, overuse or abuse of any part of normal action affects the mastication process. Patients with temporomandibular disorder pain dysfunction syndrome have toothaches or facial pains, which often lead to food intake problems (Irving et al., 1999).

Women between the ages of 30 and 60 account for 75% of all cases. Signs and symptoms include pain, clicking noise, stiffness of neck, face, or shoulders, locking of affected joint, trismus, and mandibular deviation—often from repetitive overloading (stress or habit such as gum chewing, grinding), from functional masseter muscle coordination problems, or from incorrect occlusion (as with missing teeth). Structural problems are treated by surgery (e.g., fusion can be treated by removing the area of fused bone and replacing it with silicon rubber). Sometimes an artificial joint is the answer; but surgery is recommended for only a few patients. Undue muscle tension causes most TMJ, with some other problems stemming from inadequate bite (as from a high filling or a malocclusion). People with TMJ will benefit from a visit to their dentist or other specialists (e.g., ear-nose-throat specialists).

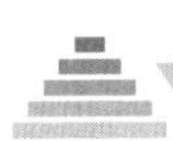

OBJECTIVES

- Reduce repetitive overloading by use of a splint or by breaking bad habits such as grinding.
- Reduce stress with relaxation techniques. Relieve pain and muscle spasms.
- Prevent or correct malnutrition or weight loss.
- Ensure adequate intake of soft, nonchewy sources of fiber.
- Reduce any existing inflammation and prevent complications such as mitral valve prolapse.

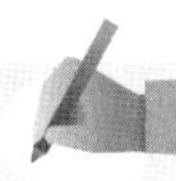

DIETARY AND NUTRITIONAL RECOMMENDATIONS

- Use a normal diet with soft foods to prevent pain while chewing.
- Cut food into small, bite-sized pieces. Avoid chewy foods such as caramel, nuts, toffee, chewy candies, and gummy bread and rolls.
- Avoid opening mouth widely, as for large and thick sandwiches. Grate vegetables (e.g., carrots) to reduce chewing.
- Use adequate sources of vitamin C for adequate gingival health.
- For some, a low-caffeine diet may be useful, although this has not been confirmed by research.

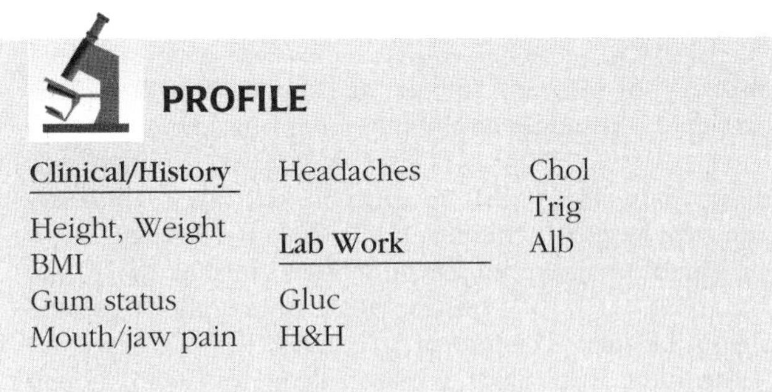

PROFILE

Clinical/History		
Height, Weight	Headaches	Chol
BMI	**Lab Work**	Trig
Gum status	Gluc	Alb
Mouth/jaw pain	H&H	

Herbs, Botanicals and Supplements

- Herbs and botanicals may be used; identify and monitor side effects.
- Counsel about use of herbal teas, especially regarding toxic substances.

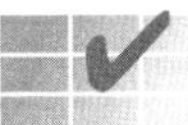

PATIENT EDUCATION

- Discuss the role of dental care in maintaining adequate health.
- Monitor for any tooth or gum soreness; advise the dentist as necessary. Regular oral hygiene must be continued despite mouth pain.
- Physical therapy may be needed to correct functioning of muscles and joints.
- Nail biting, gum chewing, use of teeth to cut thread, or similar habits should be stopped.

For More Information

- Temporomandibular Joint Disorder
  http://www.tmj.org/

SKIN DISORDERS

NUTRITIONAL ACUITY RANKING: LEVEL 1

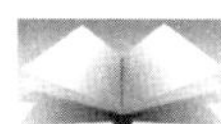

DEFINITIONS AND BACKGROUND

The skin is affected by both internal and external influences, which may lead to photo aging, inflammation, immune dysfunction, imbalanced epidermal homeostasis, and other skin disorders (Boelsma et al., 2001). The skin often reflects problems such as GI disturbances, alcoholism, or general malnutrition. In many respects, human skin fulfills the requirements for being the largest, independent peripheral endocrine organ of the body (Zouboulis, 2000).

Retinoids are a group of naturally occurring and synthetic compounds with vitamin A biologic activity; they have benefits in dealing with skin diseases such as acne, psoriasis, ichthyoses, keratodermas, skin cancers and their precursors, and reversal of photo aging (Futoryan and Gilcrest, 1994). Supplementation with vitamins, carotenoids, and polyunsaturated fatty acids have been shown, in one study, to provide protection against ultraviolet light; sunscreens are much more important overall (Boelsma et al., 2001). Nutritional factors should continue to be studied for their impact on properties such as hydration, sebum production, and elasticity and on prevention of skin cancer (Greenwald, 2001).

The first indications that a high-fat diet might promote damage from ultraviolet light were identified in animal studies back in 1939 (Black, 1998). Switching from a high-fat to a low-fat diet may be protective against nonmelanoma skin cancer (NMSC) and actinic keratoses (Black, 1998; Lamberg, 1998). Antioxidant supplements may help protect against sensitivity of the skin to UV light. Erythema was measured in one study; those taking carotenoids plus vitamin E had less redness than those not taking any or taking carotenoids alone (Stahl et al., 2000).

Eczema is a skin condition manifested by itching, blistering, oozing, and scaling skin rash. Some types of atopic dermatitis respond to primrose oil with linoleic and linolenic acids (Soyland and Drevon, 1993). Nickel sensitivity affects 8–15% of women and 1% of men; a low-nickel diet may be warranted in these cases. Epidermolysis bullosa is a hereditary condition in which blistering of the skin occurs with even slight trauma. In this condition, protein–calorie malnutrition, anemia, and vitamin–mineral deficiencies may occur (Birge, 1995). Because essential fatty acids (EFAs) form an important component of cell membranes, are eicosanoid precursors, and are required for both the structure and function of every cell, EFAs appear to be of benefit in atopic eczema and psoriasis (Das, 1999).

Rosacea is an age-related disorder of the central portion of the facial skin whose peak onset occurs when the patient is in his/her 40s or 50s (Litt, 1997). A chronic and progressive condition of flare-ups and remissions, rosacea can be disfiguring if left untreated. Rosacea resembles other dermatologic conditions, especially acne vulgaris. Oral and topical antibiotic therapy usually brings about remission; the tetracycline family is the drug of choice. It affects 1 in 20 people, or 13 million in the U.S. Members of the same family tend to be affected; fair-skinned individuals of Northern and Eastern European descent (e.g., English, Scottish, Welsh or Scandinavian) are most commonly affected (Litt, 1997).

The association of dermatitis herpetiformis (DH or Durhing's disease) with gluten-sensitive enteropathy (GSE) is supported by the presence of villous atrophy and endomysial antibodies (EMAs); EMAs are found to be a marker of GSE both in celiac disease (CD) and in DH (Kumar et al., 2001). A gluten-restricted diet is used in these conditions.

OBJECTIVES

- Reduce inflammation, redness, and edema where present.
- Apply nutritional principles according to the particular condition.
- Prevent further exacerbations of the condition.
- Identify any offending foods and omit from the diet where relevant (such as with allergies).

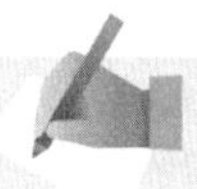

DIETARY AND NUTRITIONAL RECOMMENDATIONS

- Acne. Encourage intake of adequate zinc and vitamin A. This condition is hormone dependent.
- Psoriasis. Vitamins D (DeLuca, 1993) and E may have some benefit. Increase use of zinc from meats, seafood, and whole grains. Psoriasis may precede arthritis by months or years, because both are inflammatory processes. Studies are not yet conclusive about omega-3 fatty acids, but inclusion of more seafood in the diet may be useful (Soyland and Drevon, 1993). Careful inclusion of essential fatty acids is important (Das, 1999).
- Chronic urticaria. Reduce salicylates and aspirin use or penicillin and food molds. Berries and dried fruits are high in salicylates, as are some herbs and spices. FD&C Yellow 5 should be omitted from the diet; check labels.
- Infantile eczema. A familial tendency may be noted in this condition, which may result from hypersensitivity to milk, egg albumin, or wheat. There may be a linoleic acid metabolic defect as well. Control caloric excess in obese infants.
- Acrodermatitis enteropathica. Supplement with zinc because absorption of zinc is impaired in this condition. Use protein of high biologic value. Decrease excess fiber, if necessary, to normalize bowel function.
- Dermatitis herpetiformis. A gluten-free diet is quite successful in treating this condition.
- Hypercarotenemia. Reduce dietary and supplementary carotene (carrots, tomatoes, etc.).
- Nickel dermatitis. Avoid canned fish, tomatoes, corn, spinach, other canned vegetables, and nuts. Do not cook with stainless steel utensils. Use chocolate, nuts, dried beans or peas, and whole grains sparingly because they are naturally high in nickel.

- Epidermolysis bullosa. Gastrostomy feeding may be needed in severe cases.
- Rosacea. Consumption of alcoholic beverages, spicy foods, hot beverages, some fruits and vegetables, or dairy products may trigger flare-ups. Avoid as needed.

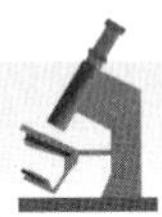

PROFILE

Clinical/History	Lab Work	
Height Weight BMI Growth pattern in infants/ children	Alb (decreased in exfoliative dermatitis) Prealbumin Serum zinc Histamine H&H Serum Fe Gluc	Chol Trig Serum carotene Retinol-binding protein (RBP) Uric acid (increased in chronic eczema)

Common Drugs Used and Potential Side Effects

- Topical corticosteroids (such as Aclovate) usually have a mild effect on the nutritional status of the patient. Stronger brands or dosages may act like oral steroids.
- Isotretinoin (Accutane) may be used for acne or psoriasis. Watch for a decrease in high-density lipoprotein (HDL) and an increase in triglycerides and avoid vitamin A supplementation. Dry mouth can occur. Avoid during pregnancy.
- Retin A (retinoic acid) is useful for moderate cases of acne.
- Antibiotics are used in acne for their anti-inflammatory effect, not for their antibacterial impact. Tetracycline should not be taken with milk or calcium supplements. Excesses of vitamin A can cause headaches or hypertension (HPN). Use more riboflavin, vitamin C, and calcium in the diet. Beware of general protein and iron malabsorption. Diarrhea is the major GI effect. Minocycline is another form; it causes less GI distress and does not affect calcium metabolism as dramatically.
- Erythromycin/Benzamycin may be used. Take with a full glass of water on an empty stomach. Sore mouth, diarrhea, and nausea are common side effects.
- Methotrexate may be used in psoriasis to reduce inflammation of skin and joints. Side effects such as nausea, anemia, folate depletion, stomatitis, or vomiting must be addressed with long-term use.
- Vitamin and mineral supplementation should be free from tartrazine for chronic urticaria patients.

Herbs, Botanicals and Supplements

- Herbs and botanicals may be used; identify and monitor side effects. For dermatoses: avocado, camomile, evening primrose, and calendula may be recommended but have not been proven effective. For psoriasis: bishop's weed, avocado, licorice, red pepper, Brazil nut, and purslane have been suggested without studies. For scabies: evening primrose, onion, neem, mountain mint, and tree oil have been proposed. For sunburn: tea, eggplant, plantain, and calendula have been proposed for use in addition to aloe; no confirming studies are on record.
- Counsel about use of herbal teas, especially regarding toxic substances.
- Red clover is sometimes used for eczema or psoriasis. Do not use with warfarin or hormone replacement therapy.
- Aloe is sometimes used for abrasions, sunburn, and mild burns. It may cause GI cramping and hypokalemia if ingested.
- There is insufficient evidence to make recommendations on maternal allergen avoidance for prevention of atopic eczema through use of oral antihistamines, Chinese herbs, dietary restriction in established atopic eczema, homeopathy, house dust mite reduction, massage therapy, hypnotherapy, evening primrose oil, emollients, topical coal tar, and topical doxepin (Hoare et al., 2000).

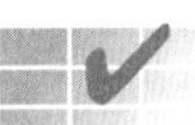

PATIENT EDUCATION

- Encourage the patient to read food, medication, and supplement labels.
- Help the patient modify his or her diet as specifically indicated by the condition.
- Encourage adequate fluid intake but not excess.
- Discuss avoidance of topical or specialty products, except as prescribed by the doctor.
- Discuss the roles of nutrients in skin care. Sunscreens may prevent vitamin D from penetrating the skin, especially formulas with higher protective factors; if dietary intakes are poor for vitamin D, a supplement may be needed. Other nutrients such as protein, vitamin A, and zinc are also important in balanced amounts from the diet; describe good sources.
- Discuss the role of essential fatty acids on membrane function and how to include them in the diet.

For More Information

- Acne Hotline
  800-235-ACNE
- American Academy of Dermatology
  930 N. Meacham Rd.
  Schaumburg, IL 60173

847-330-0230
888-462-DERM
http://www.aad.org/

- National Eczema Foundation for Science and Education
  1220 SW Morrison, Suite 433
  Portland, OR 97205
  503-228-4430
  800-818-7546
  http://www.eczema-assn.org/
- National Psoriasis Foundation
  6600 SW 92nd Avenue, Suite 300
  Portland, OR 97223
  http://www.psoriasis.org/

PRESSURE ULCER

NUTRITIONAL ACUITY RANKING: LEVEL 2 (STAGES 1–2) LEVEL 3 (STAGES 3 OR 4)

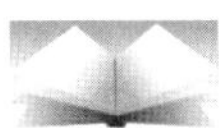

DEFINITIONS AND BACKGROUND

A pressure plus friction or shear and a lack of oxygen and nutrition to the affected area cause pressure ulcers. Pressure ulcers often occur over bone or cartilaginous prominences (e.g., hip, sacrum, elbow, or heels). They are common among patients with protein–calorie malnutrition (PCM) (as in HIV infection or cancers) and among bedridden or paralyzed patients. Medicare costs attributable to pressure ulcer treatment are as high as $2 billion annually. Mean length of treating pressure ulcers in one study was 116 days at a cost of $2,731 per ulcer, including hospital costs; $489 without hospital treatment (Allman, 1997).

Many patients with pressure ulcers are elderly, below their usual body weight, have a low prealbumin level, and are not taking in enough nutrition to meet their needs; aggressive nutritional therapy may be warranted (Guenter et al., 2000). Poorer nutritional status and decreased oxygen perfusion are predictors of pressure ulcers on admission; nutritional status and length of stay are predictors of ulcer severity (Williams et al., 2000).

Risk factors for pressure ulcer development include immobility, poor circulation (as in diabetes, peripheral vascular disease, or anemia), infection, poor nutritional status, prolonged pressure, drugs, and serum albumin below 3.5 g/dL. Reduced functional ability, poor oral intake of less than 50% of meals over 3 days compared with usual intakes, chewing problems, low serum albumin with normal hydration, and low cholesterol levels are also commonly found. Patients fed low-fat tube feedings are often found to be hypocholesterolemic. There is a strong association with pressure ulcers in this group; low cholesterol levels are often more predictive of pressure ulcer development than low albumin levels (Braden, 1996).

Mortality, usually secondary to sepsis, has been estimated to be as high as 60% in patients with pressure ulcers. In most cases, it is difficult to determine whether a pressure ulcer led to a terminal event such as sepsis or whether the process of dying (i.e., decreased cardiac output, severe catabolic state) led to an unpreventable pressure ulcer (Braden, 1996).

Staging of pressure ulcers is found in Table 2–4.

TABLE 2–4 Staging of Pressure Ulcers (Bergstrom, 1987; Durr, 1986; Hunan and Schesle, 1991)

Stage I—redness and warmth
Stage II—shallow ulcer with distinct edges
Stage III—full-thickness loss of skin
Stage IV—involvement of fascia, connective tissue, muscle, and bone
Stage V—area covered with black eschar

OBJECTIVES

- Restore normal calorie, protein, and nutrient status. Correct PCM. Protein and calories are of paramount importance.
- Monitor scores on the Braden scale (sensory perception, skin moisture, activity, mobility, nutritional status, friction, shear). The nutrition subscale is intended to measure the person's usual food intake pattern; intake of 3–5 days should be assessed. Persons "protected" from pressure ulcer development usually have dietary intakes of nearly 120% of the RDA for protein (Braden, 1996).
- Heal the pressure ulcer and prevent further tissue breakdown. Assess risk status using the Braden scale (Bergstrom et al., 1987). Table 2–4 indicates staging. Assess healing status using the Sessing scale (see Table 2–5).
- Improve low-grade infections, fever, diarrhea, and vomiting.
- Assess nutritional intake via calorie counts.
- Maintain intact skin once healing has occurred.
- Support the patient's immune system to prevent infections.

DIETARY AND NUTRITIONAL RECOMMENDATIONS

- Provide a high-protein diet: 1.25–1.5 g protein/kg body weight (higher levels for higher stages). A deep ulcer may require up to 2 g/kg. It may be necessary to add protein powders to beverages, casseroles, tube feedings, and liquid supplements to get the adequate amount. Individuals given 24% protein formulas heal faster than those receiving standard 14% protein formulas (Breslow et al., 1993). Products such as NutriFocusR (Ross Labs) contain 14.8 grams of protein per serving, 2% as arginine; it also contains fructooligosaccharides to support beneficial bacteria in the gut.

TABLE 2–5 Sessing Scale of Healing (Ferrell et al., 1995)

0 = normal skin, but at risk
1 = skin completely closed, but may lack pigmentation or may be reddened
2 = wound edges and center are filled in
3 = wound bed filling with pink granulating tissue; slough present; free of necrotic tissue; minimal drainage and odor
4 = moderate-to-minimal granulating tissue; slough and minimal necrotic tissue; moderate drainage and odor
5 = presence of heavy drainage and odor, eschar, and slough; surrounding skin reddened or discolored
6 = breaks in skin around primary ulcer; purulent discharge; foul odor; necrotic tissue and/or eschar; may have sepsis

- Provide calories at the rate of 25–35 kcal/kg current weight. Use lower levels for obese patients and higher levels to gain weight.
- Feed by tube if necessary. With a large sacral pressure ulcer, total parenteral nutrition (TPN) may be the only way to feed if incontinence of bowel is a concern.
- Provide small, frequent feedings if oral intake is poor, 4–6 times daily.
- Supplement diet with multivitamins, especially vitamin A and 120–240 mg of vitamin C, extra thiamine, and 30–60 mg of zinc. Excesses are wasteful and do not necessarily speed the healing process.

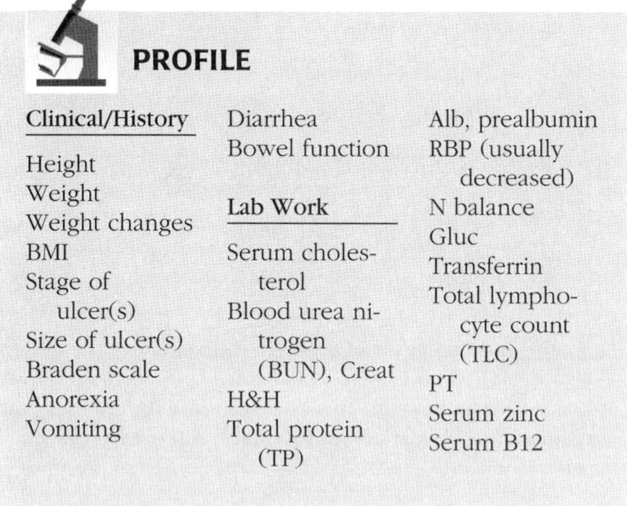

PROFILE

Clinical/History		
Height Weight Weight changes BMI Stage of ulcer(s) Size of ulcer(s) Braden scale Anorexia Vomiting	Diarrhea Bowel function **Lab Work** Serum cholesterol Blood urea nitrogen (BUN), Creat H&H Total protein (TP)	Alb, prealbumin RBP (usually decreased) N balance Gluc Transferrin Total lymphocyte count (TLC) PT Serum zinc Serum B12

Common Drugs Used and Potential Side Effects

- Monitor the drug profile for potential side effects, depletion of serum proteins, and blood-forming nutrients.
- Antibiotics may be needed in sepsis; monitor specific effects.

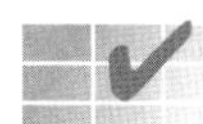

PATIENT EDUCATION

- ✓ Instruct nursing personnel and patient's family about the importance of adequate nutrition for healing of tissues.
- ✓ Discuss importance of maintaining healthy, intact skin. Keep skin clean and dry; avoid excessive massage over bony prominences.
- ✓ Provide teaching tools in regard to high-protein diets and the appropriate calorie level.
- ✓ Where possible, improve ambulation and circulation to all tissues.
- ✓ Discuss the role of nutrition in wound healing (i.e., collagen and fibroblasts require protein, zinc, and vitamin C for proper formation). See Table 2–5 for the Sessing scale of healing.

Herbs, Botanicals and Supplements

- Herbs and botanicals may be used; identify and monitor side effects.
- Counsel about use of herbal teas, especially regarding toxic substances.

For More Information

- Agency for Healthcare Research and Quality
  Clinical Practice Guidelines – Pressure Ulcer Treatment
  2101 E. Jefferson St., Suite 501
  Rockville, MD 20852
  301-594-1364
  http://www.ahcpr.gov/
- National Pressure Ulcer Advisory Panel
  11250 Roger Bacon Dr., Suite 8
  Reston, VA 20190-5202
  703-464-4849
  http://www.npuap.org/Default.htm

VITAMIN DEFICIENCIES (VITAMIN A, BERIBERI, SCURVY, RIBOFLAVIN, PELLAGRA)

NUTRITIONAL ACUITY RANKING: LEVEL 3

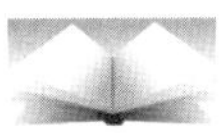

DEFINITIONS AND BACKGROUND

Vitamins are a part of a healthy diet. If a person eats a variety of foods, deficiency is unlikely. However, people who follow restricted diets may not get enough of a particular nutrient. Deficiencies may be primary (self-induced by inadequate diet) or secondary to disease process. They are especially common in diet faddists, alcoholics, and people who live alone and eat poorly. Vegetarians are also susceptible, especially for B12 deficiency.

Vitamin A deficiency is common among children. Night blindness and eye changes are often early signs. There is evidence now that many infections (such as measles) may cause vitamin A deficiency.

Vitamin D deficiency—(see Osteomalacia). Nutritional rickets in children is rare. Treatment consists of giving adequate vitamin D3 and ensuring adequate exposure to sunlight. Vitamin D is shunted to fat cells rather than to circulation in obese persons; they may need extra intake of vitamin D or sun exposure.

Vitamin E deficiency—rare; problems can occur with fat malabsorption (especially in children). Abetalipoproteinemia is the most severe deficiency and occurs mainly in premature and sick children. Aquasol E has no adverse side effects if used within RDA dosage.

Vitamin K deficiency—rare except in intestinal problems and short gut syndromes. Intestinal bacteria in the gut can make Vitamin K.

Thiamine deficiency—commonly occurs in alcoholics, patients with heart failure, and persons with poor diets.

Niacin and riboflavin deficiencies often occur in conjunction with other B-complex vitamin deficiencies.

Folacin and vitamin B12 deficiencies—megaloblastic anemias can result. Peripheral neuropathy and a positive Schilling test are needed to indicate B12 deficiency. Treat both conditions with adequate vitamin supplementation (see Anemia section). Studies now indicate that folic acid deficiency plays a role in formation of neural tube defects.

Vitamin B6 deficiency—decreases conversion of tryptophan to niacin. It can occur after surgery or as a result of poor diet.

Pantothenic acid and biotin deficiencies are rare.

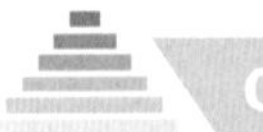

OBJECTIVES

- Replenish the deficient nutrient and restore normal serum levels.
- Prevent or correct side effects of nutrient deficiency:
  Vitamin A. Reduced growth, night blindness leading progressively to xerophthalmia, changes in epithelial tissue, failure of tooth enamel and/or degeneration, and loss of taste and smell.
  Vitamin D. Abnormal bone growth and repair; rickets in children, osteomalacia in adults; muscle spasms.
  Vitamin E. Rupture of red blood cells; nerve damage.
  Vitamin K. Poor wound healing may occur because of the role in blood clotting.
  Thiamine. Impairment of cardiovascular, nervous, and gastrointestinal systems.
  Riboflavin. Magenta tongue, angular stomatitis, and cheilosis.
  Niacin. Dermatitis, diarrhea, depression, and (sometimes) death.
  Folic Acid. Decrease in number of all types of blood cells; large red blood cells.
  Vitamin B6. Convulsions in infants; anemias; nerve and skin disorders.
  Vitamin B12. Pernicious anemia and other anemias; poor vision; some psychiatric disorders.
  Biotin. Inflammation of the lips and skin.
  Vitamin C. Changes in oral cavity (gums, teeth), easy bruising. Anemia may also be a common finding with petechiae and circulatory problems. Delay in wound healing can occur.

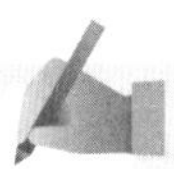

DIETARY AND NUTRITIONAL RECOMMENDATIONS

- Vitamin A deficiency. Use a diet including foods high in vitamin A and carotene: carrots, sweet potatoes, squash, apricots, collards, broccoli, cabbage, dark leafy greens, liver, kidney, cream, butter, and egg yolk.
- Vitamin D deficiency. Use fortified milk, fish liver oils, and egg yolks. Expose skin to sunlight if possible.
- Vitamin E deficiency. Use vegetable oil, wheat germ, leafy vegetables, egg yolks, margarine, and legumes.
- Vitamin K deficiency. Use a diet high in leafy vegetables, pork, liver, and vegetable oils.
- Thiamine deficiency or beriberi. Use a diet including foods high in thiamine: pork, whole grains, enriched cereal grains, nuts, potatoes, legumes, green vegetables, fish, meat, fruit, and milk in quantity. A high-protein/high-carbohydrate (CHO) intake should be included.
- Riboflavin deficiency. Use a diet including foods high in riboflavin: milk, eggs, liver, kidney, and heart. Caution against losses resulting from cooking and exposure to sunlight.
- Niacin deficiency or pellagra. Use a diet including foods high in niacin and other B vitamins: yeast, milk, meat, peanuts, cereal bran, and wheat germ.
- Folic acid deficiency. Use fresh, leafy green vegetables, fruits such as oranges and orange juice, liver and other organ meats, and dried yeast.
- Vitamin B6 deficiency. Use dried yeast, liver, organ meats, whole-grain cereals, fish, and legumes.

- Vitamin B12 deficiency. Use liver, beef, pork, organ meats, eggs, milk, and dairy products.
- Biotin deficiency. Use liver, kidney, egg yolks, yeast, cauliflower, nuts, and legumes.
- Pantothenic acid deficiency. Use live yeast and vegetables.
- Vitamin C deficiency or scurvy. Use a diet high in citrus fruits, tomatoes, strawberries, green peppers, cantaloupe, and baked potatoes.

PROFILE

Clinical/History

Height
Weight
BMI
Neurological changes
Signs of malnutrition (hair, eyes, skin, mouth, gums, tongue, teeth)

Lab Work

H&H, Serum Fe
Serum levels of specific nutrients (only as needed; they are costly)
Aspartate aminotransaminase (AST) (decreased in beriberi)

Common Drugs Used and Potential Side Effects

- Vitamin A. Absorption of vitamin A depends on bile salts in the intestinal tract. Also, beware of doses greater than 1,000–3,000 IU per kg body weight/day. This is especially true for children. Controlled 25,000 IU/day doses may be prescribed.
- Vitamin D. Calderol, Rocaltrol, Hytakerol, and Calciferol are common drug sources.
- Vitamin K. Vitamin K is usually injected to correct deficiency rather than using diet alone. Synkayvite, Mephyton, and Konakion are trade names.
- Thiamine. A common dose is 5–10 mg/day thiamine; anorexia and nausea may be common at the beginning of treatment. Intravenous therapy may be better tolerated.
- Riboflavin. Achlorhydria may precipitate a deficiency and may preclude successful correction. Alkaline substances destroy riboflavin.
- Niacin. Treatment with niacin may cause flushing. Niacinamide is a better choice. 200–400 mg niacin or niacin equivalents may be used. Nicotinic acid can cause nausea, vomiting, and diarrhea.
- Vitamin B6. Vita-Bee 6 is a pyridoxine hydrochloride drug.
- Vitamin C. Excesses can cause false–positive glucosuria tests. Cevalin or Cevita are drug sources. 50–300 mg/day may be given to correct scurvy. Excesses may have an antihistamine effect or cause diarrhea.
- Pantothenic acid. Pantholin is a drug that is prescribed as needed.

Herbs, Botanicals and Supplements

- Herbs and botanicals may be used; identify and monitor side effects.
- Counsel about use of herbal teas, especially regarding toxic substances.

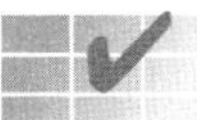

PATIENT EDUCATION

- ✓ Explain where sources of the specific nutrient may be found.
- ✓ Demonstrate methods of cooking, storage, etc. that prevent losses.
- ✓ Help the patient plan a menu incorporating his/her preferences.
- ✓ Discuss the use of vitamin and mineral supplements. About 40% of Americans take at least one vitamin or mineral supplement daily and another 20% take them occasionally (WebMD, visited 7/5/01). Though they may be appropriate to correct a deficiency state, they may not be warranted for continuous or long-term use.

For More Information

- American Heart Association—Vitamin Supplementation
  http://www.americanheart.org/Heart_and_Stroke_A_Z_Guide/vitamin.html
- Federation of American Societies for Experimental Biology
  http://faseb.org/ain/intro.html
- NIH Office of Dietary Supplements
  http://www.cc.nih.gov/ccc/supplements/intro.html
- Vitamin Nutrition Information Service
  Hoffman-LaRoche Inc.
  Nutley, NJ 07110
  (201) 909-8470
- U.S. Department of Health and Human Services
  200 Independence Ave. SW
  Washington, DC 20201
  877-696-6775
  http://www.dhhs.gov/

FOOD ALLERGY

NUTRITIONAL ACUITY RANKING: LEVEL 2 (SIMPLE); LEVEL 3 (COMPLEX)

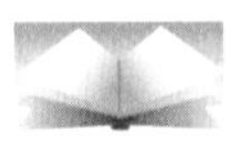

DEFINITIONS AND BACKGROUND

True food allergy is an immune response, generally from immunoglobulin E (IgE); a reaction usually occurs within 2 hours. Immediate (1 minute–2 hours) or delayed reactions (2–48 hours) may occur. A food allergy results from hypersensitivity to an antigen of food source (usually protein). The manifestations of the allergy are caused by the release of histamine and serotonin. It is important to distinguish intolerances caused by toxins, drugs, or metabolic disorders (such as lactase deficiency) from true food allergy (American Gastroenterological Association, 2001).

Ingestion is the principal route for food allergens, yet some highly sensitive individuals may also react through skin contact or inhalation (Tan et al., 2001). Over 90% of food allergies are caused by eight foods—egg, milk, wheat, soy, fish, shellfish, peanuts, and tree nuts. Children with atopic dermatitis could have a food allergy that can be diagnosed using a skin prick test. These 8 foods account for about 89% of the positive food challenge responses; skin prick tests can identify 99% of the patients with a food allergy (Burks et al., 1998). Cow's milk formulas and cow milk allergies (CMA) are becoming progressively more common; children with CMA can get adequate nutrition through a hypoallergenic substitute (Cantani, 1999). Casein is the major allergen in CMA.

Allergic tendencies are inherited but not necessarily to a specific antigen (i.e., a parent with a genetic predisposition to severe bee sting reactions could have a child with a food or other allergy). People who have a tendency toward allergy may develop sensitivity to new foods. Approximately 6% of children younger than age 3 and 1.5% of the general population have true food allergies; about 4 million people suffer from allergies (FDA, 2001). Careful clinical history, diagnostic studies, endoscopy, or biopsy may be needed. The main therapy remains avoidance of incriminating foods and education to deal with inadvertent exposures. Treatment strategies include use of plasmid DNA vaccines to treat these disorders (Sampson, 1997).

The most common symptoms (70%) of food allergies are gastrointestinal: diarrhea, nausea, vomiting, cramping, and abdominal distention and pain; 24% of results are skin-related, 4% are respiratory, and 2% involve other systemic responses. Oral allergy syndrome (OAS) may occur from eating tomatoes and some other vegetables. Patients with OAS may react against stable allergens (lipid transfer proteins) that are shared by botanically unrelated fruits such as nuts, peanuts, legumes, tomato, and plum (Asero, 1999).

The greatest danger in food allergy comes from anaphylaxis, a violent allergic reaction that involves many parts of the body. Anaphylaxis occurs after a person is exposed to an allergen after being sensitized by a previous exposure. Peanuts, tree nuts, shellfish, milk, eggs, and fish are the most common causes; even miniscule amounts of the offending food have caused deaths. A nonallergic reaction may occur from spoiled fish, which tends to be high in histamine and may cause a reaction similar to anaphylaxis. Histamine appears to play a role in chronic idiopathic urticaria (CIU), or hives. Persons with CIU may have a subclinical impairment of small bowel enterocyte function that could induce higher sensitivity to histamine-producing foods (Guida et al., 2000).

Nutritional consequences of food allergy by allergen are listed in Table 2–6.

OBJECTIVES

- Exclude or avoid the offending allergen. If it is not known, use an elimination diet to discover the cause. Rotation diets are not effective and are potentially dangerous.
- Monitor the onset of the reaction, which may be delayed or immediate. If delayed, the onset of the reaction may take from several hours to as long as 5 days. An imme-

TABLE 2–6 Major Food Allergens and Nutritional Consequences

Most Common:

Milk. Check for deficiencies in protein, riboflavin, calcium, and vitamins A and D. Be wary of early introduction of cow's milk in infancy.

Eggs. Check for iron deficiency. Egg albumin is used in marshmallows, frozen dinners, and many other food mixes. Yolks are generally tolerated.

Wheat. Check for B vitamins and iron. Read labels on packaged soups and sauces.

Fish. Other protein sources will be needed.

Shellfish (e.g., crab, lobster, shrimp). Protein and omega-3 fatty acids will be needed from other sources.

Soy. Protein and other nutrients may be needed from other sources. Read labels for lecithin and other soy additives.

Tree Nuts. Avoid nut butters also. Aflatoxins can cause an allergic-like reaction.

Peanuts. Protein and other nutrients will be needed from other sources in the diet.

Less Common:

Spices. Sesame is a fairly common allergen.

Sulfites. Foods such as wine, beers, dried fruits and vegetables, maraschino cherries, and dried or frozen potatoes may contain sulfites. Although not an IgE-mediated allergic response and thus not a true food allergen, sulfites can produce life-threatening reactions similar to the major food allergens. To help sulfite-sensitive people avoid problems, FDA requires the presence of sulfites in processed foods to be declared on the label and prohibits the use of sulfites on fresh produce intended to be sold or served raw to consumers (FDA Consumer at http://vm.cfsan.fda.gov/~dms/wh-alrg1.html).

Artificial food dyes. Many foods and prescription or over-the-counter drugs contain tartrazine (FD&C Yellow No. 5). This may cause itching or hives in sensitive individuals.

diate response is more common with raw foods; patient history may include diarrhea, urticaria, eczema, rhinitis, and asthma.

- Treat nutritional deficiencies or ensure adequate supplementation.
- For patients with asthma, use a normal diet with small meals. Nothing should be eaten after dinner, to lessen GI reflux. (See the Asthma entry in Section 5.)
- Keep food diaries to track reactions to food.
- Ensure extensive nutrition counseling and health education with food allergies to avoid nutrient deficiencies and unnecessary restrictions and to prevent reactions.
- Breastfeeding (BF) should be promoted for primary prevention of allergic infants (Isolauri et al., 1999).

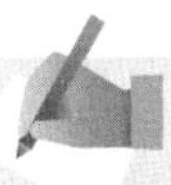

DIETARY AND NUTRITIONAL RECOMMENDATIONS

- For the elimination diet, use an unflavored elemental diet as a hypoallergenic base to which other foods are added as test challenges. Foods that seldom cause an allergic reaction and may be used readily include apples, artichokes, carrots, gelatin, lamb, lettuce, peaches, pears, and rice.
- Read labels of foods prepared for the patient. Check all menus served to the patient. Monitor food preparation methods to exclude possible cross contact with the allergen.
- Monitor nutrient needs specific for the patient's age.
- The most common allergens in infants are eggs, wheat, milk, and fish. For children, cow's milk, eggs, soy, peanuts, wheat, tree nuts, and fish are often a problem. For adults, common allergens include shellfish, peanuts, and tree nuts. Peanuts are implicated in approximately one-third of all cases of anaphylaxis; be aware of the use of peanut oil in foods. See Table 2–7.
- For infants, exclusive breastfeeding is best (American Academy of Pediatrics, 2000). Breast milk generally is nonallergenic.
- Mothers may need to omit cow's milk from their own diets, as well as eggs, fish, and nuts. Infants with CMA may exhibit eczema, rhinorrhea, abdominal pain, diarrhea, and otitis media appearing from 2–80 hours after their mothers have drunk cow's milk (Jarvinen et al., 1999). Infants who are allergic to cow's milk and soy may need Nutramigen or another hydrolyzed formula.

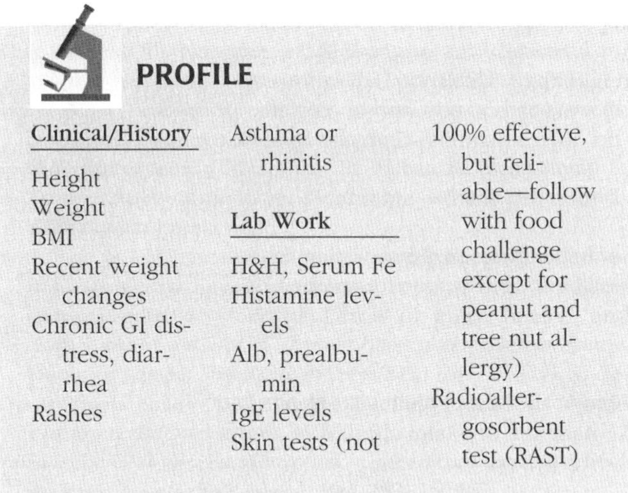

PROFILE

Clinical/History

Height
Weight
BMI
Recent weight changes
Chronic GI distress, diarrhea
Rashes
Asthma or rhinitis

Lab Work

H&H, Serum Fe
Histamine levels
Alb, prealbumin
IgE levels
Skin tests (not 100% effective, but reliable—follow with food challenge except for peanut and tree nut allergy)
Radioallergosorbent test (RAST)

Common Drugs Used and Potential Side Effects

- Benadryl should be taken with food. Dry mouth, constipation, or GI distress is a potential side effect.
- Atarax (Vistaril) is an antihistamine that reduces swelling and itching. Dry mouth or nausea is a common side effect.
- Injectable epinephrine is a synthetic version of a naturally occurring adrenaline and should be carried by those who are prone to allergic reactions to food and other allergens. An Epi-Pen provides a single dose; the Ana-Kit provides two doses.

TABLE 2–7 Food Processing Concerns

The food industry has taken steps to address the needs of food allergic consumers, including changes to manufacturing processes to reduce the potential for cross contact with major food allergens. Under existing good manufacturing practice (GMP) regulations, reasonable precautions must be taken to prevent cross contact with major allergenic proteins. In instances when cross contact cannot be avoided, even when complying, food and ingredient manufacturers use labeling that informs the food allergic consumer of the possible presence of allergens in the food. Food manufacturers label the ingredients in their products in accordance with existing regulatory requirements. The Food Allergy Issues Alliance has set Food Allergen Labeling Guidelines (http://www.nfpa-food.org/science/FoodAllergenLabelingGuidelines.htm)

Most oils used in food processing and for sale to the public contain no protein and are extracted from the oilseed or nut using solvents and then are degummed, refined, bleached, and deodorized. Some oils are mechanically extracted (cold pressed) and left unrefined to purposely maintain the flavor; these oils may contain protein and be allergenic. Of the 8 commonly allergenic foods, peanuts, soybeans, and tree nuts are used as oil sources. In the U.S., virtually all oils made from allergenic sources are solvent-extracted and refined. The level of protein needed to cause an allergic reaction is unknown and may vary between individuals. The majority of well-performed studies support the position that refined oils are safe for consumption by food-allergic individuals (Hefle and Taylor, 1999).

Herbs, Botanicals and Supplements

- Food/plant sensitivities are common (e.g., melon/ragweed, apple/birch, wheat/grasses). Be wary of herbal teas.
- Bee pollen does not prevent allergies and may, in fact, cause asthma, urticaria, rhinitis, or anaphylaxis after eating plants that cross-react with ragweed, such as sunflowers or dandelion greens.
- Other herbs and botanicals may be used; identify and monitor side effects. For allergies: garlic, stinging nettle, gingko, chamomile, and feverfew have been proposed for use, but no long-term studies prove efficacy. For hives: jewelweed, parsley, ginger, stinging nettle, and amaranth have been suggested but not studied for effectiveness.
- Counsel about use of herbal teas, especially regarding toxic substances.

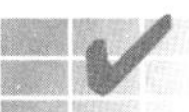

PATIENT EDUCATION

- ✓ Encourage the patient to keep a food diary and to read all labels every time a food is purchased and used.
- ✓ Persons with a milk allergy can add vanilla or other flavorings to soy milk.
- ✓ Explain to patients taking goat's milk that it has less lactalbumin, vitamin D, and folacin than cow's milk and that supplements may be required. Some people may also be allergic to goat's milk, so caution must be used.
- ✓ Persons with milk allergy can receive sufficient calcium from greens, broccoli, clams, oysters, shrimp, and salmon. Calcium supplementation may also be warranted.
- ✓ Recipe books are available from formula companies, food manufacturers, the Food Allergy and Anaphylaxis Network, and from registered dietitians.
- ✓ Cytotoxic testing, sublingual provocative tests, pulse tests, kinesiologic testing, yeast hypersensitivity, and brain allergy theories should be dismissed entirely.
- ✓ Early infection may protect against allergies in later life (Kramer et al., 1999).
- ✓ For **Latex Allergy:** Natural rubber latex contains more than 35 proteins that may be related to Type IgE-mediated allergy (Perkin, 2000). Latex-specific IgF may be responsible. Cross-reactivity has been documented with banana, avocado, potato, sweet pepper, kiwi, and chestnuts; less concern with papaya, watermelon, pineapple, and figs. Individuals with latex allergy also tend to report food allergies, including fish and shellfish (Kim and Hussain, 1999). Children with atopic dermatitis are a high-risk group for latex sensitization. Increasing age, additional sensitization to ubiquitous inhaled allergens, and enhanced total serum IgE values seem to be important variables for latex sensitization and further sensitization to the latex-associated foods (Tucke et al., 1999).
- ✓ After reviewing scientific studies, FDA determined in 1981 that aspartame is not allergenic and is safe for use in foods; those persons with phenylketonuria (PKU) should not use it because it is made from phenylalanine (http://vm.cfsan.fda.gov).
- ✓ Corn allergy, although rare, may be severe. Studies are on going at Tulane University (http://www.foodallergy.org/.)
- ✓ Schools need to educate their entire staff, improve prevention and avoidance measures, make sure epinephrine is readily available and that the staff knows how to administer it, and use consumer agency resources. Students should be encouraged to wear a Medic-Alert bracelet.
- ✓ For genetically modified (GM) foods, possible allergenicity of expressed proteins is evaluated by comparison of their amino acid sequence with that of known allergens and determination of their stability to digestion and food processing (Martens, 2000).
- ✓ Some individuals have headaches and relate them to monosodium glutamate or "Chinese Restaurant Syndrome." See Table 2–8.

For More Information

- ✦ American Academy of Allergy, Asthma, and Immunology
  85 West Algonquin Road, Suite 550
  Arlington Heights, IL 60005
  800-822-2762
  http://www.aaaai.org/
  Food Allergy: http://allergy.mcg.edu/Advice/foods.html
- ✦ American College of Allergy, Asthma, and Immunology
  http://www.acaai.org/
- ✦ The Asthma and Allergy Foundation of America
  1233 20th St., NW, Suite 402
  Washington, DC 20036
  800-7-ASTHMA
  http://www.aafa.org/
- ✦ Food Allergy and Anaphylaxis Network
  http://www.foodallergy.org/
- ✦ Food Allergies Database
  http://allergyadvisor.com/

TABLE 2–8 Glutamate, MSG, and "Chinese Restaurant Syndrome"

Glutamate, a nonessential amino acid, has a role as a neurotransmitter with intracellular nitrogen transfer reactions being a major action (Fernstrom and Garattini, 2000). Glutamate is found naturally in foods such as tomatoes and cheeses. It is also released in protein hydrolysis during meat and fish stock or soup preparation or added to foods in crystalline form as MSG. MSG, which is 14% sodium, is used as a flavor enhancer. The flavor contributed by MSG is different from that provided by sweet, salty, bitter, or sour foods; it is called "umami." Glutamate helps to stimulate the vagus nerve and helps to facilitate digestion and nutrient absorption (Fermstrom and Garattini, 2000). Dietary glutamate is also a major energy source for the intestines and placenta. The brain is well protected against a flux of glutamate, and it is not toxic. Adverse reactions have been reported but not confirmed in double-blind studies.

Chinese restaurant syndrome—Sensitivity to MSG has been suspected to be the cause of "Chinese restaurant syndrome," which causes a temporary burning sensation in the neck and forearms, chest tightness, and headache. In double-blind studies no adverse reactions were seen from MSG given with food (Geha et al., 2000).

- Food and Nutrition Information Center
  National Agricultural Library/USDA
  10301 Baltimore Avenue, Room 304
  Beltsville, MD 20705-2351
  http://www.nal.usda.gov/fnic/pubs/bibs/gen/allergy.htm
- FDA Consumer –Food allergy page
  http://vm.cfsan.fda.gov/~dms/wh-alrg1.html
- International Food Information Council Foundation
  1100 Connecticut Avenue, NW, Suite 430
  Washington, DC 20036
  http://ific.org
- Mayo Clinic
  http://mayohealth.org
- National Food Processors Association
  http://www.nfpa-food.org/
- National Institute on Allergy and Infectious Diseases
  http://www.niaid.nih.gov/

MIGRAINE HEADACHE AND VASCULAR RESPONSES

NUTRITIONAL ACUITY RANKING: LEVEL 2

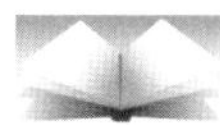

DEFINITIONS AND BACKGROUND

Migraine involves paroxysmal attacks of headache, vasospasm, and increased coagulation, often preceded by visual disturbances. Approximately 8% of the population is affected.

Investigators now believe that migraine is caused by inherited abnormalities in certain cell populations in the brain (http://www.ninds.nih.gov/health_and_medical/pubs/migraine update.htm). Using new imaging technologies, scientists can see changes in the brain during migraine attacks; they believe there is a migraine pain center located in the brainstem. As neurons fire, surrounding blood vessels dilate and become inflamed, causing the characteristic pain of a migraine.

Low blood levels of serotonin may bring on migraine attacks. 5-Hydroxytryptamine (5-HT) is also thought to be involved in migraine headache (Hoel et al., 2001). A drop in serotonin or estrogen or use of vasodilators (found in some foods) may cause blood vessels to swell and may contribute to migraines in sensitive individuals. Reactions are often within 24 hours after an implicated food has been consumed. Nausea, vomiting, and acute sensitivity to light or sound may occur. Vascular-amine toxicity causes a rapid increase in blood pressure when high-tyramine foods such as cheese, wine, beer, chocolate, and bananas are eaten in combination with medications such as MAO inhibitors; death may even result (Young and Buchbinder, 1995).

Lack of food or sleep, exposure to light, anxiety, stress, fatigue, or hormonal irregularities in women can set off a migraine attack in individuals with the disorder. Exercise, relaxation, biofeedback, and other therapies designed to help limit discomfort have a role in migraine treatment.

OBJECTIVES

- Eliminate stressors and other triggers, such as crowds, bright lights, and noises, at vulnerable times.
- Reduce or eliminate use of foods that cause migraines in sensitive individuals.
- Encourage adequate meal spacing to prevent fasting or skipping of meals.

DIETARY AND NUTRITIONAL RECOMMENDATIONS

- Promote regular mealtimes and adequate relaxation.
- Magnesium and fish oil capsules have been recommended for some cases, especially to curb onset quickly.
- Monitor for cross-reactivity in foods, even if never eaten before.
- Methyl-xanthine toxicity may occur in sensitive individuals. For some people, caffeine and theobromine in coffee, tea, chocolate, and cocoa may cause symptoms such as migraine-like headaches (Young and Buchbinder, 1995). For others, use of caffeine (130 mg) may help to reduce migraines. It is an individual response.
- Omit trigger foods if identified; see Table 2–9.

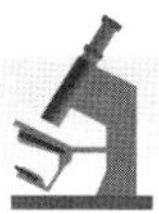

PROFILE

Clinical/History		Lab Work
Headache symptoms and duration	History of similar reactions	Histamine
Foods eaten in past 24 hours	Recent illnesses	PT
		Na+, K+
		Ca++, Mg++

Common Drugs Used and Potential Side Effects

- Medicines can be used to relieve pain and restore function during attacks. The most promising of these are drugs called *triptans*. Drugs such as eletriptan, naratriptan, rizatriptan, sumatriptan, and zolmitriptan may be used to enhance the effects of serotonin.
- For some women suffering from migraines, hormone therapy may help.
- If sedatives, tranquilizers, antidepressants, and diuretics are used, alter diet accordingly.

TABLE 2–9 Foods Implicated in Various Types of Headaches

- ✦ Histamine-containing foods—scombroid or spiny-finned fish such as tuna, mackerel, or mahi-mahi (Young and Buchbinder, 1995)
- ✦ Fermented foods—chicken livers, aged cheese such as cheddar, red wine, pickled herring, chocolate, broad beans, and beer contain tyramine
- ✦ Alcohol—champagne and red wine contain both phenols and tyramine; sulfites may also be involved as a trigger
- ✦ Hot dogs, bacon, ham, and salami—contain sodium nitrate and also may contain tyramine
- ✦ Coffee, tea, and cola—can trigger caffeine-withdrawal headache from methyl xanthines (18 hours after withdrawal); taper withdrawal gradually
- ✦ Chocolate—contains phenylethylamine
- ✦ Nuts—some contain vasodilators

- Capsaicin from hot chili peppers may eventually be used as a source of relief for cluster headache pain.
- If effective medicines are not found to treat headache with its onset, daily preventive medicines are sometimes used: anticonvulsants, beta-blockers, calcium channel blockers, NSAIDS, tricyclic antidepressants, and serotonergic agents (http://www.achenet.org/women/menst/prevent.php). Propanolol (Inderal) and calcium channel blockers such as verapamil and diltiazem may be used; constipation is one possible side effect.
- An older remedy, Cafergot (ergotamine) contains 100 mg of caffeine per tablet. It can cause nausea, vomiting, drowsiness, edema, high blood pressure, or vertigo in some individuals.

Herbs, Botanicals and Supplements

- Feverfew may have some usefulness. Side effects include decreased platelet aggregation if used with warfarin, aspirin, and ticlopidine. Nonsteroidal anti-inflammatory drugs (e.g., ibuprofen, indomethacin, etc.) decrease the herb's anti-inflammatory action; do not use together.
- Food/plant sensitivities may exist (e.g., melon/ragweed, carrot/potato, apple/birch, wheat/grasses). Monitor herbal products.
- Bee pollen does not prevent allergies and may, in fact, cause asthma, urticaria, rhinitis, or anaphylaxis after eating plants that cross-react with ragweed, such as sunflowers or dandelion greens.
- Other herbs and botanicals may be used; identify and monitor side effects. Evening primrose, red pepper, willow, and ginger have been recommended but no studies prove efficacy.
- Counsel about use of herbal teas, especially regarding toxic substances.
- Omega-3 fatty acids are being studied for their effect on migraines.

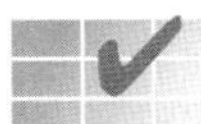

PATIENT EDUCATION

- ✓ Teach the importance of not skipping meals because fasting can increase likelihood of a headache. Regular mealtimes are important.
- ✓ Teach the patient how to keep an accurate food diary if food sensitivities are implicated. Read food labels. Avoid packaged items containing foods that are problematic.
- ✓ Monitor drugs taken in correlation with headache sensitivity.
- ✓ Investigate underlying conditions such as hypertension, glaucoma, and eye and ear problems.
- ✓ Psychotherapy may be useful for emotional distress.

For More Information

- ✦ American Council for Headache Education
  800-255-ACHE
  http://www.achenet.org
- ✦ American Headache Society
  856-423-0043
  http://www.ahsnet.org
- ✦ Migraine Information Center
  http://www.ama-assn.org/special/migraine/migraine.htm
- ✦ National Headache Foundation
  888-643-5552
  http://www.headaches.org/
- ✦ National Institute of Neurological Disorders and Stroke—Brain Resources and Information Network
  http://www.ninds.nih.gov

MÉNIÈRE'S SYNDROME

NUTRITIONAL ACUITY RANKING: LEVEL 1

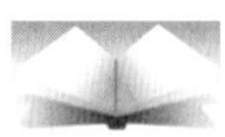

DEFINITIONS AND BACKGROUND

A rare disease of unknown origin, Ménière's syndrome affects the inner ear and causes disturbed balance. Signs and symptoms include rapid onset, recurrent deafness, tinnitus with roaring sensation, vertigo, nausea and vomiting, and blurred vision. Patient may have a history of otitis media, smoking, allergies, leukemia, or atherosclerosis. Attacks may last from a few hours to several days. Vertigo causes disability in many patients with Ménière's disease and may be the result of the effects of endolymphatic hydrops on the semicircular canals.

Sodium restriction and diuretic treatment response are correlated to clinical measures of Ménière's disease (Devaiah and Ator, 2000). Patients with possible Ménière's disease should be treated with aggressive medical therapy to prevent disease progression.

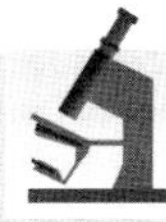

PROFILE

Clinical/History		
Height	Temp	IgE
Weight	BP	H&H
BMI	**Lab Work**	Alb
Known allergies	Chol, Triglycerides (TG)	Electrocochleography

OBJECTIVES

- Correct nausea and vomiting; replace any necessary electrolytes.
- Avoid or decrease edema.
- Decrease fluid retention, which can aggravate an attack.
- Omit any known food allergens from the diet.

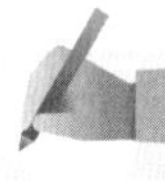

DIETARY AND NUTRITIONAL RECOMMENDATIONS

- Low-sodium diet, as tolerated, may be necessary.
- Restrict fluid to reduce pressure on the labyrinth, unless contraindicated for other reasons (such as history of dehydration).
- Use supplements and foods that are nutrient dense. Intakes of vitamins A and C, riboflavin, and niacin may have been low.
- Provide a diet that is free of known allergens and is specific for the individual.

Common Drugs Used and Potential Side Effects

- Diuretics are used to reduce edema in the ear.
- Anticholinergics such as atropine or epinephrine may be used. Cardiac output is increased through an increased heart rate.
- Diazepam (Valium) may cause nausea, fatigue, and other effects. Limit caffeine.
- Antihistamines may be used. Antivert (Meclizine HCl) is an antihistamine that helps with dizziness. Dry mouth may result.
- Vasodilators may be used to dilate the blood vessels.

Herbs, Botanicals and Supplements

- Herbs and botanicals may be used; identify and monitor side effects. For earache: ephedra, goldenseal, forsythia, gentian, garlic, honeysuckle, and Echinacea are sometimes recommended but have not been proven as effective. For tinnitus: black cohosh, sesame, goldenseal, and spinach have been suggested; no long-term studies are on record that prove effectiveness; one study in England proved that gingko biloba is not effective for tinnitus, but audiometry was not used as a valid assessment. More studies are needed.
- Counsel about use of herbal teas, especially regarding toxic substances.

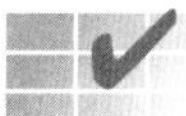

PATIENT EDUCATION

- Discuss how a balanced diet can affect general health status.
- Discuss sources of sodium and hidden ingredients that could aggravate the condition.

FOOD-BORNE ILLNESS (FOOD POISONING)

NUTRITIONAL ACUITY RANKING: LEVEL 1 (PREVENTIVE COUNSELING) LEVEL 2 (CORRECTIVE THERAPY)

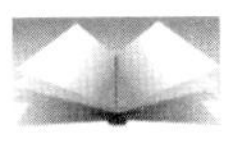

DEFINITIONS AND BACKGROUND

True cases of food-borne illness are gastrointestinal insults or infections/intoxications resulting from contaminated beverages or food. Millions of cases occur annually, but only a few hundred are reported. There are thousands of related deaths annually.

The Centers for Disease Control reported that during 1993–1997, a total of 2,751 outbreaks of food-borne disease were reported; they caused a reported 86,058 persons to become ill (Olsen et al., 2000). In this same report, it was noted that bacterial pathogens caused the largest percentage of outbreaks (75%); *Salmonella enteritidis* accounted for the largest number of outbreaks, cases, and deaths, mostly attributed to eating eggs. Chemical agents caused 17% of outbreaks and 1% of cases; viruses, 6% of outbreaks and 8% of cases; and parasites, 2% of outbreaks and 5% of cases. In addition, multistate outbreaks caused by contaminated produce and outbreaks caused by *Escherichia coli* O157:H7 remained prominent.

Pathogens often transmitted via food contaminated by infected food handlers are *Salmonella typhi* and other species, *Shigella, Staphylococcus aureus, Streptococcus pyogenes,* hepatitis A virus, and Norwalk viruses (Ollinger-Snyder and Matthews, 1996). *Listeria* and *E. coli* O157:H7 are also important sources from food handling. Salads are often sources of *Shigella; Staph aureus* may occur from nose and throat. Moist, high-protein foods and salty, cooked foods are often sources of *Staphylococcus* outbreaks. Milk, eggs, and meat are often sources of *Strep pyogenes*. Personal hygiene is one of the most important steps in food safety.

An outbreak is when two or more individuals develop the same symptoms over the same time period. Infants and children younger than age 6, people with chronic illnesses (such as AIDS or cancer), pregnant women, and elderly individuals are most at risk. Nausea, vomiting, diarrhea, abdominal cramping, vision problems, fever, chills, dizziness, and headaches may occur. Some people attribute their symptoms mistakenly to "flu."

Although sanitation and Hazard Analysis and Critical Control Points program (HACCP) share the common goal of producing safe food products, the focus of sanitation is on the environment surrounding the food to prevent contamination, whereas HACCP focuses on controlling hazards intrinsic to food materials. An integrated system has a better chance of controlling all hazards than either system by itself (Setiabuhdi et al., 1997).

Common types of food-borne illnesses in the U.S. are described in Table 2–10.

TABLE 2–10 Types of Food-Borne Illness http://www.cdc.gov/health/diseases.htm

Campylobacter. Diarrhea (often bloody), fever, and abdominal cramping are the key symptoms within 2–5 days after exposure. It may be acquired by drinking raw milk or by eating raw or undercooked meat, shellfish, or poultry. Some people develop antibodies to it, but others do not. In persons with compromised immune systems, *Campylobacter* occasionally spreads to the bloodstream and causes a serious life-threatening infection. Some people may have arthritis following campylobacteriosis. Others may develop a rare disease, Guillain-Barré syndrome, that affects the nerves of the body beginning several weeks after the diarrheal illness, can lead to paralysis that lasts several weeks and usually requires intensive care. It is estimated that approximately one in every 1,000 reported campylobacteriosis cases leads to Guillain-Barré syndrome; 40% of Guillain-Barré syndrome cases in this country may be triggered by campylobacteriosis. To prevent exposure, avoid raw milk and cook all meats and poultry thoroughly. It is safest to drink only pasteurized milk. The bacteria may also be found in tofu or raw vegetables. Handwashing is important for prevention; wash hands with soap before handling raw foods of animal origin, after handling raw foods of animal origin, and before touching anything else. Prevent cross contamination in the kitchen. Proper refrigeration and sanitation are also essential.

Clostridium botulinum. Symptoms of botulism are related to muscle paralysis caused by the bacterial toxin: double or blurred vision, drooping eyelids, slurred speech, difficulty swallowing, dry mouth, and muscle weakness. Infants with botulism appear lethargic, feed poorly, are constipated, and have a weak cry and poor muscle tone. If untreated, these symptoms may progress to cause paralysis of the arms, legs, trunk, and respiratory muscles; long-term ventilator support may be needed. In food-borne botulism, symptoms generally begin 18–36 hours after eating contaminated food but can occur as early as 6 hours or as late as 10 days. Food-borne botulism is often caused by home-canned foods with low acid content, such as asparagus, green beans, beets, and corn. Outbreaks have occurred from more unusual sources such as chopped garlic in oil, chile peppers, tomatoes, improperly handled baked potatoes wrapped in aluminum foil, and home-canned or fermented fish. Persons who do home canning should follow strict hygienic procedures to reduce contamination of foods. Oils infused with garlic or herbs should be refrigerated. Potatoes that have been baked while wrapped in aluminum foil should be kept hot until served or refrigerated. Because high temperatures destroy the botulism toxin, persons who eat home-canned foods should boil the food for 10 minutes before eating. Throw out bulging, leaking, or dented cans and jars that are leaking. Safe home canning can be obtained from county extension services or from the U.S. Department of Agriculture. Honey can contain spores of *Clostridium botulinum* and has been a source of infection for infants; children younger than 12-months-old should not be fed honey.

(continued)

TABLE 2–10 Types of Food-Borne Illness http://www.cdc.gov/health/diseases.htm (*Continued*)

Clostridium perfringens. Symptoms include nausea with vomiting, diarrhea, and signs of acute gastroenteritis lasting 1 day. Illness usually results within 6–24 hours from the ingestion of canned meats, contaminated dried mixes, gravy, stews, refried beans, meat products, and unwashed vegetables. Leftovers must be reheated properly or discarded. Thorough cooking is also important.

Cryptosporidium parvum. This is a protozoan cause of diarrhea among immunocompromised patients. Watery stools, diarrhea, nausea, vomiting, slight fever, and stomach cramps often result. Symptoms generally begin 2–10 days after being infected. Handwashing is important.

Escherichia coli:O157:H7. This causes painful, bloody diarrhea, usually from undercooked ground beef and meats, from unprocessed apple cider, or from unwashed fruits and vegetables. It has even been found in water sources. Onset is slow, usually approximately 3–8 days after the meal. Antibiotics are not used because they spread the toxin further. The condition may progress to hemolytic anemia, thrombocytopenia, and acute renal failure requiring dialysis and transfusions. HUS can be fatal, especially in young children. To avoid the condition, cook meats thoroughly, use only pasteurized milk, and wash all produce well. There are several outbreaks each year, particularly from catering operations, church events, and family picnics. *Escherichia coli* O157:H7 survival in acid foods such as unpasteurized apple cider and fermented sausage is well documented; researchers have determined that *E. coli* O157:H7 can survive in refrigerated acid foods for weeks (Mayerhauser, 2001).

Listeria monocytogenes. Symptoms include mild fever, headache, vomiting, and severe illness in pregnancy; sepsis in the immunocompromised patient; meningoencephalitis in infants; and febrile gastroenteritis in adults. Lm is found in processed, ready-to-eat products such as hot dogs, lunchmeats, and some dairy products. Postpasteurization contamination of soft cheeses such as feta or Brie, milk, and commercial coleslaw has also been implicated. Cross contamination between food surfaces has also been a problem. Onset is 2–30 days, and the condition may be fatal. Use pasteurized milk and cheeses; wash produce before use. Reheat foods to proper temperatures. Wash hands with hot, soapy water after handling these ready-to-eat foods. Discard foods by their expiration dates. Caution must be used by pregnant women, who may pass the infection on to their unborn child (Wotecki, 2001).

Salmonella. There are many different kinds of *Salmonella* bacteria. *Salmonella typhimurium* and *Salmonella enteritidis* are the most common in the United States. Most people infected with *Salmonella* develop diarrhea, fever, and abdominal cramps 12–72 hours after infection; it usually lasts 4–7 days. Most people recover without treatment, but some have diarrhea that is so severe that the patient needs to be hospitalized. This patient must be treated promptly with antibiotics. The elderly, infants, and those with impaired immune systems are more likely to have a severe illness. This type of food-borne illness is usually caused by ingestion of raw or undercooked meat, poultry, fish, eggs, or unpasteurized dairy products. Fruits and raw vegetables may also be sources (be wary of melons and sprouts). Salmonella reacts within 8–48 hours and can be prevented by thorough cooking, proper sanitation, and hygiene.

Shigellosis. This is caused by a group of bacteria called *Shigella.* Most who are infected with *Shigella* develop bloody diarrhea, fever, and stomach cramps starting a day or two after they are exposed to the bacterium. Shigellosis usually resolves in 5–7 days but may be severe in young children and the elderly. Severe infection with high fever may be associated with seizures in children younger than 2-years-old. Milk and dairy products may be sources. Cold mixed salads such as egg, tuna, chicken, potato, and meat salads should also be suspect. Proper cooking, reheating, and maintenance of holding temperatures should aid in prevention; careful handwashing is essential.

Staphylococcus aureus. Meat, pork, eggs, poultry, tuna salad, prepared salads, gravy, and stuffing are often sources. *Staphylococcus* poisoning begins within 1–6 hours but is rarely fatal. Cooking does not destroy the toxin. Proper handling and hygiene are crucial for prevention. Refrigerate foods promptly during preparation and after meal service.

Vibrio vulnificus. This is a bacterium in the same family as those that cause cholera; it yields a Norwalk-like virus, symptoms of vomiting, diarrhea, or both. The illness is mild, with symptoms lasting 12–48 hours. Incubation is 31 hours average after eating seafood, especially raw clams and oysters, that has been contaminated with human pathogens. It may be fatal in immunocompromised individuals. Although oysters can only be harvested legally from waters free from fecal contamination, even these can be contaminated with *V. vulnificus* because the bacterium is naturally present.

Yersinia enterocolitica. Yersiniosis is an infectious disease caused by the bacterium *Yersinia.* In the United States, most human illness is caused *Y. enterocolitica.* Infection with *Y. enterocolitica* occurs most often in young children. Common symptoms in children are fever, abdominal pain, and diarrhea, which is often bloody. Symptoms typically develop 4–7 days after exposure and may last 1–3 weeks or longer. In older children and adults, right-sided abdominal pain and fever may be the predominant symptoms and may be confused with appendicitis. In a small proportion of cases, complications such as skin rash, joint pains, or spread of bacteria to the bloodstream can occur. Infection is most often acquired by eating contaminated food, especially raw or undercooked pork products (e.g., chitterlings). Postpasteurization contamination of chocolate milk, reconstituted dry milk, pasteurized milk, and tofu are also high-risk foods. Cold storage does not kill the bacteria. Onset is 1–7 days after consumption. Cook meats thoroughly; use only pasteurized milk. Proper handwashing is also important.

OBJECTIVES

- Allow the GI tract to rest after rehydration.
- Progress as tolerated.
- Prepare and store all foods using safe food-handling practices and good personal hygiene. Temperatures should be maintained below 40° or above 140° for safe handling, storage, and holding.
- Teach the importance of handwashing, care of food contact surfaces, and insect or rodent extermination. Sanitize all surfaces before food preparation; sanitize after each food item is prepared when using the same surface (e.g., cutting boards and slicers). See Table 2–11.

DIETARY AND NUTRITIONAL RECOMMENDATIONS

- For patients with extreme diarrhea or vomiting, feed with intravenous glucose (NPO) until progress has been made.

TABLE 2–11 Food Safety Guidelines

- Cook foods thoroughly; cook beef to proper internal temperature of 160°, pork to 165°, and poultry to 175°. Monitor internal temperatures with an accurate food thermometer, placed correctly into the meat or poultry.
- Cook hamburger to the proper temperature of 165°. "If pink in the middle, it is cooked too little."
- Boil water used for drinking when necessary; hold at boiling temperature for 1 minute.
- Hold and serve foods at 140–165° during meal service.
- Reheat foods to at least 165°. Discard leftovers after the first reheating process.
- Keep hot foods above 140° and cold foods below 40°.
- Discard cooked foods that are left at room temperature more than 2 hours.
- Demonstrate safe food preparation techniques. For example, discard cracked eggs and reheat home-canned foods appropriately. In institutional settings, do not allow home cooked foods at all.
- Keep pet foods and utensils separate from those for human use.
- Use clean plates and separate utensils between raw and cooked foods.
- Sanitize work surfaces and sponges daily with a mild bleach solution (2 teaspoons per quart of water is sufficient). However, if a work surface comes into contact with raw food, it should be sanitized after contact with each food, just like cutting boards.
- Sanitize others after each food. Ideally, keep one board for poultry, another for meats, and another for produce to prevent cross contamination. Discard cutting boards that are badly damaged.
- Thaw meats and poultry properly—in the refrigerator, not at room temperature. If necessary, thaw in a sink with cold running water that allows continuous drainage or thaw quickly in the microwave and use immediately.
- Do not partially cook meat or poultry in advance of final preparation. Bacteria may still grow rampantly.
- Cool foods quickly in shallow pans (2–4 inches deep). Temperature should reach 70° within 2 hours. If food has not cooled to that level, place in the freezer for a short time. Then, wrap lightly and return to refrigerator.
- Reports of food-borne illness have been associated with oils and vinegars that have garlic, herbs, or other intact pieces in them related to growth of either aerobic or anaerobic bacteria entering from the flavoring agent.

Oral rehydration therapy may be a useful adjunct treatment in the recovery process.

- Start with bland or soft foods and then progress to a normal diet. Prolonged inability to eat orally may require tube feeding.

PROFILE

Clinical/History		
Height	Vomiting	symptoms after suspected meal
Weight	Diarrhea	
BMI	Nausea	**Lab Work**
Usual weight	Abdominal cramps	K+
Weight loss/ changes during illness	Temperature/ fever	Na+
	Timing of	Cl−

Common Drugs Used and Potential Side Effects

- Octreotide (Sandostatin) may be used, parenterally only. It may alter fat absorption and fat-soluble vitamin absorption.
- Paromycin, erythromycin, or a fluoroquinolone may be prescribed.
- For salmonella, ampicillin, gentamicin, trimethoprim/sulfamethoxazole, or ciprofloxacin may be used.
- *V. vulnificus* infection is treated with doxycycline or ceftazidime.

Herbs, Botanicals and Supplements

- Note that herbs and botanicals themselves could be a source of food-borne bacteria and thus exacerbate an existing food-borne infection. If herbs and botanicals are used, identify and monitor for potential contamination and side effects.
- Counsel about use of herbal teas, especially regarding toxic substances.

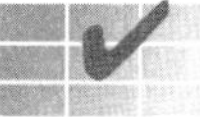

PATIENT EDUCATION

- ✓ Encourage safe methods of food handling.
- ✓ Discuss ways to prevent further episodes of food-borne illness. See Table 2–11 for food safety guidelines.
- ✓ Teach awareness that commercial mayonnaise, salad dressings, and sauces appear to be safe due to their content of acetic acid and lesser amounts of citric or lactic acids (Smittle, 2000).

For More Information

- American Dietetic Association Home Food Safety Program http://www.homefoodsafety.com/index.html/
- Food borne Diseases Active Surveillance Network CDC's Emerging Infections Program http://www.cdc.gov/foodnet/

- Food and Drug Administration
  Center for Food Safety & Applied Nutrition (CFSAN)
  200 C Street SW; Washington, DC 20204 USA
  http://www.cfsan.fda.gov/
- FDA Seafood Hotline:
  800-FDA-4010
- Fight BAC
  http://www.fightbac.org/
  http://www.pueblo.gsa.gov/cic_text/food/fight-back/fightbac.htm
- Federal USDA—Food Safety Research
  http://www.nal.usda.gov/fsrio/new/release.htm
- Government Food Safety Website
  http://www.foodsafety.gov/
- International Food Safety sites
  http://www.foodsafety.gov/˜7Efsg/fsgintl.html
- National Food Safety Database
  http://www.foodsafety.ufl.edu/index.html
- North Carolina State University
  http://www.ces.ncsu.edu/depts/foodsci/agentinfo/
- USDA Food borne Illness Education Information Center
  http://www.nal.usda.gov/fnic/foodborne/about.html
- USDA Meat & Poultry Hotline
  http://www.fsis.usda.gov/OA/programs/mphotlin.htm
- US Food Safety and Inspection Service (FSIS)
  http://www.fsis.usda.gov/
- Water Quality Association
  708-505-0160

REFERENCES

General Nutritional Practices, Cultural Issues, and Vegetarianism–Cited references

American Dietetic Association. *Ethnic and regional food practices: Indian and Pakistani food practices, customs, and holidays.* Chicago: The American Dietetic Association, 1996.

American Dietetic Association. *Ethnic and regional food practices: Hmong American food practices, customs, and holidays.* Chicago: The American Dietetic Association, 1999.

American Dietetic Association. Position of The American Dietetic Association: functional foods. *J Am Diet Assoc.* 1999;99:1278.

American Dietetic Association. Position of The American Dietetic Association: vegetarian diets. *J Am Diet Assoc.* 1997;97:1317.

Bederova A, et al. Comparison of nutrient intake and corresponding biochemical parameters in adolescent vegetarians and nonvegetarians. *Cas Lek Cesk.* 2000;139:396.

Bermudez O, et al. Intake and food sources of macronutrients among older Hispanic adults: association with ethnicity, acculturation, and length of residence in the United States. *J Am Diet Assoc.* 2000;100:665.

Dulloo A, et al. Efficacy of a green tea extract rich in catechin polyphenols and caffeine in increasing 24-hr energy expenditure and fat oxidation in humans. *Am J Clin Nutri.* 1999;70:1040.

Earl R, Borra S. Guidelines for dietary planning. In: Mahan K, Escott-Stump S. *Krause's food, nutrition, and diet therapy.* 10th ed. Philadelphia: WB Saunders, 2000.

Kennedy E, et al. Popular diets: correlation to health, nutrition, and obesity. *J Am Diet Assoc.* 2001;101:411.

Kim K, et al. Nutritional status of Korean Americans: implications for cancer risk. *Oncol Nurs Forum.* 2000;27:1573.

Mangels A, Messina V. Considerations in planning vegan diets: infants. *J Am Diet Assoc.* 2001;101:670.

Messina M, Messina V. *The dietitian's guide to vegetarian diets: issues and applications.* Gaithersburg, MD: Aspen Publishers; 1996.

Satia J, et al. Development of scales to measure dietary acculturation among Chinese-Americans and Chinese-Canadians. *J Am Diet Assoc.* 2001,101:548.

Scali J, et al. Diet profiles in a population sample from Mediterranean southern France. *Public Health Nutri.* 2001;4:173.

Young V, Pellett P. Plant proteins in relation to human protein and amino acid nutrition. *Am J Clin Nutri.* 1994;59:1203S.

Suggested Readings

American Dietetic Association. *Ethnic and regional food practices: northern plains Indian food practices, customs, and holidays.* Chicago: The American Dietetic Association, 1999.

American Dietetic Association. *Ethnic and regional food practices: Cajun and Creole food practices, customs, and holidays.* Chicago: The American Dietetic Association, 1996.

American Dietetic Association. Position of The American Dietetic Association: health implications of dietary fiber. *J Am Diet Assoc.* 1997;97:1157.

American Dietetic Association. Translating the science behind the Dietary Reference Intakes. *J Am Diet Assoc.* 1998;98:7.

Barnard N, et al. Effectiveness of a low-fat vegetarian diet in altering serum lipids in healthy premenopausal women. *Am J Cardiol.* 2000;85:969.

Devine C, et al. Life course influences on fruit and vegetable trajectories: qualitative analysis of food choices. *J Nutr Ed.* 1998;30:361.

Geiger C. Health claims: history, current regulatory status, and consumer research. *J Am Diet Assoc.* 1998;98:1312.

Dental/Oral–Cited References

American Dietetic Association. Position of The American Dietetic Association: the impact of fluoride on health. *J Am Diet Assoc.* 2000;100:1208.

Bruerd B, Jones C. Preventing baby bottle tooth decay. *Pub Health Reports.* 1996;111:63.

Faine M, Oberg D. Survey of dental nutrition knowledge of WIC nutritionists and public health dental hygienists. *J Am Diet Assoc.* 1995;95:190.

Garg A, Malo M. Manifestations and treatment of xerostomia and associated oral effects secondary to head and neck radiation therapy. *J Am Dental Assoc.* 1997;97:1128.

Irving J, et al. Does temporomandibular disorder pain dysfunction syndrome affect dietary intake? *Dent Update.* 1999;26:405.

Katz J. Elevated blood glucose levels in patients with severe periodontal disease. *J Clin Periodontal.* 2001;28:710.

Scully C. Advances in oral medicine. *Prim Dent Care.* 2000;7:55.

Sheiham A, et al. The relationship among dental status, nutrient intake, and nutritional status in older people. *J Dent Res.* 2001;80:408.

Spolarich A. Managing the side effects of medications. *J Dent Hyg.* 2000;74:57.

Tonetti M. Advances in periodontology. *Prim Dent Care.* 2000;7:149.

Touger-Decker R. Oral and dental health. In: Mahan K, Escott-Stump S. *Krause's food, nutrition, and diet therapy.* 10th ed. Philadelphia: WB Saunders, 2000.

Suggested Readings

American Dietetic Association. Position of The American Dietetic Association: oral health and nutrition. *J Am Diet Assoc.* 1996;96:184.

Barr S, Broughton T. Relative weight, weight loss efforts, and nutrient intakes among health-conscious vegetarian, past vegetarian and nonvegetarian women ages 18–50. *J Am Col Nutri.* 2000;19:781.

Dyment H, Casas, M. Dental care for children fed by tube: a critical review. *Spec Care Dentist.* 1999;19:220.

Fitzsimmons D, et al. Nutrition and oral health guidelines for pregnant women, infants, and children. *J Am Diet Assoc.* 1998;98:182.

Fowler J Jr. Systemic contact dermatitis caused by oral chromium picolinate. *Cutis.* February, 2000;65:116.

Milgrom P, et al. Dental caries and its relationship to bacterial infection, hypoplasia, diet, and oral hygiene in 6- to 36-month-old children. *Community Dent Oral Epidemiol.* 2000;228:295.

Mobley C, Saunders M. Oral health screening guidelines for nondental healthcare providers. *J Am Diet Assoc.* 1997;97:S123.

Moneret-Vautrin D. Cow's milk allergy. *Allerg Immuno.* June, 1999; 31:201–210.

Niggemann B, et al. The atopy patch test (APT)–a useful tool for the diagnosis of food allergy in children with atopic dermatitis. *Allergy*. 2000;55:281.

Olsen S, et al. Surveillance for food borne-disease outbreaks–United States, 1993–1997. *Mor Mortal Wkly Rep CDC Surveil Sum*. March, 2000;49:1.

Palmer J, et al. Evaluation and treatment of swallowing impairments. *Am Fam Physician*. 2000;61:2453.

Pendrys D, et al. Risk factors for enamel fluorosis in a fluoridated community. *Am J Epid*. 1994;140:461.

Plaut A. Clinical pathology of food borne diseases: notes on the patient with food borne gastrointestinal illness. *J Food Prot*. 2000;63: 822.

Nutrition and Vision/Blindness, Self-feeding Problems, Miscellaneous–Cited References

Ajemian M, et al. Routine fiberoptic endoscopic evaluation of swallowing following prolonged intubation: implications for management. *Arch Surg*. 2001;136:434.

Age-related eye disease research group. A randomized, placebo-controlled, clinical trial of high-dose supplementation with vitamins C and E, beta-carotene, and zinc for age-related cataract and vision loss. AREDS Report No. 9. *Arch Ophthalmol*. 2001;119:1439–1452.

Cho E, et al. Prospective study of dietary fat and the risk of age-related macular degeneration. *Am J Clin Nutri*. 2001;73:209.

Cumming R, et al. Dietary sodium intake and cataract: the Blue Mountains Eye Study. *Am J Epid*. 2000;151:624.

Devaiah A, Ator G. Clinical indicators useful in predicting response to the medical management of Ménière's disease. *Laryngoscope*. 2000;110:1861.

Jacques P, et al. Long-term vitamin C supplement use and prevalence of early age-related lens opacities. *Am J Clin Nutri*. 1997;66:911.

Perlman A. Dysphagia: populations at risk and methods of diagnosis. *Nutr in Clin Pract*. 1999;14:2S.

Smith W, et al. Dietary fat and fish intake and age-related maculopathy. *Arch Ophthalmol*. 2000;118:401.

Skin Disorders and Pressure Ulcers–Cited References

Allman R. Pressure ulcer prevalence, incidence, risk factors, and impact. *Clinics in Geriatric Med*. 1997;13:421.

Black H. Influence of dietary factors on actinically induced skin cancer. *Mutat Res*. 1998;422:185.

Boelsma E, et al. Nutritional skin care: health effects of micronutrients and fatty acids (review). *Am J Clin Nutr*. 2001;73:853.

Braden B. Using the Braden scale for predicting pressure sore risk. *Support Line*. 1996;XVIII:14.

Greenwald P. From carcinogenesis to clinical interventions for cancer prevention. *Toxicology*. 2001;166:37.

Guenter P, et al. Survey of nutritional status in newly hospitalized patients with stage III or stage IV pressure ulcers. *Adv Skin Wound Care*. 2000;13:164.

Lamberg L. Diet may affect skin cancer prevention. *JAMA*. 1998;279: 1427.

Litt J. Rosacea: how to recognize and treat an age-related skin disease. *Geriatrics*. 1997;52:39.

Stahl W, et al. Carotenoids and carotenoids plus vitamin E protect against ultraviolet light-induced erythema in humans. *Am J Clin Nutr*. 2000;71:795.

Williams D, et al. Patients with existing pressure ulcers admitted to acute care. *J Wound Ostomy Continence Nurs*. 2000;27:216.

Zouboulis C. Human skin: an independent peripheral endocrine organ. *Horm Res*. 2000;54:230.

Suggested Readings

Bergstrom N, et al. Strategies for preventing pressure ulcers. *Clinics in Geriatric Med*. 1997;13:437.

Cruse J, et al. Review of immune function, healing of pressure ulcers, and nutritional status in patients with spinal cord injury. *J Spinal Cord Med*. 2000;23:129.

Efron D, Barbul A. Role of arginine in immunonutrition. *J Gastroenterol*. 2000;35:20.

Ferguson M, et al. Pressure ulcer management: the importance of nutrition. *Med Surg Nurs*. 2000;9:163.

Gupta S, Mukhtar H. Chemoprevention of skin cancer through natural agents. *Skin Pharmacol Appl Skin Physiol*. 2001;14:373.

Hardman C, et al. Absence of toxicity of oats in patients with dermatitis herpetiformis. *N Engl J Med*. 1997;337:1884.

Thomas D. The role of nutrition in prevention and healing of pressure ulcers. *Clinics in Geriatric Med*. 1997;13:497.

Xakellis G. Quality assurance programs for pressure ulcers. *Clinics in Geriatric Med*. 1997;13:599.

Food Allergies, Sensitivities, Headaches, and Glutamate Sensitivity–Cited References

American Academy of Pediatrics, Committee on Nutrition. Hypoallergenic infants' formulas. *Pediatr*. 2000;106:346.

Clinical Practice and Practice Economics Committee. American Gastroenterological Association medical position statement: guidelines for the evaluation of food allergies. *Gastroenterology*. 2001;120:1023.

Asero R. Detection and clinical characterization of patients with oral allergy syndrome caused by stable allergens in Rosaceae and nuts. *Ann Allergy Asthma Immunol*. 1999;83:377.

Birmingham P, Suresh S. Latex allergy in children: diagnosis and management. *Indian J Pediatr*. 1999;66:717.

Burks A, et al. Atopic dermatitis and food hypersensitivity reactions. *J Pediatr*. 1998;132:132.

Cantani A. Feeding high-risk infants with family history of allergy. *Eur Rev Med Pharmacol Sci*. 1999;3:143.

Chiu A, Zacharisen M. Anaphylaxis to dill. *Ann Allergy Asthma Immunol*. 2000;84:559.

Das U. Essential fatty acids in health and disease. *J Assoc Physicians India*. 1999;47:906.

Fernstrom J, Garattini S. International symposium on glutamate: proceedings of a symposium held October 12–14, 1998 in Bergamo, Italy. *J Nutri*. 2000;130:891S.

FDA. *Food allergies: when food becomes the enemy*. FDA Consumer Magazine. Washington, DC: USDA Food and Drug Administration. July–August, 2001.

Geha R, et al. Review of alleged reaction to monosodium glutamate and outcome of a multicenter double-blind placebo-controlled study. *J Nutri*. 2000;130:1058S.

Guida B, et al. Histamine plasma levels and elimination diet in chronic idiopathic urticaria. *Euro J Clin Nutri*. 2000;54:155.

Hefle S, Taylor S. Allergenicity of edible oils. *Food Technology*. 1999;53:62.

Hoare C, et al. Systematic review of treatments for atopic eczema. *Health Technol Assess*. 2000;4:1.

Hoel N, et al. Selective up-regulation of 5-HT(1B/1D) receptors during organ culture of cerebral arteries. *Neuroreport*. 2001;12:1605.

Hubbard-Wilson S. Nutritional care in food allergy and food intolerance. In: Mahan K, Escott-Stump S. *Krause's food, nutrition, and diet therapy*. 10th ed. Philadelphia: WB Saunders, 2000.

Isolauri E, et al. Breastfeeding of allergic infants. *J Pediatr*. 1999;134:27.

Jarvinen K, et al. Cow's milk challenge through human milk evokes immune responses in infants with cow's milk allergy. *J Pediatr*. 1999;135:506.

Kim K, Hussain H. Prevalence of food allergy in 137 latex-allergic patients. *Allergy Asthma Proc*. 1999;20:95.

Kramer U, et al. Age of entry to day nursery and allergy in later childhood. *Lancet*. 1999;353:450.

Kumar V, et al. Tissue transglutaminase and endomysial antibodies-diagnostic markers of gluten-sensitive enteropathy in dermatitis herpetiformis. *Clin Immunol*. 2001;98:378.

Martens M. Safety evaluation of genetically modified foods. *Int Arch Occup Environ Health*. 2000;73:S14.

Perkin J. The latex and food allergy connection. *J Am Diet Assoc*. 2000;100:1381.

Sampson H. Food allergy. *J Am Med Assoc*. 1997;278:1888.

Tan B, et al. Severe food allergies by skin contact. *Ann Allergy Asthma Immunol*. 2001;86:583.

Tucke J, et al. Latex type I sensitization and allergy in children with atopic dermatitis. Evaluation of cross-reactivity to some foods. *Pediatr Allergy Immunol*. 1999;10:160.

Varjonen E, et al. Antigliadin IgE–indicator of wheat allergy in atopic dermatitis. *Allergy*. 2000;55:386.

Zeiger R. Dietary aspects of food allergy prevention in infants and children. *J Pediatr Gastroenterol Nutri*. 2000;30:77S.

Suggested Readings

Asero R. Fennel, cucumber, and melon allergy successfully treated with pollen-specific injection immunotherapy. *Ann Allergy Asthma Immunol*. 2000;84: 460.

Caballero T, Martin-Esteban M. Association between pollen hypersensitivity and edible vegetable allergy: a review. *J Investig Allergol Clin Immunol*. 1998;8:6.

De Boissieu D, Dupont C. Time course of allergy to extensively hydrolyzed cow's milk proteins in infants. *J Pediatr*. 2000;136:119.

Fuchs R, Astwood J. Allergenicity assessment of foods derived from genetically modified plants. *Food Technology*. 1996;50:83.

Hagan L, et al. Sudden infant death syndrome: a search for allergen hypersensitivity. *Ann Allergy Asthma Immunol*. 1998;80:227.

Hodge L, et al. Assessment of food chemical intolerance in adult asthmatic subjects. *Thorax*. 1996;51:805.

Isolauri E, et al. Elimination diet in cow's milk allergy: risk for impaired growth in young children. *J Peds*. 1998;132:100.

Koerner C, Munoz-Furlong A. *Food allergies: tips from the nutrition experts*. New York: John Wiley and Sons, 1998.

Lolinger J. Function and importance of glutamate for savory foods. *J Nutri*. 2000;130: 915S.

Martin B. Skin manifestations of food allergies. *J Am Osteopath Assoc*. 1999;99:15S.

Pham T, Rudner E. Peanut allergy. *Cutis*. 2000;65:285.

Solvoll K, et al. Dietary habits among patients with atopic dermatitis. *Eur J Clin Nutr*. February, 2000;54:93–97.

Taylor J, et al. Assessing adherence to a rotary diversified diet, a treatment for "environmental illness." *J Am Diet Assoc*. 1998;98:439.

Tsai P, et al. Circadian variations in plasma and erythrocyte concentrations of glutamate, glutamine, and alanine in men on a diet without and with added monosodium glutamate. *Metabolism: Clin and Experi*. 1999;48:1455.

Walker R, Lupien J. The safety evaluation of monosodium glutamate. *J Nutri*. 2000;130:1049S.

Worm M, et al. Clinical relevance of food additives in adult patients with atopic dermatitis. *Clin Exp Allergy*. 2000;30:407.

Yang W, et al. The monosodium glutamate symptom complex: assessment in a double-blind, placebo-controlled, randomized study. *J Allergy Clin Immunol*. 1997;99:757.

Yunginger J, et al. Quantitative IgE antibody assays in allergic diseases. *J Allergy Clin Immunol*. 2000;105:1077.

Food Safety–Cited References

Mayerhauser C. Survival of enterohemorrhagic *Escherichia coli* O157:H7 in retail mustard. *J Food Prot*. 2001;64:783.

Ollinger-Snyder P, Matthews E. Food safety: review and implications for dietitians and diet technicians. *J Am Diet Assoc*. 1996;96:163.

Olsen S, et al. Surveillance for food borne disease outbreaks–United States, 1993–1997. *Mor Mortal Wkly Rep CDC Surveil Sum*. March, 2000;49:1.

Setiabuhdi M, et al. Integrating Hazard Analysis and Critical Control Point (HACCP) and sanitation for verifiable food safety. *J Am Diet Assoc*. 1997;97:889.

Smittle R. Microbiological safety of mayonnaise, salad dressings, and sauces produced in the United States. *J Food Protection*. 2000;63: 1144.

Woteki C. Dietitians can prevent listeriosis. *J Am Diet Assoc*. 2001;101:285.

Suggested Readings

Altekruse S, et al. Consumer knowledge of food borne microbial hazards and food-handling practices. *J Food Protection*. 1996;59:287.

American Medical Association, Centers for Disease Control and Prevention, Center for Food Safety and Applied Nutrition, Food and Drug Administration, Food Safety and Inspection Service, U.S. Department of Agriculture. Diagnosis and management of food borne illnesses: a primer for physicians. *MMWR Morb Mortal Wkly Rep*. January, 2001;2:1.

Bayerl C. Nutrition in the community. In: Mahan K, Escott-Stump S. *Krause's food, nutrition, and diet therapy*. 10th ed. Philadelphia: WB Saunders, 2000.

Blaser M. How safe is our food? Lessons from an outbreak of Salmonellosis. *N Engl J Med*. 1996;334:1324.

Borra S, et al. Paucity of nutrition and food safety "news you can use" reveals opportunity for dietetics practitioners. *J Am Diet Assoc*. 1998;98:190.

Evans A, Brachman P, eds. *Bacterial infections of humans*. New York: Plenum Medical, 1998.

Hennessy T, et al. A national outbreak of *Salmonella enteritidis* infections from ice cream. *N Engl J Med*. 1996;334:1281.

Puzo D. Food safety: the thin blue line. *Restaurants and Institutions*. 1998;108:94.

Reichler G, Dalton S. Chefs' attitudes toward healthful food preparation are more positive than their food science knowledge and practices. *J Am Diet Assoc*. 1998;98:165.

Woodburn M, Raab C. Household food preparers' food safety knowledge and practices following widely publicized outbreaks of food borne illness. *J Food Protection*. 1997;60:1105.

Woteki C, et al. Keep food safe to eat: healthful food must be safe as well as nutritious. *J Nutri*. 2001;131:502S.

SECTION 3

Special Pediatric Conditions

CHIEF ASSESSMENT FACTORS

Anthropometric:

- BIRTH DATA (WEIGHT, LENGTH, HEAD CIRCUMFERENCE, SIZE, GESTATIONAL AGE)
- CURRENT WEIGHT AND HEIGHT, ESPECIALLY IF BELOW 5% OR ABOVE 95% FOR AGE
- UNINTENTIONAL WEIGHT LOSSES
- PUBERTAL STAGING, SKELETAL MATURITY STAGING

Clinical:

- CONGENITAL OR CHROMOSOMAL ABNORMALITIES, INBORN ERRORS OF METABOLISM
- CHRONIC ILLNESSES (DIABETES, FAILURE TO THRIVE [FTT], DEVELOPMENTAL DELAY, KIDNEY DISEASE, MALABSORPTION, SYNDROMES, HIV/AIDS, TRAUMA)
- ORAL LESIONS
- RECENT TRAUMA, SURGERY, HOSPITALIZATIONS, AND ACUTE ILLNESSES
- RECENT CHEMOTHERAPY, RADIATION, ETC.
- MEDICATIONS, ESPECIALLY CHRONIC (SUCH AS DILANTIN, RITALIN)
- PROTEIN–CALORIE MALNUTRITION (APPROXIMATELY 25–33% OF HOSPITALIZED CHILDREN)
- GASTROINTESTINAL FUNCTIONING, NAUSEA, VOMITING, DIARRHEA, AND CONSTIPATION

Dietary Issues & Feeding Skill:

- FEEDING: PERSONS INVOLVED, LENGTH OF TIME, FEEDING METHOD, SKILL LEVEL
- AVOIDANCE OF FOODS THAT ARE READILY ASPIRATED
- TEXTURE MODIFICATIONS
- COORDINATION FOR SAFE AND PROPER CHEWING, SUCKING, SWALLOWING
- FOOD INTAKE
- PREFERENCES, INTOLERANCES
- MULTIPLE OR SEVERE FOOD ALLERGIES
- SPECIAL FORMULA OR SUPPLEMENTS, TUBE FEEDING OR TOTAL PARENTERAL NUTRITION (TPN)

Behavioral:

- GROWTH AND DEVELOPMENT MILESTONES
- USE OF FOOD FOR REWARD OR AS PACIFIER

TABLE 3–1 Overview of Pediatric Disorders

Newborn Screening:

Mandated state newborn screening programs for the approximately 4 million infants born each year in the United States involve components of: 1) initial screening, 2) immediate follow-up testing of the screen-positive newborn, 3) diagnosis confirmation (true positive versus false positive), 4) immediate and long-term care, and 5) evaluation of process and outcomes measures (Desposito et al., 2001).

Nutritional Assessment of Hospitalized Children:

Nutritional status affects a child's response to illness. Good nutrition is important for achieving normal growth and development; nutritional assessment, therefore, should be an integral part of the care for every pediatric patient (Mascarenhas et al., 1998). About 10–15% of children in the United States have special healthcare needs that require medical attention. Pediatric nutritional assessment is essential in identifying children at risk. Simple nutritional risk screening tools can help identify children at risk for malnutrition during hospital stays—weight, length or height, head circumference; food intake, ability to eat and retain food; medical condition; and symptoms interfering with feedings, such as depression, pain, and dyspnea (Sermet-Gaudelus et al., 2000). Nutritionally at risk patients may benefit from determination of resting energy expenditure by indirect calorimetry (Mascarenhas et al., 1998). Use of the new CDC age, gender, and disease-specific growth charts is essential in assessing nutritional status and monitoring nutrition interventions; accuracy is better when using trained personnel and appropriate equipment. Proper interventions and referrals are important for growth and optimal development. Efforts should be made to enhance appetite and intake in children who cannot eat at home with their families. Familiarity is important; hospitalized children enjoy home-like meals.

Chronic Diarrhea:

Chronic diarrhea in infants under age 3 months may indicate inappropriate formulas, infection, use of too much juice, disaccharide deficiency, cow's milk or soymilk protein intolerance, cystic fibrosis, or immunodeficiency state. In ages 3–18, it might mean celiac disease, lactose deficiency, or inflammatory bowel disease. But gastrointestinal (GI) infection is the most common cause in children of all ages. Watery, explosive stools indicate sugar intolerance; foul-smelling, bulky stools indicate fat malabsorption. Marked weight loss indicates malabsorption, inflammatory bowel disease (IBD), hyperthyroidism, or malignancy. Neutrophils or red blood cell counts (RBCs) in the stool suggest bacterial gastroenteritis (GE) or IBD; eosinophils suggest protein intolerance or parasitic infestation (Leung and Robson, 1996).

Developmental Disabilities:

Proper assessment of nutritional status, feeding skills, and feeding behaviors, including positioning, is important. Various disability-screening tools have been developed, which should screen for all major disabilities (i.e., physical, motor, sensory, and mental retardation). Gradually rewarding behaviors as they begin to match desired behaviors is known as "shaping" and is used commonly for these children. Catch-up growth is important with an emphasis on energy and protein. For those in whom measurement of height is difficult, arm span may be a reasonable substitute. Three developmental disabilities do not have mental retardation as a component—cerebral palsy, autism, and epilepsy.

Otitis Media:

Otitis media with effusions (OME) can lead to significant hearing loss in childhood (Gok et al., 2001). Breast milk is more protective than formula. Artificially fed breast milk provides some protection against otitis media in infants with cleft palate (Paradise et al., 1994). In older children, chewing xylitol gum or lozenges helps to prevent dental caries by preventing growth of pneumococci and may also help prevent acute otitis media (Uhari et al., 1998).

(continued)

TABLE 3–1 Overview of Pediatric Disorders (*Continued*)

Pediatric Tube Feedings and TPN:

Home tube feeding promotes catch-up growth in most children (Kang et al., 1998). Pedia-Sure (Ross) is a complete tube feeding (TF) formula for children; it contains 237 kcal/250 mL and is free of lactose and gluten; Kinder-Cal TF (Mead Johnson) and other pediatric tube feedings are available. A percutaneous endoscopic gastrostomy may be a good alternative to a nasogastric tube in children with cholestasis and mild portal hypertension (Duche et al., 1999). Mothers of children with tube feedings expressed greater stress than mothers who did not have tube feedings to provide; they also received less support from family and friends. Include fathers, friends, etc. in training so this can be changed (Adams et al., 1999). For TPN, special pediatric solutions are available.

TABLE 3–2 Inborn Errors of Metabolism and Suggested Dietary Management

Inborn Error of Metabolism	*Suggested Dietary Management*
Arginosuccinic Aciduria (Urea Cycle Disorders)	Low protein diet, use of special formulas and supplements of arginine
Galactosemia	Galactose elimination diet
Glutaric Aciduria Type 1 Note: *alpha* Ketoadipic Aciduria has no treatment	Restrictions of amino acids
Glycogen Storage Disease	Prevent hypoglycemia by use of a carbohydrate-controlled diet
Homocystinuria	Restriction of amino acids, use of formulas such as Hominex (Ross) if vitamin B6 nonresponsive
Isovaleric Acidemia	Restriction of protein
Maple Syrup Urine Disease (MSUD)	Restrictions of amino acids leucine, isoleucine, and valine; use of special formulas MSUD diet powder
Ornithine Transcarbamylase Deficiency (Urea Cycle Acid disorder)	Low-protein diet; additives such as Moducal (Mead Johnson) may be added to give CHO calories
Phenylketonuria	Phenylalanine-restricted diet; use of formulas such as Lofenalac or Phenyl-Free (Mead Johnson) and Phenex (Ross)
Propionic Acidemia and Methylmalonic Acidemia	Low protein diet
Tyrosinemia	Restrictions of tyrosine, phenylalanine, and methionine; use of special formulas

TABLE 3–3 Nutritional Risk Factors Associated with Selected Pediatric Disorders

X = common problems	*Underweight*	*Overweight*	*Short Stature*	*Low Energy Needs*	*High Energy Needs*	*Feeding Problems*	*Constipation*	*Chronic Meds*
Autism	X					X		X
Bronchopulmonary dysplasia	X				X			
Cerebral palsy	X	X	X	X	X	X	X	X
Cystic fibrosis	X		X		X			
Down syndrome		X		X		X		
Fetal alcohol syndrome	X		X					
Heart disease, congenital	X				X			
HIV/AIDS	X				X			X
Prader Willi syndrome		X	X	X				
Prematurity	X		X		X	X		
Seizure disorder								X
Spina bifida	X	X	X	X			X	X

Based on data from: Baer and Harris, 1997.

For More Information About Birth Defects and Genetic Disorders

- March of Dimes
  1275 Mamaroneck Ave.
  White Plains, NY 10605
  1-888-MODIMES
  http://www.modimes.org/
- Clinical Genetic Services
  Children's Service
  Massachusetts General Hospital
  Boston, MA 02114
- National Center for Education in Maternal and Child Health
  http://www.ncemch.georgetown.edu/

- Producers of metabolic formulae:
  Ross Laboratories-800-986-8510
  SHS (Scientific Hospital Supply)-800-636-2283
  Mead Johnson-800-429-6399
  Applied Nutrition-800-605-0410

- Low-Protein Foods:
  Loprofin-888-567-7646
  Dietary Specialties-888-640-2800
  Ener-G Foods-800-331-5222
  Cambrooke Foods-508-279-1800
  MedDiet-800-633-5550
  Glutino-800-363-3438
  Kingsmill Foods-416-755-1124

For More Information About Feeding Problems

- American Occupational Therapy Association, Inc.
  http://www.aota.org/
- The Oley Foundation for Special Foods, Dietary Needs, Home Enteral/Parenteral Therapy
  214 Hun Memorial, A-23
  Albany Medical Center
  Albany, NY 12208
  1-800-776-OLEY
  http://www.wizvax.net/oleyfdn

For More Information About Health Laws Affecting Families/Children with Special Healthcare Needs

- National Health Law Program
  1101 14th Street, NW, Suite 405
  Washington, DC 20005
  (202) 289-7661
  http://www.healthlaw.org

For More Information About Pediatric Journals

- http://www.angelfire.com/in/pedscapes/index.html

For More Information About Rare Disorders

- FDA—National Information Center for Orphan Drugs and Rare Diseases
  http://www.fda.gov/orphan/rdid/index.htm
- National Organization for Rare Disorders, Inc.
  P.O. Box 8923, New Fairfield, CT 06812-8923
  http://www.rarediseases.org/
- Office of Rare Diseases
  National Institutes of Health
  Building 31, Room 1B03
  Bethesda, MD 20892-2082
  301-402-4336
  FAX: (301) 402-0420
  http://www.rarediseases.info.nih.gov/ord

For More Information About Tube Feeding Products

- Mead Johnson
  1-800-BABY123
  http://www.meadjohnson.com
- Novartis
  http://www.novartis.com
- Ross Laboratories
  1-800-551-5838
  http://www.rosslabs.com
- SHS North America
  PO BOX 117
  Gaithersburg MD 20884-0117
  1-800-365-7354
  http://www.shsna.com

ADRENOLEUKODYSTROPHY

NUTRITIONAL ACUITY RANKING: LEVEL 3

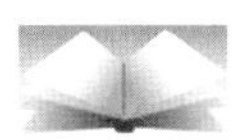

DEFINITIONS AND BACKGROUND

Peroxisome biogenesis disorders (PBDs) are severe neurological diseases, of which the most severe is Zellweger syndrome; neonatal adrenoleukodystrophy and infantile Refsum disease are milder phenotypes (Suzuki et al., 2001). Adrenoleukodystrophy (ALD) is an autosomal recessive disorder characterized by demyelination, adrenal insufficiency, and accumulation of saturated very long-chain fatty acids (VLFA), especially hexacosanoate (C26:0). The protein that is missing or defective to process that fatty acid is called ALDP (ALD protein).

An enzymatic defect in VLFA oxidation, abundant in sphingomyelin, is suspected. Ultimately, the myelin sheath surrounding the nerves is destroyed causing neurologic problems, and the adrenal gland malfunction causes Addison's disease.

The onset of ALD is usually in childhood, with a rapid, progressive demyelination of the central nervous system (CNS), hypotonia, and psychomotor retardation. An adult form is usually manifested as an adrenomyeloneuropathy (AMN). Studies have shown that dietary fatty acids and environmental factors can be involved in CNS myelinogenesis (DiBiase and Salvati, 1997). The observation that dietary fatty acids can affect membrane composition has led to the use of modified diets in these conditions. During treatment, C22:6 content increases in red blood cells and probably in the brain membranes, as considerable neurologic and electrophysiological improvement suggests. The course of the fatal childhood form is generally from 1–10 years with nervous system deterioration leaving the patient bedridden (http://www.ulf.org/).

A 2-year trial of glycerol trioleate and glycerol trierucate (Lorenzo's oil) had no clinically relevant effect in preventing the myelopathy or demyelination in adults with AMN (Auborg et al., 1993). Lymphocytopenia and depression of natural killer cells have been observed in patients with ALD treated with Lorenzo's oil, an indication of increased reactivity of cellular immunity to unspecific immunological stimuli (Pour et al., 2000). The effects on cellular immunoreactivity must, therefore, be considered in ALD patients treated with Lorenzo's oil. Early initiation is needed (Suzuki et al., 2001).

An omega-3 fatty acid, DHA, is present in large amounts in infant brains. DHA is present in fatty fish (e.g., salmon, tuna, mackerel) and mother's milk but is not usually present in infant formulas. Because DHA deficiencies have been noted in adrenoleukodystrophy (Horrocks and Yeo, 1999), intake of omega-3 fatty acids may be beneficial. For some prospective parents, preventive measures can be recommended: dietary supplementation with monounsaturated fatty acids in symptomatic carriers for X-linked ALD (Endres, 1997).

Genetic and biochemical analysis, neuroimaging, and the ability to create animal models have led to advances in the field of leukodystrophy research (Berger et al., 2001). Although definitive treatments are not available for ALD, studies are being done with bone marrow transplant, lovastatin, and 4 phenylbutyrate; gene therapy is under investigation (http://www.ulf.org/).

OBJECTIVES

- Decrease rapid progression of demyelination of CNS.
- Prevent or lessen complications of the disorder.
- Alter type of dietary fat to limit progression of the disease. Use more omega-3 fatty acids.
- Overall, maintain total VLFA levels while altering sources.

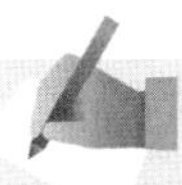

DIETARY AND NUTRITIONAL RECOMMENDATIONS

- Increase endogenous VLFA synthesis of monounsaturated fatty acids by restricting exogenous (dietary) VLFA (C26:0) to less than 3 mg and by increasing oleic acid (C18:1). The typical American diet yields 35–40% total energy from fat with 12–40 mg C26:0 daily.
- Dietary therapy, low-VLFA diet and supplementation with unsaturated fatty acids such as glyceryl trioleate (GTO) and glyceryl trierucate (GTE), commonly called Lorenzo's oil, has been used without significant clinical improvement in the cerebral forms. For this diet, use the VLFA C26:0-restricted diet, with the addition of 60 mL of GTO oil for oleic acid. GTO is similar to olive oil (87% C18:1, 4.8% linoleic acid) but lacks measurable fatty acids with a chain length greater than C20. GTO is available from Capital Cities Products, Inc. (Columbus, OH). GTO can be used in cooking, as a supplement in juice, or as an oil consumed directly. GTO replaces oils, margarine, butter, mayonnaise, and shortening in food preparation.
- If the patient requires tube feeding, a formula can be developed that contains nonfat milk, GTO, corn syrup or sugar, and a vitamin-mineral supplement.
- Studies are not conclusive regarding vitamin E, selenium, and carnitine requirements.
- Include sources of omega-3 fatty acids, such as salmon, tuna, or mackerel for older children and adults.
- To reduce the need to digest C26:0 present in fatty foods and in cutin (outer layer of plants, fruits, vegetables, and nuts), use these items less often in the diet. For example, peel fruits and vegetables before serving.

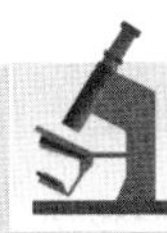

PROFILE

Clinical/History	Lab Work	
Height Weight Growth chart Bronzing of skin (Addison's disease)	Plasma phosphatidylcholine Fatty acid profile Albumin (alb) Cholesterol	(chol), Triglycerides (Trig) Plasma sphingomyelin Hemoglobin and hematocrit (H&H)

Herbs, Botanicals and Supplements

- Herbs and botanicals should not be used for this condition because there are no clinical trials proving efficacy.

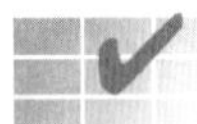

PATIENT EDUCATION

- ✔ The whole family can be instrumental in accepting the diet; it can be adapted for everyone.
- ✔ Restaurant dining can be a problem. Some special meals may have to be developed for travel.
- ✔ If nausea occurs, the oil can be taken in an emulsion.

For More Information

- United Leukodystrophy Association
  2304 Highland Dr.
  Sycamore, IL 60178
  1-800-728-5483
  http://www.ulf.org/

BILIARY ATRESIA

NUTRITIONAL ACUITY RANKING: LEVEL 4

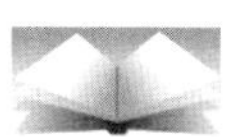

DEFINITIONS AND BACKGROUND

Unconjugated hyperbilirubinemia occurs in approximately 60% of normal term infants and in 80% of preterm infants; persistence beyond 2 weeks of age demands evaluation (Gubernick et al., 2000). Biliary atresia (neonatal hepatitis) is a serious condition with an unknown etiology. Complete degeneration or incomplete development of one or more of the bile duct components, due to arrested fetal development, occurs. It results in persistent jaundice, liver damage, and portal hypertension, with pale stools, dark urine, and swollen abdomen. It is evident between 2 and 6 weeks after birth. This is the most common disease in childhood that requires liver transplantation.

Progressive destruction of intrahepatic bile ducts may determine outcome in biliary atresia; CD4(+) lymphocytes and CD56(+) (NK cells) predominate in the liver of infants with extra-hepatic biliary atresia (EHBA) (Davenport et al., 2001). If a donor is available, the patient may be a candidate for a liver transplant. Malnutrition is a critical predictor of mortality and morbidity in children with biliary atresia who undergo orthotopic liver transplantation (Bucuvalas et al., 1996). Immunosuppressive drugs are necessary to overcome organ rejection after transplantation.

OBJECTIVES

- Correct malabsorption and alleviate steatorrhea from decreased bile.
- Prevent hemorrhage from high blood pressure.
- Correct malnutrition of fat-soluble vitamins and zinc.
- Prevent rickets, visual disturbances, peripheral neuropathy, and coagulopathies.
- Prepare for potential surgery (Kasai procedure removes damaged tubes) or transplantation.
- Postoperatively, promote normal growth and development.
- Correct increased protein oxidation; decreased branched chain fatty acids and increased aromatic amino acids occur.
- Provide regular nutritional assessments to evaluate progress and improvement or decline.

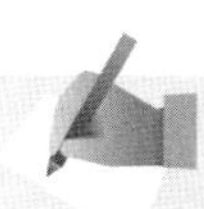

DIETARY AND NUTRITIONAL RECOMMENDATIONS

Pretransplant:

- Infants need 1.5–3 g protein/kg dry weight to avoid protein catabolism, dependent on enteral versus parenteral source. Check for products enriched with branched chain amino acids. Small, frequent feedings may be useful.
- Use a low-total-fat diet. Supplement with oil high in medium-chain triglycerides (MCT). Add essential fatty acids (EFAs) for age and body size.
- Portagen is available for infants but provides only minimal EFAs. Pregestimil or Alimentum may be used.
- When edema exists, restrict the intake of sodium to 1–2 g.
- Decrease fiber intake to prevent hemorrhage from anywhere along the GI tract.
- Supplement with vitamins A, D, E, and K. Intravenous supplementation may be necessary, or water-miscible forms can be used. Selenium tends to be low also. Avoid use of copper in TPN or supplements; extra zinc and iron will be needed.
- Tube feed especially if recurrent or prolonged bleeding from the GI tract occurs. If nasogastric (NG) feeding is not tolerated, a percutaneous gastrostomy (PEG) tube may be used (Duche et al., 1999). Some evidence suggests that special attention to protein and branched chain amino acids may be needed (Kawahara et al., 1999).

Posttransplant:

- For needed catch-up growth, tube feeding may be beneficial (Holt et al., 2000).
- Control sodium, protein, and other nutrients only if necessary based on symptoms such as edema, renal failure, etc.
- Carefully monitor vitamin and mineral requirements.

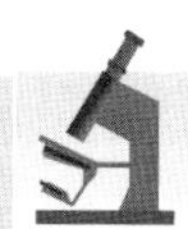

PROFILE

Clinical/History	Lab Work	
Birth weight	Alb	Aspartate aminotransaminase (AST)
Height	Prealbumin	Alanine aminotransferase (ALT)
Growth (%)	H&H	Physical therapy (PT)
Dark urine	Chol	Serum zinc
Steatorrhea	Trig	Serum copper
Edema	Transferrin	
Jaundice	Blood urea nitrogen (BUN)	

Common Drugs Used and Potential Side Effects

- Antacids may be helpful for biliary atresia.
- Phenobarbital and cholestyramine are often used to control the hyperlipidemia of this disorder, as well as pruritus. Increase vitamin D and calcium intakes; also increase vitamin B12 and folate. Constipation can result.
- Diuretics may be used; monitor carefully.
- Growth hormone may be useful to promote catch-up growth.

Herbs, Botanicals and Supplements

- Herbs and botanicals should not be used for this condition because the liver is not able to perform its usual role of detoxification.

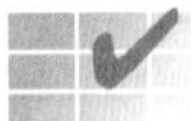

PATIENT EDUCATION

- ✔ Teach parents about proper feedings and supplements.
- ✔ If bile flow improves after surgery or transplantation, a regular diet may be used.

For More Information

- American Liver Foundation
  http://www.liverfoundation.org/indexnew.htm
- Children's Liver Association for Support Services
  1-877-679-8256
  http://www.classkids.org/library/biliaryatresia.htm

BRONCHOPULMONARY DYSPLASIA

NUTRITIONAL ACUITY RANKING: LEVEL 3 (NOT FORMALLY RANKED)

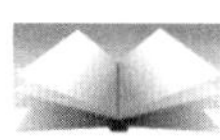

DEFINITIONS AND BACKGROUND

Bronchopulmonary dysplasia (BPD) is a chronic lung disease with abnormal growth of the lungs, usually following respiratory distress syndrome of prematurity. Mechanical ventilation, oxygen use, endotracheal intubation, and congenital heart disease may play a part in the etiology (Mueller, 2000). Slow growth occurs as a result, and feeding problems are common. Long-term chronic care is required. Infants with BPD may benefit from comprehensive postdischarge nutrition therapy and feeding therapy, which provides adequate energy, parental support and education, and feeding evaluation (Johnson et al., 1998).

Extremely low-birth-weight infants, who develop severe respiratory disease, may have special nutrient requirements to enhance utilization of nutrients for epithelial cell repair and to support catch-up growth (Atkinson, 2001). Vitamin A provides benefit in these patients (Darlow and Graham, 2000). Inositol, free fatty acids, and vitamin E are proposed nutrients for which infants at risk of chronic pulmonary insufficiency may have special requirements; further research is needed. Antioxidant therapy may also be beneficial.

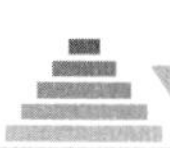

OBJECTIVES

- Achieve desirable growth. Infants with BPD tend to have delayed development (Abrams, 2001). High energy needs persist (approximately 25–50% above normal needs). Correct malnutrition and anorexia from respiratory distress and ventilator support.
- Provide optimal amounts of protein for linear growth, development, and resistance to infection. Increase lean body mass if depleted.
- Spare protein by providing extra energy from fat and carbohydrate. Need to be careful here, too much carbohydrate (CHO) can increase CO_2 and prevent extubation if too high; calculate needs carefully.
- Replace lost electrolytes, especially chloride, which may lead to death if not corrected.
- Provide essential fatty acids and inositol.
- Correct gastroesophageal reflux, which is common, especially if too high a fat formulation is given.
- Avoid overfeeding, which can lead to too rapid a weight gain for length and result in obesity.
- Prevent progressive pulmonary disease and complications such as aspiration pneumonia or choking during feeding.
- Improve tolerance for therapies and medications.
- Fluid restriction may be needed; monitor closely.
- Prevent metabolic bone disease.

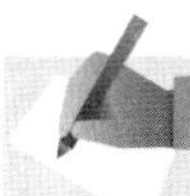

DIETARY AND NUTRITIONAL RECOMMENDATIONS

- Protein should be 7–10% of total energy for infants.
- Energy requirements will be 25% above normal; intake should be 120–160 kcal/kg to achieve optimal weight. Within the first few days of life TPN or tube feeding may be required, if possible.
- Decrease total CHO intake if glucose intolerance develops.
- Provide at least the normal recommended dietary allowances (RDAs) for antioxidant and other important nutrients. Include vitamins A, D, and E (use water-miscible sources if necessary); provide adequate calcium, phosphorus, and iron if needed. Enriched infant formula may be needed for catch-up growth.
- Fluid intake (may be restricted to less than 150 cc/kg/day) and sodium levels may need to be restricted if there is pulmonary edema or hypertension. Infants with BPD may have improved protein status with careful formula management (Puangco and Schanler, 2000).
- Infants can tolerate most formulas. Nocturnal tube feeding may be useful, especially with growth failures. With GE reflux, a gastrostomy feeding tube may be more comfortable than an NG tube.
- Increase fat:CHO ratio with respiratory distress. To meet essential fatty acid needs, start with 0.5–1 g/kg and progress to 3 g/kg.
- Omega-3 fatty acids and carnitine have been suggested, but further studies are needed. Inositol, free fatty acids, and vitamins A and E have been suggested for use with infants who have chronic pulmonary insufficiency, but only vitamin A has evidence suggestive of special requirements (Atkinson, 2001).
- When ready to progress to oral diet, use of solids may be better tolerated than liquids. If necessary, thicken liquids or formula (e.g., with baby cereal or other thickeners). Use a supine position to avoid aspiration.

Common Drugs Used and Potential Side Effects

- Exogenous steroid therapy (dexamethasone or methylprednisone) is often used to improve pulmonary compliance in ventilated premature infants; it may compromise vitamin A status and restrict somatic and bone mineral growth (Atkinson et al., 2001). Sodium retention, anorexia, edema, hypertension, and potassium losses are common side effects. Take with food to de-

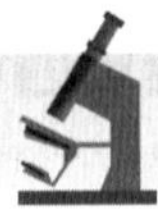

PROFILE

Clinical/History

Gestational age
Length
Body mass index (BMI)
Growth chart for height and weight (LBW and VLBW charts are available)
Size for gestational age (use intrauterine growth chart if available)
Head circumference
Emesis
Stool pattern
Urinary output
Pulmonary hypertension (HPN)

Lab Work

H&H
pH
Chol, Trig
K+ (tends to be low)
Na+
Cl (tends to be low)
Alb
Serum phosphorus; Alkaline phosphatase (alk phos)
White blood cell count (WBC)
PT
Glucose (gluc)
Oxygen saturation levels
Partial pressure of carbon dioxide (pCO2), partial pressure of oxygen (pO2)
Mg++
Urine-specific gravity

crease GI effects. Use more protein and less sodium; enhance potassium if needed.

- Antibiotics are needed during infections. Check magnesium levels.
- Bronchodilators or caffeine may be used for apnea of prematurity. Anorexia can occur.
- Diuretics may be needed to lessen pulmonary edema. Monitor those that deplete serum K+ such as furosemide (Lasix).
- Antiarrhythmics may be used.

Herbs, Botanicals and Supplements

- Herbs and botanicals should not be used for BPD because the lungs are not able to perform their role in oxygenation of cells.

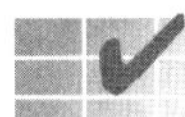

PATIENT EDUCATION

- ✓ Diet must be reevaluated periodically to reflect growth and disease process.
- ✓ New foods may be introduced gradually; thicken as needed to avoid aspiration.
- ✓ Fluid intake should be adequate to meet needs but not excessive.
- ✓ Ensure that all foods and beverages are nutrient dense.
- ✓ Discuss signs of overhydration and dehydration with the parent/caregiver.
- ✓ Oral-motor skills may be delayed from long-term ventilator use; discuss how to make adjustments with caregiver.

For More Information

- National Blood, Heart, and Lung Institute http://www.nhlbi.nih.gov/health/public/lung/other/bpd/toc.htm

CEREBRAL PALSY

NUTRITIONAL ACUITY RANKING: LEVEL 3

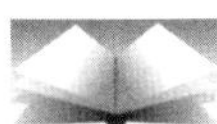

DEFINITIONS AND BACKGROUND

Cerebral palsy (CP) is a neurologic dysfunction resulting from brain damage to motor centers before, during, or after birth. Human epidemiologic data suggest a relationship between cerebral palsy and chorioamnionitis mediated by cytokines; evidence suggests this damage is the result of a fetal inflammatory response initiated in response to placental inflammation (Gaudet and Smith, 2001).

CP causes physical and mental disabilities and is considered to be nonprogressive. Seizures, mental retardation, hyperactive gag reflex, tongue thrust, poor lip closure, and inability to chew properly are common problems. Behavioral problems and visual or auditory problems may occur. Infants may present with early abnormal rolling, stiffness, irritability, and developmental delays. Symptoms may be mild or more severe and vary from one person to the next. Skeletal maturation is frequently delayed in children with cerebral palsy, a result of disrupted embryologic skeletal development due to hypoxic attack (Ihkkan ands Yalcin, 2001).

Types of palsy include spastic paralysis (difficult, stiff movement), choreoathetosis (involuntary worm-like movement), ataxia (impaired coordination and balance), and flaccidity (decreased muscle tone). Approximately, 70–80% of those with CP have the spastic form with uncontrolled shaking and stiffness; 10–20% have athetosis with continuous worm-like movement; 5–10% have ataxia; and many have mixed forms (Ekvall, 1993). Two out of 1,000 live births may be affected.

In adults with CP, athetosis may increase calorie needs as much as 524 kcal/day (Johnson et al., 1995).

OBJECTIVES

- ▲ Alleviate malnutrition resulting from the patient's inability to close lips, suck, bite, chew, or swallow.
- ▲ Promote independence through use of special feeding devices. Eye-hand coordination is often lacking, and grasp may not be strong.
- ▲ Assess appropriate energy and nutrient needs.
- ▲ Promote mealtimes in a quiet, unhurried environment.
- ▲ Correct nutritional deficits, altered growth rate, developmental delays, or retardation.
- ▲ Correct constipation and/or diarrhea.
- ▲ Prevent aspiration pneumonia and gastroesophageal reflux.
- ▲ Prevent or correct pressure ulcers.

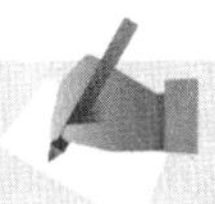

DIETARY AND NUTRITIONAL RECOMMENDATIONS

- For chewing problems, eliminate coarse, stringy foods. Puree foods as needed.
- For frequent vomiting, assess actual intake (take a calorie count). Medications may be needed.
- For constant dribbling, add cereal or yogurt to fluids.
- For constipation, use laxative foods, high fiber, or bran in the diet. Provide extra fluids. In younger children, too much fiber can displace intake of adequate nutrition; Milk of Magnesia can be used safely.
- For swallowing problems, tube feed if necessary.
- Reduce caloric intake for the spastic patient, 11 kcal/cm ages 5–11. For moderately active patients, use 14 kcal/cm.
- Increase caloric intake (45 kcal/kg) to accommodate the added movements of the older athetoid patient. Use tube feeding if needed to correct malnutrition; night feedings may allow more normal daytime routines.
- Supplement with a general multivitamin-mineral supplement, especially for B-complex vitamins.

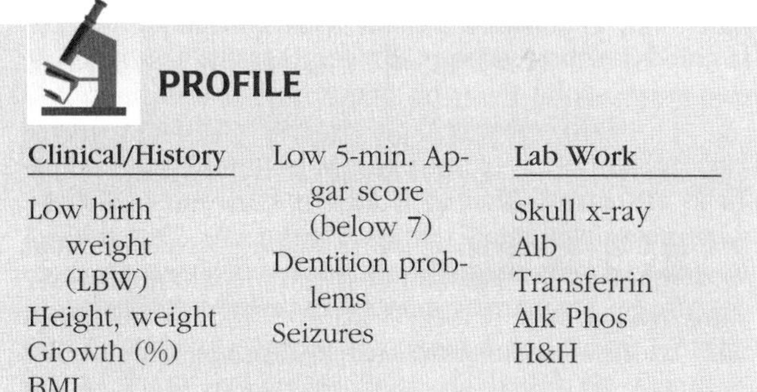

PROFILE

Clinical/History		Lab Work
Low birth weight (LBW)	Low 5-min. Apgar score (below 7)	Skull x-ray
Height, weight	Dentition problems	Alb
Growth (%)	Seizures	Transferrin
BMI		Alk Phos
		H&H

Common Drugs Used and Potential Side Effects

- Dantrolene (Dantrium) is used to control muscle spasms and cramps. It inhibits the release of calcium in muscle and skeletal tissue preventing muscle cramping and spasms. Diarrhea, changes in blood pressure, weight loss, and constipation may all occur.
- Klonopin (clonazepam) is a benzodiazepine used to slow down the central nervous system (CNS) in the treatment of spasticity. Side effects may include constipation or diarrhea, dizziness, drowsiness, clumsiness or unsteadiness, a "hangover" effect, headache, nausea, and vomiting.
- Antibiotics such as Baclofen may cause or aggravate diarrhea.
- Laxatives may often be needed; monitor for fiber and fluid needs.
- Anticonvulsants may increase risk of osteomalacia if calcium and vitamin D are insufficiently supplemented. Nutrient deficiencies are common.

Herbs, Botanicals and Supplements

- Herbs and botanicals should not be used for CP because there are no controlled trials to prove efficacy.

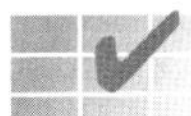

PATIENT EDUCATION

- ✓ Remind patients to keep lips closed to avoid losing food from their mouths as they try to chew.
- ✓ Fortify the diet with dry or evaporated milk, wheat germ, and other foods when intake is inadequate.
- ✓ If special training is needed for a specific feeding procedure (e.g., a preemie nipple for poor sucking), it should be provided.
- ✓ Help parent or caretaker with problems relating to dental caries, drugs, constipation, pica, or weight.
- ✓ Allow extra time for feedings.

For More Information

- American Cerebral Palsy Information Center
  http://www.cerebralpalsy.org
- United Cerebral Palsy Association, Inc.
  1660 L St., Suite 700
  Washington, DC 20036
  http://www.ucpa.org/
- Easter Seals
  230 W. Monroe Street, Ste. 1800
  Chicago, IL 60606
  312-726-6200
  http://www.easter-seals.org

CLEFT PALATE

NUTRITIONAL ACUITY RANKING: LEVEL 3

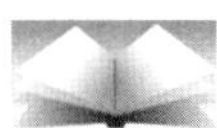

DEFINITIONS AND BACKGROUND

Cleft palate is a congenital malformation occurring during the embryonic period of development. It results in a fissure in the roof of the mouth, which may be unilateral or bilateral. Some cleft palates are complete; some are incomplete. Incidence is approximately 150 in 100,000 births.

Recently, folic acid was tested for its antiteratogenic effects on experimentally induced cleft palate; it has a partial ameliorating effect on the teratogenicity of procarbazine given to pregnant rats. Additional studies are necessary in different species (Bienengraber et al., 2001). In other studies, it was found that infants with cleft palate were often smaller in size and weight (Spyropoulos and Burdi, 2001).

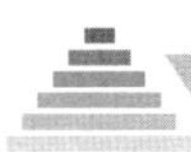

OBJECTIVES

- Compensate for the patient's inability to suck.
- Prevent choking, air swallowing, coughing, and fatigue as much as possible.
- For surgery, allow extra energy and protein for healing; use a multivitamin supplement.
- Encourage breastfeeding where possible to prevent otitis media.

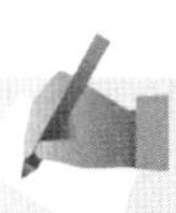

DIETARY AND NUTRITIONAL RECOMMENDATIONS

- Provide a normal diet in accordance with the patient's age (RDAs should be fulfilled, etc.).
- For feeding, use a medicine dropper or plastic bottle with a soft nipple and enlarged hole. Release formula or milk a little at a time, in coordination with the infant's chewing movements. Burp infant frequently to release swallowed air.
- In one study, squeezable and rigid feeding bottles were tested on babies with cleft palate. There was increased growth in the squeezable bottle group, and this method was found to require less support after initial instruction (Shaw et al., 1999). Haberman feeder is designed for cleft palate available through websites: www.widesmiles.org or www.medela.com.
- When the infant is 6 months of age, begin to use solids in the diet. Pureed baby foods can be used with milk in the bottle; or the infant can be spoon fed with milk used to dilute the baby foods.
- Avoid fruit peelings, nuts, peanut butter, leafy vegetables, heavy cream dishes, popcorn, grapes, biscuits, cookies, and chewing gum.
- Feed the infant in an upright position.
- If irritating, avoid spicy, acidic foods.

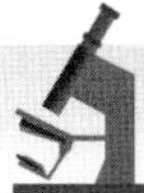

PROFILE

Clinical/History		Lab Work
Length (height)	Weight changes	Alb
Growth (%)	Head circumference	H&H
Weight	Palate type	

Herbs, Botanicals and Supplements

- Herbs and botanicals should not be used for cleft palate because there are no controlled trials to prove efficacy.

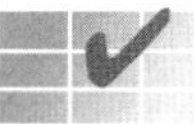

PATIENT EDUCATION

- Explain how to feed the infant with a special nipple.
- Indicate at what age the infant may be fed solids.
- Tell the parents to supplement the infant's diet with vitamin C if citrus juices are not taken well.
- Have the parents use small amounts of liquid when they are feeding the infant. To prevent choking, slow swallowing should be encouraged.

For More Information

- AboutFace USA
  http://www.aboutfaceusa.org/
- American Cleft Palate-Craniofacial Association
  http://www.cleftline.org/
- Cleft Lip and Palate Resource
  http://www.widesmiles.org/
- FACES: The National Cranio-Facial Organization
  http://www.faces-cranio.org/
- Johns Hopkins Center for Craniofacial Development & Disorders
  http://omie.med.jhmi.edu/craniofacial
- Minnesota Dietetic Association
  "Feeding Young Children with Cleft Lip and Palate"
  http://www.eatrightmn.org/
- Forward Face: The Charity for Children with Craniofacial Conditions
  317 East 34th Street, Suite 901
  New York, NY 10016
  (212) 684-5860
  (800) 393-FACE
- NYU School of Medicine
  Forward Face Support Group
  Institute of Reconstructive Plastic Surgery
  New York, NY
  (212) 263-8209
  http://www.med.nyu.edu/index.cgi

CONGENITAL HEART DISEASE

NUTRITIONAL ACUITY RANKING: LEVEL 2

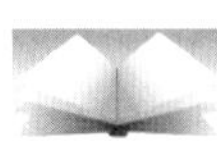

DEFINITIONS AND BACKGROUND

Persons born with congenital heart disease may have associated noncardiac anomalies (25%); a small percentage (6%) are small for gestational age at birth. Usually, some developmental defect occurred between weeks 5 and 8 of pregnancy, e.g., from rubella. Incidence is approximately 700 of 100,000 births. Patients with congenital heart disease are at increased risk for malnutrition and growth failure. Pulmonary hypertension seems to be the key factor (Varan et al., 1999).

Growth disturbance is generally related to an anatomical lesion and is most severe in infants and children with congestive heart failure (Leitch, 2001). Cyanotic congenital heart disease causes more growth retardation than acyanotic. Chronic hypoxemia may reduce serum IGF-I concentrations and cause growth retardation. Malnourished patients had the lowest IGF-I levels, and IGF-I levels rose with improvement in the oxygen saturation of patients (Dundar et al., 2000).

Energy expenditure appears to be significantly elevated in this population (Leitch, 2001). Feeding difficulties are related to the organic condition; professional support may be required for mothers of infants with cardiac heart disease (CHD) to maintain feeding routines and to deal with the difficulties that arise (Clemente et al., 2001). Supplementary oxygen is often needed, and the child will not grow if oxygen is inadequate. During feeding, many desaturate and need oxygen.

Presently, surgical repair in this population is often delayed in order to permit increased weight gain. Surgery is performed when a patient reaches an ideal weight and age or when failure to thrive precludes further waiting.

OBJECTIVES

- Support normal growth and weight gains. These infants or children tend to have growth failure, especially with associated congestive heart failure.
- Improve oral intake. Poor sucking may occur in infants.
- Lessen fatigue associated with mealtimes.
- Meet caloric needs from increased metabolic rate and from need for catch-up growth, without creating excessive cardiac burden.
- Avoid excessive renal solute overload.
- Assure adequate oxygen replacement, especially during feeding.

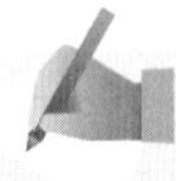

DIETARY AND NUTRITIONAL RECOMMENDATIONS

- Use calorie needs for age (e.g., 100 kcal/kg in second year of life, etc.). See RDA tables. For infants, a formula containing 90–100 kcal/dL can be used while carefully monitoring adequacy of fluid ingestion. Most formulas contain 67 kcal/dL or 20 kcal/oz.
- PEG tube feeding can be a useful adjunctive therapy, especially formulas with a lower mineral:protein ratio (e.g., partially demineralized whey).
- Energy should contain approximately 10% protein (avoid overloading), 35–50% fat as vegetable oils (known to be readily absorbed), and 40–55% CHO.
- Sodium intake should be approximately 6–8 mEq daily, dependent on diuretic use and cardiopulmonary status.
- Continuous 24-hour NG tube feeding may be useful.

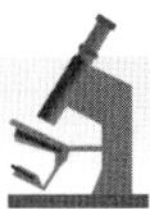

PROFILE

Clinical/History		Lab Work
Height	Blood pressure (BP)	Urinary Osm
Weight	Weight changes	Na+, K+
Head circumference	Intake and output (I & O)	BUN, Creatinine
Growth		

Common Drugs Used and Potential Side Effects

- Drugs are specific to the individual patient's requirements.

Herbs, Botanicals and Supplements

- Herbs and botanicals should not be used for congenital heart disease because there are no controlled trials to prove efficacy.

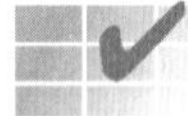

PATIENT EDUCATION

- Discuss the role of nutrition in achieving adequate growth and controlling heart disease.
- Discuss growth patterns and goals.

For More Information

- Kids with Heart, National Association for Children's Heart Disorders, Inc
  http://www.execpc.com/~kdswhrt/index.html

CYSTINOSIS AND FANCONI'S SYNDROME

NUTRITIONAL ACUITY RANKING: LEVEL 3

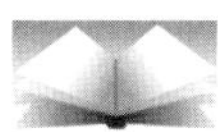

DEFINITIONS AND BACKGROUND

There are 3 distinct forms of Cystinosis. Infantile Nephropathic Cystinosis is the most severe form and is a lysosomal membrane transport defect. Failure to thrive and unexplained glucosuria of renal tubular origin may occur. Abnormal sensitivity to light and loss of color in the retina of the eyes can appear as early as 6–12 months of age. Crystals of cystine are deposited throughout the body. The affected gene is known as CTNS; molecular studies are underway. If left untreated, this form of the disease may lead to kidney failure by age 10. Toxic accumulations of copper in the brain and kidney account for neurologic symptoms. Manifestations are also seen in hereditary fructose intolerance.

In people with Intermediate Cystinosis (juvenile/adolescent), kidney and eye symptoms typically become apparent during the teenage years or early adulthood. Polyuria, growth retardation, rickets, acidosis, and vomiting are present. In Benign or Adult Cystinosis, crystalline cystine accumulates primarily in the cornea of the eyes. Adults also present with acidosis, hypokalemia, polyuria, and osteomalacia. Cystinosis may also be caused by lead poisoning.

Fanconi's syndrome is generalized tubular dysfunction and can be acquired or inherited. Renal Fanconi syndrome demonstrates impaired kidney function with excessive urination (polyuria), excessive thirst (polydipsia), and abnormally low levels of potassium in the blood (hypokalemia). Myopathy in nephropathic cystinosis results in restrictive lung disease in adults who have not received long-term cystine depletion; whether or not oral cystamine therapy can prevent this complication remains to be determined (Anikster et al., 2001).

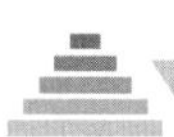

OBJECTIVES

- Prevent bone demineralization and kidney failure.
- Correct hypokalemia.
- Adapt to swallowing dysfunction.
- Support growth, which tends to be stunted in infants and children.
- Prevent or delay corneal damage.
- Provide large volumes of water and supplemental nutrients.

DIETARY AND NUTRITIONAL RECOMMENDATIONS

- Use a diet low in cystine, with Product 80056 (Mead Johnson).
- Provide sufficient fluid intake. Input and output should be checked by standards for age.
- Supplement with vitamin D (cannot convert 25-dihydroxycholecalciferol to the 1,25 form); give phosphate and calcium as appropriate. Bicarbonate is also needed.
- Provide sufficient sodium and potassium replacements.
- Alter consistency (liquids, solids) as needed.
- Monitor serum copper levels and adjust diet if needed.

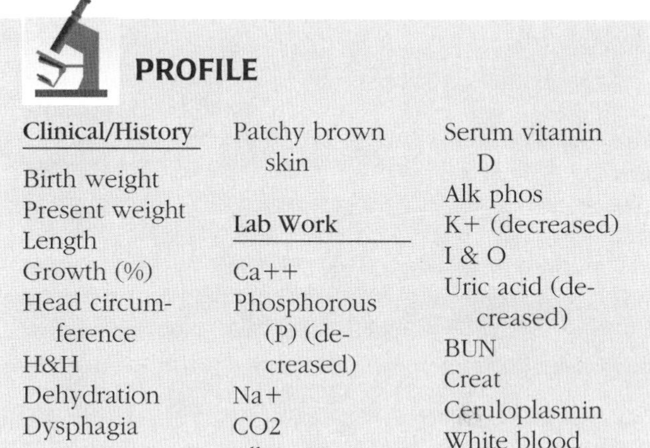

PROFILE

Clinical/History

- Birth weight
- Present weight
- Length
- Growth (%)
- Head circumference
- H&H
- Dehydration
- Dysphagia
- Patchy brown skin

Lab Work

- Ca++
- Phosphorous (P) (decreased)
- Na+
- CO2
- Alb
- Serum vitamin D
- Alk phos
- K+ (decreased)
- I & O
- Uric acid (decreased)
- BUN
- Creat
- Ceruloplasmin
- White blood cells

Common Drugs Used and Potential Side Effects

- Sodium bicarbonate or citrate should be used to correct acidosis. Take separately from iron supplements. Edema is one side effect for some patients.
- Cystamine, administered orally, can halt glomerular destruction.
- Long-term growth hormone treatment can be safe and effective in young children with nephropathic cystinosis; it should be started early in the course of the disease (Wuhl et al., 2001).

Herbs, Botanicals and Supplements

- Herbs and botanicals should not be used for this condition because there are no controlled trials to prove efficacy.

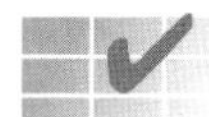

PATIENT EDUCATION

- Emphasize the importance of correcting fluid and electrolyte imbalances.
- Discuss any necessary changes in consistency.
- Discuss diet for managing renal failure if necessary.

For More Information

- American Foundation for Urologic Disease
  1128 North Charles Street
  Baltimore, MD 21201
  800-242-2383
  http://www.afud.org
- Cystinosis Central
  http://medicine.ucsd.edu/cystinosis/INDEX.htm
- Cystinosis Foundation
  http://www.cystinosisfoundation.org/
- Cystinosis Research Foundation
  http://www.cystinosis.org/

DOWN SYNDROME (MONGOLISM)

NUTRITIONAL ACUITY RANKING: LEVEL 2

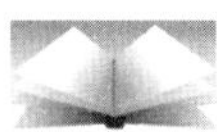

DEFINITIONS AND BACKGROUND

Down syndrome (DS) is a congenital defect, in which patients carry altered chromosomes; Trisomy 21 patients are those with an extra chromosome 21. There is a direct correlation between the incidence of the syndrome and maternal age. Children with this condition have short stature, decreased muscle tone, constipation, intestinal defects, weight changes, and mental retardation. There is a higher risk for congenital heart disease, celiac disease, Hirschsprung disease, hypothyroidism, and gastroesophageal reflux.

There is convincing epidemiologic evidence of chronic oxidative stress in individuals with DS; these individuals develop Alzheimer-like changes in the brain in their 30s and 40s, autoimmune diseases, and cataracts (Jovanovic et al., 1998). Antioxidants, such as vitamins C and E, are under study.

Recent research suggests that folate may also have a relationship to DS; folate does not cure DS (James et al., 1999). Any woman of childbearing age should consume a food source or supplement of 400 mg folic acid daily (Trissler, 2000). The Human Genome Study may point out that supplementation may help prevent this condition (Rosenblatt, 1999).

OBJECTIVES

- Provide adequate energy and nutrients for growth. Use Down's growth charts; shortness is not caused by nutritional deficiencies.
- To avoid lowering already inadequate intakes of several vitamins and minerals, treatment of obesity in children with DS should combine a balanced diet without energy restriction, vitamin and mineral supplementation, and increased physical activity (Luke et al., 1996).
- Assist with feeding problems. Tongue thrust is common.
- Prevent emotional problems that may lead to overeating.
- Counteract constipation, diarrhea, and urinary tract infections (UTIs).
- Correct gum disease, which is common.
- Monitor introduction of solid food, which is often delayed. Fruits and vegetables may not be consumed in adequate amounts (Hopman et al., 1998).

DIETARY AND NUTRITIONAL RECOMMENDATIONS

- Tube feed if the patient is unable to eat orally. Gradually wean to solids when possible.
- Supply adequate amounts of energy and protein for age. 1–1.5 g protein/kg (age-dependent) may be needed. Boys usually are given 16 kcal/cm, girls 14 kcal/cm.
- Monitor for pica, overeating, and idiosyncrasies.
- Provide supplemental sources of folate, vitamin A, vitamin E, zinc, iron, and calcium (Hopman, 1998) if intake of fruits, vegetables, meats, dairy products, or whole grains is limited.
- Provide feeding assistance if needed.
- Provide extra fluid for losses in drooling, diarrhea, or spillage.
- Encourage complex carbohydrates, prune juice, etc. if constipation is a problem.

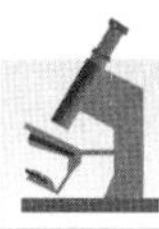

PROFILE

Clinical/History

- Length or height
- Birth weight
- Present weight
- BMI
- Head circumference
- Down syndrome growth chart
- Growth (%)
- Eye slant
- Hyperextensibility of joints
- History (hx) of prematurity
- Large tongue
- Endocardial defects
- Developmental delay
- Small nose with flat bridge
- I & O

Lab Work

- Gluc
- Uric acid (increased)
- Plasma Zn
- Chol
- Trig

Herbs, Botanicals and Supplements

- Herbs and botanicals should not be used for DS because there are no controlled trials to prove efficacy.

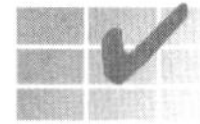

PATIENT EDUCATION

- Explain feeding techniques.
- Help control or increase caloric intake and physical activity.
- Discuss use of self-feeding utensils.
- Never rush mealtime.
- Encourage socialization.

For More Information

- Down Syndrome Health Issues
  http://www.ds-health.com
- Down Syndrome Quarterly
  http://www.denison.edu/dsq
- Drexel University
  Down Syndrome Growth Charts
  http://www.growthcharts.com/
- National Down Syndrome Society
  121 Fifth Avenue
  New York, NY 10010
  1 (800) 221-4602 or 1 (800) 232-NDSC
  http://www.ndss.org/

FAILURE TO THRIVE (GROWTH DEFICIENCY)

NUTRITIONAL ACUITY RANKING: LEVEL 4

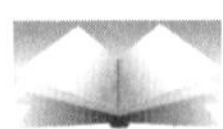

DEFINITIONS AND BACKGROUND

Failure to thrive (FTT) is a diagnostic term used to describe infants and children who fail to grow and develop at a normal rate; it is also another term for protein–calorie malnutrition. In many pediatric centers, one-third of the referred children are malnourished. Vitamin–mineral depletion is also found with protein–calorie malnutrition. Adequate hydration is needed.

Feeding disorders can lead to FTT, susceptibility to chronic illness, and death. It is a complex problem that can be caused by many factors. Prevention is suggested by giving children a wide range of foods before reaching 15–18 months, keeping healthy foods available, teaching children to communicate hunger by relating food intake to appetite, and reinforcing good mealtime behaviors (Stein, 2000).

The growth percentiles of an infant or child who fails to thrive are at the fifth percentile or below for weight and length of infants the same age. Other indices include a small head circumference, muscular wasting, apathy, weight loss, or poor weight gain. Learning failure (e.g., slow to talk, behavior problems) can occur in children with FTT. Weight is the most reliable marker for FTT and its associated problems (Raynor and Rudolf, 2000).

Primary FTT is from social/environmental deficits, inadequate feeding procedures, or caretaker behaviors. Adolescent mothers may need a lot of support and teaching. If FTT results from a problematic infant–mother interaction, there may also be a physiologic basis to the behaviors that are exhibited by these infants (Steward et al., 2001). Early interventions by trained home visitors can promote a more nurturing environment and reduce developmental delays in primary FTT (Black et al., 1995).

Secondary FTT is caused by some disease state (e.g., cancer, allergies, chronic infections, CF, cleft lip or palate, or physical or mental disability). Growth failure plus fever of unknown origin and anemia in older children or teens may suggest the onset of Crohn's disease; evaluation may be useful.

The American Dietetic Association recommends 5 medical nutrition therapy visits for infants and children with pediatric FTT (http://www.knowledgelinc.com/ada/mntguides/).

OBJECTIVES

- Provide optimal nutrition compatible with normal growth pattern. Evaluate actual versus ideal height/length and set a goal. Achieve daily gains (30 g for young infants is about average weight gain; extra may be desirable for catch-up).
- Identify and correct causes, which may include decreased intake, increased nutrient losses, increased metabolic demands, and decreased growth efficiency. Determine if malnutrition is primary (from faulty feeding patterns or dietary inadequacy) or secondary (from disease process interfering with intake).
- Teach the parent or caretaker how to properly feed and how to determine needs. Parenting advice is often useful.
- Provide adequate schedule of feeding for infant's age.
- Support catch-up growth.

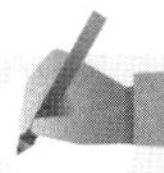

DIETARY AND NUTRITIONAL RECOMMENDATIONS

- Conduct a calorie count and full assessment with actual food intake records. Evaluate the infant's nutritional history and growth in comparison to the percentiles of normal infants. Discuss with caretaker.
- Calculate diet according to infant's age for kilocalories and protein. Energy is estimated at ideal weight for length times the RDA divided by the actual weight. By using the ideal weight for length divided by the actual weight you are including kilocalories for catch-up. Protein needs are calculated using the same method.
- Check RDAs for nutrients and provide adequate zinc and vitamin B6, as determined by the infant's age. Using slightly higher levels (such as 130%) is a common practice.
- Monitor growth (weight) and feeding behaviors. Weekly weights may be needed, especially in young infants.
- If the infant is in a state of dehydration, provide adequate amounts of water.
- FTT can be aggravated by excessive consumption of fruit juice and sweetened beverages (often 12–30 oz daily). Limit to 4–6 oz daily until overall dietary quality and growth rate have improved.
- Tube feeding may be useful or necessary as a supplemental or alternative feeding method to oral intake.

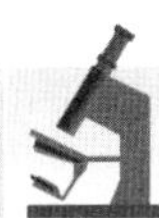

PROFILE

Clinical/History

Height
Birth weight
Weight, goal weight
BMI
Growth grid
Percent height for age (actual height/expected height)
Head circumference
Skinfold thickness
Apgar scores
Food allergies
Medical history
Prematurity? Small for gestational age (SGA)?
Breastfed or bottle-fed?
Solid food introduction pattern
Diarrhea
Vomiting
Constipation
Sources of income for food
Feeding schedule and timing

Lab Work

H&H
Alb
Gluc
Chol, Trig
BUN

Common Drugs Used and Potential Side Effects

- Evaluate all medications given for any reason to determine if some or all affect nutritional intake. Adjust diet as needed.

Herbs, Botanicals and Supplements

- Herbs and botanicals should not be used for FTT because there are no controlled trials to prove efficacy.

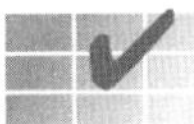

PATIENT EDUCATION

- ✓ Describe the appropriate nutritional intake according to age of the child. Describe the predisposing organic conditions when appropriate.
- ✓ Encourage the use of appropriate growth charts at home to monitor success.
- ✓ Explain proper use of over-the-counter vitamin–mineral supplements.
- ✓ Develop progress chart for developmental milestones. Growth spurts follow sustained weight gains.
- ✓ Offer simple, specific instructions such as mechanics of breastfeeding and typical intakes for children of same age.
- ✓ Practical suggestions should be offered regarding emotional support for the child. Parenting classes may be beneficial.
- ✓ Follow-up should be provided at outpatient clinics or by home visits. Refer to WIC programs if possible.
- ✓ Discuss nutrient density (e.g., milk versus soda pop).

For More Information

- ✦ American Dietetic Association
  Failure to thrive protocol
  www.eatright.org

FETAL ALCOHOL SYNDROME

NUTRITIONAL ACUITY RANKING: LEVEL 3–4

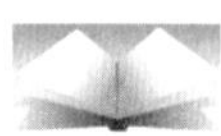

DEFINITIONS AND BACKGROUND

Generally noted shortly after birth, fetal alcohol syndrome (FAS) is a syndrome in infants with developmental delay, ocular anomalies, LBW, tremors, short stature, retardation of intellect, seizures, and microcephaly. FAS is the third leading cause of mental retardation in the United States. Children with fetal alcohol effects (FAE) perform better on motor abilities than those with FAS and have a slightly better weight status (Alvear et al., 1998).

Exposure to alcohol during brain development can permanently alter the physiology of the hippocampal formation, thus promoting epileptic activity and facilitating spreading of depression (Bonthius et al., 2001).

Sometimes blood tests are better to detect at-risk pregnant women rather than self-reported alcohol intakes (Stoler et al., 1998). Acetaldehyde may play a role in the damage that is done (Eriksson, 2001). Heavy prenatal alcohol exposure with or without physical features of FAS leads to IQ defects (Mattson et al., 1997). The steady concurrent use of tobacco and alcohol by young women emphasizes the need for enhanced efforts to reduce initial tobacco and alcohol use by young people. Women who report abuse of tobacco or alcohol should be evaluated for abuse of both substances, and interventions should address abuse of both substances, especially to prevent FAS (Ebrahim et al., 2000).

OBJECTIVES

- ▲ Promote effective family coping skills.
- ▲ Prevent additional retardation and developmental delays, blindness, etc.
- ▲ Improve intake and nutritional status.
- ▲ Prevent or correct vomiting and other problems.
- ▲ Improve cardiac symptoms.
- ▲ Promote effective parental bonding.
- ▲ Encourage normal growth patterns.

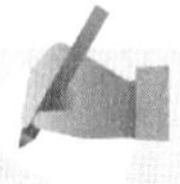

DIETARY AND NUTRITIONAL RECOMMENDATIONS

- Provide a diet appropriate for age and status (see Low Birth Weight entry).
- Ensure adequate protein and energy for catch-up growth.
- If necessary, provide tube feeding or TPN while hospitalized. Some infants may require additional attention in the home setting to promote normalized development.

Common Drugs Used and Potential Side Effects

- Anticonvulsants may be needed to correct seizures. Monitor for depletion of vitamins C, D, B12, or folic acid.

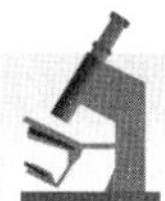

PROFILE

Clinical/History		Lab Work
Birth weight	Growth (%)	Alb
Current weight	Head circumference	Na+, K+
Length	Seizures	Gluc
		H&H

Herbs, Botanicals and Supplements

- Herbs and botanicals should not be used for FAS because there are no controlled trials to prove efficacy.

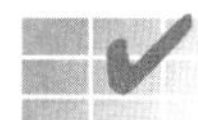

PATIENT EDUCATION

- ✓ Encourage mother's participation in alcohol rehabilitation if needed.
- ✓ Discuss appropriate feeding techniques for age of infant.
- ✓ Discuss importance of diet in aiding normal growth and development.

For More Information

- ✦ CDC-Division of Birth Defects and Developmental Disabilities
  Fetal Alcohol Syndrome Prevention Section
  4770 Buford Hwy. NE, Bldg. 101
  Atlanta, GA 30341-3724
  770-488-7370
  http://www.cdc.gov/
- ✦ Fetal Alcohol and Drug Unit
  http://depts.washington.edu/fadu
- ✦ Fetal Alcohol Syndrome websites
  http://www.come-over.to/FAS/faslinks.htm
- ✦ FAS Community Resource Center
  http://www.azstarnet.com/~tjk/fashome.htm
- ✦ National Council on Alcoholism and Drug Dependence (NCADD)
  20 Exchange Place, Suite 2902
  New York, NY 10005
  212-269-7797
  Fax: (212) 269-7510
  http://www.ncadd.org/
- ✦ National Clearinghouse for Alcohol and Drug Information (NCADI)
  11426 Rockville Pike
  Rockville, MD 20852
  1-800-729-6686
  http://www.health.org/
- ✦ National Organization of Fetal Alcohol Syndrome
  http://www.nofas.org/

HIRSCHSPRUNG'S DISEASE (MEGACOLON)

NUTRITIONAL ACUITY RANKING: LEVEL 4

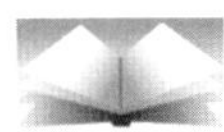

DEFINITIONS AND BACKGROUND

Hirschsprung's disease (HD) is characterized by the absence of ganglion cells and the presence of hypertrophic nerve trunks in the distal bowel (Yoneda et al., 2001). HD is also known as jejunal gangliosus or megacolon in infancy. It is a congenital malformation; this results in interference with normal mass peristalsis and functional obstruction. Treatment includes enemas and laxatives for chronic constipation. Surgical removal may be required and may be followed by a colostomy. The usual complications after a definitive pull-through procedure for HD include stricture formation, enterocolitis, bowel obstruction, and occasionally, wound infection (Finck et al., 2001).

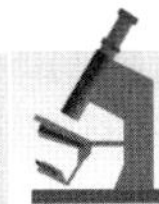

PROFILE

Clinical/History		Lab Work
Birth weight	Growth (%)	H&H
Length	Diarrhea	Alb
Present weight	Temperature	Na+
BMI	Vomiting	Gluc
FTT	Dehydration	K+
	I & O	

OBJECTIVES

- Replace electrolytes and fluids.
- Compensate for poor absorption.
- Provide adequate nutrition for the patient's age and development. Growth may be inhibited.
- Prevent complications after surgery, if that is planned.

DIETARY AND NUTRITIONAL RECOMMENDATIONS

- Use a high-calorie/high-protein diet. Enteral products or oral supplements can be used if required. In some extreme cases, TPN may be required.
- Monitor levels of potassium if laxatives are used.
- Provide total parenteral nutrition, if large sections of the bowel are removed. Gradually progress to soft/bland foods.
- Provide fluids adequate for the patient's age.
- Monitor calcium needs with long-term TPN.

Common Drugs Used and Potential Side Effects

- Laxatives can deplete numerous nutrient reserves; monitor carefully.
- If steroids are used, there are numerous nutritional consequences.

Herbs, Botanicals and Supplements

- Herbs and botanicals should not be used for megacolon because there are no controlled trials to prove efficacy.

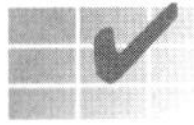

PATIENT EDUCATION

- ✓ Teach patient about sources of protein, calories, and potassium from diet.
- ✓ Discuss wound healing or colostomy, if surgery was completed.

For More Information

- American Pseudo-obstruction and Hirschsprung's Disease Society (APHS) http://www.tiac.net/users/aphs/med.htm
- The Hirschsprung's & Motility Disorders Support Network http://www.theguardiansociety.org/

HOMOCYSTINURIA

NUTRITIONAL ACUITY RANKING: LEVEL 4

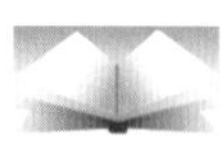

DEFINITIONS AND BACKGROUND

Homocystinuria (HCU) is an autosomal-recessive metabolic disorder, a disorder of amino acid metabolism caused by a missing cystathionine enzyme. There are three forms of HCU: cystathionine B-synthase (CBS) deficiency, defective cobalamin coenzyme synthesis, and N5,10-methylene-tetrahydrofolatedreductase deficiency. Therefore, depending on the type, use of the appropriate vitamin becomes important. Dietary restriction of methionine is only helpful in the CBS deficiency; in the others it is harmful to restrict.

Human CBS is an S-adenosylmethionine-regulated enzyme that plays a key role in the metabolism of HCU (Shan et al., 2001). Deranged vitamin B6 metabolism or low levels of reductase enzyme may also cause HCU (methionine to cysteine conversion). It occurs in 1 in 20,000 to 1 in 200,000 births in the U.S. If untreated, it may lead to mental retardation, seizures, altered growth, hepatic disease, osteoporosis, thromboses, glaucoma, cataracts, or strokes. Urinary excretion of homocystine occurs but is an unusual condition. A single biochemical test is not available; abnormal urinary tHcy response after methionine loading is the most sensitive test (Guttormsen et al., 2001).

Inborn errors of cobalamin transport and metabolism present with HCU and methylmalonic aciduria, either alone or in combination; they share many of the clinical features of nutritional cobalamin deficiency (Rosenblatt and Whitehead, 1999). Patients may have dramatic reduction of plasma-free homocystine and urine methylmalonic acid excretion after initiation of therapy with carnitine, intramuscular hydroxocobalamin, and, in two cases, oral betaine; growth and microcephaly may also be improved (Anderssin et al., 1999).

Tall stature is almost invariably seen in homocystinuric patients, suggesting that overgrowth is directly mediated by homocysteine and that it may be prevented by optimal metabolic control (Topaloglu et al., 2001).

OBJECTIVES

- Reduce methionine in the diet to prevent accumulation of homocystine only in CBS deficiency.
- Prevent further mental retardation and growth delays, etc. Fractures are common because of defective collagen formation; eye is affected and so lens may become dislocated in CBS deficiency
- Prevent cardiovascular complications (arterial and venous thrombosis).
- Supplement with essential nutrients. It is possible that low folic acid intakes aggravate the symptoms.

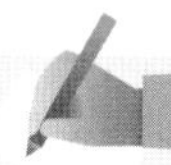

DIETARY AND NUTRITIONAL RECOMMENDATIONS

- **For B6 nonresponsive group,** dietary control of methionine intake is the mainstay of therapy. Use a low-protein diet with a supplement of cystine to supply sulfur. Reduce intake of methionine (only in CBS deficiency), no meat, poultry, fish, or eggs. Soy products (e.g., Isomil, ProSobee, Soyalac) can be used. XMET Maxamaid (SHS North America, Gaithersburg, MD), Hominex 1 for infants or Hominex 2 for children (Ross Laboratories), or Product HOM 1 or HOM 2 (Mead Johnson) are also useful.
- The doctor may prescribe large doses of vitamin B6. Also supplement with folic acid. Monitor needs carefully.
- Increase fluid intake.

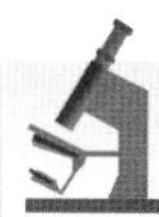

PROFILE

Clinical/History	Lab Work	
Birth weight	ALT, AST	Serum folate
Present weight	Gluc	Serum and urinary homocystine
BMI	Serum B12	Plasma methionine (increases more than 1 mg/dL)
Length	Urinary methylmalonic acid	
FTT		
Growth (%)		
Hepatomegaly		
Pale complexion		
Seizures		

Common Drugs Used and Potential Side Effects

- Dipyridamole may be used to decrease thrombosis.
- Pyridoxine therapy (vitamin B6) for longer than 1 month is useful for some patients. The doctor may prescribe 100–500 mg or higher. Folic acid and vitamin B12 should be supplied if low serum levels are detected.

Herbs, Botanicals and Supplements

- Herbs and botanicals should not be used for HCU because there are no controlled trials to prove efficacy.

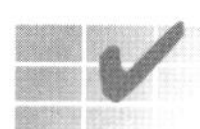

PATIENT EDUCATION

- Emphasize the importance of controlling diet, snacks, etc.
- Discuss good food sources of folic acid and other B-complex vitamins.

INBORN ERRORS OF CARBOHYDRATE METABOLISM

NUTRITIONAL ACUITY RANKING: LEVEL 4

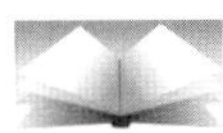

DEFINITIONS AND BACKGROUND

A defective gene that prevents a normal step in carbohydrate metabolism is the cause of these inborn error disorders. Diagnosis of these conditions is usually during infancy or childhood, with hypoglycemia, hepatomegaly, poor physical growth, and deranged biochemical profiles. Those with delayed development, seizures, stroke-like episodes, cerebellar hypoplasia, and demyelinating neuropathy should be assessed for CHO-deficient syndromes (Patterson, 1999).

Fructosemia results from a defect in the enzyme converting fructose to glucose.

Sucrose/maltose intolerance requires omission of sucrose and maltose from the diet.

Galactosemia results from a lack of galactose-1-phosphate uridyltransferase (GALT), possibly in combination with high levels of galactitol (Ning et al., 2001). Cataracts can occur if untreated.

For congenital glucose–galactose malabsorption (CGGM), a rare disorder thought to be an autosomal-recessive trait, watery, profuse diarrhea occurs because of the defective sodium-coupled cotransport of glucose and galactose in the intestinal mucosa. A CHO-free formula, to which fructose is incrementally added, may be tolerated. (Abad-Sinden et al., 1997).

Hepatic glycogen storage diseases (GSDs) are rare genetic disorders in which glycogen cannot be metabolized to glucose in the liver because of enzyme deficits. GSD type I (glucose-6-phosphatase deficiency, Von Gierke's disease) is caused by a deficiency of the enzyme, which normally converts glycogen to glucose. Treatment of GSD type 1 by portacaval shunt may need to be considered in patients with height-for-age below the 3rd percentile (Corbeel et al., 2000). GSD type II is alpha glucosidase deficiency, Pompe's disease. GSD type III is debrancher enzyme deficiency, Cori disease. GSD type IV is brancher enzyme deficiency, Anderson's disease. GSD type V (muscle glucagon phosphorylase deficiency, McArdle's disease) is an X-linked liver glycogenosis (XLG) and is one of the most common forms of glycogen storage disease (Burwinkel et al., 1998). GSD type VI is liver phosphorylase deficiency, Hers disease. GSD type VII is muscle phosphofructokinase deficiency, Tauri disease. GSD type IX is liver glycogen phosphorylase kinase deficiency. Liver transplantation results in normal fasting glucose production, normal glucose and insulin concentrations, and mildly elevated glucagon concentrations in patients.

OBJECTIVES

- Prevent hypoglycemia, where indicated.
- Eliminate the offending nutrient that cannot be digested. Alter other nutrient intakes to promote growth and maintenance.
- Read labels carefully. Note that galactose is not reported on labels (Gropper et al., 1993).
- For persons with galactosemia, correct diet to prevent physical and mental retardation, cataracts, portal hypertension, and cirrhosis. Vitamin E is being studied for its positive, protective effects.
- For persons with glycogen storage disease, maintain glucose homeostasis, prevent hypoglycemia, promote positive nitrogen balance and growth, and correct or prevent fatty liver.
- Sucrose intolerance occurs rarely as a genetic defect or temporarily after GI flu or irritable bowel distress. Sucrase deficiency may be combined with maltase deficiency. Eliminate the carbohydrate(s) to decrease osmotic diarrhea.
- Fructose intolerance is rare and can cause GI discomfort, nausea, malaise, and growth failure.

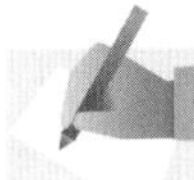

DIETARY AND NUTRITIONAL RECOMMENDATIONS

Fructosemia:

- Diet must exclude fructose, sucrose, sorbitol, invert sugar, maple syrup, honey, and molasses.
- Read labels carefully.
- Be careful when using tube feedings or intravenous solutions that may contain sources of fructose.

Galactosemia:

- Use a lactose and galactose-free diet—no milk, milk products, soybeans, peaches, lentils, liver, brains, or breads or cereals containing milk or cream cheese. Fresh blueberries and honeydew melon should be excluded from the diets of these persons; however, fresh cherries, citrus, mango, red plums, and strawberries are allowed (Stepnick-Gropper et al., 2000).
- For infants with the condition, try formulas such as Isomil or ProSobee, Elecare, Nutramigen, or formulas containing casein hydrolysate.
- Supplement with calcium, vitamin D, vitamin E, and riboflavin. In some forms of galactosemia, galactose can often be reintroduced later in life.
- Be careful when using tube feedings or intravenous solutions that may contain sources of lactose.
- Read labels carefully; galactose is not reported on labels (Gropper et al., 1993). Formulas labeled "low lactose" are <u>not</u> good substitutes; they contain lactose in amounts that can seriously harm patients with galactosemia.

Glycogen storage disease:

- Increase protein intake (for most types).
- Use small, frequent feedings and, if steroids are used in treatment, a 2-g sodium diet.

- Avoid lactose and sucrose. Glucose may be used; check labels. Cornstarch is used to prevent hypoglycemia.
- Concentrated sweets may be restricted.
- Sometimes, night feedings with additional daytime meals work effectively. Giving Vivonex or cornstarch/uncooked starch at night may help the liver to maintain a normal blood glucose level (sometimes allowing omission of parenteral nutrition).
- A multivitamin–mineral supplement with vitamin C, iron, and calcium may be needed because fruits and milk are limited.

Sucrose/maltose intolerance:
- Omit sucrose and maltose from the diet.
- For nongenetic form, gradually add these sugars back into the diet.
- Be careful when using tube feedings or intravenous solutions, which may contain sources of sucrose or maltose.

PROFILE

Clinical/History		
Height or Length	Edema	Gluc (may drop in fructosemia)
Weight	**Lab Work**	Acetone
BMI	Trig and Chol (elevated in Von Gierke's)	Serum phosphate
Growth (%)	Fructose or lactose tests	Serum lactate
Infections	Urinary & serum galactose or fructose	Serum ammonia
Nausea and vomiting		Uric acid
Jaundice		Alb
Head circumference		

Common Drugs Used and Potential Side Effects

- For persons with galactosemia, eliminate drugs containing lactose and supplement with calcium and riboflavin.
- Sucrose and maltose are added to many drugs; check carefully.
- All vitamin–mineral supplements must be free of the nontolerated carbohydrates.

Herbs, Botanicals and Supplements

- Herbs and botanicals should not be used for these conditions because there are no controlled trials to prove efficacy.

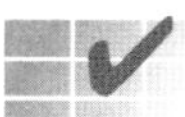

PATIENT EDUCATION

- ✓ Explain which sources of carbohydrate are allowed specific to the disorder.
- ✓ Read labels carefully. Many foods contain milk solids, galactose (e.g., luncheon meats, hot dogs), and other sugars. Omit according to the disorders.
- ✓ Contact formula companies regarding special product updates. More research is being conducted regarding these conditions.

For More Information

- Association for Glycogen Storage Disease
  http://www.agsd.org.UK/

LARGE-FOR-GESTATIONAL-AGE INFANT

NUTRITIONAL ACUITY RANKING: LEVEL 2

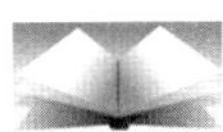

DEFINITIONS AND BACKGROUND

High birth weight (3,300–4,000+ g) at 40 weeks is termed "large for gestational age." These infants are considered to be over the 90th percentile of appropriate weight for gestational age. Common problems often include hypoglycemia, respiratory distress, aspiration pneumonia, bronchial paralysis, macrosomia, and facial paralysis. They are often born to mothers who are obese or have diabetes, multiparous women, or mothers with genetic predispositions for excessive birth weight.

Fetal growth standards are more appropriate in predicting the impact of birth weight category on the risk of spontaneous preterm delivery than are neonatal growth standards; the risks of preterm birth in LGA infants are 2- to 3-fold greater than the risk among appropriate-for-gestational-age (AGA) infants (Lackman et al., 2001). LGA neonates have higher body fat and lower lean body mass than AGA infants; impaired maternal glucose tolerance exaggerates these body composition changes (Hammami et al., 2001).

OBJECTIVES

- Allow adequate growth rate and development.
- Prevent hypoglycemia.
- Maintain calories at lowest possible level while allowing adequate growth to prevent obesity and its consequences.
- Monitor serum lipid levels as deemed necessary.

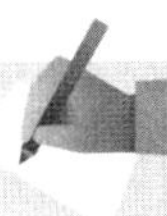

DIETARY AND NUTRITIONAL RECOMMENDATIONS

- Feed often or with larger amounts, as indicated by infant's appetite.
- Control source of calories, avoiding excessive glucose intake if infant shows signs of hyperglycemia.
- Alter intake of fat as determined by a lipid profile.

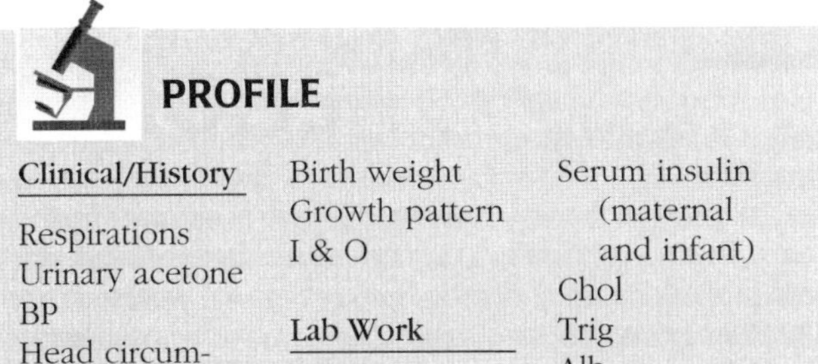

PROFILE

Clinical/History	Lab Work	
Birth weight	Serum gluc (maternal and infant)	Chol
Growth pattern	Serum insulin (maternal and infant)	Trig
I & O		Alb
Respirations		H&H
Urinary acetone		
BP		
Head circumference		
Length		

Common Drugs Used and Potential Side Effects

- Insulin may be necessary to control hyperglycemia. Beware of any excesses, which could aggravate hypoglycemia.

Herbs, Botanicals and Supplements

- Herbs and botanicals should not be used for LGA infants because there are no controlled trials to prove efficacy for any related problems.

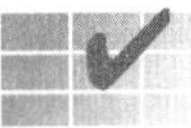

PATIENT EDUCATION

- Signs of hyperglycemia and hypoglycemia should be discussed.
- Discuss normal growth patterns as appropriate for the larger infant.
- Review risks inherent in another pregnancy, especially if the mother has diabetes.

LOW BIRTH WEIGHT OR PREMATURITY

NUTRITIONAL ACUITY RANKING: LEVEL 3

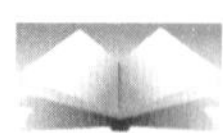

DEFINITIONS AND BACKGROUND

Low-birth-weight (LBW) infants weigh less than 2,500 g or 5.5 lb (below 10th percentile for gestational age) at birth. Very-low-birth-weight (VLBW) infants (lower than 1,300–1,500 g) are especially prone to nutritional deficits. For this group, a slower pace of feeding may be needed if respiratory instability occurs (Blondheim et al., 1993). Infants who weigh 1,000 g are sometimes called "micropreemies." Typical problems include hypoglycemia, hypothermia, jaundice, dry skin, decreased subcutaneous fat, and anemia. Admission to neonatal ICUs is common.

LBW infants comprise 6–7% of all live births; 20% are born to mothers younger than 15 years of age. LBW infants may be small for date or have intrauterine growth retardation or dysmaturity. Early motherhood is associated with LBW infants, and because this is avoidable, public health strategies need to be developed to educate women about delaying pregnancy (Okosun et al., 2000). Infants of women with hypertension, preeclampsia, smoking, or use of an antihypertensive agent or prednisone during pregnancy are at increased risk of LBW, preterm birth, diseases of prematurity, and death (Ray et al., 2001).

Premature infants are infants younger than 36 weeks of gestational age. The usual gestational age is 40 weeks. Prematurity is often correlated with LBW. For premature infants, the immunologic and GI benefits of human milk compared with those of preterm infant formula outweigh the risks associated with slower growth (Schanler et al., 1999). Loss of body water is the same with healthy preterm babies and those with respiratory distress syndrome; adequate nutrition support almost immediately after birth is important (Tang et al., 1997).

Interventions to support BF in the hospital and at home are indicated to improve brainstem maturation (Amin et al., 2000), as is an increased emphasis on monitoring growth among LBW infants to prevent developmental delays. If weight gain by 4 months is not adequate, aggressive nutritional therapy should be offered (Kennedy et al., 1999). For VLBW babies, during the first months after discharge, they need to have nutrition support to help promote early catch-up growth and mineralization. These babies are at risk of postnatal growth deficiency and osteopenia (Rigo et al., 2000).

Early feeding increases intestinal lactase activity in preterm infants; lactase activity is a marker of intestinal maturity and may influence clinical outcomes. Infants who begin enteral feedings early have 100% greater lactase activity at age 10 days and 60% greater levels at age 28 days than those who start at traditional times (Shulman et al., 1998). Enteral glutamine supplementation for VLBW infants decreases morbidity and sepsis in particular (Neu et al., 1997). Hospital costs are lower when VLBW infants receive enteral glutamine supplements than when they do not (Dallas et al., 1998).

In LBW infants, although the full-term sucking pattern is not necessary for successful oral feeding, an infant's feeding proficiency and efficiency at the first oral feeding are reliable predictors of early independent oral feeding (Lau et al., 1997). Non-nutritive sucking before bottle feedings may improve oxygen saturation, behavior state, and feeding behavior of preterm infants (Pickler et al., 1996). Premature breast milk has higher electrolyte, protein, and MCT than mature breast milk.

Table 3–4 lists the nutritional deficits found in premature or LBW infants. The American Dietetic Association recommends 5 medical nutrition therapy visits for high-risk, premature infants (http://www.knowledgelinc.com/ada/mntguides/).

OBJECTIVES

- Begin feedings of distilled water or colostrum as soon as possible for infants without respiratory distress. Early feeding (3–5 days after birth) tends to allow babies to mature faster than those fed later. Early-fed babies have fewer days of intolerance, a shorter hospital length-of-stay, and earlier tolerance of full feedings.
- Encourage the mother to breastfeed, especially to provide milk with the higher preterm protein level.
- Supplement the infant's diet as needed with formula or MCT; ensure intake of EFAs.
- Gradually increase energy and protein to meet the needs of rapid growth.
- Promote normal growth and development. Prevent illness, rickets, respiratory distress, hypoglycemia or hyperglycemia, necrotizing enterocolitis, infections, obstructive jaundice, and tyrosinemia.
- Ensure proper whey:casein ratio.
- Include amino acids in proper amounts, especially cysteine, taurine, tyrosine, and glycine. American McGaw makes intravenous TrophAmine for parenteral nutrition (PN).

TABLE 3–4 Nutritional Deficits in the Premature or LBW Infant

1. Marginal nutrient stores at birth, fat, glycogen, and minerals such as calcium and phosphorus.
2. Limited ability to consume adequate amounts of nutrient caused by delayed oral neuromuscular development and small gastric capacity.
3. Immaturity at the cellular level with consequent alteration of biochemical needs.
4. Higher metabolic demands and rate of growth.
5. Malabsorption from underdeveloped digestive/absorptive abilities.
6. Risk from poor nutritional intake of the mother where relevant. Mothers who are folate deficient are more likely to give birth to LBW infants.
7. Risk of EFA deficiency with less growth, more renal and lung changes, fatty liver, impaired water balance, RBC fragility, and dermatitis.

- ▲ Advance oral or tube feedings to reduce cholestasis and osteopenia.
- ▲ EFA deficiency increases antioxidative susceptibility of RBCs in VLBW infants (Tomsits et al., 2000).
- ▲ Assure adequate intake of folate and vitamin B12 to reduce severe anemias.
- ▲ Prolonged IV feeding with solutions containing aluminum is associated with impaired neurologic development (Bishop, 1997). Bayley Scales of Mental Development are used to assess neurologic development; those infants exposed to aluminum are more likely to have an index below 85 (more likely to have increased risk of subsequent educational problems).

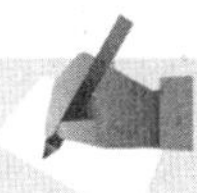

DIETARY AND NUTRITIONAL RECOMMENDATIONS

- While in the radiant warmer, feed the infant 60–80 mL/kg body weight (BW)/day of water. Gradually increase to 150 mL/kg BW. Add electrolytes (Na+, Cl−, K+ on at least the second day).
- Day 1—breastfeed or give glucose at 6–8 mg/kg/min. Progress to special formulas such as Similac Special Care 24, SMA "Preemie," Enfamil Premature Formula (24 kcal/oz) to yield 120–150 mL/kg up to 180–200 mL/kg/day. Use TPN if not fed by day 3; infusion rate in the neonatal intensive care unit (NICU) is often 15 mg/kg per minute. Use 100 kcal/kg, 2–3 g/kg for amino acids, and 70 kcal/kg nonprotein calories.
- Special needs: Extra energy may be needed for fever (7% per 1° elevation), for cardiac failure (15–25%), for major surgery (20–30%), for severe sepsis (40–50%), for protein–calorie malnutrition (PCM) (50–100%), for burns (100%), or for growth failure (60%).
- TPN needs are similar to enteral nutrition (EN) needs. Modern crystalline amino acid infusions promote positive nitrogen balance by use of 1 g/kg/day as soon as possible.
- Tube feeding initiation: Start at 10–15 mL/hour at one-quarter strength. Progress as tolerated to desired rate.
- Within 7 days, the diet should provide 120–150 kcal/kg BW daily. Carbohydrate should be 40–45% total kcal (10–30 g/kg). Protein should be age specific. Nonprotein:protein kcal should be 150–200:1. Advance by no more than 20 mL/kg daily.
- If poor sucking or swallowing instincts exist, the infant may need gavage feeding. Feed every 2 hours or use a continuous drip feeding and change to bolus feedings when full strength is tolerated.
- Feeding style: If infant weighs 1,000–1,750 g, feed more vigorously; if infant weighs 1,750 g or more, feed as a normal term infant.
- The nutrient needs of an LBW infant may be as follows: high levels of calcium (140–160 mg/100 kcal), 25 international units (IU) of vitamin E (water soluble) daily, 2.5 mg iron/100 kcal in formula (necessary only if stores are depleted), 300–500 IU of vitamin D, adequate folic acid, adequate sodium (3 mEq/day) to avoid hyponatremia, 30–50 mg vitamin C/day, and 95–108 mg phosphorus per 100 kcal given. Monitor need for vitamin B12.
- Other nutrients should be provided according to the RDAs for the newborn: Magnesium, zinc, selenium, and copper may be low. New evidence suggests that Vitamin A should be supplemented (Wardle et al., 2001; Shenai et al., 2000).
- Total fat should be 2–3 g/kg, to meet energy needs without excess carbohydrate. Soybean oil can give EFAs (1–2% EFAs needed) in linoleic acid form. Exogenous carnitine may be needed to take EFAs into the mitochondria. Inositol (in membrane phospholipids) may also be needed to decrease respiratory distress, but this is still under study.
- With TPN, use up to 3 mg/kg/day lipid infused continuously or early enteral feeding to prevent cholestatic liver disease. Carnitine deficiency may also occur with PN therapy (Bonner et al., 1995).

TABLE 3–5 Enteral Needs (Premature Infant):

Basal needs = 40–50 kcal/kg
+ activity 5–15 kcal/kg
+ cold stress 0–10 kcal/kg
+ fecal losses 10–15 kcal/kg
+ SDA 10 kcal/kg
+ growth 20–30 kcal/kg
Total = 85–130 kcal/kg

PROFILE

Clinical/History		
Birth weight	Apgar scores	Transferrin (8-day half-life)
Gestational age	I & O	ALT, AST
Birth length	**Lab Work**	Serum folacin and B12
Percentage of weight/length	H&H	PO4
Swallowing reflex	Alb	Total lymphocyte count (TLC)
Temperature (often decreases)	Ca++	Gluc
Sucking reflex	Respiratory distress syndrome (RDS)	Lecithin-sphingomyelin ratio (L:S ratio)
	Prealbumin (7-day half-life)	Bilirubin

Common Drugs Used and Potential Side Effects

- VLBW babies often experience hyperkalemia and hyperglycemia and are given insulin to manage these problems (Ditzenberger et al., 1999). Insulin may also be needed if hyperglycemia results from TPN. Continuous intravenous infusion is best tolerated.
- Other medications may be used for underlying disease states.

Herbs, Botanicals and Supplements

- Herbs and botanicals should not be used for LBW or prematurity because there are no controlled trials to prove efficacy for any related problems.

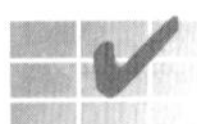

PATIENT EDUCATION

- ✓ Teach the caretaker or parent about increased nutrient needs of infant. Special formulas have 80 kcal/dL compared with the usual 67 kcal/dL and have MCT, extra protein, calcium, phosphorus, and sodium.
- ✓ Chronic lung disease, prolonged parenteral nutrition, delayed initiation of enteral feeding, severe intraventricular hemorrhage, necrotizing enterocolitis, or late-onset sepsis delays weight gain in VLBW infants (Ehrenkrantz, 1999). Emphasize the normal progression of infant feeding after the infant achieves adequate growth pattern and weight. Catch-up is common by 2–3 years.
- ✓ Emphasize the importance of zinc, vitamin B6, and vitamin E in small infants (for growth).
- ✓ Monitor for the tendency to aspirate, for lactose intolerance, and for other problems.
- ✓ Decrease use of supplements when 300 kcal/day can be consumed.
- ✓ Follow-up clinic or home visits are recommended.
- ✓ The child may benefit from the WIC program if available.
- ✓ VLBW infants experience catch-up growth and attain predicted genetic height during adolescence, if they were not small for gestational age (Hirata and Bosque, 1998).
- ✓ VLBW infants (i.e., less than 1,000 g), who survive without major neurodevelopmental disability, attain lower growth during adolescence than normal-birth-weight infants; sexual maturation and relative body composition will be similar (Peralta-Carcelen et al., 2000).
- ✓ Do not overfeed.

For More Information:

- ✦ The American Dietetic Association
  High Risk Premature Infant protocol
  http://www.eatright.org

MAPLE SYRUP URINE DISEASE

NUTRITIONAL ACUITY RANKING: LEVEL 4

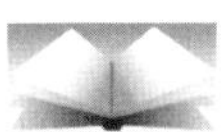

DEFINITIONS AND BACKGROUND

Maple syrup urine disease (MSUD) results from an autosomal recessive trait, causing an inborn error of metabolism in which branched-chain amino acids (BCAAs—leucine, isoleucine, valine) are not degraded through decarboxylation to simple acids. MSUD occurs in 1 in 225,000 births. Onset of disease occurs in children aged 1–8 years. The name of the disease reflects the maple syrup odor of the urine and sweat of affected children. The Mennonite population from eastern Pennsylvania is at high risk for this disorder.

If the disease is left untreated, it leads to retardation and peripheral neuropathy. Thiamine is the coenzyme for BCAAs. Alpha-keto acids also have a role in MSUD along with transport of glutamate (Reis et al., 2000).

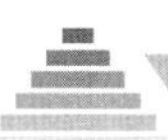

OBJECTIVES

- Feed despite difficulty with sucking and swallowing reflexes.
- Replace needed electrolytes if prolonged vomiting occurs.
- Control intake of BCAAs for life. As the child grows, add BCAAs individually in a controlled manner.
- Prevent tissue catabolism. Support normal growth and development.
- Prevent toxic buildup of abnormal metabolites, which may cause retardation.

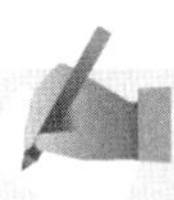

DIETARY AND NUTRITIONAL RECOMMENDATIONS

- Restrict intake of BCAAs in the diet. Use Mead Johnson's MSUD powder or Ross Laboratories' Maxamaid MSUD. Use the latter with Product 80056 (Mead Johnson) because it contains no cholesterol or fat.
- Use patient support to alleviate feeding problems.
- Use small amounts of milk in the diet to support growth.
- Gelatin, a form of protein low in BCAAs, may be used in the diet.
- Replace needed electrolytes.
- The doctor may prescribe large doses of thiamine for children who are thiamine responsive.
- Provide adequate caloric intake to spare protein.

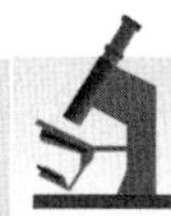

PROFILE

Clinical/History	Lab Work	
Length (height)	Plasma leucine, isoleucine, valine	Urinary excretion of ketoacids
Birth weight	Plasma L-alloisoleucine >5 micromol/L (most specific and most sensitive for MSUD)	Urinary odor
Present weight		Alb
Growth (%)		Globulin
BMI		Uric acid (increase)
Grand mal seizures		
Hypertonicity		

Herbs, Botanicals and Supplements

- Herbs and botanicals should not be used for MSUD because there are no controlled trials to prove efficacy for any related problems.

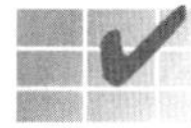

PATIENT EDUCATION

- Tell the patient that the diet must be maintained for life.
- Make sure that the diet's total calorie and protein intake is appropriate for the patient's age and stage of development.
- Cow's milk contains 350 mg of leucine, 228 mg of isoleucine, and 245 mg of valine per 100 mL.

For More Information

- MSUD Family Support Group
  http://www.msud-support.org/

MYELOMENINGOCELE

NUTRITIONAL ACUITY RANKING: LEVEL 2

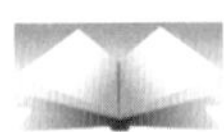

DEFINITIONS AND BACKGROUND

Myelomeningocele (MMC) is one of the most severe forms of birth defects of the brain and spinal cord. The bones of the spine do not completely form, and the spinal canal is incomplete. This allows the spinal cord and meninges (the membranes covering the spinal cord) to protrude from the child's back. MMC is a severe malformation that includes external protrusion of meninges, spinal fluid and cord, and the nerve roots. Neural tube defects (NTDs) may be caused by a variety of genetically caused defects in developmental mechanisms that are responsible for elevation of the neural folds (Harris and Juriloff, 1999). The cause of MMC is unknown. However, folic acid deficiency is thought to play a part in all NTDs. Daily consumption of 400 micrograms of folic acid before conception and during early pregnancy dramatically reduces the occurrence of NTDs (Honein et al., 2001).

MMC is a congenital CNS defect with myelodysplasia and cystic distention of the meninges. Patients are usually wheelchair-bound or will wear braces or be on crutches. Patients with MMC are often overweight; this may occur because of complex interactive factors that are not strictly related to energy intake (Fiore et al., 1998). Obesity may occur because of decreased active muscle tissue. Obesity can increase likelihood of pressure ulcers or make ambulation and surgery more difficult (see also Spina Bifida and Neural Tube Defects).

Protrusion of the spinal cord and meninges damages the spinal cord and nerve roots, causing a decrease or lack of function of body areas controlled at or below the defect. Symptoms are related to the anatomic level of the defect. Most defects occur in the lower lumbar or sacral areas of the back (the lowest areas of the back), because this area is normally the last part of the spine to close. Symptoms include partial or complete paralysis of the legs with corresponding partial or complete lack of sensation and loss of bowel or bladder control. The exposed spinal cord is susceptible to infections such as meningitis. Congenital disorders such as hydrocephalus and hip dislocation may also be present.

OBJECTIVES

- Control weight; metabolic rate may only be 50% usual rate for age.
- Prevent or heal pressure ulcers.
- Promote any and all possible ambulation or activity.
- Correct infections; prevent or correct sepsis.
- Correct nutrient deficiencies.
- Alter diet to prevent or correct constipation, obesity, and urinary tract infections.
- Manage feeding problems, which are common.

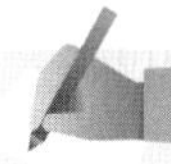

DIETARY AND NUTRITIONAL RECOMMENDATIONS

- Decrease energy to control weight; as low as 7 kcal/cm may be needed. Use of standard CDC growth charts is not beneficial in this population.
- Low-calorie snacks should be the only between-meal snacks allowed.
- For healing of any pressure ulcers, adequate zinc, vitamins A and C, and protein are required.
- Ensure adequate fiber intake and fluid to prevent or correct problems with diarrhea or constipation.

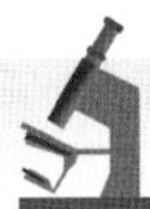

PROFILE

Clinical/History		
Height, weight	Constipation	Chol
Birth weight/length	Skin integrity	Na+
BMI	Triceps skinfold (TSF)	K+
Weight changes	Hydrocephaly	Mg++
Temperature	**Lab Work**	Ca++
Diarrhea	H&H	Gluc
		Alb, prealbumin
		Serum Fe

Common Drugs Used and Potential Side Effects

- No specific drugs are used in this condition. Monitor individual prescriptions.
- Be cautious when using zinc and iron (especially with parenteral administration) with infections or sepsis; these are bacterial nutrients.

Herbs, Botanicals and Supplements

- Herbs and botanicals should not be used for MMC because there are no controlled trials to prove efficacy for any related problems.

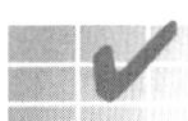

PATIENT EDUCATION

- Behavior modification, low-calorie food and snack preparation, rewards, and activity/exercise factors should be reviewed with the parent/caretaker.

- ✔ Food lists with green "go" foods, red "stop" foods, and yellow "caution" foods have been used with some success for weight management.
- ✔ Parental/caretaker motivation and attitude are important.

For More Information

- ✦ Information and Resources
  http://neurosurgery.mgh.harvard.edu/hyd-rsrc.htm

NECROTIZING ENTEROCOLITIS

NUTRITIONAL ACUITY RANKING: LEVEL 4

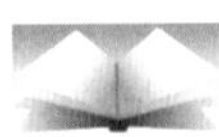

DEFINITIONS AND BACKGROUND

Necrotizing enterocolitis (NEC) involves ischemia of the intestinal tract and invasion of the mucosa with enteric pathogens. Age is important because this problem can occur in preterm infants. Symptoms and signs include a distended abdomen, lethargy, RDS, pallor, hyperbilirubinemia, vomiting, diarrhea, grossly bloody stools, and sepsis. NEC is the leading cause of short bowel syndrome in infancy. This is a medical emergency.

NEC is a serious GI disease that mainly affects premature infants but has been seen in infants with congenital heart disease. Cases of NEC in those with heart disease after cardiac procedures may have resulted from mesenteric ischemia (Fatica et al., 2000). It also occurs in small, asphyxiated preterm infants after exchange transfusions or in infants with Hirschsprung's disease.

Feeding intolerance can be rather significant. It seems to be beneficial to use breast milk rather than formula in the prevention of NEC. Infants with colitis induced by protein in their infant formula may not respond to casein hydrolysate formula; symptoms may resolve when given amino acid hydrolysate infant formula (Vanderhoof et al., 1997).

NEC affects about 1–5% of all admissions to NICUs. Decreased IL-12 levels may contribute to the pathogenesis of NEC by allowing bacteria to escape host defenses (Nadler et al., 2001).

OBJECTIVES

- Allow bowel to rest; avoid stimulants. These measures are usually temporary.
- Prevent or correct starvation, diarrhea, and further malnutrition.
- Prepare patient for bowel surgery and for wound healing if surgery becomes necessary, as for perforation.
- Prevent or correct hypoglycemia.
- Breastfeeding is more protective than formula feeding. Promote and encourage breastfeeding when possible.

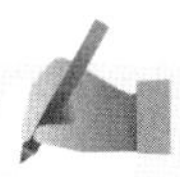

DIETARY AND NUTRITIONAL RECOMMENDATIONS

- Acute: Nil per os (NPO or nothing by mouth) with IVs and TPN as appropriate.
- Recovery: Use 2 times RDA of protein; 25% more kcal than normal for age; frequent feedings.
- If formula is used, review intolerances. Some partially elemental formulas are available such as Pregestimil or Nutramigen. Simple nutrients may be required if the digestive tract has not recovered fully.
- Omit milk, if lactose is not tolerated. Provide a replacement for calcium and riboflavin, if milk will be omitted for an extended period of time.
- Ensure adequate intake of iron but not in excess while infection is extensive (especially parenteral iron). Zinc should also be monitored during acute stages because it contributes to bacterial nutriture.
- Occasionally, a colostomy or ileostomy must be performed, and tube feeding may be needed.

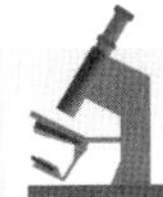

PROFILE

Clinical/History	Lab Work	
Height/length	H&H (decreased)	Na+ (decreased)
Weight/birth weight	Abdominal x-ray	Platelets (decreased)
Head circumference	PT (increased)	K+ (increased)
Vomiting	Guaiac test for blood in stools	Glucose
Diarrhea		Elevated WBCs
		Lactic acidosis

Common Drugs Used and Potential Side Effects

- Antidiarrheal medications may be used as appropriate for age.

Herbs, Botanicals and Supplements

- Herbs and botanicals should not be used for NEC because there are no controlled trials to prove efficacy for any related problems.

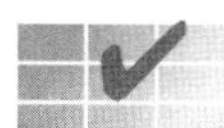

PATIENT EDUCATION

- Promote continuation of breastfeeding when possible.
- Monitor weight and stool changes; advise physician when necessary.
- Ensure that the parent/caretaker understands the differences between ready-to-feed and concentrated formula (i.e., hypertonicity of the solution).

OBESITY IN CHILDHOOD

NUTRITIONAL ACUITY RANKING: LEVEL 3 (COUNSELING)

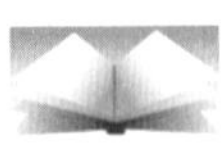

DEFINITIONS AND BACKGROUND

Obesity does not have one set definition, and different ages use different indicators. In young children, 120% above ideal body weight for length is used as a criterion. While there is no generally accepted definition for obesity as distinct from *overweight* in children and adolescents, the prevalence of overweight is increasing for children and adolescents in the United States. Approximately 11% of children (ages 6–11) and 11% of adolescents (ages 12–17) were overweight in 1994—up from approximately 5% in the 1960s and 1970s (www.NIDDK.nih.gov). Overweight is defined by the sex- and age-specific 85th percentile cutoff points of the revised NCHS/CDC growth charts; obese if above the 95th percentile.

BMI increases during the first year of life and then decreases; it begins to rise again at 6–6 ½ years of age. BMI is not useful in infancy; it is a screening tool and does not reflect body composition. The preferred weight gain history in childhood is as follows: Usual weight gain is that an infant doubles birth weight by 6 months, triples birth weight at 12 months. Tripling birth weight before one year is associated with increased risk of obesity. In year 2, gain is 3.5–4.5 kg; year 3 is gain of 2–3 kg; annually thereafter, gain is 2–3 kg. Until 6 years of age, the number of fat cells increases (hyperplasia). After 6 years of age, the size of fat cells increases (hypertrophy).

Evidence that poor nutrition in early life is a risk factor for increased fatness later in life is not confirmed. Overfeeding for catch-up growth can contribute to obesity; weight gain proceeds at a rate that is too fast for linear growth. Overnutrition, resulting from high birth weight or gestational diabetes, is associated with subsequent fatness. Several large, well-conducted studies in developed countries suggest that breastfeeding has a protective effect against obesity later in life (Gillman et al., 2001) and that early nutritional intake has an impact on adult obesity (Martorell et al., 2001).

Clearly, both genetics and environment play a role. Social factors in childhood are strongly influential on obesity in adulthood. Three critical periods for prevention of adult obesity are: ages 5–7 years, adolescence, and during pregnancy (women).

Obesity tracks from childhood into adulthood, and the persistence of obesity rises with age among obese children (Maffeis and Tato, 2001). Clinical syndromes of concern related to childhood obesity include asthma, sleep apnea, maturity onset diabetes of youth (MODY), Cushing syndrome, hyperinsulinemia, hypothyroidism, polycystic ovary syndrome, Prader-Willi syndrome, and hypothalamic dysfunction or tumor. Treatment of preadolescent obesity seems to be most successful when it is started during preschool years and includes frequent clinic visits (Davis and Kaufer, 1994).

OBJECTIVES

- Gradually reduce excess food intake and increase activity. Allow the child to "grow" into his or her weight.
- Discourage the use of sweets and foods to reward behavior.
- Determine the extent of dental caries; offer appropriate suggestions.
- Evaluate the types of entrees used as well as the use of vegetables, sweets, snacks, and milk in the daily diet.
- Counsel family about good nutrition in general and, in particular, the caloric needs for different age groups. Avoid the "clean plate" theory.
- Help the child "find" the right body for him or her.
- Be wary about withholding food; it can have the opposite effect.
- Encourage self-recognition of hunger cues, e.g., stop eating when feeling "full."

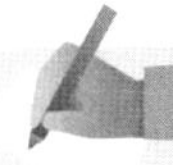

DIETARY AND NUTRITIONAL RECOMMENDATIONS

- Determine the RDAs for the child's age group: kcal, protein, and other nutrients. Protein should be 15–20%, fat should be 30–35%, CHO should be 50%.
- Ensure that the family has adequate fluoride protection.
- Decrease the use of sweets as snack foods or dessert. Decrease fatty or fried foods.
- Plan a diet with basal calories. Do not provide a reduction diet per se. The diet should be calculated according to the patient's age, required needs, activity, and growth spurts.
- Check for anemia; correct diet accordingly.
- Limit milk to a reasonable amount daily; use low-fat or skim milk after 2 years of age.
- Good snacks include fresh fruit or vegetables, plain crackers, pretzels, plain popcorn, cooked egg slices, unsweetened fruit or vegetable juices, and low-fat cheese cubes. Age appropriateness of snacks is important; younger children can choke on popcorn and fresh carrots etc.
- Avoid grazing, control between-meal snacks, give small helpings, and allow more small helpings until "full."

Common Drugs Used and Potential Side Effects

- Discourage the use of drugs for weight loss in childhood.
- Antidepressants are sometimes prescribed for childhood depression, which is more common than once

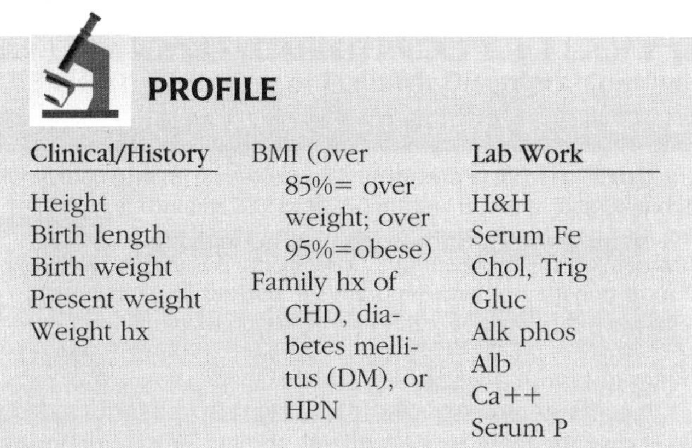

PROFILE

Clinical/History		Lab Work
Height Birth length Birth weight Present weight Weight hx	BMI (over 85%= over weight; over 95%=obese) Family hx of CHD, diabetes mellitus (DM), or HPN	H&H Serum Fe Chol, Trig Gluc Alk phos Alb Ca++ Serum P

realized. Monitor for side effects such as changes in metabolism and appetite, which can contribute to obesity in some cases.

Herbs, Botanicals and Supplements

- Herbs and botanicals should not be used for obesity in children because there are no controlled trials to prove efficacy.

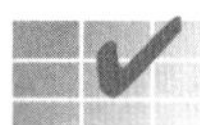

PATIENT EDUCATION

- ✔ Explain to parents that obese parents may tend to overfeed their children. Discuss hereditary and environmental factors, including age-appropriate portions and snacks.
- ✔ One-fourth of children who enter adolescence overweight will be overweight or obese as adults. Encourage healthy eating habits and increased physical activity. Limit time in front of the television and computer.
- ✔ Help the family to carefully monitor menu planning and snacking patterns. Encourage regular meals; limit unplanned snacking.
- ✔ Encourage activity: jogging, ball games, swimming, and bike riding are all good examples. Demonstrate the relationship of food, weight, and energy balance. Metabolic rates tend to be quite low while watching television (Klesges et al., 1993).
- ✔ Discourage risk-filled weight-control schemes or practices.
- ✔ Try to eliminate one "problem food" per visit such as regular soda pop or sugar-sweetened fruit punch. Offer an acceptable alternative.
- ✔ While weight loss is occurring, maintain the child's self-image through positive reinforcement. Stress nonfood-related achievements; do not nag.
- ✔ A good example should be set in the home by the parent/caretaker.
- ✔ Between meals, ice water should be offered as a special beverage instead of soda pop or fruit drinks.
- ✔ A system for "traffic light" foods can be used—green "go" foods, yellow "caution" foods, red "stop" foods.
- ✔ Responsibilities should be shared—parents are responsible for a proper emotional setting and for what is offered; the child is responsible for what and how much is eaten (Satter, 1986).
- ✔ Parents who practice restrained eating with their children tend to be overly indulgent later (fast/feast); the result is chronic anxiety. Eating can become very controlled, inconsistent, and emotional.

For More Information

- ✦ Activate: Childhood Obesity Prevention Initiative
  International Food Information Council
  202-296-6540
  http://ificinfo.health.org/
- ✦ American Academy of Family Physicians
  http://www.aafp.org/afp/990215ap/861.html
- ✦ Centers for Disease Control
  http://www.cdc.gov/nccdphp/dnpa/dnpaaag.htm
- ✦ Kidsource
  http://www.kidsource.com/kidsource/content2/obesity.html
- ✦ NIDDK Weight Control Network
  http://www.niddk.nih.gov/health/nutrit/pubs/helpchld.htm
- ✦ Pediatrics – Recommendations for Managing Obesity in Children
  http://www.pediatrics.org/cgi/reprint/102/3/e29.pdf

PHENYLKETONURIA

NUTRITIONAL ACUITY RANKING: LEVEL 4

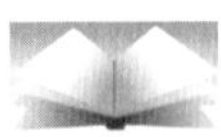

DEFINITIONS AND BACKGROUND

Phenylketonuria (PKU) is caused by an inborn error that results from a mutation in the phenylalanine hydroxylase gene. As a result, phenylalanine (Phe) is not metabolized to tyrosine. The mutations are inherited in an autosomal-recessive manner.

Infants are tested for this disorder after birth and the first feeding, and again if levels of phenylalanine are above given cutoff levels. Children with PKU who follow their special diet for life have fewer intellectual and neurologic deficits (Weglage et al., 2001). The diet should not be totally discontinued at any age. Referral to a metabolic dietitian and special programs at the state level may be required.

Ubiquinone-10 is a lipid that has an important role in energy metabolism in mitochondria and, in its reduced form, protects cells from peroxidative damage. Patients with PKU eat a diet that is restricted in natural proteins; therefore, they are limited in their intake of ubiquinone-10. Research is needed to see whether or not ubiquinone-10 has significant effects (Artuch et al., 1999).

Tyrosine is an essential amino acid in patients with PKU because of the limited Phe converted to tyrosine, but the recommendations for tyrosine intake appear to be overestimated by five times what is needed (Bross et al., 2000). Importance of complete or almost-complete intake of recommended Phe-free amino acid mixture (AAM) for control of blood Phe levels for patients with PKU has not been universally appreciated (Duran et al., 1999). Hospitalization may be needed to get this control from time to time. About 87% of PKU centers favor lifelong dietary control of Phe (Fisch et al., 1997).

Patients who are not under strict dietary control may be at risk for B12 deficiency; therefore, patients with PKU should be seen often by medical and dietetic professionals and have their B12 status checked (Robinson et al., 2000). Individuals who follow diets low in natural proteins (as in PKU) should be advised to take selenium supplements (van Bakel et al., 2000).

There is international consensus that patients with Phe levels <360 microM on a free diet do not need Phe-lowering dietary treatment, whereas patients with levels >600 microM do; different recommendations exist for patients with mild hyperphenylalaninemia (Weglage et al., 2001). In general, however, "diet for life" is the rule, especially for women with PKU who are considering pregnancy (de la Cruz and Koch, 2001).

Women with untreated PKU often have poor reproductive outcomes. Early maintenance of maternal plasma Phe concentrations at <360 micromol/L and mean protein intake greater than RDA with adequate energy intake results in the best reproductive outcomes (Acosta et al., 2001). Women with PKU seem to have a higher number of babies who are born with congenital heart disease; prevention requires initiation of the low Phe diet before conception or early in pregnancy with metabolic control no later than the eighth gestational week (Levy et al., 2001).

Desirable serum Phe levels are below 10 mg/dL. Higher levels are associated with declining IQ.

OBJECTIVES

- ▲ Establish the child's daily requirement for Phe, protein, and energy according to age. The appropriate Phe intake for age is as follows: infants, 0–3 months, 60–90 mg/kg; infants 4–6 months, 40 mg/kg; infants 7–9 months, 35 mg/kg; infants 10–12 months, 30 mg/kg; children 1–2 years, 25 mg/kg; children 2–5 years, 20 mg/kg BW; children older than 5 years of age, 15 mg/kg BW. Inadequate intake of Phe can result in anorexia, fever, vomiting, lethargy, bone changes, and stunted growth.
- ▲ Prevent mental retardation. Promote normal intellectual development.
- ▲ Provide a diet aiding growth and development. A high energy:protein ratio is needed.
- ▲ Provide adequate protein sparing. A high energy:protein ratio is needed.
- ▲ Introduce solids and textures at usual ages. Encourage self-feeding when it is possible for the infant to do so.
- ▲ Allow intellectually normal patients with PKU to develop a normal social life.
- ▲ Develop a positive attitude toward the diet in the parent or caretaker and in the child.
- ▲ Prevent toxic buildup of abnormal metabolites.
- ▲ Monitor for any nutrient deficiency.

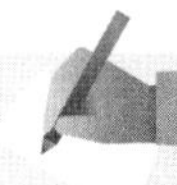

DIETARY AND NUTRITIONAL RECOMMENDATIONS

- Use a diet low in Phe. The average diet provides 5% Phe in a protein food. The Lofenalac formula, Phenyl-free or Maxamaid XP can be used. Lofenalac contains 454 calories in 100 g of powder: protein, 15 g; CHO, 60 g; fat, 18 g. Lofenalac is a milk substitute made from casein hydrolysate, corn oil, corn syrup, tapioca starch, minerals, and vitamins. Phenyl-free does not provide total nutritional needs.
- Omit meat, fish, poultry, bread, milk, cheese, legumes, and peanut butter. Use Lofenalac for 85–100% of an infant's needs. Some milk and Lofenalac formula should be used to provide for the infant's needs. Flavors can be added to the formula.
- Initially, the infant's tolerance must be assessed individually, and progress in treatment must develop accordingly.
- Determine if serum iron or other nutrient levels are low and correct as needed.

- Monitor serum pyridoxine because turnover seems to be reduced in PKU and excesses may be retained (Prince and Leklem, 1994).
- Introduce solids and textures at the appropriate ages.
- Subtract Phe requirement in formula from total needs (the difference is that which is provided by solid foods).
- To add calories, try jam, jelly, sugar, honey, molasses, syrups, cornstarch, and oils that are Phe-free.

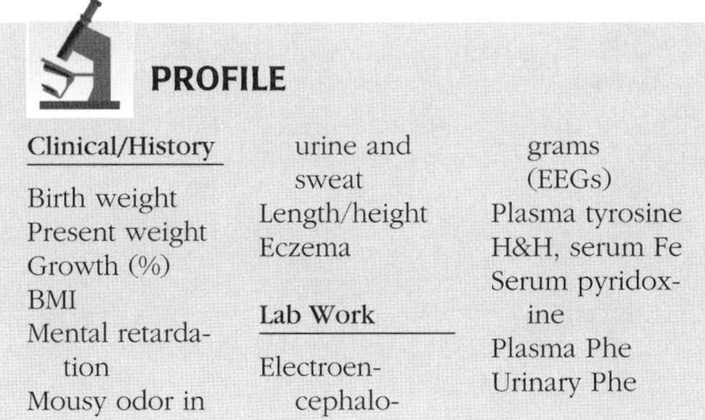

PROFILE

Clinical/History

Birth weight
Present weight
Growth (%)
BMI
Mental retardation
Mousy odor in urine and sweat
Length/height
Eczema

Lab Work

Electroencephalograms (EEGs)
Plasma tyrosine
H&H, serum Fe
Serum pyridoxine
Plasma Phe
Urinary Phe

Herbs, Botanicals and Supplements

- Herbs and botanicals should not be used for PKU because there are no controlled trials to prove efficacy.

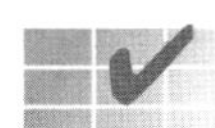

PATIENT EDUCATION

- Because initial acceptance of Lofenalac may be poor due to its strong taste, the mother should be careful not to express her own distaste. Recommend appropriate recipes and cookbooks.
- Monitor the presence of Phe in the diet.
- Avoid items sweetened with aspartame (Nutra-Sweet), including diet sodas.
- Self-management should begin by 7–8 years of age, at least for formula preparation. By 12 years of age, the child should begin calculating his or her own intake of Phe from foods.
- For women of childbearing age, it is important to note that women who have PKU tend to give birth to children with microcephaly, mental retardation, congenital heart defects, and intrauterine growth retardation with LBW (Rouse et al., 2000). Metabolic control by the end of the first trimester is, therefore, important as a goal. Treatment at any time during pregnancy may reduce the severity of delayed development (Waisbren et al., 2000).

For More Information

- Children's PKU Network
  1520 State St., Suite 240
  San Diego, CA 92101
  619-233-3202
  http://www.kumc.edu/gec/support/pku.html
- National Coalition for PKU and Allied Disorders
  http://www.pku-allieddisorders.org/
- PKU News
  www.pkunews.org

PRADER-WILLI SYNDROME

NUTRITIONAL ACUITY RANKING: LEVEL 3

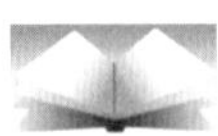

DEFINITIONS AND BACKGROUND

Prader-Willi syndrome (PWS) is a disorder caused by DNA abnormalities of chromosome 15. Major characteristics are infant hypotonia, hypogonadism, mental retardation, a short stature, small hands and feet, atypical facial features, and obesity because of insatiable hunger in early childhood. Short stature is part of the syndrome and is not nutritional in origin.

The incidence of PWS is 1 in 15,000 births in the United States. Onset occurs at birth, but symptoms begin by 1–4 years of age. These children often have poor suck, FTT, and floppy muscle tone (hypotonia) as infants. Learning disability or retardation may occur.

Individuals with PWS are not able to control food sneaking, stealing, and gorging behaviors (Hoffman et al., 1992). Those with PWS sometimes eat contaminated food and highly unusual edible and inedible food combinations (Dykens, 2000). Because they are difficult to manage, approximately 75% of these patients live in group homes. Bilio-pancreatic diversion is not an adequate treatment alone for weight loss for those with this syndrome (Grugni et al., 2000).

OBJECTIVES

- Reduce excess weight. Monitor weight weekly.
- Maintain RDAs for all nutrients and protein to promote growth and development.
- Provide feeding assistance if needed.
- Prevent complications like CHD, HPN, DM, sleep apnea, and pneumonia.
- Correct pica and related nutritional deficits.
- Correct or maintain normal serum lipid levels.
- Minimize unusual food-seeking behaviors such as eating food from the trash or eating inappropriate or unpalatable food combinations.

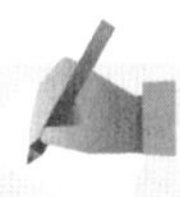

DIETARY AND NUTRITIONAL RECOMMENDATIONS

- Often, these children start with FTT and then become obese; know where the child is in this continuum.
- Use a low-calorie diet to reduce weight: 10–11 kcal/cm height to maintain; 8–9 kcal/cm for weight loss. For older teens, reduce the total calorie level to 800–1,200 a day; lower levels will provide for weight loss or maintenance for patients', whose needs are about 60% of those without PWS.
- Ensure that the diet provides adequate protein and nutrients. Follow RDAs for age. A Prader-Willi Food pyramid is available at http://www.pwsausa.org/foodpyramid.htm.
- Consider gastric bypass if hyperphagia becomes a problem.
- Reduce use of high-fat foods.

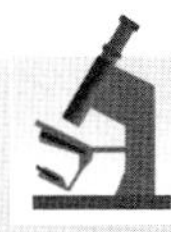

PROFILE

Clinical/History		
Height	Mental retardation	Gluc
Birth weight	Small head	Alb
Present weight		BP
BMI	**Lab Work**	Chol, Trig
Goal weight	H&H	pCO2, pO2

Herbs, Botanicals and Supplements

- Herbs and botanicals should not be used for PWS because there are no controlled trials to prove efficacy.

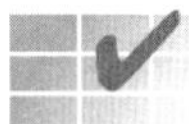

PATIENT EDUCATION

- Encourage the patient to be active and to exercise daily.
- Help the patient lose weight with behavior modification techniques. Effective systems promote a green/yellow/red method of food choices: go/caution/stop.
- Main elements of concern in the diet are sugars and fats.
- Discuss feeding practices plus activity factors.
- Record-keeping and calorie-counting are generally better than use of exchange systems. Control of excess intake is the main goal.
- Gastroplasty generally is not a successful solution.
- An interdisciplinary approach is useful: There is a need to reduce guilt and depression. Self-monitoring is the eventual goal.
- Behavior modification is an important part of treatment.

For More Information

- The Prader-Willi Syndrome Association
  5700 Midnight Pass Rd.
  Sarasota, FL 34242
  1-800-926-4797
  http://www.pwsausa.org/
- Diagnostic Tool for Prader Willi
  http://www.pwsausa.org/Diagnos.htm
- Prader-Will Food Pyramid
  http://www.pwsausa.org/foodpyramid.htm.

RICKETS OF NUTRITIONAL ORIGIN

NUTRITIONAL ACUITY RANKING: LEVEL 3

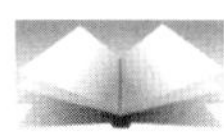

DEFINITIONS AND BACKGROUND

Rickets is relatively uncommon in modern medicine but is becoming a problem in some populations. Nutritional rickets is seen in breastfed children of multiparous mothers; those living in higher latitudes with greater skin pigmentation are at increased risk (Pugliese et al., 1998). Factors that may have contributed to the increase in referrals of children with nutritional rickets include: more African American women breastfeeding, fewer infants receiving vitamin D supplements, and mothers and children exposed to less sunlight (Kreiter et al., 2000).

Features of nutritional rickets include leg bowing, poor linear growth, seizures, abnormal serum calcium and phosphorus, and abnormal alkaline phosphatase levels. Nutritional rickets is caused by calcium, phosphorus, and vitamin D deficiency. It is usually seen in children or infants (often premature), including up to 30–70% of LBW and VLBW infants. The condition may also occur in breastfed infants who do not receive adequate supplementation, exposure to sunlight, or vitamin D-fortified milk. Because vitamin D is fat soluble, malabsorption syndromes decrease the ability of vitamin D to be absorbed from the intestines. Sunlight is important to skin production of vitamin D, and environmental conditions where sunlight exposure is limited may reduce access. Rickets may also be secondary to steatorrhea, anticonvulsant use, or renal failure or biliary cirrhosis.

Signs and symptoms include weakness, inability to stand or walk, slow growth, seizures, and irritability. Vitamin D supplementation and sunlight are effective treatments (Kaper et al., 2000). Therapy for hypophosphatemic rickets is different from that for common nutritional rickets, where treatment needs to be started early to prevent development of irreversible renal insufficiency (Garg and Tandon, 1999). Dark-skinned, breastfed infants should be given vitamin D supplements to prevent nutritional rickets (Kreiter et al., 2000).

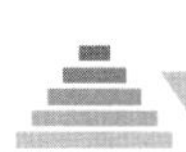

OBJECTIVES

- Correct body mineral status; prevent further problems and deformity. Vitamin D participates in mineral homeostasis, regulation of gene expression, and cell differentiation. Complement drug therapy with adequate diet; usually, a single large dose of vitamin D is given for 3 months.
- Prevent or correct tetany, hypocalcemia, and other complications.
- Identify and treat other problems such as dental caries or bone fractures, which may also be common.
- Promote growth, since short stature can result if not treated early enough.

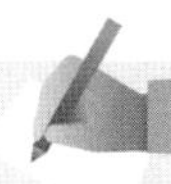

DIETARY AND NUTRITIONAL RECOMMENDATIONS

- Use a balanced diet appropriate for age and sex. If diet is inadequate in the specific nutrients, ensure intake of at least 500 mg/day of calcium, RDA levels/day for vitamin D, and 100 mg/Kg daily for phosphorus. Ensure that phytate intake is not excessive.
- Use milk if no milk or lactose intolerances exist; increase appropriately while monitoring serum values.
- There may be additional use of such calcium-containing foods as cheeses, yogurt, ice cream, etc., if milk is not tolerated.
- If necessary, early TF with extra calcium and phosphorus may be useful.
- With PN, there may be inadequate use of calcium and phosphorus; monitor carefully.
- With steatorrhea, check serum levels of vitamin D and calcium and supplement appropriately.

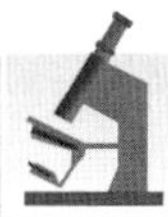

PROFILE

Clinical/History

Height
Weight
BMI
Growth (%)
Decreased linear growth
Steatorrhea
Muscle spasm
Chvostek's sign (facial spasm)
Metabolic acidosis

Lab Work

Wrist radiographs
Radiographs for fractures
Urinary Ca++ (elevated)
Urinary P
Alk Phos (increased)
Ca++ (often low)
Serum phosphorus (decreased)

Common Drugs Used and Potential Side Effects

- Calciferol: 1,500–3,000 IU daily by mouth helps in 2–4 weeks; some maintenance doses may also be required over time. Monitor use with dietary calcium. Calcitriol may be needed in renal disorders that cause deficiency.
- Vitamin D: A large dose may be given upon diagnosis, with long-term usage given according to causative factors. Be wary of toxic effects of vitamin D (hypercalcemia, nausea, vomiting, anorexia, malaise, renal problems, or hypertensive problems). For anticonvulsant use, vitamin D will be supplemented at 1,000–2,000 IU/day.

- Furosemide (Lasix): May cause the problem in some cases; hypercalciuria may occur.
- Antacid excess may cause a phosphorus deficiency; monitor carefully and correct. Use alternative measures.

Herbs, Botanicals and Supplements

- Herbs and botanicals should not be used for rickets because there are no controlled trials to prove efficacy.

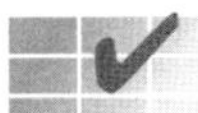

PATIENT EDUCATION

- ✔ Discuss needed alterations of the diet in conjunction with drug therapy.
- ✔ Discuss the role of sunlight in vitamin D metabolism.
- ✔ Good posture and positioning are important aspects of treatment.

SPINA BIFIDA AND NEURAL TUBE DEFECTS

NUTRITIONAL ACUITY RANKING: LEVEL 3

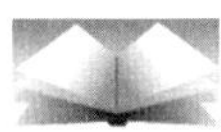

DEFINITIONS AND BACKGROUND

Spina bifida includes any congenital defect involving insufficient closure of the spine (usually laminae of the vertebrae). Approximately 2,500–3,000 children are born each year with either spina bifida or anencephaly. MMC accounts for about 75% of all cases of spina bifida and may affect as many as 1 out of every 800 infants (see that entry also). The rest of the cases are most commonly spina bifida occulta (where the bones of the spine do not close, the spinal cord and meninges remain in place, and skin usually covers the defect) and meningoceles (where the meninges protrude through the vertebral defect but the spinal cord remains in place).

Spina bifida occurs in 150 in 100,000 births; the lumbar section generally is affected. Clubfoot, dislocated hip, scoliosis, and other musculoskeletal deformities may also be present. Spina bifida cystica is more severe. Spina bifida occulta is seen in approximately 10% of children and adults; the defect is usually discovered accidentally on x-ray.

A majority of serious birth defects of the spine and brain could be prevented if women consumed adequate daily amounts of folate in their diets, especially in the months preceding pregnancy. Women who plan to become pregnant should be certain that their diets contain sufficient amounts of folate. Clinical trials indicate that periconceptual use of folic acid supplements (400–800 ug/day) can reduce up to 70% of these neural tube defects (Gross et al., 2001). Use of folic acid supplements and fortified foods are even more effective than eating high-folate foods (Cuskelly et al., 1996). There may be a diverse range of disability in adults with spina bifida (McDonnell and McCann, 2000).

A study published in the June 20, 2001 *Journal of the American Medical Association* found that the number of children born each year with NTDs had dropped by 19% since the government mandated the addition of folic acid to enriched grain products, starting in January 1998.

OBJECTIVES

- ▲ Control side effects (i.e., hydrocephalus and possibly sepsis).
- ▲ Increase independence and self-care potentials.
- ▲ Improve nutritional status.
- ▲ Achieve and maintain ideal body mass index for age.
- ▲ Preserve brain function, as far as possible, with hydrocephalus.
- ▲ Initiate treatment or surgical intervention as appropriate.
- ▲ Correct constipation, pressure ulcers, and other complications.

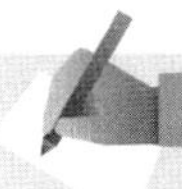

DIETARY AND NUTRITIONAL RECOMMENDATIONS

- Individualize diet for proper nutrition to achieve a desirable weight, and monitor carefully.
- Provide adequate protein, calories, B-complex, zinc, and other nutrients for age. Folic acid has been implicated in etiology.
- Provide adequate nutrients for wound healing if surgery has been performed.

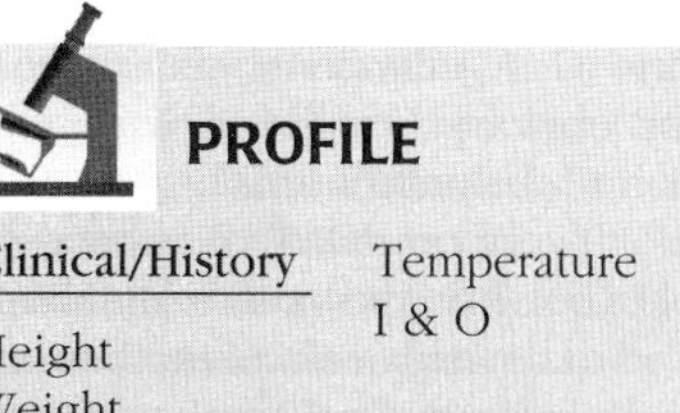

PROFILE

Clinical/History	Temperature	Serum folic acid
Height	I & O	Gluc
Weight		Alb
BMI or growth percentile	**Lab Work**	H&H
	TLC	

Common Drugs Used and Potential Side Effects

- Antibiotics may be required if the patient develops sepsis.
- Use of oral contraceptives depletes folic acid; change diet and supplement as needed.

Herbs, Botanicals and Supplements

- Herbs and botanicals should not be used for spina bifida because there are no controlled trials to prove efficacy.

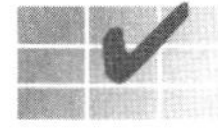

PATIENT EDUCATION

- ✔ Family counseling may be needed in preparation for future pregnancies.
- ✔ Referral to a local chapter of the March of Dimes may be beneficial.

For More Information

- Centers for Disease Control
  Folic Acid National Campaign
  http://www.cdc.gov/ncbddd/Folicacid
- Food and Drug Administration
  "How Folate Can Help Prevent Birth Defects"
  http://www.cfsan.fda.gov/~dms/fdafolic.html
- Spina Bifida Association of America
  4590 MacArthur Blvd., NW, Suite 250
  Washington, DC 20007-4226
  1-800-621-3141
  http://www.sbaa.org/

TYROSINEMIA

NUTRITIONAL ACUITY RANKING: LEVEL 4

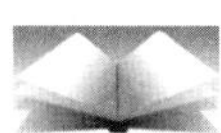

DEFINITIONS AND BACKGROUND

Tyrosinemia is a hereditary disorder in which a deficiency of parahydroxyphenyl-pyruvic acid oxidase blocks the conversion of tyrosine to homogentisic acid. This condition results in liver failure or severe nodular cirrhosis with renal tubular involvement. Tyrosine accumulation can be aggravated by vitamin C deficiency, a high-protein diet, and liver immaturity.

Tyrosinemia type I is a recessive hepatorenal disease involving enzyme deficiency of fumarylacetoacetate hydrolase (FAH). Increased tyrosine, Phe, and methionine occur. The condition is acute, often causing death within the first year of life. In tyrosinemia type II, dietary therapy alone prevents complication; type I needs to be treated with diet for life and is a much more severe disease.

OBJECTIVES

- ▲ Restrict Phe and tyrosine from the diet.
- ▲ Promote normal growth and development for age.
- ▲ Provide adequate vitamin C for conversion processes.

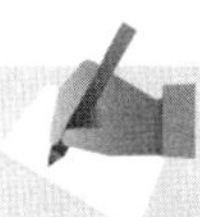

DIETARY AND NUTRITIONAL RECOMMENDATIONS

- Initially, feed a Phe/tyrosine hydrolysate to infants, with small amounts of milk added to provide the minimum requirements of tyrosine and Phe. Mead Johnson product TYROS and 3200-AB; Ross product Maxamaid XPHEN, TYR; or TYROMEX-1 or TYREX from SHS can be used.
- If blood methionine levels are elevated, try Product 80056 (Mead Johnson). Use carbohydrate supplements such as Polycose plus vitamins and minerals.
- Supplement with vitamin C appropriate to the patient's age.

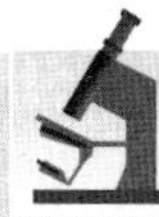

PROFILE

Clinical/History

Birth weight, present weight
Growth (%)
BMI
Abdominal distention
Hyperpigmentation
Dermatitis
"Cabbage-like" odor
Rancid butter-like odor (type I)
FTT

Lab Work

Phosphate
Gluc
Alb (often low)
Fumarylacetoacetate hydrolase (FAH)-low
Plasma Phe
Methionine
H&H
Plasma tyrosine

Common Drugs Used and Potential Side Effects

- Antibiotics may be needed to correct infections.

Herbs, Botanicals and Supplements

- Herbs and botanicals should not be used for tyrosinemia because there are no controlled trials to prove efficacy.

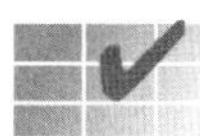

PATIENT EDUCATION

- ✓ Provide sources of tyrosine and Phe in the diet determined appropriately for age and body size.
- ✓ Adjust intake of energy and nutrients according to the patient's age.

For More Information

- ✦ American Liver Foundation
1425 Pompton Avenue, Cedar Grove, NJ 07009
1-800-223-0179

UREA CYCLE DISORDERS

NUTRITIONAL ACUITY RANKING: 3 OR 4

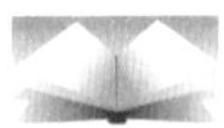

DEFINITIONS AND BACKGROUND

The urea cycle disorders are manifested most often in the newborn between ages 1 and 5 days and are often initially thought to be septic. Early onset occurs in the newborn; with late onset, patients have partial enzyme deficiencies and are recognized after a clinical episode months or years later.

Urea acid cycle disorders are caused by defects in the following enzymes: Carbamyl phosphate synthetase I (CPS); Ornithine transcarbamylase (OTC); Argininosuccinate synthetase (citrullinemia) (ASS); Argininosuccinate lyase (argininosuccinic aciduria) (ASL); Arginase (hyperargininemia); N-acetylglutamate synthase. Except for OTC, which is X-linked, all others are autosomal recessive.

When they present in childhood, adolescence, and adulthood there is often FTT, persistent vomiting, developmental delay, and behavioral changes. Signs and symptoms include hyperammonemia, irritability, somnolence, vomiting, seizures, and coma; if not treated rapidly, it may cause irreversible neuronal damage (Mathias et al., 2001). The outcome of untreated or poorly treated patients with urea cycle disorders is universally bad (Summar, 2001). Hemodialysis may be needed to bring down ammonia levels rapidly (Mathias et al., 2001).

Statewide newborn screening does not always screen for these conditions. However, screening is important for all newborns, especially if there is a family history of any of these disorders. It is believed that some cases of sudden infant death syndrome may be related to these urea cycle disorders. The prospect of gene therapy "cures" for these diseases, striving for the best possible outcome in the critical newborn period, is a worthy goal (Summar, 2001).

OBJECTIVES

- Restrict total protein from the diet to minimize endogenous ammonia production and protein catabolism.
- Promote anabolism with normal growth and development for age. Give calories from nonprotein sources in amounts to promote anabolism.
- Normalize blood ammonia levels and reduce the effects of hyperammonemia, which may cause neuronal damage. Elevated levels of ammonia can come from muscle breakdown or diet; situations can be made worse if not evaluated to determine which process is the problem.
- Administer desired substrates of the urea cycle. Limit one or more essential amino acids while providing adequate energy and nutrients (Trahms, 2000).
- If necessary, support dialysis if blood ammonia levels are 3–4 times above normal.

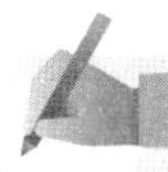

DIETARY AND NUTRITIONAL RECOMMENDATIONS

- Initially, feed a low-protein diet (often 1.0–1.5 g/kg daily) with use of special formulas. For example, Cyclinex (Ross Labs) with specific supplements of arginine or Product 80056 (Mead Johnson) is used for arginosuccinic aciduria. For ornithine transcarbamylase deficiency, a low-protein diet is needed, with additives such as Moducal (Mead Johnson) to give extra energy.
- Add extra energy sources if needed to support growth and development. Weight gain is the best measure of success in infants and children.
- If dehydration occurs, intravenous fluids and glucose may be needed.

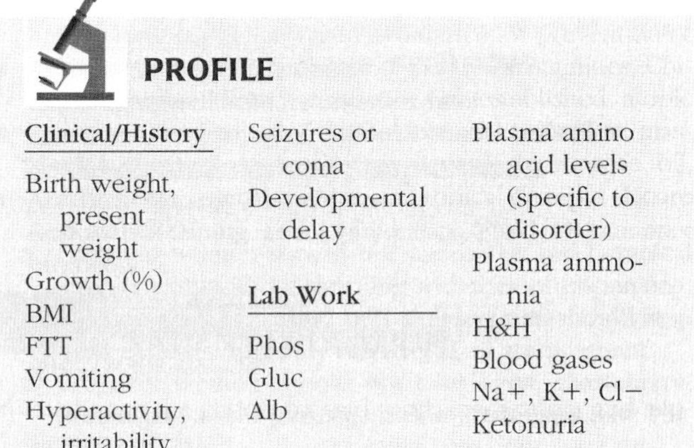

PROFILE

Clinical/History		
Birth weight, present weight	Seizures or coma	Plasma amino acid levels (specific to disorder)
Growth (%)	Developmental delay	Plasma ammonia
BMI	**Lab Work**	H&H
FTT	Phos	Blood gases
Vomiting	Gluc	Na+, K+, Cl−
Hyperactivity, irritability	Alb	Ketonuria

Common Drugs Used and Potential Side Effects

- Provide alternative route for ammonia; what is given depends on where the defect in the urea cycle has occurred. Arginine is often supplemented, 400–700 mg/day, except for arginine deficiency (Trahms, 2000). For ASS and ASL deficiencies, 0.4–0.7 gm arginine/kg/d; 0.17 g/kg/d of citrulline is given for CPS deficiency
- Phenylbutyrate may also be used to normalize serum ammonia.

Herbs, Botanicals and Supplements

- Herbs and botanicals should not be used for urea cycle disorders because there are no controlled trials to prove efficacy.

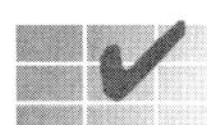

PATIENT EDUCATION

- ✔ Provide sources of all essential amino acids in the diet, determined appropriately for age and body size. There are tables available for these purposes (Trahms, 2000).
- ✔ Adjust intake of energy and nutrients according to the patient's age.

For More Information

- ✦ National Urea Cycle Disorders Foundation
  4841 Hill Street
  La Canada, CA 91011
  1-800-38NUCDF
  http://www.nucdf.org

WILSON'S DISEASE (HEPATOLENTICULAR DEGENERATION)

NUTRITIONAL ACUITY RANKING: LEVEL 3

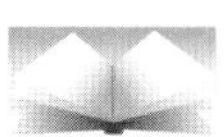

DEFINITIONS AND BACKGROUND

An autosomal recessive disorder, Wilson's disease causes abnormal transport and storage of copper, resulting in hepatolenticular degeneration, neurologic damage, and damage to the kidney, brain, and cornea. Onset occurs at birth but symptoms may appear from 5–40-years-old.

The major physiological role of copper is to serve as a cofactor to a number of key metabolic enzymes. Copper is a trace element essential for normal cell homeostasis, promoting iron absorption for hemoglobin synthesis and for formation of bone and myelin sheath. In hepatic tissues, 90% of the copper in the copper/albumin complex is converted to ceruloplasmin. Tissue deposition occurs instead of formation of ceruloplasmin in Wilson's disease.

Genetic defects of copper distribution, such as Wilson's disease, lead to severe pathologies, including neurodegeneration, liver lesions, and behavior abnormalities. A low-copper diet is implemented when other therapies are unsuccessful (e.g., copper-chelating agents.) If not diagnosed until onset of fulminant failure, the patient will die. Liver transplantation is the requirement at that point.

OBJECTIVES

- Keep optimal balance of copper in patient.
- Decrease serum copper levels, generally with drug chelation. Enhance urinary excretion of excesses.
- Prevent or reverse damage to body tissues and liver.
- Watch caloric intake to prevent obesity.
- Monitor changes in gag reflex or dysphagia.
- Provide sufficient zinc to chelate excess copper under doctor's supervision.
- Prepare for transplantation if necessary.

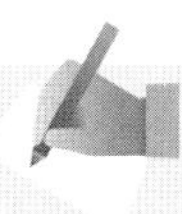

DIETARY AND NUTRITIONAL RECOMMENDATIONS

- A normal diet provides 2–5 mg/day of copper. A low-copper diet (1–2 mg) may be needed. Limit dietary sources of copper: liver, kidney, shellfish, nuts, raisins and other dried fruits, dried legumes, brain, oysters, mushrooms, chocolate, poultry, and whole-grain cereals.
- A lacto-ovo vegetarian diet may be useful to increase content of fiber and phytates. Copper is also less available in vegetarian diets (Brewer et al., 1993).
- Control calories, food textures, and other nutrients if necessary.
- Increase fluid intake but avoid alcoholic beverages.
- Increase zinc from meat, poultry, fish, eggs, and milk if deemed appropriate for the patient.

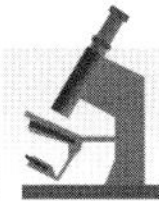

PROFILE

Clinical/History

Height
Weight, BMI
Swallowing difficulty
Easy bruising
ceruloplasmin (often low)
Kayser-Fleischer ring (eye)

Lab Work

Alb
H&H
BUN/Creat
Serum P
PT
Serum Cu (increased)
Liver tests
Urinary Cu
ALT, AST
Alk phos
Serum zinc

Common Drugs Used and Potential Side Effects

- D-penicillamine (Cuprimine or Depen), a copper-chelating agent, should be taken orally before meals. A vitamin B6 supplement is needed with this drug; usually a dose of 25 mg. Zinc may also be necessary.
- Laxatives or stool softeners may be needed.
- Zinc acetate may be used to chelate copper with fewer side effects than D-penicillamine. Doses of 75–150 mg are often prescribed.

Herbs, Botanicals and Supplements

- Herbs and botanicals should not be used for Wilson's disease because there are no controlled trials to prove efficacy.

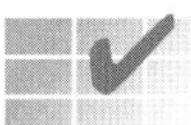

PATIENT EDUCATION

- Teach the patient about the copper and zinc content of foods.
- Explain that breast milk has higher copper levels than cow's milk to those individuals who need to know.
- Help the patient with feeding at mealtimes, if poor muscular control is demonstrated.
- Discuss effective coping mechanisms, community resources, and genetic counseling.

For More Information

- Wilson's Disease
  432 W. 58th St., Suite 614
  New York, NY 10019
  1-888-638-6928
  http://www.wilsonsdiseasecenter.org/

REFERENCES

CLEFT PALATE—Cited References

Bianchi F, et al. Environment and genetics in the etiology of cleft lip and cleft palate with reference to the role of folic acid. *Epidemiol Prev.* 2000;24(1):21.

Paradise J, et al. Evidence in infants with cleft palate that breast milk protects against otitis media. *Pediatrics.* 1994;94:853.

Spyropoulos M, Burdi A. Patterns of body and visceral growth in human prenates with clefts of the lip and palate. *Cleft Palate Craniofac J.* 2001;38:341.

Shaw W, et al. Assisted feeding is more reliable for infants with clefts—a randomized trial. *Cleft Palate Craniofac J.* 1999;36:262.

DOWN SYNDROME—Cited References

Hopman E, et al. Eating habits of young children with Down syndrome in The Netherlands: adequate nutrient intakes but delayed introduction of solid food. *J Am Diet Assoc.* 1998;98:79.

James S, et al. Abnormal folate metabolism and mutation in the methylenetetrahydrofolate reductase gene may be maternal risk factors for Down syndrome. *Am J Clin Nutri.* 1999;70:495.

Jovanovic S, et al. Biomarkers of oxidative stress are significantly elevated in Down syndrome. *Free Radic Biol Med.* 1998;25:1044.

Rosenblatt D. Folate and homocysteine metabolism and gene polymorphisms in the etiology of Down syndrome. *Am J Clin Nutri.* 1999;70:429.

Trissler R. Folic acid and Down syndrome. *J Am Diet Assoc.* 2000; 100:159.

NEURAL TUBE DEFECTS—Cited References

Cuskelly G, et al. Effect of increasing dietary folate on red-cell folate: implications for prevention of neural tube defects. *Lancet.* 1996;347:657.

Fiore P, et al. Nutritional survey of children and adolescents with myelomeningocele (MMC): overweight associated with reduced energy intake. *Eur J Pediatr Surg.* 1998;1:34S.

Gross S, et al. Inadequate folic acid intakes are prevalent among young women with neural tube defects. *J Am Diet Assoc.* 2001;101:342.

Harris M, Juriloff D. Mini-review: toward understanding mechanisms of genetic neural tube defects in mice. *Teratology.* 1999;60:292.

McDonnell G, McCann J. Issues of medical management in adults with spina bifida. *Childs Nerv Syst.* 2000;16:222.

PHENYLKETONURIA—Cited References

Acosta P, et al. Intake of major nutrients by women in the Maternal Phenylketonuria (MPKU) Study and effects on plasma phenylalanine concentrations. *Am J Clin Nutri.* 2001;73:792.

Artuch R, et al. Decreased serum ubiquinone-10 concentrations in phenylketonuria. *Am J Clin Nutri.* 1999;70:892.

Bross R, et al. Tyrosine requirements in children with classical PKU determined by indicator amino acid oxidation. *Am J Physiol Endocrinol Metab.* 2000;278:195.

de la Cruz F, Koch R. Genetic implications for newborn screening for phenylketonuria. *Clin Perinatol.* 2001;28:419.

Duran G, et al. Necessity of complete intake of phenylalanine-free amino acid mixture for metabolic control of phenylketonuria. *J Am Diet Assoc.* 1999;99:1559.

Fisch R, et al. Phenylketonuria: current dietary treatment practices in the United States. *J Am College Nutri.* 1997;16:147.

Levy H, et al. Congenital heart disease in maternal phenylketonuria: report from the Maternal PKU Collaborative Study. *Pediatr Res.* 2001;49:636.

Prince A, Leklem J. Vitamin B6-status of school-aged patients with phenylketonuria. *Am J Clin Nutri.* 1994;60:249.

Robinson M, et al. Increased risk of vitamin B12 deficiency in patients with phenylketonuria on an unrestricted or relaxed diet. *J Pediatr.* 2000;136:545.

Rouse B, et al. Maternal phenylketonuria syndrome: congenital heart defects, microcephaly, and developmental outcomes. *J Pediatr.* 2000;136:57.

Van Bakel M, et al. Antioxidant and thyroid hormone status in selenium-deficient phenylketonuric and hyperphenylalaninemic patients. *Am J Clin Nutri.* 2000;72:976.

Waisbren S, et al. Outcome at age 4 years in offspring of women with maternal phenylketonuria: the Maternal PKU Collaborative Study. *JAMA.* 2000;283:756.

Weglage, et al. Normal clinical outcome in untreated subjects with mild hyperphenylalaninemia. *Pediatr Res.* 2001;49:532.

PREMATURITY AND LOW-BIRTH-WEIGHT INFANTS—Cited References

Anderson D. Nutrition in the care of the low-birth-weight infant. In: Mahan K, Escott-Stump S, eds. *Krause's Food, Nutrition, and Diet Therapy.* 10th ed. Philadelphia: WB Saunders, 2000.

Amin S, et al. Brainstem maturation in premature infants as a function of enteral feeding type. *Pediatr.* 2000;106:318.

Bienengraber V, et al. Is it possible to prevent cleft palate by prenatal administration of folic acid? An experimental study. *Cleft Palate Craniofac J.* 2001;38:393.

Bishop N, et al. Aluminum neurotoxicity in preterm infants receiving intravenous-feeding solutions. *N Engl J Med.* 1997;336: 1557.

Bonner C, et al. Effects of parenteral L-carnitine supplementation on fat metabolism and nutrition in premature neonates. *J Pediatr.* 1995;126:287.

Dallas M, et al. Enteral glutamine supplementation for very-low-birth-weight infants decreases hospital costs. *J Parenter Enter Nutri.* 1998;22:353.

Darlow B, Graham P. Vitamin A supplementation for preventing morbidity and mortality in very-low-birth-weight infants. *Cochrane Database Syst Rev.* 2000;2:CD000501.

Ditzenberger G, et al. Continuous insulin intravenous infusion therapy for VLBW infants. *J Perinat Neonatal Nurs.* 1999;13:70.

Ehrenkrantz R, et al. Longitudinal growth of hospitalized very low birth weight infants. *Pediatrics.* 1999;104:280.

Gok U, et al. Bacteriological and PCR analysis of clinical material aspirated from otitis media with effusions. *Int J Pediatr Otorhinolaryngol.* 2001;60:49.

Hirata T, Bosque E. When they grow up: the growth of extremely low birth weight (under 1000 gm) infants at adolescence. *J Peds.* 1998;132:1033.

Kennedy T, et al. Growth patterns and nutritional factors associated with increased head circumference at 18 months in normally developing, low-birth-weight infants. *J Am Diet Assoc.* 1999;99:1522.

Lau C, et al. Oral feeding in low birth weight infants. *J Pediatr.* 1997;130:561.

Neu J, et al. Enteral glutamine supplementation for very low birthweight infants decreases morbidity. *J Pediatrics.* 1997;131:691.

Okosun I, et al. Ethnic differences in the rates of low birth weight attributable to differences in early motherhood: a study from the Third National Health and Nutrition Examination Survey. *J Perinatol.* 2000;20:105.

Peralta-Carcelen M, et al. Growth of adolescents who were born at extremely low birthweight without major disability. *J Pediatr.* 2000;136:633.

Pickler R, et al. Effects of nonnutritive sucking on behavioral organization and feeding performance in preterm infants. *Nurs Res.* 1996;45:132.

Rigo J, et al. Bone mineral metabolism in the micropreemie. *Clin Perinatol.* 2000;27:147.

Schanler R, et al. Feeding strategies for premature infants: beneficial outcomes of feeding fortified human milk versus preterm formula. *Pediatrics.* 1999;103:1150.

Shulman R, et al. Early feeding, feeding tolerance, and lactase activity in preterm infants. *J Pediatr.* 1998;133:645.

Tang W, et al. Influence of respiratory distress syndrome on body composition after preterm birth. *Arch Dis Child Fetal Neonatal Ed.* 1997;77:28.

Tomsits E, et al. Effects of early nutrition on free radical formation in VLBW infants with respiratory distress. *J Am Col Nutr.* 2000;19:237.

OTHER PEDIATRIC CONDITIONS—Cited References

Abad-Sinden A, et al. Nutrition management of congenital glucose-galactose malabsorption: a case study. *J Am Diet Assoc.* 1997;97:1417.

Abrams S. Chronic pulmonary insufficiency in children and its effects on growth and development. *J Nutri.* 2001;131:938S.

Adams R, et al. Maternal stress in caring for children with feeding disabilities: implications for health care providers. *J Am Diet Assoc.* 1999;99:962.

Alvear J, et al. Fetal alcohol syndrome and fetal alcohol effects: importance of early diagnosis and nutritional treatment. *Rev Med Chil.* 1998;126:407.

Andersson H, et al. Long-term outcome in treated combined methylmalonic acidemia and homocystinemia. *Genet Med.* 1999;1:146.

Anikster Y, et al. Pulmonary dysfunction in adults with nephropathic cystinosis. *Chest.* 2001;119:394.

Atkinson S. Special nutritional needs of infants for prevention of and recovery from bronchopulmonary dysplasia. *J Nutri.* 2001;131:942S.

Auborg P, et al. A two-year trial of oleic acid and erucic acids (Lorenzo's oil) as treatment for adrenomyeloneuropathy. *N Engl J Med.* 1993;329:745.

Baer M, Harris A. Pediatric nutrition assessment: identifying children at risk. *J Am Diet Assoc.* 1997;97:107A.

Berger J, et al. Leukodystrophies: recent developments in genetics, molecular biology, pathogenesis and treatment. *Curr Opin Neurol.* 2001;14:305.

Black M, et al. A randomized clinical trial of home intervention for children with failure to thrive. *Pediatrics.* 1995;95:807.

Bonthius D, et al. Alcohol exposure during the brain growth spurt promotes hippocampal seizures, rapid kindling, and spreading depression. *Alcohol Clin Exp Res.* 2001;25:734.

Brewer G, et al. Does a vegetarian diet control Wilson's disease? *J Am Col Nutri.* 1993;12:527.

Bucuvalas J, et al. Growth hormone insensitivity in children with biliary atresia. *J Pediatr Gastroenterol Nutri.* 1996;23:135.

Burwinkel B, et al. Variability of biochemical and clinical phenotype in X-linked liver glycogenosis with mutations in the phosphorylase kinase PHKA2 gene. *Hum Genet.* 1998;102:423.

Clemente C, et al. Are infant behavioral feeding difficulties associated with congenital heart disease? *Child Care Health Dev.* 2001;27:47.

Corbeel L, et al. Long-term follow-up of portacaval shunt in glycogen storage disease type 1B. *Eur J Pediatr.* 2000;159:268.

Davenport M, et al. Immunohistochemistry of the liver and biliary tree in extrahepatic biliary atresia. *J Pediatr Surg.* 2001;36:1017.

Desposito F, et al. Survey of pediatrician practices in retrieving statewide authorized newborn screening results. *Pediatrics.* 2001; 108:22.

Di Biase A, Salvati S. Exogenous lipids in myelination and myelination. *Kaohsiung J Med Sci.* 1997;13:19.

Duche M, et al. Percutaneous endoscopic gastrostomy for continuous feeding in children with chronic cholestasis. *J Pediatr Gastroenterol Nutri.* 1999;29:42.

Dundar B, et al. Chronic hypoxemia leads to reduced serum IGF-I levels in cyanotic congenital heart disease. *J Pediatr Endocrinol Metab.* 2000;13:431.

Dykens, E. Contaminated and unusual food combinations: what do people with Prader-Willi syndrome choose? *Ment Retard.* 2000; 38:163.

Ebrahim S, et al. Combined tobacco and alcohol use by pregnant and reproductive-aged women in the United States. *Obstet Gynecol.* 2000;96:767.

Ekvall S. *Pediatric Nutrition in Chronic Diseases and Developmental Disorders.* New York: Oxford University Press, 1993.

Endres W. Inherited metabolic diseases affecting the carrier. *J Inherit Metab Dis.* 1997;20:9.

Eriksson C. The role of acetaldehyde in the actions of alcohol (update 2000). *Alcohol Clin Exp Res.* 2001;25:15S.

Fatica C, et al. A cluster of necrotizing enterocolitis in term infants undergoing open heart surgery. *Am J Infect Control.* 2000;28:130.

Finck C, et al. Presentation of carcinoma in a patient with a previous operation for Hirschsprung's disease. *J Pediatr Surg.* 2001;36:E5.

Garg R, Tandon N. Hypophosphatemic rickets: easy to diagnose, difficult to treat. *Indian J Pediatr.* 1999;66:849.

Gaudet L, Smith G. Cerebral palsy and chorioamnionitis: the inflammatory cytokine link. *Obstet Gynecol Surv.* 2001;56:433.

Gillman M, et al. Risk of overweight among adolescents who were breastfed as infants. *JAMA.* 2001;285:2461.

Gubernick J, et al. U.S. approach to jaundice in infants and children. *Radiographics.* 2000;20:173.

Ihkkan D, Yalcin E. Changes in skeletal maturation and mineralization in children with cerebral palsy and evaluation of related factors. *J Child Neurol.* 2001;16:425.

Johnson R, et al. Athetosis increases resting metabolic rate in adults with cerebral palsy. *J Am Diet Assoc.* 1995;95:145.

Johnson D, et al. Nutrition and feeding in infants with bronchopulmonary dysplasia after initial hospital discharge: Risk factors for growth failure. *J Am Diet Assoc.* 1998;98:649.

Grugni G, et al. Failure of biliopancreatic diversion in Prader-Willi syndrome. *Obes Surg.* 2000;10:179.

Guttormsen A, et al. Disposition of homocysteine in subjects heterozygous for homocystinuria due to cystathionine beta-synthase deficiency: relationship between genotype and phenotype. *Am J Med Genet.* 2001;100:204.

Hammami M, et al. Disproportionate alterations in body composition of large for gestational age neonates. *J Pediatr.* 2001;138:817.

Holt R, et al. Nasogastric feeding enhances nutritional status in pediatric liver disease but does not alter circulating levels of IGF-I and IGF binding proteins. *Clin Endocrinol.* 2000;52:217.

Honein M, et al. Impact of folic acid fortification of the U.S. food supply on the occurrence of neural tube defects. *JAMA.* 2001;285:2981.

Horrocks L, Yeo Y. Health benefits of docosahexaenoic acid (DHA). *Pharmacol Res.* 1999;40:211.

Kang A, et al. Catch-up growth in children treated with home enteral nutrition. *Pediatr.* 1998;102:951.

Kaper B, et al. Nutritional rickets: report of four cases diagnosed at orthopedic evaluation. *Am J Orthop.* 2000;29:214.

Kawahara H, et al. The importance of the plasma amino acid molar ratio in patients with biliary atresia. *Surgery.* 1999;125:487.

Klesges R, et al. Effects of television on metabolic rate: potential implications for childhood obesity. *Pediatrics.* 1993;91:281.

Kreiter S, et al. Nutritional rickets in African American breastfed infants. *J Pediatr.* 2000;137:153.

Lackman F, et al. The risks of spontaneous preterm delivery and perinatal mortality in relation to size at birth according to fetal versus neonatal growth standards. *Am J Obstet Gynecol.* 2001;184:946.

Leitch C. Growth, nutrition and energy expenditure in pediatric heart failure. *Prog Pediatr Cardiol.* 2001;11:195.

Maffeis C, Tato L. Long-term effects of childhood obesity on morbidity and mortality. *Horm Res.* 2001;55:42S.

Martorell R, et al. Early nutrition and later adiposity. *J Nutri.* 2001;131:874S.

Mascarenhas M, Zemel B, Stallings V. Nutritional assessment in pediatrics. *Nutrition.* 1998;14:105.

Mathias R, et al. Hyperammonemia in urea cycle disorders: role of the nephrologist. *Am J Kidney Dis.* 2001;37:1069.

Mattson S, et al. Heavy prenatal alcohol exposure with or without physical features of fetal alcohol syndrome leads to IQ defects. *J Pediatrics.* 1997;131:718.

Nadler E, et al. Intestinal cytokine gene expression in infants with acute necrotizing enterocolitis: interleukin-11 mRNA expression inversely correlates with extent of disease. *J Pediatr Surg.* 2001;36:1122.

Ning C, et al. Galactose metabolism in mice with galactose-1-phosphate uridyltransferase deficiency: sucklings and 7-week-old animals fed a high-galactose diet. *Mol Genet Metab.* 2001;72:306.

Patterson, M. Screening for "prelysosomal disorders": carbohydrate-deficient glycoprotein syndromes. *J Child Neurol.* 1999;14:S16.

Pour R, et al. Enhanced lymphocyte proliferation in patients with adrenoleukodystrophy treated with erucic acid (22:1)-rich triglycerides. *J Inherit Metab Dis.* 2000;23:113.

Puangco M, Schanler R. Clinical experience in enteral nutrition support for premature infants with bronchopulmonary dysplasia. *J Perinatol.* 2000;20:87.

Pugliese M, et al. Nutritional rickets in suburbia. *J Am Col Nutri.* 1998;17:637.

Ray J, et al. MOS HIP: McMaster outcome study of hypertension in pregnancy. *Early Hum Dev.* 2001;64:129.

Raynor P, Rudolf M. Anthropometric indices of failure to thrive. *Arch Dis Child.* 2000;82:364.

Reis M, et al. Chloride-dependent inhibition of vesicular glutamate uptake by alpha-keto acids accumulated in maple syrup urine disease. *Biochem Biophys Acta.* 2000;1475:114.

Rosenblatt D, Whitehead V. Cobalamin and folate deficiency: acquired and hereditary disorders in children. *Semin Hematol.* 1999;36:19.

Satter E. *Child of Mine.* 2nd ed. Palo Alto: Bull Publishing, 1986.

Shan X, et al. Mutations in the regulatory domain of cystathionine beta synthase can functionally suppress patient-derived mutations in cis. *Hum Mol Genet.* 2001;10:635.

Shenai J, et al. Vitamin A status and postnatal dexamethasone treatment in bronchopulmonary dysplasia. *Pediatrics.* 2000;106:547.

Stein K. Children with feeding disorders: an emerging issue. *J Am Diet Assoc.* 2000;100:1000.

Stepnick-Gropper S, et al. Free galactose content of fresh fruits and strained fruit and vegetable baby foods: more foods to consider for the galactose-restricted diet. *J Am Diet Assoc.* 2000;100:573.

Steward D, et al. Biobehavioral characteristics of infants with failure to thrive. *J Pediatr Nurs.* 2001;16:162.

Stoler J, et al. The prenatal detection of significant alcohol exposure with maternal blood markers. *J Pediatr.* 1998;133:346.

Summar M. Current strategies for the management of neonatal urea cycle disorders. *J Pediatr.* 2001;138:S30.

Suzuki Y, et al. Clinical, biochemical, and genetic aspects and neuronal migration in peroxisome biogenesis disorders. *J Inherit Metab Dis.* 2001;24:151.

Suzuki Y. The clinical course of childhood and adolescent adrenoleukodystrophy before and after Lorenzo's oil. *Brain Dev.* 2001;23:30.

Topaloglu A, et al. Influence of metabolic control on growth in homocystinuria due to cystathionine b-synthase deficiency. *Pediatr Res.* 2001;49:796.

Trahms C. Metabolic disorders. In: Mahan K, Escott-Stump S, eds. *Krause's Food, Nutrition, and Diet Therapy.* 10th ed. Philadelphia: WB Saunders, 2000.

Uhari M, et al. A novel use of xylitol sugar in preventing acute otitis media. *Pediatr.* 1998;102:879.

Vanderhoof J, et al. Intolerances to protein hydrolysate infant formulas: an unrecognized cause of gastrointestinal symptoms in infants. *J Pediatrics.* 1997;131:741.

Varan B, et al. Malnutrition and growth failure in cyanotic and acyanotic congenital heart disease with and without pulmonary hypertension. *Arch Dis Child.* 1999;81:49.

Wardle S, et al. Randomized controlled trial of oral vitamin A supplementation in preterm infants to prevent chronic lung disease. *Arch Dis Child Fetal Neonatal Ed.* 2001;84:F9.

Wuhl E, et al. Long-term treatment with growth hormone in short children with nephropathic cystinosis. *J Pediatr.* 2001;138:880.

Yoneda A, et al. Cell-adhesion molecules and fibroblast growth factor signaling in Hirschsprung's disease. *Pediatr Surg Int.* 2001;17:299.

Suggested References

Bartonek A, Saraste H. Factors influencing ambulation in myelomeningocele: a cross-sectional study. *Dev Med Child Neurol.* 2001;43:253.

Botto L, et al. Neural tube defects. *N Engl J Med.* 1999;341:1509.

Cloud H. Developmental disabilities. In: Samour P, Helm K, Lang C. *Handbook of Pediatric Nutrition*. 2nd ed Gaithersburg, MD: Aspen Publication, 1999.

Iqbal M. Prevention of neural tube defects by periconceptional use of folic acid. *Pediatr Rev*. 2000;21:58.

Pass K, et al. 2000 US Newborn Screening System Guidelines II Follow-up of children diagnosis and management and evaluation. Statement of the council of regional networks for genetic services (CONR). *J Pediatr*. 2001;137:1S.

Summar M, Tuchman M. Proceedings of a consensus conference for the management of patients with urea cycle disorders. *J Pediatr*. 2001;138:S6.

SECTION 4

NEUROLOGICAL, MENTAL HEALTH, AND PSYCHIATRIC CONDITIONS

CHIEF ASSESSMENT FACTORS

- LOSS OF CONSCIOUSNESS, SEIZURES
- DIZZINESS, VERTIGO, WEAKNESS, DROWSINESS
- HEADACHES, PAIN
- NUMBNESS, PARALYSIS, SENSORY PAIN
- BOWEL OR BLADDER DYSFUNCTION
- DISTURBED TASTE, SMELL, VISION
- DYSPHAGIA; COUGHING OR CHOKING WHILE EATING/SWALLOWING
- STATUS OF FOOD IN ORAL CAVITY
- EASY ASPIRATION OF FOOD INTO LUNGS
- HALLUCINATIONS, TREMORS; TICS, SPASMS, ATAXIA
- NERVOUSNESS, IRRITABILITY
- DEPRESSION, ANXIETY
- CONFUSION, MEMORY LOSS; DISORIENTATION REGARDING PLACE AND TIME
- PROBLEMS WITH ABSTRACT THINKING, PERSONALITY CHANGES
- POOR OR WEAKER JUDGMENT; DIFFICULTY PERFORMING FAMILIAR TASKS
- MOOD OR BEHAVIORAL CHANGES
- EXTREMITIES: COLDNESS, STIFFNESS, LIMITED MOVEMENT, DISCOLORATION, PAIN

OVERVIEW OF NEUROLOGICAL AND PSYCHIATRIC DISORDERS

This chapter provides an overview of many neurological and psychiatric disorders that have nutritional implications. A few disorders, however, are found in other relevant sections (e.g., migraine headache is found near food allergies in section 2; mental retardation and developmental disorders are found in section 3; cerebrovascular disease/stroke is found in cardiovascular disorders in section 6; dysphagia is found in section 7; effects of anesthesia because of surgery are found in section 14).

The primary neurological disorders are separated from those indicated as psychiatric disorders because there is often a need for referral to a qualified psychologist or psychiatrist for the latter. A multidisciplinary approach is often more effective for psychiatric conditions. Note that nearly one of five Americans will experience a mental disorder during a lifetime. Table 4–1 describes goals in the treatment of psychiatric patients, and Tables 4–2 to 4–5 provide other information on neurological function relative to nutrition.

For More Information

- American Academy of Neurology
  1-800-879-1960
  http://www.aan.com
- AAN Education & Research Foundation
  www.thebrainmatters.org
- American Association of Neuroscience Nurses
  1-888-557-2266
  http://www.aann.org
- American Neurological Association
  612-545-6284
  http://www.aneuroa.org
- American Society of Neurorehabilitation
  612-545-6324
  http://www.asnr.com
- Brain Research Foundation
  343 South Dearborn Street
  Chicago, IL 60604
- Child Neurology Society
  651-486-9447
  http://www.umn.edu
- Society for Neuroscience
  202-462-6688
  http://www.sfn.org

TABLE 4–1 Goals in Nutritional Treatment of Psychiatric Patients

Careful review of history and assessments, including all medications and treatments
Positive approach
Prevention of malnutrition
Team-concept treatment
Restoration of feeding abilities and satisfaction

TABLE 4–2 CNS and Neuromuscular Conditions Impairing Ability to Self-Feed

Altered consciousness
Cerebral lesions
Cerebral palsy with either spasticity or ataxia
Dyskinesias
Mental retardation, severe
Motor weakness from demyelinating and related diseases such as ALS and multiple sclerosis
Myopathies
Organic brain syndrome
Paralysis from stroke
Peripheral neuropathy
Psychotic states such as paranoia
Tremor

TABLE 4–3 Food, Nutrition, and Neurotransmitters

The substrates of neuronal communication are called neurotransmitters (serotonin, dopamine, norepinephrine, and acetylcholine), which are subject to dietary manipulation. Increases or decreases in dietary precursors will affect nervous tissue functioning: choline affects acetylcholine production. Aromatic amino acids (tryptophan, tyrosine, and phenylalanine) are the precursors of serotonin, dopamine, and norepinephrine; acidic amino acids (glutamate and aspartate) are brain neurotransmitters but do not have dietary precursors in the same way (Fernstrom, 1994). Different combinations of meal content and/or drugs will alter substrate availability for neuron activity. Tryptophan can induce sleep from high-carbohydrate (CHO) meals, whereas, high-protein meals can increase alertness.

Although etiology and pathogenesis of the major neurodegenerative and neuroinflammatory disorders (i.e., Alzheimer's disease, amyotrophic lateral sclerosis, Parkinson's disease, Huntington's disease, and multiple sclerosis) are unknown, numerous recent studies strongly suggest that reactive nitrogen species play an important role. Nitric oxide and other reactive nitrogen species play crucial roles in the brain, including normal processes such as neuromodulation, neurotransmission, and synaptic plasticity and pathological processes such as neurodegeneration and neuroinflammation (Calabrese et al., 2000). Cytoprotective proteins such as heat shock proteins (HSPs) appear to be critically involved in protection from nitrosative and oxidative stress (Calabrese, 2000).

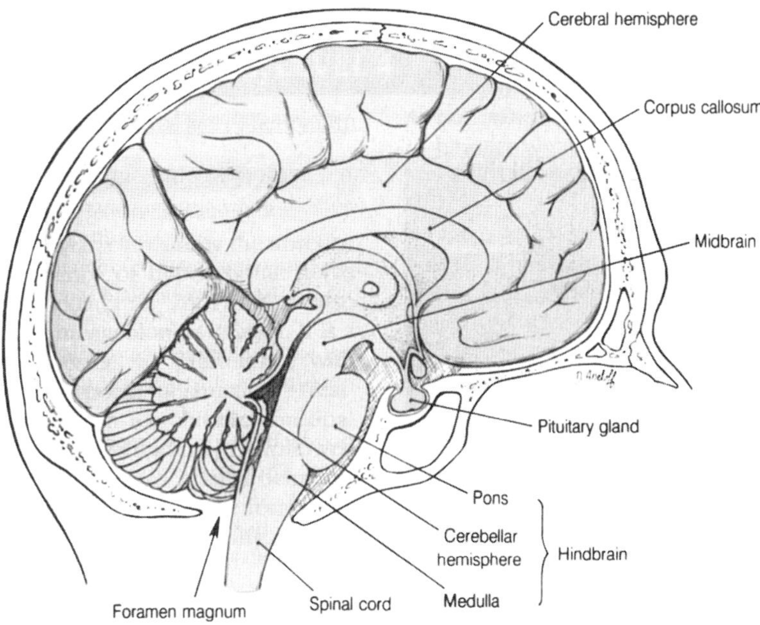

Figure 4–1

TABLE 4–4 Brain Parts and Functions

Medulla oblongata (8th–12th cranial nerves here)
Midbrain
Cerebellum (3rd–5th cranial nerves here)
Cerebrum
Pons (6th cranial nerve here)

BRAIN FUNCTIONS:

Hippocampus–important for learning and memory
Temporal lobe–controls thinking, ability to learn new things, expressive language, music and rhythm, and processing of memory
Frontal lobe–controls personality, mood, behavior, reasoning, emotional control, and cognition
Parietal lobe–comprehension of written language and oral speech; sensory stimulation such as pain, touch, smell, hearing, and heat; body image
Occipital lobe–vision
Cerebellum–voluntary movements such as sitting, standing, and walking
Pons–breathing
Medulla–involuntary functions such as heartbeat, temperature regulation, digestion, swallowing, and blinking
Spinal cord–sends and receives messages to and from brain and body parts

Note: A normal brain weighs 45 ounces, with steady growth until 20 years of age, then loses weight for the rest of life.

TABLE 4–5 Cranial Nerves Affecting Mastication and Swallowing

Nerve	*Function*
Trigeminal (V)	Controls some tongue and jaw muscles
Facial (VII)	Controls facial muscles
Glossopharyngeal (IX)	Controls muscles of pharynx; affects taste
Hypoglossal (XII)	Controls tongue muscles

ALZHEIMER'S DISEASE AND DEMENTIAS

NUTRITIONAL ACUITY RANKING: LEVEL 2

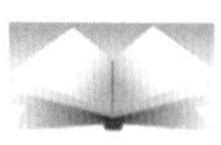

DEFINITIONS AND BACKGROUND

Dementias include multiple cognitive defects with memory loss; they also include aphasia, apraxia, agnosia, and disturbed daily functioning (Nutrition Screening Initiative, 2002). Risk factors for dementia include diatbetes, cardiovascular diseases such as stroke and hypertension, head injury, aging, depression, and family history. Of over 50 common dementias, Alzheimer's disease (AD) involves a progressive deterioration of intellect, memory, personality, and self-care, leading to severe dementia from degeneration of nerve cells. Acetylcholine-containing neurons are especially affected. Acetylcholine normally triggers breakdown of a b-amyloid precursor protein (APP) in brain cells; this factor is missing in Alzheimer's disease.

Cognitive function can be measured using the Mattis dementia rating scale (MDRS). Cerebrospinal fluid lactate and pyruvate levels provide a reliable measure of cerebral glucose metabolism, which affects neuronal health (Parnetti et al., 1995).

Memory, thinking ability, judgment, and learning ability are impaired; personality may also deteriorate. Some dementias are reversible, but AD is not. Dementias that develop in very old age are not always associated with malnutrition and decreased life expectancy (Franzoni et al., 1996).

Early stages of Alzheimer's disease manifest with short-term memory loss and no later recall; problems finding the appropriate word; asking the same questions over and over; difficulty making decisions and planning; suspiciousness; changes in smell, taste, and vision; claims that nothing is wrong; depression; loss of initiative; personality changes; and problems with abstract thinking.

Evidence from preclinical and clinical studies supports the hypothesis that oxidative stress may be associated with the onset and progression of AD (Pitchumoni, 1998). Elements that have been implicated in free-radical-induced oxidative stress in AD have been measured by instrumental neutron activation analysis (INAA); a significant elevation of iron and zinc was observed in multiple regions of the AD brain (Cornett et al., 1998). Mercury was elevated but not significantly; selenium, a protective agent against mercury toxicity, was significantly elevated. The elevation of iron and zinc in the AD brain may augment neuron degeneration through free radical processes. The way zinc is metabolized in the brain may accelerate progression of amyloid/plaque formation.

Noncognitive behavioral changes such as depression, aggressive behavior, psychosis, and overactivity occur frequently in patients with dementia, in addition to cognitive impairment, and often determine the need for institutionalization. The biochemical basis of such changes is poorly understood, but clinical trials indicate that cholinomimetics improve noncognitive behaviors (Minger et al., 2000). Choline acetyltransferase activity (ChAT) is reduced in AD compared with controls correlated with cognitive impairment and increasing overactivity. Disturbance of the cholinergic system may underlie both cognitive and some noncognitive behavioral changes in dementia.

Medications or vitamins that increase the levels of brain catecholamines and protect against oxidative damage may reduce the neuronal damage and slow the progression of AD. Decreasing levels of vitamin E per unit of cholesterol is associated with poor memory, while vitamins A and C, beta-carotene, and selenium are not (Pitchumoni, 1998). Either monoamine oxidase (MAO), selegiline, or vitamin E (10,000 units) can slow the progression of disease (Miller, 2000; Sano et al., 1997).

High dietary intake of vitamin C and vitamin E may lower the risk of this disorder (Engelhart et al, 2002). Adequate vitamin E or selenium and other antioxidants may be identified as essential in management of this disorder (Reichman, 2000; Leszek, 1999). Vitamin D supplements have been useful for some individuals (Kipen et al., 1995). Vitamins B6, B12, and folate lower elevated levels of homocysteine, which can clog arteries in the brain; include dietary sources.

Patients with AD may have dysfunctional mechanisms of body weight regulation. Risk of weight loss tends to increase with severity and progression of AD. Weight loss is a predictor of mortality among subjects with AD (White et al., 1998). Weight gain or losses are common up to 5% in one year (White et al., 1996).

Comprehensive treatment of AD requires thorough caregiver support and a thoughtful and informed use of medications for cognition enhancement, neuroprotection, and the treatment of disturbed behavior (Reichman, 2000). The current prognosis for AD is poor, with death most often from renal, pulmonary, or cardiac complications after 2–20 years.

The future of Alzheimer's research is aimed at developing lifestyle activity and dietary interventions to maintain adequate energy intake, restore energy balance, and maintain skeletal muscle mass, because these patients have high daily energy expenditures and low energy intakes (Poehlman & Dvorak, 2000). The way the brain uses energy is another area of further research. The disease affects primarily the frontal lobe of the cerebral cortex, the temporal lobe, and the parietal lobe. See Table 4–4 and Figure 4–1.

OBJECTIVES

- Prevent weight loss or excessive gains from altered activity levels, eating habits, depression, tardive dyskinesia, impaired memory, and self-feeding behaviors. Dementia does not necessarily cause undernutrition; it may be necessary for caregivers to prioritize the feeding process (Morley, 1996).
- Avoid constipation or impaction. Promote continence as long as possible.
- Encourage self-feeding at mealtimes.
- Nourish by appropriate methods (tube, if necessary). The terminal stage of the disease is initiated by the inability to

swallow. No published trials exist which demonstrate that tube feeding (TF) is better than oral feeding (Finucane et al., 1999).

- Prevent or correct dehydration.
- Monitor dysphagia and aspiration.
- Protect patient from injury; provide emotional support.
- Offer frequent snacks, even at night if desired. Use creative feeding strategies (Nutrition Screening Initiative, 2002).
- Prevent pressure ulcers and other signs of nutritional decline.

DIETARY AND NUTRITIONAL RECOMMENDATIONS

- Ensure an adequate diet, including protein and increased calories for age, sex, and activity, especially for "wanderers" and those who pace. Persons with Alzheimer's may need 35 kcal/kg of body weight (Spindler et al., 1996).
- Adequate vitamin E or selenium and other antioxidants may be identified as essential in management of this disorder (Reichman, 2000; Leszek, 1999). Vitamin D supplements have been useful for some individuals (Kipen et al., 1995). Vitamins B6, B12, and folate lower elevated levels of homocysteine, which can clog arteries in the brain; include dietary sources.
- Offer one course at a time (first salad, then entree, etc.) to prevent confusion. Avoid distractions and allow extra time for meals. Cueing is also useful.
- Finger foods, such as sandwiches cut into four, chicken strips, julienne vegetables, and brownie versus apple pie, may be easier to eat, helping the patient to maintain weight (Soltesz and Dayton, 1993).
- Because sweets are well liked, offer nutrient-dense desserts.
- Tube feed or use thick, pureed foods if needed to counteract dysphagia.
- Choline may be beneficial (Minger et al., 2000). Use of foods such as soybeans or eggs will provide choline in the form useful to the body; lecithin tablets do not increase acetylcholine levels adequately.
- Adequate fluid intake is essential.
- Cut back on saturated fats, which may increase brain beta-amyloid levels and the effects of AD.

Common Drugs Used and Potential Side Effects

- Cholinesterase inhibitors donepezil and rivastigmine can slow the progression of cognitive and functional deficits in AD over the short term. Rivastigmine tartrate (Exelon) improves cognitive function, behavior, and daily functioning. Reminyl (galanthamine) blocks acetylcholine breakdown and shows promise. Nausea or diarrhea may occur.
- Although antioxidant, anti-inflammatory, and other treatment strategies are promising, recent studies of the treatment of AD with estrogen or prednisone have produced disappointing results. For managing the behavioral symptoms that commonly accompany AD (e.g., delusions, aggression, depression, anxiety, irritability), various antipsychotics, antidepressants, and anticonvulsants have been effective in carefully selected patients. Select those without causing dry mouth or constipation.
- Treatment with 2,000 IU alpha-tocopherol (vitamin E) has been shown to delay the progression of nursing home admission in patients with mild-to-moderate AD (Reichman, 2000; Nutrition Screening Initiative, 2002).
- Cognex (tacrine hydrochloride) may cause abdominal pain, increased liver function tests, constipation, diarrhea, indigestion, anorexia, vomiting, or weight loss. To date, no strongly proven effectiveness has been identified (Davis et al., 1992).
- Hydergine relieves symptoms of declining mental capacity. Nausea and gastrointestinal (GI) distress are common side effects.
- Laxatives may be used to control constipation. Offer high-fiber foods whenever possible. Ensure adequate fluid intake.
- Ibuprofen and other nonsteroidal, anti-inflammatory drugs may reduce the risk of development of AD, according to studies at Johns Hopkins; reduction of the inflammatory process occurs.
- Methanesulfonyl fluoride (MSF), a long-acting CNS-selective acetylcholinesterase (AChE) inhibitor, has been tested as a palliative treatment for AD. Most of the improvement in cognition was maintained 8 weeks after ending MSF. There were no toxic or adverse drug-related side effects. MSF may be a safe and effective palliative treatment for AD, and further clinical trials in larger groups of patients are warranted (Moss et al., 1999).

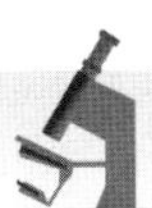

PROFILE

Clinical/History

Height, weight
BMI
Weight changes
Anorexia
Nausea, vomiting
Diarrhea
Bowel incontinence
Intake and output (I & O)
Cognitive performance (Mini-Mental State Examination)
Behavior (Present Behavioral Examination).

Lab Work

Choline acetyltransferase activity (ChAT)
Serum hormone levels (estrogen, etc.)
Serum glucose
Hemoglobin and hematocrit (H&H)
Electroencephalogram (EEG)
Serum zinc
Alanine aminotransferase (ALT), Aspartate aminotransaminase (AST)
Dopamine (DA)
Na+, K+
Blood urea nitrogen (BUN), Creat
Serum Fe
Albumin (alb)
Computed tomography (CT) scan or MRI
CSF pyruvate and lactate levels

Herbs, Botanicals and Supplements

- Gingko biloba has some evidence of efficacy in reducing memory decline, possibly by inhibiting cellular oxidation and enhancing circulation. It interacts with anticoagulants and antiplatelets such as aspirin, warfarin, and dipyridamole.
- Coenzyme Q10, choline, and lecithin may be useful. More studies are planned.
- Huperzine A (Chinese club moss) may prevent breakdown of acetylcholine. Research is underway.
- Phosphatidylserine, acetyl-L-carnitine, horse balm, Brazil nut, rosemary, dandelion, and sage have been promoted but have not been proven for efficacy; side effects have not been clearly identified.
- Selegiline (Eldepryl) should not be used with ginseng, ma huang (ephedra,) yohimbe, or St. John's wort.

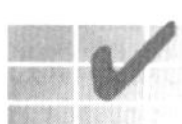

PATIENT EDUCATION

- ✓ Consider need for home services or nursing home placement.
- ✓ Encourage routines such as regular mealtimes, good mouth care, etc. Reduce distractions at mealtime.
- ✓ Refer family or caretakers to support groups.
- ✓ Aluminum toxicity studies are still controversial; discuss with empathy. Data from a study in France suggest long-term exposure to aluminum and silica from drinking water may be somewhat relevant (Rondeau et al., 2000).
- ✓ Special feeding methods may be needed.
- ✓ If the patient must be spoon-fed, gently holding his or her nose will force the mouth open.
- ✓ Products like Carnation Instant Breakfast can add extra calories and protein without excessive expense. Baking nutritious cookie bars or snacks enhances calorie intake and addresses the need for sensory stimulation.
- ✓ Use unbreakable dishes and utensils to avoid injury. Cutting and preparing foods for the patient are useful.

For More Information

- Alzheimer's Association
  919 North Michigan Avenue, Suite 1000
  Chicago, IL 60611-1676
  1-800-272-3900
  http://www.alz.org/
- Alzheimer's Disease Education and Referral Center
  1-800-438-4380
  http://alzheimers.org
- National Hotline – Alzheimer's Association
  919 N. Michigan Ave., Suite 1000
  Chicago, IL 60611
  1-800-272-3900
  http://www.icfs.org/bluebook/bb000301.htm

AMYOTROPHIC LATERAL SCLEROSIS

NUTRITIONAL ACUITY RANKING: LEVEL 3

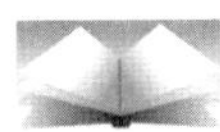

DEFINITIONS AND BACKGROUND

Amyotrophic lateral sclerosis (ALS) is a progressive neuron disease of adult life that destroys nerve cells from the spinal cord to muscle cells. Men are more often affected than women; the disease affects 20,000 people in the U.S., usually after age 40. It is also known as a motor neuron disease, progressive spinal muscular atrophy, or Lou Gehrig's disease.

The optimal management of nutrition in early ALS has not been established. Malnutrition is present in 16–50% of ALS patients and is an independent prognostic factor for worsened survival (Desport et al., 2001). It is caused primarily by swallowing dysfunction from involvement of the lower sets of cranial nerves. Hypermetabolism is also implicated. Malnutrition produces neuromuscular weakness and adversely affect patients' quality of life. In later stages of the disease, percutaneous endoscopic gastrostomy (PEG) confers a significant survival benefit in selected patients (Hardiman, 2000). While enteral nutrition support can improve the respiratory status of ALS patients, the effect on survival remains to be confirmed (Desport et al., 2001).

Dietary factors have long been suspected of being risk factors for ALS, but few human studies have been reported; a major study found that lycopene and magnesium are most useful (Longnecker et al., 2001). Energy metabolism by the brain is affected. There is a positive association between glutamate intake and ALS that is consistent with the theory that implicates glutamate excitotoxicity in the pathogenesis of ALS and the negative impact of fiber intake (Nelson et al., 2000).

Familial amyotrophic lateral sclerosis (FALS) shows mutations in the gene for superoxide dismutase-1 (Shibata, 2001). Proposed mechanisms of motor neuron degeneration have been suggested such as oxidative injury, peroxynitrite toxicity, cytoskeletal disorganization, glutamate excitotoxicity, disrupted calcium homeostasis, superoxide dismutase-1 aggregation, carbonyl stress, and apoptosis. Over-expression of mutant superoxide dismutase-1 in mice seems to enhance oxidative stress generation. Creatine significantly increases longevity and motor performance of mice and improves function of the glutamate transport system, which has a high demand for energy and is susceptible to oxidative stress (Andreassen et al., 2001).

Table 4–5 lists nerves affected in ALS. Symptoms and signs of ALS include muscular wasting and atrophy, drooling, loss of reflexes, respiratory infections or failure, spastic gait, and weakness. Respiratory failure occurs as a result of bulbar, cervical, and thoracic loss of motor neurons; inspiratory muscles are affected. Management of respiratory failure includes the use of strategies that limit aspiration pneumonia, the reduction in secretions, positioning of the patient to a maximal mechanical advantage, and use of noninvasive positive pressure ventilation. The decision to undertake invasive mechanical ventilation should be made prior to the development of symptoms that might warrant this intervention (Hardiman, 2000). For 50% of cases, ALS is usually fatal within 3–4 years from pneumonia or renal failure; 10% live 10 years or longer. There is no known cure at this time.

Research with AIDS patients has shown some evidence that a form of ALS can improve or disappear with some of the antiviral drug therapies (McGowan et al., 2001).

OBJECTIVES

- Maintain good nutrition to prevent further complications.
- Reduce difficulties in chewing and swallowing. Monitor gag reflex.
- Reduce the patient's fear of aspiration; test swallowing reflexes with water and feed slowly.
- Minimize the possibility of urinary tract infection and constipation.
- Correct negative nitrogen balance and nutritional deficiencies that exist.
- Ease symptoms to try to maintain independence.
- Reduce fatigue from the mealtime process; provide a slower pace to avoid choking.

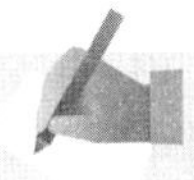

DIETARY AND NUTRITIONAL RECOMMENDATIONS

- Use a soft diet. Provide adequate fiber in the diet. Flaky fish, ground meats, and casseroles should be encouraged, along with foods moistened with gravies and sauces.
- The diet should include 2–3 L of water daily. Thicken liquids as needed with commercial thickeners, gelatin powder, or mashed potato flakes.
- Place food at side of mouth and tilt head forward to facilitate swallowing, when possible.
- Caloric intake should be normal to high. Five to six small meals should be scheduled daily. Increase protein intake to counteract wasting.
- Diet and supplemental feedings should provide an adequate intake of zinc, magnesium, potassium, amino acids, and phosphorus.
- Inclusion of foods rich in magnesium and lycopene may prove to be adjunctive treatments.
- Foods should be moistened and not dry or crumbly. Cake and crackers should not be served plain, whereas yogurt, applesauce, and pudding generally are acceptable.
- Sips of liquid are best tolerated between bites of food.
- PEG tube placement is well-tolerated and provides more efficient enteral nutrition than nasogastric tube feeding when dysphagia becomes severe (Desport et al., 2001). Percutaneous gastrojejunostomy (PEJ) is also well-tolerated in patients with ALS and is a safe alternative (Strong et al., 1999).

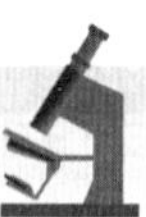

PROFILE

Clinical/History		
Weight	Difficulty in swallowing	Alb, prealbumin
Weight changes	Temperature	Transferrin
BMI (below 18–20 indicates malnutrition)	I& O	BUN, Creat
Height	Gag reflex	Nitrogen (N) balance
	Lab Work	Electromyogram (EMG)
	H&H, serum Fe	Glucose
	Na+, K+	

Common Drugs Used and Potential Side Effects

- Riluzole (a glutamate release inhibitor, membrane stabilizer) has been used to block nerve cell destruction. It seems to slow the disease but not curb its progress. Side effects are not yet noted. Reports from patient databases describe experience with increased survival with riluzole over time.
- Myotrophin, which is a muscle protein, is used experimentally to slow progression of symptoms.
- Antiviral drugs such as nelfinavir, zidovudine, and lamivudine have shown evidence of being effective in one patient with HIV infection (MacGowan et al., 2001).
- Studies suggest that magnesium, lycopene, and anti-inflammatory drugs may be beneficial.
- Minocycline may slow progression of ALS by blocking capases.
- Baclofen reduces muscle spasm and may lessen muscle cramping.

Herbs, Botanicals and Supplements

- No specific herbs and botanical products have been proven for efficacy for ALS in clinical trials.
- Creatine significantly increases longevity and motor performance of mice and improves function of the glutamate transport system (Andreassen et al., 2001). It is not clear that supplemental use is indicated.

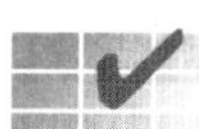

PATIENT EDUCATION

- ✓ Dietary counseling is important but rapidly becomes insufficient, particularly in bulbar-onset ALS, where enteral nutritional support is then necessary (Desport et al., 2001). Discuss care plan in front of patient; include the patient as much as possible.
- ✓ In early stages, discuss adding fiber to the diet to prevent constipation. Explain which foods have fiber.
- ✓ Encourage the planning of small, adequately balanced meals.
- ✓ Carefully monitor the patient's weight loss. A weight loss of 10% is common.
- ✓ Lightweight utensils are beneficial. A referral to an occupational therapist is recommended.
- ✓ Minimize chewing, but avoid use of baby food, which can be insulting. Puree adult foods, especially preferred foods that are seasoned as usual for the individual.
- ✓ In later stages, decide if enteral nutrition will be used.

For More Information

- ALS Association
  Woodland Hills, CA 91364
  818-880-9007
  1-800-782-4747 for patients
  http://www.alsa.org/

CEREBRAL ANEURYSM

NUTRITIONAL ACUITY RANKING: LEVEL 2

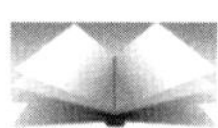

DEFINITIONS AND BACKGROUND

A cerebral aneurysm may involve the dilation of a cerebral artery resulting from a weakness of the blood vessel wall. Symptoms and signs include altered consciousness, drowsiness, confusion, stupor, sometimes coma, headache, facial pain, eye pain, blurred vision, vertigo, tinnitus, hemiparesis, elevated blood pressure, and dilated pupils.

Aneurysms may burst and cause hemorrhage. An intracranial hemorrhage is bleeding inside the skull. Head injury is the most common cause. Bleeding within the brain is intracerebral; those between the brain and the subarachnoid space are called subarachnoid hemorrhages. Those between the meninges are subdural hemorrhages; those between the skull and covering of the brain are called epidural hemorrhages. Hemorrhagic stroke may occur (see section 6 for more information about stroke).

OBJECTIVES

- ▲ Omit fluids if necessary to reduce cerebral edema.
- ▲ Rest is essential. Avoid constipation and straining at stool.
- ▲ Lower hypertension if possible.
- ▲ Prevent further complications or problems such as lingering neurological problems.
- ▲ Prepare for surgery if safe and possible.

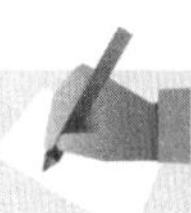

DIETARY AND NUTRITIONAL RECOMMENDATIONS

- Nil per os (NPO or nothing by mouth) unless otherwise ordered. Appropriate IVs should be used.
- Upon verification of progress, the physician should order a diet appropriate for condition. Assist with self-feeding measures.
- Restrict sodium and dietary cholesterol if deemed necessary.
- Alter dietary fiber intake, as appropriate.
- Control fluid if required.

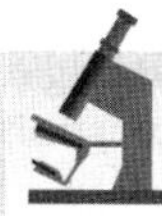

PROFILE

Clinical/History

Height
Weight
BMI
Weight changes
I & O
Blood pressure (BP) (increased)

Lab Work

Cholesterol (chol)
Trig
Alb, prealbumin
Glucose (gluc)
Na+, K+
H&H
MRI
CT scan results

Common Drugs Used and Potential Side Effects

- Cardiovascular drugs are usually ordered according to significant parameters. Adjust dietary intake accordingly.
- Diuretics may be used. Monitor need for potassium replacement if Lasix is prescribed.

Herbs, Botanicals and Supplements

- No specific herbs and botanical products have been used for cerebral aneurysm in any clinical trials.

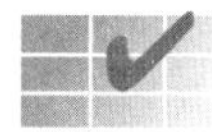

PATIENT EDUCATION

- ✔ Discuss fiber sources from the diet. Foods such as prune juice or bran added to cereal can be helpful in alleviating constipation.
- ✔ Counsel regarding self-feeding techniques.
- ✔ Discuss role of nutrition in preventing further cardiovascular or neurological problems.

COMA

NUTRITIONAL ACUITY RANKING: LEVEL 3

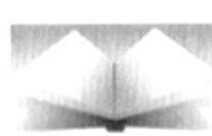

DEFINITIONS AND BACKGROUND

Impaired consciousness or coma can occur from a stroke, head injury, meningitis, encephalitis, sepsis, lack of oxygen, epileptic seizure, toxic effects of alcohol or drugs, liver or kidney failure, high or low blood glucose levels, or altered body temperature. Coma is the unconscious state in which the patient is unresponsive to verbal or painful stimuli. Medical staff can use the Glasgow Coma Scale to determine levels of unconsciousness and prognosis.

In the U.S., there are 14,000–35,000 people in a permanently unconscious state. A patient in a permanently vegetative state (PVS) does not have the ability to request or refuse treatment. The doctor determines the diagnosis of PVS. According to the American Dietetic Association position on legal and ethical issues in feeding permanently unconscious patients (1995), the meaning of nutrition, hydration, and the definition of death are central to the dilemma of feeding permanently unconscious patients. Dietitians serve an integral role with other members of the team in developing and implementing ethical guidelines for feeding permanently unconscious patients. Most are tube fed because it is safer and more practical than hand feeding. Nutritional support is associated with improved survival in coma (Borum et al., 2000).

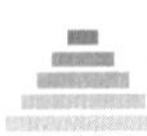

OBJECTIVES

- Maintain standards for primary condition.
- Where possible, elevate head to prevent aspiration during feeding process.
- Assess daily calorie and fluid requirements.
- Prevent or treat pressure ulcers, constipation, and other complications of immobility.

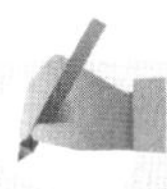

DIETARY AND NUTRITIONAL RECOMMENDATIONS

- Immediately, give intravenous glucose until the cause is better identified.
- Tube feed (increased calories and protein as appropriate) every 2–3 hours or as ordered by the physician. Parenteral fluids may also be appropriate at this time.
- Total parenteral nutrition (TPN) or use of intravenous fat solutions can be appropriate for some persons dependent on evaluations of original disorder, sepsis, or other complicating factors.
- A formula with fiber can be helpful in preventing or easing constipation because of the added fiber content.
- Progress, when or if possible, to oral feedings.

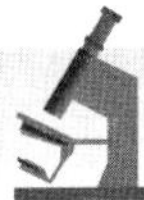

PROFILE

Clinical/History

Height/weight
BMI
Weight changes (bed scale)
Glasgow Coma Scale (4–7 = coma; measures eye opening, motor, and verbal responses)
BP

Lab Work

H&H
Partial pressure of carbon dioxide (pCO2)
Partial pressure of oxygen (pO2)
Chol
Trig
Alb
Gluc
BUN, Creat
CT scan or MRI
Serum Fe
I & O
Urine tests for chemicals, glucose
Serum alcohol level

Common Drugs Used and Potential Side Effects

- Anticonvulsants, such as phenytoin (Dilantin), may aggravate folic acid metabolism and cause decreased serum levels over time. Avoid use with evening primrose oil, gingko biloba, and kava.
- Steroids may be used with side effects such as increased sodium retention, increased potassium, calcium and magnesium losses, and increased nitrogen depletion.
- Antacids may be needed to prevent stress ulcers.
- Cathartics are often used. Monitor for electrolyte imbalances.

Herbs, Botanicals and Supplements

- No specific herbs and botanical products have been used in comatose patients in any clinical trials.
- With phenytoin (Dilantin), avoid use with evening primrose oil, gingko biloba, and kava.

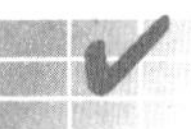

PATIENT EDUCATION

- Discuss with caretaker or family any necessary measures that are completed to provide adequate nourishment. Explain importance of prevention of complications such as aspiration.
- Evaluate self-feeding potentials over time.
- A Medic Alert bracelet or other ID may be useful for persons with disorders that may lead to unconsciousness.

EPILEPSY/SEIZURE DISORDERS

NUTRITIONAL ACUITY RANKING: LEVEL 1

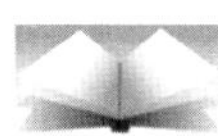

DEFINITIONS AND BACKGROUND

Epilepsy, a paroxysmal disturbance of the nervous system, results in recurrent attacks of loss of consciousness, convulsions, motor activity, or behavioral abnormalities. The seizures result from excessive neuronal discharges in the brain. A grand mal seizure involves an aura, a tonic phase, and a clonic phase. A petit mal seizure involves momentary loss of consciousness. Patients with protein–calorie malnutrition are sometimes found to have some neurologic deficits or signs of epilepsy (Dike, 1999).

There are many forms of epilepsy, each with its own symptoms. In two-thirds of cases, no structural abnormality is found. A single seizure does not imply epilepsy. Incidence is 2–6 in 1,000 people. It is common with cerebral palsy and spina bifida.

A ketogenic diet should be considered for children ages 1–10 with refractory epilepsy whose seizures are difficult to control (Freeman et al., 1998). Several modifications of the original diet have been used (e.g., the medium-chain triglycerides [MCT] diet) in an attempt to overcome the obstacles of compliance and acceptance. A ketogenic diet is 70–90% fat with remainder as protein and CHO; in most patients, this produces a ketosis, and seizure activity is reduced or eliminated (Couch et al., 1999). Modern ketogenic diets have been used with better success as compared with previous attempts (Carroll and Koenigsberger, 1998). Medical nutrition therapy (MNT) with the ketogenic diet for seizure control requires an average of 16 hours per patient (MacCracken and Scalisi, 1999). Seizure reduction and improved behavior control occurs; substantial financial savings are likely (Mandel et al., 2002.)

OBJECTIVES

- Minimize seizures via medications or lesionectomy surgery.
- Provide a well-balanced diet that avoids excess of food or fluid intake.
- If drug therapy does not work (as in the case of intractable myoclonic or akinetic seizures of infancy), a ketogenic diet may be used to produce ketosis. Ketosis stabilizes convulsions by decreasing restlessness and irritability. Reverse the usual ratio of cholesterol and fat. Beware of changing the diet abruptly; a gradual approach is preferred. This approach works best for children aged 2–5 years. If hyperuricemia or hypercalciuria occurs, increase fluid intake and consider use of diuretics.
- Monitor need for key nutrients.
- Correct nutritional deficits from long-term anticonvulsant medication use (disorders of vitamin D, calcium, and bone metabolism). Phenytoin therapy (PHT) decreases serum folate by 50%, thereby increasing risk of deficiency (Berg, 1995).
- Monitor for possible long-term cardiac implications while following the ketogenic diet (Best et al., 2000). Growth retardation in children should also be prevented.

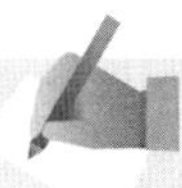

DIETARY AND NUTRITIONAL RECOMMENDATIONS

- Provide a diet reflecting the patient's age and activity.
- A ketogenic diet is unpalatable. The diet follows a ratio of 3:1 or 4:1 fat to carbohydrate and protein. MCTs are more ketogenic, having more rapid metabolism and absorption. If used in this way, MCTs would provide 60% of kcal (the rest of the diet would consist of 10% other fats, 10% protein, and 20% carbohydrates). Protein should meet basal needs (e.g., 1 g/kg body weight).
- Stimulants such as tea, coffee, colas, and alcohol are not permitted.
- Supplements may be needed, especially for calcium, vitamin D, folacin, and vitamins B6 and B12.
- Add fiber and fluid for constipation.

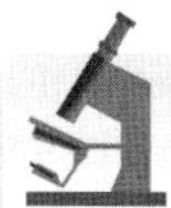

PROFILE

Clinical/History	Lab Work	
Height	Urinary acetone (AM levels)	CT scan
Weight	EEG	H&H
BMI	Serum Ca++	Alkaline phosphatase (Alk phos)
BP	Alb, prealbumin	Chol, Trig
I & O		Skull x-ray
		Serum folate

Common Drugs Used and Potential Side Effects

- Anticonvulsant therapy can cause interference with vitamin D metabolism, leading to a calcium imbalance and possibly rickets or osteomalacia. Therapy with 25-hydroxy vitamin D is recommended. Common anticonvulsants include:
  - Carbamazepine (Tegretol) causes dry mouth, vomiting, nausea, anorexia, low red blood cell and white cell counts.
  - Depakote/Depakene (Valproic acid) may cause nausea, vomiting, anorexia, weight gain, or hair loss.
  - Ethosuximide (Zarontin), trimethadione (Tridione), and primidone (Mysoline) can cause gastrointestinal upset, anemia, and weight loss. Take with food or milk.

  - Felbatol (Felbamate) is effective against seizures but can cause constipation, nausea, vomiting, and anorexia.
  - Phenytoin (Dilantin) causes gum hyperplasia and carbohydrate intolerance. It also binds serum proteins and decreases folate and vitamin B12 absorption. Patients will also need more vitamin C and magnesium. Be careful with vitamin B6; excess supplementation can reduce effectiveness. With tube feedings, it usually is necessary to stop feedings 30 minutes before and after administration of the medication; nutritional intake may need to be calculated over 21 versus 24 hours. PHT therapy to control seizures decreases serum folate levels in half of epileptic patients, thus increasing risk of folate depletion. Supplementation prevents deficiency but also changes PHT pharmacokinetics (Berg et al., 1995).
  - Phenobarbital depletes vitamins D, K, B12, B6, folate, and calcium. Nausea, vomiting, sedation, and anorexia can occur.
- Cough syrups, laxatives, and other medications contain a high CHO content; monitor drug–drug interactions (McGhee and Katyal, 2001).
- Mysoline is similar to a barbiturate; vomiting may occur.

Herbs, Botanicals and Supplements

- Vitamin B6 is the vitamin associated with neuronal function. High doses of pyridoxine should not be taken with phenobarbital or phenytoin, where seizure control might be compromised. If B6 is added to either drug regimen, keep it at the lowest effective dose and monitor serum drug levels.
- St John's wort is used as a natural antidepressant. Do not use with monoamine oxidase inhibitors (MAOI) antidepressants, selective serotonin reuptake inhibitors (SSRI) antidepressants, cyclosporine, digoxin, oral contraceptives, HIV protease inhibitors, theophylline, warfarin, or calcium channel blockers such as amlodipine, diltiazem, or verapamil. No studies have been conducted for efficacy in seizure patients.
- Psyllium and ginseng should not be used with Depakote and lithium.
- With dilantin (phenytoin), avoid use with evening primrose oil, gingko biloba, and kava.

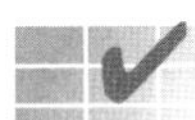

PATIENT EDUCATION

- ✓ Ketogenic diets cause nausea and vomiting; a small drink of fruit juice can help relieve the symptoms. Regular monitoring of the diet is crucial.
- ✓ An ID tag, such as Medic-Alert, is recommended.
- ✓ Alcohol should be avoided. A balanced diet is needed.
- ✓ To alter fats, the following tips may be helpful: to increase long-chain triglycerides (LCT)—add sour cream, whipped cream, butter, margarine, or oils to casseroles, desserts, or other foods. To use MCT—add to salad dressings, fruit juice, casseroles, and sandwich spreads.
- ✓ Pseudo ice cream may be made with frozen, flavored whipped cream.

For More Information

- American Epilepsy Society
  860-586-7505
  http://aesnet.org
- Epilepsy Foundation
  1-800-332-1000
  http://www.EpilepsyFoundation.org
- Citizens United for Research in Epilepsy (CURE)
  630-734-9957
  http://www.CUREepilepsy.org

GUILLAIN-BARRÉ SYNDROME

NUTRITIONAL ACUITY RANKING: LEVEL 3

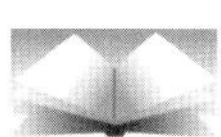

DEFINITIONS AND BACKGROUND

Guillain-Barré syndrome (GBS), also known as acute postinfectious polyneuritis, is a neurological syndrome of increasing weakness, numbness, pain, and paralysis, often after recent surgery, a viral infection (*Campylobacter jejuni* from undercooked meat, poultry, or contaminated milk), or immunization. Bloody diarrhea, fever, cramping, and headache occur with *C. jejuni*.

Symptoms and signs include muscular weakness of lower extremities progressing to arms, trunk, face, and head, respiratory failure, paralysis of lower extremities or quadriplegia, unstable blood pressure, aspiration, dysphagia, difficulty in chewing, impaired speech, muscular pain, low-grade fever, tachycardia, weight loss, anorexia, urinary tract infections (UTIs), or personality changes. Patients with GBS develop ileus rarely.

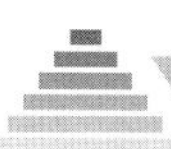

OBJECTIVES

- Prevent or correct weight loss and resulting malnutrition.
- Adjust diet for chewing and swallowing problems.
- Meet added calorie requirements from any fever.
- Wean, as possible, from ventilator dependency.
- Improve neurological functioning and overall prognosis.

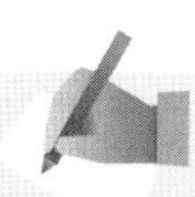

DIETARY AND NUTRITIONAL RECOMMENDATIONS

- Acute: Intravenous fluids will be required. Tube feeding or TPN may be necessary while patient is acutely ill over a period of time. Increased calories and protein may be necessary. Alter fat intake as appropriate to reduce production of carbon dioxide, especially on ventilator.
- Progression: When tolerated, the individual can use a soft or general diet. For some, a thick, pureed diet may be beneficial with dysphagia.
- Supplement oral intake with frequent snacks such as shakes or eggnogs.
- A vitamin–mineral supplement may be beneficial, if intake has been poor.

Common Drugs Used and Potential Side Effects

- Antibiotics may be needed if UTIs or other problems are identified.
- Autoimmune globulin may be given.
- Analgesics are used to reduce pain and inflammation.
- Steroids are seldom used except for chronic relapsing polyneuropathy; their effects can be deleterious over time.
- Vasopressors may be used.

Herbs, Botanicals and Supplements

- Vitamin B6 is the vitamin associated with neuronal function. High doses of pyridoxine should not be taken with phenobarbital or phenytoin, where seizure control might be compromised. If B6 is added to either drug regimen, keep it at the lowest effective dose and monitor serum drug levels.
- St. John's wort is used as a natural antidepressant. Do not use with MAOI antidepressants, SSRI antidepressants, cyclosporine, digoxin, oral contraceptives, HIV protease inhibitors, theophylline, warfarin, or calcium channel blockers such as amlodipine or diltiazem or verapamil. No studies have been conducted for efficacy in Guillain-Barré syndrome.

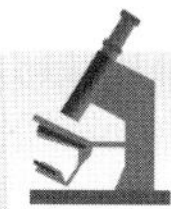

PROFILE

Clinical/History

Height
Weight
Weight changes
BMI
BP
Temperature
Dysphagia
Vomiting
Diarrhea

Lab Work

Complete blood count (CBC)
H&H
Serum Fe
Alb
pO2
pCO2
CSF protein levels
Gluc

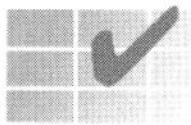

PATIENT EDUCATION

- Encourage self-feeding, if possible.
- Maintain adequacy of calorie and protein intake to improve weight status and nutritional health.
- Avoid upper respiratory infections and exposure to other illnesses.
- Arrange for special feeding utensils, if needed by the individual.
- Avoid constipation through use of fruits, vegetables, crushed bran, prune juice, and adequate fluid intake.

For More Information

- National Chronic Care Organization
  952-814-2652
  http://www.nccconline.org
- National Organization for Rare Disorders (NORD)
  1-800-999-6673
  http://www.rarediseases.org

HUNTINGTON'S DISEASE

NUTRITIONAL ACUITY RANKING: LEVEL 3

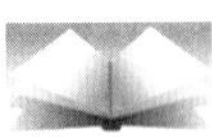

DEFINITIONS AND BACKGROUND

Huntington's disease (HD) is a genetic, autosomal dominant, neurodegenerative disorder for which there is no known cure (Sullivan et al., 2001). There is a defective gene on chromosome 4. HD develops in middle-to-late life with involuntary, spasmodic, irregular movements (chorea) and cerebral degeneration. Cognitive decline and speech difficulties occur. HD differs from AD in that there is loss of control of voluntary movements.

Behavioral changes begin 10 years before movement disorder, which often begins at ages 35–40. Remotivation therapy may be beneficial; it leads to increased self-awareness, self-esteem, and an improved quality of life, even in late-stage HD (Sullivan et al., 2001). Duration of HD is generally 13–15 years before death, which often results from pneumonia or a fatal fall.

OBJECTIVES

- Promote normal nutritional status, despite tissue degeneration.
- Encourage the patient to self-feed until this is no longer possible.
- Improve brain levels of dopamine and acetylcholine, which tend to be low.
- Avoid aspiration of solids and liquids.

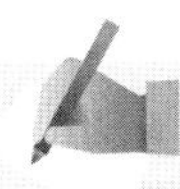

DIETARY AND NUTRITIONAL RECOMMENDATIONS

- Provide a high-calorie, high-protein diet: Usually 1.2–1.5 g/kg protein is recommended.
- Use a thick, pureed or chopped diet as appropriate. Tube feed when necessary; bolus feedings are usually tolerated.
- Feed slowly to prevent choking. Small, frequent meals are suggested.
- Provide adequate fiber (e.g., prune juice) for normal elimination.
- Supplement with a multivitamin/mineral supplement if needed.

Common Drugs Used and Potential Side Effects

- Anti-inflammatory drugs such as ibuprofen may be useful.
- Supplemental vitamin E and antioxidants may be suggested.
- Minocycline may slow the disease process. It blocks capases from entering the brain.
- Riluzole has been used with some success and few side effects. It is a membrane stabilizer, a glutamate-release inhibitor.

Herbs, Botanicals and Supplements

- Vitamin B6 is the vitamin associated with neuronal function. High doses of pyridoxine should not be taken with phenobarbital or phenytoin, where seizure control might be compromised. If B6 is added to either drug regimen, keep it at the lowest effective dose and monitor serum drug levels.
- St. John's wort is used as a natural antidepressant. Do not use with MAOI antidepressants, SSRI antidepressants, cyclosporine, digoxin, oral contraceptives, HIV protease inhibitors, theophylline, warfarin, or calcium channel blockers such as amlodipine or diltiazem or verapamil. No studies have been conducted for efficacy in seizure patients.

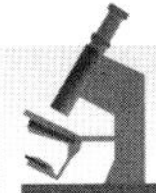

PROFILE

Clinical/History

Height
Weight
BMI
Weight changes
Ability to self-feed
Chewing or swallowing difficulties
I & O

Lab Work

BUN/Creat
Serum glucose
H&H
Acetylcholine levels
Dopamine levels
Alb, prealbumin
CT scan for changes in the brain

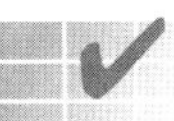

PATIENT EDUCATION

- Semisolid foods may be easier to swallow than thin liquids.
- Provide genetic counseling—each child of an affected parent has a 50% chance of inheriting the disease.
- Teach family or caretakers about the Heimlich maneuver.
- Adding protein and kcal through supplements or nutritionally dense foods may be essential.

For More Information

- Huntington's Disease Society of America http://www.hdsa.org/

MULTIPLE SCLEROSIS

NUTRITIONAL ACUITY RANKING: LEVEL 2

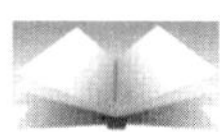

DEFINITIONS AND BACKGROUND

Multiple sclerosis (MS) involves scarring and the loss of myelin sheath, the insulating material around nerve fibers. The disease causes progressive or episodic nerve degeneration and disability. The cause is not known, but possibly a virus or some unknown antigen that triggers an autoimmune response early in life may be responsible. There is circumstantial evidence implicating proinflammatory cytokines such as tumor necrosis factor-alpha (TNFalpha) in the pathogenesis of multiple sclerosis (Mikova et al., 2001).

Onset is usually between 20 and 40 years of age (average age, 27-years-old); women have MS more often than men (ratio of women to men = 3:2). MS has a much higher incidence among Caucasians than in any other race; white females living in colder, wetter areas are more susceptible than those living in warmer areas (Johnson, 2000). One study proposed a hypothesis linking geographic latitude with mortality from MS (Esparza et al., 1995). Heredity also seems to play a role.

The Nurses' Health Study found no differences between intake of specific types of fat and risk for MS, although this had been proposed in the past (Zhang et al., 2000). Proinflammatory cytokines, pathological iron deposition, and oxidative stress have been implicated in the pathogenesis of MS (Mehindate et al., 2001). Antioxidants may play a role; it is speculated that supplementation with magnesium, vitamin B6, vitamin B12, zinc, vitamin D, vitamin E, selenium, and omega-3 fatty acids may help to prevent MS (Johnson, 2000).

Symptoms and signs include tingling, numbness in arms, legs, trunk, or face, double vision, fatigue, weakness, clumsiness, tremor, stiffness, sensory impairment, loss of position sense, and respiratory problems. Dysphagia is common in MS patients but is not a major complaint and does not cause nutritional failure of these patients (Thomas and Wiles, 1999). Spasticity and bladder dysfunction are also common (Klewer et al., 2001). After diagnosis, 70% of persons with MS are as active as previously. The courses of MS are shown in Table 4–6.

TABLE 4–6 Courses of Multiple Sclerosis

Benign—few, mild early exacerbations with normal life expectancy and minimal disability (20% of cases)

Exacerbating/remitting—more frequent early attacks with less complete clearing; long periods of stability, some disability (25% of cases)

Chronic/relapsing—fewer and less complete remissions after attacks; greater disability that may plateau after many years (20% will be ambulatory, 20% will be nonambulatory)

Chronic/progressive—onset is more insidious and more slowly progressive than chronic/relapsing (15% of cases)

OBJECTIVES

- During the active phase of the disease, corticosteroids are used to decrease symptoms. Alter diet accordingly.
- During the chronic phase of the disease, treatment centers on reducing the incidence of respiratory infections and UTIs, managing bowel problems, controlling muscle spasms, preventing contractures and pressure ulcers, and correcting constipation and fecal impactions.
- Adjust caloric intake to avoid excessive weight gain, if this becomes a problem.
- Maintain good nutritional status.
- Reduce fatigue associated with mealtimes.

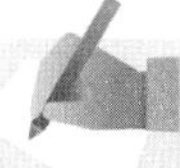

DIETARY AND NUTRITIONAL RECOMMENDATIONS

- No special diet is necessary, although some persons suggest use of a low-fat diet (less than 30 g), with 10 g of saturated fats, normal protein levels, and adequate carbohydrates to complete caloric needs. Use olive oil and ω-3 fatty acids more frequently in the diet.
- As swallowing difficulties increase and coordination decreases, foods may need to be liquefied or provided by tube feeding.
- Laxative foods and liquids may ease constipation.
- Reduce sodium intake during use of steroid therapy. Otherwise, sodium plays a role in lipid/protein transport in myelin tissues.
- Provide adequate intake of vitamin C and multivitamins, especially B complex. Vitamin E may also prove to be useful.
- Small, frequent meals may be better tolerated than large meals.
- To prevent UTIs, 10 oz of cranberry juice daily (low calorie if needed) may be useful (Avorn et al., 1994).

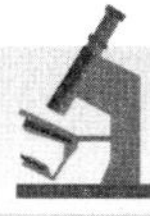

PROFILE

Clinical/History	Lab Work	
Height	Alb	Evoked potentials test
Weight	Chol	CSF (WBC, g-globulin are increased)
BMI	K+	Serum Fe
BP	Trig	EEG
I & O	H&H	L:S ratio
Edema	Gluc	
Temperature	MRI scan	

Common Drugs Used and Potential Side Effects

- Interferon injections are the latest treatment. Beta 1a-interferon (Avonex) may cause nausea, diarrhea, flu-like symptoms, headache, infections, or anemia. Beta 1b-interferon (Betaseron) may cause weight changes, abdominal pain, diarrhea, constipation, fever, headache, hypertension, or tachycardia.
- Corticosteroids require controlled sodium intake while these drugs are being used. Glucose intolerance, negative nitrogen balance, and decreased serum zinc, calcium, and potassium may occur.
- Antispasticity drugs such as baclofen (Lioresal) may cause nausea, diarrhea, and constipation.
- Muscle relaxants may be used.
- Newer drugs such as Avonex, Betaseron, and Copaxone are intended to work by causing the body to attack the drug instead of the myelin. Precise actions are not yet known. Side effects may include chest tightness.

Herbs, Botanicals and Supplements

- Vitamin B6 is the vitamin associated with neuronal function. High doses of pyridoxine should not be taken with phenobarbital or phenytoin, where seizure control might be compromised. If B6 is added to either drug regimen, keep it at the lowest effective dose and monitor serum drug levels.
- St. John's wort is used as a natural antidepressant. Do not use with MAOI antidepressants, SSRI antidepressants, cyclosporine, digoxin, oral contraceptives, HIV protease inhibitors, theophylline, warfarin, or calcium channel blockers such as amlodipine or diltiazem or verapamil. No studies have been conducted for efficacy in MS patients.
- Stinging nettle, blueberry, pineapple, black currant, evening primrose, and purslane have been recommended, but no clinical trials have proven efficacy.

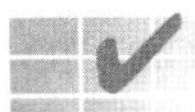

PATIENT EDUCATION

- ✔ Teach the patient how to control caloric intake.
- ✔ Teach the patient about sources of linoleic acid and v-3 fatty acids in the diet.
- ✔ Describe the role of fat and vitamin E in myelin sheath formation and maintenance.
- ✔ Teach the patient about foods high in fiber.
- ✔ Avoid total inactivity.
- ✔ Utensils with large handles may be useful in food preparation and self-feeding.
- ✔ At a restaurant, foods may need to be cut before serving.
- ✔ Use tabletop cooking methods and equipment to avoid lifting.
- ✔ Past trials of diets such as allergen-free, gluten-free, pectin-free, fructose-restricted, raw foods, Cambridge liquid diets, and specific vitamin or mineral therapies have been ineffective (Wozniak-Wowk, 1993).

For More Information

- Consortium of Multiple Sclerosis Centers
  1-877-700-CMSC
  http://www.mscare.org
- Multiple Sclerosis Association of America
  1-800-532-7667
  http://www.msaa.com
- National Multiple Sclerosis Society
  733 3rd Ave.
  New York, NY 10017
  1-800-Fight-MS
  http://www.nmss.org/

MYASTHENIA GRAVIS

NUTRITIONAL ACUITY RANKING: LEVEL 3

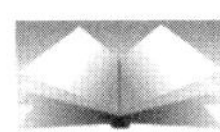

DEFINITIONS AND BACKGROUND

Myasthenia gravis (MG) is an autoimmune disease resulting from the production of antibodies against the acetylcholine (ACh) receptors of the neuromuscular synapse (Baraka, 2001). The thymus gland is involved in the autosensitization process, and the disease frequently is associated with thymic morphologic abnormalities. Etiology is not known, but there is a genetic predisposition.

Symptoms and signs include drooping eyelids, double vision, fatigue, general weakness, dysphagia, weak voice, inability to walk on heels, and pneumonia. MG occurs in 50–125 in 1,000,000 individuals (approximately 25,000 affected people in the United States). One peak occurs in women ages 20–40; a second peak occurs in men between 60 and 80 years of age (Drachman, 1994). Plasmapheresis can be used during a crisis to remove the abnormal antibodies.

A myasthenic crisis is defined as the need for mechanical ventilatory support; approximately 16% of all patients experience a crisis with progressive weakness, oropharyngeal symptoms, refractoriness to anticholinesterase medication, intercurrent infection, and invasive procedures including needle biopsies of thymic gland masses (Young and Raksadawan, 2001).

There is consensus that removal of the thymus gland is imperative in MG. An early, safe, and complete thymectomy offers benefits to a patient with MG with minimal risk for morbidity and postoperative pain (Meyers and Cooper, 2001).

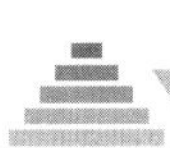

OBJECTIVES

- Increase the likelihood of obtaining adequate nutrition by altering the consistency of foods. This is necessary when muscles used in chewing and swallowing are weakened.
- Feedings should be small to reduce fatigue.
- Prevent permanent structural damage to the neuromuscular system.
- Allow adequate time to complete meals.

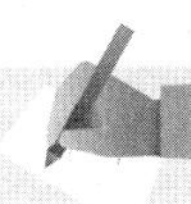

DIETARY AND NUTRITIONAL RECOMMENDATIONS

- Diet should include frequent, small feedings of easily masticated foods.
- Provide tube feeding when needed.
- Provide adequate potassium supplements.
- If corticosteroids are part of treatment, use a low-sodium diet.
- Use a high-protein/high-carbohydrate diet.
- The use of lecithin and choline has been successful in some cases but has not been documented consistently.
- Avoid giving medications with coffee or fruit juice; give with milk and crackers or bread.

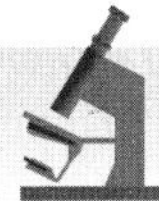

PROFILE

Clinical/History

Height
Weight
BMI
I & O
Edrophonium test–drug injected by IV (temporarily improves muscle strength)
Weight changes

Lab Work

K+
Alb
H&H
CT scan of the chest for thymoma
Tensilon test
BP
Acetylcholine antibodies test
Electromyogram
Gluc
Mg++, Ca++

Common Drugs Used and Potential Side Effects

- Short-acting anticholinesterase compounds (neostigmine [Prostigmin] or pyridostigmine [Mestinon]) or corticosteroids (prednisone, etc.) may require limiting sodium intake. Anorexia, abdominal cramps, diarrhea, and weakness may result from use of these drugs. They increase levels of acetylcholine. Long-acting capsules may be needed if morning weakness is persistent.
- Long-term use of antacids negatively affects calcium and magnesium metabolism.
- Azathioprine (Imuran) and cyclosporine are also used for antibody suppression in some patients. GI distress, nausea, vomiting, or anorexia may occur.

Herbs, Botanicals and Supplements

- No studies have been conducted for efficacy of herbs or botanicals in MG patients.

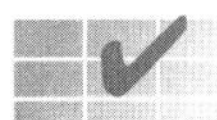

PATIENT EDUCATION

- Show the patient how to prepare foods with the use of a blender, if necessary.
- Indicate how to take medication with food or milk. Discuss potential side effects.
- Avoidance of alcohol is important.
- Food and utensils should be arranged within reach of the patient.

For More Information

- Myasthenia Gravis Foundation
  222 S Riverside Plaza, Suite 1540
  Chicago, IL 60606
  1-800-541-5454
  http://www.med.unc.edu.mgfa

NEUROLOGICAL TRAUMA (SPINAL CORD INJURY)

NUTRITIONAL ACUITY RANKING: LEVEL 3

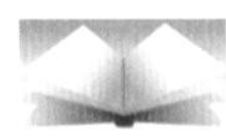

DEFINITIONS AND BACKGROUND

Spinal cord injury (SCI) is often caused by traffic accidents, falls, diving accidents, sports injury, or gunshot wounds. Partial versus total self-care deficits depend on resulting hemiplegia, diplegia, paraplegia (thoracic or lumbar cord), or quadriplegia (cervical cord). Classification usually includes cause, direction of injury, level of injury, stability of vertebral column, and degree of cord involvement. The nervous system of a patient with neurologic trauma is vulnerable to glucose and oxygen variations, and variations in other nutrients. Osteoporosis and risk of fracture increases in this population (Lazo et al., 2001).

OBJECTIVES

- Control acid-base and electrolyte balances. Assess needs on admission and then daily thereafter.
- Reduce the danger of aspiration by avoiding oral feedings if patient has been vomiting.
- Ensure adequate fluid intake to prevent urinary calculi.
- Increase opportunities for rehabilitation by monitoring weight changes. Weight loss of 10–30% in the first month is common.
- Prevent UTIs, paralytic ileus, pneumonia, malnutrition, pressure ulcer, constipation, stress ulcer, and fecal impaction.
- Long term: Mobilize, prevent complications, and regain independence as far as possible. Monitor for weight gain since excessive weight gain can lead to pressure ulcers and make transfers more difficult for oneself and family; maintain an ideal body weight.

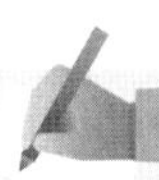

DIETARY AND NUTRITIONAL RECOMMENDATIONS

- Provide patient with intravenous solutions as soon as possible after injury. Check blood gas measurements and chemistries. Once peristalsis returns, patient may be tube fed. Elevate head of bed 30–45°, if possible, to prevent aspiration.
- Ensure adequate intake of thiamine, niacin, vitamin B6, and amino acids. Monitor iron stores and adjust diet as needed.
- Paraplegics initially need 1.5–1.7 g protein/kg. Progression to more normal intake, such as 1.2–1.5 g/kg, can occur when nitrogen balance returns.
- Monitor weight: Male paraplegics should be 10–15% below ideal body weight (IBW); male quadriplegics should be 15–20 lb below IBW. Calculations for women are equivalent. Ensure adequate CHO and fat intake, including 1–2% essential fatty acids (EFA).
- Encourage adequate fluid and fiber. Be careful about gas-forming foods; monitor tolerance.
- Provide adequate vitamin D and calcium intake to prevent osteoporosis.

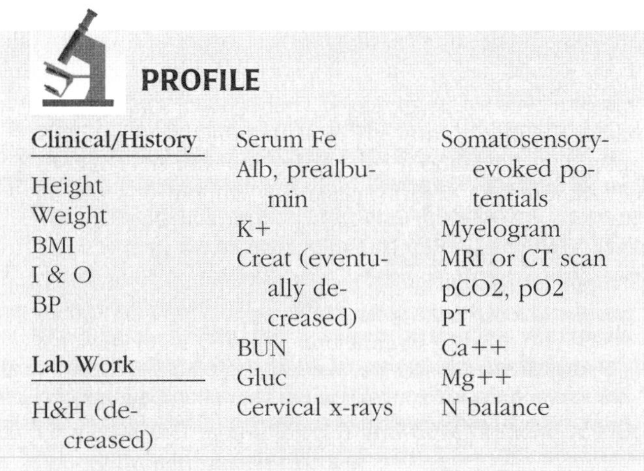

PROFILE

Clinical/History		
Height	Serum Fe	Somatosensory-evoked potentials
Weight	Alb, prealbumin	Myelogram
BMI	K+	MRI or CT scan
I & O	Creat (eventually decreased)	pCO2, pO2
BP	BUN	PT
Lab Work	Gluc	Ca++
H&H (decreased)	Cervical x-rays	Mg++
		N balance

Common Drugs Used and Potential Side Effects

- Corticosteroids such as prednisone are used to prevent swelling. Long-term use can cause hyperglycemia and nitrogen, calcium, and potassium losses. Sodium retention occurs.
- Analgesics for pain relief (e.g., aspirin/salicylates) can prolong bleeding time. GI bleeding may eventually result. An increased intake of vitamin C and folacin is needed.
- Laxatives may be used; encourage fiber and fluid instead.

Herbs, Botanicals and Supplements

- No studies have been conducted for efficacy of herbs or botanicals in SCI patients.

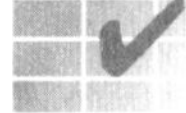

PATIENT EDUCATION

- Provide weight-control measures for rehabilitation.
- Teach patient about good sources of iron in the diet, as well as vitamins and protein.
- Help promote a structured feeding routine. Feed slowly (over 30–45 minutes). Bites of food should be small.
- Use of seat belts should be promoted to prevent future vehicular injury.
- Discuss long-term risks of heart disease.

For More Information

- Christopher Reeve Paralysis Foundation
  500 Morris Ave.
  Springfield, NJ 07081
  1-800-225-0292
  http://www.apacure.com/
- Foundation for Spinal Cord Injury Prevention, Care, & Cure
  1-800-342-0330
  http://www.fscip.org/
- National Spinal Cord Injury Association
  8701 Georgia Ave., Suite 500
  Silver Spring, MD 20910
  301-588-6959
  http://www.spinalcord.org/
- Paralysis Society of America
  801 18th St., NW
  Washington, DC 20006-3517
  202-973-8420
  1-888-772-1711
  http://www.psa.org/
- Paralyzed Veterans of America
  1-800-424-8200
  http://www.pva.org
- Spinal Cord Injury Education and Training Foundation
  801 Elizabeth Street, NW
  Washington, DC 20006-3517
  1-800-424-8200 x655
  http://www.frontpage.pva.inter.net/prof/etfgd/index.htm
- Spinal Cord Injury Information Network
  http://www.spinalcord.uab.edu/

PARKINSON'S DISEASE

NUTRITIONAL ACUITY RANKING: LEVEL 2

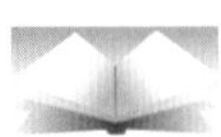

DEFINITIONS AND BACKGROUND

Parkinson's disease (PD) is a neuromuscular disorder resulting from diminished levels of dopamine at the basal ganglia of the brain that causes tremor, rigidity, abnormal gait, and difficulty in chewing, speaking, or swallowing. L-dopa must be provided. Men are affected slightly more often than women. The disease is more common after 60 years of age, and life expectancy is 12.5 years after diagnosis. Causes are not known, and pathophysiology is poorly understood (Calne, 1993). Epidemiological studies suggest that there is significant variation in the prevalence of PD between different populations, and rates are highest in populations of European origin (Muthane et al., 2001). Approximately 1–1.5 million people are affected.

Altered brain energy metabolism occurs. An association between PD and high intakes of total fat, saturated fat, cholesterol, lutein, and iron has been found (Johnson et al., 1999). Studies indicate that drinking 4–5 cups of coffee daily may be preventive; further studies are needed (Benedetti, 2000; Honig, 2000; Ross et al., 2000).

PD is a progressive neurologic disorder for which no long-term effective treatment strategies are available. Toxic elements have not been identified, but long-term exposure to manganese, Demerol, and some herbicides or pesticides may be related. Sometimes, use of medications such as major tranquilizers or Reglan can cause Parkinson-like symptoms; when doctors place the patient on Parkinson medications, further adverse effects accrue and health declines further. Cessation of those medications is warranted.

Oxidative stress could initiate or promote degeneration of neurons; antioxidant therapy may reduce the rate of progression of the disease, although this is not proven (Prasad, 1999). Neuroprotection is being studied as a means of combating PD. Results have not been verified for use of vitamin E or other specific antioxidants.

Approximately 24 conditions are categorized as Parkinson's disorders. A test for PD progression includes decline in ability to smell, depression, and speed of wrist movements. About 30% of those with PD get dementia-related symptoms (Rodriguez and Arenas, 2001).

Unintentional weight loss is a common occurrence, resulting in increased risk for morbidity and mortality. Esophageal motor abnormalities are frequent in PD and may appear at an early stage of the disease (Bassotti et al., 1998). Patients with PD are four times more likely to report weight loss greater than 10 lb (Beyer et al., 1995). Causes of weight loss include increased energy expenditure due to tremor, dyskinesias, and rigidity; reduced energy intake due to olfactory dysfunction, cognitive impairment, depression, dysphagia, disability; and medication-related side effects, including dry mouth, nausea/vomiting, appetite loss, anorexia, insomnia, fatigue, and anxiety (Holden, 2000; McIntosh and Holden, 1999). There are various treatments and algorithms for management of PD (Olanow et al., 2001).

OBJECTIVES

- Supply dopamine to the brain with drugs. Monitor diet therapy accordingly.
- Maintain optimal physical and emotional health.
- Improve the patient's ability to eat. Use semisolid foods rather than fluids if sucking/swallowing reflexes are reduced. Drooling may also be a problem. (See CVA entry regarding dysphagia.)
- Provide adequate calories to prevent weight loss; obesity should be avoided as well.
- Provide adequate hydration.
- Correct alterations in GI function (i.e., increased transit time, heartburn, and constipation).
- Preserve functioning; prevent disability as long as possible.

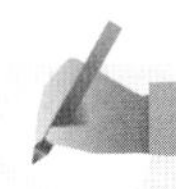

DIETARY AND NUTRITIONAL RECOMMENDATIONS

- A high intake of protein diminishes the effectiveness of levodopa; use 0.5 g/kg body weight. If unplanned weight loss is a problem, 1–1.5 g/kg may be needed. For some, a protein redistribution diet is used (i.e., low protein at breakfast and lunch, high-protein dinner and snack) but is not always effective.
- Broad beans and other legumes may be useful in reducing fluctuations of levodopa in response to protein (Lieberman et al., 1994).
- In the rare use of levodopa alone, vitamin B6 foods should be consumed: dry skim milk, peas and beans, sweet potatoes, yams, avocado, fortified cereal, bran, oatmeal, wheat germ, yeast, pork, beef organs, tuna, and fresh salmon.
- Query patient about choking. Order a swallow evaluation from a speech therapist; determine proper consistency of foods and plan diet accordingly. Cut, mince, or soften foods as required. Use small meals if needed.
- Add crushed bran to hot cereal for fiber; prune juice may be needed.

Common Drugs Used and Potential Side Effects

- Anticholinergics: Cogentin (benztropine), Artane (trihexyphenidyl), Kemadrin (procyclidine)—possible adverse effects include confusion, agitation, dizziness, sedation, euphoria, tachycardia, hypotension, dry mouth, constipation, nausea, urinary retention, and blurred vision.
- MAO-B inhibitor: Eldepryl (selegiline)—possible adverse effects include insomnia, dry mouth, confusion, hypertension, abdominal pain, and weight loss. Selegi-

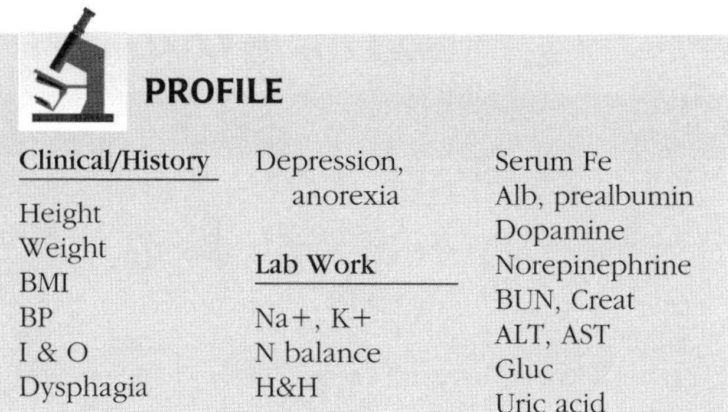

PROFILE

Clinical/History		
Height	Depression, anorexia	Serum Fe
Weight		Alb, prealbumin
BMI	**Lab Work**	Dopamine
BP	Na+, K+	Norepinephrine
I & O	N balance	BUN, Creat
Dysphagia	H&H	ALT, AST
		Gluc
		Uric acid

line should not be used with ginseng, ma huang (ephedra,) yohimbe, or St. John's wort.

- Dopamine agonists: Permax (pergolide), Parlodel (bromocriptine), Mirapex (pramipexole), Requip (ropinirole)—possible adverse effects include nausea, headache, fatigue, confusion, hallucinations, somnolence, and "sleep attacks." With Requip, fewer side effects such as dyskinesia have been identified.
- Levodopa/carbidopa: Sinemet, Sinemet CR, Atamet, Madopar—possible adverse effects include nausea, dyskinesia, weakness, hallucinations, mental confusion, orthostatic hypotension, fatigue, daytime sleepiness, insomnia, elevated serum glucose, homocysteine, and lower Hgb and Hct. The large neutral amino acids block levodopa absorption, both from the gut and at the blood-brain barrier. Levodopa preparations should be taken 30–60 minutes prior to meals, and intake of vitamin B6 should be limited to RDA levels. Today's preparations combine levodopa with carbidopa or benserazide, which prevent peripheral decarboxylation of levodopa. Up to 15 mg of B6 can be taken daily in either food or supplement form. Increase intake of B12, folate (Yasui et al., 2000) and vitamin C-rich foods.
- Tricyclic antidepressants may be ordered for depression. Weight gain, dry mouth, or nausea can result.
- Catechol-O-methyltransferase inhibitors: Tasmar (tolcapone), Comtan (entacapone)—possible adverse effects include diarrhea, orthostatic hypotension, hallucinations, sleep disturbances, dyskinesias, muscle cramping, and vivid dreams.
- Antiviral agent: Symmetrel (amantadine)—possible adverse effects include anorexia, dry mouth, nausea, constipation, dizziness, insomnia, blurred vision, depression, ataxia, confusion, fatigue, leg/ankle edema, hallucinations, anxiety, and livedo reticularis (skin discoloration).

Herbs, Botanicals and Supplements

- No studies have been conducted for efficacy of herbs or botanicals in PD patients; fava bean, evening primrose, St. John's wort, passionflower, velvet bean, and gingko have been suggested but not proven.
- Kava should not be taken in patients with PD, because it decreases effectiveness.
- Ginseng, ma huang (ephedra), yohimbe, and St. John's wort should not be used with MAO-inhibitors, including selegiline (Eldepryl).

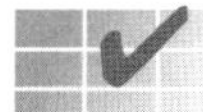

PATIENT EDUCATION

- ✔ Explain how to blenderize food.
- ✔ Help patient to control weight, which may fluctuate from reduced mobility or inability to ingest sufficient quantities.
- ✔ Place all foods within easy reach of the patient.
- ✔ Braces may help the patient control severe tremors at mealtime.
- ✔ Music therapy helps to relieve depression and improves balance.

For More Information

- ✦ American Parkinson's Disease Association
  718-981-8001
  http://www.apdaparkinson.com/
- ✦ Michael J. Fox Foundation for Parkinson's Research
  1-800-780-7644
  http://www.MichaelJFox.org/
- ✦ National Parkinson's Foundation
  1-800-327-4545
  http://www.parkinson.org/
- ✦ Parkinson's Disease Foundation, Inc.
  1-800-457-6676
  http://www.pdf.org/
- ✦ Parkinson's Web
  http://pdweb.mgh.harvard.edu
- ✦ Massachusetts General Hospital – PD Support
  http://neurosurgery.mgh.harvard.edu/pd-suprt.htm
- ✦ Parkinson's Disease: Guidelines for MNT
  http://www.nutritionucanlivewith.com/

TARDIVE DYSKINESIA

NUTRITIONAL ACUITY RANKING: LEVEL 1

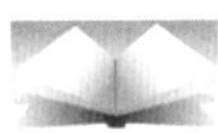

DEFINITIONS AND BACKGROUND

Tardive dyskinesia (TD) is a condition that imitates other neurologic disorders and is caused by long-term use of antipsychotic drugs. Signs and symptoms include abnormal, involuntary movements (e.g., chorea, athetosis, dystonia, tics, and facial grimacing). Tongue, face, neck, lung muscles, and extremities are usually involved. TD occurs in 20–40% of all patients receiving long-term antipsychotic drugs. Patients are often elderly and chronically institutionalized (often brain damaged), who have had extended use of such drugs as reserpine, chlorpromazine (Thorazine), thioridazine (Mellaril), haloperidol (Haldol), thiothixene (Navane), lidone, fluphenazine (Prolixin), and trifluoperazine (Stelazine).

In some cases, an acetylcholine deficiency is speculated, and brain dopamine receptors may become supersensitive with chronic use of neuroleptic drugs. Neurotoxic damage from formation of free radicals is another theory. Vitamin E treatments have been found to benefit a subgroup of patients (Boomershint et al., 1999).

OBJECTIVES

- ▲ Prevent or correct malnutrition, weight loss, and other problems.
- ▲ Identify and assist with feeding problems. Some patients have problems with sucking and puckering of the lips and difficulty in eating.
- ▲ Restore eating capacity as far as possible.
- ▲ Alter textures as necessary (eating problems are rare or occur late in the condition).
- ▲ Prevent stress, which aggravates supersensitivity psychoses.
- ▲ Free radicals may be involved in the pathogenesis of TD, and vitamin E may be effective in its treatment (Elkashef and Wyatt, 1999).

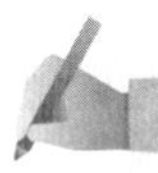

DIETARY AND NUTRITIONAL RECOMMENDATIONS

- Offer the usual diet with soft textures to reduce chewing as needed.
- Decrease calories if obese; increase if underweight.
- Decrease caffeine intake because of the effects of drug therapy.
- Carbohydrate craving is common from drugs that block histamine receptors; watch overall intake of sweets or offer nutrient-dense varieties.
- Increase dietary choline from foods such as eggs, soybeans, peanuts, and liver.
- Moisten foods with gravy, sauces, and liquids if dry mouth is a problem.
- Alter fiber intake if needed to prevent or correct constipation.
- Ensure adequate intake of antioxidants, including vitamin E.

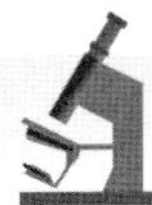

PROFILE

Clinical/History	Lab Work	
Height	BUN, Creat	(often increased)
Weight	H&H, serum Fe	Acetylcholine levels
BMI	Serum folate	Gluc
BP	Serum prolactin	Alb, prealbumin

Common Drugs Used and Potential Side Effects

- Drug therapy usually includes the same medications as normal; otherwise, withdrawal symptoms may be exacerbated with a greater effect on overall signs and symptoms of TD.
- Vitamin E therapy may be indicated: 1,200–1,600 international units (IU) have been used in some cases (Adler et al., 1993).

Herbs, Botanicals and Supplements

- No studies have been conducted for efficacy of herbs or botanicals in TD.

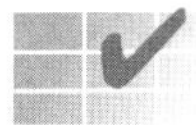

PATIENT EDUCATION

- ✓ Diet instructions should be offered directly to the patient unless this is not possible.
- ✓ Discuss major issues related to nutrition, self-feeding practices, moistening of foods, etc.
- ✓ Discuss food sources of vitamin E and foods that contain antioxidants.

For More Information

- American Psychiatric Association
  1400 K St., NW
  Washington, DC 20005
  1-888-357-7924
  http://www.psych.org/

TRAUMATIC BRAIN INJURY

NUTRITIONAL ACUITY RANKING: LEVEL 4 (NOT RANKED BY CONSENSUS)

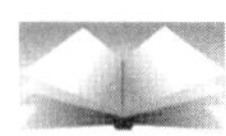

DEFINITIONS AND BACKGROUND

Traumatic brain injury (TBI) results from head injury after motor vehicle or industrial accidents, falls, fights, explosions, and gunshot wounds (with 40% involving alcohol use). Any sudden impact or blow to the head (with or without unconsciousness) may cause a TBI. Two-thirds of patients with TBI die before reaching a hospital. TBI is not used for persons who are born with a brain injury or for injuries that happen during the birth process.

Immediate signs of concussion (seen within seconds or minutes) include any loss of consciousness, impaired attention, vacant stare, delayed responses, inability to focus, slurred or incoherent speech, lack of coordination, disorientation, unusual emotional reactions, and memory problems. Later signs of concussion (hours, days, or even weeks after head injury) include persistent headache, dizziness with vertigo, poor attention or concentration, memory problems, nausea or vomiting, easy fatigue, irritability, intolerance for bright lights or loud noises, anxiety or depression, and disturbed sleep.

A TBI is classified by location, effect, and severity. Hypothalamic lesions can aggravate hyperphagia. Lateral lesions can aggravate aphasia and cachexia. Frontal lobe damage may result in loss of voluntary motor control and expressive aphasia. Occipital lobe damage may impair vision. Temporal lobe damage could result in receptive aphasia and hearing impairments.

TBI patients may exhibit dyspnea, vertigo, altered consciousness, seizures, vomiting, altered blood pressure, weakness or paralysis, aphasia, problems with physical control of hands, head, or neck with resulting difficulty in self-feeding. A TBI can change how a student learns in school, how a person acts, and how thinking and reasoning occur. There are often problems understanding words, learning and remembering things, paying attention, solving problems, thinking abstractly, talking, behaving, walking, seeing, or hearing. Headache, some irritability, and altered thought processes are a general outcome. Longitudinal psychological test results are used to explore the complex relationship between length of coma, time of testing on the recovery curve, and corresponding cognitive status after a TBI (Wong et al., 2001).

Severe head injuries tend to be associated with hypermetabolism and hypercatabolism with negative nitrogen balances. With severe head injuries (Glasgow Coma Scale < 8), there is an increased tendency for gastric feeding to regurgitate into the upper airway; keeping the patient upright and checking residuals is important in such patients. Jejunal feedings are less apt to be aspirated. If the gastrointestinal tract cannot be used to reach nutritional goals within 3 days, total parental nutrition is begun within 24–48 hours so as to reach these nutritional goals by either one or both routes by the third or fourth day (Wilson et al., 2001).

Data show that starved head-injured patients lose sufficient nitrogen to reduce weight by 15% per week (Brain Trauma Foundation, 2000). Resting energy expenditures tend to be elevated approximately 31% in mechanically ventilated patients with head trauma (Raurich and Ibanez, 1994). Patients with severe closed-head injuries receiving early versus delayed feeding show no difference in length of stay or infectious complications; severity of the head injury may be associated with infections (Minard et al., 2000).

OBJECTIVES

- Prevent life-threatening complications: aspiration pneumonia, meningitis, sepsis, UTIs, syndrome of inappropriate antidiuretic hormone (SIADH), hypertension, pressure ulcers, Curling's ulcer, and GI bleeding.
- Assess regularly the substrate needs to prevent malnutrition, cachexia, or overfeeding. Indirect calorimetry to determine the respiratory quotient and resting energy expenditure should be determined twice weekly. It has not been established that any method of feeding is better than another or that early feeding prior to 7 days improves outcome, but based on the level of nitrogen wasting and the nitrogen-sparing effect of feeding, it is a guideline that full nutritional replacement be instituted by day 7 (Brain Trauma Foundation, 2000).
- Prevent hyperglycemia by carefully regulating the glucose and insulin intake.
- Provide adequate protein for improving nitrogen balance (serum albumin tends to be low, especially if comatose, and urinary losses may be as high as twice normal). About 100–140% replacement of resting metabolism expenditure with 15–20% nitrogen calories reduces nitrogen loss (Brain Trauma Foundation, 2000).
- Monitor hydration; prevent dehydration and overhydration.
- Correct any self-feeding problems, breathing and swallowing problems, and other conditions affecting self-care.
- Prevent or reduce seizure activity, convulsions, and intracranial edema.
- Prevent cerebral edema and fluid overload with use of TPN, if necessary.
- After patient is stabilized, adapt to residual impairments.

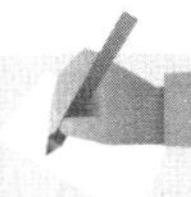

DIETARY AND NUTRITIONAL RECOMMENDATIONS

- Enteral feeding should begin as soon as the patient is hemodynamically stable, attempting to reach a nonprotein caloric intake of at least 30–35 kcal/kg on day 1 and a protein intake of 2.0–2.5 g/ kg on day 1 or as soon as possible (Wilson et al., 2001). The need for surgery or ventilation will have an effect on the ability to progress to any oral intake. Aggressive early intravenous nutrition and infusion of recombinant human insulin-like growth factor (IGF-1) may help support the normalization of T cells after head injury (Kudsk et al., 1994).

- While postpyloric feedings or TPN may be required for a long period of time, it is not always essential to use a jejunostomy feeding, if aspiration risk is carefully managed (Klodell et al., 2000).
- Patient may require 1.4–2 g protein/kg BW; 35–50 kcal/kg; and a kilocalorie:nitrogen ratio of 85–100:1 because of nitrogen losses. Monitor carefully.
- Intravenous lipids may be needed if the patient is on TPN for an extended period of time. However, tube feeding is preferable over parenteral nutrition (PN) in general.
- Patients who are immobile for a long period of time may have a 10% decrease in weight, perhaps from lowered metabolic rate. Calorie intake may need to be varied accordingly.
- Increased urinary zinc losses can occur. Otherwise, use normal RDA levels for most vitamins and minerals. Monitor K+, phosphorus, and magnesium requirements; losses are high.
- Progress, when possible, to oral intake (perhaps using a thick pureed diet with dysphagia).
- Over time, a patient may actually gain excessive weight if the brain injury affects the hypothalamus. Some patients forget that they have eaten and indicate constant hunger.

PROFILE

Clinical/History

Height
Weight
BMI
BP
Temperature
Visual field examination
Glasgow Coma Scale
Dysphagia examination
Weight changes
Intracranial pressure
I & O

Lab Work

pCO2
pO2
Alb, prealbumin
Urinary urea nitrogen (UUN) excretion (24-hour specimens 1–2 times weekly at first)
Gluc (increased with ischemia of the brain)
Serum ethanol/ethyl alcohol (ETOH) levels
CBC
Total lymphocyte count (TLC)
Transferrin
Na+, K+, Mg++
Ca++
AST (increased with brain necrosis)
BUN, Creat
CT scan
Skull x-rays
Brain scan
Cerebral angiography
EEG
Serum Phos
Alk Phos

Common Drugs Used and Potential Side Effects

- Steroids may be used to reduce swelling—these are used less frequently today.
- Analgesics are used for pain.
- Anticonvulsants may be needed to reduce seizure activity. Watch folic acid levels and other affected nutrients. Stop TF for 30–60 minutes before and after Dilantin administration.
- Albumin replacement may be needed to raise serum levels.
- Psyllium laxative (Metamucil) is often helpful in alleviating constipation. Bloating, nausea, diarrhea, or vomiting may result.
- Antacids and Pepcid may be used to reduce the onset of stress ulcers.
- Insulin may be needed if hyperglycemia occurs or persists.
- Reglan may be used as a promotility agent in tube-fed patients to assist in transit time and to decrease the risk of aspiration.

Herbs, Botanicals and Supplements

- No studies have been conducted for efficacy of herbs or botanicals in head-injured patients.
- Avoid using phenytoin (Dilantin) with evening primrose oil, gingko biloba, and kava.

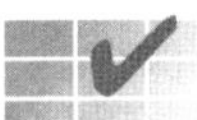

PATIENT EDUCATION

- ✓ Encourage the patient to chew and swallow slowly, if and when able to eat solids.
- ✓ Gradually relearn self-feeding techniques. Calorie counts should be completed often to evaluate intakes.
- ✓ Be wary of food temperatures, especially if patient has become less sensitized to hot and cold.
- ✓ Preparation of colorful and attractive meals is crucial to acceptance.
- ✓ The team approach is beneficial, with occupational therapists, speech therapists, psychologists, and physical therapists helping the dietitian with treatment plans.
- ✓ Use of a helmet to prevent future accidents may be suggested.
- ✓ Maintain a consistent, structured routine when possible.
- ✓ Provide written or typed instructions for review on occasion.
- ✓ Plate guards, long-handled utensils, and other adaptive feeding devices may be useful. Discuss with the occupational therapist.
- ✓ Emotional changes are common after a head injury. Family should be prepared to address changes that relate to mealtimes, eating patterns, and weight management (Hurley and Taber, 2002).

For More Information

- Brain Injury Association
  1-800-444-6443
  http://www.biausa.org
- Head Injury Awareness Foundation
  http://www.hiaf.org/
- Head Injury Hotline
  http://www.headinjury.com

TRIGEMINAL NEURALGIA

NUTRITIONAL ACUITY RANKING: LEVEL 1

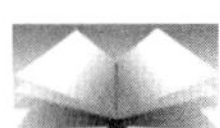

DEFINITIONS AND BACKGROUND

Trigeminal neuralgia (tic douloureux) manifests as a disorder of the fifth cranial nerve, characterized by paroxysms of excruciating pain of a burning nature. The painful periods alternate with pain-free periods. The disorder is rare before 40 years of age and is more common in elderly women. The right side of the face is affected more often; the pain can be incapacitating.

Loss of taste in patients after surgery for trigeminal neuralgia supports the existence of an accessory gustatory pathway through the trigeminal sensory root and the gasserian ganglion; Bell's palsy is the most common pathology of the peripheral gustatory pathway (Sanchez-Juan and Combarros, 2001).

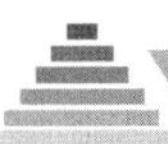

OBJECTIVES

- ▲ Control pain with medications, especially before meals.
- ▲ Provide appropriate counseling and assistance with consistency of meals (foods and beverages).
- ▲ Individualize for preferences and tolerances.
- ▲ Maintain body weight within a desirable range.
- ▲ Reduce caffeine intake.

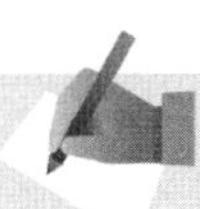

DIETARY AND NUTRITIONAL RECOMMENDATIONS

- Use a normal diet as tolerated—perhaps altering to soft or pureed foods as needed.
- Small, frequent feedings may be better tolerated than large meals.
- Liquids may be preferred if given by straw. Individualize.
- Avoid extremes in temperature.
- Use nutrient-dense foods if weight loss occurs.
- Limit caffeine to consumption of decaffeinated coffee (2–3 mg per cup).

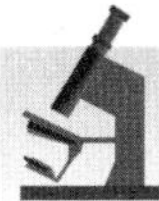

PROFILE

Clinical/History		Lab Work
Height	I & O	Alb
Weight	BP	H&H, serum Fe
BMI	Dysphagia	K+
	Temperature	BUN, Creat
	Facial pain	

Common Drugs Used and Potential Side Effects

- Carbamazepine (Tegretol) may be used as an anticonvulsant. Diarrhea, nausea, and vomiting are common.
- Phenytoin (Dilantin) may be given for seizure activity. Ensure adequate folate intake.
- Sedatives or narcotics may be used to reduce pain.
- Avoid caffeine-containing medications.
- Baclofen and antidepressants may help as well.

Herbs, Botanicals and Supplements

- No studies have been conducted for efficacy of herbs or botanicals in trigeminal neuralgia.
- With anticonvulsants such as phenytoin (Dilantin) avoid use with evening primrose oil, gingko biloba, and kava.

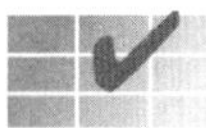

PATIENT EDUCATION

- ✔ The importance of oral and dental hygiene should be stressed, even with pain. Use pain medications as directed.
- ✔ The patient should be encouraged to avoid eating when tense or nervous.
- ✔ Relaxation therapy may be beneficial.

ANOREXIA NERVOSA

NUTRITIONAL ACUITY RANKING: LEVEL 4

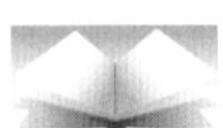

DEFINITIONS AND BACKGROUND

Anorexia nervosa (AN) is an eating disorder (ED) in which the patient severely rejects food, causing extreme weight loss, low basal metabolic rate, and exhaustion. The gene AGRP (agouti-related protein) has been linked with anorexia susceptibility in some patients (Vink et al., 2001). Insulin-like growth factor (IGF-1) represents a biochemical marker of malnutrition and a sensitive index of nutritional repletion in patients with eating disorders (Cargaro et al., 2001).

Patients with eating disorders often have dermatologic manifestations secondary to starvation; recognition of these signs can lead to early diagnosis and treatment (Glorio et al., 2000). About 6–15% of the population is affected. Two possible long-term sequelae include Cushing's disease and osteoporosis. Death occurs in extreme cases, usually from arrhythmias.

Five percent of females and 1% of males suffer from eating disorders (American Dietetic Association, 2001). AN is 10 times more common in girls, especially just after the onset of puberty, peaking at 12–13 and 19–20-years-old. Studies indicate that it also can occur at any age. Diagnosis includes signs such as the relentless pursuit of thinness, the misperception of body image, restrained eating or binge eating or purging (see Bulimia and Binge Eating entries), fear of fatness, and a codependent focus outside one's self. The intense fear of becoming fat not diminishing as weight loss progresses has no known physical cause. Weight is often 75% of former weight. There usually is amenorrhea. Length of amenorrhea, estrogen exposure (age minus age at menarche minus years of amenorrhea), and body weight have independent effects on bone densities; therefore, osteopenia is common in women with AN (Brooks et al., 1998).

Generally, cases are separated into "restricting" or "binge-purging" types. Traits include being obsessional, meticulous, compulsive, introverted, emotionally reserved, socially insecure, overly rigid in thinking, self-denying, and overly compliant. Problems most commonly found in these patients include denial, family issues, impulse control, manipulative behavior, trust issues, power issues in the family, misinformation, and other concerns (Whisenant and Smith, 1995).

Some fields promote a thin body for success (e.g., fashion, air travel, athletics, and entertainment). Up to one-third of female athletes struggle with an eating disorder (Clark, 1994). Although female athletes with subclinical eating disorders have dietary intakes of energy, protein, CHO, and certain micronutrients below RDA levels, micronutrient status is relatively unaffected, probably due to use of supplements (Beals and Manore, 1998).

Because patients deny the severity of their illness, they delay seeking psychiatric treatment (Mehler, 2001). Teens with ED often use subterfuge to give the impression that they are cooperating with treatment plans, when they in fact are not. These behaviors prolong treatment and lead to malnutrition and metabolic disturbances (Ammerman et al., 1996). Medical nutrition therapy for eating disorders is a specialization that requires training beyond entry level. All dietitians must be able to identify and refer patients with eating disorders (Whisenant and Smith, 1995). The American Dietetic Association recommends 8 medical nutrition therapy visits for adolescents or adults who have eating disorders (http://www.knowledgelinc.com/ada/mntguides/).

OBJECTIVES

- Restore normal physiologic function by correcting starvation and its associated changes, including electrolyte imbalance.
- Check growth chart and determine percentage of difference and future goals. Promote weight gain of 1–2 lb weekly to reach a weight closer to a healthy body weight (HBW).
- Promote adequate psychotherapy and use of medications to protect the heart, fluid, and electrolytes, which are the most important.
- Obtain diet history to assess bulimia, vomiting, use of diuretics, or laxatives.
- Do not force feedings. Rejection of food is part of the illness. Promote normal eating behavior.
- Gradually increase intake to a normal or high-calorie diet to reduce excessive edema.
- Reduce preoccupation with weight and food; promote adequate self-esteem.
- Nutrition education and counseling must be affiliated with the care plan.
- For young women, promote normal menstrual cycles.

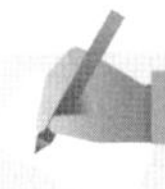

DIETARY AND NUTRITIONAL RECOMMENDATIONS

- Serve attractive, palatable meals in small amounts, observing food preferences. Small, frequent meals are useful. Encourage variety.
- Limit bulky foods during the early stages of treatment; gastrointestinal intolerance may persist for a long time.
- Diet should be called a "low-calorie diet for anorexia nervosa" to convince the patient of the counselors' good intentions. Increasing the caloric intake must be done slowly. Start at basal needs +300–400 kcal. Promote gain of 1–2 kg/week by gradually attaining intake of up to 2,500–3,000 kcals/day.
- Protein refeeding takes a long time. Repletion may not be complete until weight has returned to normal or exceeded premorbid values (Russell et al., 1994). Monitor total body nitrogen (TBN).
- While not a preferred method, use tube feeding if necessary (i.e., only if the patient weighs 40% of IBW or less).
- Have the patient measure and record food intake at first; then, gradually lessen the emphasis on food.

- Help the patient resume normal eating habits. Ensure the patient that constipation will be alleviated.
- A "no added salt" diet may reduce fluid retention.
- Avoid caffeine because of stimulant/diuretic effect.
- A vitamin–mineral supplement may be needed (zinc, etc.).

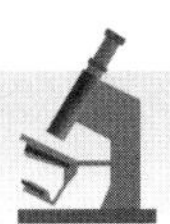

PROFILE

Clinical/History	Lab Work	
History (Hx) of bulimia	Luteinizing hormone (LH) (decreased)	Serum cortisol (high)
Laxative abuse	Follicle-stimulating hormone (FSH)	Sex-hormone binding globulin (SHBG)
Diuretic abuse	IGF-1	Alb, prealbumin
Height	Serum estrogen (low)	TBN
Present weight		Chol, Trig
Former weight		Gluc
Recent weight		H&H, serum Fe
Percentage of weight changes		thyroid-stimulating hormone (TSH)
BMI		Leukopenia
Weight goal/ timing		K+, Na+, Cl−
BP (low?)		
Amenorrhea		
Lanugo hair		
Edema		

Common Drugs Used and Potential Side Effects

- MAO inhibitors may require use of a low tyramine diet (see Depression entry).
- Other antidepressants have nutritional side effects that should be monitored carefully.

Herbs, Botanicals and Supplements

- No specific herbs and botanical products have been used for AN in clinical trials.

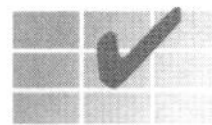

PATIENT EDUCATION

- Help the patient become an effective, independently functioning person. Convey principles rather than rigid "rules" to avoid reinforcing the patient's compulsive rituals and preoccupation with food. Positive regular habits should be encouraged. Behavioral contracting is often useful (Solanto et al., 1994).
- Encourage the patient to follow a balanced diet. Discuss weight gain, weight maintenance, and snacks.
- Discuss nutritional hunger signs.
- Include family members in positive nutrition education. Family dynamics may play a role in the disorder. A family that avoids conflict, devalues individuality, and rejects emotions and personal opinions and beliefs should receive counseling.
- Assertiveness training or transactional analysis theories may be helpful when the patient is ready. Codependent behavior generally is a problem.
- For patients with type 1 diabetes, monitor for poor control, bulimia, and skipping meals. These individuals are at high risk for hypoglycemia, hyperglycemia, and early onset of complications.
- Social pressures for thinness should be addressed. Preventive activities before middle school years are important.
- For some individuals, videotaping and playback of abnormal eating behaviors may be useful (Touyz et al., 1994).
- Two or more consecutive spontaneous menses implies resumption of menses; this is dependent on body weight but not on body fat levels (Golden, 1997).
- The majority of patients with ED make a full recovery, despite the severity of disturbances in eating patterns and poor nutritional status present at diagnosis (Rock, 1999).
- There is often relapse in eating disorder patients. It was found that recovered patients still have psychiatric abnormalities (Foppiani, 1998). Inhibiting food intake may have consequences not anticipated; starvation and self-imposed dieting appear to lead to binges once food is available. Preoccupation with food and eating, increased emotional responsiveness and dysphoria, and distractibility may result (Polivy, 1996).
- For women with AN who become pregnant, successful treatment includes appropriate pattern of weight gain, decreases in bingeing and purging behaviors, and normal infant birth weight. Special guidance is needed to achieve positive fetal outcomes.
- Eating disorders negatively affect pregnancy; therefore, a team approach is suggested for helping a pregnant woman with an eating disorder (Franko and Spurrell, 2000).

For More Information

- Academy for Eating Disorders
  http://www.aedweb.org
- American Anorexia/Bulimia Association
  http://www.aabainc.org/
- American Dietetic Association
  Eating Disorders protocol
  www.eatright.org
- Anorexia Nervosa and Related Eating Disorders (ANRED)
  http://www.anred.com/
- Eating Disorders Awareness
  http://www.eatingdisordersanonymous.org/
- International Association of Eating Disorders Professionals (IAEDP)
  407-338-6494
- National Association of AN and Associated Disorders (ANAD)
  Hotline: 847-831-3438
  http://www.anad.org/
- National Eating Disorders Association
  http://www.edap.org/
- Renfrew Centers
  1-800-RENFREW
- Yale Centers for Eating and Weight Disorders
  203-432-4610

BINGE-EATING DISORDER

NUTRITIONAL ACUITY RANKING: LEVEL 2 (NOT RANKED BY CONSENSUS)

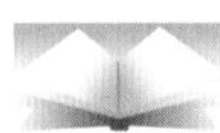

DEFINITIONS AND BACKGROUND

Recurrent episodes of binge eating (eating in a discrete period of time an amount of food larger than most people would eat in the same time) with a sense of lack of control over the eating episode are the main indicators of a binge-eating disorder. Episodes may involve any three: eating more rapidly than normal, eating until uncomfortable, eating when not physically hungry, eating these foods alone, and feeling disgusted, guilty, or depressed. Binge eating occurs an average of 2 days weekly for 6 months or longer (Berg, 1994). There is no regular purging, fasting, or excessive exercise, and binge eating does not occur as part of anorexia or bulimia nervosa. Weight cycling is weight loss followed by weight regain; binge eaters report this cycling along with psychological distress (Kensinger et al., 1998).

Obesity is a major public health problem and is now recognized as a heterogeneous condition. Treatment requires understanding of the multiple factors that contribute to the problem; binge eating is a serious problem among a subset of the obese (Bruce and Wilfley, 1996). Chronic dieting may predispose binge eating or drug abuse. Clinical depression is also a common precedent. Approximately 25–33% of patients in weight control programs binge at least twice per month. There is often a history of parental or personal alcohol abuse. A single traumatic event, several years of unusual stress or pain, an extended period of emotional pain, or mood disorders may be involved.

Fairburn (1995) suggests three stages for overcoming binge eating. Stage one: Establish self-monitoring records; establish regular pattern of eating to displace binge eating; use alternative behaviors to help resist urges; educate about food, eating, shape, and weight. Stage two: Eliminate all aspects of restrained eating; develop skills for dealing with difficulties that triggered past binges; identify and challenge problematic ways of thinking; consider the origins of the binge eating problem and the role of family/social factors. Stage three: Plan for the future—have realistic expectations and strategies to use should problems occur.

OBJECTIVES

- Support the individual's counseling and therapy to identify the causes of binges. See Fairburn's stages above.
- Encourage a return to eating that is under the control of the individual.
- Correct any imbalances that have occurred as a result of the binges (e.g., weight, electrolyte imbalances, etc.).

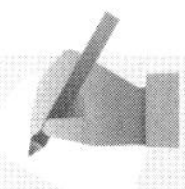

DIETARY AND NUTRITIONAL RECOMMENDATIONS

- A balanced diet should be offered, using the principles of the Food Guide Pyramid according to age, sex, height, and goal weight.
- Alter diet according to medication therapies, medical recommendations or history, and interdisciplinary care plan. This may include restriction of CHO, protein, fat, sodium, or other nutrients accordingly.

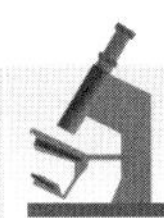

PROFILE

Clinical/History		
Height	Binge pattern and frequency	Cl−
Weight		BUN, Creat
BMI	**Lab Work**	Gluc
% Weight changes	Na+, K+	Urinary acetone
		Chol, Trig

Common Drugs Used and Potential Side Effects

- Antidepressants may be useful. Monitor specific effects.
- Topiramate could be an effective binge-eating disorder treatment; this treatment has mild side effects and helps improve the symptoms of binge-eating disorder (Shapira et al., 2000). Weight loss is one effect.

Herbs, Botanicals and Supplements

- No specific herbs and botanical products have been used for binge eating in any clinical trials.

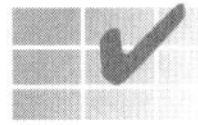

PATIENT EDUCATION

- Discuss use of a food diary to record time, place, foods eaten, cues, binge feelings, and other comments.
- Discuss exercise and its effect on sense of well-being.
- Discuss shopping, holidays, and stressors.
- Discuss not skipping breakfast and lunch and then bingeing into the night.

For More Information

- Academy for Eating Disorders
  http://www.aedweb.org
- American Dietetic Association
  Eating Disorders protocol
  www.eatright.org
- Eating Disorders Awareness
  http://www.eatingdisordersanonymous.org/
- National Association of AN and Associated Disorders (ANAD)
  Hotline: 847-831-3438
  http://www.anad.org/
- National Eating Disorders Association
  http://www.edap.org/

BULIMIA NERVOSA

NUTRITIONAL ACUITY RANKING: LEVEL 4

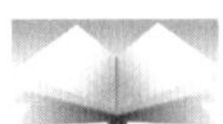

DEFINITIONS AND BACKGROUND

Bulimia nervosa is an eating disorder with food addiction as the primary coping mechanism. Criteria for diagnosis of bulimia include recurrent episodes of binge eating, sense of lack of control, self-evaluation unduly influenced by weight or body shape, and recurrent and inappropriate compensating behavior two times weekly for 3 months or longer (vomiting, use of laxatives or diuretics, fasting, excessive exercise). Purging versus nongorging types have been identified. In bulimia nervosa, repeated binge episodes increase gastric capacity, which delays emptying, blunts cholecystokinin (CCK) release, and impairs satiety response (Devlin et al., 1997).

Of the 5–30% of the population with bulimia, 85% are college-educated women. Patients with bulimia are more likely than individuals without bulimia to experience loneliness, irritability, passivity, sadness, and suicidal behavior. Usually, 60–70% have had overweight mothers, and eating may have been taught as a coping mechanism for stress. Mothers also may have been more domineering, with excessively high expectations of their children. Codependency may also be present. Codependency is a dysfunctional pattern of relating to one's own feelings, focus on others or on things outside of oneself, and denial of feelings within the family unit. Fear, shame, despair, anger, rigidity, denial, and confusion may be involved.

There are substance disorders in 9–55% of those with bulimia, 0–19% with AN, 10–44% of obese persons, and 11% who are not psychiatric patients (Varner, 1995). Disordered eating usually occurs for some time before drug or alcohol problems. ED and substance disorders may represent different expressions of the same underlying problem or predisposition to addictive behavior patterns (Varner, 1995). Other commonalities include cognitive dysfunction, use of food or substance to relieve negative affect (anxiety or depression), secretiveness about the problem, and social isolation. Denial is common; therefore concurrent therapies are recommended.

Patients with bulimia are often at normal weight or slightly above normal. Table 4–7 lists oral manifestations and issues of concern in bulimia nervosa. Chronic dieting may predispose binge eating or drug abuse. Addictive behavior patterns and impulse control are common.

OBJECTIVES

- Stabilize fluid and electrolyte imbalances.
- Assess patient thoroughly and create an individualized care plan. Include such factors as weight history, dieting behaviors, binge-eating episodes, purging behaviors, eating patterns, and exercise patterns.
- Promote effective weight control while altering life-stress management. Establish a target weight in accordance with desirable BMI, present weight, time frame for recovery, and related factors.
- Correct or prevent edema.
- Prevent any or additional tooth enamel decay or erosion (perimolysis) from vomiting and poor eating habits. About one-third of persons with this condition will have erosion.
- Counteract low metabolic rate with diet and exercise.

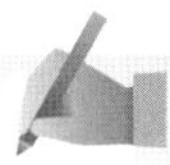

DIETARY AND NUTRITIONAL RECOMMENDATIONS

- Provide basal energy needs plus 300–400 calories above present intake.
- Use controlled portions of a regular diet, usually with three meals and two snacks.
- Decrease sugar intake over all, stressing importance of other key nutrients.

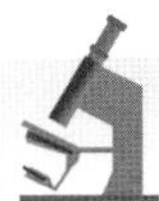

PROFILE

Clinical/History		Lab Work
Hx laxative and diuretic abuse	Weight, current	Cl−
BP	Usual weight	K+
Height	BMI	Chol, Trig
	Percentage of weight changes	Gastrin
	Oral/dental concerns	Alb
		Na+

TABLE 4–7 Assessment of Oral Manifestations in Bulimia Nervosa

Condition	*Issues of Concern*
Enamel erosion (perimolysis)	Thermal sensitivity and pain
Salivary gland swelling (sialadenosis)	Hypertrophy from regurgitation of acidic contents; malnutrition
Dry mouth (xerostomia)	From vomiting, laxative, or diuretic abuse
Increased serum amylase (hyperamylasemia)	2–4 times increased levels occur after bingeing and vomiting; used as a marker for bulimia
Mucosal trauma	Abrasions and bleeding from rapid, forceful regurgitation
Gingival recession	From frequent and rigorous tooth brushing
Dental caries	From increased intake of junk foods, candy, sweets

Common Drugs Used and Potential Side Effects

- Laxative and diuretic abuse can cause cardiac arrest and other problems.
- Phenytoin (Dilantin) is sometimes given to patients with abnormal EEGs. A supplement with folate and vitamin D is often needed. Nausea, vomiting, and constipation can occur.
- Antidepressants (e.g., Elavil, Tofranil, or Prozac) may be used. Monitor side effects such as dry mouth, constipation, increased blood pressure, abdominal cramps, and weight changes. Prozac may also cause nausea, vomiting, glucose changes, and decreased sodium. Avoid use with ma huang (ephedra), St. John's wort, and gingko biloba, because they may enhance the effects and cause restlessness.

Herbs, Botanicals and Supplements

- No specific herbs and botanical products have been used for bulimia nervosa in any clinical trials.
- Ma huang (ephedra), St. John's wort, and gingko biloba may enhance the effects of antidepressants and cause restlessness.
- With anticonvulsants such as phenytoin (Dilantin), avoid use with evening primrose oil, gingko biloba, and kava.

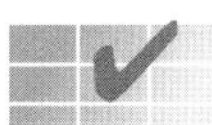

PATIENT EDUCATION

- ✓ Self-help groups such as Overeaters Anonymous or group therapy can help.
- ✓ Information, as from basic nutrition texts, can also encourage improved habits.
- ✓ Help the patient rediscover the ability to be alone without giving in to the urge to binge.
- ✓ Assertiveness training may be of great benefit.
- ✓ Discuss the outcomes of electrolyte imbalance: muscle spasms, kidney problems, or cardiac arrest.
- ✓ Assert that there is "no such thing as a forbidden food."
- ✓ Discuss the vicious cycle of bulimia: hopelessness or anxiety leading to gorging, leading to fear of fatness, leading to vomiting or drug abuse, leading to release from fear, leading to guilt, etc.
- ✓ Stringent oral hygiene after vomiting may reduce dental erosion.

For More Information

- Academy for Eating Disorders
  http://www.aedweb.org
- American Dietetic Association
  Eating Disorders protocol
  www.eatright.org
- Anorexia Nervosa and Related Eating Disorders
- http://www.anred.com/
- Bulimia Anorexia Self-Help Hotline
  1-800-762-3334
- Eating Disorders Awareness
  http://www.eatingdisordersanonymous.org/
- National Association of AN and Associated Disorders (ANAD)
  Hotline: 847-831-3438
  http://www.anad.org/
- National Eating Disorders Association
  http://www.edap.org/

DEPRESSION

NUTRITIONAL ACUITY RANKING: LEVEL 1 (MILD); LEVEL 2 (NUMEROUS MEDICATIONS)

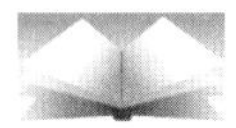

DEFINITIONS AND BACKGROUND

Depression affects approximately 2–4% of the general population at any point in time. About 39% of risk for major depression is inherited; 61% is from environmental factors such as substance abuse. In nursing homes, it is expected that about 50% of individuals will have some form of depression for which medication should be prescribed. Monitoring physical health, including nutrition, is an adjunct to psychiatric treatment or psychotherapy. 40% of persons with depression may have a deficiency of brain serotonin. A mixed diet of protein/CHO should provide tryptophan, a precursor of serotonin. Intake of dietary protein high in tryptophan increases the ratio of tryptophan to large neutral amino acids (LNAA) and improves coping ability in stress-vulnerable persons (Markus et al., 2000).

Diagnosis of depression is indicated by four of seven of the following: SIGECAPS—sleep changes, loss of interest, guilt/hopelessness, energy decline, concentration changes, appetite changes, psychomotor changes, or suicidal tendencies. For some persons for whom medications cannot be given, electroshock therapy (ECT) may be effective but may have side effects. An experimental pacemaker-like device is now being tried, which sends electrical stimulations into the vagus nerve in the neck.

Studies indicate that low levels of n-3 fatty acids correlate with increased rates of depression and depressive symptoms in alcoholism. Adequate intakes of long-chain polyunsaturated fatty acids, especially DHA, may reduce the development of depression (Hibbeln and Salem, 1995). Cholesterol levels are lower in manic and depressive phases than in mixed episodes; no differences were found in patients with unipolar or bipolar mood disorders, so cholesterol may be a state rather than a trait (Ghaemi et al., 2000).

Exogenous/reactive depression involves an unrealistic and inappropriate reaction to some event or internal conflict. Endogenous depression involves multiple factors leading to intrapsychic conflict; this is a major depression that requires antidepressants and usually psychotherapy. Seasonal affective disorder (SAD) increases with latitude; serotonin agonists may be useful in treatment (i.e., Prozac, Zoloft, or Paxil).

For treatment of resistant bipolar disorder, high-dose thyroid hormones, calcium channel blockers, electroconvulsant therapy, omega-3 fatty acids, and various psychosocial strategies are under active investigation (Gitlkin, 2001).

Women with antepartum depression have a risk of poor nutrition, substance abuse, and prenatal noncompliance (Spinelli, 1998). Careful assessment is needed.

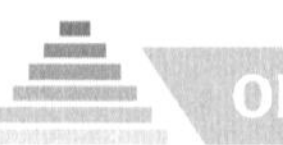

OBJECTIVES

- Provide adequate nutritional intake, e.g., excessive weight loss or shock therapy requires increased caloric intake.
- Monitor weight weekly to evaluate status.
- Detect complications as suggested by weight loss. Determine whether weight loss is caused by inadequate calorie and nutrient intake.
- Assess usual eating habits and related problems, which may include loneliness, difficulty in activities of daily living, boredom, lack of hobbies and interests, and poor sleep habits. Adequate drug therapy usually helps appetite improve.
- Centrally located body fat and obesity are found to be more prevalent in bipolar patients compared to matched population controls (Elmslie et al., 2000). Monitor calorie intake if overeating; counsel appropriately.

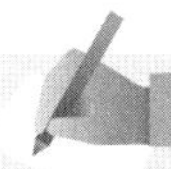

DIETARY AND NUTRITIONAL RECOMMENDATIONS

- Use a diet providing high biologic value (HBV) proteins and a high-calcium intake. Emotional stress lowers serum nitrogen and calcium levels.
- Watch for inadequate protein intake, which may lower intake of iron, thiamine, riboflavin, niacin, and vitamins B6 and B12.
- Use a tyramine-restricted diet for patients given monoamine oxidase inhibiting drugs. Such a diet excludes aged cheese, beer, red wine, ale, pickled herring, chicken liver, broad bean pods, canned figs, sausage, salami, pepperoni, commercial gravies, ripe avocado, fermented soy sauce, ripe banana, yeast concentrates, and pickled or smoked fish.
- If overeating, limit access to food and provide a low-calorie diet. Encourage physical activity.
- Drinking liquid supplements may be useful because they require less effort.
- TPN is not advised for patients who are suicidal.
- Increase intake of omega-3 fatty acid food sources because they are part of the synaptic membrane.
- Low serum folate is common in 15–38% of depressed adults; need 400 mcg daily.

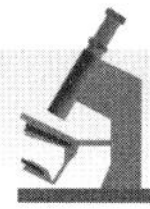

PROFILE

Clinical/History

Height
Weight
BMI
BP
Food pica
I & O
Constipation

Lab Work

H&H, serum Fe
Alb
Serum Ca++, Mg++
Gluc
Serotonin
Thyroid tests (T4)
Na+, K+
N balance

Common Drugs Used and Potential Side Effects

- Monoamine oxidase inhibitors (tranylcypromine [Parnate], phenelzine [Nardil], isocarboxazid [Marplan]) require a tyramine-restricted diet to prevent hypertensive crisis. Tyramine is a pressor amine. Spoiled, overripe, and aged products are the most problematic. Beware of Chianti wines, beer, excessive chocolate, and caffeine. Constipation, weight gain, and GI distress are common side effects. Avoid ginseng.
- Tricyclic antidepressants (such as imipramine [Tofranil], amitriptyline [Elavil], amoxapine [Asendin], Sinequan [Doxepin]) may cause dry mouth. Some may cause an increase in appetite, with potential for excessive weight gain. Others may cause nausea, vomiting, SIADH, constipation, anorexia, or stomatitis. Norpramin may cause abdominal cramps, altered blood glucose levels, and vomiting. Avoid use with ma huang (ephedra), St. John's wort, and ginkgo biloba.
- Lithium carbonate (Lithane, Lithobid, Lithotabs) requires constancy in sodium intake. Weight gain, metallic taste, nausea, vomiting, and diarrhea may occur. Limit caffeine intake. Lithium is often used for bipolar mood disorders.
- Nortriptyline (Aventyl, Pamelor) may cause increased appetite for sweets, GI distress, vomiting, and diarrhea.
- Clomipramine HCl (Anafranil) is used for obsessive-compulsive disorders. Dry mouth is common; hard sugarless candy or chewing gum may be useful. Anorexia and abdominal pain are also common.
- Panic disorders may be treated with Tofranil, Xanax, Klonopin, or Paxil. Paxil, Prozac, and Effexor (serotonin-reuptake blockers) may cause abdominal pain, anorexia, diarrhea, and weight changes; they are used to treat despair and helplessness. Prozac may also cause nausea, vomiting, glucose changes, or decreased sodium.
- Wellbutrin (bupropion) tends to have a stimulating effect but may also cause weight loss, dry mouth, nausea, and vomiting.
- Zoloft (sertraline) can cause dry mouth or diarrhea. Avoid use with St. John's wort and ma huang (ephedra).
- SAMe is 5-adenosyl-methionine and is useful for mild depression but may trigger coronary problems. A positive side effect is that it may actually help with degenerative joint disease symptoms.
- Fluvoxamine (Luvox) is an antiobsessive-compulsive SSRI medication that may cause anorexia, dry mouth, nausea, diarrhea, or constipation.
- Lamotrigine has been shown to be effective for bipolar disorder. If topiramate (an anticonvulsant) is used, weight loss is a side effect.

Herbs, Botanicals and Supplements

- L-tryptophan may be tried for insomnia or depression. Do not use with MAOI antidepressants, SSRI antidepressants, or serotonin receptor antagonists.
- St. John's wort is used as a natural antidepressant. Do not use with MAOI antidepressants, SSRI antidepressants, cyclosporine, digoxin, oral contraceptives, HIV protease inhibitors, theophylline, warfarin, or calcium channel blockers such as amlodipine, diltiazem, or verapamil.
- Kava should not be taken in patients with depression.
- Licorice, ginger, purslane, rosemary, and ginseng have been suggested, but there are no clinical trials that prove efficacy.
- SAMe is under investigation for various uses.
- Ma huang (ephedra) should not be used with antidepressants.
- Psyllium and ginseng should not be used with Depakote or lithium.
- Ginseng and yohimbe should not be used with MAOI antidepressants

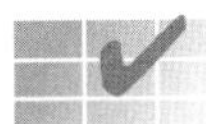

PATIENT EDUCATION

- ✓ Teach creative menu planning and food preparation methods that address the side effects and symptoms the patient is experiencing.
- ✓ Teach the patient how to moisten foods for dry mouth syndrome resulting from certain medications. Sugar-free candy may help.
- ✓ Limit caffeine-containing foods and beverages in the late evening.
- ✓ After giving birth, three postpartum mood disorders—postpartum "blues," postpartum depression, and postpartum psychosis—are common, and education is an important instrument in the treatment of these disorders (Spinelli, 1998).

For More Information

- ✦ National Depressive and Manic-Depressive Association
  730 N. Franklin, Suite 501, Chicago, IL 60610
  1-800-826-3632
- ✦ Recovery Inc.
  802 Dearborn, Chicago, IL 60610
  312-337-5661
  http://www.ed.psu.edu/~recovery

PSYCHOSIS

NUTRITIONAL ACUITY RANKING: LEVEL 2

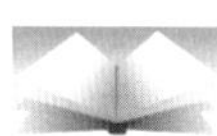

DEFINITIONS AND BACKGROUND

Psychosis is a condition in which an individual loses contact with reality; it can be either episodic or chronic and can result in irrational behaviors. It usually is best treated in a hospital setting, where the afflicted persons are less likely to hurt themselves or other people. Organic forms can cause a dazed expression, confused speech, visual hallucinations, bizarre or withdrawn behavior, low self-esteem, and appetite or sleep disturbances.

Viral infection during pregnancy promotes genetic vulnerability and is currently being studied. The finding of perinatal complications, urban/suburban residence at birth, and cat ownership in childhood as risk factors for the later development of psychoses seems to be linked (Fuller Torrey et al., 2000). Serial analysis of gene expression (SAGE) and reverse transcriptase-polymerase chain reaction are used to identify RNA transcripts that are differentially expressed in the brains of individuals with various psychiatric conditions (Johnston-Wilson et al., 2001).

Types of psychosis include the following:

Schizophrenia: group of disorders manifested by disordered thinking, hallucinations, delusions, social withdrawal, mood and behavioral disturbances (can be simple, catatonic, schizo-affective, paranoid, hebephrenic). Nearly 1% of the population develops schizophrenia during a lifetime, usually between ages 15–25. Interesting research has suggested a link to maternal herpes simplex 2 (HSV-2) with infants who later develop schizophrenia. This latter study has been conducted at the Developmental Neurovirology, Department of Pediatrics, Johns Hopkins University School of Medicine, Baltimore, Maryland by Dr. Robert Yolken.

Organic Brain Syndrome: from cerebral arteriosclerosis, chemical or toxic trauma, senile dementia, or other states. This is usually diagnosed using an OBS-scale (Organic Brain Syndrome Scale).

Delusions: can involve control, persecution, infidelity, or other abnormal fears.

Hallucinations: perceptions of an external stimulus without a source in the external world.

OBJECTIVES

- Provide adequate nourishment to prevent significant weight changes.
- Correct any nutritional deficits.
- Promote a normal pattern of dietary intake and routines.
- Develop a trusting relationship; make expectations clear to the patient.
- Prevent or correct constipation or impaction.

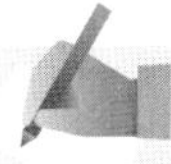

DIETARY AND NUTRITIONAL RECOMMENDATIONS

- A normal diet for age and sex can be used, unless other dietary/medical problems exist.
- Adjust calories up or down according to goal weight for patient and medications.
- Reduce potential accidents by avoiding glass containers and serving dishes.
- Vitamin C levels tend to be low in persons with schizophrenia; encourage improved and adequate intake accordingly.
- Breastfeeding mothers should avoid use of medications as much as possible. Should psychiatric medication be necessary, available information regarding the effects of these medications on the neonate should be provided. It is strongly recommended that the infant's pediatrician be involved in monitoring the infant (Burt et al., 2001).

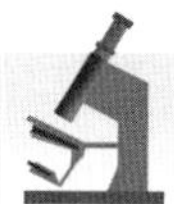

PROFILE

Clinical/History	Lab Work	
Height	Alb, prealbumin	Creatine phosphokinase (CPK) (elevated in acute episodes)
Weight	K+	
Weight changes	Na+	
BMI	H&H, serum Fe	
I & O	Gluc	
BP		

Common Drugs Used and Potential Side Effects

- Tranquilizers are often used. Triavil combines an antidepressant with a tranquilizer. Nausea, diarrhea, and vomiting may result.
- Laxatives or stool softeners may be required. Discuss potential use of higher fiber foods, fluids, etc.
- Antidepressants and medications may be used; evaluate specific drugs accordingly.
- Antipsychotics (Olanzapine, Quetiapine, Mellaril, Prolixin, Haldol, Trilafon, Navane, Risperdal, Seroquel, Zyprexa, and Clozaril) may cause dizziness, drowsiness, dry mouth, weight gain, edema, nausea, constipation, or vomiting. They help to quiet symptoms and help when the patient is resistant to other drugs and alternatives. Chlorpromazine (Thorazine) contains sulfites. It may

cause dry mouth, constipation, or weight gain. Geodon (Ziprasidone), a new drug with prolonged QT intervals, is not as likely to cause weight gain.

- In some people, drugs can cause psychiatric symptoms. The response is rare but may include confusion (acyclovir, propoxyphene [Darvon], and cimetidine [Tagamet]); depression (oral contraceptives, ibuprofen, metronidazole [Flagyl], barbiturates, cimetidine [Tagamet], and diazepam [Valium]); insomnia (acyclovir and alprazolam; paranoia [amphetamines], ibuprofen, cimetidine [Tagamet], and tricyclic antidepressants); excitement, hyperactivity, or agitation (alprazolam, amphetamines, barbiturates, metronidazole [Flagyl], and diazepam [Valium]); anxiety, mania, hallucinations, suicidal thoughts, and bizarre behavior may result from various other medications. The doctor should be contacted.
- To reduce compulsions of the obsessive-compulsive disorders, Prozac, Anafranil, Luvox, and Zoloft have been used with some success. Avoid use with ma huang (ephedra) and St. John's wort.
- To reduce anxiety, Tofranil, Xanax, Klonopin, and Paxil have been used. Sometimes, it is useful to offer a beverage or snack to reduce anxiety rather than adding more medications.

Herbs, Botanicals and Supplements

- Indian snakeroot may be used for mental illness. Do not use with digoxin, phenobarbital, levodopa, albuterol, furosemide, thiazide diuretics, MAOI antidepressants, beta-blockers such as atenolol or propanolol, or tranquilizers. Problems include potential sedation, increased blood pressure, arrhythmias, or CNS excitation.
- Some people may use ginseng. Do not use with CNS stimulants, caffeine, hormones, steroids, or antipsychotics.
- Kava and valerian should not be taken by patients with schizophrenia who are using anxiety-reducing drugs (alprazolam, diazepam, lorazepam.)

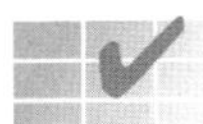

PATIENT EDUCATION

- ✔ Teach nutrition principles to the patient or the caregiver.
- ✔ Encourage self-care.
- ✔ Successfully terminate client relationship when independence is possible.
- ✔ Provide follow-up, especially with any stages of regression.

SUBSTANCE ABUSE AND WITHDRAWAL

NUTRITIONAL ACUITY RANKING: LEVEL 2 (WITHDRAWAL/REHABILITATION)

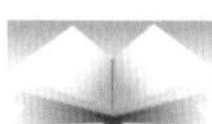

DEFINITIONS AND BACKGROUND

Abuse of chemical substances may be chronic or acute and may involve abuse of alcohol, prescription or over-the-counter drugs, or illicit drugs. Physiological problems that result are definite and are usually specific to the abused substance. Social, emotional, vocational, and legal problems may arise as a result. Addiction is a brain disorder, a chronic disorder with compulsive and relapsing behavior.

Persons with substance dependency tend to have type A personalities and are prone to perfectionism and depression. Substance abusers are codependent, neglecting their own feelings and emotions. Some studies suggest that abnormalities in the metabolism of dopamine, serotonin, and norepinephrine may contribute to the cause of substance dependency; in some cases, use of antidepressant medication has helped alleviate the dependency. The master "pleasure" molecule of addiction is dopamine (D-2 receptor gene). Heroin, amphetamines, marijuana, alcohol, nicotine, and caffeine all trigger the release of dopamine.

Eating disorders and substance disorders may represent different expressions of the same underlying problem, predisposition to addictive behavior patterns (Varner, 1995). Other commonalities include cognitive dysfunction, use of food or substance to relieve negative affect (anxiety or depression), secretiveness about the problem, and social isolation.

Polydrug use, including marijuana, nicotine, cocaine, opiates, and related drugs, may alter food intake, taste preferences, and nutrient metabolism. Denial is common and psychotherapy along with substance withdrawal is recommended.

In alcoholism, the most consistent predictor of alcohol dependency is alcoholism in a biological parent. Three predisposing factors exist: constitutional lability (biochemical), personality factor (psychological vulnerability), and social factors (environmental conditioning). Alcoholics have 2.5 times the normal death rate in similar age groups, especially from stroke or cirrhosis. An estimated 3 million children between 14 and 17 years of age are problem drinkers. The earlier the exposure, the more likely dependency will occur.

The C-A-G-E questions to ask include: "Have you tried to cut back? Has anybody ever annoyed you regarding this behavior? Have you ever felt guilty about it? Have you ever needed an early morning eye opener?" With two or more affirmative answers, there is a problem that should be addressed.

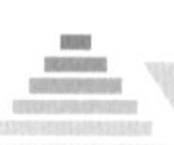

OBJECTIVES

- Protect during withdrawal (e.g., alcohol detoxification may cause tremors, hallucinations, seizures, and delirium tremens). Of persons with delirium tremens, 20% may die, even with therapy; monitor closely.
- Normalize brain levels of neurotransmitters.
- Correct fluid and electrolyte imbalances or dehydration.
- Modify diet for such problems as liver failure, cirrhosis, pancreatitis, GI bleeding, esophageal varices, renal impairment, ascites, or edema. See appropriate entries.
- Maintain homeostasis; prevent physical complications.
- Reorient to reality; develop trusting relationships between patient and care providers.
- Promote abstinence and long-term substance-abuse treatment.
- Improve nutritional status and outcome.
- Prevent or correct any related eating disorders (approximately 50% of this group). Avoid major changes in food choices and intake during recovery to prevent drastic weight fluctuations.

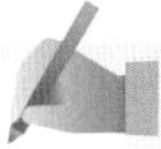

DIETARY AND NUTRITIONAL RECOMMENDATIONS

- According to I & O values, adjust fluid intake. Offer beverages that are nonalcoholic favorites.
- Encourage nutrient-dense foods. Fruits, vegetables, whole grains, and fish are important inclusions.
- Adequate intake of protein will be essential.
- Include adequate calories, especially because patients often become hypoglycemic. Feed several times daily to help regulate blood glucose.
- Adequate intake of B-complex vitamins, foods rich in L-tryptophan and L-tyrosine, and other depleted nutrients may be beneficial during recovery. Thiamine is especially important.
- Adjust diet, as appropriate, to reduce excess sweets, because many chemical abusers tend to substitute sweets for their dependency drug.
- Adequate fiber intake may be useful to correct or prevent constipation.

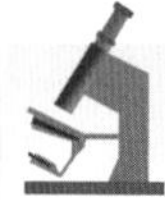

PROFILE

Clinical/History	Lab Work	
Height	Prolactin levels	Mg++
Weight	Serotonin levels	Cl−
BMI	Ca++	Gluc
Weight changes	Na+	Chol, Trig
I & O	K+	Serum thiamine
BP	H&H, serum Fe	Serum folate
Tremors, delirium	Alb, prealbumin	Serum vitamin B12

Common Drugs Used and Potential Side Effects

- Tricyclic antidepressants (imipramine, desipramine) are often beneficial with some side effects such as dry mouth.
- Bromocriptine (Parlodel) may also be used for some drug-recovery patients. Nausea, vomiting, or constipation may occur.
- Stool softeners may be beneficial if constipation results after withdrawal, as with cocaine abuse.
- Antabuse, when mixed with alcohol, can cause severe nausea, vomiting, low BP, and flushing.
- Naltrexone is a drug that decreases pleasurable sensation of alcohol; it is used for narcotic dependency after detoxification. Anorexia, weight loss, nausea, vomiting, and abdominal cramping or pain may occur.

Herbs, Botanicals and Supplements

- No studies have been conducted for efficacy of herbs or botanicals in substance abuse patients.

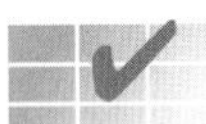

PATIENT EDUCATION

- ✓ Help the patient accept responsibility for his or her own actions. Cognitive behavioral therapy, family, group, and self-help therapies are all recommended.
- ✓ Help plan adequate discharge planning, follow-up, family therapy, or other support group interactions.
- ✓ Help to maintain abstinence. Avoid discussion of unanswerable questions such as "why" substances have been abused.
- ✓ In recovery, simple guidelines are useful: eat breakfast and regular meals daily; eat a variety of foods; make mealtimes pleasant and unhurried; choose healthy snacks; drink decaffeinated coffee; and take supplements only if prescribed (Pelican et al., 1994).
- ✓ Help dispel myths such as those related to food cravings.
- ✓ Discuss issues regarding personal "control." Coping skills will be needed to reduce helplessness.
- ✓ Include patient in decision making to increase self-esteem and confidence.
- ✓ Discuss the dangers of diet pills to control appetite and weight. Assess history of starving to lose weight or being overweight as a child or a teenager.
- ✓ Heavy drinkers tend to have higher total and HDL cholesterol levels than controls. Moderate alcohol intake does not seem to be protective against CHD through lipid control alone.
- ✓ Treatment should focus on sufficient duration, intensity, family support, after-care and follow-up, self-help groups, collaboration with social services, and a drug-free lifestyle. One of five individuals will be drug-free or sober after 5 years. New studies will include new, effective medications and evaluations of the changes that occur in the brain.

TABLE 4–8 Chocolate – Sensory Addiction?

Although addictive behavior is generally associated with drug and alcohol abuse or compulsive sexual activity, chocolate may evoke similar psychopharmacologic and behavioral reactions in susceptible persons. Hedonic appeal of chocolate (taste, texture, fat, sugar) is likely to be a predominant factor. Chocolate may also be a self-medication for low magnesium levels and to balance low neurotransmitters for mood (serotonin and dopamine). Chocolate cravings are often episodic and related to hormonal swings such as with menses. Chocolate contains methylxanthines, biogenic amines, and cannabinoid-like fatty acids, all of which cause potentially abnormal behaviors and psychologic sensations that parallel other addictions. Chocolate cravings are real and must be considered (Bruinsma and Taren, 1999).

For More Information

- Alcoholics Anonymous
  PO Box 459
  New York City, NY 10163
  212-870-3400
  http://www.alcoholics-anonymous.org
- American Society of Addiction Medicine
  (301) 656-3920
  http://www.asam.org/Frames.htm
- National Clearinghouse for Alcohol and Drug Information
  http://www.health.org
- National Council on Alcoholism and Drug Dependence
  http://www.ncadd.org
- National Institute on Drug Abuse
  6001 Executive Blvd.
  Bethesda, MD 20892-9561
  301-443-1124
  http://www.nida.nih.gov/NIDAHome1.html

REFERENCES

Alzheimer's Disease–Cited References

Davis K, et al. A double-blind, placebo-controlled multicenter study of tacrine for Alzheimer's disease. *N Engl J Med*. 1992;327:1253.

Engelhart MJ, et al. Dietary intake of antioxidants and risk of Alzheimer Disease. *JAMA*. 2002;287:3223.

Finucane T, et al. Tube feeding in patients with advanced dementia: a review of the evidence. *JAMA*. 1999;282:1365.

Franzoni S, et al. Good nutritional oral intake is associated with equal survival in demented and nondemented very old patients. *J Am Geriatr Soc*. 1996;44:1366.

Kipen E, et al. Bone density, vitamin D nutrition and parathyroid hormone levels in women with dementia. *J Am Geriatr Soc*. 1995;43:1088.

Leszek J, et al. Colostrinin: a proline-rich polypeptide (PRP) complex isolated from ovine colostrum for treatment of Alzheimer's disease. A double-blind, placebo-controlled study. *Arch Immunol Ther Exp*. 1999;47:377.

Miller J. Vitamin E and memory: is it vascular protection? *Nutr Rev*. 2000;58:109.

Minger S, et al. Cholinergic deficits contribute to behavioral disturbance in patients with dementia. *Neurology*. 2000;55:1460.

Morley J. Dementia is not necessarily a cause of undernutrition. *J Am Geriatr Soc*. 1996;44:1403.

Moss D, et al. Methanesulfonyl fluoride (MSF): a double-blind, placebo-controlled study of safety and efficacy in the treatment of senile dementia of the Alzheimer type. *Alzheimer Dis Assoc Disord*. 1999;13:20.

Nutrition Screening Initiative. A physician's guide to nutrition in chronic disease management for older adults. http://www.aafp.org/nsi/physiciansguide.pdf.

Parnetti L, et al. Increased CSF pyruvate levels as a marker of impaired energy metabolism in Alzheimer's disease. *J Am Geriatr Soc*. 1995;43:316.

Perkins A. Association of antioxidants with memory in a multiethnic elderly sample using the Third National Health and Nutrition Examination Survey. *Am J Epidemiol*. 1999;150:37.

Pitchumoni S, et al. Current status of antioxidant therapy for Alzheimer's disease (review). *J Am Geriatr Soc*. 1998;46:1566.

Poehlman E, Dvorak R. Energy expenditure, energy intake, and weight loss in Alzheimer disease. *Am J Clin Nutri*. 2000;71:650S.

Reichman W. Alzheimer's disease: clinical treatment options. *Am J Manag Care*. 2000;6:1125S.

Rondeau V, et al. Relation between aluminum concentrations in drinking water and Alzheimer's disease: an eight-year follow-up study. *J Epid*. 2000;152:59.

Sano M, et al. A controlled trial of selegiline, alpha tocopherol, or both as treatment for Alzheimer's disease. *N Engl J Med*. 1997;336:1216.

Spindler A, et al. Nutritional status of patients with Alzheimer's disease: a 1-year study. *J Am Diet Assoc*. 1996;96:1013.

Soltesz K, Dayton J. Finger foods that help those with Alzheimer's maintain weight. *J Am Diet Assoc*. 1993;93:1106.

Touyz S, et al. Videotape feedback of eating behavior in patients with anorexia nervosa: does it normalize eating behavior? *Aust J Nutr Diet*. 1994;51:79.

White H, et al. The association of weight change in Alzheimer's disease with severity of disease and mortality: a longitudinal analysis. *J Am Geriatr Soc*. 1998;46:1223.

White H, et al. Weight change in Alzheimer's disease. *J Am Geriat Soc*. 1996;44:265.

Alzheimer's Disease–Suggested Readings

Adelman A, Hersey M. Selegiline and vitamin E in Alzheimer's disease. *J Family Practice*. 1997;15:98.

Drachman D, Leger P. Treatment of Alzheimer's disease—searching for a breakthrough, settling for less. *N Engl J Med*. 1997;336:1245.

Finley B. Nutritional needs of the person with Alzheimer's disease: practical approaches to quality care. *J Am Diet Assoc*. 1997;97:177S.

Franzoni S, et al. Good nutritional oral intake is associated with equal survival in demented and nondemented very old patients. *J Am Geriat Soc*. 1996;44:1366.

Leber P. Observations and suggestions on antidementia drug development. *Alzheimer's Dis Assoc Disord*. 1996;10:31.

Spindler A, et al. Nutritional status of patients with Alzheimer's disease: a 1-year study. *J Am Diet Assoc*. 1996;96:1013.

Thomas R, et al. Analysis of longitudinal data in an Alzheimer's disease clinical trial. *Stat Med*. 2000;19:1433.

Tohgi H, Abe T, et al. Concentrations of a-tocopherol and its quinone derivative in cerebrospinal fluid from patients with vascular dementia of the Binswanger type and Alzheimer's type dementia. *Neuroscience Letters*. 1994;174:73.

Whitehouse P, et al. First International Pharmacoeconomics Conference on Alzheimer's Disease: report and summary. *Alzheimer's Dis Assoc Disord*. 1998;12:266.

Anorexia Nervosa and Eating Disorders–Cited References

Ammerman S, et al. Unique considerations for treating eating disorders in adolescents and preventive intervention. *Top Clin Nutri*. 1996;12:79.

American Dietetic Association. Position of The American Dietetic Association: nutrition intervention in the treatment of anorexia nervosa, bulimia nervosa, and eating disorders not otherwise specified (EDNOS). *J Am Diet Assoc*. 2001;101:805.

Beals K, Manore M. Nutritional status of female athletes with subclinical eating disorders. *J Am Diet Assoc*. 1998;98:419.

Berg F. Binge eating disorder: what's it all about? *Obesity and Health*. 1994;8(2):26.

Brooks E, et al. Compromised bone density 11.4 years after diagnosis of anorexia nervosa. *J Women's Health*. 1998;7:567.

Bruce B, Wilfley D. Binge eating among the overweight population: a serious and prevalent problem. *J Am Diet Assoc*. 1996;96:58.

Cargaro L, et al. Insulin-like growth factor 1 (IGF-1), a nutritional marker in patients with eating disorders. *Clin Nutri*. 2001;20:251.

Clark N. Counseling the athlete with an eating disorder. *J Am Diet Assoc*. 1994;94:656.

Devlin M, et al. Postprandial cholecystokinin release and gastric emptying in patients with bulimia nervosa. *Am J Clin Nutri*. 1997;65:114.

Fairburn C. *Overcoming binge eating*. New York: Gilford Publications, Inc., 1995.

Foppiani L, et al. Frequency of recovery from anorexia nervosa of a cohort patients re-evaluated on a long-term basis following intensive care. *Eat Weight Disord*. 1998;3:90.

Franko D, Spurrell E. Detection and management of eating disorders during pregnancy. *Obstet Gynecol*. 2000;95:942.

Glorio R, et al. Prevalence of cutaneous manifestations in 200 patients with eating disorders. *Int J Dermatol*. 2000;39:348.

Golden N, et al. Resumption of menses in anorexia nervosa. *Arch Peds & Adol Med*. 1997;151:16.

Kensinger G, et al. Psychological symptoms are greater among weight cycling with severe binge eating behavior. *J Am Diet Assoc*. 1998;98:8.

Mehler P. Diagnosis and care of patients with anorexia nervosa in primary care settings. *Ann Intern Med*. 2001;134:1048.

Polivy J. Psychological consequences of food restriction. *J Am Diet Assoc*. 1996;96:589.

Rock C. Nutritional and medical assessment and management of eating disorders. *Nutrition in Clinical Care*. 1999;2(6):332.

Shapira N, et al. Treatment of binge-eating disorder with topiramate: a clinical case series. *J Clin Psychiatry*. 2000;61:368.

Solanto M, et al. Rate of weight gain of inpatients with anorexia nervosa under two behavioral contracts. *Pediatrics*. 1994;93:989.

Varner L. Dual diagnosis: patients with eating and substance disorders. *J Am Diet Assoc*. 1995;95:224.

Vink T, et al. Association between agouti-related protein gene polymorphism and anorexia nervosa. *Molecular Psychaitr*. 2001;6:325.

Anorexia Nervosa and Eating Disorders–Suggested Readings

Faber R, et al. Two forms of compulsive consumption: comorbidity of compulsive buying and binge-eating. *J Consumer Research*. 1995;22:296.

Fisher M, et al. Hypophosphatemia secondary to oral refeeding in anorexia nervosa. *Int J Eat Disord*. 2000;28:181.

Neiderman M, et al. Enteric feeding in severe adolescent anorexia nervosa: a report of four cases. *Int J Eat Disord*. 2000;28:470.

Rees J. Eating disorders in adolescents: a model for broadening our perspective. *J Am Diet Assoc*. 1996;96:22.

Schebendach J. Eating disorders. In: Mahan K, Escott-Stump S, eds. *Krause's food, nutrition, and diet therapy*. 10th ed. Philadelphia: WB Saunders, 2000.

Vitiello B, Lederhendler I. Research on eating disorders: current status and future prospects. *Biol Psychiatry*. 2000;47:777.

Whisenant S, Smith B. Eating disorders: current nutrition therapy and perceived needs in dietetics education and research. *J Am Diet Assoc*. 1995;95:1109.

Woolsey M. When food becomes a cry for help. *J Am Diet Assoc*. 1998;98:395.

Epilepsy–Cited References

Berg M, et al. Folic acid improves phenytoin pharmacokinetics. *J Am Diet Assoc*. 1995;95:352.

Berryman M. The ketogenic diet revisited. *J Am Diet Assoc*. 1997;97:S192.

Best T, et al. Cardiac complications in pediatric patients on the ketogenic diet. *Neurology*. 2000;54:2328.

Carroll J, Koenigsberger D. The ketogenic diet: a practical guide for caregivers. *J Am Diet Assoc*. 1998;98:316.

Couch S, et al. Growth and nutritional outcomes of children treated with the ketogenic diet. *J Am Diet Assoc*. 1999;99:1573.

Dike G. Severe malnutrition due to subtle neurologic deficits and epilepsy: report of three cases. *East Afr Med J*. 1999;76:597.

Freeman J, et al. The efficacy of the ketogenic diet—1998: a prospective evaluation of intervention in 150 children. *Pediatrics*. 1998;102:1358.

MacCracken K, Scalisi J. Development and evaluation of a ketogenic diet program. *J Am Diet Assoc*. 1999;99:1554.

Mandel A, et al. Medical costs are reduced when children with intractable epilepsy are successfully treated with the ketogenic diet. *J Am Diet Assoc*. 2002;102:396.

McGhee B, Katyal N. Avoid unnecessary drug-related carbohydrates for patients consuming the ketogenic diet. *J Am Diet Assoc*. 2001;101:87.

Multiple Sclerosis–Cited References

Esparza M, et al. Nutrition, latitude, and multiple sclerosis mortality: an ecologic study. *Am J Epid*. 1995;142:733.

Johnson S. The possible role of gradual accumulation of copper, cadmium, lead and iron and gradual depletion of zinc, magnesium, selenium, vitamins B2, B6, D, and E and essential fatty acids in multiple sclerosis. *Med Hypotheses*. 2000;55:239.

Mehindate K, et al. Proinflammatory cytokines promote glial heme oxygenase-1 expression and mitochondrial iron deposition: implications for multiple sclerosis. *J Neurochem*. 2001;77:1386.

Thomas F, Wiles C. Dysphagia and nutritional status in multiple sclerosis. *J Neurol*. 1999;246:677.

Timmerman G, Stuifbergin A. Eating patterns in women with multiple sclerosis. *J Neurosci Nurs*. 1999;31:152.

Wozniak-Wowk C. Nutrition intervention in the management of multiple sclerosis. *Nutr Today*. 1993;28:12.

Parkinson's Disease–Cited References

Bassotti G, et al. Esophageal manometric abnormalities in Parkinson's disease. *Dysphagia*. 1998;13:28.

Benedetti M, et al. Smoking, alcohol, and coffee consumption preceding Parkinson's disease: a case-control study. *Neurology*. 2000;55:1350.

Beyer P, et al. Weight change and body composition in patients with Parkinson's disease. *J Am Diet Assoc*. 1995;95:979.

Calne D. Treatment of Parkinson's disease. *N Engl J Med*. 1993;329:1021.

Holden K. Unintentional weight loss. In: *Parkinson's disease: guidelines for medical nutrition therapy*. 1st ed. Ft. Collins, CO: Five Star Living, Inc., 2000.

Honig L. Relationship between caffeine intake and Parkinson's disease. *JAMA*. 2000;284:1378.

Johnson C, et al. Adult nutrient intake as a risk factor for Parkinson's disease. *Int J Epidemiol*. 1999;28:1102.

Lieberman A, et al. Protein distribution diets in the management of fluctuations in levodopa response. In: *Drugs and nutrients in neurology (special report)*. Cedar Knolls, NJ: National Medical Information Network, 1994.

McIntosh G, Holden K. Risk for malnutrition and bone fracture in Parkinson's disease. *J Nutr Elderly*. 1999;18:3.

Muthane U, et al. Hunting genes in Parkinson's disease from the roots. *Med Hypotheses*. 2001;57:51.

Olanow C, et al. An algorithm (decision tree) for the management of Parkinson's disease (2001): treatment guidelines. *Neurology*. 2001;56:S1.

Prasad K, et al. Multiple antioxidants in prevention and treatment of Parkinson's disease. *J Am Col Nutri*. 1999;8:413.

Ross G, et al. Association of coffee and caffeine intake with the risk of Parkinson's disease. *JAMA*. 2000;283:2674.

Rodriguez J, Arenas A. Variables affecting cognitive deterioration in Parkinson's disease. *Rev Neurol*. 2001;32:107–111.

Yasui K, et al. Plasma homocysteine and MTHFR C677T genotype in levodopa-treated patients with PD. *Neurology*. 2000;55:437.

Tardive Dyskinesia–Cited References

Adler A, et al. Vitamin E treatment of tardive dyskinesia. *Am J Psychiatry*. 1993;150:1405.

Boomershint K, et al. Vitamin E in the treatment of tardive dyskinesia. *Ann Pharmacother*. 1999;33:1195.

Elkashef A, Wyatt R. Tardive dyskinesia: possible involvement of free radicals and treatment with vitamin E. *Schizophr Bull*. 1999;25:731.

Other Conditions–Cited References

American Dietetic Association. Position of The American Dietetic Association: legal and ethical issues in feeding permanently unconscious patients. *J Am Diet Assoc*. 1995;95:231.

Andreassen O, et al. Increases in cortical glutamate concentrations in transgenic amyotrophic lateral sclerosis mice are attenuated by creatine supplementation. *J Neurochem*. 2001;77:383.

Avorn J, et al. Reduction of bacteriuria and pyuria after ingestion of cranberry juice. *JAMA*. 1994;271:751.

Baraka A. Anesthesia and critical care of thymectomy for myasthenia gravis. *Chest Surg Clin N Am*. 2001;11:337.

Borum M, et al. The effect of nutritional supplementation on survival in seriously ill hospitalized adults: an evaluation of the SUPPORT data. Study to Understand Prognoses and Preferences for Outcomes and Risks of Treatments. *J Am Geriatr Soc*. 2000;48:S33.

Brain Trauma Foundation. The American Association of Neurological Surgeons. The Joint Section on Neurotrauma and Critical Care: nutrition. *J Neurotrauma*. 2000;17:539.

Bruinsma K, Taren D. Chocolate: food or drug? *J Am Diet Assoc*. 1999;99:1249.

Burt V, et al. The use of psychotropic medications during breastfeeding. *Am J Psychiatry*. 2001;158:1001.

Calabrese V, et al. NO synthase and NO-dependent signal pathways in brain aging and neurodegenerative disorders: the role of oxidant/antioxidant balance. *Neurochem Res*. 2000;25:1315.

Desport J, et al. Nutritional assessment and survival in ALS patients. *Amyotroph Lateral Scler Other Motor Neuron Disord*. 2000;1:91.

Drachman D. Myasthenia gravis. *N Engl J Med*. 1994;330:1797.

Elmslie J, et al. Prevalence of overweight and obesity in bipolar patients. *J Clin Psychiatry*. 2000;61:179.

Fernstrom J. Dietary amino acids and brain function. *J Am Diet Assoc*. 1994;94:714.

Fuller-Torrey E, et al. The antecedents of psychoses: a case-control study of selected risk factors. *Schizophr Res*. 2000;46:17.

Ghaemi S, et al. Cholesterol levels in mood disorders: high or low? *Bipolar Disord*. 2000;2:60.

Gitlin M, et al. Treatment-resistant bipolar disorder. *Bull Menninger Clin*. 2001;65:26.

Hardiman O. Symptomatic treatment of respiratory and nutritional failure in amyotrophic lateral sclerosis. *J Neurol*. 2000;247:245.

Hibbeln J, Salem N. Dietary polyunsaturated fatty acids and depression: when cholesterol does not satisfy. *Am J Clin Nutri*. 1995;62:1.

Hurley R, Taber K. Emotional disturbances following traumatic brain injury. *Cur Treat Options Neurol*. 2002;4:59.

Johnston-Wilson N, et al. Emerging technologies for large-scale screening of human tissues and fluids in the study of severe psychiatric disease. *Int J Neuropsychopharmacol*. 2001;4:83.

Klewer J, et al. Problems reported by elderly patients with multiple sclerosis. *J Neurosci Nurs*. 2001;33:167.

Klodell C, et al. Routine intragastric feeding following traumatic brain injury is safe and well tolerated. *Am J Surg*. 2000;179:168.

Longnecker M, et al. Dietary intake of calcium, magnesium, and antioxidants in relation to risk of amyotrophic lateral sclerosis. *Neuroepidemiology*. 2000;19:210.

Markus C, et al. The bovine protein alpha-lactalbumin increases the ratio of tryptophan to the other large neutral amino acids, and in vulnerable subjects raises brain serotonin activity, reduces cortisol concentration, and improves mood under stress. *Am J Clin Nutri*. 2000;71:1536.

MacGowan D, et al. An ALS-like syndrome with new HIV infection and complete response to antiretroviral therapy. *Neurology*. 2001;57:1094.

Meyers B, Cooper J. Transcervical thymectomy for myasthenia gravis. *Chest Surg Clin N Am*. 2001;11:363.

Mikova O, et al. Increased serum tumor necrosis factor alpha concentrations in major depression and multiple sclerosis. *Eur Neuropsychopharmacol*. 2001;11:203.

Minard G, et al. Early versus delayed feeding with an immune-enhancing diet in patients with severe head injuries. *JPEN*. 2000;24: 1450.

Nelson L, et al. Population-based case-control study of amyotrophic lateral sclerosis in western Washington state. *Am J Epid*. 2000; 151:164.

Pelican S, et al. Nutrition services for alcohol/substance abuse clients. *J Am Diet Assoc*. 1994;94:835.

Raurich J, Ibanez J. Metabolic rate in severe head trauma. *J Parenter Enteral Nutri*. 1994;18:521.

Sanchez-Juan P, Combarros O. Gustatory nervous pathway syndromes. *Neurologia*. 2001;16:262.

Shibata N. Transgenic mouse model for familial amyotrophic lateral sclerosis with superoxide dismutase-1 mutation. *Neuropathology*. 2001;21:82.

Spiers P, et al. Aspartame: neuropsychiatric and neurophysiologic evaluation of acute and chronic effects. *Am J Clin Nutri*. 1998;68: 531.

Spinelli M. Antepartum and postpartum depression. *J Gend Specif Med*. 1998;1:33.

Strong M, et al. Percutaneous gastrojejunostomy in amyotrophic lateral sclerosis. *J Neurol Sci*. 1999;169:128.

Sullivan F, et al. Remotivation therapy and Huntington's disease. *J Neurosci Nurs*. 2001;33:136.

Wilson R, et al. The nutritional management of patients with head injuries. *Neurol Res*. 2001;23:121.

Wong P, et al. Mathematical models of cognitive recovery. *Brain Inj*. 2001;15:519.

Younger D, Raksadawan N. Medical therapies in myasthenia gravis. *Chest Surg Clin N Am*. 2001;11:329.

Other Conditions–Suggested Readings

Barefoot J, et al. Symptoms of depression and changes in body weight from adolescence to mid-life. *Int J Obesity and Related Disorders*. 1998;22:688.

Beal M. Energetics in the pathogenesis of neurodegenerative diseases. *Trends Neurosci*. 2000;23:298.

Hardiman O. Symptomatic treatment of respiratory and nutritional failure in amyotrophic lateral sclerosis. *J Neurol*. 2000;247:245.

Iacono L. Exploring the guidelines for the management of severe head injury. *J Neurosci Nurs*. 2000;32:54.

Lazo M, et al. Osteoporosis and risk of fracture in men with spinal cord injury. *Spinal Cord*. 2001;39:208.

Ragheb S, Lisak R. The thymus and myasthenia gravis. *Chest Surg Clin N Am*. 2001;11:311.

Shivley L, Connolly P. Nutrition in neurologic disease. In: Mahan K, Escott-Stump S, eds. *Krause's food, nutrition, and diet therapy*. 10th ed. Philadelphia: WB Saunders, 2000.

S E C T I O N

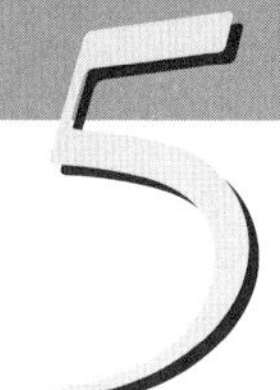

Pulmonary Disorders

CHIEF ASSESSMENT FACTORS

- COUGH, ESPECIALLY WITH CHEST PAIN, HOARSENESS, DIZZINESS
- PAIN (CHEST, ABDOMINAL)
- WHEEZING (WHISTLING, MUSICAL SOUND FROM OBSTRUCTED AIRWAYS)
- STRIDOR (CROWING SOUND ON INHALATION)
- SHORTNESS OF BREATH (DYSPNEA)
- POOR EXERCISE OR ACTIVITY TOLERANCE
- FEVER OR CHILLS
- RAPID BREATHING, EXCESSIVE PERSPIRATION
- DIZZINESS
- FLARING NOSTRILS; RED, SWOLLEN NOSE
- CYANOSIS OF LIPS, NAIL BEDS
- PALLOR; ASHEN OR GRAY COLORING
- CONFUSION, SOMNOLENCE
- ORTHOPNEA, TACHYPNEA
- CLUBBING OF NAIL BEDS
- ENGORGED EYE VEINS
- ALTERED RESPIRATIONS (NL = 14–20 PER MINUTE IN ADULTS)
- ANOREXIA
- ELEVATED BLOOD PRESSURE
- ALTERED BLOOD GASES (DECREASED PARTIAL PRESSURE OF OXYGEN [pO2], INCREASED PARTIAL PRESSURE OF CARBON DIOXIDE [pCO2])
- RESTLESSNESS, IRRITABILITY
- HEMOPTYSIS (COUGHING UP BLOOD)

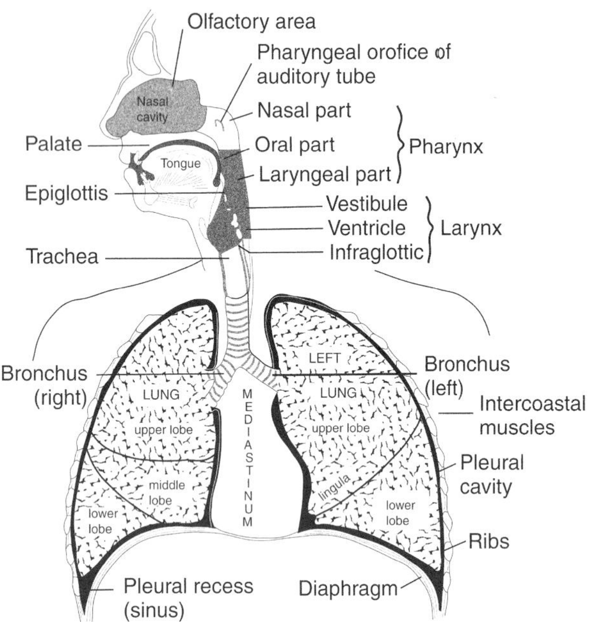

Figure 5–1 The Respiratory System. (Reprinted with permission from Longe R, Calvert J. *Physical assessment: a guide for evaluating drug therapy.* Vancouver, WA: Applied Therapeutics, Inc., 1994.)

PULMONARY NUTRITION NOTES

Pulmonary surfactant is a complex and highly active material composed of lipids and proteins and is found in the fluid lining the alveolar surface of the lungs. Surfactant prevents alveolar collapse at low lung volume and preserves bronchiolar patency during normal and forced respiration (Griese, 1999). It is also involved in protecting the lungs from injuries and infections caused by inhaled particles and micro-organisms (immunological, nonbiophysical functions).

The pathophysiological role for surfactant was first studied in premature infants with respiratory distress syndrome and hyaline membrane disease, a condition now routinely treated with exogenous surfactant replacement. Biochemical surfactant abnormalities of varying degrees have been described in obstructive lung diseases (asthma, bronchiolitis, chronic obstructive pulmonary disease, and after lung transplantation), infectious and suppurative lung diseases (cystic fibrosis, pneumonia, and human immunodeficiency virus), adult respiratory distress syndrome, pulmonary edema, other diseases specific to infants (chronic lung disease of prematurity, and surfactant protein-B deficiency), interstitial lung diseases (sarcoidosis, idiopathic pulmonary fibrosis, and hypersensitivity pneumonitis), pulmonary alveolar proteinosis following cardiopulmonary bypass, and in smokers (Griese, 1999). For some pulmonary conditions, surfactant replacement therapy is on the horizon, but for the majority, much more needs to be learned about the pathophysiological role.

Evidence for a role of diet in asthma and chronic obstructive pulmonary disease (COPD) has been accumulating. Associations have been reported between the intake of fruit, fish, antioxidant vitamins, fatty acids, sodium or magnesium, and indicators of asthma and COPD. Based on the available evidence, dietary guidelines could be proposed for the primary and secondary prevention of asthma and COPD that are in line with existing dietary guidelines for the prevention of coronary heart disease and cancer (Smit, 2001). Because antioxidant nutrients are positively corrected with lung function, vitamin C, vitamin E, beta-carotene, and selenium are important inclusions in the diets of those persons with lung disorders (Hu and Cassano, 2000). Plasma antioxidant capacity increases after drinking cranberry juice (more from the vitamin C than from phenolics); blueberry juice is higher in phenolics than vitamin C and does not have the same effect (Pedersen et al, 2000).

Tables 5–1 and 5–2 list factors that contribute to malnutrition with hypoxic cardiopulmonary disease and respiratory quotients for fats, protein, and carbohydrates.

TABLE 5–1 Factors Contributing to Malnutrition in Patients with Hypoxic Cardiopulmonary Disease

Factors affecting dietary intake:
- Anorexia of chronic illness
- Gastric hypomotility
- Difficulty in eating with continuous dyspnea
- Aerophagia
- Depression, apprehension
- Chronic debility
- Unpalatable diet
- Concurrent vitamin deficiency
- Concurrent fasting ketosis

Metabolic factors:
- Increased mechanical work of breathing
- Increased cardiac work
- Mildly elevated body temperature
- Febrile complications
- Increased sympathetic tone
- Metabolic inefficiency due to cellular hypoxia
- Hypermetabolism

Abnormal losses of nutrients:
- Therapeutic removal of body fluids
- Malabsorption
- Decreased xylose tolerance associated with degree of hypoxemia

Drug side effects:
- Anorexia and nausea
- Increased sympathetic tone

Derived from: Willard M. *Nutritional management for the practicing physician.* Reading, MA: Addison-Wesley Publishing, 1982:28.

TABLE 5–2 Respiratory Quotient (RQ)

RQ = VO2/VCO2
RQ from fat = 0.7
RQ from protein = 0.8
RQ from carbohydrates (CHO) = 1.0

For More Information

- American Lung Association
  212-315-8700
  http://www.lungusa.org/
- Canadian Lung Association
  http://www.lung.ca/
- National Heart, Lung, and Blood Institute
  http://www.nhlbi.nih.gov/
- National Jewish Center for Immunology and Respiratory Medicine
  1-800-222-LUNG
  http://www.njc.org/main.html

ASTHMA

NUTRITIONAL ACUITY RANKING: LEVEL 1

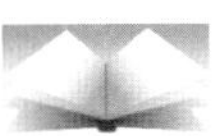

DEFINITIONS AND BACKGROUND

Bronchial asthma involves paroxysmal dyspnea accompanied by wheezing and is caused by spasm of the bronchial tubes or swelling of their mucous membranes. Bronchial asthma differs from wheezing caused by cardiac failure (cardiac asthma), in which an x-ray shows fluid in the lung.

The timing of events leading to allergic sensitization has become a very important area in the attempt to halt the dramatic increase in the prevalence of diseases such as asthma, eczema, and hay fever; research has demonstrated that events taking place during the gestational period may well play a role in determining whether or not a genetic susceptibility becomes translated into disease processes (Warner and Warner, 2000). More than 12 million Americans are affected by asthma, ranking seventh among chronic conditions. Asthma seems to be inherited in two-thirds of cases.

Most infants with wheezing have transient conditions that later clear; only a small number have asthma later in life. Among transient cases (i.e., those who possibly had an infection with wheezing at 3–4-years-old), day-care attendance and a short duration of breastfeeding resulted in increased risk; results support the hypothesis that opportunity for early infections reduces the risk of asthma (Infante-Rivard et al., 2001). Overall, there continues to be controversy over the role of breastfeeding and risk for asthma. Some studies of children breastfed exclusively for the first 4 months of life show decrease risk for asthma (Oddy, 2000), while other studies suggest that breastfeeding promotes it (Takemura et al., 2001). Longer duration of breastfeeding seems to be more protective (Dell and To, 2001).

Signs and symptoms of asthma include respiratory distress, audible wheezing, decreased breath sounds, tachycardia, cyanosis, hypotension, anxiety, pulmonary edema, dehydration, hard and dry cough, and distended neck veins. Two types of bronchial asthma are recognized: allergic (extrinsic) and nonallergic (intrinsic or infectious). Chronic poor control can lead to a serious condition, status asthmaticus, which generally requires hospitalization and can be life threatening. Brittle asthma is a rare form of asthma with repeated attacks, either with wide variation from predicted daily peak expiratory flow or with apparent good control of asthma (Baker et al., 2000). A high prevalence of food intolerances has been noted with brittle asthma.

For children 2- to 3-years-old, noninvasive viruses like the common cold virus and rhinovirus (RV) continue to be major triggers of wheezing, a pattern that also continues for adults with asthma. This appears to be unique among allergic patients. Children of smokers tend to have more asthma than children of nonsmokers (Hatch, 1995). Because treatment varies so much from one pediatrician to another, the American Academy of Allergy, Asthma, and Immunology (AAAAI), in partnership with the National Asthma Education and Prevention Program (NAEPP), coordinated by the National Heart, Lung, and Blood Institute, launched a comprehensive new initiative—Pediatric Asthma: Promoting Best Practice.

Overweight is significantly higher in children with moderate-to-severe asthma than in their healthy peers; being overweight affects severity. Studies are needed to investigate the effects of weight loss on lung function and other markers of asthma severity (Luder et al., 1998). Body mass index (BMI) is significantly positively associated with risk of adult-onset asthma; women who gain a significant amount of weight after age 18 have a much higher risk of developing asthma later in life (Camargo et al., 1999). The effects of increased BMI on asthma may be mediated by mechanical properties of the respiratory system associated with obesity or by inflammatory mechanisms rather than by allergic eosinophilic inflammation of the airway epithelium (von Mutius et al., 2001).

An early intake of cereals in the diet by infants might cause IgE sensitization to cereals, with possible grass-pollen allergy later in life (Armentia et al., 2001). Studies are needed.

OBJECTIVES

- Prevent distention of stomach from large meals, resulting in distress and perhaps aggravation of asthmatic state.
- Prevent lung infection and inflammation. Promote improved resistance against disease, especially for nonallergic type. Diet affects the pathophysiology of asthma by altered immune or antioxidant activity with consequent effects on airway inflammation.
- For allergic asthma, identify and control allergens in the environment.
- Promote adequate hydration to liquefy secretions.
- Optimize nutritional status. Vitamins C, B6, and magnesium are important (Schwartz and Weiss, 1994). Vitamin C plays a protective role against nitrogen oxides, which arise from both endogenous and exogenous sources (Hatch, 1995); however, low vitamin C levels do not seem to be specifically associated with wheezing (Mainous, 2000). Vitamin E is modestly protective against symptoms (Troisi et al., 1995). Encourage foods high in selenium also (Brown and Arthur, 2001).
- Lung function is found to be better with higher antioxidant levels (Hu and Cassano, 2000).
- Encourage a health maintenance program.
- Caffeine relaxes muscles and opens airways of the lung. About 2–3 cups of coffee daily may be useful in adults.

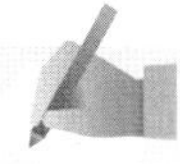

DIETARY AND NUTRITIONAL RECOMMENDATIONS

- Provide balanced, small meals that are nutrient dense (i.e., high-quality protein, calories, vitamins, and minerals), especially to reduce risk of infections and poor state of health.

- Highlight foods rich in vitamins A, B6 (Bartel et al., 1994), and zinc. Vitamin C is especially important for its antioxidant effect (Abbey et al., 1995); use more broccoli, grapefruit, oranges, sweet peppers, kiwi, tomato juice, and cauliflower.
- Other nutrients that support immunocompetence should be addressed. Quercetin in apples, onions, oranges, and berries are good; use 5 or more times per week. Include sources of selenium such as Brazil nuts and vitamin E.
- For allergic asthma, omit food allergens as identified. Only 4% of adult patients with asthma will have food allergies; the common foods to omit are milk, eggs, seafood, and fish. Sulfites may also need to be assessed carefully. Salicylates rarely are a problem but may aggravate asthma in 2% of patients.
- Encourage extra fluids unless otherwise contraindicated.
- For some individuals, salt intake may be beneficial if controlled (Mickleborough et al., 2001). This tends to be true for men more than for women (Knox, 1993); evidence in this area is still unclear.
- Saturated and monounsaturated fats may have different effects on airway inflammation; saturated fatty acids (SFAs) may aggravate and monounsaturated fatty acids (MUFAs) may be inversely related (Huang and Pan, 2001). Omega-3 fatty acids may be useful for those without fish allergy. Walnuts and flaxseed may be used if tolerated.

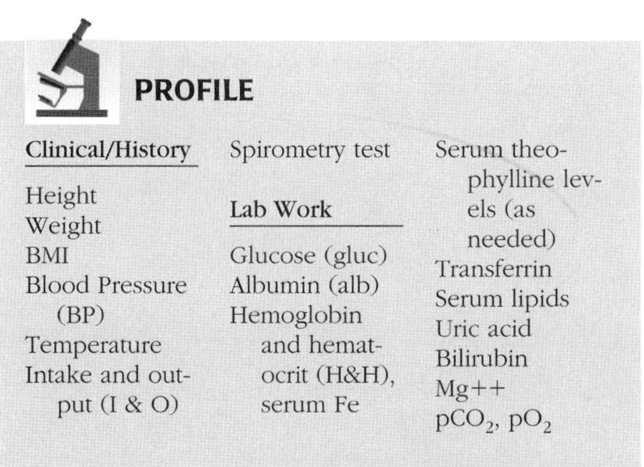

PROFILE

Clinical/History	Lab Work	
Height	Glucose (gluc)	Serum theophylline levels (as needed)
Weight	Albumin (alb)	Transferrin
BMI	Hemoglobin and hematocrit (H&H), serum Fe	Serum lipids
Blood Pressure (BP)		Uric acid
Temperature		Bilirubin
Intake and output (I & O)		Mg++
Spirometry test		pCO_2, pO_2

Common Drugs Used and Potential Side Effects

- Bronchodilators—nausea and vomiting can be a problem for some types of these drugs. Theophylline (Theo-Dur, Slo-BID, Slo-Phyllin, Theolair, Uniphyl) metabolism is affected by protein and CHO availability; avoid extreme changes in protein and CHO intake. Because it is a methylxanthine, avoid extreme changes in usual intakes of caffeine-containing foods. Theophylline depresses levels of vitamin B6. In addition, lipid levels (cholesterol, high-density lipoprotein [HDL], and HDL: low-density lipoprotein [LDL] ratios) are higher in children who are taking theophylline. No changes in risk are observed in cases of cardiac heart disease (CHD). Metaproterenol (Metaprel, Alupent) may alter taste and cause nausea or vomiting. Albuterol (Ventolin, Proventil) may have cardiac side effects or may cause nausea or diarrhea.
- Antibiotics—long-term use can cause diarrhea and other problems. Penicillin should not be taken with fruit juices.
- Epinephrine may be required for emergencies. Intravenous (IV) administration of epinephrine results in a prolonged increase in resting energy expenditure (REE) as measured by RQ; fuel for this is increased CHO oxidation. Rate of protein oxidation does not change, and REE returns to normal 24 hours after epinephrine infusion stops (Ratheiser et al., 1998).
- Potassium iodide, an expectorant, may affect existing thyroid problems.
- Corticosteroids (Medrol/Methylprednisone) have many side effects such as depleting serum potassium and retaining excess sodium, causing hyperglycemia, and other problems. Monitor carefully, especially if needed over a long period of time. AeroBid contains an anti-inflammatory steroid and is inhaled; it may cause nausea, vomiting, or diarrhea. Bone mineral density is often decreased after long-term use of inhaled corticosteroids (Sivri and Coplu, 2001). A follow-up of patients with asthma who are taking inhaled corticosteroids is needed to assess bone density, decreases in osteocalcin levels, and dietary intakes of calcium (Gagnon et al., 1997).

Herbs, Botanicals and Supplements

- Formulas with enhanced omega-3 fatty acids are being tested to reduce lung inflammation from leukotrienes. However, asthma patients should not expect supplementation of their diet with these fatty acids to help their condition (Woods et al., 2000).
- Ephedra (ma huang) is an effective bronchodilator, but it increases blood pressure significantly. Avoid taking with digoxin, hypoglycemic agents for diabetes, monoamine oxidase inhibitor (MAOI) antidepressants, antihypertensive medications, oxytocin, theophylline, caffeine, and dexamethasone steroids. Problems with blood pressure, blood glucose, arrhythmias, increased heart rate, and central nervous system (CNS) stimulation can occur.
- Stinging nettle, licorice, gingko, and anise have been suggested; efficacy and side effects must be evaluated.
- One study of massage therapy involved children with asthma. The 30-day study revealed increased relaxation, decreased anxiety, and better lung function scores.
- Insect bites that cause asthmatic attacks have no correlation with diet, although for some persons, use of thiamine hydrochloride can reduce biting of mosquitoes. Check with a physician regarding any over-the-counter or home remedies for asthma.
- St. John's wort can inhibit theophylline's effectiveness.

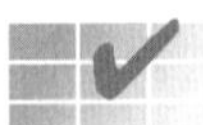

PATIENT EDUCATION

✔ Mild, chronic asthma can be a warning that, if untreated, can lead to an acute exacerbation.
✔ All medications should be taken as directed by the physician.
✔ Work with the patient/family to avoid precipitating events or triggers. Discuss exercise, rest, and nutrition.

For More Information

- Allergy and Asthma Advocate
  http://www.aaaai.org/public/publicedmat/advocate/default.stm
- Allergy and Asthma Network–Mothers of Asthmatics
  2751 Prosperity Ave., Suite 150
  Fairfax, VA 22031
  1-800-878-4403
  http://www.aanma.org/
- Jewish Center for Immunology and Respiratory Disease
  National Asthma Center
  1999 Julian Street
  Denver, CO 80204
  http://nationaljewish.org/main.html
  1-800-227-5864
- National Asthma Education and Prevention Program (NAEPP)
  http://www.nhlbi.nih.gov/about/naepp/

BRONCHIECTASIS

NUTRITIONAL ACUITY RANKING: LEVEL 1 OR 2

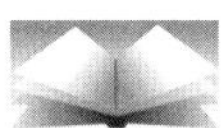

DEFINITIONS AND BACKGROUND

Bronchiectasis belongs to the family of chronic obstructive lung diseases, although it is much less common than asthma, chronic bronchitis, or emphysema (Mysliwiec and Pina, 1999). Bronchiectasis is an irreversible widening of portions of the bronchi resulting from damage to the bronchial wall. Chronic dilation of the bronchi (or a bronchus) occurs in this condition.

The triad of chronic cough, profuse, foul, and purulent sputum production, and hemoptysis is common. Other symptoms and signs include early morning paroxysmal cough, decreased breath sounds, weight loss, fatigue, anorexia, pneumonia, and fever. The most common causes are acute respiratory illness in patients with COPD. Other causes include measles, whooping cough, tuberculosis, fungal infection, inhaled object, lung tumor, cystic fibrosis, ciliary dyskinesia, immunoglobulin deficiency syndromes, rheumatoid arthritis, ulcerative colitis, HIV infection, and heroin abuse.

The relapse of bronchiectasis can be controlled with antibiotics, chest physiotherapy, inhaled bronchodilators, proper hydration, and good nutrition (Mysliwiec and Pina, 1999). In rare circumstances, surgical resection or bilateral lung transplantation may be the only option available for improving quality of life. Surgery has few complications and improves symptoms in the great majority of patients, especially when complete resection of the disease is achieved (Prieto et al., 2001). Physiological lung exclusion is sometimes used for control of massive hemoptysis in cases where lung resection is not advised.

OBJECTIVES

- Promote recovery.
- Avoid fatigue associated with mealtimes.
- Prevent or correct dehydration.
- Improve weight status, when necessary.
- Reduce fever and inflammation.
- Prevent relapse.
- Support lung function, which is found to be better with higher antioxidant levels (Hu and Cassano, 2000).
- Prevent lung collapse or atelectasis.

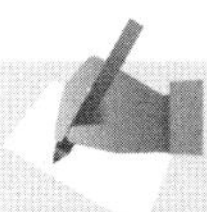

DIETARY AND NUTRITIONAL RECOMMENDATIONS

- Use a diet with 1.0–1.25 g protein/kg and sufficient calories to meet elevated metabolic requirements appropriate for age and sex.
- Small, frequent feedings may be better tolerated.
- Fluid intake of 2–3 L daily may be offered, unless contraindicated.
- Intravenous fat emulsions may be indicated (eicosanoids are inflammatory modulators, and thromboxanes and leukotrienes tend to be potent mediators of inflammation).
- Adequate antioxidant use with vitamins C, E, and selenium may be beneficial. Ensure adequate potassium intake, depending on medications used.

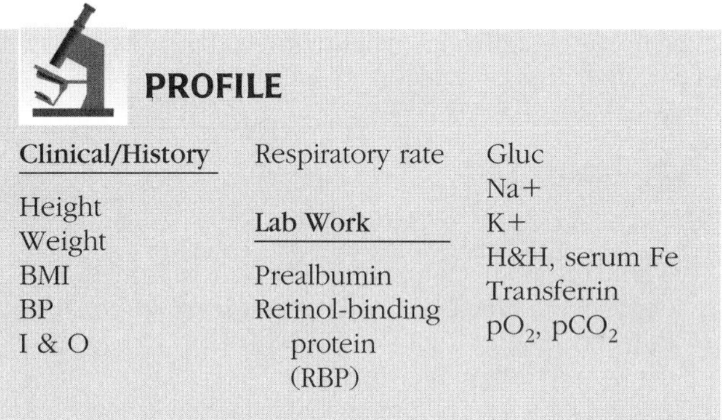

PROFILE

Clinical/History

Height
Weight
BMI
BP
I & O
Respiratory rate

Lab Work

Prealbumin
Retinol-binding protein (RBP)
Gluc
Na+
K+
H&H, serum Fe
Transferrin
pO_2, pCO_2

Common Drugs Used and Potential Side Effects

- Antibiotics are used if the condition is bacterial in origin.
- Analgesics and antipyretics may be used. Monitor side effects according to the specific drugs used.
- Dry powder mannitol has been shown to improve tracheobronchial clearance in bronchiectasis but is not yet available for clinical use.

Herbs, Botanicals and Supplements

- No clinical trials have proven efficacy for use of herbs or botanicals in bronchiectasis.

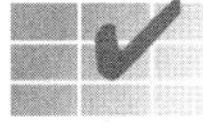

PATIENT EDUCATION

- Discuss the role of nutrition in health and recovery; emphasize quality proteins and nutrient-dense foods, especially if the patient is anorexic.
- Emphasize fluid intake, perhaps recommending juices or calorie-containing beverages instead of water.

BRONCHITIS (ACUTE)

NUTRITIONAL ACUITY RANKING: LEVEL 1

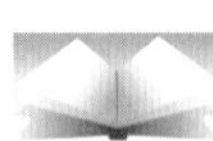

DEFINITIONS AND BACKGROUND

Bronchitis is caused by inflammation of the air passages. The acute form may follow a cold or other upper-respiratory infection, producing hemoptysis, sore throat, nasal discharge, slight fever, cough, and back and muscle pain. Causes include *Mycoplasma pneumoniae* and *Chlamydia;* exposure to strong acids, ammonia or chlorine fumes, air pollution ozone, or nitrogen dioxide. The chronic form–believed to be due mostly to cigarette smoking and air pollution–can produce breathing difficulty, wheezing, blueness, fits of coughing, and sputum production. (See COPD entry.)

OBJECTIVES

- Normalize body temperature when there is fever.
- Replenish nutrients used in respiratory distress.
- Prevent complications such as dehydration and otitis media; avoid further infections.
- Allow ample rest before and after feedings.
- Prevent dehydration. Extra fluids are needed.
- Relieve discomfort.
- Support lung function, which is found to be better with higher antioxidant levels (Hu and Cassano, 2000).

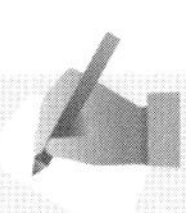

DIETARY AND NUTRITIONAL RECOMMENDATIONS

- Provide a regular or high-calorie diet, specific to the patient's needs.
- Milk gives a sensation of thickening mucus secretions, but this is anecdotal only. Skim milk may be better tolerated at this time and is important for adequate calcium consumption.
- Provide adequate amounts of vitamins C, E, selenium, and potassium.
- Increase the intake of fluids, 2–3 L unless contraindicated.
- Appropriate fatty acid intake may be beneficial to reduce inflammation.

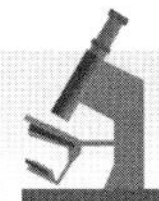

PROFILE

Clinical/History		
Height	Edema	K+
Weight	**Lab Work**	Alb, prealbumin
BMI	Na+	Total lymphocyte count (TLC)
I & O	H&H	Mg++

Common Drugs Used and Potential Side Effects

- Bronchodilators can cause gastric irritation. They should be taken with milk, food, or an antacid.
- Theophylline can be toxic if a diet high in carbohydrates and low in protein is used. Avoid large amounts of stimulant beverages, namely, coffee, tea, cocoa, and cola, unless the physician permits.
- Antibiotics may be used. Avoid taking penicillin with fruit juice.

Herbs, Botanicals and Supplements

- No clinical trials have proven efficacy for use of herbs or botanicals such as eucalyptus, mullein, horehound, stinging nettle, or marshmallow.
- Belladonna leaf and root are respiratory antispasmodic agents. They should not be used with tricyclic antidepressants, some antihistamines, phenothiazines, or quinidine. Sedation, dry mouth, and difficult urination may occur.

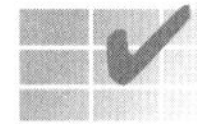

PATIENT EDUCATION

- Explain to the patient that adequate hydration is one of the best ways to liquefy secretions.
- Maintain body weight within a healthy range.

CHRONIC OBSTRUCTIVE PULMONARY DISEASES (EMPHYSEMA AND CHRONIC BRONCHITIS)

NUTRITIONAL ACUITY RANKING: LEVEL 2–3

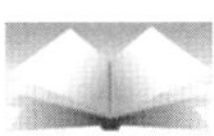

DEFINITIONS AND BACKGROUND

COPD may result from a history of emphysema, asthma, chronic bronchitis, etc. with persistent lower airway obstruction. Smoking is the most common cause. Starvation can cause emphysema, even without smoking. Symptoms and signs of COPD include dyspnea on exertion, frequent hypoxemia, decreased forced expiratory volume in one second, and destruction of alveolar capillary bed. In COPD, total air quantity is blown out much sooner. COPD is a leading cause of death in the United States.

Chronic bronchitis ("blue bloater patient") involves inflamed bronchial tubes with excess mucus production, chronic cough (for 3 months each year), shortness of breath, and no weight loss. Cardiac enlargement with failure is common. COPD and chronic heart failure are both associated with muscular impairment, nutritional depletion, and systemic inflammation (Gosker et al., 2000).

Emphysema ("pink puffer patient") causes weight loss and thinness without heart failure. It is characterized by tissue destruction, distention, and destruction of pulmonary air spaces by smoking and air pollution. Wheezing, shortness of breath (SOB), and chronic mild cough result. Nutritional depletion is significantly greater in patients who have emphysema than in those who have chronic bronchitis. Serious weight loss occurs from anorexia, secondary to significant SOB and gastrointestinal (GI) distress.

Recently, studies have shown that pulmonary inflammation may be detected in the systemic circulation. This has an important clinical consequence—loss of skeletal muscle mass, which limits exercise capacity, jeopardizes health status and has a negative impact on prognosis (Agusti, 2001). Malnutrition and tissue wasting are common in patients with COPD (Farber and Mannix, 2000). Risk of respiratory mortality is higher among patients who are malnourished than among those who are well nourished (Thorsdottir et al., 2001). Approximately 75% of patients with COPD suffer from weight loss where chronic mouth breathing, dyspnea, aerophagia, certain medications, and depression often act in concert. Malnutrition decreases ventilatory muscle strength, exercise tolerance, and immunocompetence.

Recommendations for fats, CHO, proteins, and water must be individualized (Chapman and Winter, 1996). One study suggests that a high dietary intake of omega-3 fatty acids may protect smokers against COPD because of the anti-inflammatory effects (Shahar et al., 1994). Differences in fruit and fish intake may partially explain the differences in mortality between populations who have COPD; high fruit intake is most important (Tabak et al., 1998).

Underweight subjects with COPD may have significantly higher bitter taste thresholds than normal-weight subjects, which is related to bicarbonate levels and pH (Chapman-Novakofski et al., 1999). Foods such as meats, vegetables, and coffee may be more bland to the patient than he/she has remembered; recognition of this may be important in planning meals.

OBJECTIVES

- Screen early and correct any malnutrition. Because there is less oxygen available for adenosine triphosphate (ATP) formation, the patient is less able to be active, and there is less blood flow to the GI tract and muscles. Malnutrition increases likelihood of infections.
- Overcome anorexia resulting from slowed peristalsis and digestion. Patient lethargy, poor appetite, and gastric ulceration result from inadequate oxygen to GI cells.
- Improve ventilation before meals with intermittent positive-pressure breathing and overall physical conditioning to strengthen respiratory muscles.
- Lessen work efforts by losing weight, if needed, or prevent excessive losses, which can increase morbidity.
- Prevent respiratory infections or respiratory acidosis from decreased CO_2 elimination. Decrease excess CO_2 production.
- Alleviate difficulty in chewing or swallowing from SOB.
- Prevent or correct dehydration, which thickens mucus.
- Avoid constipation and straining at stool.
- Avoid distention from large meals or gaseous foods.
- Ensure adequate flavor of foods, because appetite is often minimized.
- Improved pulmonary function after vitamin A supplementation suggests that patients with COPD have a local respiratory vitamin A deficiency (Paiva et al., 1996). In addition, lung function is found to be better with higher antioxidant levels (Hu and Cassano, 2000).

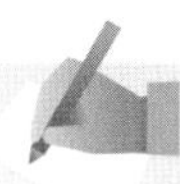

DIETARY AND NUTRITIONAL RECOMMENDATIONS

- A high-protein/high-calorie diet is necessary to correct malnutrition. Use 1.2–1.5 g protein/kg and basal energy expenditure (BEE) × 1.5–1.7 for anabolism. Promote weight loss through a calorie-controlled diet for obese patients. Diets should be 40–55% CHO, 30–40% fat, and 15–20% protein.
- A soft diet (no tough or stringy foods) and an antireflux regimen are recommended. Gas-forming vegetables are not allowed, unless tolerated well. Increase use of omega-3 fatty acids in foods such as salmon, haddock, mackerel, tuna, and other fish sources.
- To enrich the diet with antioxidants, use more citrus fruits, whole grains, salmon, mackerel, and tuna. Supplement diet with vitamins A and C to support lung function, allow healing, and improve formation of tissue. B-complex vitamins may also be needed for energy metabolism. Magnesium also plays an important role (Britton et al., 1994).
- Use small, concentrated feedings at frequent intervals to lessen fatigue. Eggnogs and shakes may be helpful.
- Fluid intake should be high, especially if the patient is

febrile. Use 1 mL/kcal as a general rule. This may translate to eight or more cups of fluid daily. For discomfort, consume liquids between meals to increase intake of nutrient-dense foods. Use caffeinated beverages in moderation, because they may increase nervousness.

- For patients with peripheral edema, restrict intake of sodium and increase levels of potassium.
- Fiber should be increased gradually, perhaps through use of crushed bran, prune juice, and extra fruits and vegetables.
- Chicken soup clears the respiratory tract better than plain water; monitor effectiveness.
- If necessary, moderate CHO is needed to avoid overload. During anabolism, dietary CHO should be less than 50% of kcal intake. Lipid intake is safe up to 55% of kcal but is only indicated with high-calorie diets.
- Pulmocare or Respalor may be useful for tube feedings.
- Limit salt intake; too much sodium can cause fluid retention that may interfere with breathing.
- See Tables 5–3 and 5–4 for ways to add extra protein or calories to a diet.

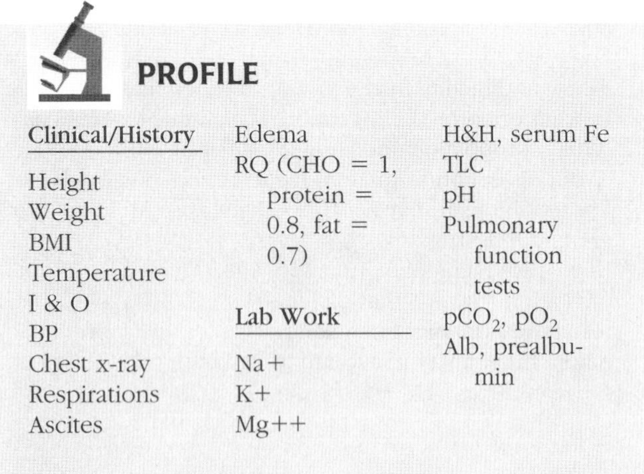

PROFILE

Clinical/History		
Height	Edema	H&H, serum Fe
Weight	RQ (CHO = 1, protein = 0.8, fat = 0.7)	TLC
BMI		pH
Temperature	**Lab Work**	Pulmonary function tests
I & O	Na+	pCO_2, pO_2
BP	K+	Alb, prealbumin
Chest x-ray	Mg++	
Respirations		
Ascites		

TABLE 5–3 Food Tips to Add Calories to a Diet

To add calories to a diet from fat and carbohydrate:

- Fats can be used, including butter or margarine, cream, sour cream, gravies, salad dressings, and shortening. Mix butter into hot foods such as soups and vegetables, mashed potatoes, cooked cereals, and rice. Serve hot bread with lots of melted butter and jelly.
- Mayonnaise can be added to salads or sandwiches.
- Sour cream or yogurt can be used on vegetables such as potatoes, beans, carrots, and squash. Try sour cream or yogurt in gravy or salad dressings for fruit.
- Spread honey on toast, in tea, or on cereal.
- Whipping cream has 60 kcal per tablespoon. Add it to pies, fruits, pudding, hot chocolate, gelatin, eggnog, and other desserts.
- Add marshmallows to hot chocolate.
- Fry the entree (e.g., chicken, meat, fish). The caloric value of fried foods is higher than that of baked or broiled foods.
- Have snacks ready to eat: nuts, dried fruits, candy, buttered popcorn, crackers and cheese, granola, ice cream, and popsicles.
- Drink milk shakes with lots of ice cream added. These will be high in calories and protein.

TABLE 5–4 Tips for Adding Protein to a Diet

- Protein can be added to many foods without having to increase the number of foods eaten.
- Add skim milk powder to the regular amount of milk used in recipes or for a beverage. Or, add 1 cup of dry powder to 1 quart of fluid milk, allow it to sit overnight. This adds 286 kcal and 15 g protein. This is "double-strength milk."
- Add protein powder to casseroles, soups, sauces, gravies, milkshakes, and eggnogs. One scoop may have 4 or 5 grams of protein, depending on the brand. Some do not stir in as well as others; some dissolve better in hot foods.
- Add milk powder to hot or cold cereals, scrambled eggs, mashed potatoes, soups, gravies, ground meats (e.g., meat patties, meatballs, meatloaf), casserole dishes, and baked goods.
- Use milk or half-and-half, instead of water, when making soups, cereals, instant puddings, cocoa, and canned soups.
- Add diced or ground meat to soups and casseroles.
- Add grated cheese or cheese chunks to sauces, vegetables, soups, casseroles, hot crab dip, and mashed potatoes. Add extra cheese to pizza.
- Choose dessert recipes that contain egg such as sponge or angel food cake, egg custard, bread pudding, or rice pudding.
- Buy instant breakfast mixes and use them instead of milk with meals or as snacks. One 8-oz glass provides 280 kcal. Formulary products that are high in protein may be useful as supplements with or between meals, or with medication pass in an institution.
- Peanut butter (1 tablespoon = 90 kcal plus some protein) can be spread on crackers, apples, celery, pears, and bananas.
- Use yogurt as a fruit dip, or add to sauces and gravies.
- Serve a chef salad that includes chunks of cheese, ham, turkey, and sliced egg.

Common Drugs Used and Potential Side Effects

- Bronchodilators (Atrovent, Theo-Dur, etc.) are used to liquefy secretions, treat infections, and dilate the bronchi. They can cause gastric irritation and ulceration.
- Antibiotics, steroids, expectorants, antihistamines, diuretics, anticholinergics, and other drugs may be used. Monitor accordingly.
- Corticosteroids may be needed for chronic bronchitis.

Herbs, Botanicals and Supplements

- No clinical trials have proven efficacy for use of herbs or botanicals such as mullein, camu-camu, licorice, red pepper, peppermint, or eucalyptus.
- Ephedra (ma huang) is an effective bronchodilator, but it increases blood pressure significantly. Avoid taking with digoxin, hypoglycemic agents for diabetes, MAOI antidepressants, antihypertensive medications, oxytocin, theophylline, caffeine, and dexamethasone steroids. Problems with blood pressure, blood glucose, arrhythmias, increased heart rate, and CNS stimulation can occur.

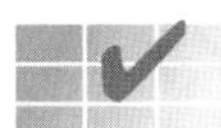

PATIENT EDUCATION

- ✓ Explain how to conserve energy while preparing meals at home. Choose foods that are easy to prepare. Try the main meal early in the day to have more energy throughout the rest of the day.
- ✓ Explain how to concentrate protein and calories in small feedings.
- ✓ Encourage rest periods before and after meals. Encourage slow eating.
- ✓ Encourage the patient to make small, attractive meals. Six small meals will prevent overfilling the stomach and causing more shortness of breath.
- ✓ Explain that excessively hot or cold foods may cause coughing spells.
- ✓ Limit fluid intake with meals to decrease early satiety and subsequent decreased food intake.
- ✓ Schedule treatments to mobilize mucus (postural drainage, aerosol treatment) 1 hour before and after meals to prevent nausea.
- ✓ Improve physical conditioning with planned exercises, especially strengthening exercises.
- ✓ Lung function in the general population is related to antioxidant vitamin intake; it plays a protective role against COPD (Britton et al., 1995).
- ✓ If using oxygen, be sure the cannula is worn during and after meals. Eating and digestion require energy, which causes the body to use more oxygen.
- ✓ Maintain a relaxed atmosphere to make meals attractive and enjoyable.
- ✓ Promote good oral hygiene; there may be a relationship with periodontal disease and COPD (Scannapieco and Ho, 2001).

For More Information

- ✦ American Dietetic Association
  COPD protocol
  www.eatright.org
- ✦ COPD
  http://www.aarc.org/patient_education/tips/copd.html
- ✦ National Emphysema Treatment Trial (Nett)
  http://www.nhlbi.nih.gov/health/prof/lung/nett/lvrsweb.htm
- ✦ National Heart Lung and Blood Institute—COPD
  http://www.nhlbi.nih.gov/health/public/lung/other/copd/index.htm

CHYLOTHORAX

NUTRITIONAL ACUITY RANKING: LEVEL 3

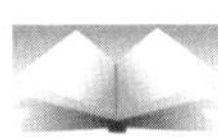

DEFINITIONS AND BACKGROUND

Chylothorax involves accumulation of clear lymph (chyle) in the pleural or thoracic space. It may be spontaneous or caused by invasion of the thoracic space. Etiologies may also include amyloidosis, congenital chylothorax, coronary artery bypass grafting (CABG), violent vomiting or coughing after heavy meals, cancer, complications of neck surgery including a radical dissection, spontaneous accumulation, thoracic cage compression after CPR, thoracic duct trauma from thoracotomy tubes, thoracic surgery affecting the heart, lungs, or esophagus, thrombosis of the subclavian vein during total parenteral nutrition (TPN), or tuberculosis.

Breast milk and/or regular infant feeding formula should be used in the congenital form before proceeding to medium-chain triglyceride (MCT)-rich formula; surgery should be considered if conservative management of congenital chylothorax fails after 4–5 weeks (Al-Tawil et al., 2001).

OBJECTIVES

- Offer continuous chest-tube drainage to decrease pleural chyle.
- Lessen consequences of a nutritional or immunological nature from drainage (e.g., sepsis, protein–calorie malnutrition (PCM), decreased TLC, and other parameters).
- Replace fat, protein, and micronutrient losses from exudates.
- Achieve a positive nitrogen balance.

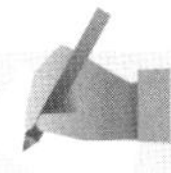

DIETARY AND NUTRITIONAL RECOMMENDATIONS

- Decrease enteral fat intake for patients who are tube fed. For patients who are fed orally, reduce total fat intake.
- For patients without sepsis, TPN may be indicated, with care to avoid aggravating the condition.
- For patients who are fed normally, a low-fat diet may be used alone or with an elemental product.
- Replace exudate losses of nutrients such as vitamin A and zinc. Check serum levels and replace with higher levels of the recommended dietary allowance (RDA) as necessary.

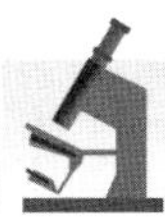

PROFILE

Clinical/History	Lab Work	
Height	Alb, prealbumin	(chol)/triglycerides (Trig)
Weight	RBP	TLC (decreased)
BMI	H&H	Gluc
Weight changes	Transferrin	Mg++
Temperature	Cholesterol	Na+, K+
I & O		

Common Drugs Used and Potential Side Effects

- Medications are given, as appropriate, for the etiology. Monitor side effects accordingly, especially in conditions such as tuberculosis (TB) or cancer in which numerous side effects are created from drug therapies.
- Bronchodilators may be used. Some nausea and vomiting may occur.

Herbs, Botanicals and Supplements

- No clinical trials have proven efficacy for use of herbs or botanicals in chylothorax.

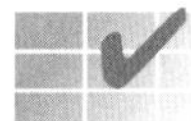

PATIENT EDUCATION

- ✔ Discuss the importance of adequate nutrition in recovery.
- ✔ Discuss interventions that are appropriate for the conditions and diagnoses involved.

COR PULMONALE

NUTRITIONAL ACUITY RANKING: LEVEL 2

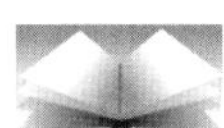

DEFINITIONS AND BACKGROUND

A heart disease following disease of the lung (end-stage emphysema, silicosis, etc.), cor pulmonale strains the right ventricle, creating hypertrophy and eventual failure. It may be acute, subacute, or chronic. Signs and symptoms include hypoxia, wheezing, cough, fatigue, weakness, cyanosis, and clubbing of the extremities.

OBJECTIVES

- ▲ Improve the patient's capacity to eat meals without straining the diaphragm.
- ▲ Correct malnourished status. Weight gain may not always be indicated, because this would increase stress on the heart.
- ▲ Reduce or prevent fluid retention and edema to lessen cardiac workload.
- ▲ Prevent additional damage to cardiac and respiratory tissues.
- ▲ Support adequate lung function, which is found to be better with higher antioxidant levels (Hu and Cassano, 2000).

DIETARY AND NUTRITIONAL RECOMMENDATIONS

- Recommend small, frequent meals.
- Use a high-calorie diet with concentrated protein sources: double-strength milk, foods with milk powder added to them, high-calorie supplements, and addition of extra gravies or sauces to meals.
- To reduce fluid retention, intake of fluids may be restricted to 500 mL plus the amount of the previous day's fluid intake. Sodium restriction may also be necessary.
- Use soft or bland foods to reduce gastric irritation and reflux.
- Provide adequate potassium intake, unless fluid retention elevates levels excessively.
- Include adequate to higher levels of vitamins C, E, and selenium.

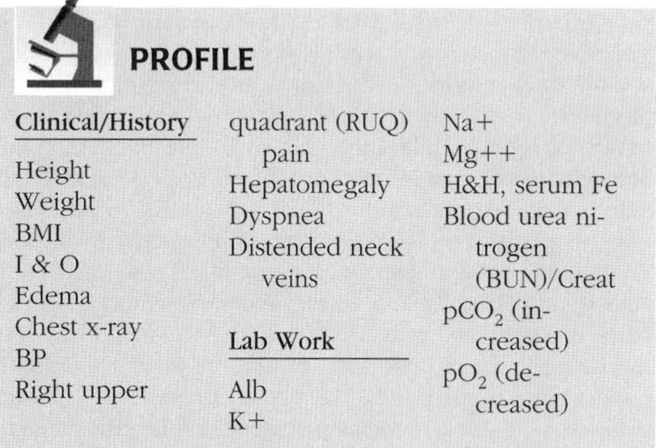

PROFILE

Clinical/History

Height
Weight
BMI
I & O
Edema
Chest x-ray
BP
Right upper quadrant (RUQ) pain
Hepatomegaly
Dyspnea
Distended neck veins

Lab Work

Alb
K+
Na+
Mg++
H&H, serum Fe
Blood urea nitrogen (BUN)/Creat
pCO_2 (increased)
pO_2 (decreased)

Common Drugs Used and Potential Side Effects

- ■ Corticosteroids can cause sodium retention, negative N balance, etc. Monitor carefully.
- ■ Diuretics can cause potassium depletion with diuresis.

Herbs, Botanicals and Supplements

- ■ No clinical trials have proven efficacy for use of herbs or botanicals in cor pulmonale.

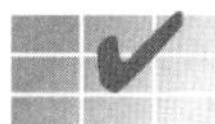

PATIENT EDUCATION

- ✓ Plan small, attractive meals that are nutrient dense.
- ✓ Emphasize the importance of eating slowly.
- ✓ Recommend snacks that are high in calories and protein but that do not provide excessive amounts of sodium.

CYSTIC FIBROSIS

NUTRITIONAL ACUITY RANKING: LEVEL 4

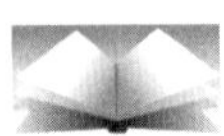

DEFINITIONS AND BACKGROUND

Cystic fibrosis (CF) or mucoviscidosis is an autosomal-recessive, inherited disease. Manifestations include general dysfunction of mucus-producing exocrine glands, high levels of sodium and chloride in the saliva and tears, high levels of electrolytes in the sweat, and highly viscous secretions in the pancreas, bronchi, bile ducts, and small intestine. Meconium ileus is a classic sign in newborn infants with CF; it is thicker than usual and passes more slowly. About one in 2,500 Caucasians is affected; 2–5% of Caucasians carry the CF gene. The median life expectancy for cystic fibrosis is now over 30 years, and it is projected that in newborn infants it will become more than 40 years (Doull, 2001). The identification of the CF gene and its product, cystic fibrosis transmembrane conductance regulator (CFTR), has widened the spectrum of the disease; there is increasing evidence of the advantages of newborn screening for CF and subsequent specialist care (Doull, 2001).

Pancreatic insufficiency occurs in 80–90%, and 85% show growth retardation. Decreased bone density and increased risk of fractures are seen in patients with CF; osteoporosis is seen due to longer life expectancy (Lambert, 2000). Nutrition problems, hypogonadism, inactivity, corticosteroid use, and cytokines may contribute to the low bone mass seen in these patients. Treatment recommendations must be individualized and may include nutrition, vitamin D, estrogen or testosterone, and exercise (Ott and Aiken, 1998).

A major goal in the management of CF patients is to maintain a good nutritional status as it improves long-term survival (Munck and Navarro, 2000). A link has been established between the degree of malnutrition and the severity of the disease. Stature is a significant prognostic indicator of CF survival (Beker et al., 2001). Careful follow-up, better knowledge of energy requirements, dietary counseling, and nutritional intervention help optimize the growth of these patients through childhood and adolescence. Today, lung transplants are being performed, and gene therapy holds great promise to replace the defective gene.

Intestinal malabsorption is severe in virtually all people who have CF. The main cause is deficiency of pancreatic enzymes, but bicarbonate deficiency, abnormalities of bile salts, mucosal transport and motility, and anatomical structural changes are other factors (Littlewood and Wolfe, 2000). Appropriate pancreatic replacement therapy achieves near normal absorption in many patients, but it is important to identify both malabsorption and any evidence of a pancreatic lesion in all patients who receive pancreatic enzymes. All who have evidence of fat malabsorption are deemed pancreatic insufficient and are candidates for enzyme replacement therapy (Littlewood and Wolfe, 2000).

Poor nutritional status in patients with CF is associated with severe lung disease. Possible causative factors include inadequate intake, malabsorption, and increased energy requirements. Body cell mass, which can be quantified by measurement of total body potassium, provides an ideal standard for measurements of energy expenditure (Shepherd et al., 2001).

Effective treatment should allow a normal diet, symptom control, malabsorption correction, and attainment of a normal nutritional state and growth. Categories of nutritional management for CF include (Creveling et al., 1997): routine care, anticipatory guidance (90% irritable bowel syndrome [IBW]), supportive intervention (85–90% of IBW), resuscitative or palliative care (below 75% IBW), and rehabilitative care (below 85% IBW consistently). Neonatal screening provides the opportunity to prevent malnutrition in infants with CF (Farrell et al., 1997). The percentage of children with CF identified as malnourished differs, depending on whether anthropometric or body composition data are used as the nutritional indicator. Weight-based indicators greatly underestimate the extent of malnutrition (McNaughton et al., 2000).

Trolox-equivalent antioxidant capacity (TEAC), as measured in CF patients, is related to nutritional status, lung function, and blood measurements of some known antioxidants. TEAC appears to represent a mixed antioxidant response, not a response to a single antioxidant (Lands et al., 2000). Patients with CF have altered copper distributions. It is not known whether this occurs because of poor copper absorption, inadequate dietary intake, or chronic inflammation. It is possible that the severity of CF and the activity of a copper-dependent enzyme are related (Percival, 1999).

The onset of CF-related diabetes mellitus (CFDM) is often associated with a decline in health and nutritional status. Energy requirements may be higher than usual for the patients with CF and CFDM during periods of recovery from mild exercise because of increased work of breathing consistent with higher ventilatory requirements (Ward et al., 1999).

Patients with CF who receive optimal nutrition have better growth, maintain better nutritional reserves, and have better pulmonary function than patients with CF who have poor nutrition (Erdman, 1999). These factors influence quality of life and survival. Metabolic and immunologic response to infection and the increased work of breathing escalate calorie requirements. No single strategy works for every patient; close monitoring of growth, symptoms, and changes in respiratory status must occur. The American Dietetic Association recommends a minimum of 4 medical nutrition therapy visits for patients who have CF (http://www.knowledgelinc.com/ada/mntguides/).

OBJECTIVES

- Achieve desirable body weight. Correct anorexia from respiratory distress.
- Provide optimal amounts of protein for growth, development, and resistance to infection. Increase lean body mass if depleted.
- Spare protein by providing up to twice the normal amount of calories.

- ▲ Decrease electrolyte losses in vomiting and steatorrhea. Replace lost electrolytes.
- ▲ Achieve adequate enzyme replacement to bring about near-normal digestion.
- ▲ Reduce excessive nutrient losses from maldigestion and malabsorption, and modify intake as required.
- ▲ Provide essential fatty acids in tolerated form. Reduce arachidonic acid to lessen inflammatory cascade.
- ▲ Correct edema, diarrhea, anemia, azotorrhea, and steatorrhea.
- ▲ Prevent progressive pulmonary disease or complications such as glucose intolerance, intestinal obstruction, cirrhosis, and pancreatic or cardiac diseases.
- ▲ Improve tolerance for therapies and medications.

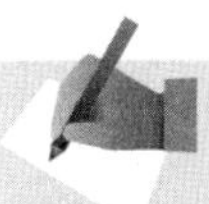

DIETARY AND NUTRITIONAL RECOMMENDATIONS

- For persons with acute disease, starch and fat will not be well tolerated unless adequate levels of pancreatic enzymes are provided.
- Protein should be 30–35% of total calories (i.e., 4 g/kg for infants, 3 g/kg for children, 2 g/kg for teens, 1.5 g/kg for adults).
- Supplement the diet with two times the normal RDAs for vitamins A, D, and E (use water-miscible sources) and iron (if needed). Use 4–6 g of sodium to replace perspiration losses. Use riboflavin for cheilosis. MCTs and safflower oil may be beneficial.
- Lactose intolerance is common, as is intolerance for gas-forming foods and concentrated sweets. Omit milk during periods of diarrhea if lactose intolerance occurs.
- Calorie intake should be 150 kcal/kg for children, 200 kcal/kg for infants, or 150% RDA for age and sex. Manage total CHO intake if glucose intolerance (CFDM) develops.
- Fluid intake should be liberal unless contraindicated.
- Replace zinc, copper, and vitamin K as needed; check serum levels regularly.
- Patients with CF are at risk for fat-soluble vitamin malabsorption. Those with low 25-OH vitamin D levels are at increased risk of low bone mineral density and long-term skeletal complications, but no recommendations exist for 25-OH vitamin D intake (Grey et al., 2000).
- Infants can tolerate most formulas (may need 24 kcal/oz) or commercial products such as Nutramigen, Probana, Pregestimil, or Portagen. Intake of protein should be higher; intake of fat should be lower. Do not add pancreatic enzymes to formula—desired amounts may not be totally consumed, or enzymes may block the opening of the nipple.
- Nocturnal tube feeding may be appropriate, especially with growth failures. Pulmocare or Ensure Plus may be beneficial. Elemental feedings such as Vivonex do not necessitate use of pancreatic enzymes (Fulton, 1995); they may be low in essential fatty acids and should be monitored carefully. If gastroenteritis (GE) reflux occurs, a gastrostomy feeding tube may be more comfortable than a nasogastric (NG) tube. Gastrostomy is a safe and effective way of improving nutritional intake in CF patients (Rosenfeld et al., 1999).
- Salt should be added to commercial baby foods; monitor carefully, especially for cor pulmonale.
- Soft foods may be useful if chewing fatigues the patient.
- Increase fat:CHO ratio with respiratory distress. Special respiratory formulas may be useful. Carnitine may be useful to correct fatty liver.
- Encourage fish intake for ω-3 fatty acids.
- Prolonged parenteral nutrition (PN) promotes weight gain in advanced CF, but effects are transient and sepsis is a risk (Allen et al., 1995).

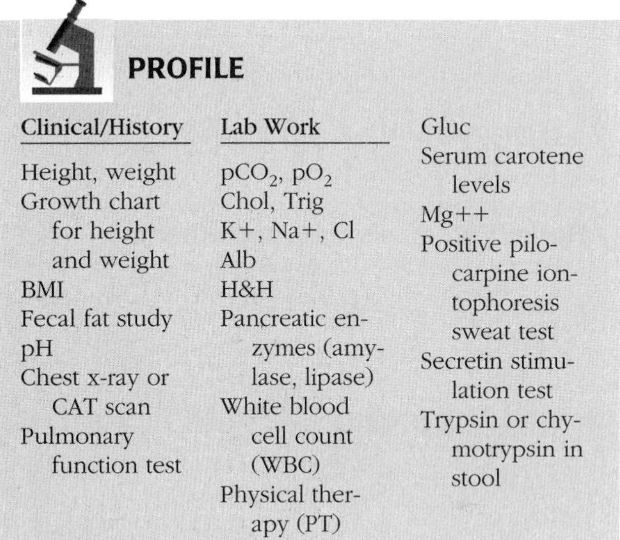

PROFILE

Clinical/History	Lab Work	
Height, weight	pCO_2, pO_2	Gluc
Growth chart for height and weight	Chol, Trig	Serum carotene levels
BMI	K+, Na+, Cl	Mg++
Fecal fat study	Alb	Positive pilocarpine iontophoresis sweat test
pH	H&H	Secretin stimulation test
Chest x-ray or CAT scan	Pancreatic enzymes (amylase, lipase)	Trypsin or chymotrypsin in stool
Pulmonary function test	White blood cell count (WBC)	
	Physical therapy (PT)	

Common Drugs Used and Potential Side Effects

The need for taking up to 40–60 pills daily is common.

- Pancreatic enzymes (pancrelipase). With modern enzymes, adequate control of gastrointestinal symptoms and absorption can be achieved at dosages up to 10,000 international units (IU) lipase/kg/day or only slightly more, and a normal nutritional state and growth rate can be maintained in most patients with CF (Littlewood and Wolfe, 2000; Fitzsimmons et al., 1997). Pancreatic granules (Viokase or Cotazym) are used to help improve digestion/absorption. Enteric preparations (Pancrease) act in the duodenum. Give before meals; for nocturnal feedings, give before, during, and after feedings. Avoid mixing with milk or ice cream. If too much is given, anorexia and constipation may result. Return of a voracious appetite and increase in stool bulk suggest an inadequate dosage. Pancreatic enzyme therapy interferes with oral iron therapy, and generic brands may not be as effective as brand names (Cowing-Cannella et al., 1993). Fibrosing colonopathy has been reported in young children with CF, the majority of whom take high-strength pancreatic enzymes to control intestinal malabsorption.
- Mucolytics such as potassium iodide liquefy secretions. Bronchodilators are used to open breathing passages. Monitor both for side effects.
- Antibiotics are needed during infections. Check magnesium levels.
- Use of ursodeoxycholic acid has a beneficial effect on primary sclerosing cholangitis, intrahepatic cholestasis

of pregnancy, liver disease associated with CF, chronic graft-versus-host disease, TPN-associated cholestasis, and various pediatric cholestatic liver diseases (Kumar and Tandon, 2001).

- In 1997, the FDA approved the drug TOBI (tobramycin solution for inhalation). In trials, a reformulated version of this common antibiotic improved lung function in people with CF and reduced the number of hospital stays. It can be delivered in a more concentrated dose directly to the site of CF lung infections and is preservative-free. The development of TOBI should lead to a long line of other aerosolized antibiotics for people with CF.
- In patients at high risk for bone fractures, calcitonin or growth hormone may be considered.

Herbs, Botanicals and Supplements

- Herbs and botanicals should not be used for CF, because there are no controlled trials to prove efficacy.
- The individual with CF should work with the CF nutritionist to maintain a healthy diet before considering adding herbal therapies. Each label on any supplement should be read carefully, because there are some ingredients that can be toxic to people with CF but not to people who do not have CF. As with all new therapies, the best course of action is to maintain close communication with the CF team for advice (http://www.nacfchighlights.com/homeframe.html).

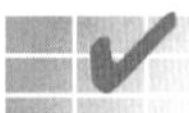

PATIENT EDUCATION

- ✔ Diet must be periodically reevaluated to reflect growth and disease process.
- ✔ New foods may be introduced gradually.
- ✔ To liquefy secretions, adequate fluid intake should be ensured.
- ✔ Bronchopulmonary drainage, three times daily, may be required. Plan meals for 1 hour before or after therapy.
- ✔ Ensure that all foods and beverages are nutrient dense.
- ✔ Discuss signs of dehydration.
- ✔ If the patient is a teen, discuss issues related to fertility (males with CF are often infertile, but females are not).
- ✔ Discuss the fact that pancreatic enzymes should not be chewed.
- ✔ In adults with CF, 40% have some glucose intolerance.
- ✔ Discuss reimbursement issues for tube feedings and pumps.
- ✔ Hypnosis may be useful in reducing the effects of pain from frequent intravenous injections or other treatments.

For More Information

- ✦ American Dietetic Association
  Cystic Fibrosis protocol
  www.eatright.org
- ✦ Cystic Fibrosis Foundation
  6931 Arlington Road
  Bethesda, MD 20814
  http://www.cff.org/
- ✦ Cystic Fibrosis Resources
  http://www.cysticfibrosis.com/
- ✦ Cystic Fibrosis Newsletters
  http://www.cysticfibrosis.com/newsletters.htm
- ✦ Cystic Fibrosis Research
  http://www.cfri.org/indexframes.htm
- ✦ International Association of Cystic Fibrosis Adults
  http://www.iacfa.org/
- ✦ National Heart, Lung and Blood Institute—CF
  http://www.nhlbi.nih.gov/health/public/lung/other/cystfib.htm

PNEUMONIA

NUTRITIONAL ACUITY RANKING: LEVEL 2

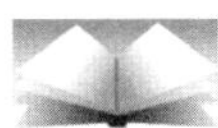

DEFINITIONS AND BACKGROUND

Pneumonia involves acute inflammation of the alveolar spaces of the lung. Lung tissue is consolidated as alveoli fill with exudate. Many types exist such as bacterial (from bacteria normally present in mouth/throat), viral, chemical, hypostatic (in bedridden persons, usually elderly individuals), aspiration (from swallowing a foreign substance), and allergic (from sensitivity to dust or pollen). It may be classified as community-acquired, hospital-acquired, or atypical.

The most common form is community-acquired pneumococcal pneumonia. Before antibiotics, pneumonia caused many deaths in elderly individuals; it now ranks sixth among causes of death in the United States (Fein and Niederman, 1994).

Signs and symptoms include difficult, painful respirations, shortness of breath, rales, rhonchi, tachypnea, chills and fever (102–106°), delirium, anorexia, malaise, abdominal distention, restlessness, cyanosis of nail beds, tachycardia, atelectasis, anxiety, and a productive cough that is painful and incessant (generally with green/yellow sputum that progresses to pink, brown, or rust color).

Enteral feeding provides nutrients for patients who require endotracheal tubes and mechanical ventilation. There is a presumed increase in the risk of ventilator-associated pneumonia (VAP) with tube feeding, but this is not always true (Kearns et al., 2000).

Elderly patients with reduced body cell mass and hypoalbuminemia are two to three times more likely to die from pneumonia than patients without nutritional impairment (LaCroix et al., 1989). Inflammation is the main reason for low serum albumin levels in elderly patients with pneumonia. Nutritional supplements are unlikely to significantly alter the clinical outcome of these patients (Hedlund et al., 1995). Lung function is found to be better with higher antioxidant levels; extra intake may be needed at this time (Hu and Cassano, 2000). The American Dietetic Association recommends 3 medical nutrition therapy visits for pneumonia (http://www.knowledgelinc.com/ada/mntguides/).

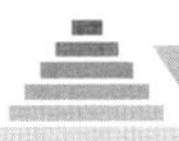

OBJECTIVES

- Prevent or correct dehydration.
- Relieve breathing difficulty and discomfort. Oxygenate all tissues.
- Prevent weight loss from hypermetabolic state.
- Avoid additional infections; prevent sepsis and multiple organ dysfunction syndrome.
- In convalescent stage, avoid constipation.
- Support diet with adequate antioxidants.

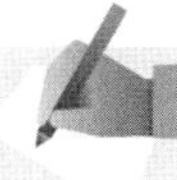

DIETARY AND NUTRITIONAL RECOMMENDATIONS

- If not contraindicated, offer 3–3.5 L fluid daily to liquefy secretions and to help lower temperature.
- Progress, as tolerated, to a high-calorie/soft diet. If overweight, allow normal calorie intake for age and sex.
- Frequent, small meals may be tolerated better.
- A multivitamin/mineral supplement may be beneficial, especially including vitamins A and C.
- When possible, add more fiber to prevent constipation.
- Ensure adequate potassium intake, as from fruits and juices.

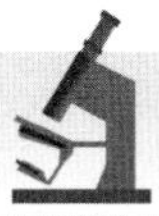

PROFILE

Clinical/History

Height
Weight
BMI
Temperature (fever, chills)
Pleuritic pain
Bronchoscopy
Productive cough (purulent, green, or rust)
Respiratory rate (increase)
I & O
BP

Lab Work

WBCs (increase)
TLC
Na+
K+
Mg++
Alb, prealbumin
RBP
H&H, serum Fe
Transferrin
Gluc
BUN, Creat
pCO_2, pO_2

Common Drugs Used and Potential Side Effects

- Antibiotics, such as clarithromycin/Biaxin, are used in bacterial conditions. Nausea, diarrhea, and abdominal pain can occur.
- Analgesics are used to reduce pain.
- Antipyretics are used to lower temperature.

Herbs, Botanicals and Supplements

- No clinical trials have proven efficacy for use of herbs or botanicals such as Echinacea, honeysuckle, garlic, dandelion, astragalus, or baikal skullcap.

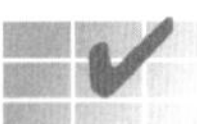

PATIENT EDUCATION

- Discuss the role of diet and fluid intake in recovery.
- In hypostatic pneumonia, suggest greater activity (within restraints of complicating disorders).
- Fruit and vegetable juices add calories, fluid, and sometimes fiber to the diet and can be available at bedside.
- A vaccine is now available to prevent the most common bacterial pneumonias.
- Protect from others who have respiratory tract infections.

For More Information

- American Dietetic Association
  Pneumonia protocol
  www.eatright.org
- American Lung Association–pneumonia
  http://www.lungusa.org/diseases/lungpneumoni.html
- Pneumonia information
  http://www.pneumonia.net/

PULMONARY EMBOLISM

NUTRITIONAL ACUITY RANKING: LEVEL 2

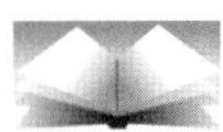

DEFINITIONS AND BACKGROUND

A pulmonary embolism is caused by a partial or complete occlusion of a pulmonary artery from a blood clot from another part of the body that has found its way to the lung. The condition can be life threatening. Sudden, sharp substernal pain, SOB, cyanosis, pallor, faintness, fever, hypotension, and wheezing can occur, sometimes followed by right heart failure. Approximately 10% suffer some form of tissue death or pulmonary infarction.

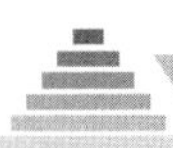

OBJECTIVES

- ▲ Normalize body temperature if fever exists.
- ▲ Replenish nutrients depleted by respiratory distress.
- ▲ Stabilize prothrombin time if warfarin (Coumadin) is used.
- ▲ Eliminate edema when present.
- ▲ Prepare for possible surgery (embolectomy).
- ▲ Prevent right-sided heart failure, atelectasis, and bleeding.
- ▲ Maintain lung function; which is found to be better with higher antioxidant levels (Hu and Cassano, 2000).

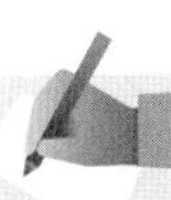

DIETARY AND NUTRITIONAL RECOMMENDATIONS

- Use a regular or high-calorie diet.
- Use a low sodium diet for patients with edema.
- Increase fluid intake as tolerated.
- Control vitamin K in diet if prothrombin time is not stabilized.
- Small meals may be needed.
- Provide sufficient antioxidants such as vitamins C, E, and selenium.

Common Drugs Used and Potential Side Effects

- Anticoagulants. Warfarin (Coumadin) increases clotting times by thinning blood. If problems in stabilizing the prothrombin time exist, the diet may need to be controlled in vitamin K. Use low-to-moderate amounts of green leafy vegetables and fish.
- Antibiotics, cardiotonic drugs, diuretics, or antiarrhythmics may be used.

Herbs, Botanicals and Supplements

- No clinical trials have proven efficacy for use of herbs or botanicals in pulmonary embolism.

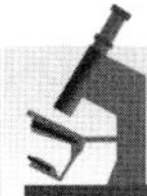

PROFILE

Clinical/History

Height
Weight
BMI
Edema
Temperature (fever)
I & O
Chest x-ray
Electrocardiogram (EKG)
Echocardiography
Perfusion scans
Pulmonary angiography
Pulse (NL = 60–100 beats)

Lab Work

Alb
Na+, K+
Mg++
PT
Lactic acid dehydrogenase (LDH) (increased)
WBCs (increased)
Bilirubin (increased)
H&H
pCO_2, pO_2

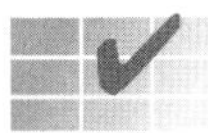

PATIENT EDUCATION

- ✓ Explain sources of vitamin K in the diet. Therapy often continues for 3–6 months.
- ✓ Discuss relaxation techniques, especially related to mealtimes.

RESPIRATORY DISTRESS SYNDROME

NUTRITIONAL ACUITY RANKING: LEVEL 2

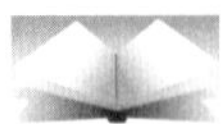

DEFINITIONS AND BACKGROUND

Adult respiratory distress syndrome (ARDS) is a secondary lung state that develops within 24–48 hours in patients who have sepsis or who are critically ill, in shock, or severely injured. Other causes include pneumonia, aspiration of food into the lung, several blood transfusions, pulmonary embolism, chest injury, burns, near drowning, cardiopulmonary bypass surgery, pancreatitis, overdose of drugs such as heroin, methadone, or aspirin.

Patients often have pulmonary edema but have normal left atrial and pulmonary venous pressures. Respiratory distress syndrome (RDS) may occur as part of systematic inflammatory response syndrome (SIRS), affecting approximately 70% of patients in the intensive care unit (ICU). In infants, RDS often occurs in low-birth-weight babies, and the condition may be called hyaline membrane disease. Such babies are often born to mothers who have diabetes.

Recent studies of sepsis-induced ARDS have shown that a low-carbohydrate, high-fat diet combining the anti-inflammatory and vasodilatory properties of eicosapentaenoic acid (EPA; fish oil), gamma-linolenic acid (GLA; borage oil) (EPA+GLA), and antioxidants improves lung microvascular permeability, oxygenation, and cardiopulmonary function and reduces proinflammatory eicosanoid synthesis and lung inflammation (Gadek et al., 1999).

Indirect calorimetry (IC) is an accurate method of estimating a patient's energy expenditure, particularly the complex critically ill patient who benefits most from nutritional support; this bedside technique measures variables related to gas exchange and replaces assumptions about physiologic stress (McCarthy, 2000). Data are valuable to the healthcare team when trying to identify reasons for weaning failure.

OBJECTIVES

- Promote rapid recovery and oxygenation of tissues.
- Prevent relapse.
- Counteract side effects of medications as ordered.
- Replace essential fatty acids, carnitine, and other nutrients as indicated.
- Restore normal oxygenation of bloodstream and tissues.
- Prevent malnutrition. CNS output for ventilatory drive may be depressed. Starvation decreases desire to breathe, causing abnormal breathing pattern, pneumonia, and atelectasis. Muscle mass (including diaphragm) varies with body weight. Refeeding may take 2–3 weeks.
- Prevent overfeeding (hepatic dysfunction, fatty liver, and CO_2 overproduction) or underfeeding (morbidity, mortality, and decreased response to therapy). Avoid refeeding syndrome.
- Prevent fluid overload.
- Support lung function, which is found to be better with higher antioxidant levels (Hu and Cassano, 2000).

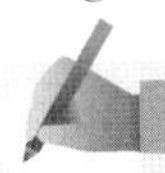

DIETARY AND NUTRITIONAL RECOMMENDATIONS

- Provide parenteral fluids as ordered. Progress, when possible, to oral feedings. Use TPN only if GI tract is nonfunctional.
- For calories, use 1–1.2 × BEE. Nonprotein calories (NPC) should be 50% glucose and 50% lipid.
- Increased fat may be required to normalize the RQ. Fat also adds extra calories and palatability to the diet.
- Ensure adequate provision of EFA and fat-soluble vitamins in appropriate forms. Low linoleic acid status in critically ill RDS infants may require IVs with a fat emulsion added. Inositol is being studied for its effects on survival of premature infants with RDS.
- Increase intake of omega-3 fatty acids to reduce arachidonic cascade from high intake of omega-6 diets. Include antioxidants such as vitamins C, E, and selenium at slightly higher than RDA levels.
- Be careful with TPN-induced changes in CO2 production.

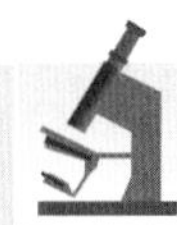

PROFILE

Clinical/History
- Height
- Weight
- BMI
- Growth profile
- Indirect Calorimetry (IC)
- I & O
- BP
- Temperature
- RQ

Lab Work
- H&H
- Transferrin
- pCO_2, pO_2
- Complete blood count (CBC)
- Prealbumin
- K+
- Na+
- Mg++
- Serum phosphorus
- BUN, Creat

Common Drugs Used and Potential Side Effects

- Corticosteroids may be used with many side effects if prolonged use is required.
- Diuretics are used in cases of pulmonary edema. Monitor serum electrolytes accordingly.

Herbs, Botanicals and Supplements

- No clinical trials have proven efficacy for use of herbs or botanicals in respiratory distress.

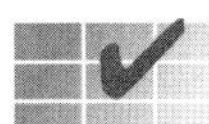

PATIENT EDUCATION

- ✔ Discuss the role of fat intake on respiratory requirements. Fat decreases CO2 production.
- ✔ Small, frequent feedings may be beneficial.

For More Information

- ✦ Acute Respiratory Distress Clinical Network http://hedwig.mgh.harvard.edu/ardsnet/

RESPIRATORY FAILURE AND VENTILATOR WEANING

NUTRITIONAL ACUITY RANKING: LEVEL 3

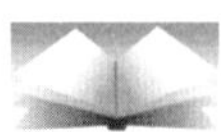

DEFINITIONS AND BACKGROUND

Acute respiratory failure (ARF) involves sudden absence of respirations, with confusion or unresponsiveness and failure of pulmonary gas exchange mechanism. Chronic pulmonary disease or an acute injury can cause acute pulmonary failure, which requires mechanical ventilation. Other causes are noted in Table 5–5.

Anabolic and catabolic hormones, muscle work, and nutritional status affect skeletal muscle mass and muscle strength. Substrate and muscle work stimulate protein synthesis. Hypermetabolic patients often have at least a 30% increase in oxygen use. In starvation, respiratory muscles are catabolized to meet energy needs. Refeeding helps ventilatory response. Lung function is found to be better with higher antioxidant levels (Hu and Cassano, 2000). Use of intravenous fat emulsions may help reduce inflammation.

Forced vital capacity (FVC) is used to measure ventilatory function; percentage of body fat and fat-free mass can be estimated from skinfold thicknesses. Handgrip strength is positively related to adjusted FVC (Lazarus et al., 1998).

Daily screening of patients requiring mechanical ventilation, followed by trials of spontaneous breathing, can reduce the duration and costs and the complications of usual care (Ely et al., 2002). Weaning from a ventilator takes a few days and requires proper refeeding. The length of ventilator dependency significantly positively correlates with calorie and carbohydrate intake (Huang et al., 2000). Also important is control of total calories rather than any singular nutrient (CHO versus fat) to avoid excess production of carbon dioxide (Talpers et al., 1992).

No matter what method is used to wean from ventilator support, careful attention must be paid to reversible factors such as electrolytes, infections, anemia, heart failure, medications, and superimposed metabolic acidosis (Weinberger and Weiss, 1995). See Table 5–6 for stages.

According to a study in Healthcare Benchmarks, enteral feedings within 3 days can reduce length of time on a ventilator and improve outcomes for critically ill patients. Such feedings, which cost only about $80 per day, would have saved Medicare as much as $1.08 billion from 1996 to 2002, according to a study by Washington, DC-based KPMG Peat Marwick (Healthcare Benchmarks, 1998). Older patients may be harder to wean from the ventilator (Ely et al., 2002).

TABLE 5–5 Causes of Respiratory Failure

Airway Obstruction—Chronic bronchitis, emphysema, bronchiectasis, cystic fibrosis, asthma, bronchiolitis, and inhaled particles
Poor Breathing—Obesity, sleep apnea, and drug intoxication
Muscle Weakness—Myasthenia gravis, muscular dystrophy, polio, Guillain-Barré syndrome, polymyositis, stroke, amyotrophic lateral sclerosis, and spinal cord injury
Abnormality of lung tissue—Acute respiratory distress, drug reaction, pulmonary fibrosis, fibrosing alveolitis, widespread tumors, radiation therapy, sarcoidosis, and burns
Abnormality of chest wall—Kyphoscoliosis and chest wound

TABLE 5–6 Ventilatory-Dependency Feeding Stages (Burns et al., 2000; Irwin and Openbrier, 1985)

1. Acute repletion—Replenish muscle glycogen stores and reverse catabolism.
2. Preweaning—Maintain positive nitrogen balance, improve visceral protein stores, improve creatinine-height index (CHI), and promote weight gain.
3. Weaning—Provide energy substrates to cover needs of respiratory muscles that are working harder; minimize CO2 production. Be careful not to overfeed, which may impair weaning.
4. Outcome or Postweaning—Maintain nutrient needs despite anorexia or dysphagia; support anabolism.

OBJECTIVES

- Promote normalized nutritional intake despite hypermetabolic status of the patient and the prohibition of oral intake due to endotracheal tubes.
- Oxygenate tissues and relieve breathlessness; decrease CO2 production.
- Monitor sensations of hunger because patients are unable to communicate their hunger and thirst.
- Prevent respiratory muscle dysfunction by ensuring that the patient is properly nourished. Achieve or maintain weight; not all patients are malnourished.
- Counteract hypotension caused by positive-pressure ventilation, acidosis, or both.
- Provide nutritional substrates that will not greatly increase CO2 production while maintaining surfactant production and keeping lean body mass (LBM).
- Prevent atelectasis, pulmonary infection, sepsis, glucose or lipid intolerance, multiple organ dysfunction syndrome, and aspiration.
- Adjust goals as appropriate. Maintain flexible approaches to patient requirements.

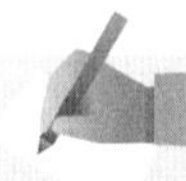

DIETARY AND NUTRITIONAL RECOMMENDATIONS

- Begin nourishing the patient as soon as possible to wean the patient from the ventilator. Start any tube feeding slowly to avoid gastric retention or diarrhea. Some institutions add blue food coloring to feedings to detect problems in tracheal secretions, but this is not universally accepted. Advance gradually and use continuous administrations unless contraindicated. Tube feedings of low osmolality are needed. Essential fatty acids are important; 2% total fat is the usual estimate. Vivonex does not contain EFAs, but most other tube feedings do.

- A diet with 35–50% CHO and 30–50% lipid (high omega-3 fatty acids) is common. Adults need a daily diet of at least 25–35 kcal/kg. Increases from labored breathing will occur; monitor using indirect calorimetry when possible. For some cases, use of specialty products such as Pulmocare or Respalor may be recommended, but they are not always necessary.
- Protein needs may be as high as 1.5–2 g/kg body weight (BW).
- Monitor TPN carefully for complications such as pneumonia. Watch use of TPN because of high-calorie loading and increased carbon dioxide production.
- Patients with pulmonary edema should have their sodium intake reduced as needed. Include adequate protein in the diet to prevent additional fluid retention because of lowered colloidal osmotic pressure.
- Supplement diet with multivitamins, especially vitamins A and C.
- Phosphorus and magnesium may be needed if stores are depleted.

PROFILE

Clinical/History

Height
Weight
BMI
REE from IC
I & O
Respiratory rate
RQ
BP
Temperature (fever is common)

Lab Work

Prealbumin (decreased)
TLC (decreased)
H&H, serum Fe
Na+
K+
Mg++
WBC (elevated)
Chol, Trig
Urinary gluc
Transferrin
Serum phosphorus (decrease can cause ARF)
pH (acidemia below 7.4, alkalemia above 7.4)

Common Drugs Used and Potential Side Effects

- Bronchodilators may be needed. Monitor side effects related to potassium, etc.
- Antibiotics are often required; monitor specific side effects.

Herbs, Botanicals and Supplements

- No clinical trials have proven efficacy for use of herbs or botanicals in respiratory failure.

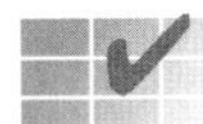

PATIENT EDUCATION

- ✓ A daily calorie count may be needed to assess the patient's nutritional status.
- ✓ The greatest danger in using enteral nutrition is aspiration. Low-osmolarity products are essential, as well as elevation of the head of the bed.
- ✓ Discuss early satiety, bloating, fatigue, dyspnea, etc. as related to food or tube feeding (TF) intake.

For More Information

- National Heart, Lung, and Blood Institute-RF http://www.nhlbi.nih.gov/health/public/lung/other/res fail.htm

SARCOIDOSIS

NUTRITIONAL ACUITY RANKING: LEVEL 2

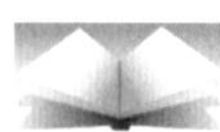

DEFINITIONS AND BACKGROUND

Sarcoidosis is a disease of undetermined origin (Aliot, 2000); it is a rare disease in which tiny patches of inflammation (granulomas) occur in almost any organ. Etiology is unknown. Pulmonary effects are most common. It develops most often between ages 20–40, more often among northern Europeans and American blacks. In most cases, it is benign; but in 10% of cases, the condition becomes chronic.

Symptoms and signs may include weight loss, fever, anorexia, weakness, aching joints, abdominal pain, lymphadenopathy, bone cysts in hands and feet, pulmonary hypertension, cor pulmonale, clubbing of fingers, dyspnea, cough, hypoxemia, iritis, glaucoma, blindness, chest pain, shortness of breath, or congestive heart failure (CHF). There is a correlation between 1 alpha-hydroxylase gene expression in alveolar macrophages with the activity of sarcoidosis and its associated disturbances in calcium metabolism (Inui et al., 2001).

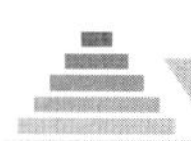

OBJECTIVES

- Reduce heart failure, bronchiectasis, and related problems.
- Correct weight loss, anorexia, fever, and abdominal pain.
- Improve ability to breathe and eat normally.
- Prevent further deterioration of organ functions with any and all affected organ systems.
- Prevent or correct fluid retention.
- High levels of calcium may accumulate in the blood and urine; control accordingly for related nausea, anorexia, vomiting, thirst, excessive urination, and potentially renal failure.

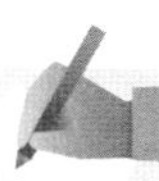

DIETARY AND NUTRITIONAL RECOMMENDATIONS

- Restrict salt if necessary for congestive heart failure or for use of corticosteroids. A 2- to 3-g sodium diet may be beneficial.
- Use a diet containing adequate to high potassium (unless medications are used).
- As needed, decrease calcium and vitamin D if bone involvement is suggested; monitor use of supplements accordingly.

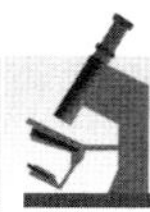

PROFILE

Clinical/History	Pulmonary function tests	Transferrin
Height		Globulin (increase is common)
Weight	**Lab Work**	Ca++ in urine (increased)
BMI	H&H (anemia common)	Na+
BP	Serum Fe	K+
Chest x-ray	Alb (decrease common)	Mg++
Biopsy	Prealbumin	Uric acid (increased)
Gallium scan	Alkaline phosphatase (alk phos)	Serum Ca++ (increased)
Tender red lumps, usually on the shins	Nitrogen (N) balance	PO_4
Uveitis		Kveim test
TB test to rule out tuberculosis		

Common Drugs Used and Potential Side Effects

- Glucocorticoids or corticosteroids may be used to suppress severe symptoms such as shortness of breath. Need to watch electrolytes, N balance, and other changes. Treatment may require several years.
- Isoniazid (INH) may be ordered for pulmonary status. Watch use of vitamin B6; increase intake accordingly of high vitamin B6 foods to prevent neuritis.
- Calcium-chelating agents may be used if hypercalcemia persists.

Herbs, Botanicals and Supplements

- No clinical trials have proven efficacy for use of herbs or botanicals in sarcoidosis.

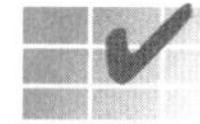

PATIENT EDUCATION

- ✔ If the patient is using steroids, antacids could also be taken to reduce GI side effects. Check with the doctor.
- ✔ Discuss the role of diet in maintaining immunocompetence and in improving tolerance for other therapies.
- ✔ Follow closely on the low calcium intake; avoid vitamin D supplements and exposure to sunlight to avoid hypercalcemia and hypercalciuria.

For More Information

- National Heart, Lung, and Blood Institute—Sarcoidosis
  http://www.nhlbi.nih.gov/health/public/lung/other/sarcoidosis/index.htm
- National Sarcoidosis Resources Center
  P.O. Box 1593
  Piscataway, NJ 08855-1593
  (908) 699-0733

- Sarcoidosis Family Aid and Research Foundation
  460A Central Avenue
  East Orange, NJ 07018

- Sarcoidosis Research Institute
  3475 Central Avenue
  Memphis, TN 38111
  (901) 327-5454

THORACIC EMPYEMA

NUTRITIONAL ACUITY RANKING: LEVEL 2

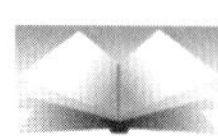

DEFINITIONS AND BACKGROUND

Thoracic empyema involves accumulation of pus in the pleural cavity, often as a complication of pneumonia. Signs and symptoms may include dyspnea, orthopnea, constant localized chest pain, productive cough, malaise, fatigue, fever, tachycardia, tachypnea, weight loss, and anorexia.

OBJECTIVES

- Lessen fatigue; promote improved well-being.
- Reduce fever. Prevent sepsis.
- Correct weight loss.
- Control and reduce anorexia.

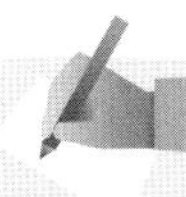

DIETARY AND NUTRITIONAL RECOMMENDATIONS

- Provide diet as ordered. Patient may need high-calorie/high-protein foods served at frequent intervals.
- Two or more liters of fluid may be needed daily, unless contraindicated.
- Meals should be served in an attractive manner to stimulate appetite.

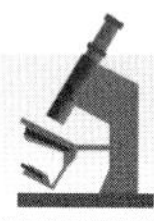

PROFILE

Clinical/History		
Height	Pleural examination	Gluc
Weight	I & O	Na+
BMI	**Lab Work**	K+
BP	Alb, Prealbumin	pO_2 (often decreased)
Temperature	H&H	pCO_2
		Transferrin

Common Drugs Used and Potential Side Effects

- Antibiotics are often provided. Monitor side effects accordingly.
- Monitor effects of other medications as prescribed.

Herbs, Botanicals and Supplements

- No clinical trials have proven efficacy for use of herbs or botanicals in thoracic empyema.

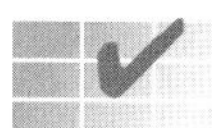

PATIENT EDUCATION

- Discuss the role of nutrition in illness and recovery, especially as it relates to immunocompetence.
- With family, discuss signs to observe for future problems or relapses.

TRANSPLANTATION, LUNG

NUTRITIONAL ACUITY RANKING: LEVEL 4

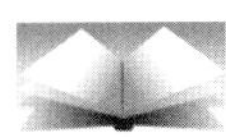

DEFINITIONS AND BACKGROUND

Lung transplantation (LTX) is an accepted treatment for end-stage pulmonary parenchymal and vascular diseases. In some cases of CF or COPD, transplants may be considered. The International Society for Heart and Lung Transplantation and the Cystic Fibrosis Foundation have uniform guidelines for transplant candidate selection. As with other types of transplants, graft-host resistance and sepsis are the major concerns. Infections are the most common cause of morbidity and mortality in lung transplant recipients; half are bacterial in origin (Speich and van Der Bij, 2001).

Proper nutrition plays a key role in preparing for lung transplantation. Therefore, the lung transplant dietitian plays an important role and meets with the patient for an initial interview. Weight and weight history, foods typically eaten, and appetite are reviewed. Being at ideal body weight range for height helps assure good physical condition for pretransplant pulmonary rehabilitation and the transplant itself. Certain patients with advanced pulmonary disease are unable to eat enough to maintain ideal body weight because of increased metabolic demands and breathlessness with eating. In such situations, it may be recommended that a percutaneous endoscopic gastrostomy (PEG) feeding tube be placed.

Proper nutrition is critical to maximize the chances of a successful transplant. Occasionally, listing for transplant will be delayed until the patient's nutritional status improves. In patients with a pretransplant BMI <17 kg/m(2) or >25 kg/m(2) the risk of dying within 90 days post-transplant was increased; patients with a pretransplant BMI of >27 kg/m(2) had significantly higher risk (Madill et al., 2001). In a group of underweight patients with lung disease assessed for lung transplantation, it is possible to increase energy intake by an intensified nutritional support to achieve a significant weight gain, compared to the regular nutritional support during a short hospital stay (Forli et al., 2001). Lean body mass depletion may be associated with more severe hypoxemia, reduced walking distance, and a higher mortality (Schwebel et al., 2001). Both undernutrition and obesity should be carefully managed before surgery.

Immunosuppressive therapy with glucocorticoids contributes to protein degradation; the nitrogen balance after LTX is negative because of high glucocorticoid requirements; aggressive nutritional intervention and increased nitrogen intake are needed to reduce protein losses in these patients.

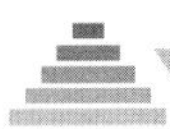

OBJECTIVES

Preoperative:

- Correct nutritional risks (loss of LBM, cachexia, vitamin or mineral deficiencies).
- Prepare for surgical procedure. Most patients will require sodium or fluid restrictions; monitor serum potassium as well.
- Allow for mild weight loss with a planned diet if the patient is obese and has time to do this.

Postoperative:

- Prevent infection.
- Promote wound healing.
- Prevent surgical complications, organ rejection, and organ failure.
- Promote weight gain but not excessive amounts.
- Reduce protein losses, support nitrogen balance, and correct hypoalbuminemia.
- Prevent aspiration.
- Wean from ventilator or oxygen when possible.

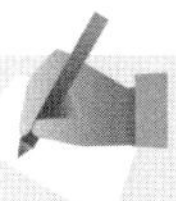

DIETARY AND NUTRITIONAL RECOMMENDATIONS

- Return to oral intake by 48–72 hours postoperatively, when possible.
- Promote adequate intake of kcal (25–30 kcal/kg) and protein (1 g/kg BW). Do not overfeed, which can aggravate ventilatory mechanisms.
- Parenteral solutions may be used if needed; include branched-chain amino acids (BCAAs) for healing.
- Calorie-dense options should be considered if fluid restriction is required. Maintain sufficient fat intake to prevent excess carbon dioxide production from a high CHO intake.
- Restrict Na+ and K+ if renal status is compromised.

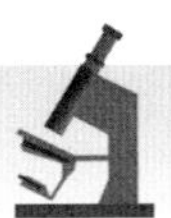

PROFILE

Clinical/History	Lab Work	
Height	Alb, prealbumin	PO_4
Weight	Transferrin	Alanine aminotransferase (ALT), aspartate aminotransaminase (AST)
BMI	Chol, Trig	Lactate
Weight changes	H&H, serum Fe	TLC
RQ	Gluc	pCO_2, pO_2
Ventilator support	BUN, Creat	
I & O	Na+, K+	
	Mg++	

Common Drugs Used and Potential Side Effects

- Corticosteroids (such as Prednisone, Solu-Cortef) are used for immunosuppression. Side effects include increased catabolism of proteins, negative nitrogen balance, hyperphagia, ulcers, decreased glucose tolerance, sodium retention, fluid retention, and impaired calcium absorption and osteoporosis. Cushing's syndrome, obesity, muscle wasting, and increased gastric secretion may result. A higher protein intake and lower intake of simple CHOs may be needed.

- Cyclosporine does not retain sodium as much as corticosteroids do. Intravenous doses are more effective than oral doses. Nausea, vomiting, and diarrhea are common side effects. Hyperlipidemia, hypertension (HPN), and hyperkalemia also may occur; decrease sodium and potassium as necessary. Elevated glucose and lipids may occur. The drug is also nephrotoxic; a controlled renal diet may be beneficial.
- Immunosuppressants such as Muromonab or Orthoclone (OKT3) and antithymocyte globulin (ATG) are less nephrotoxic than cyclosporine but can cause nausea, anorexia, diarrhea, and vomiting. Monitor carefully. Fever and stomatitis also may occur; alter diet as needed.
- Azathioprine (Imuran) may cause leukopenia, thrombocytopenia, oral and esophageal sores, macrocytic anemia, pancreatitis, vomiting, diarrhea, and other side effects that are complex. Folate supplementation and other dietary modifications (liquid or soft diet, use of oral supplements) may be needed. The drug works by lowering the number of T cells; it is often prescribed along with prednisone for conventional immunosuppression.
- Tacrolimus (Prograf, FK506) suppresses T-cell immunity; it is 100 times more potent than cyclosporine, thus requiring smaller doses. Side effects include GI distress, nausea, vomiting, hyperkalemia, and hyperglycemia.
- Diuretics such as Lasix may cause hypokalemia. Low-sodium/low-calorie diets may be indicated. If Aldactone is used, it spares potassium.

Herbs, Botanicals and Supplements

- No clinical trials have proven efficacy for use of herbs or botanicals after lung transplantation.

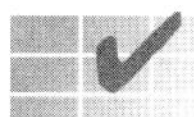

PATIENT EDUCATION

- Discuss appropriate calorie and protein levels.
- Sodium and fluid restrictions should be addressed as needed.
- Decreased fat and cholesterol intakes may be useful to decrease cardiac risks.
- Adequate fiber and vitamin E are useful.
- Slow return to activity will be important.

TUBERCULOSIS

NUTRITIONAL ACUITY RANKING: LEVEL 2

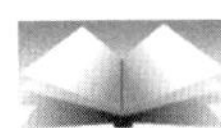

DEFINITIONS AND BACKGROUND

Tuberculosis (TB) is caused by a tubercle bacillus (*Mycobacterium tuberculosis*) invading the lungs and setting up an inflammatory process. Healing occurs with a calcification of the tubercular cavity. TB causes tissue wasting, exhaustion, hemoptysis, productive cough with green, yellow, or blood-tinged sputum, fever and profuse night sweats, and expectoration. The acute form resembles pneumonia; the chronic form causes low-grade fever. The recent increase in TB in the United States has been correlated with inadequate compliance to prescribed drug therapy. New cases are either recently acquired or reactivated latent infections (Small et al., 1994).

Immunocompromised persons are more vulnerable to the effects of TB, especially those persons who have acquired immunodeficiency syndrome (AIDS). These patients exhibit alterations in the metabolism of iron that lead to increased deposition of this element in the tissues; this may promote increased susceptibility of AIDS patients to mycobacterial infections, namely, by *Mycobacterium avium* (Gomes et al., 2001). Hypermetabolism appears to play a role in the wasting process in patients infected with both HIV and TB.

Active TB begins in the lungs but often spreads through the bloodstream as extrapulmonary TB. Fatigue, abdominal tenderness, painful urination, headache, shortness of breath, arthritis-like symptoms, kidney damage, and pain in the spine and bones can occur. Tuberculosis meningitis is a very dangerous complication, especially for the elderly.

Because many TB patients have early, unplanned readmission and often need assistance with activities of daily living, ambulatory treatment may not be appropriate for selected patients (Chu et al., 2001). They may have drug complications, the need to use a nonstandard drug regimen, and other illnesses. With high prevalence of malnutrition, relatively low utilization rate of nutritional services, and the potential effect of adverse reactions to therapeutic drugs, careful attention is needed for this patient population.

OBJECTIVES

- Maintain weight (or prevent losses). Reduce fever. The basal metabolic rate is 20–30% above normal to counteract fever of 102.2° or higher.
- Normalize calcium levels in serum. Either hypocalcemia or hypercalcemia may occur.
- Replace nutrient losses from lung hemorrhage, if present.
- Promote healing of the cavity.
- Counteract neuritis from isoniazid (INH) therapy, where used.
- Stimulate appetite.
- Prevent dehydration.
- Prevent pleurisy (lung inflammation) and complications.

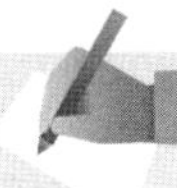

DIETARY AND NUTRITIONAL RECOMMENDATIONS

- Use a well-balanced diet containing liberal amounts of protein and adequate calories (may need up to 3,000 kcal).
- Ensure that the diet provides sufficient calcium without excess. Vitamin D is needed in controlled amounts.
- Ensure that the diet provides iron and vitamin C for proper hemoglobin formation and wound healing.
- Ensure that the diet provides vitamin B-complex, especially vitamin B6, to counteract INH therapy.
- Alcohol should not be used as a calorie replacement.
- Use supplemental vitamin A as carotene if poorly converted.
- Use adequate fluids (2 L is common), unless contraindicated.

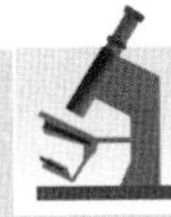

PROFILE

Clinical/History

- Height
- Weight
- BMI
- TB skin tests—tine or PPD
- Chest x-rays (irregular white areas on dark background)
- Temperature, fever
- Sputum test for *Mycobacterium tuberculosis*
- Spinal tap for polymerase chain reaction (PCR)
- I & O

Lab Work

- Alb, prealbumin
- RBP
- TLC
- Serum pyridoxine
- H&H, serum Fe
- N balance
- Chol (decreased)
- Na+, K+
- Ca++
- Mg++
- Serum folate
- Transferrin
- BUN, Creat
- Liver function tests (from medication use)

Common Drugs Used and Potential Side Effects

Therapy always involves two or more drugs because of the long-term treatment period required.

- INH can cause neuritis by depleting vitamin B6. Its bad taste can be disguised in pureed fruit or jam to make it palatable, especially for pediatric patients. Niacin, calcium, and B12 are also depleted. Nausea, vomiting, and dry mouth are common. Avoid histamine.
- Rifampin (Rifadin, Rimactane) has side effects such as anorexia and GI distress.
- Pyrazinamide (PZA) may cause anorexia, nausea, and vomiting. It can be hepatotoxic.

- Aminosalicylic acid interferes with vitamin B12 and folate absorption. Nausea and vomiting are common.
- Ethambutol (Myambutol) may cause GI distress, nausea, or anorexia. It should not be used longer than 2 months, because it can harm the eyes.
- Ethionamide (Trecator-SC) requires a B6 supplement. It may cause anorexia, metallic taste, nausea, vomiting, diarrhea, weight loss, or hypoglycemia.
- Streptomycin was one of the first drugs used to treat TB. It is given by injection. Use longer than 3 months can affect balance and hearing.
- Chemotherapy can increase serum calcium levels.
- Immunotherapy is now being tested with some positive results.

Herbs, Botanicals and Supplements

- No clinical trials have proven efficacy for use of herbs or botanicals such as eucalyptus, Echinacea, garlic, licorice, honeysuckle, or forsythia.

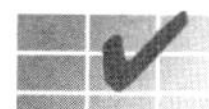

PATIENT EDUCATION

- ✓ Add nonfat dry milk to beverages, casseroles, soups, and desserts to increase protein and calcium intake, unless contraindicated.
- ✓ Encourage the preparation of appetizing meals.
- ✓ Plan rest periods before and after meals.
- ✓ Discuss anxiety related to weight loss, night sweats, loss of strength, high fever, and abnormal chest x-rays.
- ✓ Discuss communicability of TB. Family members should have x-rays and other testing. About 5% of exposures result in TB within 1 year; others may be dormant until another condition sets in such as AIDS, DM, or leukemia.
- ✓ Promote adequate rehabilitation if the patient is an alcoholic.

For More Information

- ✦ Tuberculosis Control Program
  http://www.ci.nyc.ny.us/html/doh/html/tb/tb.html

REFERENCES

Asthma–Cited References

Armentia A, et al. Early introduction of cereals into children's diets as a risk factor for grass pollen asthma. *Clin Exp Allergy*. 2001;31:1250.

Baker J, et al. Development of a standardized methodology for double-blind, placebo-controlled food challenge ion patients with brittle asthma and perceived food intolerance. *J Am Diet Assoc*. 2000;100:1361.

Bartel P, et al. Vitamin B6 supplementation and theophylline-related effects in humans. *Am J Clin Nutri*. 1994;60:93.

Britton J, et al. Dietary magnesium, lung function, wheezing, and airway hyper-reactivity in a randomized adult population sample. *Lancet*. 1994;344:357.

Camargo C, et al. Prospective study of body mass index, weight change and risk of adult-onset asthma in women. *Arch Int Med*. 1999;159:2582.

Dell S, To T. Breastfeeding and asthma in young children: findings from a population-based study. *Arch Pediatr Adolesc Med*. 2001;155:1261.

Gagnon L, et al. Influence of inhaled corticosteroids and dietary intake on bone density and metabolism in patients with moderate to severe asthma. *J Am Diet Assoc*. 1997;97:1401.

Hatch G. Asthma, inhaled oxidants, and dietary antioxidants. *Am J Clin Nutri*. 1995;61S:625S.

Huang S, Pan W. Dietary fats and asthma in teenagers: analyses of the first Nutrition and Health Survey in Taiwan (NAHSIT). *Clin Exp Allergy*. 2001;31:1875.

Infante-Rivard C, et al. Family size, day-care attendance, and breastfeeding in relation to the incidence of childhood asthma. *Am J Epidemiol*. 2001;153:653.

Knox A. Salt and asthma. *BMJ*. 1993;307:1159.

Luder E, et al. Association of being overweight with greater asthma symptoms in inner city black and Hispanic children. *J Pediatr*. 1998;132:699.

Martinez F, et al. Asthma and wheezing in the first six years of life. *N Engl J Med*. 1995;332:133.

Mainous A, et al. Serum vitamin C levels and use of health care resources for wheezing episodes. *Arch Fam Med*. 2000;9:241.

Mickleborough T, et al. Dietary salt alters pulmonary function during exercise in exercise-induced asthmatics. *J Sports Sci*. 2001;19:865.

Oddy W. Breastfeeding and asthma in children: findings from a West Australian study. *Breastfeed Rev*. 2000;8:5.

Ratheiser K, et al. Epinephrine produces a prolonged elevation in metabolic rate in humans. *Am J Clin Nutri*. 1998;68:1046.

Sivri A, Coplu L. Effect of the long-term use of inhaled corticosteroids on bone mineral density in asthmatic women. *Respirology*. 2001;6:131.

Troisi R, et al. A prospective study of diet and adult-onset asthma. *Am J Respir Crit Care Med*. 1995;151:1401.

Warner J, Warner J. Early life events in allergic sensitization. *Br Med Bull*. 2000;56:883.

Woods R, et al. Dietary marine fatty acids (fish oil) for asthma. *Cochrane Database Syst Rev*. 2000;2:CD001283.

Wright A, et al. Relationship of infant feeding to recurrent wheezing at age 6 years. *Arch Pediatr Adolesc Med*. 1995;149:758.

Chronic Obstructive Pulmonary Disease–Cited References

Agusti A. Systemic effects of chronic obstructive pulmonary disease. *Novartis Found Symp*. 2001;234:242.

Chapman K, Winter L. COPD: using nutrition to prevent respiratory function decline. *Geriatrics*. 1996;51:37.

Chapman-Novakofski K, et al. Alterations in taste thresholds in men with chronic obstructive pulmonary disease. *J Am Diet Assoc*. 1999;99:1536.

Farber M, Mannix E. Tissue wasting in patients with chronic obstructive pulmonary disease. *Neurol Clin*. 2000;18:245.

Gosker H, et al. Skeletal muscle dysfunction in chronic obstructive pulmonary disease and chronic heart failure: underlying mechanisms and therapy perspectives. *Am J Clin Nutri*. 2000;71:1033.

Paiva S, et al. Assessment of vitamin A status in chronic obstructive lung disease patients and healthy smokers. *Am J Clin Nutri*. 1996;64:928.

Scannapieco F, Ho A. Potential associations between chronic respiratory disease and periodontal disease: analysis of National Health and Nutrition Examination Survey III. *J Periodontol*. 2001;72:50.

Shahar E, et al. Dietary n-3 polyunsaturated fatty acids and smoking-related chronic obstructive pulmonary disease. *N Engl J Med*. 1994;331:228.

Tabak C, et al. Fruit and fish consumption: a possible explanation for population differences in COPD mortality (The Seven Countries Study.) *Euro J Clin Nutri*. 1998;52:819.

Thorsdottir I, et al. Screening method evaluated by nutritional status measurements can be used to detect malnourishment in chronic obstructive pulmonary disease. *J Am Diet Assoc*. 2001;101:648.

Cystic Fibrosis–Cited References

Allen E, et al. Prolonged parenteral nutrition for cystic fibrosis patients. *Nutr Clin Pract*. 1995;10:73.

Beker L, et al. Stature as a prognostic indicator in cystic fibrosis survival. *J Am Diet Assoc*. 2001;101:438.

Cowing-Cannella P, et al. Feeding practices and nutrition recommendations for infants with cystic fibrosis. *J Am Diet Assoc*. 1993;93:297.

Creveling S, et al. Cystic fibrosis, nutrition and the health care team. *J Am Diet Assoc*. 1997;97:S186.

Doull I. Recent advances in cystic fibrosis. *Arch Dis Child*. 2001;85:62.

Erdman S. Nutritional imperatives in cystic fibrosis therapy. *Pediatr Ann*. 1999;28:129.

Farrell P, et al. Nutritional benefits of neonatal screening for cystic fibrosis. *N Engl J Med*. 1997;337:963.

Fitzsimmons S, et al. High-dose pancreatic enzyme supplements and fibrosing colonopathy in children with cystic fibrosis. *N Engl J Med*. 1997;336:1283.

Fulton J, et al. Nutrition in the pediatric double lung transplant patient with cystic fibrosis. *Nutr Clin Pract*. 1995;10:67.

Grey V, et al. Monitoring of 25-OH vitamin D levels in children with cystic fibrosis. *J Pediatr Gastroenterol Nutri*. 2000;30(3):314–319.

Kumar D, Tandon R. Use of ursodeoxycholic acid in liver diseases. *J Gastroenterol Hepatol.* 2001;16:3.

Lambert J. Osteoporosis: a new challenge in cystic fibrosis. *Pharmacotherapy.* 2000;20(1):34.

Lands L, et al. Total plasma antioxidant capacity in cystic fibrosis. *Pediatr Pulmonol.* 2000;29:81.

Littlewood J, Wolfe S. Control of malabsorption in cystic fibrosis. *Pediatr Drugs.* 2000;2:205.

McNaughton S, et al. Nutritional status of children with cystic fibrosis measured by total body potassium as a maker of body cell mass: lack of sensitivity of anthropometric measures. *J Pediatr.* 2000;136:188.

Mueller D. Nutrition in pulmonary disease. In: Mahan K, Escott-Stump S, eds. *Krause's food, nutrition, and diet therapy.* 10th ed. Philadelphia: WB Saunders, 2000.

Munck A, Navarro J. Nutritional management of cystic fibrosis in children. *Arch Pediatr.* 2000;7:396.

Ott S, Aitken M. Osteoporosis in patients with cystic fibrosis. *Clin Chest Med.* 1998;19:555.

Percival S, et al. Altered copper status in adult men with cystic fibrosis. *J Am Col Nutri.* 1999;18:614.

Rosenfeld M, et al. Nutritional effects of long-term gastrostomy feedings in children with cystic fibrosis. *J Am Diet Assoc.* 1999;99:191.

Shepherd R, et al. Energy expenditure and the body cell mass in cystic fibrosis. *Nutrition.* 2001;17:22.

Ward S, et al. Energy expenditure and substrate utilization in adults with cystic fibrosis and diabetes mellitus. *Am J Clin Nutri.* 1999;69:913.

OTHER PULMONARY CONDITIONS–Cited References

Abbey M, et al. Dietary supplementation with orange and carrot juice in cigarette smokers lowers oxidation products in copper oxidized low-density lipoproteins. *J Am Diet Assoc.* 1995;95:671.

Alliot C, et al. Neurosarcoidosis associated with Hodgkin's disease; malignancy. *Hematol.* 2000;5:285.

Al-Tawil K, et al. Congenital chylothorax. *Am J Perinatol.* 2001;17:121.

Britton J, et al. Dietary antioxidant vitamin intake and lung function in the general population. *Am J Respir Crit Care Med.* 1995;151:1383.

Brown K, Arthur J. Selenium, selenoproteins, and human health: a review. *Public Health Nutri.* 2001;4:593.

Burns S, et al. The weaning continuum use of Acute Physiology and Chronic Health Evaluation III, Burns Wean Assessment Program, Therapeutic Intervention Scoring System, and Wean Index scores to establish stages of weaning. *Crit Care Med.* 2000;28:2259.

Chu C, et al. Early unplanned readmission of patients with newly diagnosed tuberculosis discharged from acute hospital to ambulatory treatment. *Respirology.* 2001;6:145.

Ely E, et al. Recovery rate and prognosis in older persons who develop acute lung injury and the acute respiratory distress syndrome. *Ann Intern Med.* 2002;136:25.

Ely E, et al. Effect on the duration of mechanical ventilation of identifying patients capable of breathing spontaneously. *N Engl J Med.* 1996;335:1864.

Fein A, Neiderman M. Severe pneumonia in the elderly. *Clin Geriatr Med.* 1994;10:121.

Forli L, et al. Dietary support to underweight patients with end-stage pulmonary disease assessed for lung transplantation. *Respiration.* 2001;68:51.

Gadek J, et al. Effect of enteral feeding with eicosapentaenoic acid, gamma-linolenic acid, and antioxidants in patients with acute respiratory distress syndrome. Enteral Nutrition in ARDS Study Group. *Crit Care Med.* 1999;27:1409.

Gomes M, et al. Role of iron in experimental Mycobacterium avium infection. *J Clin Virol.* 2001;20:117.

Griese M. Pulmonary surfactant in health and human lung diseases: state of the art. *Eur Respir J.* 1999;13:1455.

Healthcare Benchmarks. Nutrition intervention in ICU improves outcomes. *Healthcare Benchmarks.* 1998;5:175.

Hedlund J, et al. Hypoalbuminemia in hospitalized patients with community-acquired pneumonia. *Arch Int Med.* 1995;155:1438.

Hu G, Cassano P. Antioxidant nutrients and pulmonary function: the Third National Health and Nutrition Examination Survey. *Am J Epidemiol.* 2000;151: 975.

Huang Y, et al. Nutritional status of mechanically ventilated critically ill patients: comparison of different types of nutritional support. *Clin Nutri.* 2000;19:101.

Inui N, et al. Correlation between 25-hydroxyvitamin D3 1-alpha-hydroxylase gene expression in alveolar macrophages and the activity of sarcoidosis. *Am J Med.* 2001;110:687.

Irwin M, Openbrier D. A delicate balance—strategies for feeding ventilated COPD patients. *Am J Nurs.* 1985;85:274.

Kearns P, et al. The incidence of ventilator-associated pneumonia and success in nutrient delivery with gastric versus small intestinal feeding: a randomized clinical trial. *Crit Care Med.* 2000;28:1742.

LaCroix A, et al. Prospective study of pneumonia hospitalizations and mortality of U.S. older people: role of chronic conditions, health behaviors and nutritional status. *Public Health Reports.* 1989;104:350.

Lazarus R, et al. Effects of body composition and fat distribution on ventilatory function in adults. *Am J Clin Nutri.* 1998;68:35.

Madill J, et al. Nutritional assessment of the lung transplant patient: body mass index as a predictor of 90-day mortality following transplantation. *J Heart Lung Transplant.* 2001;20:288.

McCarthy M. Use of indirect calorimetry to optimize nutrition support and assess physiologic dead space in the mechanically ventilated ICU patient: a case study approach. *AACN Clin Issues.* 2000;11:619.

Mysliwiec V, Pina J. Bronchiectasis: the 'other' obstructive lung disease. *Postgrad Med.* 1999;106:123.

Pedersen C, et al. Effects of blueberry and cranberry juice consumption on the plasma antioxidant capacity of healthy female volunteers. *Euro J Clin Nutri.* 2000;54:405.

Prieto D, et al. Surgery for bronchiectasis. *Eur J Cardiothorac Surg.* 2001;20:19.

Schwartz J, Weiss S. Relationship between dietary vitamin C intake and pulmonary function in the first National Health and Nutrition Examination Survey (NHANES I). *Am J Clin Nutri.* 1994;59:110.

Schwebel C, et al. Prevalence and consequences of nutritional depletion in lung transplant candidates. *Eur Respir J.* 2000;16:1050.

Small P, et al. The epidemiology of tuberculosis in San Francisco. *N Engl J Med.* 1994;330:1703.

Smit H. Chronic obstructive pulmonary disease, asthma and protective effects of food intake: from hypothesis to evidence? *Respir Res.* 2001;2:261.

Speich R, van Der Bij W. Epidemiology and management of infections after lung transplantation. *Clin Infect Dis.* 2001;33:58S.

Takemura Y, et al. Relation between breastfeeding and the prevalence of asthma: the Tokorozawa Childhood Asthma and Pollinosis Study. *Am J Epid.* 2001;154:115.

Talpers S, et al. Nutritionally associated increased carbon dioxide production: excess total calories vs high proportion of carbohydrate calories. *Chest*. 1992;102:551.

von Mutius E, et al. Relation of body mass index to asthma and atopy in children: the National Health and Nutrition Examination Study III. *Thorax*. 2001;56:835.

Weinberger S, Weiss J. Weaning from ventilatory support. *N Engl J Med*. 1995;332:388.

Other Pulmonary Conditions–Suggested Readings

Beale R, et al. Immunonutrition in the critically ill: a systematic review of clinical outcome. *Crit Care Med*. 1999;27:2799.

Kortbeek J, et al. Duodenal versus gastric feeding in ventilated blunt trauma patients: a randomized controlled trial. *J Trauma*. 1999; 46:992.

Mannino D, et al. Obstructive lung disease and low lung function in adults in the United States: data from the National Health and Nutrition Examination Survey, 1988–1994. *Arch Intern Med*. 2000; 160:1683.

Nevins M, Epstein S. Weaning from prolonged mechanical ventilation. *Clin Chest Med*. 2001;22:13.

Pichard C, et al. Treatment of cachexia with recombinant growth hormone in a patient before lung transplantation: a case report. *Crit Care Med*. 1999;27(8):1639.

Scannapieco F, et al. Associations between oral conditions and respiratory disease in a national sample survey population. *Ann Periodontol*. 1998;3:251.

Schwartz J. Role of polyunsaturated fatty acids in lung disease. *Am J Clin Nutri*. 2000;71:393S.

SECTION

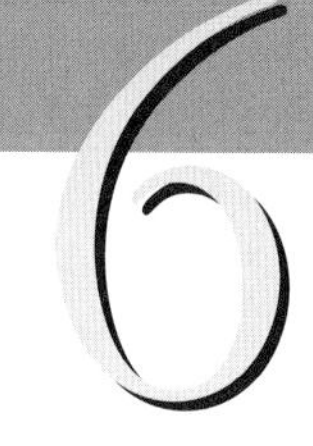

CARDIOVASCULAR DISORDERS

CHIEF ASSESSMENT FACTORS

- DECREASED CARDIAC OUTPUT: ARRHYTHMIAS, RALES, VERTIGO, PALLOR, FATIGUE, LABORED RESPIRATIONS
- CARDIOGENIC SHOCK: TACHYCARDIA, LOW SYSTOLIC BLOOD PRESSURE (BP), COOL AND MOIST SKIN, WEAK PULSES, DECREASED URINARY OUTPUT, PULMONARY EDEMA
- ASCITES, EDEMA
- CHEST PAIN
- BLOOD PRESSURE
- OBESITY; WAIST CIRCUMFERENCE OVER DESIRED RANGE FOR MEN OR WOMEN
- CHOLESTEROL AND LIPID PROFILES
- SERUM HOMOCYSTEINE
- ANGIOGRAMS, EKG, ECHOCARDIOGRAMS
- ELECTROLYTE BALANCE
- AGE, ESPECIALLY OLDER THAN 40 YEARS
- SEX (MALES, OR WOMEN AFTER MENOPAUSE)
- SMOKING HISTORY (HX) (SMOKING INCREASES HEART RATE)
- DIABETES
- EXERCISE PATTERNS
- FAMILY HX HEART DISEASE
- TYPE A PERSONALITY, STRESSFUL LIFESTYLE
- XANTHOMAS
- PANCREATITIS, OTHER COMPLICATIONS
- MEDICATIONS
- ALCOHOL USE
- LACTIC ACID DEHYDROGENASE (LDH), CREATINE PHOSPHOKINASE (CPK) LEVELS

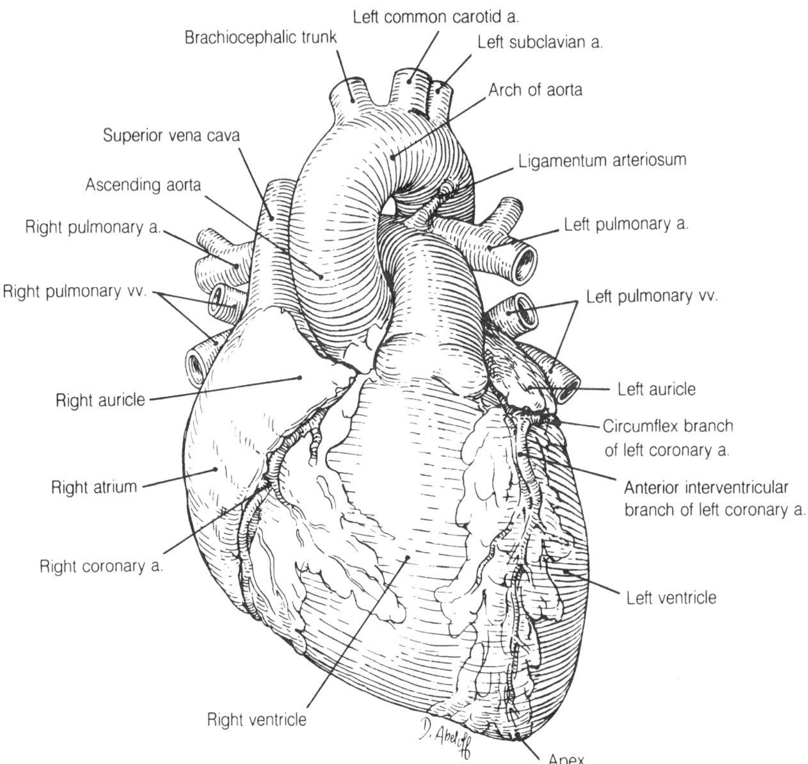

Figure 6–1 Anatomy of the Heart. (Reprinted with permission from Hall-Craggs, ECB. *Anatomy as a Basis for Clinical Medicine.* 2nd Ed. Baltimore: Urban & Schwartzenberg, 1990.)

OVERVIEW: DIET IN HEART DISEASES—LIPIDS

Atherosclerotic disease of coronary arteries (coronary artery disease, CAD) is the most common cause of death in the United States, accounting for about 600,000 deaths annually. The most recent NHANES III identified that 20% of Americans have high cholesterol (Over 240 mg/dL) and 31% have borderline levels (200–239 mg/dL). The majority of preventable deaths occur in people with serum cholesterol levels between 180–250 mg/dL (American Dietetic Association, Nutrition Fact Sheet, Dec. 2000).

The benefits of primary prevention of cardiovascular disease are greatest for people who have multiple risk factors. Secondary prevention is beneficial for high-risk and low-risk patients. Patients with 3 risk factors are considered high risk (e.g., smoking, hypertension [HPN], hyperlipidemia); patients with isolated HPN or hyperlipoproteinemia (HLP) are considered lower risk (Grover et al., 1998). Both active smoking and secondary exposure are associated with the progression of an index of atherosclerotic heart disease (ASHD); smoking is of greater concern for persons who also have diabetes mellitus (DM) and HPN (Howard et al., 1998). Reduction in smoking, improved diet, and increased use of hormone replacement therapy accounted for much decline in incidence of CAD in women between 1980 and 1994 (Hu et al., 2000). Both intermittent and continuous exercise reduces postprandial lipemia and triglycerides (Gill et al., 1998). Increased exercise is associated with a lower waist circumference and higher high-density lipoprotein cholesterol (HDL-C) level (Heim et al., 2000).

Low levels of high-density lipoprotein (HDL) cholesterol and high levels of triglycerides are independent risk factors of cardiovascular death (NHLBI, 2001). Elevated plasma lipoprotein (a) is also an independent risk factor, comparable to serum cholesterol levels over 240 mg/dL (Bostrom et al., 1996). Apo E phenotype may also influence risk of CAD because of the tendency to have higher levels of low-density lipoproteins (LDL) and lower HDLs (Howard et al., 1998). Non-HDL-C is a better predictor of mortality than low-density lipoprotein cholesterol (LDL-C) alone for CAD; it is the difference between total cholesterol and HDL-C (Cui et al., 2001).

Mean serum total cholesterol levels decreased in U.S. children and adolescents between the late 1960s and the 1990s; changes were smallest among black females (Hickman et al., 1998). Through childhood and young adulthood, a person's total plasma cholesterol (TC) and LDL-C are related to the TC levels of his or her parents (Uiterwaal, 1997). Current studies are unclear about how aggressive treatment should be for elevated cholesterol and triglycerides in children or teens; widespread screening does not seem warranted at this time, unless there is early cardiovascular morbidity and mortality in immediate family members.

Saturated fat is more important than total cholesterol intake. High intakes of saturated fats tend to increase total cholesterol levels. High intakes of saturated fatty acids (SFA), especially mystiric acid (C14:0) and palmitic acid (C16:0), are associated with high concentrations of large, cholesterol-rich LDLs and low activity of hepatic lipase (Dreon et al., 1998). National Cholesterol Education Program (NCEP) diets that have primarily lean red or lean white meat have equivalent effects on serum lipids and lipoproteins (Davidson et al., 1999). Overall control of saturated fat intake is beneficial.

Dietary cholesterol is now recognized as only one of many nutritional factors to play a role in the etiology of heart disease. Cholesterol is readily made from acetate in all animal tissues; it has many roles in the body (see Fig. 6–1).

Vitamin C has a role in cholesterol metabolism and is now known to affect levels of LDL-cholesterol. Men, smokers, elderly individuals, and persons with diabetes mellitus or hypertension tend to have lower levels of serum ascorbic acid and higher risks for heart disease; monitor closely. The cessation of ovulation in perimenopausal women tends to increase levels of serum cholesterol (van Beresteijn et al., 1993); statin drugs are now recommended (NHLBI, 2001).

The role of total fat is important to consider as well. Substitution of extra virgin olive oil for saturated fats may decrease patient need for medication to control HPN; this may be mediated by reductions in SFA, increased HDL cholesterol, lower triglycerides, and increased antioxidant polyphenols (Ferrara et al., 2000). For example, extra virgin olive oil has the most phytochemicals and strongest flavor. A specific distinction between stearic acid and other SFA does not appear to be important in dietary advice to lower risk of CAD; intake of fatty red meat versus lean red meat or poultry and fish, and high-fat compared with low-fat dairy products, results in a significant decrease in SFA (Hu et al., 1999). Interestingly, a diet higher in total fat (i.e., unsaturated fat) may be indicated for some individuals such as those with metabolic syndrome (see section 9).

There is currently no strong evidence to support a high monounsaturated fatty acid (MUFA) diet over a low-fat, high-carbohydrate (CHO) diet because of an effect on arterial elasticity (Ashton et al., 2000); other changes in diet may be needed to cause a beneficial effect on arterial elasticity—for example, consuming phytoestrogen-rich foods, vitamin E, or omega-3 fatty acids. Fish consumption is inversely related to death from CAD, especially from myocardial infarction (MI) (Davig et al., 1997). Both eicosapentanoic acid (EPA) and docosahexanoic acid (DHA) decrease serum triglycerides (TG) but have different effects on lipoprotein and fatty acid metabolism, especially on liver enzymes (Grimsgaard et al., 1997). Dietary supplementation of n-3 fatty acids decreases risk of death, MI, and stroke in patients who survive a recent MI; vitamin E has no clear effects on these risks (GISSI-Preventione investigators, 1999; Pruthi et al., 2001). Foods enriched or naturally high in omega-3 fatty acids decrease production of inflammatory mediators, which can have a preventive or therapeutic effect for patients with cardiovascular disease (Mantzioris et al., 2000).

Plant stanol or sterol esters are found in plant foods such as corn, soy, and other vegetable oils; they are derived from plant phytosterols. Plant stanol esters block intestinal absorption of dietary and biliary cholesterol (Hallikainen et al., 2000). Possibly, when less cholesterol appears to be in the diet, the body up-regulates the LDL-receptors to increase cholesterol turnover, and a net reduction occurs. Fat-soluble vitamins are not lowered significantly; neither is HDL cholesterol. Most people see a significant reduction in serum cholesterol levels within 2 weeks after starting to consume 2–3 servings of plant stanol or sterol ester foods daily.

A major goal of dietary prevention and treatment of most heart diseases is to attain and maintain weight control at an ideal body weight. Decreasing excess calories, reducing total fat intake, adding fiber, reducing excess intake of refined carbohydrates, and increasing exercise can all help achieve this goal. High glycemic load due to high intake of refined carbohydrates is positively related to CAD risk, independent of other known risk factors (Liu et al., 2000). Weight cycling does not appear to have an adverse effect on BP or lipids; excess mortality previously reported among weight cyclers is probably not attributable to effects on these risk factors (Petersnarck et al., 1999). Among morbidly obese women (body mass index [BMI] over 40), total cholesterol levels tend to be increased (Vierhapper et al., 2000).

Soluble fiber lowers lipid levels. There is substantial evidence from randomized controlled clinical trials that a mean

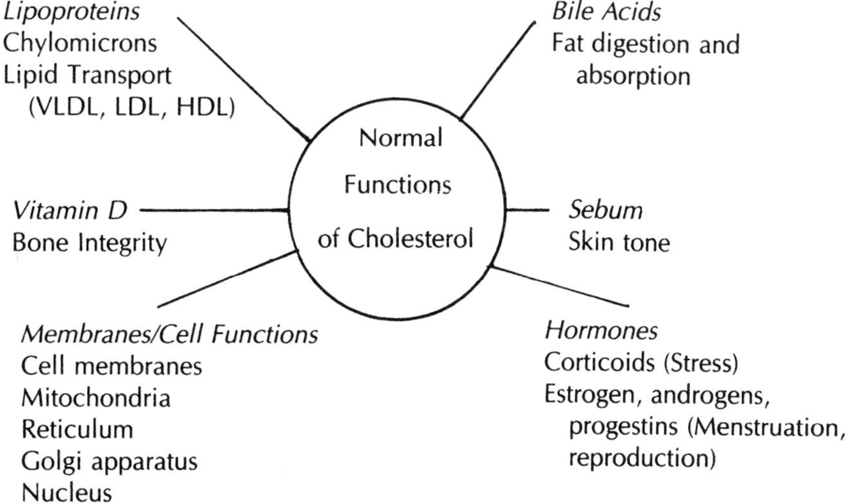

Figure 6–2 Normal Functions of Cholesterol.

reduction of 9% in LDL-cholesterol can be achieved by intake of different sources of soluble fiber. Important modifications in volume, bulk, and viscosity in the intestinal lumen, alter metabolic pathways of hepatic cholesterol and lipoprotein metabolism and result in lowering of plasma LDL-cholesterol (Fernandez, 2001).

Changes in the number and activity of bacteria in the colon may help control serum lipid risk factors for cardiovascular disease (Jenkins et al., 1999). Regular intake of yogurt containing an appropriate strain of *Lactobacillus acidophilus* may reduce risk for CAD by 6–10% (Anderson et al., 1999).

Daily intake of soy protein may improve blood lipid profiles and decrease risk of cardiovascular disease by altering quantity or activity of apo-B lipoproteins or LDL receptors (Baum et al., 1998). In October 1999, the FDA gave permission to label products high in soy protein as helpful in lowering heart disease risk; products must contain at least 6.25 grams per serving. Dietary intake of soy isoflavones improves the lipid profile of premenopausal women during all phases of the menstrual cycle; long-term intake of soy products could lower the risk of CAD (Merz-Demlow et al., 2000). Lecithin has a role in bile acid metabolism and has a small role in intestinal cholesterol absorption; it is readily made by the body.

Fruit and vegetable intake is protective against coronary heart disease, stroke, and possibly hypertension (Van Duyn and Pivonka, 2000). Risk reduction by 20–40% has been estimated. Quercetin protects against coronary heart disease, stroke, cataracts, and hypertension (Knekt et al., 2000). It is found in onions, especially red onions, apple skin, tea, berries, and red wine. Other antioxidants are also important.

While there may be a role for vitamin E to protect cell membranes from oxidation and damage, in patients at high risk for cardiac events (MI, stroke, or death from cardiac causes), daily supplementation with 400 IU natural sources of vitamin E for a mean of 4.5 years had no specific effect on cardiovascular outcomes (Heart Outcomes Prevention . . ., 2000). The Women's Health Study, the Women's Antioxidant and Cardiovascular Study, the Physician's Health Study, and the Heart Protection Study are examining the effects of vitamin E on CAD. Other studies may be warranted, especially using natural sources of this vitamin.

Note that eggs are a source of dietary cholesterol and need to be incorporated in the diet within current dietary recommendations. Healthy men and women who eat eggs are unlikely to have a higher risk of CAD or stroke than those who do not. 37,851 men aged 40–75 in the Health Professionals Follow-Up Study and 80,082 women aged 34–59, who were in the Nurses' Health Study, were studied; eating eggs was positively associated only for individuals with diabetes (Hu et al., 1999).

Aspirin and other salicylates may have contributed to the decline in mortality from cardiovascular disease over the past 3–4 decades (Ingster and Feinleib, 1997). Aspirin and other salicylates inhibit production of enzymes that influence platelet release and aggregation, vasoconstriction, and vasodilation; salicylates have analgesic, antipyretic, anti-inflammatory, and antirheumatic properties. They occur in foods, including herbs, spices, fruits, and tomatoes.

Epidemiologic studies have found a positive relation between placental vascularization, size of placenta at birth, and cardiovascular morbidity and mortality later in life. When hemoglobin levels were studied, anemic women, especially in the first trimester, had more capillaries per villous cross section than women with normal hemoglobin levels (Kadyrov et al., 1998).

Lipid-lowering therapy has been determined to be safe and beneficial with a large number of individuals at risk for CAD; cost-effective therapy is needed to extend treatment to all of those who may benefit (Jacobson et al., 2000). Nutrition counseling should receive high priority, both in medical training and in patient care; referral to registered dietitians may save billions of healthcare dollars annually (Plous et al., 1995; McGhee et al., 1995; Oster and Thompson, 1996). The American Dietetic Association identifies cost savings per cardiovascular case to be $2,496 annually with nutrition counseling, thereby reducing the need for some medications.

Moderately elevated plasma or serum homocysteine (tHcy) levels are prevalent in the general population and are associated with increased risk of cardiovascular disease, stroke, and peripheral vascular disease, independent of other classic cardiovascular disease risk factors (Bostom et al., 1999). In addition, in patients who experience acute coronary events, serum total tHcy level measured at the time of admission is an independent negative predictor of long-term survival (Omland et al., 2000). Reducing coffee intake and smoking may be useful in lowering serum tHcy (de Bree et al., 2001). Black women have higher tHcy levels and lower plasma folate levels than white women, which may contribute to a higher level of CAD in black women. More white women use multivitamin supplements on a daily basis and eat a lot more ready-to-eat cereal (Gerhard et al., 1999). The high frequency of mild B12 deficiency in the elderly is not related to poor intake but may be related to other factors (Howard et al., 1998). Simple, inexpensive, nontoxic therapy with folic acid, vitamins B6, and B12 reduces plasma tHcy levels (Eichelboom et al., 1999). For example, habitual intake of commercially fortified breakfast cereals that contain 200 ug folic acid results in significant reductions in homocysteine levels (Malinow et al., 2000). According to National Institutes of Health (NIH) studies, the blood-pressure lowering Dietary Approaches to Stop Hypertension (DASH) diet also reduces levels of homocysteine; this diet includes high quantities of fruits, vegetables, low-fat dairy products, whole grains, poultry, fish, and nuts. Use of folic acid (400 ug) and B12 (500 ug cyanocobalamin) supplements to lower elevated tHcy levels could result in substantial clinical benefits at a reasonable cost (Nallamothu et al., 2000).

Sources of folate and other important nutrients are listed in Table 6–1.

OVERVIEW: DIET IN HEART DISEASES—SODIUM

Sodium has been found to be only one factor in the development of hypertension. It has minimal and specific blood pressure effects in normotensive adults, and there are benefits and risks of sodium reduction; therefore, future public health recommendations should be based on new, carefully acquired science (McCarron, 2000). Sodium intake is independently positively associated with risk of cardiovascular disease and

TABLE 6–1 Folate and Other Key Nutrient Sources (Potassium, Calcium, and Magnesium)

Folate Sources:

Amount	Food	Micrograms of Folate
1 cup	Fortified cereals	400
1 cup	Lentils	360
1 cup	Spinach, collards	90–130
½ cup	Chick peas, pinto beans	130–145
1 cup	Pasta, cooked	100–120
¾ cup	Asparagus	110
1 cup	Rice, fortified	80
2 oz	Peanuts	80
1 cup	Broccoli	80
1 cup	Orange juice	40–60

High-Potassium Sources:
Apricots, peaches, pumpkin
Bananas
Catfish, cod, flounder
Dried beans and peas
Green beans, lima beans
Milk
Potatoes
Pork and veal, lean
Prunes, prune juice
Oranges, orange juice
Spinach
Tomatoes, stewed

High-Calcium Sources:
Broccoli, spinach, turnip greens
Cheese, Milk, Tofu made with calcium
Mackerel, Perch, Salmon

High Magnesium Sources:
Beans
Broccoli
Chard
Croaker
Mackerel
Nuts and Seeds
Okra
Oysters, scallops
Plantain
Sea Bass
Soy Milk
Spinach
Tofu
Whole Grain and Fortified Breads and Cereals

For a Healthy Heart, Eat More Often—(from http://www.awesomelibrary.org/heart-dis.html)

- Carrots
- Sweet potatoes
- Green leafy vegetables
- Pumpkin, canned or cooked
- Squash
- Fat-free chicken and turkey breast
- Low-fat tomato sauces and pasta
- Homemade pizza with fat-free chicken as meat sauce
- Foods with no or low salt for those who have high BP
- Peanuts, walnuts, almonds, other nuts in moderation
- Olive oil and canola oil substituted for other oils
- Salmon and other fish, including the skin and fat (1–5 servings per week recommended)
- Defatted soy flour (1/3 of a cup per day)
- Fat-free milk (skim)
- Oatmeal, shredded wheat; high-fiber, low-sugar cereals
- Fresh fruits
- Red or black grapes
- Grape juice (1 cup per day recommended)
- Grapefruit, especially pink (40% more beta carotene)
- Dried fruits, especially apricots, dates, prunes
- Fat-free homemade yogurt with extra-dry milk
- Salad dressings and dips with nonfat sour cream or homemade yogurt
- Baked whole wheat chips and tortillas
- Bean and chickpea dishes and dips
- Tomato salsas

mortality in overweight adults (He et al., 1999). For BMI over 27.8 for men and over 27.3 for women, NHANES I data were analyzed: Each 100-mmol increase in sodium intake had a 32% increase in stroke, 89% increase in risk of death from stroke, 44% increase risk for death from CAD, 61% increase in death from CAD, and a 39% increase risk of death from all causes. Sodium intake was not significantly related to risk of cardiovascular disease in normal-weight individuals.

Dietary sodium intake is positively related to cardiovascular disease over time. Reduction in dietary sodium intake reduces left ventricular hypertrophy (Messerli et al., 1997). Hypertension increases the risk for CAD, MI, stroke, and congestive heart failure. African Americans and Hispanics of Caribbean descent tend to have a high prevalence of hypertension with a worse prognosis than whites (Richardson and Piepho, 2000). There are no racial, age, sex, or weight differences in the effect of salt on blood pressure in salt-sensitive hypertensive patients; blood pressure is lowered significantly with a restricted diet and increased with a high-sodium diet (Chrysant et al., 1997).

A majority of Americans over age 60 have high blood pressure. Increased risk of major cardiovascular and renal diseases, morbidity and mortality, and shortened life expectancy result. The Trial of Nonpharmacologic Interventions in the Elderly (TONE) study indicated that in older patients with high

BP who received antihypertensive drugs for years and had well controlled BP (average 129/72), moderate lowering of sodium intake and moderate reduction of obesity may be beneficial (Stamler, 1998). With subsequent cessation of drug treatment and continued lifestyle counseling, sodium and weight reduction can be maintained long term. TONE results agree with those of the DASH feeding trial, showing that both high-normal and high BP can be significantly reduced by improvements in diet (Stamler, 1998).

For More Information

- Agency for Healthcare Research and Quality
  2101 E. Jefferson St., Suite 501
  Rockville, MD 20852
  http://www.ahcpr.gov/
- American Association of Cardiovascular Pulmonary Rehabilitation
  http://www.jhbmc.jhu.edu/aacvpr/aacvpr.htm
- American Dietetic Association
  Congestive Heart Failure, Hyperlipidemia, and Hypertension protocols
  www.eatright.org
- American Heart Association
  http://www.americanheart.org/
- Association of Heart Patients
  PO Box 54305
  Atlanta, GA 30308
  1-800-241-6993
- Heartlife (heart disease, pacemakers): 1-800-241-6993

ANGINA PECTORIS

NUTRITIONAL ACUITY RANKING: LEVEL 2

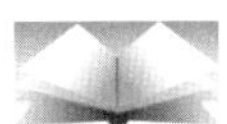

DEFINITIONS AND BACKGROUND

Angina pectoris involves retrosternal chest pain or discomfort from decreased blood flow to the myocardium from decreased oxygen supply (often during exertion). The pain frequently is correlated with hypertension or with coronary artery disease but may also occur as a result of anemia, hyperthyroidism, aortic stenosis, or vasospasm. Stable (classic) angina occurs after exertion and is relieved by rest and vasodilation; it lasts 3–5 minutes. Intractable (progressive) angina causes chronic chest pain that is not relieved by medical treatment. Variant angina is a mixed condition. Some carotenoids decrease the risk for angina pectoris (Ford and Giles, 2000).

In addition to chest pain, signs and symptoms of angina include shortness of breath, sweating, nausea, vertigo, neck, jaw, or earache, or numbness or burning sensations. If diagnosed early, the chance of living longer than 10–12 years is at least 50%.

Based upon the Framingham Disability Study, disability rates in coronary patients are highest in women, the older old, and in the presence of angina pectoris or chronic heart failure (Ades, 1999). Older coronary patients would be good candidates for cardiac rehabilitation, as it has been documented to improve aerobic exercise capacity, physical functioning, and mental depression.

OBJECTIVES

- ▲ Relieve chest pain. Improve circulation to the heart.
- ▲ Increase activity only as tolerated or prescribed.
- ▲ Maintain adequate rest periods.
- ▲ Maintain weight or lose weight if obese.
- ▲ Avoid constipation without straining.

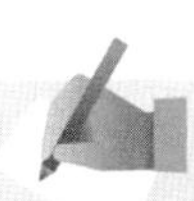

DIETARY AND NUTRITIONAL RECOMMENDATIONS

- Small, frequent feedings rather than three large meals are indicated.
- Increase fiber as tolerated; include an adequate fluid intake.
- Restrict saturated fats, dietary cholesterol, and sodium as necessary according to the individual profile.
- Limit stimulants such as caffeine to less than 5 cups of coffee or equivalent daily.
- Promote calorie control if overweight; modify by age and sex.
- It may be prudent to increase vitamin E for antioxidant effects, although supplements may not help (Rapola et al., 1996); beta carotene supplements actually seem to increase angina. Dietary sources are recommended.
- If homocysteine levels are high, add more foods with folic acid, vitamins B6 and B12, and riboflavin in the diet. Supplementation with B-group vitamins with or without antioxidants reduces total tHcy levels in men who have mildly elevated levels (Woodside et al., 1998).
- It is prudent to increase intake of olive, soybean, and canola oils and nuts such as walnuts, almonds, macadamias, pecans, peanuts, and pistachios. Walnuts contain alpha-linolenic acid; almonds are a good source of vitamin E. Nuts also contain flavonoids, phenols, sterols, saponins, elegiac acid, folic acid, magnesium, copper, potassium, and fiber.

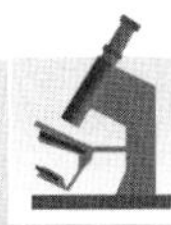

PROFILE

Clinical/History

Height
Weight
BMI
Recent weight changes (e.g., gain)
Pulse (NL = 60–100 beats/min)
BP
Intake and output (I & O)

Lab Work

Cholesterol (Chol)—LDL, HDL, total
Trig
Lactic acid dehydrogenase (LDH)
Homocysteine levels
Serum folate
Glucose (gluc)
Hemoglobin and hematocrit (H&H)
Electrocardiogram (ECG)
Radionucleotide imaging
Stress test
Coronary angiography
Serum Fe
Total iron-binding capacity (TIBC)
Aspartate aminostransaminase/alanine aminotransferase (AST/ALT)
Transferrin
Na+
K+
Ca++
Mg++
Alkaline phosphatase (Alk phos)

Common Drugs Used and Potential Side Effects

- Calcium channel blockers (verapamil [Calan], nicardipine, or diltiazem [Cardizem]) are used to dilate coronary arteries and slow down nerve impulses through the heart, thereby increasing blood flow. Nausea, edema, or constipation may be side effects. Take on an empty stomach. These drugs may also cause congestive heart failure (CHF) or dizziness. Avoid taking with aloe, buckthorn bark and berry, cascara, and senna leaf. With nifedipine (Procardia), nausea, weakness, dizziness, and flatulence may occur; take after meals.
- Dipyridamole (Persantine)—Nausea or vomiting may occur. This drug contains tartrazine. It helps to reduce blood clots.
- Norpace may cause abdominal pain, nausea, or constipation.

- Nitroglycerin (Nitro-BID, Nitrostat) is a general vasodilator. Take with water on an empty stomach; watch for headaches, nausea, vomiting, or dry mouth.
- Isosorbide (Isordil or Imdur) may cause nausea, vomiting, or dizziness. Take on an empty stomach.
- Nadolol (Corgard) is a beta-blocker; it may cause weakness.
- Grapefruit juice decreases drug metabolism in the gut (via P450-CYP3A4 inhibition) and can affect medications up to 24 hours later. Consistency of use may be more important than total quantity. Avoid taking with alprazolam, buspirone, cisapride, cyclosporine, statins, tacrolimus, and many others.

Herbs, Botanicals and Supplements

- The patient should not take herbals and botanicals without discussing with the physician.
- Danshen may be used for ischemic heart disease. Avoid large amounts with warfarin, aspirin, and other antiplatelet drugs. It can increase risks of bleeding or bruising.
- Garlic should not be taken in large amounts with warfarin, aspirin, and other antiplatelet drugs because of increased risks of bleeding or bruising. It may also increase insulin levels with hypoglycemic results; monitor carefully in patients with diabetes.
- CoEnzyme Q10 should not be used with statins, gemfibrozil, tricyclic antidepressants, or warfarin. CoQ10 may act similarly to vitamin K.
- Niacin (nicotinic acid) should not be taken with statins, antidiabetic medications, or carbamazepine because of potentially serious risks of myopathy and altered glucose control.
- Vitamin E should not be taken with warfarin because of the possibility of increased bleeding. Avoid doses greater than 400 IU per day.

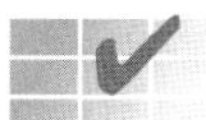

PATIENT EDUCATION

- ✓ The patient will require stress management, activity, and education about proper eating habits.
- ✓ Discuss the role of nutrition in maintenance of wellness and in cardiovascular disease. Discuss in particular: fiber, total fat intake, potassium and sodium, calcium and other nutrients, and caffeine.
- ✓ Discuss the importance of weight control in reduction of cardiovascular risks.
- ✓ Elevate the head of the bed 30–45° for greater comfort.

ARTERITIS

NUTRITIONAL ACUITY RANKING: LEVELS 1–2

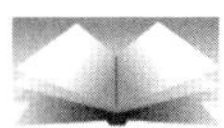

DEFINITIONS AND BACKGROUND

Arteritis involves inflammation of artery walls, with decreased blood flow. Buerger's disease includes an arteritis that causes limb pain and numbness. Periarteritis nodosa is an autoimmune disease that can affect any artery in the body. A rare form of arteritis, Takayasu's form, affects the mesenteric artery and creates local ischemia.

Temporal arteritis (cranial or giant-cell arteritis) yields chronically inflamed temporal arteries with a thickening of the lining and a reduction in blood flow; this condition is linked to polymyalgia rheumatica (PMR). Women older than 55 years of age are twice as likely to have the condition as other people. Signs and symptoms include a severe, throbbing headache at the temples or back of the head. The artery may be red, swollen, and painful. Anorexia, weight loss, mild fever, scalp tenderness, dysphagia, hearing problems, vision changes, jaw pain, and muscular aches may be indicators. The greatest danger is permanent blindness.

Tumor necrosis factor appears to influence susceptibility and interleukin (IL)-1 receptor antagonist seems to play a role in the pathogenesis. Genetic traits are being studied.

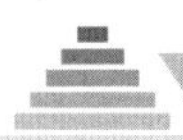

OBJECTIVES

- Prevent stroke and blindness, which are potential complications.
- Reduce inflammation.
- Promote increased blood flow through the affected vessels.
- Modify intake according to requirements and coexisting problems such as hypertension.

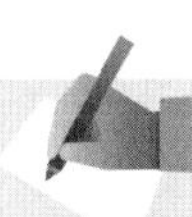

DIETARY AND NUTRITIONAL RECOMMENDATIONS

- Follow usual diet, with increased calories if patient is underweight or decreased calories if the patient is obese.
- Reduce excess sodium and total fat intake; monitor regularly.
- Patient may need to include carnitine in the diet. Although not yet proven, it may be reasonable to include in the diet more sources of vitamins E, B6, and B12, riboflavin, and folic acid or to use a multivitamin supplement that includes sufficient amounts.
- With steroids, decreased sodium intake with higher potassium intake may be needed; adequate-to-high protein may also be necessary. Monitor for glucose intolerance.
- Omega-3 fatty acids may be useful to reduce inflammatory process. Eat more salmon, tuna, mackerel, etc.

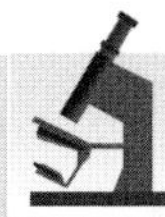

PROFILE

Clinical/History

Height
Weight
BMI
BP
Temperature

Lab Work

White blood cell count (WBC) (increased)
Na+
K+
Albumin (Alb), prealbumin
Transferrin
Biopsy
Chol—Total, HDL, LDL
Trig
H&H (often decreased)
Homocysteine level
Serum B12
Folate
Ferritin
Gluc

Common Drugs Used and Potential Side Effects

- Prednisone and other steroids may be used with numerous side effects such as elevated glucose and decreased nitrogen levels, especially with long-term use. A gradual tapering is needed, and the patient must not discontinue the medication independently.
- Other cardiovascular medications may be prescribed; monitor side effects accordingly.
- Grapefruit juice decreases drug metabolism in the gut (via P450-CYP3A4 inhibition) and can affect medications up to 24 hours later. Consistency of use may be more important than total quantity. Avoid taking with alprazolam, buspirone, cisapride, cyclosporine, statins, tacrolimus, and many others.

Herbs, Botanicals and Supplements

- The patient should not take herbals and botanicals without discussing with the physician.
- CoEnzyme Q10 should not be used with statins, gemfibrozil, tricyclic antidepressants, or warfarin. CoQ10 may act similarly to vitamin K.
- Niacin (nicotinic acid) should not be taken with statins, antidiabetic medications, or carbamazepine because of potentially serious risks of myopathy and altered glucose control.
- Vitamin E should not be taken with warfarin because of the possibility of increased bleeding. Avoid doses greater than 400 IU per day.

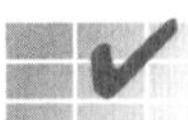

PATIENT EDUCATION

- ✔ Discuss the role of nutrition in the maintenance of health for cardiovascular disease.
- ✔ Discuss the effects of medications on nutritional status and appetite.

ATHEROSCLEROSIS, CORONARY ARTERY DISEASE, AND ISCHEMIC HEART DISEASE

NUTRITIONAL ACUITY RANKING: LEVEL 3

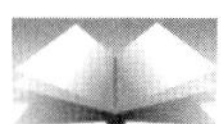

DEFINITIONS AND BACKGROUND

Atherosclerotic heart disease (ASHD) involves progressive narrowing of the arterial tree, giving rise to collateral vessels. Fat-deposit accumulations occur; the heart, brain, and leg arteries are most often affected. Sagittal abdominal diameter (height of abdomen at the umbilical level measured from exam couch in a supine position with straight legs) is more strongly correlated with cardiovascular risk factors than waist circumference, waist-to-hip ratio, and BMI (Ohrvall et al., 2000).

Major risk factors for coronary heart disease are smoking, high blood pressure, low HDL cholesterol (below 40), family history of early coronary heart disease, and age for males over 45 and females over 55 years. Obesity, elevated serum homocysteine and copper levels are lesser risk factors. Diabetes is a precursor for many individuals. In women who have had more than six pregnancies, CAD may occur as a result of insulin resistance.

Atherosclerosis is an underlying cause of CAD; arteries of the heart thicken and lose elasticity because of mineral and fibrous deposits. CAD involves plaque buildup in the arteries of the heart; gum disease may precede CAD in some cases. Clustering of atherogenic risk factors is common in men and women, positively related to weight gain, and significantly related to risk of CAD (Wilson et al., 1999). Even before menopause, the age-related increase in visceral adipose tissue makes a significant contribution to age-related CAD (Pascot et al., 1999).

Young men with high serum cholesterol concentrations are likely to have CAD later in midlife (Klag et al., 1993). Serum lipid reductions decrease CAD risk; for each 1% reduction in serum cholesterol, there is a 2% reduction in CAD risk. In men, serum triglyceride levels are not meaningful predictors of coronary heart disease beyond that noted from total cholesterol subfractions (Avins and Neuhaus, 2000). After adjustment for socioeconomic factors and years of education, HPN, overweight, physical inactivity, and type 2 diabetes are more common among high-risk groups of black and Mexican Americans (Winkleby et al., 1998).

Ischemia is a local and temporary deficiency of blood caused by obstruction (from thrombosis, etc.). Risk of ischemic heart disease is about 15% lower in subjects with very high fruit and vegetable intakes; those individuals who consume very high carotenoid intakes have over 40% less CAD (Law and Morris, 1998). Older women may also benefit from diets in which SFA is replaced by MUFA (Jeppesen et al., 1997). In some studies, a diet high in both MUFA and omega-3 fatty acids seems to correct an atherogenic profile better than a high-CHO, low-fat diet (Pieke et al., 2000).

Intake of whole grains is inversely related to death from ischemic heart disease (Jacobs et al., 1998). Whole grains and high fiber intakes, particularly from cereal sources, reduce the risk of CAD in women (Liu et al., 1999; Wolk et al., 1999). Starchy foods can prevent coronary heart disease when substituted for saturated fats; sucrose does not protect against coronary heart disease (Marckmann et al., 2000). Dietary α-tocopherol (vitamin E) and wine, vegetables, vegetable oil, and fruits seem to be preventive (Bellizzi et al., 1994) but not beta carotene (Greenberg et al., 1996).

Moderate alcohol intake appears to decrease risk of cardiovascular disease in subjects who eat a high-fat diet but not in those who consume a low-fat diet (Rumplet et al., 1999.) Compared with occasional intake (under 1 drink/week), regular intake of any type of alcoholic beverage is associated with a lower risk of CAD (Wannametheem, 1999). Benefits associated with drinking wine vs. other alcoholic beverages can be attributed to other lifestyle measures such as low rate of smoking and less obesity.

Elevated serum copper levels appear to be positively correlated with coronary heart disease; copper is a strong pro-oxidant (Ford, 2000). Studies about copper are in the early stages; data for copper are not as strong as those for homocysteine as a risk factor. In 1969, McCully made the clinical observation that linked elevated plasma homocysteine levels with cardiovascular disease; mild deficiency exists in 5–7% of the population while severe deficiency is rare (Welch and Loscalzo, 1998). In healthy siblings of patients with premature ASHD, treatment with folate and vitamin B6 to lower tHcy levels is associated with lower occurrence of abnormal exercise ECGs and fewer cardiac events (Vermeulen et al., 2000).

Angioplasty is as safe and effective as bypass surgery. Individuals who undergo the coronary artery bypass graft surgery (CABG) continue to have multiple risk factors for CAD that place them at high risk for future CAD events; other steps such as stopping smoking, following the recommended diet, and managing other risk factors must be taken (Frame et al., 2001). Other risk factors currently under study include specific lipoproteins such as Lp(a), C-reactive protein (CRP) levels, omega-3 fatty acids, prostaglandins, estrogens, and nitric oxide.

Cholesterol screening is recommended, even for older adults. When treated, risks decrease by 25–30% for those persons treated for 5 or more years (Hall and Lueopker, 2000). Early nutritional intervention is beneficial. Three or four individualized dietitian visits of 50 minutes each for a span of 7 weeks have been found to be associated with significant serum cholesterol reduction and a saving in healthcare costs (Sikand et al., 1998).

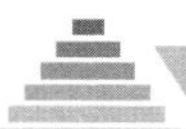

OBJECTIVES

- ▲ Lower elevated serum lipids, especially cholesterol levels higher than 200 mg/dL and triglyceride levels higher than 200 mg/dL.
- ▲ Initiate and maintain weight loss if patient is obese. Obesity with a high waist circumference is especially impor-

tant to correct in both men and women. Physical activity should be encouraged.

▲ Observe NCEP/Adult Treatment Panel III diet guidelines: Reduce intakes of saturated fatty acids to less than 7% of kcals and keep total dietary cholesterol below 200 mg/day.

▲ Improve LDL and HDL cholesterol levels. Prevent formation of new lesions.

▲ Correct high levels of homocysteine where present. Supplementation with B-group vitamins with or without antioxidants reduces total tHcy levels in men who have mildly elevated levels (Woodside et al., 1998).

▲ Intake of 1–2 g plant sterols (soybean extract) daily improves plasma lipid levels without detrimental effects on plasma carotenoid levels; sterol-enriched margarines are easily used in the diet (Hendricks et al., 1999).

▲ Flavonoids in red wine, grape juice, grapefruit, tea, onions, and apples are possible factors in risk reduction; cloves, licorice, and sage may also be beneficial (Hertog et al., 1993). The flavonoids in grape juice appear to inhibit platelet aggregation and may help decrease the risk of CAD and MI (Keevil et al., 2000). Intake of tea, a major source of flavonoids, may help prevent ASHD, especially in women (Geleijnse et al., 1999).

▲ Increase soluble fiber; use 10–25 g/day.

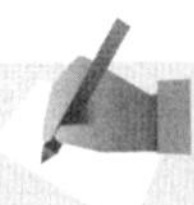

DIETARY AND NUTRITIONAL RECOMMENDATIONS

- Restrict saturated fats to 7% of total kcals and increase MUFAs and polyunsaturated fatty acids (PUFAs). Omega-3 fatty acids, more than MUFAs, may help to lower triglycerides (Howard et al., 1995). Limit cholesterol to 200 mg or less per day. Total fat should be 25–35% of total kcals; see Table 6–2 (NHLBI, 2001).
- Trans fatty acids should be used in limited amounts. Compared with butter, margarines free from trans fatty acids may be equal to or more effective than margarines that contain them in lowering LDL-C (Noakes and Clifton, 1998). Foods such as pound cake, regular microwave popcorn, snack crackers, vegetable shortening, stick margarine, vanilla wafers, snack chips, boxed chocolate chip cookies, french fries, and similar foods are sources of trans fatty acids. New food labels will likely state content of trans fatty acids as part of total saturated fatty acid amounts (Daucsh, 2002).
- Use of plant sterols can be helpful; 2 g daily has been suggested (NHLBI, 2001). Benecol or Take Control margarines may be consumed in 2 servings daily; allow at least 3 weeks for results. In addition, products made with Olestra help to lower total cholesterol (TC) levels even if weight is not lost (Patterson et al., 2000).
- Use a calorie-controlled diet with increased content of complex CHO rather than concentrated sweets and simple sugars.
- In hypertensive patients, the DASH diet may be useful. For patients with ischemia, 2 g of sodium may be needed; small amounts of alcohol may be protective by reducing insulin resistance (Hein et al., 1993).
- The diet should include fewer animal proteins and more legumes and vegetables. Fish and shellfish should be used 3–4 times weekly, especially sources rich in omega-3 fatty acids. Remove chicken skin before cooking or just before serving. Lean beef and chicken are considered to be comparable in the NCEP diet plans.
- Patients given omega-enriched eggs double their omega-3 PUFA intake; TGs become lower. The enriched eggs are affordable and easier to tolerate than fish for many (Lewis et al., 2000). However, they still provide dietary cholesterol and must be incorporated in the diet to meet the dietary cholesterol recommendation.
- Patients may want to consume less than 5 cups of coffee per day to reduce stimulant intake, even if there is no definite link with coronary heart disease (Kleemola et al., 2000).
- The diet should include an adequate fiber intake of 25–30 g daily, of which 10–25 g of soluble fiber is included. Oat bran, corn bran, apples, and legumes should be used.
- Provide vitamin C (Halfrich et al., 1994), chromium, and copper in adequate amounts from food sources.
- Vitamin E has been noted to function as an antioxidant; inclusion of nuts and other dietary sources such as oils and creamy salad dressings may be beneficial. Supplements of 100–200 IU natural vitamin E have been recommended (Hodis et al., 1995), but diet should be adapted first. In addition, intake of as little as 20 g soy daily for 6 weeks reduced non-HDL-C and apoB levels by about 2% (Teixeira, 2000).
- Garlic use may be encouraged, with parsley as a breath freshener (Stevinson et al., 2000). Avoid excesses with certain medications.
- Use more grape juice, red wine (if allowed), tea, onions, apples, cloves, licorice, and sage.
- More folic acid, vitamins B6 and B12, and riboflavin should be consumed.
- Soy products should be used in amounts equivalent to about 25 g/day. Food labels now indicate products that contain soy.

TABLE 6–2 Reducing Dietary Fat to 25–35%: Goal: Keep fat at about 3 g/100 kcals

Reducing total fat to 25% of kcals	Reducing total fat to 30% of kcals:	Reducing total fat to 35% of kcals:
28 g in 1,000 kcals	33 g in 1,000 kcals	39 g in 1,000 kcals
33 g in 1,200 kcals	40 g in 1,200 kcals	47 g in 1,200 kcals
42 g in 1,500 kcals	50 g in 1,500 kcals	59 g in 1,500 kcals
50 g in 1,800 kcals	60 g in 1,800 kcals	70 g in 1,800 kcals
56 g in 2,000 kcals	67 g in 2,000 kcals	78 g in 2,000 kcals
67 g in 2,400 kcals	80 g in 2,400 kcals	93 g in 2,400 kcals

PROFILE

Clinical/History	HDL, LDL, —ideal: 35% HDL, 65% LDL	Serum B6
Height	Homocysteine: serum and urinary	H&H
Weight	Serum and urinary folate	Serum ferritin
BMI	Serum and urinary B12	K+, Na+
BP		Ca++
Lab Work		Mg++
Trig		Gluc
Total Chol (often increased)		AST, ALT (with use of medication)

Common Drugs Used and Potential Side Effects:

"Diet First, Then Drugs" (Pedersen, 1995).

- Cardiovascular preparations such as digitalis and digoxin (Lanoxin) require the patient to avoid excessive amounts of vitamin D or natural licorice. In addition, a low potassium intake should be avoided, because these drugs could become toxic. Avoid taking with high-fiber meals and herbal teas; take drugs 30 minutes before meals. Do not take with Siberian ginseng, milkweed, hawthorn, guar gum, or St. John's wort.
- Bile acid sequestrants bind bile acids and remove them in the stool. Colestipol (Colestid) requires supplements of fat-soluble vitamins to be added to the diet. Patients taking cholestyramine (Questran) should have an increased fiber intake to alleviate constipation. Folate must also be used.
- Psyllium (Metamucil) lowers LDLs without affecting HDL levels.
- Statins or HMG-CoA reductase inhibitors such as Lovastatin (Mevacor), fluvastatin (Lescol), pravastatin (Pravachol), simvastatin (Zocor), and atorvastatin (Lipitor) reduce cholesterol production by the liver. They are better tolerated than niacin (Illingworth et al., 1994), have no effect on prothrombin (Hansen et al., 1993), and are being considered for over-the-counter use. Good nutritional practices should be followed (Kris-Etherton, 2000). Statins may lower CoEnzyme Q10 to the point of deficiency. Simvastatin may cause constipation; fluvastatin may cause nausea and abdominal cramps; pravastatin can elevate AST and ALT levels or cause nausea, vomiting, and diarrhea.
- Colestipol and nicotinic acid can be effective as vasodilators; beware of excesses. Nausea, vomiting, and cramping may result.
- Lescol (fluvastatin sodium) may cause nausea, indigestion, and abdominal pain.
- Anticoagulants (Coumadin) may be needed. Limit vitamin K-containing foods to 1 per day; consistency of intake is often more important than quantity. Decrease supplements containing vitamins A, E, and C, which counteract the medication (Harris et al., 1995).
- Children with familial hyperlipoproteinemia and hypercholesterolemia have impaired endothelium-dependent vasoregulation for which daily intakes of α-tocopherol and ascorbic acid improve arterial diameter and flow (Mietus-Snyder, 1998).
- Although not yet definitive, supplements containing folic acid, riboflavin, and vitamins B12 and B6 eventually may be recommended to correct hyperhomocystinemia.
- Hormone replacement therapy (HRT) improves plasma lipoprotein profiles in menopausal women (Vadlamudi et al., 1998). It has favorable effects on serum lipoproteins in women with normal serum lipid levels, but the effect of combined estrogen and progestin therapy on lipoproteins in women with hypercholesterolemia has not been determined.
- Grapefruit juice decreases drug metabolism in the gut (via P450-CYP3A4 inhibition) and can affect medications up to 24 hours later. Consistency of use may be more important than total quantity. Avoid taking with alprazolam, buspirone, cisapride, cyclosporine, statins, tacrolimus, and many others.
- Beta-hydoxy-b-methylbutyrate (HMB) is a metabolite of leucine and may be used as an ergogenic aid in HIV/AIDS patients to prevent muscle wasting. Significant decreases in serum total cholesterol, LDL-C, and blood pressure have been noted in this population; this may lead to decreased risk for MI or stroke (Nissen et al., 2000).

Herbs, Botanicals and Supplements

- Danshen may be used for ischemic heart disease. Avoid large amounts with warfarin, aspirin, and other antiplatelet drugs. It can increase risks of bleeding or bruising.
- Garlic should not be taken in large amounts with warfarin, aspirin, and other antiplatelet drugs because of increased risks of bleeding or bruising. It may also increase insulin levels with hypoglycemic results; monitor carefully in patients with diabetes.
- CoEnzyme Q10 should not be used with statins, gemfibrozil, tricyclic antidepressants, or warfarin. CoQ10 may act similarly to vitamin K.
- Chromium is sometimes used for dyslipidemia. Do not use excesses with insulin or hypoglycemic agents, because it may lower glucose levels.
- Niacin (nicotinic acid) should not be taken with statins, antidiabetic medications, and carbamazepine because of potentially serious risks of myopathy and altered glucose control.
- Vitamin E should not be taken with warfarin because of the possibility of increased bleeding. Avoid doses greater than 400 IU per day.
- Herbs and botanicals such as angelica, hawthorn, canola, cinchona, valerian, willow, grape, pigweed, and chicory have been recommended, but no clinical trials have proven efficacy.

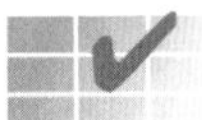

PATIENT EDUCATION

- ✔ There is no cholesterol in foods of plant origin. Encourage a plant-based diet.
- ✔ Explain which foods are sources of saturated fats and trans fatty acids. Most people eat about 3% of dietary kcals as trans fatty acids; the goal is to eat less than 1% kcals as trans fatty acids. Identify foods that are sources of polyunsaturated fats and monounsaturated fats (olive and peanut oils). An easy first step is changing to skim milk products instead of whole milk.
- ✔ Encourage the reading of labels: "free, low, reduced" cholesterol, etc.
- ✔ Help the patient to creatively include nutrient-dense foods in the diet while lowering intake of animal proteins.
- ✔ Discuss the roles of heredity, exercise, and lifestyle habits. Blood pressure, cholesterol, obesity, and diabetes are affected by dietary patterns; some control is possible.
- ✔ Note that some hearing losses and cataracts in elderly individuals are associated with ASHD.
- ✔ Although the only sterol in shellfish (lobster, crab, shrimp) is cholesterol, intake of shellfish is no longer prohibited because their saturated fat content is very low.
- ✔ Omega-3 fatty acids are found in fatter fish such as salmon, herring, tuna, mackerel, and other seafood.
- ✔ Water-soluble fibers are found in legumes (gum), fruits (pectin), and products such as oat bran.
- ✔ Relaxation should be part of the daily routine for all persons under medical guidance.
- ✔ Exercise is very useful in preventing or managing coronary heart disease; increase gradually to levels determined under the doctor's guidance.
- ✔ Family counseling may be the most beneficial to ensure adherence. Contracting with the patient is also a suggested intervention tool.
- ✔ Discuss low-fat cooking methods: baking, broiling, flame-cooking, grilling, marinating, poaching, roasting, smoking, or steaming.
- ✔ Foods such as oil-based salad dressing that contain PUFAs, including α-linolenic acid (C18:3 n03), may help reduce risk of fatal ischemic heart disease (IHD); salad with oil and vinegar (an important source of α-linolenic acid) 5–6 times per week is an effective suggestion (Dietary. . .,1999).
- ✔ Intensive lifestyle changes maintained for 5+ years can result in regression of CAD; more moderate changes are associated with progression of CAD (Ornish et al., 1998). Dr. Ornish's treatment for patients with coronary heart disease is a demanding regimen: It includes a vegetarian diet with less than 10% of calories from fat, with minimal amounts of saturated fat (the "Reversal Diet"). Moderate exercise is prescribed for each patient, usually a walking program. The treatment relies on the daily use of stress management techniques including various stretching, breathing, meditation, yoga, and relaxation exercises. Patients receive group support and psychological counseling to identify sources of stress and receive tools that help them manage stress more effectively. Smokers participate in a smoking cessation program. Patients participating in Ornish's experimental treatment program, for the most part, don't use lipid-lowering drugs.

For More Information

- ✦ American Dietetic Association
  Hyperlipidemia protocol
  www.eatright.org
- ✦ National Cholesterol Education Program (NHLBI)
  National Heart Lung & Blood Institute
  PO Box 30105
  Bethesda, MD 20892-0105
  (301) 496-0554
  http://www.nhlbi.nih.gov/guidelines/cholesterol/index.htm

CARDIAC CACHEXIA

NUTRITIONAL ACUITY RANKING: LEVEL 3

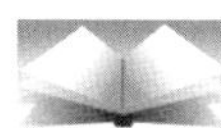

DEFINITIONS AND BACKGROUND

Cardiac cachexia involves heart failure of such severity that patients cannot eat adequately to maintain weight. The condition usually follows CHF (moderate to severe), with some valvular heart disease. Nutritional insults generally affect the heart muscle severely, and the insult may be significant. Signs and symptoms of cardiac cachexia include increased total body fluid, which occurs in an effort to improve heart function, supraclavicular and temporal muscle wasting, weight loss, anorexia, and malabsorption with steatorrhea or diarrhea. Tumor necrosis factor may be involved.

Observational studies in heart failure suggest that a moderate excess of body fat and elevated blood cholesterol may be desirable in patients with heart failure, challenging the nonevidence-based vogue for cholesterol-lowering therapy in heart failure (Louis et al., 2001). The wasting (cardiac cachexia) associated with chronic CHF leads to a worse prognosis and is an independent predictor of mortality (Adigun and Ajayi, 2001).

Data support findings that lower, rather than higher, cholesterol levels are associated with poor clinical outcome in patients with chronic heart failure. The ability of all lipoprotein fractions to bind endotoxin and to serve as natural buffer substances may explain this relationship between lower lipoprotein levels, higher cytokine concentrations, and impaired prognosis (Rauchhaus et al., 2000).

OBJECTIVES

- ▲ Improve hypoxic state and heart functioning.
- ▲ Correct malnutrition, wasting, malabsorption, and steatorrhea.
- ▲ Optimize heart function through balance of medications, fluids, and electrolytes.
- ▲ Meet hypermetabolic state with adequate calories.
- ▲ Prevent infection or sepsis, especially if tracheostomy is required.
- ▲ Provide gradual repletion to prevent overloading in a severely depleted patient.
- ▲ Treat constipation or diarrhea as necessary.

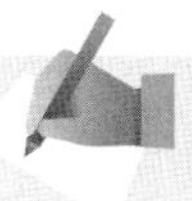

DIETARY AND NUTRITIONAL RECOMMENDATIONS

- Provide small, frequent meals to prevent overloading with high glucose levels or with rapid fat infusion.
- Provide as many preferred foods as feasible to improve appetite and intake.
- A prudent heart diet may be appropriate to lessen cardiac effects of diet, but the focus is on adequate intake at this time.
- Diet may need to be high in folate, magnesium, thiamine, zinc, and iron (depending on serum levels). Increasing vitamins E, B6, and B12 may also be beneficial.
- Thiamine should be included (Blanc and Boussuges, 2000) for cardiac beriberi.
- Calorie needs may be calculated at 1.5 times basal energy expenditure (BEE).
- Sodium may need to be restricted to 1–2 g daily; modify potassium intake as appropriate for serum levels.
- Protein should be calculated at a rate of 1.0–1.5 g/kg, increasing or decreasing, dependent on renal or hepatic status.
- Offer tube feeding or parenteral nutrition if appropriate. Sometimes, tube feedings are not well tolerated because of access to the thoracic cavity and reduced blood flow to the gastrointestinal (GI) tract. Products like Magnacal, Ensure Plus, Osmolite, Sustacal HC, and Isocal HCN have a low volume with high density of calories. They are appropriate for persons with a fluid limitation but must be monitored with renal or hepatic insufficiency.

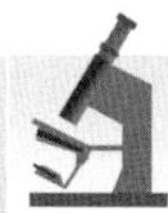

PROFILE

Clinical/History		
Height	Trig	Alb, prealbumin
Weight, current	Na+	Retinol-binding protein (RBP)
Dry weight	K+	Transferrin
BMI	Gluc	Ca++, Mg++
Edema	Fecal fat (in steatorrhea)	Homocysteine
BP	H&H, serum Fe	Serum folate
Lab Work	Total lymphocyte count (TLC)	Serum B12
Chol (total, HDL, LDL)	Serum insulin	BUN, Creat

Common Drugs Used and Potential Side Effects

- Diuretics—Side effects may include potassium depletion; review types used and alter diet accordingly.
- Insulin may be needed if patient has diabetes or becomes hyperglycemic. Alter mealtimes accordingly.
- Digoxin—Monitor potassium intake or depletion carefully, especially when combining with diuretics. Avoid excessive intakes of fiber and wheat bran. Avoid use with hawthorn, milkweed, guar gum, and St. John's wort.
- Grapefruit juice decreases drug metabolism in the gut (via P450-CYP3A4 inhibition) and can affect medications up to 24 hours later. Consistency of use may be more important than total quantity. Avoid taking with alprazolam, buspirone, cisapride, cyclosporine, statins, tacrolimus, and many others.

- Increased subcutaneous fat (increased skin-fold thickness) and greater muscle bulk (increased mid-upper arm and thigh circumferences) together with a significant elevation in plasma albumin and the hematocrit will reflect the anabolic state in patients treated with angiotensin-converting enzyme (ACE) inhibitor, digoxin, diuretic therapy in CHF (Adigun and Ajayi, 2001).

Herbs, Botanicals and Supplements

- Danshen may be used for ischemic heart disease. Avoid large amounts with warfarin, aspirin, and other antiplatelet drugs. It can increase risks of bleeding or bruising.
- Garlic should not be taken in large amounts with warfarin, aspirin, and other antiplatelet drugs because of increased risks of bleeding or bruising. It may also increase insulin levels with resulting hypoglycemic results; monitor carefully in patients with diabetes.
- CoEnzyme Q10 should not be used with statins, gemfibrozil, tricyclic antidepressants, or warfarin. CoQ10 may act similarly to vitamin K.
- Niacin (nicotinic acid) should not be taken with statins, antidiabetic medications, and carbamazepine because of potentially serious risks of myopathy and altered glucose control.
- Vitamin E should not be taken with warfarin because of the possibility of increased bleeding. Avoid doses greater than 400 IU per day.

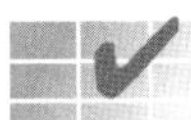

PATIENT EDUCATION

- ✔ Balance medications, fluid, and electrolytes carefully.
- ✔ Supplements may be beneficial between meals to improve total calorie intake, e.g., sherbet shakes.
- ✔ The importance of diet in cardiovascular health should be addressed. However, rapid weight loss should be prevented.

CARDIOMYOPATHIES

NUTRITIONAL ACUITY RANKING: LEVEL 3

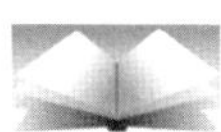

DEFINITIONS AND BACKGROUND

Cardiomyopathies may be caused by many known diseases or have no specific known cause. They are progressive disorders that impair the structure or function of the muscular wall of the lower chambers of the heart. Dilated congestive cardiomyopathy (DCC) is most commonly caused by coronary heart disease in the U.S. DCC may also occur from a viral infection such as coxsackievirus B, from diabetes or thyroid disease, or excessive alcohol, cocaine, or antidepressant use. Rarely, pregnancy or rheumatory arthritis can also trigger dilated cardiomyopathy. The first symptoms are shortness of breath on exertion and easy tiredness; sometimes, a fever and flu-like symptoms occur if triggered by a virus. Echocardiography is useful in demonstrating cardiac abnormalities seen in idiopathic cardiomyopathies, especially to differentiate constrictive pericarditis from restrictive cardiomyopathy (Nakatani and Miyatake, 2000).

Remaining heart muscle stretches to compensate for lost pumping action, and when the stretching no longer compensates, DCC occurs. Blood may pool in the swollen heart, and clots may form on the chamber walls. 70% of patients with DCC die within 5 years of the beginning of their symptoms, and the prognosis worsens as the walls become thinner and the heart valves begin to leak. Because of this, DCC is the most common cause for heart transplantation.

Hypertrophic cardiomyopathy (HCM) may occur as a birth defect, from acromegaly (excessive growth hormone in the blood), a pheochromocytoma, or a neurofibromatosis. Thickening of the heart wall causes high blood pressure, pulmonary hypertension, and chronic shortness of breath. Faintness, chest pain, irregular heartbeats and palpitations, and heart failure with dyspnea will occur. The differences in serum carnitine levels between HCM and hypertensive heart disease reflect altered myocardial fatty acid metabolic impairment, and the levels can help to distinguish between these 2 diseases (Nakamura, 2000). Preliminary studies suggest that specific polymorphism of the ACE gene influences the development of left ventricular hypertrophy (Komajda et al., 1999).

HCM is a possible cause of sudden death. Death from HCM, especially when sudden, has been reported to be largely confined to young people, but it can actually occur suddenly in all phases of life. Most patients with mild hypertrophy are at low risk and can be reassured regarding their prognosis (Spirito et al., 2000).

Treatment options for patients with hypertrophic obstructive cardiomyopathy include medical therapy, pacemaker insertion, percutaneous transluminal septal myocardial ablation, mitral valve replacement, and surgical resection of the obstructing muscle (Meisel et al., 2000). Septal myectomy reduces or abolishes left ventricular outflow tract gradient in these patients and provides long-lasting symptomatic improvement in most patients (Merrill et al., 2000). Nonsurgical septal reduction therapy is also an effective therapy for symptomatic patients with hypertrophic obstructive cardiomyopathy with persistence of the favorable outcome up to 1 year after the procedure (Lakkis et al., 2000).

OBJECTIVES

- Improve hypoxic state and heart functioning.
- Correct malnutrition, malabsorption, and steatorrhea.
- Optimize heart function through balance of medications, fluids, and electrolytes.
- Meet hypermetabolic state with adequate calories.
- Provide gradual repletion to prevent overloading in a severely depleted patient.
- Treat constipation or diarrhea as necessary.
- Prepare for surgery, if planned.

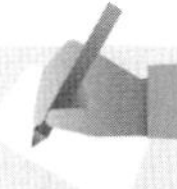

DIETARY AND NUTRITIONAL RECOMMENDATIONS

- Provide small, frequent meals to prevent overloading with high glucose or with rapid fat infusion. Provide as many preferred foods as feasible to improve appetite and intake.
- A prudent diet may be appropriate to reduce cardiac effects of diet. Follow NECP guidelines.
- Diet may need to be high in folate, magnesium, thiamine, zinc, and iron (depending on serum levels). Increasing vitamins E, B6, and B12 also may be beneficial.
- Thiamine should be included (Blanc and Boussuges, 2000) because of the likelihood of cardiac beriberi.
- Calorie intake may be calculated at 1.5 times BEE, with a calorie:nitrogen ratio of 150:1.
- Sodium may need to be restricted to 2–4 g daily; modify potassium intake as appropriate for serum levels.
- Protein should be calculated at a rate of 1.0–1.5 g/kg, increasing or decreasing, dependent on renal or hepatic status.
- Offer tube feeding or parenteral nutrition if appropriate. Sometimes, tube feedings are not well tolerated because of access to the thoracic cavity and because of reduced blood flow to the GI tract. Products like Magnacal, Ensure Plus, or Boost Plus have a low volume with high density of calories. They are appropriate for persons with a fluid limitation but must be monitored with renal or hepatic difficulty.

Common Drugs Used and Potential Side Effects

- Diuretics—Side effects may include potassium depletion; review types used and alter diet accordingly.
- Insulin may be needed if patient has diabetes or becomes hyperglycemic. Alter mealtimes accordingly.
- Digoxin—monitor potassium intake or depletion carefully, especially when combining with diuretics. Avoid

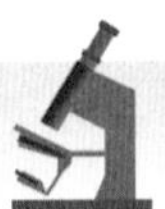

PROFILE

Clinical/History

- Height
- Weight, current
- Dry weight
- BMI
- Heart murmur
- BP (normal or low)
- Edema (common)
- Temperature

Lab Work

- Echocardiography
- ECG
- Cardiac catheterization
- Chol (total, HDL, LDL)
- Trig
- Protime therapy (PT)
- Na+
- K+
- Gluc
- H&H, serum Fe
- Serum insulin
- Alb, prealbumin
- RBP
- Transferrin
- Ca++, Mg++
- BUN, Creat
- Homocysteine, serum folate, serum B12

excessive intakes of fiber and wheat bran. Avoid use with hawthorn, milkweed, guar gum, and St. John's wort.

- Grapefruit juice decreases drug metabolism in the gut (via P450-CYP3A4 inhibition) and can affect medications up to 24 hours later. Consistency of use may be more important than total quantity. Avoid taking with alprazolam, buspirone, cisapride, cyclosporine, statins, tacrolimus, and many others.
- Anticoagulant therapy is needed to prevent clots from causing heart attacks, strokes, and other problems. With warfarin (Coumadin), use a controlled amount of vitamin K; check tube feeding (TF) products and supplements. Limit high vitamin K foods to 1 serving per day (e.g., green leafy vegetables, fish, broccoli/kale/brussels sprouts). Be wary of using supplements containing vitamins A and C with these drugs; side effects may be detrimental. Vitamin E should not be taken with warfarin because of the possibility of increased bleeding; avoid doses greater than 400 IU per day. Avoid taking with dong quai, fenugreek, feverfew, excessive garlic, ginger, ginkgo, and ginseng because of their effects.
- Beta-blockers and calcium channel blockers may be used to reduce the force of heart contractions.

Herbs, Botanicals and Supplements

- Danshen may be used for ischemic heart disease. Avoid large amounts with warfarin, aspirin, and other antiplatelet drugs. It can increase risks of bleeding or bruising.
- Garlic should not be taken in large amounts with warfarin, aspirin, and other antiplatelet drugs because of increased risks of bleeding or bruising. It may also increase insulin levels with hypoglycemic results; monitor carefully in patients with diabetes.
- CoEnzyme Q10 should not be used with statins, gemfibrozil, tricyclic antidepressants, or warfarin. CoQ10 may act similarly to vitamin K.
- Niacin (nicotinic acid) should not be taken with statins, antidiabetic medications, and carbamazepine because of potentially serious risks of myopathy and altered glucose control.

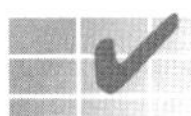

PATIENT EDUCATION

- ✓ Adequate rest is essential. Avoidance of stress is also important.
- ✓ Balance medications, fluid, and electrolytes carefully.
- ✓ Supplements may be beneficial between meals to improve total calorie intake, e.g., sherbet shakes.
- ✓ The importance of diet in cardiovascular health should be addressed.
- ✓ Because of the high risk for sudden death in hypertrophic cardiomyopathic patients, they should be advised against participation in competitive sports (DeLuca and Tak, 2000).
- ✓ For inherited forms of hypertrophic cardiomyopathy, genetic counseling may be beneficial if planning a family.

CARDIAC TAMPONADE

NUTRITIONAL ACUITY RANKING: LEVEL 1

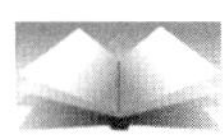

DEFINITIONS AND BACKGROUND

Cardiac tamponade involves an accumulation of fluid or blood within the pericardial sac. If uncontrolled, this condition may lead to heart failure, arrest, or shock. Decreased heart sounds, distended neck veins with inspiratory rise in venous pressure (Kussmaul's sign), decreased blood pressure, and abdominal pain may occur. It may occur as a result of a chest injury or trauma.

OBJECTIVES

- ▲ Care for ongoing disease process; prevent complications and crises.
- ▲ Prepare for possible surgery.
- ▲ Improve any poor appetite that exists.
- ▲ Normalize fluid balance.

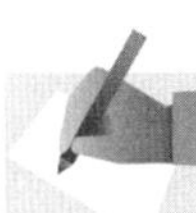

DIETARY AND NUTRITIONAL RECOMMENDATIONS

- For the first day, the patient is likely to be (nothing by mouth (NPO) with IVs.
- The diet is progressed, as tolerated, to the usual diet (perhaps reducing or increasing sodium and potassium, as appropriate, for the condition).
- Small, frequent feedings may be better tolerated.
- If surgery is required, provide an adequate diet for wound healing and prevention of infection.
- Restrict fluids only if necessary.

Common Drugs Used and Potential Side Effects

- Analgesics may be used for pain relief.
- Antiarrhythmia medications may be necessary; alter diet as needed. Quinidine (Quinaglute) should be taken with food or milk. Avoid citrus juice.
- Amiodarone may cause GI distress and nausea.
- Grapefruit juice decreases drug metabolism in the gut (via P450-CYP3A4 inhibition) and can affect medications up to 24 hours later. Consistency of use may be more important than total quantity. Avoid taking with alprazolam, buspirone, cisapride, cyclosporine, statins, tacrolimus, and many others.

Herbs, Botanicals and Supplements

- The patient should not take herbals and botanicals without discussing with the physician.
- Niacin (nicotinic acid) should not be taken with statins, antidiabetic medications, and carbamazepine because of potentially serious risks of myopathy and altered glucose control.
- Vitamin E should not be taken with warfarin because of the possibility of increased bleeding. Avoid doses greater than 400 IU per day.

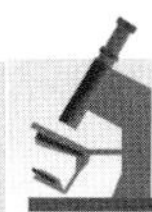

PROFILE

Clinical/History	Lab Work	
Height	H&H	Serum Fe
Weight	Partial pressure of carbon dioxide (pCO2), partial pressure of oxygen (pO2)	Alb, prealbumin
BMI		Na+
I & O		K+
BP (often low)		Chol—HDL, LDL, total
Jugular vein distention (JVD)		Trig
Muffled heart sounds		Homocysteine
Dyspnea		Serum folate
		Serum B12

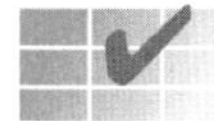

PATIENT EDUCATION

- ✔ Discuss the role of nutrition in cardiovascular disease; explain fluid and nutrient balance; include vitamins known to be protective to the heart and vessels.
- ✔ Provide lists for foods to eat or avoid, as appropriate for the condition.

CEREBROVASCULAR ACCIDENT (STROKE)

NUTRITIONAL ACUITY RANKING: LEVEL 3

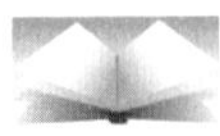

DEFINITIONS AND BACKGROUND

A cerebrovascular accident (CVA) (stroke) is caused by damage to a portion of the brain resulting from loss of blood supply resulting from a blood vessel spasm, clot, or rupture. Transient ischemic attacks (TIAs) are brief episodes of blood loss to the brain from a clot or an embolism; 10% of victims have a major CVA within a year. Stroke patients need to be seen medically within 60 minutes to begin appropriate treatment. Some people recover completely; others may be seriously disabled or die. Strokes cause 10% of all fatalities in this country.

HDL-C levels are related; high levels are more protective against ischemic stroke in the elderly (Sacco et al., 2001). Obesity and weight gain are important risk factors for ischemic and total stroke but not for hemorrhagic stroke in women, according to the Nurse's Health Study (Rexrode et al., 1997). Hypertension, smoking, diabetes mellitus, atrial fibrillation, and oral contraceptive use are key risk factors for strokes. Signs and symptoms of a stroke include sudden numbness or weakness of arm, face, or leg, especially one-sided, sudden confusion, trouble speaking or understanding speech, sudden trouble seeing in one or both eyes, sudden trouble walking, dizziness, loss of balance or coordination, or sudden excruciating headache with no known cause.

Unconsciousness, paralysis, and other problems may occur depending on the site and extent of the brain damage. Left CVA affects sight and hearing most commonly, including the ability to see where foods are placed on a plate or tray. Patients with a right-hemisphere, bilateral, or brainstem CVA have significant problems with feeding and swallowing of food; speech problems also occur.

Neurogenic deficits may include motor deficits with muscle weakness of the tongue and lips, nerve damage with resulting lack of coordination, apraxia, sensory deficits with inability to feel food in the mouth, or cognitive deficits with difficulty sustaining attention, poor short-term memory, visual field problems, impulsiveness, aphasia, and judgment problems such as not knowing how much food to take or what to do with the food once it reaches the mouth.

Among 15,000 participants in the Physicians' Health Study, there was no association between plasma Lp(a) and risk of thromboembolic stroke (Ridker et al., 1995). Lowering serum cholesterol does not seem to decrease stroke risk (Hebert et al., 1995). Intake of cruciferous and green leafy vegetables, citrus fruits, and juice may be especially protective against risk of ischemic stroke (Joshipura et al., 1999). High vitamin C intake is quite protective. Intakes of fat, SFA, and MUFA tend to be associated with reduced risk of ischemic stroke in men, whereas smoking, glucose intolerance, BMI, BP, blood cholesterol level, physical activity, and intake of alcohol do not change levels of risk (Gillman et al., 1997). Smoking and abdominal obesity appear to be independent risk factors for venous thromboembolism (Hanson et al., 1999).

Eating fish more than once per week also seems to decrease CVA risk (Gillum et al., 1996). Both fish and omega-3 fatty acids seem to prevent thrombotic strokes without increasing hemorrhagic strokes among middle-aged women (Iso et al., 2001).

Several servings daily of whole grains are also protective. Brisk walking (about 3 mph) is most protective, but any walking is good as a preventive measure. While risk reductions from controlled trials with vitamins C and E have not been consistent (Pearce et al., 2000), vitamin E may have a protective effect also; intake of mayonnaise, margarine, and nuts is useful when ingested from dietary sources (Yochum et al., 2000).

OBJECTIVES

- Immediate treatment consists of maintaining fluid-electrolyte balance for lifesaving measures.
- Ongoing treatment consists of improving residual effects such as dysphagia, hemiplegia, and aphasia and correcting side effects (i.e., constipation, urinary tract infections [UTIs], pneumonia, renal calculi, and pressure ulcers).
- If the patient is excessively overweight, weight reduction is necessary to lower elevated blood pressure and lipids and lessen workload of the cardiovascular system.
- Chewing should be minimized for dysphagia and choking should be prevented. Avoid use of straws.
- Lower serum cholesterol if high. Try to improve low levels of HDL-C.
- Promote self-help, self-esteem, and independence.

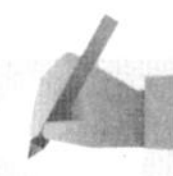

DIETARY AND NUTRITIONAL RECOMMENDATIONS

- Initial treatment—NPO with intravenous fluids for 24–48 hours. Avoid overhydration. Tube feeding may be needed, especially gastrostomy or jejunostomy. If the patient is comatose, tube feeding will be necessary; elevate head of bed to prevent aspiration, especially during feeding. Enteral sip feeding may improve nutrient intake and nutritional status of stroke patients who do not have swallowing difficulties and may improve clinical outcomes (Gariballa et al., 1998).
- Treatment should progress from NPO to liquids. After this, thick pureed liquids or a mechanical soft diet may be needed. At first, use easy-to-chew foods and spoon rather than fork foods. Progress should be made slowly.
- For dysphagia, avoid foods that cause choking or that are hard to manage (e.g., tart juices and foods, dry or crisp foods, fibrous meats, unboned fish, chewy or stringy meats, sticky peanut butter and bananas, thinly pureed foods that are easily aspirated, foods of varying consistency, excessively sweet drinks or fruits that aggravate drooling), raw vegetables, mashed potatoes or soft breads for some patients.

- Moisten foods with small amounts of liquid for people with decreased saliva production. Use thickeners to make semisolids out of soup, beverages, juices, and shakes. Test swallowing periodically. When ready, use of a syringe or training cup is beneficial.
- Limit intake of cholesterol, sodium, and saturated fats as needed. Use more olive, soybean, and canola oils and nuts such as walnuts, almonds, macadamias, pecans, and pistachios. Walnuts contain alpha-linolenic acid; almonds are a good source of vitamin E. Nuts also contain flavonoids, phenols, sterols, saponins, elegiac acid, folic acid, magnesium, copper, potassium, and fiber. Increase omega-3 fatty acids from fish as well.
- Use skim milk products whenever possible. Milk fat is negatively correlated with certain cardiovascular disease risk factors; it is not certain why. Pentadecanoic acid (C 15:0) is used as a marker for milk fat intake (Smedman et al., 1999).
- Increase potassium, pending use of diuretics. Adequate potassium may reduce stroke mortality. Fruits and vegetables are the best sources (oranges, bananas, baked potatoes, etc.).
- Provide adequate calories (patient's weight should be checked frequently). Monitor the patient's activity levels. From 25 to 45 kcal/kg and 1.2–1.5 g protein/kg may be needed, depending on weight status and loss of lean body mass.
- Six to eight cups of fluids are needed daily. They should be given at the end of the meal to prevent interference with food intake. Textures can cause problems, and liquids may not be swallowed normally, increasing risk of aspiration. Coughing is a danger sign. Liquids can be thickened with gels. Always start with small amounts of food.
- The diet should provide adequate fiber from prune juice, bran, whole grains, etc. Metamucil may be useful for persons who are unable to chew fibrous foods; try mixing with juice.
- Vitamin C and magnesium should also be provided. Vitamin E is helpful for its antioxidant properties. Include more folic acid, riboflavin, and vitamins B12 and B6.
- Flavonoids such as grapefruit, grape juice, tea, and red wine may be useful when the patient can tolerate a soft diet.
- Increase intake of whole grains (breads, cereals, oatmeal, bran, wheat germ, popcorn, brown rice).
- Compared with other nationalities, Americans tend to eat much less fish; this practice should be changed to protect against further stroke events (Iso et al., 2001).

Common Drugs Used and Potential Side Effects

- Reserpine causes cramping and diarrhea, which can be treated by using less fiber and fewer spices. Use fewer sodium-containing foods.
- With anticoagulants such as warfarin (Coumadin), use a controlled amount of vitamin K; check TF products and supplements. Limit high vitamin K foods to 1 per day (e.g., green leafy vegetables, fish, broccoli/kale/brussels sprouts). Be wary of using supplements containing vitamins A, C, and E with these drugs; side effects may be detrimental. Avoid taking with dong quai, fenugreek, feverfew, excessive garlic, ginger, ginkgo, and ginseng because of their effects.

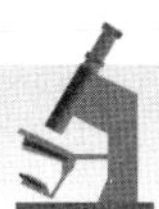

PROFILE

Clinical/History

- Height
- Weight
- BMI
- Position emission tomography (PET) scan
- Chewing ability
- Hand to mouth coordination
- Gag reflex—Present or absent?
- BP
- Temperature
- I & O

Lab Work

- Visual field scan
- Electroencephalogram (EEG)
- Carotid ultrasound
- Computed tomography (CT) scan or MRI
- Na+, K+
- Ca++, Mg++
- Chol (Total, HDL, LDL)
- Trig
- Homocysteine
- Serum folate
- Ferritin, H&H
- Gluc (often increased)
- Cerebrospinal fluid (to rule out other conditions)
- CPK
- PT

- Anticonvulsants, antifibrinolytics, and antispasmodics may be needed.
- Stool softeners may be used. Prune juice can be added to a TF or oral regimen.
- Aspirin is sometimes used to prevent future strokes as a blood thinner, often one tablet per day. Monitor for GI bleeding or other chronic side effects. Aspirin may decrease serum ferritin by increasing occult blood loss (Fleming et al., 2001).
- Grapefruit juice decreases drug metabolism in the gut (via P450-CYP3A4 inhibition) and can affect medications up to 24 hours later. Consistency of use may be more important than total quantity. Avoid taking with alprazolam, buspirone, cisapride, cyclosporine, statins, tacrolimus, and many others.
- Products containing phenylpropanolamine (PPA) are a risk for stroke. Dimetapp, Contac, Triaminic, Acutrim, and Dexatrim should be avoided.

Herbs, Botanicals and Supplements

- The patient should not take herbals and botanicals without discussing with the physician.
- CoEnzyme Q10 should not be used with statins, gemfibrozil, tricyclic antidepressants, or warfarin. CoQ10 may act similarly to vitamin K.
- Niacin (nicotinic acid) should not be taken with statins, antidiabetic medications, and carbamazepine because of potentially serious risks of myopathy and altered glucose control.
- Vitamin E should not be taken with warfarin because of the possibility of increased bleeding. Avoid doses greater than 400 IU per day.
- Herbs and botanicals such as garlic, willow, pigweed, gingko, evening primrose, and carrot have been recommended, but no clinical trials have proven efficacy.

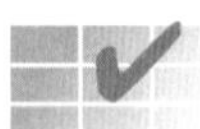

PATIENT EDUCATION

- ✔ Help the patient simplify meal preparation. Arrange food and utensils within reach. Discuss the use of appropriate assistive devices.
- ✔ Explain which sources of adequate nutrition do not aggravate the patient's condition. Discuss fat, cholesterol, sodium, potassium, calcium, magnesium, specific vitamins, and other nutrients. Correlate with drug therapy.
- ✔ Help the patient make mealtime safe and pleasant.
- ✔ Encourage small bites of food, and slow, adequate chewing.
- ✔ Discuss ways to prevent future strokes; linolenic acid from walnut, canola, and soybean oils may be protective. Increased fruit and vegetable intake is also protective.
- ✔ Physical therapy is very important in early stages after a stroke, especially to regain use of limbs such as hands and arms. EXCITE is a multicenter study that is looking at the impact of exercise in nonaffected limbs of stroke patients.

For More Information

- American Stroke Association
  Stroke Connection
  1-888-478-7653
- American Rehabilitation Foundation
  1800 Chicago Avenue
  Minneapolis, MN 55404
- National Aphasia Association
  156 Fifth Avenue, Suite 707
  New York, NY 10010
  http://www.aphasia.org
- National Institute of Neurological Disorders and Stroke
  1-800-352-9424
  http://www.ninds.nih.gov/
- National Rehabilitation Awareness Foundation
  http://www.nraf-rehabnet.org/
- National Rehabilitation Hospital
  102 Irving St., NW
  Washington, DC 20010
  202-877-1000
  http://www.nrhrehab.org/
- National Stroke Association
  8480 East Orchard Road, Suite 1000
  Englewood, CO 80111-5015
  1-800-STROKES
  http://www.stroke.org/
- Milani Foods
  Thick-It
  1-800-333-0003
- UCLA Stroke Center
  http://www.stroke.ucla.edu/

CONGESTIVE HEART FAILURE

NUTRITIONAL ACUITY RANKING: LEVEL 3

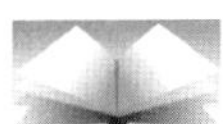

DEFINITIONS AND BACKGROUND

CHF results in reduced heart pumping efficiency in the lower two chambers, with less blood circulating to body tissues, congestion in lungs or body circulation, ankle swelling, abdominal pain, ascites, hepatic congestion, jugular vein distention, and breathing difficulty. CHF is the most common diagnosis in hospitalized patients, affecting over 4.8 million Americans and causing 400,000 new cases annually (Nutrition Screening Initiative, 2002).

CHF can be caused by coronary heart disease, previous heart attack, history of cardiomyopathy, lung disease such as chronic obstructive pulmonary disease (COPD), severe anemia, excessive alcohol consumption, or low thyroid function (see Fig. 6–2). Male sex, less education, physical inactivity, cigarette smoking, overweight, diabetes, hypertension, valvular heart disease, and coronary heart disease are all independent risk factors for CHF; more than 60% of the CHF that occurs in the U.S. is related to coronary heart disease (He et al., 2001).

Right-sided CHF yields pitting edema of extremities and fatigue. Left-sided CHF affects the lungs, with pulmonary edema, rales, and dyspnea. Decreased renal flow is common; BUN may be increased. Early adaptations to mild heart failure show susceptibility to sodium excess (Volpe et al., 1993). Treatment may include hormone therapy, implantation of a pacemaker, or cardiac transplantation. Cell therapy is being considered for conditions such as CHF. A living "cell patch" transplant from thigh muscle tissue to cardiac tissue has been successfully attempted.

Evidence suggests that advanced CHF is a multifactorial metabolic syndrome that can lead to cardiac cachexia and then carries a very poor prognosis. Joint efforts of cardiologists, endocrinologists, and immunologists are required to develop therapeutic strategies able to improve the metabolic status of CHF patients (Anker and Rauchhaus, 1999). While sometimes found in obese patients, CHF can lead to cardiac cachexia (anorexia with fat and muscle wasting and edema). In cardiac cachexia, dietary and metabolic factors and levels and activity of cytokines, thyroid hormone, catecholamines, and cortisol may be responsible for causing weight loss.

The American Dietetic Association recommends at least four medical nutrition therapy visits for patients with congestive heart failure (http://www.knowledgelinc.com/ada/mntguides/).

OBJECTIVES

- Promote rest to lessen demands on the heart. Restore hemodynamic stability; prevent cardiogenic shock or thromboembolism.
- Eliminate or reduce edema.
- Avoid distention and elevation of diaphragm, which reduces vital capacity. Prevent excessive refeeding.
- Attain ideal body weight (IBW) to decrease O2 needs and tissue demands for nutrients. Replace lean body mass (LBM), if needed.
- Limit cardiac stimulants.
- Prevent cardiac cachexia, low blood pressure, listlessness, weak pulse from K+-depleting diuretics, anorexia, nausea and vomiting, and sepsis.
- Correct any nutrient deficits.
- Prevent pressure ulcers from reduced activity levels and poor circulation.

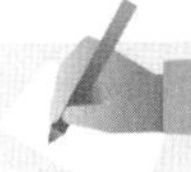

DIETARY AND NUTRITIONAL RECOMMENDATIONS

- Restrict sodium—1,000–2,400 mg. Not all patients require strict limitations; 4–6 g of sodium may be satisfactory. Consider use of the DASH diet (see Hypertension entry).

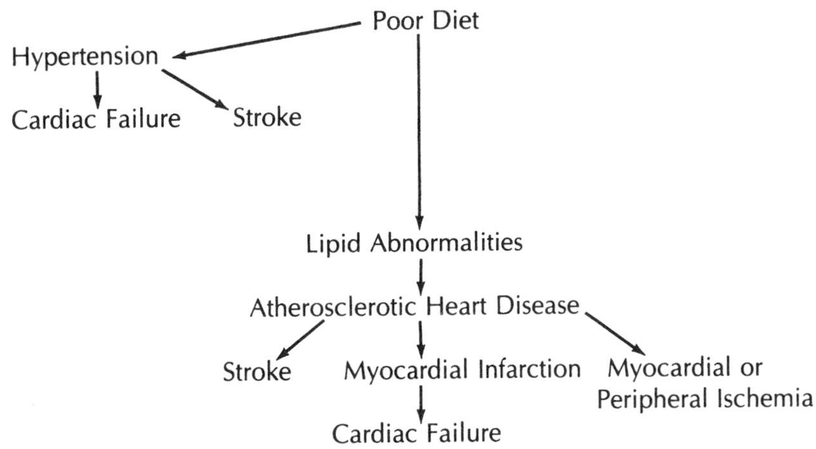

Figure 6–3 Possible Effect of Diet on Cardiac Failure.

- Diet should provide adequate potassium to replace potassium losses. Also monitor potassium supplementation.
- Provide 5–6 small meals a day, with no more than 3 L fluid per day. Patients with refractory edema should receive 0.5 mL/kcal on average.
- If patient is obese, a calorie-controlled diet is necessary.
- Restrict caffeine intake. At first, no caffeine is allowed; later, coffee intake may be limited to 5 cups of regular coffee per day to reduce stimulants.
- Use bland, low-roughage foods to lessen heartburn, distention, and flatulence. Beans, cabbage, onions, cauliflower, and Brussels sprouts may cause these problems.
- Use soft textures to reduce the amount of chewing. Add soluble fiber from apples or oat bran if tolerated.
- If total parenteral nutrition (TPN) is used, ensure adequate nutrient intake (including selenium, etc.). For TF, use a low-sodium product and increase volume gradually.
- If fat intolerance occurs, try medium-chain triglycerides (MCT).
- Ensure adequate intakes of vitamins E, B6, and B12, folic acid, and riboflavin. Thiamin levels also tend to be low and should be supplemented (Brady et al., 1995; Blanc and Boussuges, 2000). Those who are alcoholics, malnourished, elderly, or have AIDS are at special risk for thiamin deficiency. Cardiovascular problems associated with beriberi include peripheral vasodilatation with increased cardiac output, myocardial lesion, sodium and water retention, and biventricular myocardial failure; thiamin administration is the treatment (Blanc and Boussuges, 2000).
- Reduce or eliminate alcohol intake if needed (Nutrition Screening Initiative, 2002).

PROFILE

Clinical/History	Lab Work	
Height	Chest x-ray	Chol (total, HDL, LDL)
Weight	Na+, Cl−	Trig
BMI	AST, ALT	Homocysteine
BP	BNP (hormone secreted by ventricles when pressure goes up, signaling congestive heart failure)	Serum folate
Dry, hacking cough	Echocardiography	Serum B12
Skin, cyanotic or pale	ECG	K+
Abnormal breath sounds	Cardiac catheterization	Gluc
Pulse (NL = 60–100 beats/min)	Oximetry	H&H, serum Fe
Temperature	pCO2, pO2	Mg++, Ca++
Edema	Specific gravity (increased)	Serum zinc
Glomerular filtration rate (GFR)		Alk phos
Oliguria		Alb, prealbumin
I & O		BUN, Creat
		PT
		LDH (increased)
		Nitrogen (N) balance
		Uric acid

Common Drugs Used and Potential Side Effects

- Thiazide diuretics (Esidrix, Oretic, HydroDiuril) deplete potassium, which must be replaced, either orally or by medication. Furosemide (Lasix) depletes K+ and Mg++; eventually, Ca++ levels also decline. Glucose tolerance may be decreased; anorexia, nausea, or vomiting may occur. Use a low-sodium diet. Avoid use with fenugreek and ginkgo.
- Other diuretics may be used. Bumex (bumetanide) should be monitored carefully for nausea, dry mouth, weakness, and loss of potassium. Avoid use with yohimbe.
- Salt substitutes generally contain KCl, and their use could lead to hyperkalemia if potassium-sparing diuretics such as spironolactone (Aldactone) or triamterene (Dyrenium) are part of treatment.
- Digitalis can deplete potassium, especially when taken with furosemide. Beware of excesses of wheat bran, which can decrease serum drug levels. Anorexia or nausea may occur.
- Anticoagulants (Coumadin/warfarin) sometimes are used for bedridden patients. Use high vitamin K foods no more than once per day. Avoid taking with dong quai, fenugreek, feverfew, excessive garlic, ginger, ginkgo, and ginseng because of their effects.
- ACE inhibitors (captopril, enalapril [Vasotec], and lisinopril [Zestoretic, Zestril]) decrease production of angiotensin and aldosterone. Monitor for hyperkalemia, nausea, vomiting, dizziness, and abdominal pain. ACE inhibitors block angiotensin II and decrease aldosterone output, thereby decreasing sodium and water retention.
- β-adrenergic blockers (propanolol, acebutolol, nadolol, and pindolol) reduce cardiac output in competing for available receptor sites; they decrease sympathetic stimulation of the heart.
- Arterial vasodilators (hydralazine, minoxidil) reduce cardiac workload by decreasing after load of the heart. Nausea and vomiting can occur.
- Anticholinergic agents such as atropine increase cardiac output by increasing rate.
- Grapefruit juice decreases drug metabolism in the gut (via P450-CYP3A4 inhibition) and can affect medications up to 24 hours later. Consistency of use may be more important than total quantity. Avoid taking with alprazolam, buspirone, cisapride, cyclosporine, statins, tacrolimus, and many others.

Herbs, Botanicals and Supplements

- The patient should not take herbals and botanicals without discussing with the physician. It is important to stress that no supplement or diet can cure heart failure.
- A well-conducted study reported that coenzyme Q, a popular alternative remedy for heart failure patients, offers no benefits for either the heart or the quality of life (Morelli and Zoorob, 2000). CoEnzyme Q10 should not be used with statins, gemfibrozil, tricyclic antidepres-

sants, or warfarin; CoQ10 may act similarly to vitamin K.

- Chromium is sometimes used for dyslipidemia. Do not use excesses with insulin or hypoglycemic agents, because it may lower glucose levels.
- Niacin (nicotinic acid) should not be taken with statins, antidiabetic medications, and carbamazepine because of potentially serious risks of myopathy and altered glucose control.
- Vitamin E should not be taken with warfarin because of the possibility of increased bleeding. Avoid doses greater than 400 IU per day.
- L-arginine, found in health food stores, may have some benefit. This amino acid appears to reduce endothelin, a protein that causes blood vessel constriction and is found in high amounts in heart failure patients.
- Hawthorne is used in Germany for CHF, but no well-designed studies have been completed in the U.S. (Morelli and Zoorob, 2000).

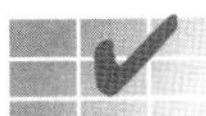

PATIENT EDUCATION

- ✓ A congested feeling may cause a poor appetite. Ensure that the patient takes smaller, more appetizing, and more frequent meals. Never force patient to eat. Allow rest before and after meals. Use high-calorie, low-volume supplements to increase nutrient density when needed.
- ✓ Check the water supply for use of softening agents. Also, have the patients monitor sodium-containing medications, toothpastes, and mouthwashes.
- ✓ Help patient plan fluid intake over waking hours, usually 75% from meals and 25% with medications and for thirst between meals.
- ✓ Alcohol should be avoided.
- ✓ Discuss spices and seasonings as salt alternatives. See Table 6–3.
- ✓ Teach label reading and tips for easy meal preparation. Freeze small meal portions for use when energy levels are low.
- ✓ Avoid excessive use of canned soups, cured or smoked meats, and commercial sauces. Many frozen dinners are high in sodium also; use healthier brands.
- ✓ Refer to local congregate meal programs or inquire about home-delivered meals for elderly individuals. Many will provide low sodium meals upon request.
- ✓ Bed rest may be required in cases of severe congestive heart failure. To reduce congestion in the lungs, the patient's upper body should be elevated; for most patients, resting in an armchair is better than lying in bed. Relaxing and contracting leg muscles is important to prevent clots. As the patient improves, progressively more activity will be recommended.
- ✓ Heart failure is associated with sleep apnea in which tissues at the back of the throat periodically collapse and become blocked, causing the sleeper to gasp for air. Sleep apnea has been associated with poorer survival in patients with congestive heart failure. A continuous positive airway pressure (CPAP) device is effective and appears to improve ejection fraction in heart failure patients.

For More Information:

- ✦ American Dietetic Association
  Congestive Heart Failure Protocol
  www.eatright.org
- ✦ NHLBI
  http://www.nhlbi.nih.gov/hbp/hbp/effect/heart.htm
- ✦ Seasonings and Spices
  http://www.nhlbi.nih.gov/hbp/prevent/sodium/flavor.htm

TABLE 6–3 Sodium Content of Typical Items

Item	*mg sodium per teaspoon*
Salt	1,938
Soda	821
Baking powder	339
Monosodium glutamate (MSG)	492

HEART VALVE DISEASES

NUTRITIONAL ACUITY RANKING: LEVEL 2

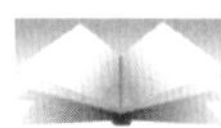

DEFINITIONS AND BACKGROUND

The heart has four valves (tricuspid, pulmonary, aortic, and mitral). Inflammation of any or several of these valves can cause stenosis with thickening (which narrows the opening) or incompetence (with distortion and inability to close fully).

Mitral stenosis can cause lung congestion, breathlessness after exercise or while lying down, hemoptysis, bronchial infections, and chest pains. In this problem, right heart failure can occur; 60% of persons with rheumatic heart disease later have heart valve problems; 75% of these persons have mitral stenosis. (See Rheumatic Heart Disease, Section 15.) Aortic stenosis can give symptoms of angina, vertigo, and fainting on exertion. Left heart failure is common. Tricuspid stenosis increases the risk of heart failure. Pulmonary stenosis is rare and occurs in only 2% of all valve disorders.

Over the long term, high cholesterol levels, high systolic blood pressure, and cigarette smoking are associated with increased risk of carotid stenosis in an elderly population (Wilson et al., 1997). Patients at high risk for valvular disease should be screened for hyperhomocystinemia; for levels over 14 and 11 umol/L for primary and secondary prevention, 400–1,000 ug folic acid and a multivitamin supplement with B6 and B12 should be taken (Stein and McBride, 1998).

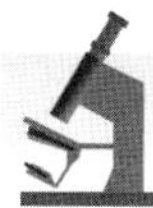

PROFILE

Clinical/History		
Height	Urinary output (decreased)	ECG
Weight	I & O	Chol (total, HDL, LDL)
BMI	**Lab Work**	Trig
Weight changes	Alb, prealbumin	BUN, Creat
Pulse	H&H, serum ferritin	Na+
Cool, moist skin	Cardiac catheterization	K+
BP		Gluc
		Homocysteine
		Serum folate
		Serum B12

OBJECTIVES

- ▲ Prevent heart failure (right- or left-sided); bacterial endocarditis; emboli or atrial fibrillation; sudden death.
- ▲ Prepare, if necessary, for valve replacement (surgery).
- ▲ Prevent or correct cardiogenic shock (tachycardia, etc.).

DIETARY AND NUTRITIONAL RECOMMENDATIONS

- Avoid excesses of calories, sodium, and fluid (as appropriate for the patient).
- If weight loss has taken place, add extra calories and snacks to return to a more desirable body weight.
- Use adequate vitamins E, B6, and B12 and folic acid.
- Encourage use of flavonoids such as grapefruit, grape juice, apples, onions, tea, and red wine (small amounts) where feasible. Flavonoids may help to reduce blood clot formation.
- Ensure adequate intake of omega-3 fatty acids.

Common Drugs Used and Potential Side Effects

- Anticoagulants are used commonly. Monitor vitamin K-rich foods carefully; use no more than 1 per day (especially green leafy vegetables). If aspirin is used, monitor for GI side effects; aspirin may also decrease serum ferritin by increasing occult blood loss (Fleming et al., 2001).
- Diuretics may be used if fluid overload occurs. Monitor potassium and sodium intake carefully.
- Fen-Phen weight reduction drug therapy was associated with valvular heart disease and pulmonary hypertension (Connolly et al., 1997). Cardiac surgical interventions that were needed found plaque-like casement like that found in carcinoid syndrome. These drugs have been removed from the market.
- Grapefruit juice decreases drug metabolism in the gut (via P450-CYP3A4 inhibition) and can affect medications up to 24 hours later. Consistency of use may be more important than total quantity. Avoid taking with alprazolam, buspirone, cisapride, cyclosporine, statins, tacrolimus, and many others.
- Digoxin may be needed to strengthen the heart's pumping action after surgery. Monitor potassium intake or depletion carefully, especially when combining with diuretics. Avoid excessive intakes of fiber and wheat bran. Avoid use with hawthorn, milkweed, guar gum, and St. John's wort.

Herbs, Botanicals and Supplements

- Danshen may be used for ischemic heart disease. Avoid large amounts with warfarin, aspirin, and other antiplatelet drugs. It can increase risks of bleeding or bruising.
- Garlic should not be taken in large amounts with warfarin, aspirin, and other antiplatelet drugs because of increased risks of bleeding or bruising. It may also increase insulin levels with hypoglycemic results; monitor carefully in patients with diabetes.
- CoEnzyme Q10 should not be used with statins, gemfibrozil, tricyclic antidepressants, or warfarin. CoQ10 may act similarly to vitamin K.

- Chromium is sometimes used for dyslipidemia. Do not use excesses with insulin or hypoglycemic agents, because it may lower glucose levels.
- Niacin (nicotinic acid) should not be taken with statins, antidiabetic medications, and carbamazepine because of potentially serious risks of myopathy and altered glucose control.
- Vitamin E should not be taken with Warfarin because of the possibility of increased bleeding. Avoid doses greater than 400 IU per day.

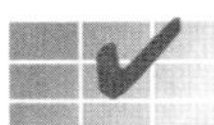

PATIENT EDUCATION

- ✓ Careful use of all prescribed medications will be essential, with adequate return visits to the physician at appropriate intervals.
- ✓ Alternative food preparation methods may be suggested to reduce sodium intake or to alter calorie levels.
- ✓ Persons with a history of heart valve abnormalities may require antibiotic therapy to prevent infections, especially before surgery or dental work.

HYPERLIPIDEMIAS: HYPERCHOLESTEROLEMIA, HYPERTRIGLYCERIDEMIA, AND HYPERLIPOPROTEINEMIAS

NUTRITIONAL ACUITY RANKING: LEVEL 3

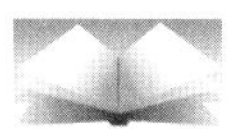

DEFINITIONS AND BACKGROUND

Hyperlipidemia refers to either elevated serum triglycerides or cholesterol. Although used less often, Frederickson's categories (types I–V) are still used to identify some of the specific familial diagnoses. There are increased levels of lipid-protein complexes attached to serum proteins. Lipoproteins are combinations of proteins and triglycerides, phospholipids, and cholesterol. (See also Atherosclerosis entry.)

Levels of HDL cholesterol (when below 40) and LDL or triglycerides (when high) are independent risk factors of cardiovascular disease death (NHLBI, 2001). Elevated plasma lipoprotein (a) is an independent factor, comparable to cholesterol levels higher than 240 (Bostrom et al., 1996). Linoleic acid concentration in adipose tissue and in platelets has been associated with degrees of heart disease, especially low levels of EPA in men and low levels of docosahexanoic acid in women (Hodgson et al., 1993). Abdominal aortic aneurysm, peripheral artery disease, symptomatic carotid artery disease, smoking, family history of premature CAD (CAD in male first-degree relative before age 55 and in female first-degree relative before age 65), hypertension (over 140/90), and age (men aged 45 and older, women aged 55 and older) are also important risk factors to consider (NHLBI, 2001).

A single high saturated-fat meal transiently reduces endothelial function for up to 4 hours in healthy, normocholesterolemic individuals, probably through the accumulation of TG-rich lipoproteins. This decrease is blocked by pretreatment with antioxidant vitamins C and E, suggesting an oxidative mechanism (Plotnick et al., 1997).

For obese persons, high levels of cholesterol ester transfer protein (CETP) may partially explain low serum HDL levels (Arai et al., 1994). Weight gain in adulthood promotes heart disease in white men and women and in black men (Stevens et al., 1998). Apo E genotype modifies the serum lipid response to changes in dietary fat and cholesterol intake in subjects with mildly elevated total cholesterol levels (Sarkkinen et al., 1998).

The effects of MCT and corn oil on plasma lipids have been evaluated; MCT was found to prevent the risk of pancreatitis due to postprandial hypertriglyceridemia but raises total cholesterol (Asakura et al., 2000).

Individuals who undergo CABG continue to have multiple risk factors for CAD that place them at high risk for future CAD events; other steps such as stopping smoking, following the recommended diet, and managing other risk factors must be taken (Frame et al., 2001).

Medical nutrition therapy (MNT) instead of statin therapy raises HDL levels by 4% (Sikand et al., 2000). After registered dietitian (RD) interventions, only 15 of 30 eligible individuals required antihyperlipidemic medication, at a cost savings of $638 per patient annually. For each dollar spent on MNT, a savings of $3 was realized. The American Dietetic Association recommends at least 4 medical nutrition therapy visits for patients with elevated lipids (http://www.knowledgelinc.com/ada/mntguides/).

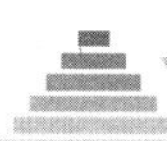

OBJECTIVES

- Initiate therapeutic lifestyle changes (TLC) if LDL is above goal (NHLBI, 2001). All types of HLP: normalize body weight. Keep cholesterol levels lower than 200 mg/dL and triglyceride levels lower than 200 mg/dL; keep HDL high and LDL low. A Mediterranean diet (olive oil, red wine, fruits and vegetables, fish) probably is beneficial for most people (Nestle, 1995). Use the NCEP guidelines for elevated lipids as well as for those persons who have the metabolic syndrome.
- Use a team approach to support the best possible outcomes: MD, RD, RN, and other therapists as needed.
- If using Frederickson's Categories of Hyperlipoproteinemia:
  - Type I: Minimize chylomicron formation. Lower triglyceride levels. Prevent abdominal pains resulting from fat ingestion. MCTs are tolerated.
  - Type IIa: Lower intake of saturated fats. Lower serum cholesterol.
  - Type IIb or III: Reduce weight; lower serum cholesterol.
  - Type IV: Reduce weight. Restrict intake of simple carbohydrates and alcohol. Intake of cholesterol should be moderate.
  - Type V: Reduce weight. Modify intake of cholesterol. Keep fat intake low.
- Treat metabolic syndrome (NHLBI, 2001): Address underlying causes (overweight/obesity and physical inactivity); intensify weight management and increase physical activity. Treat lipid and nonlipid risk factors if they persist despite these lifestyle therapies; treat hypertension; use aspirin for CAD patients to reduce prothrombotic state; help lower elevated triglycerides and/or lower HDL through diet first, then drug therapies. See Tables 6–4 and 6–5.

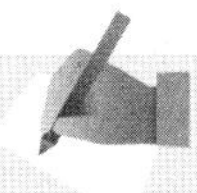

DIETARY AND NUTRITIONAL RECOMMENDATIONS

- Initiate diet if LDL level is above goal: saturated fat <7% of calories, cholesterol less than 200 mg/day; consider increased viscous (soluble) fiber (10–25 g/day) and plant stanols/ sterols (2 g/day) as therapeutic options to enhance LDL lowering, weight management, and increased

TABLE 6–4 Clinical Identification of the Metabolic Syndrome—Any 3 of the Following:

Risk Factor	*Defining Level*
Abdominal obesity*	Waist circumference**
Men	>102 cm (>40 in)
Women	>88 cm (>35 in)
Triglycerides	≥150 mg/dL
HDL cholesterol	
Men	<40 mg/dl
Women	<50 mg/dl
Blood pressure	≥130/≥85 mmHg
Fasting glucose	≥110 mg/dL

* Overweight and obesity are associated with insulin resistance and the metabolic syndrome. However, the presence of abdominal obesity is more highly correlated with the metabolic risk factors than is an elevated BMI. Therefore, the simple measure of waist circumference is recommended to identify the body weight component of the metabolic syndrome.

** Some male patients can develop multiple metabolic risk factors when the waist circumference is only marginally increased, e.g., 94–102 cm (37–39 in). Such patients may have a strong genetic contribution to insulin resistance. They should benefit from changes in life habits, similar to men with categorical increases in waist circumference.

Derived from NHLBI, 2001.

physical activity (NHLBI, 2001). Exercise helps to decrease plasma TC, LDL-C, and TG levels (Yu-Poth S et al., 1999).

- In general, use more soluble fiber (Jenkins et al., 1993). Oat bran contains "beta glucan" hemicellulose (Kelley et al., 1994); corn bran is also effective (Shane and Walker, 1995). Rice bran contains minimal soluble fiber, but rice bran oil has been shown to reduce serum lipid levels. Adding rice bran oil or oat bran to a low-fat diet lowers total serum cholesterol and LDL levels in patients with HLP (Gerhardt and Gallo, 1998). Apples and legumes are also recommended.
- Olive, canola, soybean, and peanut oils can be used (as MUFA). Substituting walnuts for part of MUFAs in a cholesterol-lowering Mediterranean diet reduces serum TC and LDL levels in men and women with hypercholesterolemia (Zambon et al., 2000).
- Pecans can be included in a healthful diet when energy intake and potential weight gain are addressed; dietary fat, MUFA and PUFA intake, insoluble fiber, Mg++, and energy were significantly higher among those who were in a study (Morgan and Clayshultze, 2000). Include nuts such as walnuts, almonds, macadamias, pecans, and pistachios. Walnuts contain alpha-linolenic acid; almonds are a good source of vitamin E. Nuts also contain flavonoids, phenols, sterols, saponins, elegiac acid, folic acid, magnesium, copper, potassium, and fiber.
- TFAs (partially hydrogenated oils in margarines) should be monitored. Use less than 1% total fat from TFAs. Compared with butter, margarines free from TFAs may be equal to or more effective than margarines containing TFAs in lowering LDL-C (Noakes and Clifton, 1998).
- Egg yolks should be limited to 3–4 per week; liver and organ meats should be limited to 1 serving per month.
- Shellfish and fish are recommended (Hodgson et al., 1993) for their omega-3 fatty acid content.
- Increased use of soy protein may also prove to be effective (Anderson et al., 1995). Substitute 25–30 g of soy protein for animal protein in several meals each week. Tofu contains 13 g of soy protein in one 4 oz serving; one soy burger contains 10–12 g of protein; ¼ cup of soy nuts and ½ cup of tempeh contain 19 g of protein each.
- Increase use of flavonoids from tea, onions, red wine, grape juice, and grapefruit, etc. for their phenolic acids and antioxidant effects (Frankel et al., 1993; Fuhrman et al., 1995).
- Increase use of vitamin E to 100 IU or more (Hodis et al., 1995). Vitamins B6 and B12, riboflavin, and folic acid should be added for general cardiac health.
- In men with hypercholesterolemia, intake of garlic supplements significantly decreases total blood cholesterol and LDL levels compared with baseline fish oil supplements, decreased TG levels, and increased LDL levels (Adler and Holub, 1997). Trials suggest that garlic has short-term benefits on levels of some blood lipids (Ackermann, 2001).
- Salatrim is the generic name for restructured TGs that contain at least one short-chain fatty acid (acetic, propionic, or butyric) and at least one long-chain fatty acid (mostly stearic); trade name is Benefat (Kosmark, 1996). Benecol and Take Control are other products that tend to quickly lower serum LDL levels by about 14%; use as a margarine substitute on breads and in cooking.
- Olestra (fat substitute) has been associated with a decrease in dietary fat and serum total cholesterol levels even if body weight does not change (Patterson et al., 2000).
- Lower elevated triglycerides to 150 mg/dL. Intensify weight management measures and increase physical activity. If triglycerides are 200 mg/dL after LDL goal is reached, set secondary goal for nonHDL cholesterol (total – HDL) 30 mg/dL higher than LDL goal. If triglycerides are 200–499 mg/dL after LDL goal is reached, omit alcohol and consider whether an added drug is needed to reach nonHDL goal; intensify therapy with LDL-lowering drug, or add nicotinic acid or fibrate to further lower VLDL. If triglycerides are 500 mg/dL, first lower triglycerides to prevent pancreatitis: very

TABLE 6–5 National Heart, Lung, and Blood Institute Recommendations

Follow the NCEP diet:
- Total fat 25–35% kcals
- Saturated fat lower than 7%
- PUFA up to 10% and MUFA up to 20%
- Cholesterol below 200 mg
- CHO 50–60% and Protein 10–20%

Comparison of LDL Cholesterol and NonHDL Cholesterol Goals for Three Risk Categories (NHLBI, 2001):

Risk Category	*LDL Goal (mg/dL)*	*NonHDL Goal (mg/dL)*
CAD and CAD Risk Equivalent (10-year risk for CAD >20%)	<100	<130
Multiple (2+) Risk Factors (and 10-year risk for CAD ≤20%)	<130	<160
0–1 Risk Factor	<160	<190

low-fat diet (15% of calories from fat), weight management and physical activity, fibrate or nicotinic acid when triglycerides <500 mg/dL, turn to LDL-lowering therapy.

- For treatment of low HDL cholesterol (<40 mg/dL), first reach LDL goal; then, intensify weight management and increase physical activity. If triglycerides are 200–499 mg/dL, achieve nonHDL goal. If triglycerides are <200 mg/dL (isolated low HDL) in CAD or CAD equivalent, consider nicotinic acid or fibrate.

PROFILE

Clinical/History

Height
Weight
BMI
BP
Pancreatitis (Type I)
Xanthomas (Type V)

Lab Work

Lipid profile after 9–12 hr fast—HDL, LDL, VLDL, chylomicrons
Trig, fasting
Lipoprotein (a) levels
Glucose tolerance test (GTT) (Types II, IV, and V)
Homocysteine (tHcy) levels
Serum folate
Serum B12
Serum B6
Gluc
H&H, serum Fe, ferritin
BUN, Creat
Uric acid (Type V)
Carotenoids (may be increased)
Mg++
Ca++
K+, Na+
Alk phos

Common Drugs Used and Potential Side Effects

- Statins such as Lesol, Lipitor, Lovastatin (Mevacor), pravastatin (Pravachol), and simvastatin (Zocor) lower LDL cholesterol and are better tolerated than niacin (Insua et al., 1994). Decreased MI and cardiovascular deaths have resulted (Shepherd et al., 1995). Abdominal cramping, altered taste, heartburn, or diarrhea may occur. RDs can help promote use of these medications along with proper nutrition (Kris-Etherton, 2000). Interestingly, statins may increase bone growth in legs and spine; they may be useful in women taking hormone replacement therapy. See Table 6–6.
- Fibric agents such as clofibrate (Atromid-S), in the treatment of type IV hyperlipidemia, can cause weight gain, diarrhea, and nausea. Gemfibrozil (Lopid) is used for elevated triglycerides when there is a risk of pancreatitis. Taste changes or abdominal pain may occur. Probucol (Lorelco) may cause nausea, vomiting, and anorexia.
- Colestipol (Colestid): Add fat-soluble vitamins. Mix with liquids. Constipation is a common side effect.
- Bile acid sequestrants such as cholestyramine (Questran): Use increased fiber to alleviate constipation and a folate supplement; vitamins A, D, E, and K may become deficient. WelChol (colesevelam HCl) can be used with statins; it is often used with type IIa HLP especially since it is not absorbed into the bloodstream and has few side effects. See Table 6–6.

TABLE 6–6 Drugs Affecting Lipoprotein Metabolism (NHLBI, 2001)

Drug Class	*Agents and Daily Doses*	*Lipid/Lipoprotein Effects*	*Side Effects*	*Contraindications*
HMG CoA reductase inhibitors (statins)	Lovastatin (20–80 mg), Pravastatin (20–40 mg), Simvastatin (20–80 mg), Fluvastatin (20–80 mg), Atorvastatin (10–80 mg), Cerivastatin (0.4–0.8 mg)	LDL-C ↓18–55% HDL-C ↑5–15% TG ↓7–30%	Myopathy Increased liver enzymes	Absolute: Active or chronic liver disease Relative: Concomitant use of certain drugs*
Bile acid Sequestrants	Cholestyramine (4–16 g) Colestipol (5–20 g) Colesevelam (2.6–3.8 g)	LDL-C ↓ 15–30% HDL-C ↑ 3–5% TG No change or increase	Gastrointestinal distress, constipation, decreased absorption of other drugs	Absolute: Dysbeta-lipoproteinemia TG >400 mg/dL Relative: TG >200 mg/dL
Nicotinic acid	Immediate release (crystalline) nicotinic acid (1.5–3 gm), extended release nicotinic acid (Niaspan ®) (1–2 g), sustained release nicotinic acid (1–2 g)	LDL-C ↓ 5–25% HDL-C ↑ 15–35% TG ↓ 20–50%	Flushing, hyperglycemia, hyperuricemia (or gout), upper GI distress, hepatotoxicity	Absolute: Chronic liver disease Severe gout Relative: Diabetes Hyperuricemia Peptic ulcer disease
Fibric acids	Gemfibrozil (600 mg BID) Fenofibrate (200 mg) Clofibrate (1,000 mg BID)	LDL-C ↓5–20% (may be increased in patients with high TG) HDL-C ↑ 10–20% TG ↓20–50%	Dyspepsia, gallstones, myopathy	Absolute: Severe renal disease Severe hepatic disease

*Cyclosporine, macrolide antibiotics, various antifungal agents, and cytochrome P450 inhibitors, fibrates and niacin should be used with appropriate caution.

- Thiazides, propranolol, estrogens, or oral contraceptives may increase lipid levels or may lower folate levels.
- Nicotinic acid (Nicobid, Nico-400) reduces glucose tolerance and may cause nausea, vomiting, diarrhea, and altered liver function tests. See Table 6–6.
- Folic acid supplements may be more effective than dietary sources (Cuskelly, 1996).
- Psyllium (Metamucil) is effective in lowering total and LDL cholesterol levels (Sprecher et al., 1993).
- Grapefruit juice decreases drug metabolism in the gut (via P450-CYP3A4 inhibition) and can affect medications up to 24 hours later. Consistency of use may be more important than total quantity. Avoid taking with alprazolam, buspirone, cisapride, cyclosporine, statins, tacrolimus, and many others.
- Aspirin may decrease serum ferritin by increasing occult blood loss (Fleming et al., 2001).

Herbs, Botanicals and Supplements

- Cholestin from red yeast extract has a drug-like effect like statins and is viewed by FDA as a drug. It helps reduce the need for other, more expensive medications (Morelli and Zoorob, 2000).
- Fenugreek may improve serum lipid levels slightly (Morelli and Zoorob, 2000). Further research is needed. Do not take with diuretics.
- Danshen may be used for ischemic heart disease. Avoid large amounts with warfarin, aspirin, and other antiplatelet drugs. It can increase risks of bleeding or bruising.
- Garlic tablets (0.6% allicin) given 3 times daily have lowered cholesterol levels and LDLs in some studies (Stevinson et al., 2000; Jain et al., 1993), but this has not been verified in all cases (Morelli and Zoorob, 2000). Large amounts should not be taken with warfarin, aspirin, and other antiplatelet drugs because of increased risks of bleeding or bruising. Garlic use may increase insulin levels with hypoglycemic results; monitor carefully in diabetes.
- CoEnzyme Q10 should not be used with statins, gemfibrozil, tricyclic antidepressants, or warfarin. CoQ10 may act similarly to vitamin K.
- Avoid high doses of omega-3 fatty acids and cod liver oil in children and pregnant or lactating women. Avoid taking with warfarin, aspirin, and other antiplatelet medications because of the risk of increased bruising or bleeding.
- Hawthorn should not be taken with digoxin, ACE inhibitors, and other cardiovascular drugs.
- Chromium is sometimes used for dyslipidemia. Do not use excesses with insulin or hypoglycemic agents, because it may lower glucose levels.
- Niacin (nicotinic acid) should not be taken with statins, antidiabetic medications, and carbamazepine because of potentially serious risks of myopathy and altered glucose control.
- Vitamin E should not be taken with warfarin because of the possibility of increased bleeding. Avoid doses greater than 400 IU per day.
- Guggul (yellowish resin from mukul myrrh tree) is used in Indian Ayurveda medicine. It lowers LDL and increases HDL because of its plant sterols; it also stimulates the thyroid and is an anti-inflammatory and an antioxidant. Gugulipid is the safest form, but a high dose is needed. GI discomfort may occur. Do not take with Inderal or Cardizem, and do not use during pregnancy or lactation.

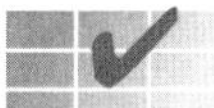

PATIENT EDUCATION

- ✔ Diets low in fat have different tastes and textures. If one changes too quickly, the diet may seem dry and unpalatable. Suggest changing gradually. Teach new ideas for moistening foods without adding excess fat (e.g., using applesauce instead of oil in some baked goods). Provide lists of resources such as cookbooks, newsletters, product samples, or coupons.
- ✔ Monitor intake of fat-soluble vitamins and iron.
- ✔ Describe food sources of saturated MUFAs and PUFAs and cholesterol; discuss olive, soybean, walnut, and peanut oil uses. Help the patient make suitable substitutions. Fish should be included several times weekly and may help to lower elevated TG levels (Schaefer et al., 1996). Eggs contain 213 mg of cholesterol in the yolk and can be planned into the diet; most guidelines recommend use of 4 whole eggs (or yolks) weekly.
- ✔ Teach the sources of soluble fiber (guar gum, pectin), as in apples, legumes, and oat and corn bran.
- ✔ Encourage the reading of food labels, including how to identify various ingredients on the label.
- ✔ Help the patient who is following a calorie-controlled diet by providing ideas. Aerobic exercise, weight loss, smoking cessation, and exogenous estrogen tend to keep HDL levels high (Rosenson, 1993).
- ✔ Discuss types of lipoproteins that carry cholesterol and triglycerides (LDL, HDL, etc.). Chylomicrons contain the most triglycerides and are lightest; HDLs are the heaviest and contain the most protein.
- ✔ Some cataracts may form in patients with hypercholesterolemia who are older than 40 years of age; corneal infiltration is a problem. Ensure adequate intake of vitamin C and encourage lowering of elevated lipid levels.
- ✔ Discuss coping skills, motivational factors, and environmental factors.
- ✔ Increase exercise. Even a single bout of low-intensity exercise reduces postprandial lipemia in young adults with normal lipid levels (Aldred et al., 1994).
- ✔ Sources of B6 include eggs, meats, fish, vegetables, yeast, whole-wheat grains, and milk. Sources of B12 include liver, meat, eggs, dairy products, and fish. Folate is found in liver, green vegetables, peas/beans, bread, bananas, and whole grain cereals. Riboflavin is found primarily in dairy products.
- ✔ Have serum lipids and lipoproteins checked as recommended by the NCEP. Note that very low cholesterol levels are not necessarily desirable; levels below 150 mg/dL may be associated with increased mortality from stroke, cancer, and other noncardiovascular disease. Decreased factor VII levels, hypoalbuminemia, and diabetes mellitus

are strongly correlated (Maniolo et al., 1993) (See Table 6–2).

For More Information

- American Dietetic Association
  Hyperlipidemia protocol
  www.eatright.org
- National Cholesterol Education Program (NHLBI)
  National Heart Lung & Blood Institute
  PO Box 30105
  Bethesda, MD 20892-0105
  (301) 496-0554
  http://www.nhlbi.nih.gov/guidelines/cholesterol/index.htm

HYPERTENSION

NUTRITIONAL ACUITY RANKING: LEVEL 2

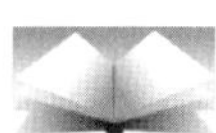

DEFINITIONS AND BACKGROUND

Hypertension results from a sustained increase in arterial diastolic or systolic pressure (160/95 mm or higher). It occurs in 15–50% of Americans. High-normal blood pressure increases the risk by 1.5–2.5 times for heart attack, stroke, and heart failure, especially for people over age 65 (NHLBI, 2001).

Blood pressure often increases with age. Hypertension is highly prevalent in elderly individuals, the most rapidly growing segment of the U.S. population (Schrier, 2001). Symptoms of hypertension include frequent headaches, impaired vision, shortness of breath, nose bleeds, chest pain, dizziness, failing memory, and GI distress. Snoring, in a young person, may lead to sleep apnea and hypertension.

Essential (primary) HPN affects 90% of all persons with HPN; an angiotensin gene may be the cause. Secondary HPN has an identifiable cause (renal disease, Cushing's syndrome, pheochromocytoma, hyperaldosteronism, use of certain medications such as steroids or oral contraceptives, pregnancy-induced HPN, and acute lead poisoning). Untreated HPN can result in stroke, CHF, renal disease, MI, accelerated bone loss and risk of fractures, or even long-term memory problems decades later; untreated malignant HPN can be fatal within 6 months. If dyspnea occurs on exertion, left-sided heart failure must be prevented. If edema of extremities occurs, right-sided heart failure must be prevented.

Early onset of type 1 diabetes mellitus increases hypertension, left ventricular mass, creatinine clearance, and microalbuminuria (Kimball et al., 1994). Oral contraceptive users and alcoholics may have BP 15–20% higher than normal. Stage 1 is mild, with BP 140–159/90–99; stage 4 is very severe, with 210/120 or higher levels. In middle-aged adults, HPN is inversely associated with plasma cholesterol levels of linoleic acid and the ratio of PUFA to SFA and positively related to plasma levels of palmitic and arachidonic acids (Zheng et al., 1999).

Reduced sodium intake and weight loss constitute a feasible, effective, and safe nonpharmacologic therapy of HPN in older persons, according to the TONE study (Whelton et al., 1998). High potassium intake should be recommended for preventing and treating HPN, especially for patients with a high sodium intake (Whelton et al., 1997). Results of a national NHANES study do not support current recommendations for population-wide sodium reductions (Alderman, 1998).

The American Dietetic Association recommends at least 3 medical nutrition therapy visits for patients with hypertension (http://www.knowledgelinc.com/ada/mntguides/).

OBJECTIVES

- Lose weight if obese (Davis et al., 1993; Denke et al., 1994). In men, there is a 6.6-mm rise in blood pressure for every 10% weight gain. Each pound requires many miles of new capillaries for nourishment.
- Control blood pressure to lessen the likelihood of congestive heart failure or stroke. Lower BP to a safe level.
- Induce negative sodium balance in the body only when this is absolutely required to lower BP rapidly. The average diet contains 6–15 g of sodium. A low-sodium diet (10 mEq) increases vascular and lymphocyte β-adrenergic responsiveness, thereby lowering BP. Only 20–50% of patients with HPN are sodium sensitive; if diet does not help within 6 months, medications will be necessary (Blake, 1994).
- Reduce excessive intake of caffeine and alcohol, which may increase blood pressure. There is no clear-cut association (Lewis et al., 1993).
- Increase calcium by 400 mg/day (Levey et al., 1995). Calcium supplementation may be useful in lowering BP in black adolescents who have lower dietary intakes of calcium (Dwyer et al., 1998).
- Increase magnesium, vitamins D, E, and K appropriately. Allow at least 2 months before monitoring outcomes.
- Force fluids unless contraindicated.
- Increase potassium intake to decrease the need for hypertensive medications (Brancati et al., 1996) but monitor current medications very carefully if some are K+-sparing.
- Educate the patient regarding follow-up care.
- Increase physical activity.

DIETARY AND NUTRITIONAL RECOMMENDATIONS

- The DASH diet has been effective, often within 14 days of initiation. A diet rich in fruits, vegetables, and low-fat dairy foods and low in SFA and total fat can prevent and reduce high BP (Appel et al., 1997). Adequate amounts of potassium from baked potatoes, grapefruit, oranges, bananas, lima beans, other fruits, and vegetables should be planned daily. Tips on eating the DASH way: Start small; make gradual changes in eating habits. Organize meals around carbohydrates such as pasta, rice, beans, or vegetables. Treat meat as one part of the whole meal, instead of the focus. Use fruits or low-fat, low-calorie foods such as sugar free gelatin for desserts and snacks.
- To rapidly decrease blood pressure, reduce intake of sodium to 200–250 mg. If diuretics are used, a diet of 2–4 g of sodium is sufficient. Be careful—sodium restriction decreases blood volume; not all persons are sodium sensitive. Table 6–7 lists common salt substitutes and their content.
- Use a calorie-controlled diet if weight loss is needed.
- Use 50% of calories as carbohydrates, preferably complex carbohydrates such as beans, oat bran, and apples (soluble fiber).
- Fat intake should be moderately low. Olive, soybean, or canola oils can be substituted for some saturated fats in cooking.
- Increase calcium—the sodium:calcium ratio should be

TABLE 6–7 Samples of Salt Substitutes and Content of Sodium and Potassium (per ½ teaspoon)

Brand Name	mg Na+	mg K+	mEq K+
Morton's	—	1,250	32
Adolph's	–	1,205	31
McCormick's	–	1,170	30
Diamond Crystal	–	1,104	28
Co-Salt	–	987	25
Adolph's Seasoned	–	849	22
Morton's Lite Salt	488	650	16
Papa Dash	180	0.03	–

1.4:4.1 (Bucher et al., 1996). Magnesium is also important (Witteman et al., 1994).

- Use caffeine-containing beverages in moderation. Drinking regular coffee may increase blood pressure in some HPN-prone subjects (Nurminen et al., 1999).
- Severely restrict alcoholic beverages.
- Use sources of omega-3 fatty acids, such as mackerel, haddock, salmon, and tuna (Appel et al., 1993; Morris et al., 1993), several times weekly.
- Increase fruits and vegetables for their flavonoids and phytochemical properties.
- Vegetarian diets tend to lower BP among blacks (Melby et al., 1993). These diets are likely to be beneficial overall.
- Increase sources of riboflavin, folic acid, B12, and B6 for overall cardiovascular health. In addition, adequate vitamin C may be important; plasma ascorbic acid is a predictor of BP and LDL-C levels (Toohey et al., 1996).

PROFILE

Clinical/History		
Height	ECG	K+
Weight	Alb, prealbumin	Cl−
BMI	Urinary albumin (elevated levels may impair arterial dilatory capacity)	Trig
Headache	Chol (HDL:LDL ratio)	Parathormone (PTH)
I & O	Ca++	AST, ALT
BP pattern	LDH	PO4, Alk phos
Lab Work	BUN	PT
Renal arteriography	Creat	Mg++
Chest x-ray	Uric acid	Gluc
Renal ultrasound	Plasma renin	Homocysteine
Intravenous pyelogram	Na+	Serum folate
		Serum B12
		Plasma ascorbic acid
		Urinary Ca++
		Urinary cortisol

Common Drugs Used and Potential Side Effects

- Diuretics—Spironolactone (Aldactone, Aldactazide) is potassium-sparing, whereas thiazides, e.g., furosemide (Lasix), deplete K+ and require supplementation; diarrhea or GI bleeding can occur. Avoid natural licorice. Long-term thiazide use alters calciotropic hormone relationships, compromising bone health (Perry et al., 1993). Hygroton (chlorthalidone) may alter blood glucose or potassium levels; it may cause anorexia, vomiting, constipation, and nausea. In general, avoid use with fenugreek, yohimbe, and ginkgo.
- Antihypertensives—Reserpine (Serpasil) requires reduced levels of Na+; consequently, a sodium-restricted diet is useful. Take hydralazine with food; use a low-sodium/low-calorie diet.
- ACE inhibitors prevent angiotensin I from conversion; they are useful in CHF. Examples include Accupril, Altace, Lotensin, Monopril, and Enalapril. Altace has been noted to prevent diabetes in hypertensive patients. Nausea, vomiting, and abdominal pain may occur; do not take with potassium supplements. Captopril (Capoten) can alter BUN/creatinine; take 1 hour before meals and reduce calories and sodium. Loss of taste can occur. Patients who take captopril and enalapril may develop zinc deficiency (Golik et al., 1998).
- Propranolol (Inderal), rauwolfia (Raudixin), and metoprolol (Lopressor) should be taken with a low-calorie/low-sodium diet. Diarrhea, nausea, vomiting, or abdominal cramps may occur.
- Estrogens and oral contraceptives (OCs) can increase BP.
- Amiloride (Moduretic) is an antihypertensive with diuretic. A low-calorie/low-sodium diet is important. Potassium loss is minimized. Avoid use with alcohol.
- Central adrenergic inhibitors such as terazosin (Hytrin) and clonidine (Catapres) require a low-sodium/low-calorie diet. Dry mouth, vomiting, nausea, constipation, or edema can occur. Avoid taking with kava, ma huang, yohimbe, fenugreek, or licorice.
- Prazosin (Minipress) may cause nausea, weight gain, anorexia, diarrhea, or constipation.
- β-blockers (atenolol/Tenormin; pindolol/Visken; propanolol/Inderal) decrease the force and rate of heart contractions, thereby decreasing blood pressure. Dizziness and nausea are common side effects.
- Drug therapy is less helpful, or even harmful, in the oldest old, i.e., individuals older than 80 years of age (Insua et al., 1994). Antihypertensive therapy is challenging in the elderly because of metabolic and physiologic alterations, comorbidities, polypharmacy, and biologic variability. Drugs with a convenient dosing schedule, minimal side effects, and the ability to impact comorbid conditions are important considerations in the treatment of HPN in the elderly (Schrier, 2001).
- Grapefruit juice decreases drug metabolism in the gut (via P450-CYP3A4 inhibition) and can affect medications up to 24 hours later. Consistency of use may be

more important than total quantity. Avoid taking with alprazolam, buspirone, cisapride, cyclosporine, statins, tacrolimus, and many others.

Herbs, Botanicals and Supplements

- Danshen may be used for ischemic heart disease. Avoid large amounts with warfarin, aspirin, and other antiplatelet drugs. It can increase risks of bleeding or bruising.
- Garlic tablets (0.6% allicin) given three times daily lower LDLs (Stevinson et al., 2000; Jain et al., 1993). Large amounts should not be taken with warfarin, aspirin, and other antiplatelet drugs because of increased risks of bleeding or bruising. It may also increase insulin levels with hypoglycemic results; monitor carefully in patients with diabetes.
- CoEnzyme Q10 should not be used with statins, gemfibrozil, tricyclic antidepressants, or warfarin. CoQ10 may act similarly to vitamin K.
- Omega-3 fatty acids in fish oil capsules can cause hypervitaminosis A and D. Avoid use in children and pregnant or lactating women. Avoid taking with warfarin, aspirin, and other antiplatelet medications because of the risk of increased bruising or bleeding.
- Hawthorn should not be taken with digoxin, ACE inhibitors, and other cardiovascular drugs.
- Yohimbe should not be used with tricyclic antidepressants, MAO inhibitors, antianxiety medications, appetite suppressants, antihypertensives, clonidine, or phenothiazides because of effects of blood pressure.
- Indian snakeroot should not be taken with digoxin, barbiturates, levodopa, neuroleptic tranquilizers, albuterol, furosemide, thiazides, MAO inhibitors, and beta-blockers such as atenolol and propranolol because of increased or decreased sedation and changed effects on blood pressure.
- Niacin (nicotinic acid) should not be taken with statins, antidiabetic medications, and carbamazepine because of potentially serious risks of myopathy and altered glucose control.
- Vitamin E should not be taken with warfarin because of the possibility of increased bleeding. Avoid doses greater than 400 IU per day.

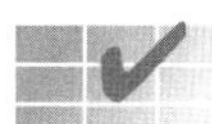

PATIENT EDUCATION

- ✔ Encourage patience; it takes 2–8 weeks to see the results of dietary changes.
- ✔ Encourage the adequate intake of fruits and vegetables.
- ✔ Remove the salt shaker from the table. Have the patient taste food before salting further. Avoid excesses of processed and canned foods.
- ✔ Interesting food flavors are often hidden by salt. Discuss other seasonings and recipes. Monitor potassium in salt substitutes and medications to prevent either hypokalemia or hyperkalemia. Read all labels carefully.
- ✔ Discuss caffeine sources (coffee, tea, cola, chocolate).
- ✔ Increase physical activity when possible; walk briskly 30–45 minutes 3–5 times weekly.
- ✔ Omit or reduce alcohol intake severely when possible.
- ✔ Weight loss reduces BP more in those who require the most weight loss (Stevens et al., 1993).
- ✔ The normal adult needs only 1/10 of a teaspoon of sodium (200 mg) per day. Greater amounts of salt are required only in hot, humid conditions or during lactation (or other salt-losing states). In such conditions, 2,000 mg of salt would be sufficient (See Table 6–3).

For More Information

- American Dietetic Association
  Hypertension protocol
  www.eatright.org
- DASH Diet
  http://dash.bwh.harvard.edu/dashdiet.html
- National High Blood Pressure Education Program
  120/80 National Institutes of Health
  Bethesda, MD 20892
  http://www.nhlbi.nih.gov/about/nhbpep/index.htm
- National High Blood Pressure Coordinating Committee
  Building 3, Room 4A05
  31 Center Drive
  Bethesda, MD 20891
  (301) 496-0554
- Papa Dash, c/o Alberto-Culver
  Melrose, IL 60160
  (708) 450-3282
- World Hypertension League
  http://www.mco.edu/whl/

MYOCARDIAL INFARCTION (ACUTE)

NUTRITIONAL ACUITY RANKING: LEVEL 2

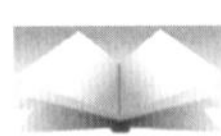

DEFINITIONS AND BACKGROUND

Myocardial infarction (MI) is necrosis in the heart muscle caused by prolonged inadequate blood supply or O2 deficit. A coronary occlusion is the closing of a coronary artery feeding heart muscle by fatty deposits or a blood clot. Commonly called a "heart attack," a coronary occlusion manifests with heavy squeezing pain, nausea and vomiting, and weakness. Rest does not relieve symptoms. Stages include critical (first 48 hours) to acute (3–14 days) to convalescent (15–90 days).

Treatment with cholesterol-lowering medications (such as Probucol) and antioxidants may decrease myocardial ischemia and may reduce adverse coronary events (Anderson et al., 1995). Plasma antioxidant vitamins are significantly lower among subjects who experienced acute MI within the previous 24 hours than among healthy control subjects (Levy et al., 1998). Recent studies relate exposure to wine/resveratrol with reduction in myocardial damage during ischemia-reperfusion, modulation of vascular cell functions, inhibition of LDL oxidation, and suppression of platelet aggregation (Wu et al., 2001).

For vitamin C and folic acid supplements, controlled trials and evidence are lacking; use of beta carotene supplements are actually discouraged for prevention of MI (Pearce et al., 2000). Fruit and vegetable intake should be encouraged (Joshipura et al., 2001).

Low magnesium levels may be a concern (Salonen et al., 1992). Magnesium in drinking water helps to protect against death from acute MI (Rubenowitz et al., 1996). Intake of black tea but not coffee seems to be inversely related to MI risk (Sesso et al., 1999).

Nonfatal MIs may be reduced by use of antioxidant vitamin E at levels of 400–800 IU (Stephens et al., 1996); but controlled clinical trials have not been consistent (Pearce et al., 2000). In older adults who have other risk factors, serum ferritin level may be positively correlated to risk of MI; serum iron and transferrin are not associated (Klipstein-Grobusch et al., 1999). Risk factors for MI are found in Table 6–8.

An arrhythmia is a variation from normal heartbeat rhythm. Among its many forms is a slowing of the heartbeat to less than 60 beats per minute (bradycardia), a speedup to more than 100 beats per minute (tachycardia), and premature or "skipped" beats. Post-MI patients will need to be aware.

TABLE 6–8 Risk Factors for Myocardial Infarction

Family history of heart disease
Patient history of heart disease
Diabetes
Hypertension
Advanced age
High Lp(a) lipids
African-American ethnicity
Stress, smoking, sedentary lifestyle, compulsive personality
Poor diet (high energy, sodium, alcohol, fat; low potassium, magnesium, folate, vitamin B12, calcium; low consumption of fruits and vegetables)

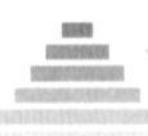

OBJECTIVES

- Promote rest to reduce heart strain. Avoid the distention of heavy meals.
- Prevent arrhythmias by serving food at body temperature.
- Avoid both constipation and flatulence.
- Avoid excessive heart stimulation from caffeine.
- Reduce elevated levels of lipids: keep cholesterol below 200 mg/dL, triglycerides below 200 mg/dL, HDL between 40–60 mg/dL, and LDL between 100–129 mg/dL.
- Decrease energy required to chew, prepare meals, etc.
- Initiate healing and promote convalescence.
- Decrease excess weight to reduce stress on the heart.
- Identify modifiable risk factors and reduce when possible.
- Consume more fish, which may reduce the risk of sudden cardiac death in men if eaten weekly (Albert, 1998).

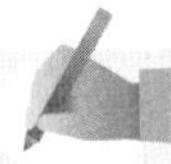

DIETARY AND NUTRITIONAL RECOMMENDATIONS

- Initially, use clear to full liquids to promote rest while reducing the dangers of aspiration or vomiting. Reduce fluid and caffeine intake to that recommended by the physician.
- As treatment progresses, diet should include soft, easily digested foods that are low in saturated fats or cholesterol. Diet should exclude gas-forming foods. Limit diet to 2 g of sodium or remove salt from the table. Schedule 3–6 small meals daily. Avoid stimulants such as caffeine.
- The diet of a patient whose condition has been stabilized, or who is at home, should be: carbohydrates, 50%; protein, 20%; fat, 30% (to be taken mostly in the form of PUFAs and MUFAs). Salt should be removed from the table. If needed, use a low-calorie diet to reduce the heart's workload.
- Increase intake of fish, oat bran, corn bran, and use of olive, canola, or soybean oil. Onions, tea, apples, grape juice, and grapefruit, which contain flavonoids, should be used often; red wine is recommended, if approved by the physician.
- Adequate calcium, magnesium, and potassium will be needed. Avoid excessive amounts.
- Decrease intake of whole milk products, red meats, visible fat on meat/poultry, and commercial baked goods. Use only 4–5 egg yolks weekly.
- Increase vitamin E, perhaps in supplemental form. Increase dietary sources of folic acid, riboflavin, and vitamins B6 and B12, if serum homocysteine levels are high.
- Fiber is especially important as a protector—choose vegetables, fruits, and cereal grains (Rimm et al., 1996).
- Include judicious use of nuts such as walnuts, almonds, macadamias, pecans, and pistachios. Walnuts contain

alpha-linolenic acid; almonds are a good source of vitamin E. Nuts also contain flavonoids, phenols, sterols, saponins, elegiac acid, folic acid, magnesium, copper, potassium, and fiber.

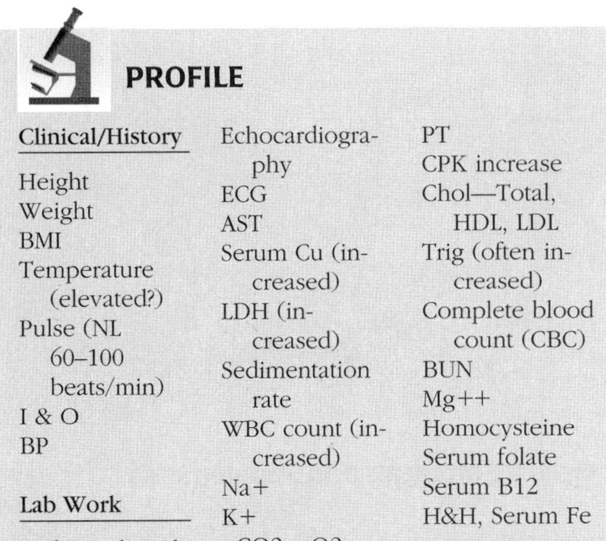

PROFILE

Clinical/History

Height
Weight
BMI
Temperature (elevated?)
Pulse (NL 60–100 beats/min)
I & O
BP

Lab Work

Radionucleotide imaging
Echocardiography
ECG
AST
Serum Cu (increased)
LDH (increased)
Sedimentation rate
WBC count (increased)
Na+
K+
pCO2, pO2
PT
CPK increase
Chol—Total, HDL, LDL
Trig (often increased)
Complete blood count (CBC)
BUN
Mg++
Homocysteine
Serum folate
Serum B12
H&H, Serum Fe

Common Drugs Used and Potential Side Effects

- Appropriate drugs are provided according to needs established by the profile (elevated blood pressure, serum cholesterol, etc.). Review specific drugs given to the patients and treat accordingly: nitrates, β-blockers, and calcium channel blockers are commonly used.
- Morphine—Used for relief of pain, morphine should be used in minimal amounts to prevent hypotension.
- Anticoagulant and thrombolytic therapy—Warfarin (Coumadin) or heparin may be given in some cases, e.g., when bleeding tendencies do not exist. Watch for excessive intake of foods high in vitamin K (green leafy vegetables such as kale, broccoli, spinach, or turnip greens), because they may alter PT values; use no more than one per day. Avoid taking with dong quai, fenugreek, feverfew, excessive garlic, ginger, ginkgo, and ginseng because of their effects.
- Aspirin is often recommended later to prevent recurrent MIs. Watch for GI bleeding or other side effects. Aspirin may decrease serum ferritin by increasing occult blood loss (Fleming et al., 2001).
- Mexitil and Rythmol are used to treat arrhythmias. Nausea, vomiting, or constipation may occur. Procan (procainamide) is also used commonly; it may give a bitter taste, nausea, anorexia, or diarrhea.

Herbs, Botanicals and Supplements

- Danshen may be used for ischemic heart disease. Avoid large amounts with warfarin, aspirin, and other antiplatelet drugs. It can increase risks of bleeding or bruising.
- Garlic tablets (0.6% allicin) given three times daily have lowered cholesterol levels and LDLs greatly (Stevinson et al., 2000; Jain et al., 1993). Large amounts should not be taken with warfarin, aspirin, and other antiplatelet drugs because of increased risks of bleeding or bruising. It may also increase insulin levels with hypoglycemic results; monitor carefully in patients with diabetes.
- CoEnzyme Q10 should not be used with statins, gemfibrozil, tricyclic antidepressants, or warfarin. CoQ10 may act similarly to vitamin K.
- Omega-3 fatty acids in fish oil capsules can cause hypervitaminosis A and D. Avoid use in children and pregnant or lactating women. Avoid taking with warfarin, aspirin, and other antiplatelet medications because of the risk of increased bruising or bleeding.
- Hawthorn should not be taken with digoxin, ACE inhibitors, and other cardiovascular drugs.
- Chromium is sometimes used for dyslipidemia. Do not use excesses with insulin or hypoglycemic agents, because it may lower glucose levels.
- Gingko biloba should not be taken with warfarin and other anticoagulant drugs.
- Niacin (nicotinic acid) should not be taken with statins, antidiabetic medications, and carbamazepine because of potentially serious risks of myopathy and altered glucose control.
- Vitamin E should not be taken with warfarin because of the possibility of increased bleeding. Avoid doses greater than 400 IU per day.

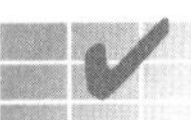

PATIENT EDUCATION

- ✓ Position patient and arrange utensils to avoid or to lessen fatigue.
- ✓ If needed, use a weight control diet.
- ✓ Encourage relaxation, especially at mealtimes.
- ✓ Discuss roles of fats, cholesterol, sodium, potassium, calcium, magnesium, and fiber in the diet.
- ✓ Avoid simple sugars and alcohol, especially with diabetes or HLP.
- ✓ Discuss convalescence regarding progression of atherosclerosis, preventing CHF, and working with cardiac rehabilitation.
- ✓ A positive attitude toward the modified diet is essential for changing food behaviors (Barnes and Terry, 1991).
- ✓ Discuss activity (gradual increase).
- ✓ Discuss saturated fats and related risks with children of post-MI patients (Russell et al., 1994) (see Table 6–4).
- ✓ Individuals who undergo the CABG continue to have multiple risk factors for CAD that place them at high risk for future CAD events; other steps, such as stopping smoking, following the recommended diet, and managing other risk factors must be taken (Frame et al., 2001).

PERICARDITIS

NUTRITIONAL ACUITY RANKING: LEVEL 2

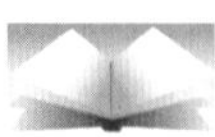

DEFINITIONS AND BACKGROUND

Pericarditis is the inflammation of the pericardium due to AIDS, MI, rheumatoid disease, radiation treatment, viral infection, trauma, neoplasm, chronic renal failure, or systemic lupus. Substernal chest pain that is severe, dyspnea, shortness of breath, fever, chills, diaphoresis, nausea, fatigue, and anxiety are common symptoms of the acute stage. The most serious complication is cardiac tamponade.

The chronic stage, often resulting from TB, may involve ascites, CHF, edema of the extremities, and shrinkage of the pericardium. Shortness of breath, coughing, fatigue, ascites, and leg edema may result.

The only possible cure is surgical removal of the pericardium. Risk of dying is 5–10%, so it is not always chosen. If this is not done, control of symptoms through diuretics is the usual treatment.

OBJECTIVES

- Maintain bed rest during acute stages.
- Promote improved cardiac function.
- Prevent sepsis.
- Decrease fever and inflammation, which may last 10–14 days in acute form.
- Reduce nausea and anorexic state.

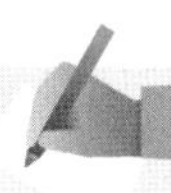

DIETARY AND NUTRITIONAL RECOMMENDATIONS

- Maintain an adequate diet as needed for any underlying conditions; increase protein and calories if tolerated and if needed to prevent loss of LBM.
- Increase fluids unless contraindicated.
- Small, frequent feedings to reduce nausea may be indicated.
- Thiamine for the heart muscle and potassium may be especially necessary. Monitor diet and supplements adequately.
- Vitamins B6 and B12, riboflavin, and folic acid may be needed if homocysteine levels are elevated.
- It may be prudent to increase vitamin E levels.

Common Drugs Used and Potential Side Effects

- Nonsteroidal anti-inflammatory drugs are often used. GI distress may result.
- Analgesics of other composition may also be used. Monitor for specific side effects.
- Antibiotics are needed for bacterial infections.

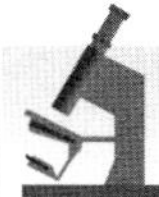

PROFILE

Clinical/History	Lab Work	
Height	Alb, prealbumin	MRI or CT scan
Weight	BP	Transferrin
BMI	H&H, Serum Fe	K+
Weight changes	ECG	Na+
Temperature	Cardiac catheterization	WBC
		Homocysteine
		Serum folate
		Serum B12

Herbs, Botanicals and Supplements

- Danshen may be used for ischemic heart disease. Avoid large amounts with warfarin, aspirin, and other antiplatelet drugs. It can increase risks of bleeding or bruising.
- Garlic tablets (0.6% allicin) given three times daily have lowered cholesterol levels and LDLs greatly (Jain et al., 1993). Large amounts should not be taken with warfarin, aspirin, and other antiplatelet drugs because of increased risks of bleeding or bruising. It also may increase insulin levels with hypoglycemic results; monitor carefully in patients with diabetes.
- CoEnzyme Q10 should not be used with statins, gemfibrozil, tricyclic antidepressants, or warfarin. CoQ10 may act similarly to vitamin K.
- Omega-3 fatty acids in fish oil capsules can cause hypervitaminosis A and D. Avoid use in children and pregnant or lactating women. Avoid taking with warfarin, aspirin, and other antiplatelet medications because of the risk of increased bruising or bleeding.
- Hawthorn should not be taken with digoxin, ACE inhibitors, and other cardiovascular drugs.
- Niacin (nicotinic acid) should not be taken with statins, antidiabetic medications, and carbamazepine because of potentially serious risks of myopathy and altered glucose control.
- Vitamin E should not be taken with warfarin because of the possibility of increased bleeding. Avoid doses greater than 400 IU per day.

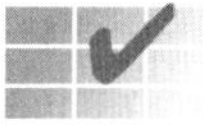

PATIENT EDUCATION

- ✔ Discuss the importance of avoiding fatigue.
- ✔ The patient should plan rest periods before and after activities and meals.
- ✔ Highlight the importance of nutrition in immunocompetence.

PERIPHERAL VASCULAR DISEASE

NUTRITIONAL ACUITY RANKING: LEVEL 2

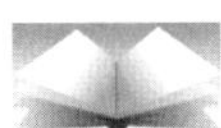

DEFINITIONS AND BACKGROUND

Peripheral vascular disease (PVD) is caused by occlusion of an artery by a clot or by plaque buildup in the extremities, such as the hands and feet. Complications of PVD can include gangrene with potential amputation. Numbness, tingling in lower extremities, pain, difficult ambulation, and tissue death can occur. Causes of PVD include heavy smoking, arterial embolism, obesity, diabetes mellitus, poor circulation, or ASHD. PVD may lead to increased risks of heart attack and stroke.

Buerger's disease is the obstruction of small- and medium-sized arteries by inflammation triggered by smoking. This is more common among men aged 20–40 who smoke. Skin ulcers or gangrene may result if smoking is not discontinued. Walking is important, unless the person has gangrene, sores, or pain at rest.

Raynaud's syndrome allows small arterioles in the fingers and toes to go into spasm, and the skin turns pale or patchy red to blue. Sometimes the underlying cause is not known. Approximately 60–90% of cases occur in young women. Scleroderma, rheumatoid arthritis, atherosclerosis, nerve disorders, hypothyroidism, injury, and reactions to certain drugs may be potential causes. Some people also have migraine headaches and pulmonary hypertension. These individuals must protect their extremities from the cold or take mild sedatives.

Hyperhomocystinemia caused by cystathionine β-synthase deficiency may occur (Clarke et al., 1991). Fish oils alter vascularity favorably and may protect arterial walls in patients with type 2 diabetes (McVeigh et al., 1994). Elevated levels of C-reactive protein may occur, which indicates that there is inflammation in the blood vessels. There seems to be a role for vitamin C as an antioxidant; excesses are not warranted because these supplements may function as peroxidants.

Angioplasty may be needed to clear the obstruction. Surgery often relieves symptoms, heals ulcers, and prevents amputation.

OBJECTIVES

- Reduce symptoms and side effects, i.e., severe leg cramps on walking, angina, heart failure, heart attack, stroke, renal failure, ulcerative disease, gangrene of lower extremities or toes, slow-healing foot ulcers, cold extremities, and paresthesia.
- Attain desirable body weight.
- Prevent sepsis, pressure ulcers, and other complications.
- Correct high levels of homocysteine.

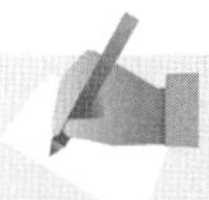

DIETARY AND NUTRITIONAL RECOMMENDATIONS

- If patient is obese, use a low-calorie diet. Use a low-fat, high-soluble fiber diet.
- Diet should provide adequate intake for wound healing when ulcers exist.
- Vitamin E also is suggested (Ubbink et al., 1994). Almonds, filberts, avocados, sunflower seeds, vegetable oils, margarine, mayonnaise, and wheat germ are the best dietary sources. Because of their high fat content, supplements may be useful.
- Diet should provide adequate protein, especially from fish.
- Increase folic acid, riboflavin, vitamins B6 and B12. In some cases, niacin may serve as a vasodilator; do not use excesses because of flushing.
- Olive oil consumption along with a dietary supplement of fish oil may be helpful in the nutritional management of peripheral vascular disease by increasing plasma omega-3 long-chain PUFA and decreasing susceptibility to LDL oxidation (Ramirez-Tortosa et al., 1999). Extra virgin olive oil may protect LDL against oxidation more than does refined olive oil in men with PVD; it has a higher antioxidant level (Ramirez-Tortosa et al., 1999).

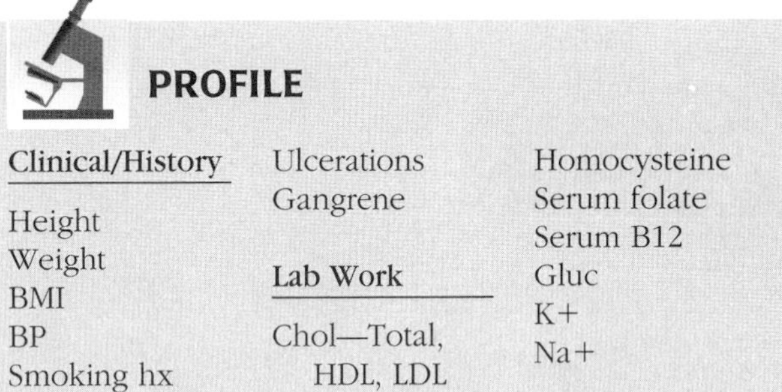

PROFILE

Clinical/History		
Height	Ulcerations	Homocysteine
Weight	Gangrene	Serum folate
BMI	**Lab Work**	Serum B12
BP	Chol—Total, HDL, LDL	Gluc
Smoking hx	Trig	K+
Exercise tolerance		Na+

Common Drugs Used and Potential Side Effects

- Isoxsuprine (Vasodilan) may be used to dilate the vessels.
- Antibiotics may be used to control infections.
- Anticoagulants such as Coumadin/warfarin may be used. Use no more than one high vitamin K food source daily. Avoid taking with dong quai, fenugreek, feverfew, excessive garlic, ginger, ginkgo, or ginseng because of their effects.
- Pentoxifylline (Trental) improves blood flow. GI distress, nausea, or anorexia may occur; take with meals.

Herbs, Botanicals and Supplements

- Danshen may be used for ischemic heart disease. Avoid large amounts with warfarin, aspirin, and other antiplatelet drugs. It can increase risks of bleeding or bruising.

- Garlic tablets (0.6% allicin) given three times daily have lowered cholesterol levels and LDLs greatly (Jain et al., 1993). Large amounts should not be taken with warfarin, aspirin, and other antiplatelet drugs because of increased risks of bleeding or bruising. It may also increase insulin levels with hypoglycemic results; monitor carefully in patients with diabetes.
- CoEnzyme Q10 should not be used with statins, gemfibrozil, tricyclic antidepressants, or warfarin. CoQ10 may act similarly to vitamin K.
- Omega-3 fatty acids in fish oil capsules can cause hypervitaminosis A and D. Avoid use in children and pregnant or lactating women. Avoid taking with warfarin, aspirin, and other antiplatelet medications because of the risk of increased bruising or bleeding.
- Hawthorn should not be taken with digoxin, ACE inhibitors, and other cardiovascular drugs.
- Chromium is sometimes used for dyslipidemia. Do not use excesses with insulin or hypoglycemic agents, because it may lower glucose levels.
- Niacin (nicotinic acid) should not be taken with statins, antidiabetic medications, and carbamazepine because of potentially serious risks of myopathy and altered glucose control.
- Vitamin E should not be taken with warfarin because of the possibility of increased bleeding. Avoid doses greater than 400 IU per day.
- Herbs and botanicals such as ginger, purslane, and gingko have been recommended, but no clinical trials have proven efficacy.

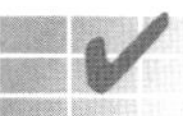

PATIENT EDUCATION

- ✔ Emphasize the importance of weight control and exercise.
- ✔ Reduce alcohol consumption, especially if triglycerides are elevated.
- ✔ Fish and meatless meals should be used 3–4 times weekly.
- ✔ Hyperbaric oxygen treatments may be needed to heal lesions. Oxygen permeates the flesh, and anaerobic bacteria cannot survive.
- ✔ Encourage a stop-smoking program.

THROMBOPHLEBITIS

NUTRITIONAL ACUITY RANKING: LEVEL 1

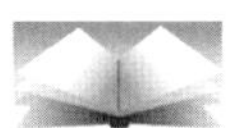

DEFINITIONS AND BACKGROUND

Phlebitis is inflammation of a vein that usually is caused by infection or injury. Blood flow may be disturbed, with blood clots (thrombi) adhering to the wall of the inflamed vein. This condition usually occurs in leg veins, especially in varicose veins. Signs and symptoms include pain, redness, tenderness, itching, and hard or cord-like swelling along the affected vein.

Fatty acids have been implicated in the etiology of thrombophlebitis, but there is no clearly demonstrated and plausible mechanism by which SFAs have a thrombotic effect on the body (Hoak, 1992). Stearic acid in cocoa butter or in milk chocolate has no effect compared with diets high in dairy butter and lauric acid (Mustad et al., 1993).

OBJECTIVES

- Reduce inflammation and swelling; reduce fever when present.
- Prevent septicemia, deep vein thrombosis, and related complications.

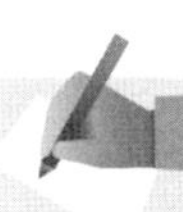

DIETARY AND NUTRITIONAL RECOMMENDATIONS

- No special diet is warranted, but weight control diet may be needed if the patient is obese. A prudent NCEP diet may also be useful.
- Sodium restriction may be beneficial for persons with a generally high salt or sodium intake. Monitor carefully.
- For general cardiovascular health, adequate vitamin E, B6, B12, folic acid, riboflavin, and thiamine should be enhanced in the diet. Be careful not to overdo vitamin E if anticoagulants are used.

PROFILE

Clinical/History	Lab Work	
Height	BP	H&H
Weight	Alb, prealbumin	Gluc
BMI	Chol—Total, HDL, LDL	TLC
Recent weight changes	Trig	Na+
Temperature	WBC	K+
I & O		Homocysteine
		Serum folate
		Serum B12

Common Drugs Used and Potential Side Effects

- Warfarin (Coumadin) may be used, with side effects that alter use of vitamin K. Monitor intake carefully. Avoid supplements that are high in vitamins E, C, or A during use. Avoid taking with dong quai, fenugreek, feverfew, excessive garlic, ginger, ginkgo, and ginseng because of their effects.
- Antibiotics are used in bacterial infections.
- Aspirin or acetaminophen may be used to reduce fever or pain. Aspirin may decrease serum ferritin by increasing occult blood loss (Fleming et al., 2001).

Herbs, Botanicals and Supplements

- Danshen may be used for ischemic heart disease. Avoid large amounts with warfarin, aspirin, and other antiplatelet drugs. It can increase risks of bleeding or bruising.
- Garlic tablets (0.6% allicin) given three times daily have lowered cholesterol levels and LDLs greatly (Jain et al., 1993). Large amounts should not be taken with warfarin, aspirin, and other antiplatelet drugs because of increased risks of bleeding or bruising. It may also increase insulin levels with hypoglycemic results; monitor carefully in patients with diabetes.
- CoEnzyme Q10 should not be used with statins, gemfibrozil, tricyclic antidepressants, or warfarin. CoQ10 may act similarly to vitamin K.
- Omega-3 fatty acids in fish oil capsules can cause hypervitaminosis A and D. Avoid use in children and pregnant or lactating women. Avoid taking with warfarin, aspirin, and other antiplatelet medications because of the risk of increased bruising or bleeding.
- Hawthorn should not be taken with digoxin, ACE inhibitors, and other cardiovascular drugs.
- Chromium is sometimes used for dyslipidemia. Do not use excesses with insulin or hypoglycemic agents, because it may lower glucose levels.
- Niacin (nicotinic acid) should not be taken with statins, antidiabetic medications, and carbamazepine because of potentially serious risks of myopathy and altered glucose control.
- Vitamin E should not be taken with warfarin because of the possibility of increased bleeding. Avoid doses greater than 400 IU per day.

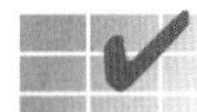

PATIENT EDUCATION

✔ Bed rest may be important during acute stages. Leg and foot elevation may be required. Monitor side effects of immobility if patient will be immobilized for a long period of time.

- ✓ Zinc ointment may relieve itching.
- ✓ Flavonoids (including tannins, quercetin, and phenols) in grapes, strawberries, blueberries, apples, kale, broccoli, tea, beer, and red wine may reduce platelet activity and prevent clots. Grapefruit and garlic may also be useful flavonoids.

TRANSPLANTATION (CARDIAC)

NUTRITIONAL ACUITY RANKING: LEVEL 4

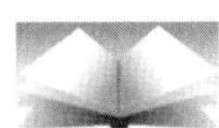

DEFINITIONS AND BACKGROUND

Cardiac transplantation is usually performed for terminal CHF, often after cardiomyopathies. Usually, the transplant will be a Jarvik-7 or a live donor heart. Screening includes evaluations for chronic, coexisting illness, psychosocial stability, and normal or reversible cardiac status. The best candidates are younger than 55 years of age with normal hepatic and renal functioning, free of diabetes mellitus and pulmonary problems, peptic ulcers, and peripheral heart disorders. Five-year survival rate is approximately 69%.

The mechanisms for regulating blood pressure in transplanted patients are very sodium sensitive; low-sodium diets are needed (Singer et al., 1994).

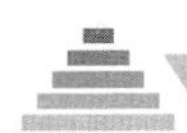

OBJECTIVES

- Normalize heart functioning; prevent morbidity and death.
- Prevent infection or sepsis.
- Decrease potential of graft rejection/failure; increase survival rate.
- Protect against further ASHD, which usually recurs within a few years of transplant.
- Prevent complications such as hypertension, hepatic or renal failure, and diabetes mellitus.
- Control side effects of steroid and immunosuppressive therapy.
- Promote adequate wound healing; prevent or correct wound dehiscence.
- Maintain or improve nutritional status and fluid balance.

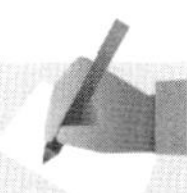

DIETARY AND NUTRITIONAL RECOMMENDATIONS

- Control calories, protein, sodium, potassium, fat, and cholesterol as appropriate for specific underlying condition (see appropriate sections). Keep in mind the role of nutrients needed for wound healing, including adequate calories.
- Fluid overload must be avoided; limit to 1 L daily, using a nutrient-dense product if needed.
- Avoid alcohol, which can aggravate cardiomyopathies.
- Increase use of garlic, fish and fish oils, and fiber (such as oat bran) when tolerance permits. Increase use of cardiac-protective agents such as vitamins E, B6 and B12, riboflavin, and folic acid.
- Reduce cardiac stimulants until fully recovered (e.g., caffeine).
- After transplantation, increase diet as tolerated and as appropriate for status. Alter as needed.
- For TF, use a low-sodium product and advance gradually.
- Include appropriate levels of calcium, magnesium, and fiber.
- It would be prudent to use more olive, soybean, and canola oils; nuts such as walnuts, almonds, macadamias, pecans, and pistachios should also be used in the diet. Walnuts contain alpha-linolenic acid; almonds are a good source of vitamin E. Nuts also contain flavonoids, phenols, sterols, saponins, elegaic acid, folic acid, magnesium, copper, potassium, and fiber.

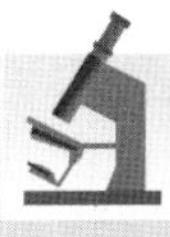

PROFILE

Clinical/History		
Height	K+	Chol—HDL, LDL, total
Weight	H&H	Trig
BMI	Transferrin	Gluc
Edema	CBC	Homocysteine
BP	BUN/Creat	Serum folate
Lab Work	AST, ALT	Serum B12
Urinary and serum Na+	ECG	
	pCO2, pO2	
	Alb, prealbumin	
	Ca++, Mg++	

Common Drugs Used and Potential Side Effects

- Corticosteroids such as Prednisone and Solu-Cortef are used for immunosuppression. Side effects include increased catabolism of proteins, negative nitrogen balance, hyperphagia, ulcers, decreased glucose tolerance, sodium retention, fluid retention, and impaired calcium absorption and osteoporosis. Cushing's syndrome, obesity, muscle wasting, and increased gastric secretion may result. A higher protein intake and lower intake of simple CHOs may be needed.
- Cyclosporine does not retain sodium as much as corticosteroids do. Intravenous doses are more effective than oral doses. Nausea, vomiting, and diarrhea are common side effects. Hyperlipidemia, HPN, and hyperkalemia may also occur; decrease sodium and potassium as necessary. Elevated glucose and lipids may occur. The drug is also nephrotoxic; a controlled renal diet may be beneficial.
- Immunosuppressants such as Muromonab or Orthoclone (OKT3) and antithymocyte globulin (ATG) are less nephrotoxic than cyclosporine but can cause nausea, anorexia, diarrhea, and vomiting. Monitor carefully. Fever and stomatitis also may occur; alter diet as needed.
- Azathioprine (Imuran) may cause leukopenia, thrombocytopenia, oral and esophageal sores, macrocytic anemia, pancreatitis, vomiting, diarrhea, and other complex side effects. Folate supplementation and other dietary modifications (liquid or soft diet, use of oral supplements) may be needed. The drug works by lowering the

number of T cells; it is often prescribed along with prednisone for conventional immunosuppression.

- Tacrolimus (Prograf, FK506) suppresses T-cell immunity; it is 100 times more potent than cyclosporine, thus requiring smaller doses. Side effects include GI distress, nausea, vomiting, hyperkalemia, and hyperglycemia.
- Diuretics such as Lasix may cause hypokalemia. Aldactone actually spares potassium; monitor drug changes closely. In general, avoid use with fenugreek, yohimbe, and ginkgo.
- Analgesics are also used to reduce pain. Long-term use may affect such nutrients as vitamin C and folacin; monitor carefully for each specific medication.
- Antihypertensive, antilipemics, diuretics, and potassium supplements may be used. Monitor side effects accordingly.
- Grapefruit juice decreases drug metabolism in the gut (via P450-CYP3A4 inhibition) and can affect medications up to 24 hours later. Consistency of use may be more important than total quantity. Avoid taking with alprazolam, buspirone, cisapride, cyclosporine, statins, tacrolimus, and many others.

Herbs, Botanicals and Supplements

- The patient should not take herbals and botanicals without discussing with the physician.
- Niacin (nicotinic acid) should not be taken with statins, antidiabetic medications, and carbamazepine because of potentially serious risks of myopathy and altered glucose control.
- Vitamin E should not be taken with warfarin because of the possibility of increased bleeding. Avoid doses greater than 400 IU per day.

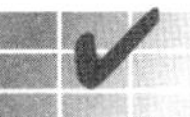

PATIENT EDUCATION

- ✔ Discuss the role of nutrition in wound healing, immunocompetence, and cardiovascular health. Specify nutrients that are known to be protective.
- ✔ Discuss how exercise affects the use of calories.
- ✔ Discuss, as appropriate, fiber intake and sources of fat and cholesterol. Highlight the importance of maintaining an adequate diet to reduce risks of further heart disease and complications. Transplant CAD proceeds at an accelerated rate; the patient must not see this procedure as a permanent cure.

TRANSPLANTATION (HEART-LUNG)

NUTRITIONAL ACUITY RANKING: LEVEL 4

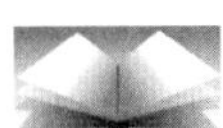

DEFINITIONS AND BACKGROUND

Heart-lung transplantation is performed rarely, as in complex cases of cystic fibrosis, pulmonary fibrosis, emphysema, Eisenmenger's syndrome, and primary pulmonary HPN. As with other types of transplants, graft-host resistance and sepsis are the major concerns.

OBJECTIVES

- ▲ Preoperative: Correct nutritional risks (loss of LBM, cardiac cachexia, vitamin or mineral deficiencies, CHF). Correct side effects of medication.
- ▲ Postoperative: Prevent surgical complications, organ rejection, and organ failure. Promote weight gain but not excessive amounts. Support nitrogen balance and correct hypoalbuminemia. Prevent aspiration. Support wound healing, and prevent infection.

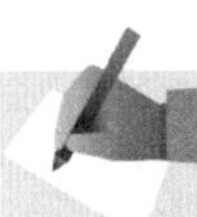

DIETARY AND NUTRITIONAL RECOMMENDATIONS

- Return to oral intake by 48–72 hours postoperatively, when possible.
- Promote adequate intake of kcal (25 kcal/kg) and protein (1 g/kg BW).
- Parenteral solutions may be used if needed; use high BCAAs for healing.
- Calorie-dense options should be considered if fluid restriction is required.
- Restrict Na+ and K+ if renal status is compromised. A soft, renal diet (70 g of protein, 2 g of Na+, and 3 g of K+) may be ordered.
- Increase intake of fruits, vegetables, whole grains, nuts, vitamins, and minerals in appropriate amounts for cardiovascular health. Monitor carefully with side effects of medications that are used.
- Adjust fluid intake according to I & O, BUN and creatinine, and lung congestion. Monitor closely to avoid overhydration and dehydration.

Common Drugs Used and Potential Side Effects

- Corticosteroids such as Prednisone and Solu-Cortef are used for immunosuppression. Side effects include increased catabolism of proteins, negative nitrogen balance, hyperphagia, ulcers, decreased glucose tolerance, sodium retention, fluid retention, and impaired calcium absorption and osteoporosis. Cushing's syndrome, obesity, muscle wasting, and increased gastric secretion may result. A higher protein intake and lower intake of simple CHOs may be needed.
- Cyclosporine does not retain sodium as much as corticosteroids do. Intravenous doses are more effective than oral doses. Nausea, vomiting, and diarrhea are common side effects. Hyperlipidemia, HPN, and hyperkalemia may also occur; decrease sodium and potassium as necessary. Elevated glucose and lipids may occur. The drug is also nephrotoxic; a controlled renal diet may be beneficial.
- Immunosuppressants such as Muromonab or Orthoclone (OKT3) and antithymocyte globulin (ATG) are less nephrotoxic than cyclosporine but can cause nausea, anorexia, diarrhea, and vomiting. Monitor carefully. Fever and stomatitis may also occur; alter diet as needed.
- Azathioprine (Imuran) may cause leukopenia, thrombocytopenia, oral and esophageal sores, macrocytic anemia, pancreatitis, vomiting, diarrhea, and other complex side effects. Folate supplementation and other dietary modifications (liquid or soft diet, use of oral supplements) may be needed. The drug works by lowering the number of T cells; it is often prescribed along with prednisone for conventional immunosuppression.
- Tacrolimus (Prograf, FK506) suppresses T-cell immunity; it is 100 times more potent than cyclosporine, thus requiring smaller doses. Side effects include GI distress, nausea, vomiting, hyperkalemia, and hyperglycemia.
- Diuretics such as Lasix may cause hypokalemia. Aldactone actually spares potassium; monitor drug changes closely. In general, avoid use with fenugreek, yohimbe, and ginkgo.
- Grapefruit juice decreases drug metabolism in the gut (via P450-CYP3A4 inhibition) and can affect medications up to 24 hours later. Consistency of use may be more important than total quantity. Avoid taking with alprazolam, buspirone, cisapride, cyclosporine, statins, tacrolimus, and many others.

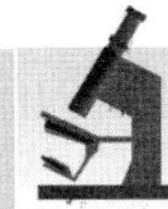

PROFILE

Clinical/History	Lab Work	
Height	Alb, prealbumin	Serum B12
Weight	Transferrin	H&H, Serum Fe
BMI	Chol	Gluc
Weight changes	Trig	BUN, Creat
Respiratory Quotient (RQ)	Homocysteine	Na+, K+
Ventilator support	Serum folate	PO4
	pCO2, pO2	ALT, AST
		Lactate
		TLC

Herbs, Botanicals and Supplements

- Danshen may be used for ischemic heart disease. Avoid large amounts with warfarin, aspirin, and other antiplatelet drugs. It can increase risks of bleeding or bruising.
- Garlic tablets (0.6% allicin) given three times daily have lowered cholesterol levels and LDLs greatly (Jain et al., 1993). Large amounts should not be taken with warfarin, aspirin, and other antiplatelet drugs because of increased risks of bleeding or bruising. It may also increase insulin levels with hypoglycemic results; monitor carefully in patients with diabetes.
- CoEnzyme Q10 should not be used with statins, gemfibrozil, tricyclic antidepressants, or warfarin. CoQ10 may act similarly to vitamin K.
- Omega-3 fatty acids in fish oil capsules can cause hypervitaminosis A and D. Avoid use in children and pregnant or lactating women. Avoid taking with warfarin, aspirin, and other antiplatelet medications because of the risk of increased bruising or bleeding.
- Hawthorn should not be taken with digoxin, ACE inhibitors, and other cardiovascular drugs.
- Chromium is sometimes used for dyslipidemia. Do not use excesses with insulin or hypoglycemic agents, because it may lower glucose levels.
- Niacin (nicotinic acid) should not be taken with statins, antidiabetic medications, and carbamazepine because of potentially serious risks of myopathy and altered glucose control.
- Vitamin E should not be taken with warfarin because of the possibility of increased bleeding. Avoid doses greater than 400 IU per day.

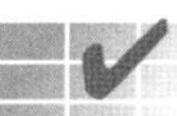

PATIENT EDUCATION

- ✔ Discuss appropriate calorie and protein levels.
- ✔ Sodium and fluid restrictions should be addressed as needed.
- ✔ Decreased fat and cholesterol intakes may be useful to decrease cardiac risks.
- ✔ Adequate fiber and vitamin E are useful.
- ✔ Restrict fresh fruits and vegetables for the first few months if a low-bacteria diet is needed.

REFERENCES

CITED REFERENCES

Ackermann R, et al. Garlic shows some promise for improving some cardiovascular risk factors. *Arch Int Med.* 2001;161:813.

Ades P. Introduction—the elderly in cardiac rehabilitation. *Am J Geriatr Cardiol.* 1999;8:61.

Adigun A, Ajayi A. The effects of enalapril-digoxin-diuretic combination therapy on nutritional and anthropometric indices in chronic congestive heart failure: preliminary findings in cardiac cachexia. *Eur J Heart Fail.* 2001;3:359.

Adler A, Holub B. Effect of garlic and fish-oil supplementation on serum lipid and lipoprotein concentrations in hypercholesterolemic men. *Am J Clin Nutri.* 1997;65:445.

Albert C, et al. Fish consumption and risk of sudden cardiac death. *J Am Med Assoc.* 1998;279:23.

Alderman M, et al. Dietary sodium intake and mortality: The National Health and Nutrition Examination Survey (NHANES I). *Lancet.* 1998;351:781.

Aldred H, et al. The effect of a single bout of brisk walking on postprandial lipemia in normolipidemic young adults. *Metabolism.* 1994;43:836.

Anderson J, et al. Meta-analysis of the effects of soy protein intake on serum lipids. *N Engl J Med.* 1995;333:276.

Anderson J, et al. Effect of fermented milk (yogurt) containing Lactobacillus L1 on serum cholesterol in hypercholesterolemic humans. *J Am Col Nutri.* 1999;18:43.

Anderson T, et al. The effect of cholesterol-lowering and antioxidant therapy on endothelium-dependent coronary vasomotion. *N Engl J Med.* 1995;332:488.

Anker S, Rauchhaus M. Heart failure as a metabolic problem. *Eur J Heart Fail.* 1999;1:127.

Appel L, et al. A clinical trial of the effects of dietary patterns on blood pressure: DASH Collaborative Research Group. *N Engl J Med.* 1997;336:1117.

Appel L, et al. Does supplementation of diet with "fish oil" reduce blood pressure? A meta-analysis of controlled clinical trials. *Arch Intern Med.* 1993;153:1429.

Arai T, et al. Increased plasma cholesterol ester transfer protein in obese subjects: possible mechanism for the reduction of serum HDL cholesterol levels in obesity. *Arterioscler Thromb.* 1994;14:1129.

Asakura L, et al. Dietary medium-chain triacylglycerol prevents the postprandial rise of plasma triacylglycerols but induces hypercholesterolemia in primary hypertriglyceridemic subjects. *Am J Clin Nutri.* 2000;71:701.

Ashton E, et al. Diet high in monounsaturated fat does not have a different effect on arterial elasticity than a low-fat, high-carbohydrate diet. *J Am Diet Assoc.* 2000;100:537.

Avins A, Neuhaus J. Do triglycerides provide meaningful information about heart disease? *Arch Int Med.* 2000;160:1937.

Barnes M, Terry R. Adherence to the cardiac diet: attitudes of patients after myocardial infarction. *J Am Diet Assoc.* 1991;91:1435.

Baum J, et al. Long-term intake of soy protein improves blood lipid profiles and increases mononuclear cell low density-lipoprotein receptor messenger RNA in hypercholesterolemic, postmenopausal women. *AJCN.* 1998;68:545.

Bellizzi M, et al. Vitamin E and coronary heart disease: the European paradox. *Eur J Clin Nutri.* 1994;48:822.

Blanc P, Boussuges A. Cardiac beriberi. *Arch Mal Coeur Vaiss.* 2000;93:371.

Blake G. Primary hypertension: the role of individualized therapy. *Am Fam Physician.* 1994;50:138.

Bostom A, et al. Nonfasting plasma total homocysteine levels and stroke incidence in elderly persons: the Framingham Study. *Ann Int Med.* 1999;131:352.

Bostrom A, et al. Elevated plasma lipoprotein(a) and coronary heart disease in men aged 55 years and younger. *JAMA.* 1996;276:544.

Brady J, et al. Thiamin status, diuretic medications, and the management of congestive heart failure. *J Am Diet Assoc.* 1995;95:541.

Brancati F, et al. Effect of potassium supplementation on blood pressure in African Americans on a low-potassium diet. *Arch Intern Med.* 1996;156:61.

Bucher H, et al. Effects of dietary calcium supplementation on blood pressure. *JAMA.* 1996;275:1016.

Chrysant S, et al. There are no racial, age, sex or weight differences in the effect of salt on blood pressure in salt-sensitive hypertensive patients. *Arch Int Med.* 1997;157:2489.

Clarke R, et al. Hyperhomocystinemia: an independent risk factor for vascular disease. *N Engl J Med.* 1991;324:1149.

Connolly H, et al. Valvular heart disease associated with fenfluramine-phentermine. *N Engl J Med.* 1997;337:581.

Daucsh J. Trans-fatty acids: a regulatory update. *J Am Diet Assoc.* 2002;18:293.

Davidson M, et al. Comparison of the effects of lean red meat vs lean white meat on serum lipid levels among free-living persons with hypercholesterolemia. *Arch Int Med.* 1999;159:1331.

Daviglus M, et al. Fish consumption and the 30-year risk of fatal myocardial infarction. *N Engl J Med.* 1997;336:1046.

Davis B, et al. Reduction in long-term antihypertensive medication requirements: effects of weight reduction by dietary intervention in overweight persons with mild hypertension. *Arch Intern Med.* 1993;153:1773.

de Bree A, et al. Lifestyle factors and plasma homocysteine concentrations in a general population sample. *Am J Epid.* 2001;154:150.

DeLuca M, Tak T. Hypertrophic cardiomyopathy. Tools for identifying risk and alleviating symptoms. *Postgrad Med.* 2000;107:127.

Denke M, et al. Excess body weight: an underrecognized contributor to dyslipidemia in white American women. *Arch Intern Med.* 1994;154:401.

Dreon D, et al. Change in dietary saturated fat intake is correlated with change in mass of large low-density lipoprotein particles in men. *Am J Clin Nutri.* 1998;67:821.

Dwyer J, et al. Dietary calcium, calcium supplementation and blood pressure in African American adolescents. *Am J Clin Nutri.* 1998;68:648.

Eichelboom J, et al. Homocysteine and cardiovascular disease: a critical review of the epidemiologic evidence. *Ann Int Med.* 1999;131:363.

Expert Panel on Detection, Evaluation, and Treatment of High Blood Cholesterol in Adults. Summary of the second report of the National Cholesterol Education Program (NCEP) Expert

Panel on Detection, Evaluation, and Treatment of High Blood Cholesterol in Adults. *JAMA*. 1993;269:3015.

Fernandez M. Soluble fiber and nondigestible carbohydrate effects on plasma lipids and cardiovascular risk. *Curr Opin Lipidol*. 2001;12:35.

Ferrara L, et al. Olive oil and reduced need for antihypertensive medications. *Arch Int Med*. 2000;160:837.

Fleming D, et al. Aspirin intake and the use of serum ferritin as a measure of iron status. *Am J Clin Nutri*. 2001;74:219.

Ford E. Serum copper concentrations and coronary heart disease among U.S. adults. *Am J Epid*. 2000;151:1182.

Ford E, Giles W. Serum vitamins, carotenoids, and angina pectoris: findings from the National Health and Nutrition Examination Survey III. *Ann Epidemiol*. 2000; 10:106.

Frame C, et al. The stages of change for dietary fat and fruit and vegetable intake of patients at the outset of a cardiac rehabilitation program. *Am J Health Promotion*. 2001;15:405.

Frankel E, et al. Inhibition of oxidation of human low-density lipoprotein by phenolic substances in red wine. *Lancet*. 1993;341:454.

Fuhrman B, et al. Consumption of red wine with meals reduces the susceptibility of human plasma and low-density lipoprotein to lipid peroxidation. *Am J Clin Nutri*. 1995;61:549.

Gariballa S, et al. A randomized, controlled single-blind trial of nutritional supplementation after acute stroke. *JPEN*. 1998;22:315.

Geleijnse J, et al. Tea flavonoids may protect against atherosclerosis: The Rotterdam Study. *Arch Int Med*. 1999;159:2170.

Gerhardt A, Gallo N. Full-fat rice bran and oat bran similarly reduce hypercholesterolemia in humans. *J Nutri*. 1998;128:865.

Gill J, et al. Postprandial lipemia: effects of intermittent versus continuous exercise. *Med & Sci in Sports & Exercise*. 1998;30:1515.

Gillman M, et al. Protective effects of fruits and vegetables on development of stroke in men. *JAMA*. 1995;273:1113.

Gillman M, et al. Inverse association of dietary fat with development of ischemic stroke in men. *J Am Med Assoc*. 1997;278:2145.

Gillum R, et al. The relationship between fish consumption and stroke incidence: the NHANES I Epidemiologic Follow-Up Study. *Arch Intern Med*. 1996;156:537.

GISSI-Preventione investigators. Dietary supplementation with n-3 polyunsaturated fatty acids and vitamin E after myocardial infarction: results of the GISSI-Preventione trial. *Lancet*. 1999;354:447.

Golik A, et al. Effects of captopril and enalapril on zinc metabolism in hypertensive patients. *J Am Col Nutri*. 1998;17:75.

Greenberg E, et al. Mortality associated with low plasma concentration of beta carotene and the effect of oral supplementation. *JAMA*. 1996;275:699.

Grimsgaard S, et al. Highly purified eicosapentaenoic acid and docosahexanoic acid in humans have similar triacylglycerol-lowering effects but divergent effects on serum fatty acids. *Am J Clin Nutri*. 1997;66:649.

Grover S, et al. Estimating the benefits of modifying risk factors of cardiovascular disease: a comparison of primary vs secondary prevention. *Arch Int Med*. 1998;158:655.

Halfrisch J, et al. High plasma vitamin C associated with high plasma HDL- and HDL2 cholesterol. *Am J Clin Nutri*. 1994;60:100.

Hall K, Luepker R. Is hypercholesterolemia a risk factor and should it be treated in the elderly (review)? *Am J Health Promotion*. 2000;14:347.

Hallikainen M, et al. Plant stanol esters affect serum cholesterol concentrations of hypercholesterolemic men and women in a dose-dependent manner. *J Nutri*. 2000;130:767.

Hansen J, et al. Inhibition of exercise-induced shortening of bleeding time by fish oil in familial hypercholesterolemia (type IIa). *Arterioscler Thromb*. 1993;13:98.

Hanson P, et al. Smoking and abdominal obesity. Risk factors for venous thromboembolism among middle-aged men: the Study of Men Born in 1913. *Arch Int Med*. 1999;159:1886.

Harris J. Interaction of dietary factors with oral anticoagulants: review and applications. *J Am Diet Assoc*. 1995;95:580.

He J, et al. Dietary sodium intake and subsequent risk of cardiovascular disease in overweight adults. *J Am Med Assoc*. 1999;282:2027.

He J, et al. Risk factors for congestive heart failure in U.S. men and women: NHANES I epidemiologic follow-up study. *Arch Intern Med*. 2001;161:996.

Heart Outcomes Prevention Evaluation Study Investigators. The vitamin E supplementation and cardiovascular events in high-risk patients. *N Engl J Med*. 2000;342:154.

Hebert P, et al. An overview of trials of cholesterol lowering and risk of stroke. *Arch Intern Med*. 1995;155:50.

Hickman T, et al. Distributions and trends of serum lipid levels among United States children and adolescents aged 4–19 years: data from the third National Health and Nutrition Examination Survey. *Preventive Medicine*. 1998;27:879.

Heim D, et al. Exercise mitigates the association of abdominal obesity with high-density lipoprotein cholesterol in premenopausal women: results from the third National Health and Nutrition Examination Survey. *J Am Diet Assoc*. 2000;100:1347.

Hein H, et al. Alcohol consumption, Lewis phenotypes, and risk of ischemic heart disease. *Lancet*. 1993;341:392.

Hertog M, et al. Dietary antioxidant flavonoids and risk of coronary heart disease: the Zutphen elderly study. *Lancet*. 1993;342:1007.

Hoak J. Workshop on dietary fatty acids and thrombosis. *Am J Clin Nutri*. 1992;56:783S.

Hodgson J, et al. Can linoleic acid contribute to coronary artery disease? *Am J Clin Nutri*. 1993;58:228.

Hodis H, et al. Serial coronary angiographic evidence that antioxidant vitamin intake reduces progression of coronary artery atherosclerosis. *JAMA*. 1995;273:1849.

Howard B, et al. Polyunsaturated fatty acids result in greater cholesterol lowering and less triacylglycerol elevation than do monounsaturated fatty acids in a dose-response comparison in a multiracial study group. *Am J Clin Nutri*. 1995;62:392.

Howard B, et al. Association of apolipoprotein E phenotype and plasma lipoproteins in African-American and white young adults: the CARDIA Study. *Am J Epid*. 1998;148:859.

Howard G, et al. Cigarette smoking and progression of atherosclerosis. *J Am Med Assoc*. 1998;279:119.

Howard M, et al. Dietary intake of cobalamin in elderly people who have abnormal serum cobalamin, methylmalonic acid and homocysteine levels. *Euro J Clin Nutri*. 1998;52:582.

Hu F, et al. A prospective study of egg consumption and risk of cardiovascular disease in men and women. *J Am Med Assoc*. 1999;281:1387.

Hu F, et al. Dietary intake of α-linolenic acid and risk of fatal ischemic heart disease among women. *Am J Clin Nutri*. 1999;69:890.

Hu F, et al. Dietary saturated fats and their food sources in relation to the risk of coronary heart disease in women. *Am J Clin Nutri*. 1999;70:1001.

Hu F, et al. Trends in the incidence of coronary heart disease and changes in diet and lifestyle in women. *N Engl J Med*. 2000;343:530.

Illingworth D, et al. Comparative effects of lovastatin and niacin in primary hypercholesterolemia: a prospective trial. *Arch Intern Med*. 1994;154:1586.

Insua J, et al. Drug treatment of hypertension in the elderly: a meta-analysis. *Ann Intern Med*. 1994;121:355.

Iso H, et al. Intake of fish and omega-3 fatty acids and risk of stroke in women. *JAMA*. 2001;285:304.

Jacobs D, et al. Whole-grain intake may reduce the risk of ischemic heart disease death in post-menopausal women: the Iowa Women's Health Study. *Am J Clin Nutri.* 1998;68:248.

Jacobson T, et al. Impact of evidence-based "clinical judgment" on the number of American adults requiring lipid-lowering therapy based on updated NHANES III data. National Health and Nutrition Examination Survey. *Arch Intern Med.* 2000;160:1361.

Jenkins D, et al. Colonic bacterial activity and serum lipid risk factors for cardiovascular disease. *Metabolism: Clin & Experimental.* 1999;48:264.

Jenkins D, et al. Effect on blood lipids of very high intakes of fiber in diets low in saturated fat and cholesterol. *N Engl J Med.* 1993;329:21.

Jeppesen J, et al. Effects of low-fat, high-carbohydrate diets on risk factors for ischemic heart disease in postmenopausal women. *Am J Clin Nutri.* 1997;65:1027.

Joshipura K, et al. Fruit and vegetable intake in relation to risk of ischemic stroke. *JAMA.* 1999;282:1233.

Joshipura K, et al. The effect of fruit and vegetable intake on risk for coronary heart disease. *Ann Intern Med.* 2001;134:1106.

Kadyrov M, et al. Increased fetoplacental angiogenesis during first trimester in anemic women. *Lancet.* 1998;352:1747.

Keevil J, et al. Grape juice, but not orange or grapefruit juice, inhibits human platelet aggregation. *J Nutri.* 2000;130:53.

Kelley M, et al. Oat bran lowers total and low-density lipoprotein cholesterol but not lipoprotein (a) in exercising adults with borderline hypercholesterolemia. *J Am Diet Assoc.* 1994;94:1419.

Kimball T, et al. Cardiovascular status in young patients with insulin-dependent diabetes mellitus. *Circulation.* 1994;90:357.

Klag M, et al. Serum cholesterol in young men and subsequent cardiovascular disease. *N Engl J Med.* 1993;328:313.

Kleemola P, et al. Coffee consumption and the risk of coronary heart disease and death. *Arch Int Med.* 2000;160:3393.

Klipstein-Grobusch K, et al. Serum ferritin and risk of myocardial infarction in the elderly: the Rotterdam Study. *Am J Clin Nutri.* 1999;69:1231.

Knekt P, et al. Quercetin intake and the incidence of cerebrovascular disease. *Euro J Nutri.* 2000;54:415.

Komajda M, et al. Genetic aspects of heart failure. *Eur J Heart Fail.* 1999;1:121.

Kosmark R. Salatrim: properties and applications. *Food Technology.* 1996;50:98.

Kris-Etherton P. Over-the-counter statin medications: emerging opportunities for RDs. *JAMA.* 2000;100:1126.

Lakkis N, et al. Nonsurgical septal reduction therapy for hypertrophic obstructive cardiomyopathy: one-year follow-up. *J Am Col Cardiol.* 2000;36:852.

Law M, Morris J. By how much does fruit and vegetable consumption reduce the risk of ischemic heart disease? *Euro J Clin Nutri.* 1998;52:549.

Lewis N, et al. Serum lipid response to n-3 fatty acid enriched eggs in persons with hypercholesterolemia. *J Am Diet Assoc.* 2000;100: 365.

Lewis C, et al. Inconsistent associations of caffeine-containing beverages with blood pressure and with lipoproteins. *Am J Epidemiol.* 1993;138:502.

Levey W, et al. Blood pressure responses of white men with hypertension to two low-sodium metabolic diets with different levels of dietary calcium. *J Am Diet Assoc.* 1995;95:1280.

Levy Y, et al. Plasma antioxidants and lipid peroxidation in acute myocardial infarction and thrombolysis. *J Am Col Nutri.* 1998;17:337.

Lichtenstein A, et al. Effects of canola, corn and olive oils on fasting and postprandial plasma lipoproteins in humans as part of a National Cholesterol Education Program step 2 diet. *Arterioscler Thromb.* 1993;13:1533.

Liu S, et al. A prospective study of dietary glycemic load, carbohydrate intake, and risk of coronary heart disease in U.S. women. *Am J Clin Nutri.* 2000;71:1455.

Liu S, et al. Whole-grain consumption and risk of coronary heart disease: results from the Nurses' Health Study. *Am J Clin Nutri.* 1999;70:412.

Louis A, et al. Clinical Trials Update: CAPRICORN, COPERNICUS, MIRACLE, STAF, RITZ-2, RECOVER and RENAISSANCE and cachexia and cholesterol in heart failure. Highlights of the Scientific Sessions of the American College of Cardiology, 2001. *Eur J Heart Fail.* 2001;3:381.

Lowe L, et al. Impact of major cardiovascular disease risk factors, particular in combination on 22-year mortality in women and men. *Arch Int Med.* 1998;158:2007.

Malinow M, et al. Increased plasma homocystine after withdrawal of ready-to-eat breakfast cereal from the diet: prevention by breakfast cereal providing 200 µg folic acid. *J Am Col Nutri.* 2000;19:452.

Maniolo T, et al. Epidemiology of low cholesterol levels in older adults: the cardiovascular health study. *Circulation.* 1993;87:728.

Mantzioris E, et al. Biochemical effects of a diet containing foods enriched with n-3 fatty acids. *Am J Clin Nutri.* 2000;72:42.

Marckmann P, et al. Ad libitum intake of low-fat diets rich in either starchy foods or sucrose: effects on blood lipids, factor VII coagulant activity, and fibrinogen. *Metab: Clin and Experimental.* 2000;49:731.

Maron B, et al. Epidemiology of hypertrophic cardiomyopathy-related death: revisited in a large nonreferral-based patient population. *Circulation.* 2000;102:858.

McCarron D. The dietary guideline for sodium: should we shake it up? Yes! *Am J Clin Nutri.* 2000;71:1013.

McGhee M, et al. Benefits and costs of medical nutrition therapy by registered dietitians for patients with hypercholesterolemia. *J Am Diet Assoc.* 1995;95:1041.

McVeigh G, et al. Fish oil improves arterial compliance in noninsulin diabetes mellitus. *Arterioscler Thromb.* 1994;14:1425.

Meisel E, et al. Pacemaker therapy of hypertrophic obstructive cardiomyopathy. PIC (Pacing in Cardiomyopathy) Study Group. *Herz.* 2000;25:461.

Melby C, et al. Blood pressure differences in older black and white long-term vegetarians and nonvegetarians. *J Am Col Nutri.* 1993;12:262.

Merrill W, et al. Long-lasting improvement after septal myectomy for hypertrophic obstructive cardiomyopathy. *Ann Thorac Surg.* 2000;69:1732.

Merz-Demlow B, et al. Soy isoflavones improve plasma lipids in normocholesterolemic premenopausal women. *Am J Clin Nutri.* 2000;71:1462.

Messerli F, et al. Salt: a perpetrator of hypertensive target organ disease? *Arch Int Med.* 1997;157:2449.

Morelli V, Zoorob R. Alternative therapies: part II. Congestive heart failure and hypercholesterolemia. *Am Fam Phys.* 2000;62:1325.

Morgan W, Clayshultze B. Pecans lower low-density lipoprotein cholesterol in people with normal lipid levels. *J Am Diet Assoc.* 2000;100:312.

Morris M, et al. Does fish oil lower blood pressure? *Circulation.* 1993;88:523.

Mustad V, et al. Comparison of the effects of diets rich in stearic acid versus myristic acid and lauric acid on platelet fatty acids and excretion of thromboxane A2 and PGI2 metabolites in healthy young men. *Metabolism.* 1993;42:463.

Nakamura T, et al. Can serum carnitine levels distinguish hypertrophic cardiomyopathy from hypertensive hearts? *Hypertension*. 2000;36:215.

Nakatani S, Miyatake K. Echocardiography of idiopathic cardiomyopathies. *Nippon Rinsho*. 2000;58:37.

Nallamothu B, et al. Potential clinical and economic effects of homocysteine lowering. *Arch Int Med*. 2000;160:3406.

Nestle M. Mediterranean diets: science and policy implications. *Am J Clin Nutri*. 1995;61S:1313S.

NHLBI. Third Report of the Expert Panel on Detection, Evaluation, and Treatment of High Blood Cholesterol in Adults (Adult Treatment Panel III). http://www.nhlbi.nih.gov/guidelines/cholesterol/atglance.htm; visited May 17, 2001.

Nissen S, et al. B-Hydroxy-B-methylbutyrate (HMB) supplementation in humans is safe and may decrease cardiovascular risk factors. *J Nutri*. 2000;130:1937.

Nurminen M, et al. Coffee, caffeine, and blood pressure: a critical review. *Euro J Clin Nutri*. 1999;53:831.

Nutrition Screening Initiative. A physician's guide to nutrition in chronic disease management for older adults. http://www.aafp.org/nsi/physiciansguide.pdf.

Omland T, et al. Serum homocysteine concentration as an indicator of survival in patients with acute coronary syndromes. *Arch Int Med*. 2000;160:1834.

Ornish D, et al. Intensive lifestyle changes for reversal of coronary heart disease. *J Am Med Assoc*. 1998;280:2001.

Ohrvall M, et al. Sagittal abdominal diameter compared with other anthropometric measurements in relation to cardiovascular risk. *Int J Obesity & Related Metab Disorders*. 2000;24:497.

Oster G, Thompson D. Estimated effects of reducing dietary saturated fat intake on the incidence and costs of coronary heart disease in the United States. *J Am Diet Assoc*. 1996;96:127.

Pascot A, et al. Age-related increase in visceral adipose tissue and body fat and the metabolic risk profile of premenopausal women. *Diab care*. 1999;22:1471.

Pedersen T. Lowering cholesterol with drugs and diet. *N Engl J Med*. 1995;333:1350.

Perry H, et al. The effects of thiazide diuretics on calcium metabolism in the aged. *J Am Geriatr Soc*. 1993;41:818.

Petersmarck K, et al. The effect of weight cycling on blood lipids and blood pressure in the Multiple Risk Factor Intervention Trial Special Intervention group. *Int J Obesity & Related Metabolic Disorders*. 1999;23:1246.

Pieke B, et al. Treatment of hypertriglyceridemia by two diets rich either in unsaturated fatty acids or in carbohydrates: effects on lipoprotein subclasses, lipolytic enzymes, and lipid transfer proteins, insulin and leptin. *Int J Obesity and Related Metabolic Disorders*. 2000;24:1286.

Plous S, et al. Nutrition knowledge and attitudes of cardiac patients. *J Am Diet Assoc*. 1995;95:442.

Pruthi S, et al. Vitamin E supplementation in the prevention of coronary heart disease. *Mayo Clinic Proceedings*. 2001;76:1131.

Ramirez-Tortosa M, et al. Extra virgin olive oil increases the resistance of LDL to oxidation more than refined olive oil in free-living men with peripheral vascular disease. *J Nutri*. 1999;129: 2177.

Ramirez-Tortosa C, et al. Olive oil- and fish oil-enriched diets modify plasma lipids and susceptibility of LDL to oxidative modification in free-living make patients with peripheral vascular disease: the Spanish Nutrition Study. *Br J Nutri*. 1999;82:31.

Rapola J, et al. Effect of vitamin E and beta carotene on the incidence of angina pectoris. *JAMA*. 1996;275:693.

Rauchhaus M, et al. Inflammatory cytokines and the possible immunological role for lipoproteins in chronic heart failure. *Int J Cardiol*. 2000;76:125.

Rexrode K, et al. A prospective study of body mass index, weight change, and risk of stroke in women. *J Am Med Assoc*. 1997;277: 1539.

Richardson A, Piepho R. Effect of race on hypertension and antihypertensive therapy. *Int J Clin Pharmacol Ther*. 2000;38:75.

Ridker P, et al. Plasma concentration of lipoprotein(a) and the risk of future stroke. *JAMA*. 1995;273:1269.

Rimm E, et al. Vegetable, fruit, and cereal fiber intake and risk of coronary heart disease among men. *JAMA*. 1996;275:447.

Rosenson R. Low levels of high-density lipoprotein cholesterol (hypoalpha-lipoproteinemia): an approach to management. *Arch Intern Med*. 1993;153:1528.

Rubenowitz G, et al. Magnesium in drinking water and death from acute myocardial infarction. *Am J Epidemiol*. 1996;143:456.

Rumpler W, et al. Changes in women's plasma lipid and lipoprotein concentrations due to moderate consumption of alcohol are affected by dietary fat level. *J Nutri*. 1999;129:1713.

Russell B, et al. Effect of premature myocardial infarction in men on the eating habits of spouses and offspring. *J Am Diet Assoc*. 1994;94:859.

Sacco R, et al. High-density lipoprotein cholesterol and ischemic stroke in the elderly. *JAMA*. 2001;285:2729.

Salonen J, et al. High stored iron levels are associated with excess risk of myocardial infarction in Eastern Finnish men. *Circulation*. 1992;86:803.

Schaefer E, et al. Effects of National Cholesterol Education Program step 2 diets relatively high or relatively low in fish-derived fatty acids on plasma lipoproteins in middle-aged and elderly subjects. *Am J Clin Nutri*. 1996;63:234.

Schrier R. Treating hypertension in the elderly. *Am J Geriatr Cardiol*. 2001;10:355.

Shane J, Walker P. Corn bran supplementation of a low-fat controlled diet lowers serum lipids in men with hypercholesterolemia. *J Am Diet Assoc*. 1995;95:40.

Shepherd J, et al. Prevention of coronary heart disease with pravastatin in men with hypercholesterolemia. *N Engl J Med*. 1995;333: 1301.

Singer D, et al. Blood pressure and endocrine responses to changes in dietary sodium in cardiac transplant recipients: implications for the control of sodium balance. *Circulation*. 1994;89:1153.

Spirito P, et al. Magnitude of left ventricular hypertrophy and risk of sudden death in hypertrophic cardiomyopathy. *N Engl J Med*. 2000;342:1778.

Sprecher D, et al. Efficacy of psyllium in reducing serum cholesterol levels in hypercholesterolemia patients on high- or low-fat diets. *Ann Intern Med*. 1993;119:545.

Stamler J. Setting the TONE for ending the hypertension epidemic (editorial). *J Am Med Assoc*. 1998;279:878.

Stephens N, et al. Randomized controlled trial of vitamin E in patients with coronary disease: Cambridge Heart Antioxidant Study (CHAOS). *Lancet*. 1996;347:781.

Stevens V, et al. Weight loss intervention in phase I of the Trials of Hypertension Prevention. *Arch Intern Med*. 1993;153:849.

Stevinson C, et al. Garlic for treating hypercholesterolemia: a meta analysis of randomized clinical trials. *Ann Int Med*. 2000;133:411.

Toohey L, et al. Plasma ascorbic acid concentrations are related to cardiovascular risk factors in African-Americans. *J Nutri*. 1996;126:121.

Ubbink J, et al. Vitamin requirements for the treatment of hyperhomocystinemia in humans. *J Nutri*. 1994;124:1927.

Uiterwaal C, et al. Families and natural history of lipids in childhood: an 18-year follow-up study. *Am J Epid.* 1997;145:777.

Vadlamudi S, et al. Effects of oral combined hormone replacement therapy on plasma lipids and lipoproteins. *Metab: Clinical and Experimental.* 1998;47:1222.

van Beresteijn E, et al. Perimenopausal increase in serum cholesterol: a 10-year longitudinal study. *Am J Epidemiol.* 1993;137:383.

Van Duyn M, Pivonka E. Overview of the health benefits of fruit and vegetable consumption for the dietetics professional: selected literature. *J Am Diet Assoc.* 2000;100:1511.

Vasan R, et al. Impact of high-normal blood pressure on the risk of cardiovascular disease. *N Engl J Med.* 2001;345:1291.

Vermeulen E, et al. Effect of homocysteine-lowering treatment with folic acid plus vitamin B-6 on progression of subclinical atherosclerosis: a randomized, placebo-controlled trial. *Lancet.* 2000; 355:517.

Vierhapper H, et al. Prevalence of paradoxically normal serum cholesterol in morbidly obese women. *Metabolism: Clin and Experimental.* 2000;49:607.

Volpe M, et al. Abnormalities of sodium handling and of cardiovascular adaptations during high salt diet in patients with mild heart failure. *Circulation.* 1993;88:1620.

Wannamethee S, et al. Type of alcoholic drink and risk of major coronary heart disease events and all-cause mortality. *Am J Public Health.* 1999;89:685.

Welch G, Loscalzo J. Homocysteine and atherosclerosis. *N Engl J Med.* 1998;338:1042.

Whelton P, et al. Effects of oral potassium on blood pressure: meta analysis of randomized controlled clinical trials. *J Am Med Assoc.* 1997;277:1624.

Whelton P, et al. Sodium contributions and weight loss in the treatment of hypertension in older persons. *J Am Med Assoc.* 1998; 279:839.

Wilson P, et al. Clustering of metabolic factors and coronary heart disease. *Arch Int Med.* 1999;159:1104.

Wilson P, et al. Cumulative effects of high cholesterol levels, high blood pressure, and cigarette smoking on carotid stenosis. *N Engl J Med.* 1997;337:516.

Winkleby M, et al. Ethnic and socioeconomic differences in cardiovascular disease risk factors: findings for women from the third National Health and Nutrition Examination Survey, 1988–1994. *J Am Med Assoc.* 1998;280:356.

Witteman J, et al. Reduction of blood pressure with oral magnesium supplementation in women with mild to moderate hypertension. *Am J Clin Nutri.* 1994;60:129.

Wolk A, et al. Long-term intake of dietary fiber and decreased risk of coronary heart disease among women. *J Am Med Assoc.* 1999;281:1998.

Woodside J, et al. Effect of B-group vitamins and antioxidant vitamins on hyperhomocystinemia: a double-blind, randomized factorial-design, controlled trial. *Am J Clin Nutri.* 1998;67:858.

Wu J, et al. Mechanism of cardioprotection by resveratrol, a phenolic antioxidant present in red wine (Review). *Int J Mol Med.* 2001;8:3.

Yochum L, et al. Intake of antioxidant vitamins and risk of death from stroke in postmenopausal women. *Am J Clin Nutri.* 2000;72:476.

Yu-Poth S, et al. Effects of the National Cholesterol Education Program's Step I and Step II dietary intervention programs on cardiovascular disease risk factors. *Am J Clin Nutri.* 1999;69:632.

Zambon D, et al. Substituting walnuts for monounsaturated fat improves serum lipid profile of hypercholesterolemic men and women: a randomized cross-over trial. *Ann Int Med.* 2000;132:538.

Zheng Z, et al. Plasma fatty acid composition and 6-year incidence of hypertension in middle-aged adults: the Atherosclerosis Risk in Communities (ARIC) Study. *Am J Epid.* 1999;150:492.

SUGGESTED READINGS

Alexander H, et al. Risk factors for cardiovascular disease and diabetes in two groups of Hispanic Americans with differing dietary habits. *J Am Col Nutri.* 1999;18:127.

Allen J, et al. Coronary risk factors in women one year after coronary artery bypass grafting. *J Women's Health & Gender-Based Medicine.* 1999;8:617.

Allison D, et al. Estimated intakes of trans fatty and other fatty acids in the U.S. population. *J Am Diet Assoc.* 1999;99:166.

Appel L, et al. Effects of reduced sodium intake on hypertension control in older individuals: results from the Trial of Nonpharmacologic Interventions in the Elderly (TONE). *Arch Int Med.* 2001;161:685.

Barr S, et al. Effects of increased consumption of fluid milk on energy and nutrient intake, body weight, and cardiovascular risk factors in healthy older adults. *J Am Diet Assoc.* 2000;100:810.

Beard T, et al. Association between blood pressure and dietary factors in the Dietary and Nutritional Survey of British Adults. *Arch Int Med.* 1997;157:234.

Berglund L, et al. HDL-subpopulation patterns in response to reduction in dietary total fat and saturated fat intakes in healthy subjects. *Am J Clin Nutri.* 1999;70:992.

Berthold H, et al. Effect of garlic oil preparation on serum lipoproteins and cholesterol metabolism. *J Am Med Assoc.* 1998;279:1900.

Bjornholt J, et al. Fasting blood glucose: an underestimated risk factor for cardiovascular disease. *Diab Care.* 1999;22:10.

Bots M, et al. Homocysteine and short-term risk of myocardial infarction and stroke in the elderly: the Rotterdam Study. *Arch Int Med.* 1999;159:38.

Bourdon I, et al. Postprandial lipid, glucose, insulin and cholecystokinin responses in men fed barley pasta enriched with B-glucan. *Am J Clin Nutri.* 1999;69:55.

Bronstrup A, et al. Effects of folic acid and combinations of folic acid and vitamin B-12 on plasma homocysteine concentrations in healthy, young women. *Am J Clin Nutri.* 1998;68:1104.

Brown L, et al. Cholesterol-lowering effects of dietary fiber: a meta-analysis. *Am J Clin Nutri.* 1999;69:30.

Cao G, et al. Increases in human plasma antioxidant capacity after consumption of controlled diets high in fruits and vegetables. *Am J Clin Nutri.* 1998;68:1081.

Carmichael H, et al. Lower fat intake as a predictor of initial and sustained weight loss in obese subjects consuming an otherwise ad libitum diet. *J Am Diet Assoc.* 1998;98:35.

Connor S. The healthy heart—challenges and opportunities for dietetics professionals in the 21st century. *J Am Diet Assoc.* 1999; 99:164.

Cook N, et al. Effect of change in sodium excretion on change in blood pressure corrected for measurement error: the Trials of Hypertension Prevention, Phase 1. *Am J Epid.* 1998;148:431.

De Lorgeril M, et al. Mediterranean diet, traditional risk factors, and the rate of cardiovascular complications after myocardial infarction: final report of the Lyon Diet Heart Study. *Circulation.* 1999;99:779.

De Winther M, Hofker M. Scavenging new insights into atherogenesis. *J Clin Invest.* 2000;105:1039.

Donovan J, et al. Catechin is present as metabolites in human plasma after consumption of red wine. *J Nutri*. 1999;129:1662.

Douglas M, et al. Benefit of a favorable cardiovascular risk-factor profile in middle age with respect to Medicare costs. *N Engl J Med*. 1998;339:1122.

Duthie G, et al. The effect of whisky and wine consumption on total phenol content and antioxidant capacity of plasma from healthy volunteers. *Euro J Clin Nutri*. 1998;52:733.

Ellison R, et al. Effects of similarities in lifestyle habits on familial aggregation of high-density lipoprotein and low density lipoprotein cholesterol: the NHLBI Family Heart Study. *Am J Epid*. 1999;150:910.

Engelman D, et al. Impact of body mass index and albumin on morbidity and mortality after cardiac surgery. *J Thorac Cardiovasc Surg*. 1999;118:866.

Finckenor M, Byrd-Bredbrenner C. Nutrition intervention group program based on preaction-stage oriented change processes of the Transtheoretical Model promotes long-term reduction in dietary fat intake. *J Am Diet Assoc*. 2000;100:335.

Galloe A, Garred P. Effects of sodium restriction on blood pressure, renin, and aldosterone, catecholamines, cholesterols, and triglyceride: a meta analysis. *J Am Med Assoc*. 1998;279:1383.

Gerhard G, et al. Higher total homocysteine concentrations and lower folate concentrations in premenopausal black women than in premenopausal white women. *Am J Clin Nutri*. 1999;70:252.

Giles W, et al. Association between total homocysteine and the likelihood for a history of acute myocardial infarction by race and ethnicity: results from the Third National Health and Nutrition Examination Survey. *Am Heart J*. 2000;139:446.

Haapanen-Niemi N, et al. Public health burden of coronary heart disease risk factors among middle-aged and elderly men. *Preventive Medicine*. 1999;28:343.

Hargreaves M, et al. Stages of change and the intake of dietary fat in African-American women: improving stage assessment using the Eating Styles Questionnaire. *J Am Diet Assoc*. 1999;99:1392.

Haynes R, Kris-Etherton P, et al. Nutritionally complete prepared meal plan to reduce cardiovascular risk factors: a randomized clinical trial. *J Am Diet Assoc*. 1999;99:1077.

Hodgson J, et al. Supplementation with isoflavonoid phytoestrogens does not alter serum lipid concentrations: a randomized controlled trial in humans. *J Nutri*. 1998;128:728.

Jacob R, et al. Moderate folate depletion increases plasma homocysteine and decreases lymphocyte DNA methylation in postmenopausal women. *J Nutri*. 1998;128:1204.

Kafato A, et al. Mediterranean diet of Crete: foods and nutrient content. *J Am Diet Assoc*. 2000;100:1487.

Kamath S, et al. Cardiovascular disease risk factors in two distinct ethnic groups: Indian and Pakistani compared with American premenopausal women. *Am J Clin Nutri*. 1999;69:621.

Karpe F, et al. Differences in postprandial concentrations of very-low-density lipoprotein and chylomicron remnants between normotriglyceridemic and hypertriglyceridemic men with and without coronary heart disease. *Metab: Clinical and Experimental*. 1999;48:301.

Koikkalainen M, et al. Difficulties in changing the diet in relation to dietary fat intake among patients with coronary heart disease. *Eur J Clin Nutri*. 1999;53:120.

Krummel D. Nutrition in cardiovascular disease. In: Mahan K, Escott-Stump S, eds. *Krause's food, nutrition, and diet therapy*. 10th ed. Philadelphia: WB Saunders, 2000.

Kumanyika S, et al. Outcomes of a cardiovascular nutrition-counseling program in African-Americans with elevated blood pressure or cholesterol level. *J Am Diet Assoc*. 1999;99:1380.

Lagstrom H, et al. Nutrient intakes and cholesterol values of the parents in a prospective randomized child-targeted coronary heart disease risk factor intervention trial—the STRIP project. *Euro J Clin Nutri*. 1999;53:654.

Luepker R, Leyasmeyer E. Proceedings from the International Symposium on Primordial Prevention of Cardiovascular Disease Risk Factors. *Prevent Med*. 1999;9:1.

Lussier-Cacan S, et al. Sources of variation in plasma lipid and lipoprotein traits in a sample selected for health. *Am J Epid*. 1999;150:1229.

Malinow M, et al. Reduction of plasma homocysteine levels by breakfast cereal fortified with folic acid in patients with coronary heart disease. *N Engl J Med*. 1998;338:1009.

Markus R, et al. Influence of lifestyle modification on atherosclerotic progression determined by ultrasonographic change in the common carotid intima-media thickness. *Am J Clin Nutri*. 1997;65:1000.

Mandel C, et al. Dietary intake and plasma concentrations of vitamin E, vitamin C, and beta carotene in patients with coronary artery disease. *J Am Diet Assoc*. 1997;97:655.

Mansfield E, et al. Diet and waist-to-hip ratio: important predictors of lipoprotein levels in sedentary and active young men with no evidence of cardiovascular disease. *J Am Diet Assoc*. 1999;99:1373.

Mark E, et al. Fatal pulmonary hypertension associated with short-term use of fenfluramine and phentermine. *N Engl J Med*. 1997; 337:602.

Mayer-Davis E, et al. Vitamin C intake and cardiovascular disease risk factors in persons with non-insulin dependent diabetes mellitus: from the Insulin Resistance Atherosclerosis Study and the San Luis Valley Diabetes Study. *Preventive Med*. 1997;26:277.

McBride P, et al. Primary care practice adherence to National Cholesterol Education Program guidelines for patients with coronary heart disease. *Arch Int Med*. 1998;158:1181.

Meydani S, et al. Vitamin E supplementation and in vivo immune response in healthy elderly subjects: a randomized, controlled trial. *J Am Med Assoc*. 1997;277:1380.

Miettinen T, et al. Serum, biliary, and fecal cholesterol and plant sterols in colectomized patients before and during consumption of stanol ester margarine. *Am J Clin Nutri*. 2000;71:1095.

Mietus-Snyder M, Malloy M. Endothelial dysfunction occurs in children with two genetic hyperlipidemias: improvement with antioxidant vitamin therapy. *J Peds*. 1998;133:35.

Mihic S, et al. Acute creatine loading increases fat-free mass, but does not affect blood pressure, plasma creatinine, or CK activity in men and women. *Med & Sci in Sports & Exercise*. 2000;32:291.

Mori T, et al. Effect of dietary fish and exercise training on urinary F2-isoprostane excretion in non-insulin dependent diabetic patients. *Metabolism: Clin and Experi*. 1999;48:1402.

Naglak M, et al. Nutrient adequacy of diets of adults with hypercholesteremia after a cholesterol-lowering intervention: long-term assessment. *J Am Diet Assoc*. 2000;100:1385.

Newman T, Garber A. Cholesterol screening in children and adolescents. *Pediatr*. 2000;105:637.

Noakes M, Clifton P. Oil blends containing partially hydrogenated or interesterified fats: differential effect on plasma lipids. *Am J Clin Nutri*. 1998;68:242.

Ockene I, et al. Effect of physician-delivered nutrition counseling training and an office-support program on saturated fat intake, weight, and serum lipid measurements in a hyperlipidemic population: Worcester Area Trial for Counseling in Hyperlipidemia (WATCH.) *Arch Int Med*. 1999;159:725.

Parks E, et al. Reduced oxidative susceptibility of LDL from patients participating in intensive atherosclerosis treatment program. *Am J Clin Nutri.* 1998;68:778.

Perry A, et al. Clinical predictability of the waist-to-hip ratio in assessment of cardiovascular disease risk factors in overweight, premenopausal women. *Am J Clin Nutri.* 1998;68:1022.

Plotnick G, et al. Effect of antioxidant vitamins on the transient impairment of endothelium-dependent brachial artery vasoactivity following a single high-fat meal. *J Am Med Assoc.* 1997;278:1682.

Pownall H, et al. Effect of moderate alcohol consumption on hypertriglyceridemia: a study in the fasting state. *Arch Int Med.* 1999;159:981.

Retzlaff BM, et al. Nutritional intake of women and men on the NCEP Step I and Step II diets. *J Am Coll Nutr.* 1997;16:52.

Riemersma R, et al. Vitamin C and the risk of acute myocardial infarction. *Am J Clin Nutri.* 2000;71:1181.

Rimm E, et al. Folate and vitamin B6 from diet and supplements in relation to risk of coronary heart disease among women. *J Am Med Assoc.* 1998;279:359.

Rosamond W, et al. Trends in the incidence of myocardial infarction and in mortality due to coronary heart disease. *N Engl J Med.* 1998;339:861.

Salo P, et al. Effect of low-saturated fat, low-cholesterol dietary intervention on fatty acid compositions in serum lipid fractions in 5-year old children. The STRIP Project. *Euro J Clin Nutri.* 1999;53:927.

Sarkkinen E, et al. Effect of apolipoprotein E polymorphism on serum lipid response to the separate modification of dietary fat and dietary cholesterol. *Am J Clin Nutri.* 1998;68:1215.

Selhub J, et al. Serum total homocysteine concentrations in the Third National Health and Nutrition Examination Survey (1991–1994): population reference ranges and contribution of vitamin status to high serum concentrations. *Ann Int Med.* 1999;131:331.

Sesso H, et al. Coffee and tea intake and the risk of myocardial infarction. *Am J Epid.* 1999;149:62.

Sikand G, et al. Dietitian intervention improves lipid values and saves medication costs in men with combined hyperlipidemia and a history of niacin noncompliance. *J Am Diet Assoc.* 2000;100:218.

Sikand G, et al. Medical nutrition therapy lowers serum cholesterol and saves medication costs in men with hypercholesterolemia. *J Am Diet Assoc.* 1998;98:8.

Sixth Report of the Joint National Committee on Prevention, Detection and Evaluation and Treatment of High Blood Pressure. *Arch Int Med.* 1997;157:2413.

Smedman A, et al. Pentadecanoic acid in serum as a marker for intake of milk fat: relations between intake of milk fat and metabolic risk factors. *Am J Clin Nutri.* 1999;69:22.

Stefanik M, et al. Effects of diet and exercise in men and postmenopausal women with low levels of HDL cholesterol and high levels of LDL cholesterol. *N Engl J Med.* 1998;339:12.

Stevens J, et al. Body weight change and carotid artery wall thickness: the Atherosclerotic Risk in Communities (ARIC) Study. *Am J Epid.* 1998;147:563.

Szklo M, et al. Trends in plasma cholesterol levels in the Atherosclerosis Risk in Communities (ARIC) Study. *Prevent Med.* 2000;30:252.

Teixeira S, et al. Effects of feeding 4 levels of soy protein for 3 and 6 wk on blood lipids and apolipoproteins in moderately hypercholesterolemic men. *Am J Clin Nutri.* 2000;71:1077.

Tershakovec A, et al. Growth of hypercholesterolemic children completing physician-initiated low-fat dietary intervention. *J Peds.* 1998;133:28.

Toohey L, et al. Cardiovascular disease risk factors are lower in African-American vegans compared to lacto-ovo vegetarians. *J Am Col Nutri.* 1998;17:425.

Valmadrid C, et al. Alcohol intake and the risk of coronary heart disease mortality in persons with older-onset diabetes mellitus. *J Am Med Assoc.* 1999;282:239.

Wald D, et al. Randomized trial of folic acid supplementation and serum homocysteine levels. *Arch Int Med.* 2001;161:695.

SECTION 7

Gastrointestinal Disorders

CHIEF ASSESSMENT FACTORS

- FEEDING MODALITY
- DENTITION
- PAINFUL ORAL TISSUES, TONGUE
- DYSPHAGIA
- APPETITE, ANOREXIA, WEIGHT LOSS
- INDIGESTION, HEARTBURN
- NAUSEA, VOMITING, REFLUX
- ABDOMINAL PAIN OR DISTENTION, ASCITES, JAUNDICE
- PAINFUL OR CRAMPING ABDOMEN, FLATULENCE
- EASY FATIGUE
- CHANGE IN EATING OR BOWEL HABITS
- CHANGE IN STOOLS, CONSISTENCY AND FREQUENCY
- CONSTIPATION, DIARRHEA, HEMORRHOIDS, RECTAL BLEEDING
- EDEMA OF EXTREMITIES
- USE OF GASTROINTESTINAL (GI) MEDICATIONS—ANTACIDS, STOOL SOFTENERS, DIURETICS, LAXATIVES, HISTAMINE BLOCKERS

TABLE 7–1 Digestion and Absorption Issues

Digestion: Processes that physically and chemically break down food in preparation for absorption. Digestion begins with mastication and mixing of food with salivary fluid and enzymes (oral phase). In the gastric phase, pepsin, gastric acid, salivary amylase, and lipase begin to work. Chyme is then delivered to the small intestine for mixing with pancreatic and biliary juices; the pancreatic phase involves pancreatic amylase and lipase, proteases, and phospholipase; the intestinal phase involves disaccharidases (maltase, lactase, sucrase), peptidases, and cholecystokinin for bile salts. Maldigestion involves the interference at any of these stages, including abnormal emptying of the stomach and pancreatic insufficiency.

Absorption: Passage of molecular nutrients into the bloodstream from the intestinal cells, mostly starting in the duodenum, with monosaccharides, amino acids and small peptides, monoglycerides, and free fatty acids. Water is also absorbed to maintain isotonicity of blood and cells. Bile and fat are needed to absorb fat-soluble vitamins A, D, E, and K. Water-soluble vitamin C- and B-complex are usually absorbed in the intestinal mucosa with some storage in the liver. Malabsorption can result from dysfunction from any of the above steps.

The entire process of digestion/absorption takes 24 hours.

A diet high in whole and unrefined foods (whole grains, dark green and yellow/orange vegetables and fruits, legumes, nuts, and seeds) is high in antioxidant phenolic compounds, fibers, and other phytochemicals. This has a beneficial effect on lipoprotein levels, decreases the need for oxidative defense mechanisms, and improves colon function (Bruce et al., 2000).

As a general test for absorptive capacity, Shils recommends testing with 25 g of *d*-xylose (urinary xylose values of 1.2–1.6 g suggest that enteral feeding is possible). Fecal fat is a valuable test of lipid digestion and absorption.

Small intestine, approximately 3.8 cm in diameter and 4.8 m long, covered with villi projections to increase absorptive surface. Villi cells have a rapid turnover rate of 2–5 days.

Large intestine is approximately 5 cm in diameter and 1.5 m long, with two sections (colon and rectum) forming a frame around a highly convoluted small intestine. The rectum is approximately 12 cm long. The area is susceptible to polyps and tumors.

Dietary fiber = Nonstarch polysaccharides + Lignin + Resistant starch. Research about resistant starch suggests that it may play a role in prevention of colorectal cancer (Cassidy et al., 1994).

TABLE 7–2 Gastrointestinal Conditions That May Lead to Malnutrition

Malabsorption:
- Celiac disease
- Disaccharidase deficiencies
- Pancreatic insufficiency
- Dumping syndrome
- Short bowel syndrome
- Crohn's disease
- Ulcerative colitis
- HIV infection or AIDS

Mechanical Function:
- Esophageal stricture
- Esophageal obstruction
- Achalasia or esophageal hypomotility
- Tracheoesophageal fistula
- Pyloric stenosis
- Adynamic ileus
- Bowel obstruction
- Hirschsprung's disease
- Infantile achalasia

Conditions That May Cause Fear of Eating:
- Diarrhea
- Ill-fitting dentures
- Dental disease
- Esophageal spasm
- Reflux esophagitis
- Gastritis
- Dumping syndrome
- Crohn's disease
- Ulcerative colitis
- Flatulence
- Peptic ulcer
- Postgastrectomy dumping syndrome
- Pancreatitis (acute or chronic)
- Cholelithiasis and other biliary diseases
- Food allergies
- Lactose intolerance
- Irritable bowel syndrome (IBS)
- Diverticulitis
- Rectal fissures

Table updated by Peter Beyer, 2/5/02.

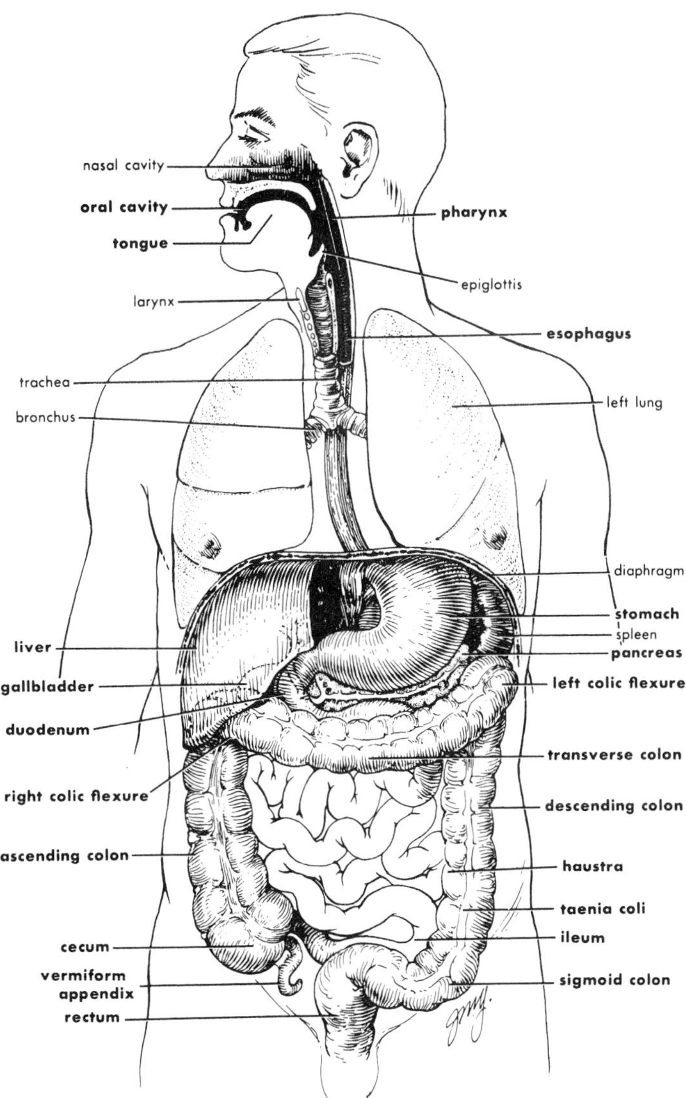

FIGURE 7–1 The digestive system: absorption sites.

TABLE 7–3 Role of Enteral Nutrition in GI Tract Function

When an oral diet is not feasible, enteral nutrition (EN) is needed to avoid prolonged starvation, to prevent deterioration of intestinal integrity, and to avoid translocation of gut bacteria. One or two basic formulas can meet most patients' needs.

EN is important to maintain GI integrity and host defense. For example, glutamine (an amino acid [AA] needed in stress/sepsis) requires GI processing to become effective. Multidisciplinary nutrition support teams are likely to offer better and more cost-effective patient care with fewer complications (American Gastroenterology Association, 1995).

Prebiotics: "Many low-digestible carbohydrates are not digested in the upper GI tract and become fermented in the large intestine; they have physiological benefits similar to those of dietary fiber. For some of these materials, the fermentation process leads to the selective stimulation and growth of beneficial gut bacteria, e.g. bifidobacteria (prebiotics), which are defined as nutrients fermented in the large bowel that favor the growth of desirable large bowel microflora. This activity has been demonstrated for insulin and oligofructose. Two other carbohydrates with low digestibility that offer desirable physiological properties are resistant starch (RS) and polydextrose (PD). These functional benefits have led to considerable interest from the food industry leading to the use of these ingredients in the development of new 'healthy' products" (Murphy, 2001).

Probiotics are live microbial food supplements that support balance in the intestinal tract (Kopp-Hoolihan, 2001). Probiotics have been studied for their reports of having the ability to modify gut pH, antagonize pathogens, produce lactase, and stimulate immunomodulatory cells. Functional foods such as yogurt with live cultures may provide these probiotics and may, therefore, help to decrease the incidence of cancer, allergic reactions, and lactose intolerance. Further research is ongoing at this time.

TABLE 7–4 Conditions That May Benefit from Use of Intestinal Fuels

Glutamine, short-chain fatty acids, soy, fermentable fiber, and/or bulk may be useful for:
Dumping syndrome
Inflammatory bowel disease
Bowel resection
Constipation
Diarrhea
Diverticulosis
Irritable bowel syndrome
Radiation/chemotherapy
Total parenteral nutrition (TPN)-induced bowel atrophy
Tube feeding

TABLE 7–5 Knowledge and Skills of Dietetics Practitioners for GI Disorders (Beyer, 1998)

Recognizes extremes of dietary intake and the effects of diet on GI function and symptoms
Knows normal secretion, digestion, and absorption of foods
Knows sites of digestion and absorption of foods
Knows sites of digestion and absorption of macronutrients and micronutrients
Understands how GI dysfunction, surgical resections, and diseases affect nutrition
Understands consequences of eating patterns in healthy persons and in those with GI disease
Can identify screening factors for persons with GI disease
Can explain relative strength of association between diet and other therapies in treating GI disorders
Knows value and limitations of EN and parenteral nutrition (PN) formulas and common nutraceuticals

For More Information

- American College of Gastroenterology
  http://www.acg.gi.org/
- American Digestive Health Foundation
  7272 Wisconsin Avenue, Suite 300
  Bethesda, MD 20814-3015
  301-941-1931 (phone); 301-941-1275 (fax)
  http://www.adhf.org
- American Gastroenterological Association
  7910 Woodmont Ave., Seventh Floor
  Bethesda, MD 20814
  Phone 301-654-2055; Fax: (301)652-3890
  http://www.gastro.org
- American Society of Gastrointestinal Endoscopy
  http://www.asge.org
- Atlas of Gastroenterology & Hepatology, Mark Feldman MD, ed.
  www.gastroamerica.com
- The Cleveland Clinic Foundation
  http://www.clevelandclinic.org
  - For Inflammatory Bowel Disease, www.clevelandclinic.org/ gastro/IBD/IBD.html
  - For colorectal surgery, www.clevelandclinic.org/ CORS
- Colon and Rectal Cancer (see section 13)
  http://www.patientcenters.com/colon
- The Digestive Disorders Foundation
  http://www.digestivedisorders.org.uk
- Gastrolab
  http://gastrolab.net
- GastroOnline
  http://www.gastronews.com
- Gastroenterology Therapy OnLine
  http://www.gastrotherapy.com/gd/
- Gutfeelings
  http://www.gutfeelings.com
- North American Society for Pediatric Gastroenterology and Nutrition
  http://www.naspgn.org
- The Online Journal of Digestive Health
  http://www.ojdh.org
- Society of American Gastrointestinal Endoscopic Surgeons
  http://www.sages.org
- Society of Gastroenterology Nurses and Associates
  http://www.sgna.org
- Gastroenterology (Websites for specialists)
  http://www.vgastroenterology.com
- World Organization for Digestive Endoscopy
  http://www.omed.org

DYSPHAGIA

NUTRITIONAL ACUITY RANKING: LEVEL 3

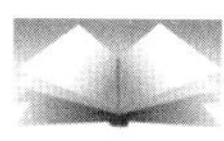

DEFINITIONS AND BACKGROUND

Anatomic or physiologic swallowing problems of dysphagia create a disturbance in the normal transfer of food from the oral cavity to the stomach. Swallowing requires 5–10 seconds and three phases for completion—oral phase, pharyngeal phase, and esophageal phase. All must be adequate to prevent choking and/or aspiration into the lung.

Watch for signs such as coughing, choking, drooling, and pocketing of foods. Consult speech therapist for a full evaluation; progression of diet is made when possible, under guidance of the therapist. A barium swallow may reveal silent aspiration. Inadequate dietary intake, weight loss, nutrient deficiencies, protein–calorie malnutrition (PCM), and dehydration may result from prolonged dysphagia.

A structured approach is needed. In children with developmental disabilities, diagnosis-specific treatment of feeding disorders results in significantly improved energy consumption and nutritional status. These data also indicate that decreased morbidity and a lower acute-care hospitalization rate may be related, at least in part, to successful management of feeding problems (Schwarz et al., 2001).

TABLE 7–6 Common Causes of Dysphagia

Achalasia	Head or neck cancer
Aging	Head/skull injuries
Alzheimer's disease, dementia	Hiatal hernia
Amyotrophic lateral sclerosis (ALS)	Huntington's disease
Anoxia	Lung cancer
Cerebral palsy	Meningitis
Cerebrovascular accident (stroke)	Muscular dystrophy
Chronic obstructive lung disease	Multiple sclerosis
Cleft lip or palate	Myasthenia gravis
Closed head injury	Myotonic dystonia
Congestive heart failure	Parkinson's disease
Dehydration from diuretics, many other medications	Pneumonia with aspiration history
Dermatomyositis	Poliomyelitis
Diabetes, type 1 after long-term	Prematurity
Encephalopathy	Pulmonary disorders
Esophageal inflammation	Radiation treatment to head/neck
Esophageal stricture or obstruction	Sjögren's disease
Esophageal trauma	Spinal cord injury
Gastroparesis	Throat cancer or injury
Gastroesophageal reflux	Tongue cancer
Goiter	Tracheoesophageal fistula
Guillain-Barré syndrome	Zenker's diverticulum

OBJECTIVES

- Prevent choking and aspiration of foods and beverages.
- Provide foods that stimulate the swallowing reflex.
- Promote weight maintenance or gain if decline has occurred.
- Individualize diet based on patient needs and preferences. Refer to speech therapist, who will help to determine the level of consistency that is required (i.e., nectar or syrup, honey, pudding). Monitor for pocketing of food. For some patients, thin liquids may be needed. Modify levels of dysphagia diets as impairment level changes; upgrade when and if safe for the patient.
- Support independence in eating, where possible.
- Provide moistened foods or thickened beverages for adequate hydration.
- Correct any nutrient deficits.
- Prevent pressure ulcers from poor nutritional status and weight loss, where relevant.
- For persons who have viscous oral secretions or dry mouth, liquefy foods before serving by adding broth, juice, or water.

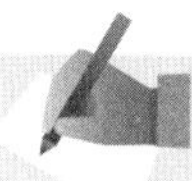

DIETARY AND NUTRITIONAL RECOMMENDATIONS

- The patient may be ordered nothing by mouth (NPO), if needed. Provide TPN, gastrostomy, or jejunostomy feedings as appropriate for the patient's condition. Home tube feeding may be needed, depending on medical condition and cause of dysphagia.
- Calculate needs at approximately 1.5 times basal energy expenditure (BEE) with 2 g of protein/kg if tolerated. Monitor cardiac, hepatic, and renal status.
- Prevent aspiration by careful selection of foods, such as thick, soft, pureed foods instead of thin liquids. Thickening may be at honey, nectar, or pudding consistency; the label on the thickener will indicate the amount required for the differing levels. When a thickened liquid diet is ordered, foods such as gelatin should not be used because they liquefy at body temperature. Thickened foods and beverages with special products such as Thick-It, Thicken-Up, and Thick 'n Easy use thickeners to make semisolids out of coffee, soup, beverages, juices, and shakes. It is possible to use mashed potato flakes to thicken some meat and casserole dishes. Baby rice cereal is an inexpensive thickener as well.
- Progress over time to a soft diet. Avoid alcoholic beverages, extremely hot liquids and beverages, caffeine, and spicy foods. Avoid foods that cause choking or that are hard to manage—tart juices and foods, dry or crisp foods such as crackers, bony fish, fibrous or chewy meats such as steak, sticky peanut butter, bananas, thinly pureed

foods that are easily aspirated, foods with varying consistency, and excessively sweet drinks or fruits that aggravate drooling.

- For decreased saliva production, moisten foods with small amounts of liquid. Extra butter, mild sauces, and gravies may be useful as well.
- Monitor for deficiencies in fiber and vitamins A and C, if whole grains, fruits, and vegetables are not consumed.
- Avoid foods that are easily aspirated such as popcorn, bran cereals, nuts, dry mashed potatoes, cottage cheese, fruits with skins, corn, celery, pineapple, and other fruits or vegetables with fibrous pulp. Sometimes dry bread in sandwiches can also be a problem. Chewy meats such as steak, crumbly foods like crackers or cake, dry foods like chips, or sticky foods such as peanut butter or bananas should also be avoided at this time.
- For reduced oral sensation, position food in the most sensitive area and use colder foods.
- To form a more cohesive bolus of food in the mouth, serve semi-solid consistencies.
- For a severely sore mouth, avoid acidic foods and use soft foods at moderate temperatures.
- For delayed or absent swallowing reflex, use of temperature extremes and spicy foods may help excite the nerves necessary to function better. Some thickening of liquids may actually be beneficial. Use of cohesive foods that do not fall apart is also recommended.
- Crushed bran on cereal or high-fiber tube-feeding products can help alleviate constipation.

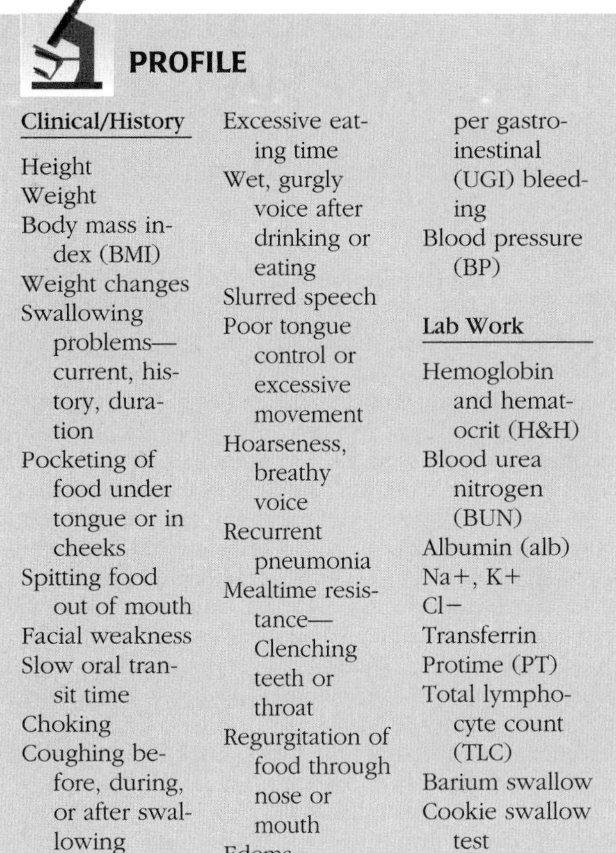

PROFILE

Clinical/History

Height
Weight
Body mass index (BMI)
Weight changes
Swallowing problems—current, history, duration
Pocketing of food under tongue or in cheeks
Spitting food out of mouth
Facial weakness
Slow oral transit time
Choking
Coughing before, during, or after swallowing
Excessive eating time
Wet, gurgly voice after drinking or eating
Slurred speech
Poor tongue control or excessive movement
Hoarseness, breathy voice
Recurrent pneumonia
Mealtime resistance—Clenching teeth or throat
Regurgitation of food through nose or mouth
Edema
Presence of upper gastroinestinal (UGI) bleeding
Blood pressure (BP)

Lab Work

Hemoglobin and hematocrit (H&H)
Blood urea nitrogen (BUN)
Albumin (alb)
Na+, K+
Cl−
Transferrin
Protime (PT)
Total lymphocyte count (TLC)
Barium swallow
Cookie swallow test
Esophagoscopy

Common Drugs Used and Potential Side Effects

- For thick saliva and gagging, artificial saliva such as lemon glycerin may be useful. Papain or citrus juices may be useful for thinning sections.

Herbs, Botanicals and Supplements

- Herbs and botanical supplements should not be used without discussing with the physician.
- It is important to stress that no supplement or diet can cure dysphagia.

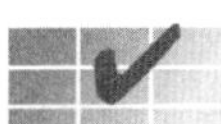

PATIENT EDUCATION

✔ Follow meals by brushing teeth to reduce dental caries; encourage optimal mouth care.

✔ Offer suggestions for specific changes in food preparation (e.g., adding moistening sauces, gravies, etc.) and cutting or mincing foods to increase control of the swallowing process.

✔ Encourage regular review of changes in swallowing abilities to identify early decline or to lessen restrictions when possible.

ESOPHAGEAL STRICTURE, ESOPHAGEAL SPASM, OR ACHALASIA

NUTRITIONAL ACUITY RANKING: LEVEL 3 (STRICTURE/SPASM); LEVEL 2 (ACHALASIA)

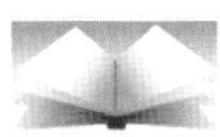

DEFINITIONS AND BACKGROUND

Dysphagia, odynophagia, heartburn, and reflux are symptoms related to the esophagus (Abell and Werkman, 1996). Esophageal stricture is normally caused by chemical ingestion, sliding hiatal hernia, neoplasm, or reflux esophagitis. In esophageal spasm, segmented, concentric contractions occur simultaneously in the lower two-thirds of the esophagus.

Achalasia is caused by failure of the cardiac sphincter to relax with obstruction of food passage into the stomach. In addition, the esophagus does not demonstrate normal waves of contraction after swallowing. Signs and symptoms include dysphagia, substernal pain after meals, weight loss, regurgitation, and halitosis. Patients with long-standing achalasia seem to be at risk of developing squamous cell carcinoma of the esophagus (Bozymski and Isaacs, 1991). Esophageal dilatation with a bougienage may be helpful; surgical myotomy may be required.

Zenker's diverticulum generally presents after 60 years of age, but patients may have years of symptoms. Regurgitation of undigested food when patient bends over or lies down may occur and may lead to aspiration pneumonia. Diagnosis is by barium swallow, and treatment is surgical resection. Esophagodiverticulostomy is an excellent method of surgically correcting Zenker's diverticulum in many patients (Thaler et al., 2001).

OBJECTIVES

- Esophageal stricture: Avoid large boluses of food. Provide adequate nutrition. Prevent weight loss. Remove cause or dilate, if necessary.
- Esophageal spasm: Avoid either very cold or hot foods or beverages. Monitor dysphagia.
- Achalasia: Individualize diet according to patient tolerances and preferences. Monitor chronic dysphagia. Avoid aspiration.

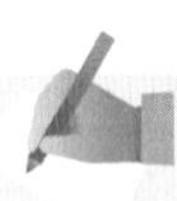

DIETARY AND NUTRITIONAL RECOMMENDATIONS

- Esophageal stricture. Begin with liquid diet and progress to soft diet as tolerance increases. Adequate calories are needed. Gastrostomy may be needed. Antireflux regimen (no alcohol, weight loss) may be helpful. Avoid sticky and dry foods. Use thin liquids and pureed or soft foods.
- Esophageal spasm. Use diet as tolerated with modified temperatures for foods and beverages.
- Achalasia: Provide large volumes of fluids with each meal, unless dysphagia prevents appropriate swallowing of liquids. Tube feed if needed; may need to use a gastrostomy feeding.

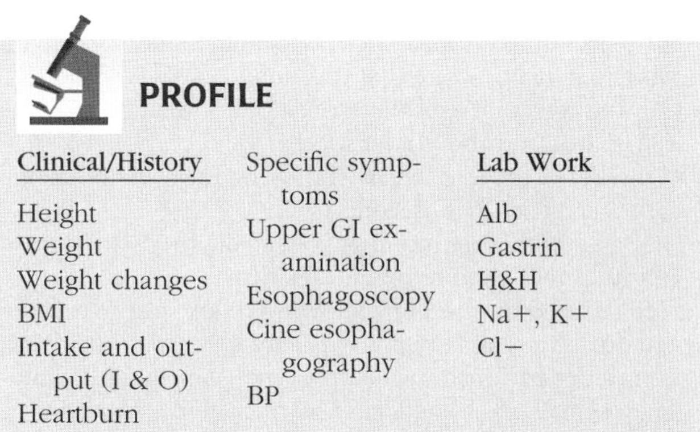

PROFILE

Clinical/History		Lab Work
Height Weight Weight changes BMI Intake and output (I & O) Heartburn	Specific symptoms Upper GI examination Esophagoscopy Cine esophagography BP	Alb Gastrin H&H Na+, K+ Cl−

Common Drugs Used and Potential Side Effects

- Antacids. Check the label for aluminum, calcium, magnesium, or sodium if other medical problems exist. Beware of long-term side effects.
- Nitroglycerin often helps spasm. Headache is one possible side effect.
- Isosorbide dinitrate and calcium-channel blockers such as nifedipine may be needed 30 minutes before meals.

Herbs, Botanicals and Supplements

- Herbs and botanical supplements should not be used without discussing with the physician.

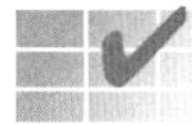

PATIENT EDUCATION

- ✓ Emphasize the importance of spacing meals and achieving relaxation. Recommend intake of food at moderate temperature only.
- ✓ Elevate head of bed for 30–45 minutes after meals and at bedtime.
- ✓ Encourage fluids at mealtimes.
- ✓ Avoid foods that aggravate dysphagia.
- ✓ Bland foods are not clearly beneficial and not required.

ESOPHAGEAL TRAUMA

NUTRITIONAL ACUITY RANKING: LEVEL 3

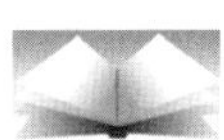

DEFINITIONS AND BACKGROUND

Esophageal trauma is a major traumatic condition that affects the esophagus, often from chemical burns, ingestion of foreign bodies, or injury. Signs and symptoms include nausea, vomiting, loss of consciousness, dysphagia, respiratory distress, shock, and esophageal perforation.

OBJECTIVES

- Emergency care, such as adequate ventilation or shock therapy, is given as needed.
- Allow the esophagus to rest and heal.
- Prepare for esophageal surgery, as necessary.
- Keep the patient adequately hydrated.
- Improve swallowing capacity as rapidly as possible; prevent aspiration.
- Prevent malnutrition, weight loss, sepsis, constipation, fluid loss from exudates, and other complications.
- For serious injuries with permanent damage, it may be necessary for a gastrostomy tube feeding to be used.

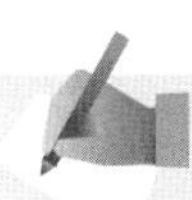

DIETARY AND NUTRITIONAL RECOMMENDATIONS

- NPO as needed. Provide TPN, gastrostomy, or jejunostomy feedings as appropriate for the patient's condition. Home tube feeding may be needed, for which a gastrostomy or jejunostomy will be important.
- Calculate needs at approximately 1.5 times BEE with 2 g of protein/kg if tolerated. Monitor cardiac, hepatic, and renal status.
- Progress over time to a soft diet. Avoid alcoholic beverages, extremely hot liquids and beverages, caffeine, and spicy foods.
- Force fluids unless overhydration is a problem or unless dysphagia prevents use of thin liquids.
- If the patient has dysphagia, use appropriately thick liquids or pureed foods until swallowing ability improves. Work with a speech therapist for proper consistency evaluations.

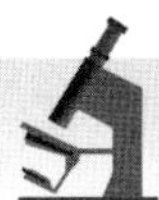

PROFILE

Clinical/History		
Height	Dysphagia	TLC
Weight	Temperature	H&H, Serum Fe
BMI	**Lab Work**	Alb or prealbumin
Weight changes	Glucose (gluc)	Transferrin
Barium swallow	BUN/Creat	
I & O	Na+, K+	

Common Drugs Used and Potential Side Effects

- Liquid topical anesthetizing agents (such as lidocaine) may be used before meals to reduce pain.
- Antibiotics may be used in bacterial infections.

Herbs, Botanicals and Supplements

- Herbs and botanical supplements should not be used without discussing with the physician.

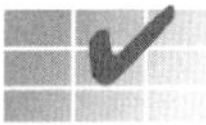

PATIENT EDUCATION

- When the patient can swallow, discuss the need to chew well and swallow carefully. The patient should also learn to eat slowly to prevent aspiration.
- Discuss the appropriate food textures for different stages of progress. This plan will be in accordance with the speech therapist and the physician.

ESOPHAGEAL VARICES

NUTRITIONAL ACUITY RANKING: LEVEL 3

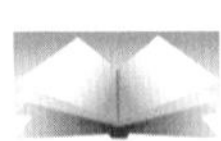

DEFINITIONS AND BACKGROUND

In esophageal varices (EV), small esophageal veins become distended and may rupture due to increased pressure in the portal system. This condition is usually caused by cirrhosis and portal hypertension. Current medical management dictates that all cirrhotic patients without a history of variceal hemorrhage undergo endoscopic screening to detect large varices (Zaman et al., 2001). Signs and symptoms include respiratory distress, aspiration of emesis, shock, hemorrhage, confusion, abdominal distention, melena, jaundice, and hepatic coma. Thrombocytopenia and splenomegaly are independent predictors of large EV in cirrhosis. Further prospective studies might result in a discriminating algorithm to predict which patients with cirrhosis would benefit from early or regular endoscopy to detect clinically significant varices (Madhotra et al., 2002). Death can occur if the condition worsens.

OBJECTIVES

- Promote healing, recovery. Prevent worsening of symptoms.
- Prevent constipation and straining with stool.
- Prevent or correct hepatic encephalopathy or coma. (See appropriate disorder sections, such as Cirrhosis and Hepatic Encephalopathy in section 8.)

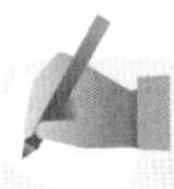

DIETARY AND NUTRITIONAL RECOMMENDATIONS

- Generally, unless comatose, the patient can tolerate 5–6 small meals of soft foods. Avoid foods such as taco chips or large pieces of raw fruits and vegetables.
- Alter carbohydrate, protein, and fat intake according to hepatic function and state of consciousness.
- Provide adequate fluid as allowed or controlled.
- To prevent constipation and straining, foods such as prune juice or formulas with fiber added can help normalize bowel function.

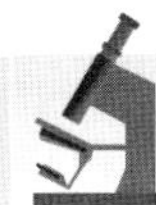

PROFILE

Clinical/History		
Height	Upper GI bleeding	BUN
Weight	BP	Alb
BMI	**Lab Work**	Ascites
Weight changes	H&H	Na+, K+
Esophagoscopy	Ammonia (NH_3)	Cl−
Edema		Transferrin
Melena		PT
		TLC

Common Drugs Used and Potential Side Effects

- Propanolol therapy reduces risk of variceal bleeding, especially in patients with cirrhosis (Abraczinskas et al., 2001).
- Antacids may be beneficial to buffer gastric acidity. Extended use can cause problems with pH, altered mineral and nutrient use, and other imbalances.
- Antibiotics may be used for infections. Monitor for specific side effects.
- Vitamin K may be needed to help with adequate clotting.
- Vasopressin may be used.

Herbs, Botanicals and Supplements

- Herbs and botanical supplements should not be used without discussing with the physician.

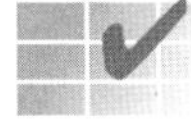

PATIENT EDUCATION

- ✓ The role of alcohol in the disease process should be discussed with the patient and family.
- ✓ The importance of good nutrition in adequate consistency should be addressed.
- ✓ Teach the patient to avoid rough or crunchy foods that are fibrous or sharp and to chew all foods well before swallowing.

HEARTBURN, HIATAL HERNIA, ESOPHAGITIS, AND GASTROESOPHAGEAL REFLUX DISEASE

NUTRITIONAL ACUITY RANKING: LEVEL 2

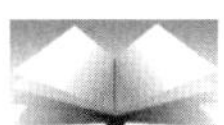

DEFINITIONS AND BACKGROUND

Hiatal hernia is caused by protrusion of part of the stomach above the diaphragm muscle, which separates the chest from the abdomen. This causes an enlarged diaphragm opening (hiatus) through which the esophagus passes to join the stomach. Hiatal hernia may show no symptoms or may cause heartburn, swallowing difficulty, reflux, or vomiting of blood.

Esophagitis results from gastric juice being forced into the esophagus from the stomach; 20% of persons who take nonsteroidal anti-inflammatory drugs (NSAIDs) develop esophagitis (Mendez et al., 1991). There seems to be a role for gastric acid suppression in treatment of gastroesophageal reflux disease (GERD) (Bell and Hunt, 1992). Gastroesophageal reflux and peptic ulcer disease are seen more commonly in elderly individuals than in other age groups; approximately 20% of the population has esophageal reflux with heartburn as a primary symptom (Bozymski and Isaacs, 1991).

GERD affects approximately 19 million Americans. GE reflux can be as high as 80% among asthma patients; medical-surgical therapy can improve asthma in about 70% of cases. About 50–90% of patients with GERD also have hiatal hernias. Gastroesophageal reflux is a frequent, nonspecific phenomenon in infants and children. Altered thresholds for pain have been noted among women with current complaints of GE reflux (Scarinci et al., 1994); pain management should be included in the treatment plan. Intractable disease may require minor surgery to strengthen a weak sphincter.

In infants, gastroesophageal reflux is common, and usually resolves by 6–12 months of age; management involves thickened feedings, positional treatment, and parental reassurance (Jung, 2001). GERD is a less common, more serious pathologic process. GERD diagnosis in children includes review for upper GI tract disorders, cow's milk allergy, or metabolic, infectious, renal, or central nervous system diseases. The recommended approach for infants with uncomplicated regurgitation is the reassurance of the parents about the physiological nature of excessive regurgitation, and if necessary, completed with dietary recommendations for formula-fed infants. In life-threatening situations, or in patients who are resistant to or dependent on acid suppressive medication, a surgical procedure such as laparoscopic fundoplication should be considered (Vandenplas, 2000).

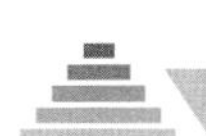

OBJECTIVES

- Eliminate reflux into the esophagus.
- Achieve and maintain desirable body weight to improve mechanical and postural states.
- Neutralize gastric acidity, when possible. Alcoholic beverages, coffee, and tea are associated with heartburn more than plain water (Feldman and Barnett, 1995).
- Avoid large meals that increase gastric pressure and alter pressure on the lower esophageal sphincter (LES), thereby allowing reflux to occur. The LES limits aspiration of gastric contents when functioning properly.
- Provide an individual diet reflecting patient needs. Assess intake of fat, alcohol, spices, caffeine, etc.
- Patients should avoid garments that fit tightly around the abdomen.

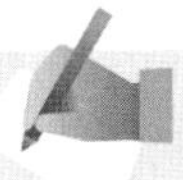

DIETARY AND NUTRITIONAL RECOMMENDATIONS

- During acute episodes, provide small, frequent feedings of soft foods.
- Instruct the patient to remain upright for 2 hours after meals and avoid intake of food (especially fatty foods) for several hours before bedtime. If needed, elevate the head of the bed.
- Diet should be high in protein to stimulate gastrin secretion and to increase lower esophageal sphincter pressure.
- Diet should be low in fat–less fried food, cream sauces, gravies, fatty meats, pastries, nuts, potato chips, butter and margarine, etc.
- Avoid foods that decrease LES pressure, including chocolate, regular and decaffeinated coffee, peppermint, onions, garlic, spearmint, after-dinner liqueurs, and alcohol (DeVault and Castell, 1995). Instruct the patient to limit or stop smoking.
- Avoid foods that may irritate the esophagus–citrus juices, tomatoes, and tomato sauce.
- Other spicy foods are to be eliminated according to individual experience.
- If needed, a low-calorie diet should be used to promote weight loss.
- Fluids can be taken between meals if consumption with meals causes abdominal distention.

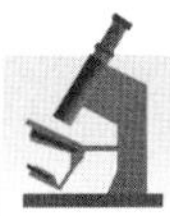

PROFILE

Clinical/History

Height
Weight
BMI

Lab Work

H&H
Mean cell volume (MCV)
Gluc
Gastrin
Alb, prealbumin
Cholesterol (chol), triglycerides (trig)
Transferrin, total iron-binding capacity (TIBC)
Bernstein test—HCl solution is dripped into the distal esophagus; positive test reproduces patient symptoms
Upper GI endoscopy
Esophagoscopy
Manometry

Common Drugs Used and Potential Side Effects

- Antacids. Used to neutralize gastric contents; antacids destroy thiamine and may provide excess sodium for the body. Check labels carefully. If the antacid contains calcium (e.g., Tums, which contains calcium carbonate), excess calcium may cause decreased levels of magnesium and phosphorus. Aluminum hydroxide (Maalox) depletes phosphorus, which is acceptable for patients with certain types of renal diseases, but which otherwise must be observed. When used as an antacid, sodium bicarbonate can decrease iron absorption and causes sodium retention; use with caution.
- Reglan may be used. Nausea or diarrhea may occur.
- Pharmacologic management of GERD includes a prokinetic agent such as metoclopramide or cisapride and a histamine-receptor type 2 antagonist such as cimetidine or ranitidine when esophagitis is suspected (Jung 2001).
- Propulsid (cisapride) may cause nausea, pain, constipation, diarrhea, or headache. It tends to be safe and the drug of choice for children, infants, or adults. Cholinergic blocking agents like cimetidine reduce the amount of gastric secretions; malabsorption can result if used for long periods.
- Pill-induced esophageal injury may occur from use of aspirin, tetracycline, vitamin C, ferrous sulfate, potassium chloride, or NSAIDs. Take with plenty of liquid.
- Omeprazole is useful for refractory reflux esophagitis, especially that which is resistant to H2 antagonist therapy (Klinkenberg-Knol et al., 1994).
- An over-the-counter (OTC) product, Prelief (calcium glycerophosphate) is somewhat useful for relief of heartburn by neutralizing the acid in foods.
- Proton pump inhibitors (PPIs) are becoming a more popular treatment (Thomson, 2001). Where clarithromycin-resistant *Helicobacter pylori* (CRHP) occur, PPIs tend to inhibit the growth and motility of CRHP.

Herbs, Botanicals and Supplements

- Herbs and botanical supplements should not be used without discussing with the physician.
- Camomile, peppermint, fennel, cardamom, cinnamon, dill and licorice have been recommended for this condition but no clinical trials have proven efficacy.

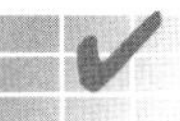

PATIENT EDUCATION

- ✔ Encourage the patient to avoid late evening meals and snacks.
- ✔ Teach the proper measures for controlling weight, including small, frequent feedings.
- ✔ Instruct the patient to maintain an upright position for 2 hours after eating. Elevating the head of the bed at night may also be beneficial. Patients with heartburn probably should not sleep in a waterbed.
- ✔ Chewing gum may help to reduce heartburn. Saliva may lessen the effect of acid.

For More Information

- GERD.com
  http://www.gerd.com
- Prelief
  1-888-773-5433
  http://www.akpharma.com/prelief/preliefhome.htm
- Pediatric and Adolescent Gastroesophageal Reflux Association
  http:// www.reflux.org

DYSPEPSIA/INDIGESTION

NUTRITIONAL ACUITY RANKING: LEVEL 2

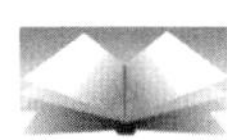

DEFINITIONS AND BACKGROUND

Indigestion (dyspepsia) may be secondary to other systemic disorders such as atherosclerotic heart disease, hypertension, liver disease, or renal disease. Dyspepsia is not necessarily synonymous with gastritis. Separation of dyspepsia, its subgroups, and irritable bowel syndrome (IBS) seems to be unnecessary; they tend to represent one entity: the "irritable gut" (Agreus et al., 1995).

The concept of gastric hypersensitivity is an important factor in the pathophysiology of functional dyspepsia (FD), but it is unclear which symptoms can predict the presence of gastric hypersensitivity (Rhee et al., 2000). Individual symptoms such as early satiety, postprandial fullness, feeling of delayed emptying, nausea, vomiting, and epigastric soreness are graded as mild to severe. While basal tone, gastric compliance, and postprandial receptive relaxation are similar in controls and patients, the threshold of abdominal discomfort is lower in FD patients than in controls. In conclusion, simple evaluation of individual symptoms does not predict the presence of gastric hypersensitivity (Rhee et al., 2000).

OBJECTIVES

- ▲ Determine whether the problem is psychogenic or organic in etiology.
- ▲ Do not oversimplify the patient's discomfort.
- ▲ As appropriate, review and discuss IBS as well; they are often related.

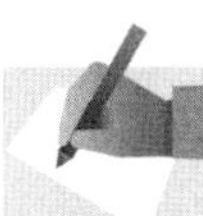

DIETARY AND NUTRITIONAL RECOMMENDATIONS

- Diet should make use of well-cooked foods, adequate in amount but not overly seasoned.
- A relaxed atmosphere is helpful.
- Small meals are best tolerated.
- If the dyspepsia is organic in etiology, a soft, low-fat diet may be helpful. If there is irritable bowel as well, discuss fiber (especially fruits and vegetables; bran is not always well tolerated—see IBS entry).
- If the dyspepsia is psychogenic in etiology, removing the cause often results in the disappearance of the dyspepsia.

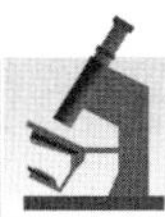

PROFILE

Clinical/History		Lab Work
Height	tests	H&H, Serum Fe
Weight	Nausea	MCV
BMI	Heartburn	Alb, prealbumin
Weight changes	Stool consistency	Gluc
Anorexia	I & O	BUN/Creat
Gastric barostat		

Common Drugs Used and Potential Side Effects

- Antacids. Beware of nutritional side effects resulting from dependency. (See Heartburn entry for more information.)
- Proton pump inhibitors may be used, especially if reflux also exists (Ligumsky et al., 2001).

Herbs, Botanicals and Supplements

- Herbs and botanical supplements should not be used without discussing with the physician.
- Ginger is often used as an antinauseant. Do not use large doses with warfarin, aspirin, other antiplatelet drugs, antihypertensive drugs, and hypoglycemic drugs. Additive effects can cause unpredictable changes in blood pressure, decreases in blood glucose levels, and may decrease platelet aggregation and therefore, increase bleeding. Ginger ale has few side effects.
- Camomile, peppermint, red pepper, angelica, and coriander have been recommended, but no clinical trials have proven efficacy.

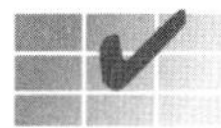

PATIENT EDUCATION

- ✔ Encourage the patient to eat in a relaxed atmosphere.
- ✔ Discuss the role of fiber in maintaining bowel regularity.

GASTRIC RETENTION

NUTRITIONAL ACUITY RANKING: LEVEL 3

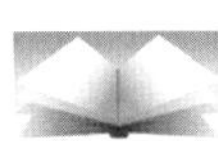

DEFINITIONS AND BACKGROUND

Gastric retention is caused by partial obstruction at the outlet of the stomach into the small bowel.

OBJECTIVES

- Use liquids or foods that liquefy at body temperature so they are able to pass by a partial obstruction before or during digestion.
- Bypass or correct obstruction or other causes of retention.
- If diabetes is also a problem, manage blood glucose levels to ensure that control is maintained. (See Gastroparesis entry.)

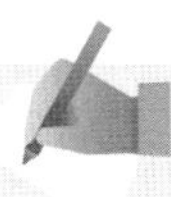

DIETARY AND NUTRITIONAL RECOMMENDATIONS

- Diet should start with full liquids. Feedings should be small and frequent.
- For patients with a lesser obstruction of the stomach, progress to a mechanical soft diet. For patients with greater obstruction of the stomach, use a low-fiber diet or tube feed, checking residuals frequently. For persistent problems, a chemically defined diet or feeding product may be needed.
- Monitor kilocalorie and protein intake carefully to ensure adequacy of the diet, because it may be difficult to obtain orally.

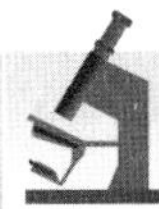

PROFILE

Clinical/History	Lab Work	
Height Weight BMI I & O	H&H BUN, Creat Alb, prealbumin Gluc	Gastrin Cl− Na+, K+ Serum vitamin B12 Gastric x-rays

Common Drugs Used and Potential Side Effects

- Reglan may be used with some positive results; monitor closely for tolerance and any negative side effects such as nausea or diarrhea.
- If there is hyperglycemia, oral agents and insulin may be needed.

Herbs, Botanicals and Supplements

- Herbs and botanical supplements should not be used without discussing with the physician.

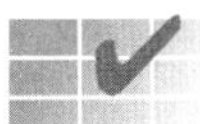

PATIENT EDUCATION

- ✔ Help the patient determine a specific dietary regimen.
- ✔ Discuss methods for liquefying foods as needed.

GASTRITIS OR GASTROENTERITIS

NUTRITIONAL ACUITY RANKING: LEVEL 2

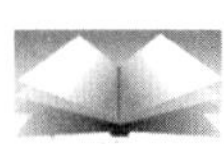

DEFINITIONS AND BACKGROUND

Gastritis involves inflammation of the stomach. Types of gastritis include idiopathic (acute or chronic), specific (acute or chronic, as in granulomatous or postirradiation), allergic, or embolic. Occult GI bleeding is common in Yupik Eskimos living in Alaska; an atypical gastritis associated with *H. pylori* infection is almost universal in this population and may cause blood loss (Yip et al., 1997). *H. pylori* seem to be the cause in the development of B12 deficiency, and eradication of *H. pylori* may be the best treatment for the deficiency (Kaptan et al., 2000).

Atrophic gastritis (AG) is chronic inflammation of the gastric mucosa without erosion but with hypochlorhydria or achlorhydria; it is important to monitor B_{12}, Ca++, and ferric iron intake. People who get their vitamin B_{12} from dairy products, fortified cereals, and supplements are better protected than those who eat mostly meats.

Gastroenteritis is an inflammation of the stomach and intestinal lining. Eating chemical toxins in food (such as seafood, mushrooms, arsenic, lead), drinking excessive alcohol, food allergies, food-borne illness, intestinal viruses, cathartics, and other drugs can cause gastroenteritis. Gastroenteritis produces malaise, nausea, vomiting, intestinal rumbles, diarrhea with or without blood and mucus, and sometimes fever and prostration. In the past century, more than 79% of gastroenteritis cases caused by contaminated shellfish were due to an unknown agent; raw oysters seem to be a major contributor (Graczyk and Schwab, 2000).

Hemorrhagic colitis may result from eating undercooked beef or drinking unpasteurized milk; *E. coli* 0157:H7 is the agent and may cause diarrhea for 1–8 days and slight fever. In vulnerable populations, 5% develop hemolytic-uremic syndrome, seizures, strokes, or may even die.

OBJECTIVES

- ▲ Prevent or correct dehydration, shock, hypokalemia, and hyponatremia.
- ▲ Allow the stomach and GI tract to rest, but relieve thirst with water and tolerated fluids.
- ▲ Empty stomach to permit mucous lining to heal.
- ▲ Omit lactose if not tolerated in gastroenteritis.
- ▲ If hemorrhage occurs, it is a medical emergency.
- ▲ Monitor for maldigestion with idiopathic gastritis.

DIETARY AND NUTRITIONAL RECOMMENDATIONS

- Gastritis: Omit foods that are poorly tolerated. Provide adequate hydration. If chronic, mucosal atrophy can lead to nutritional deficits (pernicious anemia, achlorhydria, and functional pancreatitis). Alter diet accordingly.
- Acute gastroenteritis: Patient will be NPO or on total or partial parenteral nutrition (PPN/TPN) for the first 24–48 hours to rest stomach. Use crushed ice to relieve thirst. Progress to a soft diet, if desired. Alcohol is prohibited. Omit lactose if needed. Gradually add fiber-containing foods as tolerance improves. Rehydration solutions may be effective.
- Chronic gastroenteritis: Use small, frequent feedings of easily tolerated foods. Progress with larger amounts and greater variety of foods, as tolerated. Restrict fat intake, which depresses food motility, and alcohol intake. Monitor lactose intolerance. Add fiber-containing foods as tolerated.

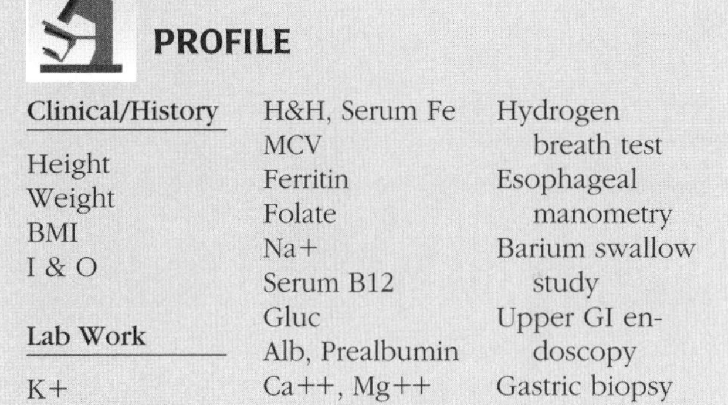

PROFILE

Clinical/History

Height
Weight
BMI
I & O

Lab Work

K+
Cl−
H&H, Serum Fe
MCV
Ferritin
Folate
Na+
Serum B12
Gluc
Alb, Prealbumin
Ca++, Mg++
Hydrogen breath test
Esophageal manometry
Barium swallow study
Upper GI endoscopy
Gastric biopsy

Common Drugs Used and Potential Side Effects

- Antacids. Watch for constipation caused by aluminum and calcium agents. Watch for diarrhea caused by magnesium agents. (See Heartburn entry for other tips.)
- Antibiotics in excess over a long time may cause or aggravate gastroenteritis. Monitor carefully.

- Sucralfate may be useful for healing ulcerations. Take separately from calcium or magnesium supplements by 30 minutes. Constipation may occur.
- In healthy volunteers, psyllium before meals reduces subsequent feelings of hunger and energy intake; it does not delay gastric emptying but results in flattened curves for serum glucose, insulin, and triglyceride (TG) levels against time after a meal, suggesting slower absorption of nutrients from the intestine (Rigaud et al., 1998). Monitor intake in patients.

Herbs, Botanicals and Supplements

- Herbs and botanical supplements should not be used without discussing with the physician.

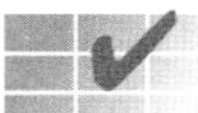

PATIENT EDUCATION

- ✓ Omit offenders in chronic conditions: alcohol, caffeine, and aspirin.
- ✓ Patients with chronic gastritis should be assessed for folate and vitamin B_{12} status. Atrophy of the stomach and intestinal lining interferes with folate and vitamin B_{12} absorption.
- ✓ Discuss calcium and riboflavin sources if dairy products must be omitted.
- ✓ Discuss the role of fiber in achieving or maintaining bowel integrity.
- ✓ Discuss food-borne illness and its prevention (e.g., avoiding raw shellfish).

HYPERTROPHIC GASTRITIS (MÉNÉTRIÈR'S DISEASE)

NUTRITIONAL ACUITY RANKING: LEVEL 3

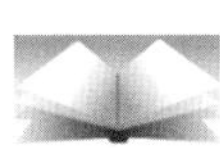

DEFINITIONS AND BACKGROUND

Ménétrièr's disease (hypertrophic gastritis) is a pathologic condition with increased loss of plasma proteins, resulting in hydrolysis by the proteolytic enzymes of the gut. The hydrolyzed proteins are then reabsorbed as amino acids. Ascites or edema may occur if the liver cannot produce sufficient albumin rapidly enough. Ménétrièr's disease is rare, diagnosed in patients with giant gastric folds, dyspeptic symptoms, and hypoalbuminemia due to gastrointestinal protein loss.

Etiology is unknown, but Ménétrièr's disease is often associated with *Helicobacter pylori* (HP) infection. It was found that complete normalization of the gastric mucosa and gastrointestinal protein loss following eradication therapy has been reported in several cases (Madsen et al., 2000).

Transient protein-losing hypertrophic gastropathy with similarity to Ménétrièr's disease may occur with acute infection with cytomegalovirus (CMV). CMV infection should be considered in patients with acute and symptomatic protein loss of gastrointestinal origin (Suter et al., 2000).

OBJECTIVES

- Replace protein; maintain adequate nitrogen balance.
- Reduce edema.
- Spare protein for tissue synthesis and repair.
- Promote normal dietary intake with a return to wellness.
- Gastric juice ascorbic acid is lower in individuals with *H. pylori* infections (Fraser and Woollard, 1999); increase intake.

DIETARY AND NUTRITIONAL RECOMMENDATIONS

- Use a high-protein/high-calorie diet. The protein level should be approximately 20% total kilocalories unless contraindicated for renal or hepatic problems.
- Sodium should be maintained at 4–6 g to help normalize edematous tissues.
- Omit any food intolerances.
- Include adequate sources of vitamin C in the diet; a supplement may be warranted.

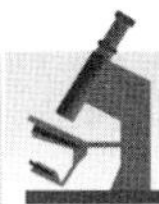

PROFILE

Clinical/History

Height
Weight
BMI
Weight changes

Lab Work

Alb, prealbumin
Retinol binding protein (RBP)
Globulin
A:G ratio
Na+
K+
Nitrogen (N) balance
Transferrin
Pepsin levels
H&H, Serum Fe
Serum folate
Serum B12
BUN, Creat
Gastroscopy
Gastric biopsy

Common Drugs Used and Potential Side Effects

- For eradication of *H. pylori,* 2 weeks of treatment with an acid-suppressing drug (one time daily), Pepto-Bismol (four times daily), and antibiotics (3–4 times daily) are prescribed. This therapy often must be used more than once. Other combinations may include antibiotic Prilosec, Biaxin, and Tritec (bismuth).

Herbs, Botanicals and Supplements

- Herbs and botanical supplements should not be used without discussing with the physician.

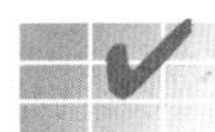

PATIENT EDUCATION

- ✓ Elimination of aggravating foods specific to the patient is warranted.
- ✓ Teach the patient about use of high-biologic-value (HBV) proteins to replenish serum protein levels.

PERNICIOUS VOMITING

NUTRITIONAL ACUITY RANKING: LEVEL 3 (LONGER THAN 7 DAYS)

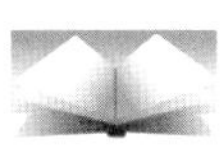

DEFINITIONS AND BACKGROUND

Pernicious (uncontrolled) vomiting may occur in any of several disorders, including cancers, gastroparesis, and pregnancy (hyperemesis gravidarum, see Pregnancy entry in section 1). Nutritional deficits are possible when the condition is prolonged.

OBJECTIVES

- Correct electrolyte and fluid imbalances.
- Eliminate oral intake until vomiting ends.
- Prevent weight loss.
- Distinguish symptoms that could be related to bulimia.
- If there is hyperglycemia or diabetes, return to normal blood glucose levels as quickly as possible; insulin may be needed.

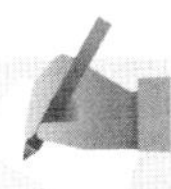

DIETARY AND NUTRITIONAL RECOMMENDATIONS

- For patients with an acute condition, NPO for 24 hours with intravenous glucose is common.
- When tolerated, gastrostomy tube feeding or jejunostomy may be warranted. An isotonic formula is desirable to reduce imbalances between solute and solvent.
- TPN may also be a consideration.
- As the patient progresses to an oral diet, toast, crackers, jelly, and simple carbohydrates in small, frequent meals may be used. Give fluids between meals (a "dry diet").
- Avoid acidic fruit and vegetable juices if not tolerated. Consider avoiding foods that delay gastric emptying (high-fat, hypertonic, or highly fibrous foods).
- Gradually have the patient resume a normal diet, but decrease fats if not tolerated.

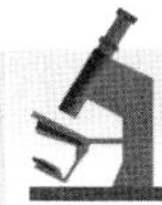

PROFILE

Clinical/History	Lab Work	
Height	Na+	Gluc
Weight	Cl−	H&H, Serum Fe
BMI	K+	Serum folate
Weight changes	Alb, prealbumin	Serum B12
	BUN, Creat	Gastric emptying tests
	N balance	

Common Drugs Used and Potential Side Effects

- Peristaltic agents may be used for gastroparesis.
- Antiemetic agents may be indicated for some conditions but not for all.
- Insulin or oral agents may be needed if diabetes is also present.

Herbs, Botanicals and Supplements

- Herbs and botanical supplements should not be used without discussing with the physician.
- Ginger is often used as an antinauseant. Do not use large doses with warfarin, aspirin, other antiplatelet drugs, antihypertensive drugs, and hypoglycemic drugs. Additive effects can cause unpredictable changes in blood pressure, decreases in blood glucose levels, and may decrease platelet aggregation and therefore, increase bleeding. Ginger ale is commonly used and generally has few side effects.

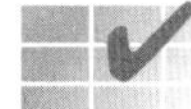

PATIENT EDUCATION

- ✓ Explain why fluids should be taken between meals.
- ✓ Discuss the role of carbohydrates and fiber in maintaining blood glucose levels.

PEPTIC ULCER

NUTRITIONAL ACUITY RANKING: LEVEL 2

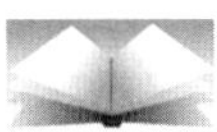

DEFINITIONS AND BACKGROUND

A peptic ulcer is an area of the GI tract that is eroded by gastric acid and pepsin, leaving exposed nerves. Of ulcers, 15% are gastric (often later correlated to stomach cancer) and 85% are duodenal, usually in the first 25–30 cm. Melena is a common initial sign of peptic ulcer disease in elderly individuals (Shamburek and Farrar, 1990).

Helicobacter pylori (HP) play a role in the etiology of most ulcers (Hentschel et al., 1993), especially in elderly individuals. Many people have HP bacteria; few have ulcers. Water or poor handwashing (as per fecal-oral route) may be a concern. Monitor for vitamin B_{12} deficiency where *H. pylori* have been found.

While the main cause of duodenal ulcer is the *H. pylori* bacterium, more than 80% of HP-infected people never develop an ulcer. Diet may be one of the most important environmental factors contributing to duodenal ulcer (Misciagna et al., 2000). Soluble fiber from fruit and vegetables seems to be protective and refined sugars a risk; the role of fiber in the treatment and prevention of recurrence of duodenal ulcers is uncertain, as is that of essential fatty acids (Misciagna et al., 2000). High intakes of vitamin A, fruits and vegetables, and dietary fiber reduce the risk (Aldoori et al., 1997). Drug therapy is most effective in preventing ulcer recurrence.

Treatment is primarily antibiotics and antacids. No single, optimal antibiotic therapy currently exists; conventional therapy should continue only with complicated or refractory ulcers, at least until eradication of *H. pylori* are confirmed (Soll, 1996). No evidence exists that bland diets affect the healing of an ulcer or a decrease in gastric acid secretion. *H. pylori* infection seems to be associated with low gastric juice ascorbic acid concentrations, often secondary to infection and corrected with successful treatment (Banerjee et al., 1994; Fraser and Woollard, 1999). There is a tentative link with gastric cancer.

The decline in duodenal ulcer disease and the established relation of peptic ulcer to *H. pylori* have eliminated the need for elective ulcer surgery (von Holstein, 2000).

OBJECTIVES

- Eradicate any *H. pylori* infection.
- Take medications as directed. Rest during healing stages. Reduce pain.
- Avoid distention from large meals.
- Dilute stomach contents and provide buffering action.
- Assess and modify detrimental habits (e.g., rushed meals, excessive use of alcohol and caffeine, and cigarette smoking, which decreases the normal pancreatic bicarbonate buffer system).
- Correct anemia, if present. Vitamin B_{12} deficiency is often corrected after effective *H. pylori* treatment.
- Monitor steatorrhea, bone disease, dumping syndrome, and other problems.
- Prevent other complications such as perforation and obstruction.
- Ensure adequate intake of vitamin C from the diet.

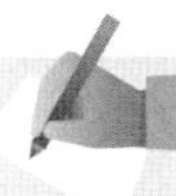

DIETARY AND NUTRITIONAL RECOMMENDATIONS

- Use small feedings, frequently if preferred. Include some high-protein foods and vitamin C to speed healing.
- Avoid personal intolerances.
- Limit gastric stimulants if not tolerated: caffeine, alcohol, peppermint, black pepper, garlic, cloves, and chili powder—sometimes called a "Liberal Bland" diet. If a particular food bothers an individual, it should be avoided.
- Use fewer saturated fats and more polyunsaturated fats if increased lipid levels are found. Arachidonic acid metabolites may play a role in peptic ulcer disease (PUD).
- Supplement with vitamin C-rich foods or an oral supplement if necessary. Citrus foods may not be tolerated.
- See Table 7–7 regarding caffeine.

TABLE 7–7 Typical Caffeine Content of Beverages and Medications

Beverages:	mg Caffeine
8 oz espresso coffee	30–50, (average 40)
8 oz coffee, brewed	65–120 (average 85)
8 oz coffee, instant	60–85 (average 75)
1 oz espresso coffee	30–50 (average 40)
8 oz decaffeinated coffee	2–4
8 oz black tea, brewed (most U.S. brands)	20–90 (average 40)
8 oz black tea, brewed (imported)	25–110 (average 60)
6 oz tea, instant	28–30
8 oz cola drinks	20–40 (average 24)
8 oz Ovaltine	0
8 oz cocoa beverage	3–32 (average 6)
8 oz chocolate milk	2–7 (average 5)
1 oz milk chocolate	1–15 (average 6)
1 oz dark chocolate	5–35 (average 20)
1 oz baker's chocolate	26
1 oz chocolate syrup	4
Medications Containing Caffeine:	
1 tablet cold preparations	30
1 tablet analgesics	30–66

Based on data from: Leonard T, et al. The effects of caffeine on various body systems: a review. *J Am Diet Assoc.* 1987;87:1048. Also: International Food Information Council, http://www.ificinfo.health.org.

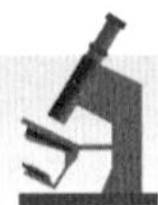

PROFILE

Clinical/History

- Height
- Weight
- BMI
- Blood loss

Lab Work

- Red blood cell count (RBC)
- Blood test for *H. pylori*
- Urea breath test
- Endoscopy
- Chol, Trig
- BUN, Creat
- Alb, prealbumin
- Alanine aminotransferase (ALT), aspartate aminotransaminase (AST)
- Blood guaiac
- Amylase (if perforated, increased)
- H&H, Serum Fe
- Serum folate
- PT
- Transferrin
- Ca++
- Serum B12
- Alk phos (increased)
- TIBC
- Na+, K+
- Cl−
- Serum gastrin (increased)

Common Drugs Used and Potential Side Effects

- For eradication of *H. pylori,* 2 weeks of treatment with an acid-suppressing drug (one time daily), Pepto-Bismol (four times daily), and antibiotics (3–4 times daily) are prescribed. This therapy often must be used more than once. Some other combinations may include antibiotic Prilosec, Biaxin, and Tritec (bismuth).
- Antacids such as aluminum hydroxide (Mylanta) may cause nausea, vomiting, and lowered vitamin A, calcium, and phosphate absorption. Milk of magnesia (magnesium hydroxide) is a laxative-antacid and can deplete phosphorus and calcium over time. Magaldrate (Riopan) decreases serum vitamin A but can be used on a low-sodium diet.
- Histamine H2 blockers such as cimetidine (Tagamet), nizatidine (Axid), and famotidine (Pepcid) should be taken with food. This drug can elevate AST/ALT and creatinine, cause confusion in elderly individuals, and cause diarrhea, constipation, or urticaria.
- Analgesics and corticosteroids. When taken over a long time, analgesics and corticosteroids may cause gastrointestinal bleeding and ulceration; take with food.
- Ranitidine (Zantac) can cause nausea, constipation, and vitamin B_{12} malabsorption.
- Vitamin B_{12} may be needed as an injection, in some cases.
- Sodium bicarbonate, used as an antacid, can precipitate milk-alkali syndrome, if taken with calcium-containing drugs and food.
- Aluminum hydroxide (Amphojel) should be taken between meals, followed by water. It binds with phosphate and may lead to constipation and anorexia. Gaviscon contains magnesium as well as aluminum and may decrease absorption of thiamine, phosphate, and vitamin A. Gelusil contains magnesium, aluminum, and simethicone; it may have side effects similar to those of Gaviscon.
- Omeprazole (Prilosec) inhibits acid secretion completely (Hosking et al., 1994). Abdominal pain, diarrhea, nausea, and vomiting are common side effects. In patients with bleeding peptic ulcers and signs of recent bleeding, treatment with omeprazole decreases the rate of further bleeding and the need for surgery (Elta 2002).
- Carafate (sucralfate) helps some ulcers heal by forming a protective coating; constipation is one side effect.

Herbs, Botanicals and Supplements

- Herbs and botanical supplements should not be used without discussing with the physician.
- Ginger may be used as an antinauseant. Do not use large doses with warfarin, aspirin, other antiplatelet drugs, antihypertensive drugs, and hypoglycemic drugs. Additive effects can cause unpredictable changes in blood pressure, decreases in blood glucose levels, and may decrease platelet aggregation and therefore, increase bleeding. Ginger ale is commonly used with few side effects.
- Licorice root may be recommended for gastric and duodenal ulcers. Do not take with digoxin, because it may cause potassium loss and digoxin toxicity. Licorice root may potentiate the effects of steroids, especially hydrocortisone, progesterone, and estrogens. Also avoid taking with thiazide diuretics and antihypertensive medications because of increased sodium and water retention, along with potential hypokalemia; spironolactone is especially antagonized by licorice root.
- Banana, garlic, cabbage and yellow root have been recommended for this condition, but no clinical trials have proven efficacy.

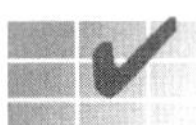

PATIENT EDUCATION

- ✓ Discuss that perfectionism and a stressful lifestyle may increase the pain of an ulcer.
- ✓ Discuss the role of any fluid in increasing gastric acidity and the flow of pepsin, as well as the importance of not skipping meals.
- ✓ As needed by the individual, offer guidance about dietary alterations that may be useful.
- ✓ Discuss the need to complete treatments for eradication of *H. pylori* bacteria, where present. One treatment is usually not sufficient.

For More Information

- American Digestive Health Foundation
  7910 Woodmont Ave., Suite 700
  Bethesda, MD 20814-3015
  301-654-2635
  1-800-NO-ULCER
  http://www.gastro.org/adhf.html
- Helicobacter Foundation
  PO Box 7965
  Charlottesville, VA 22906-7965
  http://www.helico.com/

GASTRECTOMY AND/OR VAGOTOMY

NUTRITIONAL ACUITY RANKING: LEVEL 3

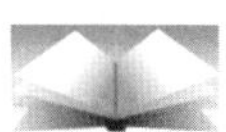

DEFINITIONS AND BACKGROUND

Gastrectomy and vagotomy are surgical procedures that are used for gastric carcinoma or when medical management for peptic ulcer has not worked. Perforation is one of the main reasons why the surgery must be done. Surgery for peptic ulcer is associated with an increased risk of later development of gastric carcinoma occurring in the distal stomach (MacDonald and Owen, 2001).

Billroth I (gastroduodenostomy) is an anastomosis between the stomach and duodenum after removal of the distal portion of the stomach. Billroth II (gastrojejunostomy) is an anastomosis between the stomach and jejunum after removal of two-thirds and three-fourths of the stomach. Iron loss can occur.

Vagotomy is a procedure in which the vagus nerve is cut to reduce pain. Much less nutritional intervention is required for the vagotomy than for the other two procedures. However, gastrectomy or vagotomy may result in reactive hypoglycemia, which may reduce the plasma glucose levels as low as 30–40 mg/dL due to rapid digestion and absorption of food, especially carbohydrates.

Partial gastrectomy usually leads to fast emptying, but if performed after vagotomy, it may lead to gastric stasis in patients (Mistiaen, 2001). Gastric emptying rate for solids may increase in a few of these patients. In most of them, however, there is a normal to decreased emptying rate. When vagotomy precedes the resective procedure, gastric emptying rate decreases significantly (Mistiaen et al., 2001).

OBJECTIVES

Preoperative:

- ▲ Empty the stomach and upper intestines.
- ▲ Ensure high-calorie intake for glycogen stores and weight maintenance or weight gain if needed.
- ▲ Maintain normal fluid and electrolyte balance.
- ▲ Ensure adequate nutrient storage to promote postoperative wound healing.

Postoperative:

- ▲ Prevent distention and pain. Reduce the likelihood of the dumping syndrome: nausea, vomiting, abdominal distention, diarrhea, malaise, profuse sweating, hypoglycemia, hypotension, increased bowel sounds, and vertigo. Additional use of soy and fermentable fiber may be useful. Liquid fiber (such as pectin products) also may be considered to prolong gastric emptying time if needed (Brown et al., 1993).
- ▲ Compensate for loss of storage/holding space and lessen dumping of large amounts of chyme into the duodenum/jejunum at one time.
- ▲ Overcome negative nitrogen balance from surgery. Restore nutritional status.
- ▲ Overcome effects of decreased hormonal output (secretin, pancreozymin, cholecystokinin) from changes in chyme and timing.
- ▲ Prevent or correct iron malabsorption (Billroth II): weight loss, steatorrhea, calcium malabsorption, and vitamin B_{12} or folacin anemias.

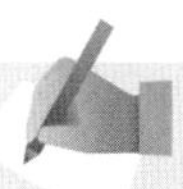

DIETARY AND NUTRITIONAL RECOMMENDATIONS

Preoperative:

- Use a soft diet that is high in calories with adequate protein and vitamins C and K.
- Regress to full liquids, then NPO.

Postoperative:

- Intake of complex carbohydrates such as bread, rice, and vegetables should be liberal (50–60%). To lessen the hyperosmolar load, use only 0–15% simple sugars (i.e., sucrose, fructose, glucose). A total calorie increase will be needed for repletion.
- Lactose intolerance is common in patients with these conditions; use less milk or omit if needed. Monitor calcium intake carefully.
- Moderate fat intake (30% of total kilocalories). Use less cholesterol. MCTs may be beneficial.
- Diet should provide moderate sodium intake; excess salt draws fluid into the duodenum. If there is diarrhea, losses of sodium in the stool may occur.
- Fluids should be taken 1 hour before or after meals, rather than with meals; assure adequate fluid intake overall.
- Avoid extremes in food temperature.
- Diet should provide frequent, small meals.
- Diet should provide adequate fiber, chromium, vitamin B_{12}, riboflavin, iron, and folacin.

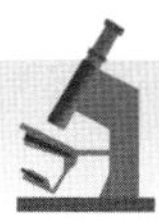

PROFILE

Clinical/History

Height
Weight
BMI
Gluc
BP

Lab Work

H&H, Serum Fe
Serum ferritin
Chol, Trig
PT
K+, Na+, Cl−
GTT
Blood guaiac
Urine acetone
White blood cell count (WBC)
BUN
Alb, prealbumin
RBP
Amylase
Transferrin
Serum B_{12}
Ca++
Serum folate
TIBC

Common Drugs Used and Potential Side Effects

- Cholinergic blocking agents (such as dicyclomine, Pro-Banthine) may cause dry mouth. Rinse mouth with water before meals. These agents are used to delay gastric emptying.
- Drugs that slow GI activity should be taken before meals.
- Antibiotics may be used to control bacterial overgrowth.
- Antidiarrheals such as Kaopectate and loperamide may be useful. Dry mouth, nausea, vomiting, and bloating may occur. Use plenty of fluids.
- For the reactive hypoglycemia, use of an alpha-glucosidase inhibitor, acarbose, may be beneficial.

Herbs, Botanicals and Supplements

- Herbs and botanical supplements should not be used without discussing with the physician.

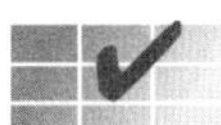

PATIENT EDUCATION

- ✔ Stress the importance of self-care and optimal functioning—what to do for illness, stress, eating away from home, and how to read labels.
- ✔ Discuss the use of artificial sweeteners.
- ✔ Instruct the patient to eat slowly in an upright position and to relax after meals.
- ✔ Discuss the social significance of food and alcohol with the patient.
- ✔ Help the patient to overcome reluctance and the fear of pain with eating.
- ✔ Discuss the dumping syndrome and its effects on nutrient absorption if untreated. If late dumping syndrome with postprandial hypoglycemia occurs, use of fast-acting carbohydrate (CHO) should be discussed (e.g., orange juice, sugar).

DIARRHEA OR ACUTE ENTERITIS

NUTRITIONAL ACUITY RANKING: LEVEL 2

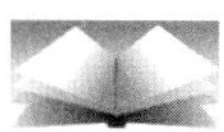

DEFINITIONS AND BACKGROUND

Diarrhea (acute enteritis) is a symptom of many disorders in which there is usually an increased peristalsis with decreased transit time through the GI tract; see Table 7–8. Reduced reabsorption of water and watery stools result. Diarrhea may be functional (from irritation or stress), organic (from intestinal lesion), osmotic (from carbohydrate intolerance), or secretory (from bacteria, viruses, bile acids, laxatives, or hormones). The secretory type is typically more serious.

Chronic diarrhea is production of loose stools with or without increased frequency for more than 4 weeks; it affects 3–5% of the U.S. population (American Gastroenterology Association, 1999). Etiologic factors for chronic diarrhea include celiac disease, cow's milk allergy, bacterial and parasitic factors, cystic fibrosis, and postinfectious gastroenteritis (Altuntas, 1999).

Rotavirus or Norwalk viruses commonly affect infants and school-aged children; vomiting and watery diarrhea may occur. Some stool specimens from nursing home residents, who become ill during outbreaks of gastroenteritis, are positive for Norwalk-like viruses (NLVs); there may be a major role for NLVs as etiologic agents of gastroenteritis in elderly persons (Green et al., 2002).

Bacteria such as *Salmonella, Shigella, Campylobacter, Yersinia, Escherichia coli,* and *Vibrio cholerae* cause varying degrees of diarrhea. Parasites such as *Giardia lamblia* are common in children 1–5-years-old, with flatulence, watery and foul-smelling stools, and abdominal pain. *Giardia lamblia* is the best-known cause of protozoal disease in North America; diagnosis is a challenge, but treatment is usually a success (Juckett, 1996). *Entamoeba histolytica* causes severe dysentery. *Cryptosporidium parvum, Balantidium coli, Isospora belli, Sarcocystis,* and other newly described protozoa may cause diarrhea in healthy persons or intractable life-threatening illness in immunosuppressed persons (Juckett, 1996). Many of these protozoa are transmitted through contaminated water supplies.

In severe protein–calorie malnutrition (PCM), diarrhea and other infections are common. Weight loss also can be caused by diarrhea. Hypoglycemia is a potentially fatal complication of infectious diarrhea in children. Dehydration is a common problem; watch for decreased skin turgor, dry mucous membranes, thirst, 2% weight loss or more, low blood pressure, postural hypotension, increased BUN and hematocrit (Hct), or decreased urinary output.

Malnutrition may be a major consequence of early childhood diarrhea and enteric infections, because enteric infections may critically impair intestinal absorptive function with potential long-term consequences for growth and development. The potentially huge, largely undefined DALY (disability-adjusted life years) impact of early childhood diarrheal illnesses demonstrates the importance of quantifying the long-term functional impact of largely preventable nutritional and infectious diseases, especially in children in developing areas (Guerrant et al., 2000). Early rehydration may prevent many deaths in high-risk infants if mothers seek medical attention and offer proper rehydration solutions as soon as diarrhea begins (Kilgore et al., 1995). New rice-electrolyte oral rehydration solutions (ORS) are well tolerated (Lebenthal et al., 1995) and shorten illness and decrease fluid losses by 20–30%.

Clostridium difficile is a gram-positive anaerobic bacterium most often responsible for antibiotic-associated diarrhea. The infection clinically ranges from asymptomatic carrier states to severe colitis. Ther may be profuse watery diarrhea that may be foul smelling, abdominal pain, cramping, and tenderness; stools that may be guaiac positive and occasionally grossly bloody; fever and white blood cell count 12,000–20,000. In severe cases, toxic megacolon, colonic perforation, and peritonitis may develop. Other complications include electrolyte abnormalities, hypovolemic shock, anasarca caused by hypoalbuminemia, sepsis, and hemorrhage. Although classically associated with clindamycin or cephalosporin use, *C. difficile* colitis can be caused by almost any antibiotic. Symptoms may develop within a few days or even 6–10 weeks after antibiotic therapy is completed. Toxin detection by latex agglutination, immunobinding assay, or Enzyme linked immunosorbent assay (ELISA) make the diagnosis. Because *C. difficile* may be a normal bowel organism (especially in children), simply culturing the organism does not mean that diarrhea is caused by *C. difficile*. Those patients with mild symptoms will usually resolve infection spontaneously once the causative antibiotic is withdrawn. More severe cases warrant therapy with oral antibiotic therapy. Both vancomycin and metronidazole for 10 days are effective therapies.

OBJECTIVES

- Determine causation and treatment.
- Prevent or alleviate dehydration, electrolyte imbalances, anemia, weight loss, and hypoglycemia. Avoid cautious refeeding, which leads to reduction in nutrient intake and atrophy of the gut (Booth, 1993; Meyers, 1993).
- Alter stool consistency and quantity. Up to 200 g of stool per day is normal.
- Restore normal bowel motility. Alimentary tract feeding maintains gut integrity; bowel rest (TPN) results in atrophy.
- Avoid extremes in temperatures, which stimulate colonic activity.
- Correct intolerances for CHO and protein. Ensure adequate fat intake.
- Short-chain fatty acids enhance sodium reabsorption; include adequate fiber.
- Probiotics may be useful, with friendly, live active cultures that help deter further diarrhea.

TABLE 7–8 Acute Diarrhea of Infectious Origin

Infectious Agent	*Age*	*Pathogenic Mechanism*	*Signs and Symptoms*
Viruses:			
Rotavirus	4–24 mos	Enteroinvasive	Vomiting, low-grade fever 1–2 days; watery diarrhea up to 1 week; dehydration; respiratory symptoms
Norwalk virus	School age; elderly	Enteroinvasive	24–48 hours of vomiting, diarrhea, nausea, cramps, headache, low-grade fever, anorexia, malaise, myalgia
Bacteria:			
Escherichia coli	<2 yrs	Enterotoxigenic	Voluminous, watery, green, foul-smelling stools, dehydration
Escherichia coli	All ages	Enteroinvasive	Small-volume watery or dysentery-like stools; fever; abdominal pain; tenesmus
Salmonella	<1 yr	Enteroinvasive	Fever; abdominal pain; tenesmus; vomiting for about 1 week; leukocytes in the stools
Shigella	6 mos–3 yrs	Enteroinvasive	Fever, abdominal pain, tenesmus; voluminous watery and bloody stools for 14 days; convulsions
Vibrio cholera	All ages	Enterotoxigenic	Voluminous, watery stools; dehydration
Campylobacter	<5 yrs	Enteroinvasive	Mild diarrhea with liquid, foul-smelling bloody stools; fever, abdominal pain, vomiting lasting 7–12 days
Yersinia	All ages	Enteroinvasive	Watery diarrhea, occasionally bloody stools; abdominal pain, fever, vomiting; may be mistaken for appendicitis
Parasites:			
Giardia lamblia	1–5 yrs	Mucosal adhesion	Flatulence; watery, foul-smelling stools; abdominal pain; symptoms acute or chronic

Based on data from: Ross Laboratories. *Acute diarrhea in infants and children*. Ross Laboratories: Columbus, OH, 1986.

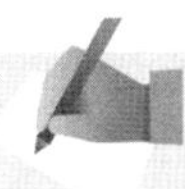

DIETARY AND NUTRITIONAL RECOMMENDATIONS

- NPO for 12 hours with intravenous fluids and electrolytes; start oral fluids as soon as allowed. Oral rehydration therapy (ORT) should be used; use Ceralyte or the WHO solution, which contains 2% glucose, some sodium, potassium, and citrate as a base. (See Table 7–9.) The addition of resistant starch to a standard ORT solution reduces fecal fluid loss and shortens duration of diarrhea in patients with cholera (Ramakrishna et al., 2000).

TABLE 7–9 Oral Rehydration Formula

⅓–⅔ table salt
¾ t sodium bicarbonate
⅓ t potassium chloride
3–⅓ T sugar
1 L boiled or sterile water
Source: World Health Organization.

Fluid repletion. A simple oral rehydration solution may be composed of 1 level teaspoon of salt and 4 heaping teaspoons of sugar added to 1 liter of water. Bottled flavored mineral water with saltine crackers is an acceptable alternative. Another option: Ceralyte All-Natural Oral Rehydration Solution – rice-based lytes and CHO powder.

- Use TPN only for intractable diarrhea. Osmotic diarrhea abates with NPO.
- As stools are formed, reintroduce small amounts of food. Temporarily omit lactose, test tolerance; in infants, full-strength formula should be used. Some fiber or pectins may help. Potassium should be replenished.
  - Adults. Start with broth, tea, toast, and gradually add foods to a normal diet as tolerance progresses. Three to four small meals may be better tolerated. Products such as Gatorade may be useful. Banana flakes may be a safe, cost-effective treatment for diarrhea in critically ill patients on tube feedings (TF), even while waiting for results of *C. difficile* testing (Emery et al., 1997). Use products containing probiotics, such as yogurt with live cultures. For fluid repletion see Table 7–9.
  - Infants. Use 50% strength formula (low in fat and CHO) or use Nutramigen for 24 hours. A mixture of 5–10% apple powder, banana flakes, or pectin-sugar can be added to the formula. Or, use rehydration solutions if allowed. Breastfeeding may be continued, or return to lactose-containing formula when feasible. Cut back on use of Sorbitol (as in apple juice, peaches).
- If TF is being used, check tube placement. Assessment of diarrhea in enterally fed patients includes checking medications, bloody stools, and endoscopic exams. Treatment includes changing medications, decreasing rate of feeding, changing formula, antibiotic therapy, or using anti-

diarrheal medications (Williams et al., 1998). High-fiber products are recommended in many cases. A jejunal placement may be too far for some patients.

- Short-chain fatty acids from high-fiber sources may be useful as intestinal fuels.
- High-sugar, clear-liquid diets are prescribed inappropriately for diarrhea (Goepp and Katz, 1993).

PROFILE

Clinical/History

Height
Weight
BMI
Weight changes
Stool consistency
BP
I & O; dehydration?
Temperature
Abdominal pain

Lab Work

Na+ (decreased)
K+, Cl−
Stool culture such as for *C. difficile*
Biopsy
BUN/Creat ratio
Gluc
Alb, prealbumin
Serum copper
N balance
Transferrin
H&H, Serum Fe
Lactose tolerance test
H-breath test

Common Drugs Used and Potential Side Effects

- Antidiarrheal drugs are used to slow peristalsis or thicken stools. Kaolin (Kaopectate) has no major side effects but is not useful with infants. Lomotil should be taken with food. Lomotil may cause bloating, constipation, dry mouth, swollen gums, dizziness, nausea, and vomiting. Psyllium ingestion reduces stool looseness without changing the percentage of water (Wenzl et al., 1995).
- Infants may benefit from smectite (mineral clay), soluble fiber (soy polysaccharide), or bismuth subsalicylate (e.g., Pepto-Bismol). Monitor carefully.
- Antibiotics are used if shigellae or amoebae are causing the problem.
- Cholestyramine (Questran) may be used for bile acid diarrhea. Nausea, belching, or constipation may result. Replace fat-soluble vitamins.
- Opiates such as Imodium (loperamide HCl) can decrease propulsive diarrhea action. They also may cause abdominal pain, nausea, vomiting, and dry mouth; they are not to be used for children.
- Multivitamin/mineral supplements may be needed to replace vitamins A and C, zinc, iron, and other nutrients. Megadoses of vitamin C actually may cause diarrhea (e.g., more than 1 g daily).
- Sorbitol may cause diarrhea; it is found in many medications.
- Flagyl or Vancomycin is used for treating *C. difficile*. Anorexia, GI distress, diarrhea, and nausea may result.
- Intestinal flora modifiers (e.g., Lactobacillus acidophilus, Lactinex, Bacid) help recolonize normal intestinal flora in people on antibiotics. A common order is 3–4 packages every day for 3 days for adults. It may be mixed with water for tube feedings.
- Magnesium-containing antacids, digoxin, broad-spectrum antibiotics, antifungal agents, colchicine, thiazide diuretics and other antihypertensives, Azulfidine, methotrexate and other anticancer agents, cholinergic stimulants, antiemetics such as Reglan, and laxatives such as mineral oil or methylcellulose may cause drug-induced diarrhea. Every patient should receive a careful medication review.

Herbs, Botanicals and Supplements

- Herbs and botanical supplements should not be used without discussing with the physician.
- Apple, carrot, blackberry, carob, bilberry, and tea have been recommended, but no clinical trials have proven efficacy.

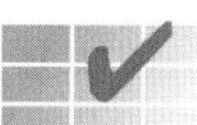

PATIENT EDUCATION

- ✔ Describe the effects of pectin as a thickening agent (in apples and bananas).
- ✔ Avoid carbonated beverages. Electrolyte content is low; osmolality is high.
- ✔ Avoid alcoholic beverages when using Lomotil.
- ✔ Caffeine can aggravate diarrhea; omit until the problem clears.
- ✔ After diarrhea improves, gradually return to milk, if tolerated.
- ✔ Omit apple juice until tolerance is established. The average child consumes 5–21 oz of fruit juice each day. Some CHO malabsorption may aggravate the condition.
- ✔ "Probiotics" can help to maintain good bacteria in the GI tract of those taking antibiotics. *Lactobacillus casei GG* may be a useful strain of bacteria; research is ongoing.
- ✔ Yogurt may also help to reculture the GI tract; check labels for active cultures. Acidophilus milk is also useful.

For More Information

- Ceralyte
  http://www.ceralyte.com
- CDC Division of Parasitic Diseases
  http://www.cdc.gov/ncidod/dpd/parasiticpathways/diarrhea.htm
- Giardiasis
  http://www.dpd.cdc.gov/dpdx/HTML/Giardiasis.htm
- Rehydration Formula
  http://www.rehydrate.org/

DYSENTERY OR TRAVELER'S DIARRHEA

NUTRITIONAL ACUITY RANKING: LEVEL 2

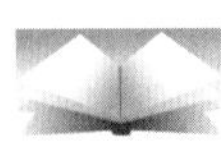

DEFINITIONS AND BACKGROUND

Dysentery, inflammation of the bowel, results from poor sanitation; causes range from contact with feces to contamination by houseflies. Symptoms include diarrhea, often with blood and mucus, intestinal rumbling, cramps, fever, and pus in stools. (See Food-borne Illness and Diarrhea entries as well.)

Traveler's diarrhea (TD) is usually caused by enterotoxic bacteria (*E. coli, Campylobacter, shigella, salmonella,* or *yersinia*) or viruses or protozoa (Juckett 1999) from contaminated food or water; *Giardia* is less common. The Norwalk virus causes vomiting, headache, and muscle pain. *Entamoeba histolytica* causes severe dysentery. Prophylaxis is not routinely recommended because of the risk of adverse effects from the drugs (i.e., rash, anaphylaxis, vaginal candidiasis) and the development of resistant gut flora. Possible regimens for prophylaxis include bismuth subsalicylate (Pepto-Bismol) with meals.

According to the CDC, high-risk destinations include most countries in Latin America, Africa, the Middle East, and Asia. Both cooked and uncooked foods are a concern if they have been improperly handled; risky foods include raw or undercooked meat and seafood and raw fruits and vegetables. Tap water, ice, and unpasteurized milk and dairy products can be associated with increased risk.

OBJECTIVES

- Reduce irritation and inflammation of the GI tract.
- Prevent dehydration.
- Reintroduce fiber as quickly as tolerated to restore bowel motility.
- Address sanitation issues regarding food and water supplies; prevent reinfection. Use safe, bottled water for drinking and brushing teeth; wash hands before eating using antiseptic gel or hand wipes; avoid ice in drinks; do not eat raw vegetables or salads, raw fruits, or unpasteurized dairy products. Avoid swimming in streams and lakes.

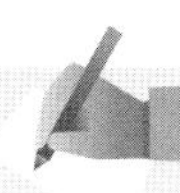

DIETARY AND NUTRITIONAL RECOMMENDATIONS

- Extra amounts of clear liquids (e.g., broth, tea, plain gelatin) should be taken during the acute stages. Oral rehydration therapy solutions may be useful.
- Quickly add nonirritating, low-fiber foods (such as rice, bread, potatoes, plain crackers, and bananas). Water-soluble fiber from apples, oranges, and oatmeal may be helpful to add pectin.

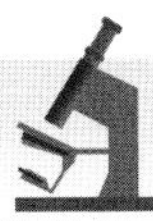

PROFILE

Clinical/History

Height
Weight
Weight changes
BMI
Stool—number, consistency
I & O

Lab Work

K+, Na+
Cl−
Alb
H&H, Serum Fe
Gluc
Serum folate
BUN, Creat
Stool examination

- If the patient is unable to consume oral products, consider tube feeding. Use products that contain fiber and glutamine whenever possible. If diarrhea persists for longer than 1 week, TPN may be needed; review with physician.
- Safe beverages include bottled carbonated beverages (especially flavored beverages), beer, wine, hot boiled coffee or tea, or water boiled and appropriately treated with iodine or chlorine. Purified bottled water is acceptable.
- Include probiotics such as yogurt with live cultures.

Common Drugs Used and Potential Side Effects

- Ciprofloxacin is used; one dose is often sufficient. It is a quinolone-class antibiotic. Avoid milk or yogurt. Nausea is one side effect.
- Antibiotics are not used in mild cases unless there is fever or bloody stools. Tetracycline, chloramphenicol, or co-trimoxazole should be taken with food to reduce GI distress. Use 3 hours separately from vitamin–mineral supplements.
- Lomotil may be used. Dry mouth can occur. Avoid alcohol.
- Nonprescription loperamide (Imodium) may be useful. Dry mouth or nausea may result. It can be added to the fluoroquinolones when treating TD; continue for 1 or 2 days after patient returns home.
- Flagyl (Protostat, metronidazole) can cause abdominal cramps, constipation, diarrhea, nausea, vomiting, and anorexia. Avoid use of alcoholic beverages.

Herbs, Botanicals and Supplements

- Herbs and botanical supplements should not be used without discussing with the physician.

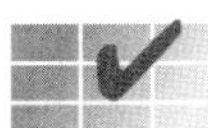

PATIENT EDUCATION

- ✔ Use only cooked foods and bottled beverages (e.g., water, juices, beer, etc.).
- ✔ Instruct the patient to brush his/her teeth with bottled water only.
- ✔ Instruct the patient concerning the possible danger of fresh foods, that may have been washed in contaminated water, foods prepared with unheated water (e.g., jello), and ice cubes added to beverages.
- ✔ If symptoms persist, medical attention should be sought.
- ✔ Bismuth subsalicylate may be protective.

For More Information

- ✦ CDC's Travelers Health
  1-888-232-3228
  http://www.cdc.gov/travel/diarrhea.htm

FAT MALABSORPTION SYNDROME

NUTRITIONAL ACUITY RANKING: LEVEL 3

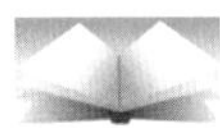

DEFINITIONS AND BACKGROUND

Fat malabsorption syndrome is caused by functional or organic causes. Symptoms and signs include fatigue, weight changes, altered bowel movements, and laboratory abnormalities. Causes may include: GI tract—postgastrectomy, blind loop syndrome, or small bowel resection; pancreas—cystic fibrosis, chronic pancreatitis, or pancreatectomy; biliary—biliary atresia; other causes—gluten enteropathy, lipoprotein deficiency, or diabetic steatorrhea.

Intake of olestra can cause false-positive results on tests for steatorrhea and can lead to an erroneous diagnosis of malabsorption syndrome. A 40-gram intake of olestra daily for 6 days was found to mimic the malabsorption syndrome (Balasekaran et al., 2000).

Low total cholesterol (under 120 mg/dL) or low serum carotene levels may be typical of fat malabsorption but are not necessarily diagnostic. Altered stools characterize different types of malabsorption (see Table 7–10); a fecal fat study may be useful (see Table 7–11).

OBJECTIVES

- Alleviate steatorrhea and reduce intake of fat sources that are not tolerated. Medium-chain triglycerides (MCT) are useful. See Table 7–12.
- Correct vitamin E deficiency, which may enhance cellular immunity (T cells).

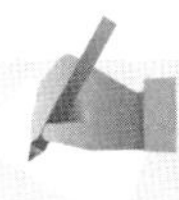

DIETARY AND NUTRITIONAL RECOMMENDATIONS

- Initial treatment should consist of parenteral solutions or liquid formula emulsions (carbohydrates, 45%; protein, 15%; MCTs, 40%) such as Portagen. MCTs alleviate steatorrhea in some cases; start with 20–60 g and increase gradually.
- For moderate to severe cases, tube feed if necessary (50 mL/hr full strength initially; advance gradually).
- For mild cases, oral feeding is preferred because it stimulates brush-border activity.
- Dietary fat may be limited to one egg and 4–6 oz of meat, poultry, or fish. Gradually check tolerance for LCTs and work up to 30–40 g.
- Increase intake of protein, which may be in the form of skim milk, egg white, cereals, or legumes.
- Complex carbohydrates may be better tolerated than simple sugars. Lactose may not be tolerated.
- A multivitamin/mineral supplement may be necessary to offset fecal losses of nutrients, vitamins, and water in patients with malabsorption syndromes—especially zinc, folate, vitamin B12, calcium, magnesium, iron, and fat-soluble vitamins. Vitamin E deficiency is common (Kowdley et al., 1992).
- Monitor oxalate intake to prevent renal stones; decrease dietary sources as needed.

TABLE 7–10 Altered Stool/Nutrients Involved

Characteristic	*Disorder*
Yellow or silver color	Fat malabsorption
Pale, foamy, mushy, or floating	Pan malabsorption
Formed in AM	Diarrhea
Formed in PM	Bile salt malabsorption

TABLE 7–11 Fecal Fat Study

Fat absorption is tested by quantitative measurement of total fat in the stool.
Preparation = 100 g of long-chain triglycerides (LCT) × 3 days should be consumed.
Normal excretion = 3.5 g (5% of a 60–100 g intake)
Mild malabsorption = less than 25 g (defects in micelle formation)
Moderate malabsorption = 25–30 g (intestinal mucosal disease)
Severe malabsorption = more than 40 g (massive ileal resection or pancreatic disease)

Source: Hermann-Zaidins M. Malabsorption. *J Am Diet Assoc.* 1986;86:1171.

TABLE 7–12 Medium-Chain Triglycerides

Medium-chain triglycerides use portal rather than lymphatic system transport (as albumin-free fatty acids) and absorption (using less lipase and bile). Many products now contain MCTs as the primary fat source; Osmolite and Isocal contain MCTs for tube feedings.
MCTs have an 8- to 10-carbon source of fat when longer-chain fats (16–18 carbons) cannot be efficiently digested or absorbed. MCTs have concentrated calories made from coconut oil for adjunct therapy.
MCT oil has 230 kcal/30 mL (6–7 kcal/g). Use instead of vegetable oil in recipes. One cup of Portagen powder has 240 kcal (MCTs, 10 g; protein, vitamins, and minerals, 8.4 g); 1 T of the powder (14 g) has 116 kcal.

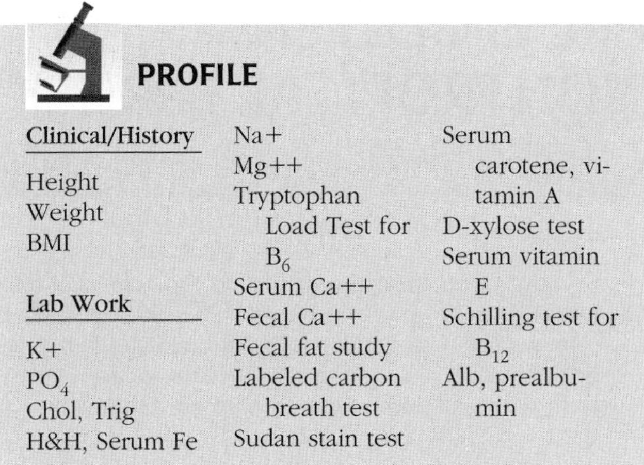

PROFILE

Clinical/History		
Height	Na+	Serum carotene, vitamin A
Weight	Mg++	D-xylose test
BMI	Tryptophan Load Test for B_6	Serum vitamin E
	Serum Ca++	Schilling test for B_{12}
Lab Work	Fecal Ca++	Alb, prealbumin
K+	Fecal fat study	
PO_4	Labeled carbon breath test	
Chol, Trig	Sudan stain test	
H&H, Serum Fe		

Common Drugs Used and Potential Side Effects

- Antibiotics are used for bacterial overgrowth.
- Pancreatic enzymes may be needed for pancreatic insufficiencies.
- Cholestyramine may be needed for bile-salt diarrhea. Fat-soluble vitamins can be depleted.
- Antidiarrheals may be used such as Kaolin (Kaopectate).

Herbs, Botanicals and Supplements

- Herbs and botanical supplements should not be used without discussing with the physician.

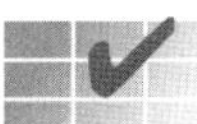

PATIENT EDUCATION

- ✔ Caution the patient about rapid consumption of MCTs; if they are consumed too rapidly, hyperosmolar diarrhea may result.
- ✔ Remember that a source of essential fatty acids may be needed if MCTs are used with a low-fat diet.
- ✔ Abdominal discomfort, flatulence, diarrhea, or steatorrhea may indicate continued malabsorption; the physician should be contacted.

CELIAC DISEASE (CELIAC SPRUE, GLUTEN-INDUCED ENTEROPATHY, NONTROPICAL SPRUE)

NUTRITIONAL ACUITY RANKING: LEVEL 4

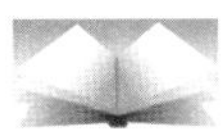

DEFINITIONS AND BACKGROUND

Celiac disease (celiac sprue) is a lifelong inflammatory condition of the GI tract that affects the small intestine; it affects genetically predisposed individuals (American Gastroenterological Association, 2001). The condition is more common than previously believed, affecting 1 out of every 120–300 persons in Europe and North America (Farrell and Kelly, 2002).

Celiac sprue results from an inappropriate T-cell–mediated immune response against ingested gluten in genetically predisposed people (Farrell and Kelly, 2002). People who have celiac disease (CD) do not tolerate amino acid sequences found in the prolamin fraction of wheat, rye, and barley (Thompson, 2000). When these grains are consumed, they damage the mucosa of the small intestine, which eventually leads to malabsorption of nutrients. Moderate amounts of oats can be consumed (Thompson, 1997); however, much of the commercially available oat flour is contaminated with wheat gluten (American Gastroenterological Association, 2001).

CD involves mucosal malabsorption and is caused either by an inborn error of metabolism or immunologic sensitivity to gliadin by the small intestines. Villi are decreased in number, with less absorptive surface and fewer enzymes in the damaged cells; crypts are markedly elongated. Symptoms and signs include frequent, foul-smelling stools that are pale and foamy, diarrhea, irritability, a distended abdomen, easy fatigue, pallor, weight loss, vomiting, and anemia. Dyspepsia occurs in 30–40% of these individuals (Bardella et al., 2000).

Immunoglobulin M antibodies and immunoglobulin A antigliadin (AGA-IgA) antibodies in gut secretions may be markers for latent CD; a high intraepithelial lymphocyte (IEL) count may also be indicative (Arranz and Ferguson, 1993). Immunoglobulin G antigliadin (AGA-IgG), AGA-IgA, and antiendomysium (EMA) antibodies are useful markers for identifying patients who should undergo a small-intestinal biopsy (Hill et al., 2000).

Many patients with CD continue to experience chronic diarrhea after treatment with a gluten-free diet; other causes should be explored (Fine et al., 1997). Microscopic colitis, steatorrhea secondary to exocrine pancreatic insufficiency, dietary lactose or fructose malabsorption, anal sphincter dysfunction causing fecal incontinence, and inflammatory bowel disease may cause diarrhea that will not subside.

Diagnosis can occur at any age (infancy through old age), often after stress, pregnancy, or viral infections. Infants may present with impaired growth, diarrhea, abdominal distention, pallor, edema, or vomiting; untreated celiac sprue may lead to short stature, pubertal delay, iron or folate deficiencies with anemia, and rickets (Farrell and Kelly, 2002). Pica and growth failure often precede diagnosis in infants or children. In pregnant women, severe anemia may persist; other adults may have episodic or nocturnal diarrhea, flatulence, intestinal bloating, which mimics irritable bowel syndrome, steatorrhea, weight loss, recurrent aphthous stomatitis, or anemias (Farrell and Kelly, 2002).

Early diagnosis is important, because it is harder to normalize body composition when CD is diagnosed in adulthood (Barera et al., 2000). Fecal chymotrypsin level (an index of exocrine pancreatic function) can predict weight recovery in the first months after diagnosis of CD and may be used to select patients for enzyme supplementation therapy (Carroccio et al., 1997). Dermatitis herpetiformis is characterized by intensely pruritic papulovesicular lesions that occur over the surface of the arm, legs, buttocks, trunk, neck, or scalp (Farrell and Kelly, 2002). It may be useful to monitor closely for thyroid disorders in this population as well (Hakanen, 2001).

If the defect is permanent, diet also must be permanent. It may be helpful to add new foods to the diet gradually, closely monitoring the patient's responses. In 50–60% of celiac patients who follow a strict diet, there are eventually few or no symptoms; the term gluten sensitivity is then used for patients with regular, atypical, or latent disease (Marsh, 1993).

CD should be considered in patients, even older patients, who have unexplained metabolic bone disease or hypocalcemia, especially because GI symptoms may be absent or mild (Shaker et al., 1997). Children and teens with CD have lower bone density of the lumbar spine and whole body than healthy children (Mora et al., 1998). Careful attention to bone health will be essential; bone fractures may be more common in this population (Farrell and Kelly, 2002). Gastroenterologists should follow patients with this condition, which is a form of inflammatory bowel disease, to reduce morbidity and mortality (Abdulkarim and Murray, 2002).

OBJECTIVES

- Remove the offending protein (gliadin fraction) from the diet. Glutenin is harmless. Improvement is noted within 4–5 days.
- Improve the patient's nutritional status. Deficiencies of iron, folate, calcium, and vitamin D may be found in patients with untreated disease. Combined iron and folate deficiency is a characteristic consequence of enteropathy of the proximal portion of the small bowel but is less frequent than iron-deficiency anemia (Farrell and Kelly, 2002).
- Replace nutrients (magnesium, calcium, and vitamins A, D, E, and K) lost from diarrhea and steatorrhea.

- Overcome anorexia with pleasant meals.
- Reverse bone demineralization. Calcium malabsorption in CD does not result from absence of vitamin D receptors but from reduction in vitamin D-regulated proteins located in the enterocytes of the villi that are essential for calcium absorption (Colston et al., 1994). The patient may need calcium supplements (Corazza et al., 1995).
- Correct hypoalbuminemia and hypoprothrombinemia if present. A dramatic increase in whole-body protein breakdown is common in CD, contributing to a high level of PCM; glutamine is an important fuel for the health of intestinal epithelial cells (Lima Dutra et al., 1999).

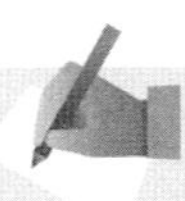

DIETARY AND NUTRITIONAL RECOMMENDATIONS

- A gliadin-free/gluten-restricted diet excludes wheat, buckwheat, rye, and barley. Oats do not damage the small-cell mucosa; include small-to-moderate amounts without adverse effects (Thompson, 1997). However, oats are sometimes contaminated with wheat during processing and should be avoided in initial stages of treatment (Farrell and Kelly, 2002).
- Corn, rice, tapioca, potato, arrowroot, cassava, and gluten-free bread can be used freely. There are many resources available for recipe adaptations.
- For infants with diarrhea, provide fluids, electrolytes, and a low-fat formula.
- Diet should provide 1–2 g of protein per kilogram body weight (adult intake, 120 g) from lean meat, whole milk, etc.
- Diet should provide 35–40 kcal/kg body weight for adults. Infants may tolerate banana powder; adults may use simple carbohydrates, gelatin, fruit juice, peanut butter, simple cornstarch pudding, and bananas.
- MCTs often are used with good results, especially in adults.
- Initially, the diet should include low amounts of fiber because of flattening of the mucosal villi. Intake can be increased as tolerated. If tube feeding is used, use a glutamine-enriched product.
- Watch for lactose intolerances that are temporary or permanent. Initially, dairy products should be avoided because these patients often have secondary lactase deficiency, but after 3–6 months of treatment, dairy products may be gradually reintroduced (Farrell and Kelly, 2002).
- Supplements to the diet should include water-miscible vitamins A, D, E, and K, iron, calcium, folic acid, and vitamin B_{12}, thiamine, and other B-complex vitamins. Many of the gluten-free products are lower than typical grains in B vitamins, iron, and dietary fiber (Thompson, 2000).
- Foods that often are not tolerated include cream soups, creamed vegetables, ice cream (labels should be checked for thickening agents), oatmeal (tolerated by some people—check with the physician before using), cakes, cookies, breads (unless made with rice, corn, or potato flours), wheat starch, mixed infant dinners and junior dinners that contain flour thickeners, spaghetti, macaroni, and other pastas.

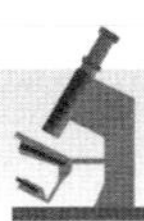

PROFILE

Clinical/History		
Height	Ca++	Antiendomysial antibody (EMA) test
Weight	Mg++	AGA-IgG antibodies
BMI	PO4 (decreased)	IEL count (increased)
Growth pattern (child)	Transferrin, TIBC	Folate tests
Steatorrhea, diarrhea	Serum copper (decreased)	Endoscopy with biopsies
Dermatitis herpetiformis	Lactic acid dehydrogenase (LDH) (increased)	Abdominal CT or MRI scan
Lab Work	Xylose absorption	DEXA scan
Alb, prealbumin	Immunoglobulin M antibodies	Fecal chymotrypsin level
Serum carotene	AGA-IgA antibodies	Fecal fat study
H&H		Liver function tests (mildly abnormal)
Serum Fe and ferritin		
K+, Na+		

Common Drugs Used and Potential Side Effects

No drug therapy has been proven to suppress the disease (Abdulkarim and Murray, 2002).

- Gluten-free laxatives include psyllium seed laxatives (Metamucil, Naturacil), docusate sodium (Surfak), and bisacodyl (Dulcolax).
- Check all labels for gluten-containing ingredients.
- Gliadins are often impurities in medications, including acetaminophen; check carefully.
- Corticosteroids may be used with numerous side effects. Take with food. Weight gain is common. Monitor for negative nitrogen or calcium balances.
- Octreotide may be needed parenterally. Nausea, vomiting, abdominal pain, or diarrhea may occur.
- Correction of vitamin and mineral deficiencies may be helpful in aiding recovery; vitamin D and calcium supplementation is often recommended (Abdulkarim and Murray, 2002).

Herbs, Botanicals and Supplements

- Herbs and botanical supplements should not be used without discussing with the physician.
- With use of bisacodyl, avoid aloe, cascara, senna, and yellow dock because of enhancing effects.

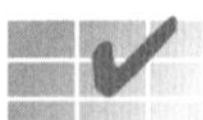

PATIENT EDUCATION

- ✔ The execution and maintenance of the "theoretically simple" exclusion of gluten is difficult; patient education and motivation are crucial to a successful outcome (Abdulkarim and Murray, 2002). An effective gluten-free diet requires extensive, repeated counseling and instruction of the patient by the physician and dietitian (Farrell and Kelly, 2002).
- ✔ Instruct the patient to read food labels for cereal, starch, flour, thickening agents, emulsifiers, gluten, stabilizers, hydrolyzed vegetable proteins, etc. Wheat starch is acceptable because the gliadin/gluten has been removed. Caramel coloring and monosodium glutamate (MSG) may not be tolerated. A gluten-free symbol is used widely by food manufacturers in Europe but, unfortunately, less so in the United States (Farrell and Kelly, 2002).
- ✔ Carefully check the ingredients of all recipes.
- ✔ Because of possible contamination with wheat, oats should be avoided in all patients with newly diagnosed celiac sprue until remission is achieved through the use of a gluten-free diet; then, up to 2 oz of oats from a reliable source can be eaten every day, if the patient has no ill effects (Farrell and Kelly, 2002).
- ✔ Strict lifelong dietary adherence is essential for those persons with true diagnosis of celiac sprue.

For More Information

- American Celiac Society (ACS)
  45 Gifford Avenue
  Jersey City, NJ 07304
  (201) 432-1207
- Celiac Disease and Gluten-Free Diet Support Group
  http://www.celiac.com/
- Celiac Disease Foundation
  13251 Ventura Blvd.
  Studio City, CA 91604-1038
  http://www.celiac.org
- CSA-USA
  PO Box 31700
  Omaha, NE 68131-0700
  402-558-0600
  http://www.csaceliacs.org/
- Gluten Intolerance Group of North America
  P.O. Box 23053
  Seattle, WA 98102-0353
  (206) 325-6980
- National Celiac-Sprue Society
  5 Jeffrey Road
  Wayland, MA 01778
  (617) 358-5150
  (617) 651-3230

TROPICAL SPRUE

NUTRITIONAL ACUITY RANKING: LEVEL 3–4

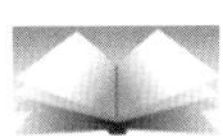

DEFINITIONS AND BACKGROUND

Tropical sprue is an acquired disorder where abnormalities of the small intestine lead to prolonged diarrhea and malabsorption. It occurs after traveling to tropical areas such as the Caribbean, southern India, and Southeast Asia. Villi of the small intestinal mucosa become scalloped in appearance, blunted, or obliterated (Shah et al., 2000). Reduced absorptive area and malabsorption occur (Morales et al., 2001).

Etiology is not known, but bacterial, viral, parasitic infections, or toxins in spoiled food have been suspected; folic acid deficiency may also play a role. Symptoms include light-colored stools, diarrhea, weight loss, pallor, sore tongue from B_{12} deficiency, and easy bruising from vitamin K deficiency.

OBJECTIVES

- Improve nutrient absorption with gradual addition of foods.
- Differentiate between tropical and nontropical sprue.
- Improve or correct folic acid, B_{12}, and vitamin K deficiencies, among others.
- Control diarrhea, which could lead to malabsorption and malnutrition over time.

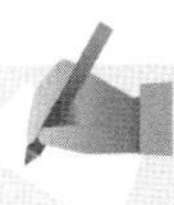

DIETARY AND NUTRITIONAL RECOMMENDATIONS

- Use a regular diet with supplements of vitamin B_{12} and folic acid. Good sources of folacin include liver, kidney, yeast, leafy greens, lean beef, and eggs. Good sources of vitamin B_{12} include meat, poultry, fish, dairy products, and eggs.
- Diet should provide sufficient amounts of calories, protein, calcium, iron, and vitamins.
- In its early phase, diet should include high protein and low fat until absorption improves. Fats may include MCTs.
- No gluten restriction applies.
- Include extra fluids to correct any dehydration.

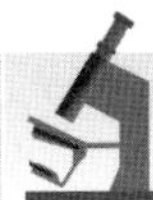

PROFILE

Clinical/History

Height
Weight
BMI
I & O; dehydration?
Malabsorption, especially for xylose

Lab Work

Gluc
H&H, Serum Fe (decreased)
Alb, prealbumin (decreased)
Serum B12 (decreased)
Serum folate (decreased)
Serum Ca++ (decreased)
PT (altered)
X-rays

Common Drugs Used and Potential Side Effects

- Vitamin supplements may be required, especially for B_{12}, folate, and vitamin K. Avoid excesses of any single nutrient for an extended time period. Calcium may also be needed.
- Tetracycline may be used; do not take within 2 hours of a calcium-containing supplement or meal, because calcium makes the drug less effective.

Herbs, Botanicals and Supplements

- Herbs and botanical supplements should not be used without discussing with the physician.

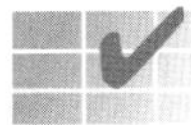

PATIENT EDUCATION

- ✓ Explain to the patient which foods are good sources of folic acid and vitamin B_{12}.
- ✓ Describe good sources of protein and calories from the diet.
- ✓ Describe how to follow a low-fat diet, and how to use MCT oil, ect.

LACTOSE MALABSORPTION (LACTASE DEFICIENCY)

NUTRITIONAL ACUITY RANKING: LEVEL 2

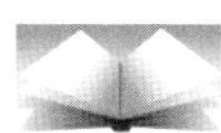

DEFINITIONS AND BACKGROUND

Lactose is a disaccharide (glucose + galactose) found in milk. If lactase is missing, lactose passes into the colon, where it is fermented to gasses and organic acids by colonic bacteria, resulting in bloating and/or cramping. Diarrhea may occur in some individuals who ingest large amounts of lactose.

Types of lactose malabsorption are congenital (rare, present at birth), primary or genetic (low incidence in children), and secondary or acquired (from GI disease, food allergy, antibiotics, or intestinal trauma). Lactase decline, which occurs after weaning, is known as hypolactasia. Typically, lactase activity declines in all people to approximately 10% of neonatal values, and levels remain lower than that for other saccharides such as sucrase or glucoamylase (Gray, 1993). Lactase "nonpersistence" is common in people of African (70%) or Asian descent (up to 95%) and is less common in Caucasians (6–10%) and in Hispanics. Adult-type hypolactasia is the most common type seen; in children, it may occur after secondary conditions such as diarrhea, HIV/AIDS, or giardiasis (Montes and Perman, 1989). Rectal bleeding in infancy is often caused by cow's milk enteropathy; therefore, excluding cow's milk from the diet should be tried before surgery (Willetts, 1999).

About 70% of the world's population are lactose maldigesters, but even those maldigesters who believe they are lactose intolerant can consume dairy products such as yogurt and lactose-hydrolyzed milk (Suarez and Saviano, 1997). Symptoms caused by lactose maldigestion need not hinder ingestion of a diet rich in dairy products that supplies around 1,500 mg calcium daily (i.e., 2 cups of milk, 1 cup yogurt, and several ounces of cheese.) Bloating, abdominal pain, diarrhea, and global perception of overall symptom severity are often tolerable (Suarez et al., 1998). Decreases in breath hydrogen suggest that colonic adaptation to the high-lactose diet occurs over several weeks of intakes of 1,200 mg calcium and 33 g lactose (Pribela et al., 2000). Lactose maldigestion should not be a contradiction in developing adequate calcium diets for susceptible populations; lactose intolerance will not result.

The American Dietetic Association recommends at least 3 medical nutrition therapy visits for adults who have lactose maldigestion (http://www.knowledgelinc.com/ada/mntguides/).

OBJECTIVES

- Omit or control lactose intake (lactose comprises 10% of the carbohydrate found in the American diet). Regular consumption of milk by lactase-deficient persons may increase the threshold at which diarrhea occurs; individual differences may reflect the state of colonic adaptation (Flourie et al., 1993).
- Check for actual tolerance by monitoring intake. Most people can tolerate 1/2 cup milk (6 g of lactose) with a meal, eventually if not immediately. Whole milk may be better tolerated than skim because it slows gastric emptying more effectively.
- Offer calcium and riboflavin from other foods and sources.
- Reduce severity of symptoms, including flatulence.

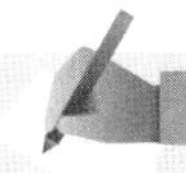

DIETARY AND NUTRITIONAL RECOMMENDATIONS

- Most people can tolerate up to 6 g of lactose, which is found in 4 oz of milk. If small amounts are gradually added over approximately 3 months, most adults can ultimately adapt to 12+ g/day, equal to one 8 oz glass of regular milk. Milk is best tolerated after other foods have been consumed at a meal.
- Lactase supplements (e.g., Lactaid, Lactrase, Dairy Ease) may be taken 30 minutes before the consumption of a lactose-containing product. Two capsules provide enough lactase to hydrolyze the lactose in an 8 oz glass of whole milk. Lactose-hydrolyzed milk is generally tolerated for other meals. Note that not all preparations are equally effective; Lactrase was the best in one study (Ramirez et al., 1994).
- Persons on a lactose-free diet can use lactate, casein (curds), lactalbumin, and calcium. If the patient is highly sensitive, check labels of foods for fillers, whey protein, milk, whey solids, and milk solids; most people can tolerate small amounts in mashed potatoes, breads, medications, etc.
- If tolerated, fermented products (buttermilk, natural or aged cheese, yogurt with active cultures, cottage cheese, or sour cream) can be used. Yogurt with active cultures

may be better tolerated than milk by many children (Shermak et al., 1995). Frozen yogurt has little or no lactase activity.

- For infants with the condition, try Nutramigen, ProSobee, Isomil, or other milk-free formulas; gradually introduce foods that contain milk or lactose.
- Beware of processed cheese or cheese foods that have nonfat dry milk solids.
- Carnation Instant Breakfast with lactose-reduced milk can be a potential supplement or tube feeding.

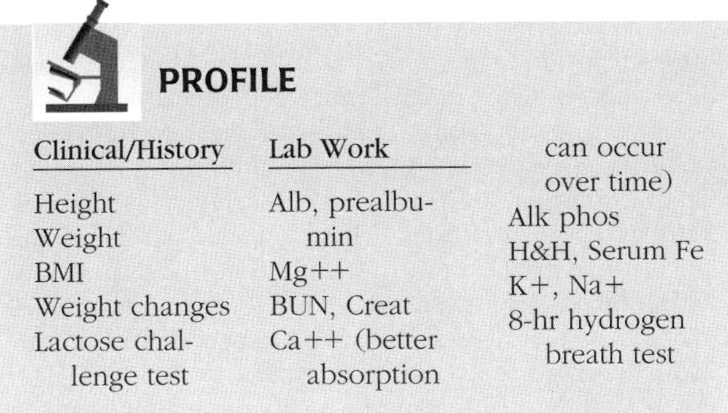

PROFILE

Clinical/History	Lab Work	
Height	Alb, prealbumin	can occur over time)
Weight	Mg++	Alk phos
BMI	BUN, Creat	H&H, Serum Fe
Weight changes	Ca++ (better absorption	K+, Na+
Lactose challenge test		8-hr hydrogen breath test

Common Drugs Used and Potential Side Effects

- Many drugs contain lactose (e.g., Premarin, Maalox, Contact cold medicine). However, this is rarely over 500 mg and should be well tolerated.

Herbs, Botanicals and Supplements

- Herbs and botanical supplements should not be used without discussing with the physician.

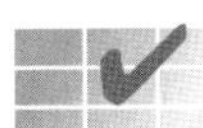

PATIENT EDUCATION

- ✓ Pregnant women should receive a calcium supplement.
- ✓ Home-cooked meals and recipes may be useful. Heating milk does not change lactose.
- ✓ Kosher foods are often acceptable if they are pareve (nonmilk, nonmeat).
- ✓ Indicate foods that are lactose-free and foods that are lactose-free sources of calcium.
- ✓ Recipes are available for use of lactose-free formulas in products such as meat loaf.
- ✓ Discuss how to use LactAid drops to allow the enzyme to hydrolyze the lactose.
- ✓ Drink milk with meals rather than alone to decrease symptoms.
- ✓ Acidophilus milk provides no specific relief of symptoms.
- ✓ Dairy foods contain approximately 1–8% lactose by weight (milk, 4–5%; yogurt, 4%; ice cream, 3–4%; milk chocolate, 8%; cottage cheese, 1–2%).

For More Information

- American Dietetic Association
  Lactose Maldigestion protocol
  http://www.eatright.org
- Dairy-Ease
  1-800-331-4536
- Lactose Intolerant Medications
  http://www.planetrx.com/product/nonrx/shelf/add_info/100600042_introduction.html
- LactAid (McNeil Consumer Products)
  1-800-435-7548
  http://www.lactaid.com/

CONSTIPATION

NUTRITIONAL ACUITY RANKING: LEVEL 1

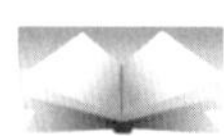

DEFINITIONS AND BACKGROUND

Constipation occurs when the fecal mass remains in the colon longer than the normal 24–72 hours after meal ingestion or when the patient strains to defecate. For chronic problems, bowel retraining may be necessary, and soy fiber currently is being investigated for its useful properties. Although fiber supplements may reduce constipation, they do not improve pelvic floor dyssynergia in elderly individuals (Cheskin, 1995). Stool type and frequency should be used to determine a problem; individuals who are constipated have a high prevalence of IBS (Probert et al., 1994).

Constipation and fecal incontinence are common symptoms in patients with cerebral palsy, traumatic spinal cord injuries, spina bifida, multiple sclerosis, diabetic polyneuropathy, Parkinson's disease, and stroke. New treatment modalities are: prokinetic agents, enemas administered through the enema continence catheter, and biofeedback.

Spastic constipation entails increased narrowing of the colon with small, ribbon-like stools caused by inactivity, immobility, or obstruction; increasing physical activity may be useful. Atonic constipation ("lazy bowel") occurs when musculature of the bowel no longer functions properly, sometimes from laxative overuse or poor bowel habits. Tube-feeding constipation is related to use of low-fiber products or other medications or conditions. In infants and children, chronic constipation is a concern, with encopresis from poor bowel habits and poor fiber intake. There may be some food allergies, such as to milk or to wheat, which should also be addressed.

Water-soluble fiber (pectins, gums, mucilages, and some hemicelluloses) delay intestinal transit, delay gastric emptying, and decrease cholesterol and glucose absorption; water-insoluble fiber in lignin, cellulose, and remaining hemicelluloses accelerate intestinal transit, increase fecal weight, slow starch hydrolysis, and delay glucose absorption; an adequate diet provides a 3:1 ratio of insoluble to soluble fiber (Gorman and Bowman, 1993).

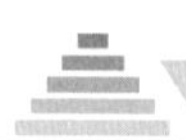

OBJECTIVES

- Atonic constipation ("lazy bowel"): Stimulate peristalsis, provide bulk, and retain water in the feces.
- Spastic constipation: Undue distention and stimulation of the bowel should be prevented during exacerbations. After the patient is well, fiber should be increased.
- Tube-feeding constipation: Check for obstruction (nausea, vomiting, distention). Record intake and output, along with activity levels.
- Constipation and encopresis in pediatrics: Provide laxatives and lubricants initially, followed by improved fiber and fluid intakes (McClung et al., 1993).

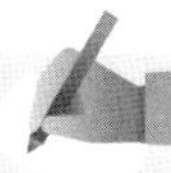

DIETARY AND NUTRITIONAL RECOMMENDATIONS

- In general, consume five servings of fruits and vegetables and six or more servings from the bread/cereal group each day, especially whole grains. Gradually increase fiber from all sources. Also increase fluids.
- Atonic constipation: The diet should be high in fiber, with liberal use of whole grains, fruits, and vegetables. Adding a few carrots and some bran to the diet can be an easy solution. Use adequate fluid, 8–10 cups daily.
- Spastic constipation: The diet should be decreased in fiber during painful episodes. Then, increase use of prune juice, dried fruits, raw fruits and vegetables, nuts, and whole grains. Be aware that some studies now suggest that wheat allergy actually may be a concern for some patients; do not use excesses of bran.
- Tube-feeding constipation: Use a fiber-containing formula if appropriate. Use adequate flushes.
- Constipation and encopresis in pediatrics. Add more fruits and vegetables to the diet; increase whole grain fiber and fluid intake.

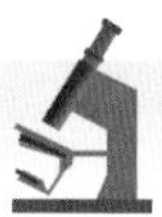

PROFILE

Clinical/History		Lab Work
Height	Stool color and number	Alb, prealbumin
Weight	I & O	BUN, Creat
BMI	BP	H&H, Serum Fe
Recent weight changes	Headaches	Ferritin
Bowel habits	Abdominal distention	Gluc
		Stool guaiac

Common Drugs Used and Potential Side Effects

- Narcotics such as morphine are common contributors to constipation and should not be used for a long period.
- Antacids containing iron, aluminum, or calcium often cause problems with constipation. In addition, narcotics (codeine and morphine), NSAIDs (such as ibuprofen), verapamil, monoamine oxidase (MAO) inhibitors and tricyclic antidepressant agents (Nardil, Elavil, Endep), phenobarbital, Benadryl, clonidine (Catapres), vincristine (Oncovin), Artane and Cogentin, Haldol, Thorazine, Questran and Colestid, furosemide (Lasix), and iron preparations (ferrous fumarate, gluconate or sulfate) may be constipating. Changes in bowel motility and tone, bloating, or sensations of "fullness" often occur.

- Suppositories, enemas, and laxatives are used to relieve constipation. Beware of using mineral oil as a laxative because decreased absorption of calcium and fat-soluble vitamins will occur. Some products may contain excessive amounts of sodium—Sal Hepatica contains 1 g of sodium per dose! Long-term use can alter fluid and electrolyte balance. Avoid using bisacodyl (Dulcolax) with dairy products; take with a high-fiber diet.
- Psyllium, a plant fiber sold as Metamucil, Syllact, etc., must be taken with plenty of water or juice (8 oz per teaspoonful). Results may require 1–4 teaspoons of the product. Taste, as well as the cost of the product, must be considered. Calcium is still available to the cells when psyllium is used (Heany and Weaver, 1995).
- Chronulac (lactulose) treats constipation by increasing the number and frequency of stools. Cramping, flatulence, nausea, vomiting, and potassium losses may occur. Lactulose contains galactose; avoid use of this product with a galactose-free diet.
- Colace (docusate sodium) is a stool softener, which is only a short-term solution. Take with milk or juice.
- Prokinetic agents are newer treatments; erythromycin may serve this role in pediatric populations.

Herbs, Botanicals and Supplements

- Herbs and botanical supplements should not be used without discussing with the physician.
- Flax, aloe (anthraquinones), fenugreek, and rhubarb have been recommended for this condition, but no clinical trials have proven efficacy.
- With use of bisacodyl, avoid aloe, cascara, senna, and yellow dock because of enhancing effects.

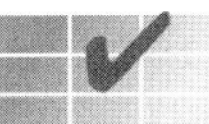

PATIENT EDUCATION

- ✔ Explain that proper diet can produce relief but cannot cure the condition.
- ✔ Explain that a normal bowel routine is needed but that daily fecal evacuation is not needed for everyone.
- ✔ Specifically identify foods that have a laxative effect for the patient. Explain that fiber may be increased on a gradual basis only and that prune juice may help. For every gram of cereal fiber, stool weight increases by 3–9 g.
- ✔ Have the patient drink 8–10 glasses of water daily, as permitted. Warm fluids are especially useful.
- ✔ Exercise may be beneficial in maintaining regularity, especially abdominal strengthening exercises.
- ✔ Discuss overuse of laxatives and cathartics.
- ✔ Discuss foods that have caused constipation, flatus, and GI distress in the past. Offer relevant suggestions.
- ✔ Discuss the need for medical assistance for diarrhea, bleeding, infection, and change in bowel habits.
- ✔ For some individuals, a cup of hot prune juice may be effective.

ACQUIRED MEGACOLON

NUTRITIONAL ACUITY RANKING: LEVEL 2

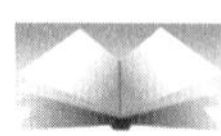

DEFINITIONS AND BACKGROUND

Acquired megacolon is a chronic disease associated with constipation and malnutrition and possibly surgical intervention (Vieira et al., 1996). The enlarged bowel results from an abnormal colonic dilatation, often reaching 8–10 cm in diameter. It is often present in elderly persons who have a long history of elimination problems created by laxative abuse or constipation. Persons with diabetes, hypothyroidism, scleroderma, multiple sclerosis, electrolyte imbalances, and other conditions may be affected. Obstruction could be caused by tumor, stricture, etc.

Signs and symptoms of megacolon involve abdominal distention, flatus, absence of stool, smearing or bowel incontinence, nausea, anorexia, fatigue, and headache. Note that the colon provides reabsorption of water and electrolytes as well as elimination of waste and regulation of bacterial homeostasis. Motility is crucial in these roles. Normal urges to defecate are affected by physical activity, neurological status, chemical/drug use, and bowel condition. Normal reflexes are needed for muscular and sphincter control.

OBJECTIVES

- ▲ Prevent complications such as lung atelectasis from distention, sepsis, ulceration with hemorrhage or perforation, or sigmoid volvulus.
- ▲ Evaluate bowel pattern by history and at present, including drug use and abuse (laxatives, etc.).
- ▲ Identify and correct any nutrient deficiencies, electrolyte imbalances, or PCM.
- ▲ Normalize bowel function as far as possible.
- ▲ Position the patient in whatever is most comfortable.

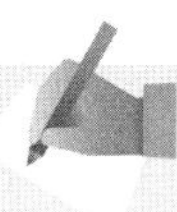

DIETARY AND NUTRITIONAL RECOMMENDATIONS

- Use adequate fluid and fiber, pending status and other conditions (such as congestive heart failure [CHF]). Prune juice added to hot cereal may help normalize bowel function.
- Raw fruits and vegetables should be used only as tolerated; progress over time.
- Avoid excesses of refined foods and concentrated sweets to the exclusion of desirable foods.
- Tube feeding deserves consideration in selected patients. Nutritional status tends to improve after surgery, with normalization of bowel function (Vieira et al., 1996).

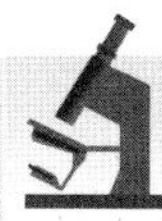

PROFILE

Clinical/History		
Height	Abdominal girth	H&H, Serum Fe
Weight	Stool consistency	Na+, K+, Cl−
BMI	**Lab Work**	Endoscopy
Stool pattern	BUN, Creat	Barium x-rays
BP		Thyroid function
I & O		Stool guaiac

Common Drugs Used and Potential Side Effects

- Anticholinergics, opiates, and antidepressants may increase or aggravate constipation. Watch use carefully.
- Suppositories and stool softeners may be used or may have been used excessively. Monitor specific medications accordingly.
- Colonic irrigations may be used (Harris Flush—800 mL of warm water slowly introduced into the rectum to relieve flatus). This may alleviate the problem temporarily but is not a permanent solution.

Herbs, Botanicals and Supplements

- Herbs and botanical supplements should not be used without discussing with the physician.

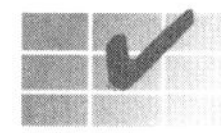

PATIENT EDUCATION

- ✓ Discuss the role of exercise in maintaining normal bowel function.
- ✓ Discuss the role of fluid and fiber in bowel regularity. For example, drinking cup of hot prune juice may be effective for some patients.

IRRITABLE BOWEL SYNDROME

NUTRITIONAL ACUITY RANKING: LEVEL 2

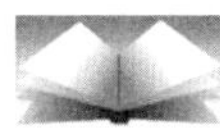

DEFINITIONS AND BACKGROUND

IBS is found in 15–20% of children and adults. IBS has been called by many names—colitis, mucous colitis, spastic colon, spastic bowel, and functional bowel disease; these terms are inaccurate. Colitis means inflammation of the large intestine (colon); IBS does not cause inflammation and should not be confused with ulcerative colitis. IBS is the most common reason why people seek medical attention; 40% of these patients also have some form of lactose intolerance (Spellett, 1994). Women are affected twice as often as men. Prevalence decreases with age.

Diagnostic criteria for IBS include at least 3 months of continuous or recurrent symptoms of: abdominal pain or discomfort relieved with defecation or associated with change in frequency of stool or changed consistency of stool; 2 or more: altered stool frequency (more than 3 per day or less than 3 per week), altered stool form (lumpy/hard or loose/watery), altered stool passage such as straining/urgency/feeling of incomplete evacuation, passage of mucus in the stool, or bloating and feeling of abdominal distention (Drossman et al., 1997).

Altered responsiveness of smooth muscle to hormones and medications may occur. In some IBS patients, the presence of dyspepsia is associated with *H. pylori* infection, female gender, and perceived stress (Su et al., 2000). Inadequate fiber intake is also common, but cause or consequence is not clear. Excessive amounts of bacteria in the small intestine have been found; antibiotic use to reduce bacterial overload may prove to be a useful treatment. Environmental and social factors may also play a role; see Table 7–13.

Signs and symptoms of IBS include belching, flatulence, heartburn, mucus in the stool, cramp-like pain, constipation (sometimes alternating with diarrhea), and nausea. There is an association between functional GI symptoms and a family history of abdominal pain or bowel problems. Having a first-degree relative with abdominal pain or bowel problems is significantly associated with reporting of IBS and dyspepsia (Locke et al., 2000).

Carbohydrate malabsorption of lactose, fructose and sorbitol has been described in normal volunteers and in patients with functional bowel complaints including IBS. Reduction or elimination of the offending sugar(s) should result in clinical improvement; dietary restriction of the offending sugar(s) should be implemented before drug therapy is initiated (Goldstein et al., 2000). Lactose is most commonly problematic; fructose and sorbitol are less problematic.

Present therapies for functional GI disorders are symptomatic and mainly treat altered bowel habits. New therapies are focused on nerve-gut communication dysfunction: 5-HT3 antagonists and 5-HT4 agonists have demonstrated activity in clinical trials. Antibiotics are being evaluated. The American Dietetic Association recommends 3 medical nutrition therapy visits for patients who have IBS (http://www.knowledgelinc.com/ada/mntguides/).

TABLE 7–13 Psychosocial Issues in Functional Gastrointestinal Disorders

Detecting psychologic disturbance and eliciting a history of physical or sexual abuse are critical in suggesting comprehensive and efficacious treatment strategies for IBS patients (Olden and Drossman, 2000). A multicomponent treatment program delivered by a team of caregivers, each bringing their unique skills (internist, psychiatrist, psychologist, and others) to patients, may be beneficial.

OBJECTIVES

- ▲ Encourage regular eating patterns, regular bowel hygiene, adequate rest, and relaxation.
- ▲ Avoid constipation.
- ▲ Use adequate fluid intake.
- ▲ Monitor for lactose intolerance, food allergies (chocolate, dairy products, wheat, yeast, and eggs have been cited), and gluten intolerance.
- ▲ Alleviate pain, symptoms, and flatulence. Production of colonic gas, especially hydrogen, is greater in IBS patients.
- ▲ Individualize diet management to the patient's needs.

DIETARY AND NUTRITIONAL RECOMMENDATIONS

- Provide an elemental diet for persons with IBS in its acute form.
- As treatment progresses, use adequate but not excessive fiber; ensure that fluid intake is high. Avoid high fat, which may increase cholecystokinin release; avoid high sugar intake, which increases osmolarity.
- Liberal amounts of fruits and vegetables are important.
- Omit milk, if lactose is not tolerated. Add calcium in other forms.
- Omit spicy foods or gas-forming oligosaccharides (beans, barley, Brussels sprouts, cabbage, nuts, figs, and soybeans), if not tolerated. Some patients benefit from exclusion of beef, dairy, cereals other than rice, yeast, citrus fruits, and caffeinated beverages (King et al., 1998). Wheat may also cause problems; omit as necessary (Francis and Whorwell, 1994).
- Gluten products may not be tolerated; limit or omit for those individuals. Be aware that supplementation of B-complex vitamins will be needed.

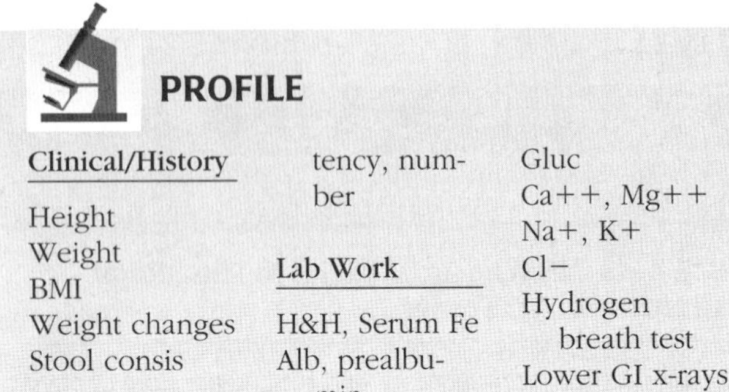

PROFILE

Clinical/History

Height
Weight
BMI
Weight changes
Stool consistency, number

Lab Work

H&H, Serum Fe
Alb, prealbumin
Gluc
Ca++, Mg++
Na+, K+
Cl−
Hydrogen breath test
Lower GI x-rays

Common Drugs Used and Potential Side Effects

- Methylcellulose (Metamucil) and other bulking agents always must be taken with large amounts of water. Generally, 1 tablespoon is sufficient per day. Increased peristalsis occurs.
- Antispasmodic drugs can be used to alleviate abdominal pains. Donnatal is one that contains phenobarbital.
- If tranquilizers such as Xanax are used, abdominal pain, nausea and vomiting, or weight changes may result.
- Antidepressants may be prescribed if there is depression (Jackson et al., 2000; Olden and Drossman, 2000).
- Alosetron (Lotronex) reduces diarrhea by blocking serotonin 5-HT3 receptors. Because of severe side effects that include the possibility of ischemic colitis and severe, painful constipation, FDA withdrew it. Some patients have lobbied for its cautious return to the market.
- Upper gut dysmotility drugs include motilin and cholecystokinin A receptors (Chovet, 2000). Tachykinins, calcitonin gene-related peptide, or glutamate antagonists are being evaluated for visceral pain.

Herbs, Botanicals and Supplements

- Herbs and botanical supplements should not be used without discussing with the physician.

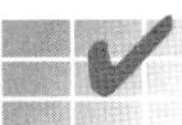

PATIENT EDUCATION

- ✔ Slowly increase dietary fiber to prevent discomfort. Bran may aggravate IBS; assess individually.
- ✔ Explain that regular times for bowel evacuation should be planned.
- ✔ Ensure the patient has adequate food intake.
- ✔ Help the patient devise adequate methods for coping with stress.
- ✔ A food diary may help to identify any food sensitivities.
- ✔ Regular exercise also may be important.
- ✔ To prevent intestinal gas from forming, try Bean-O (1-800-257-8650) and other products now available on the market. Bean-O does significantly improve flatulence, bloating, and pain (Ganiats et al., 1994).
- ✔ Red flags requiring medical attention include: anemia, fever, persistent diarrhea, rectal bleeding, weight loss, and nocturnal symptoms. Any of these symptoms require further diagnostic work-up.

For More Information

- American Dietetic Association
  Irritable bowel syndrome protocol
  www.eatright.org
- National Digestive Diseases Information Clearinghouse
  2 Information Way
  Bethesda, MD 20892
  http://www.niddk.nih.gov/health/digest/pubs/irrbowel/irrbowel.htm

DIVERTICULAR DISEASES

NUTRITIONAL ACUITY RANKING: LEVEL 2

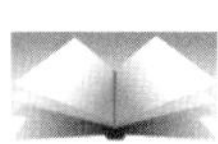

DEFINITIONS AND BACKGROUND

Diverticulitis results from inflammation of small pouches (diverticula) formed in the colon wall and lining due to chronic constipation. Diverticular disease has been increasing in occurrence in Westernized countries because of low-fiber diet and may be classified as asymptomatic, atypical, acute or uncomplicated, and complicated (Wolff and Devine, 2000).

Inflammation develops when bacteria or other irritants are trapped in pouches, causing spasm and pain in the lower left side of the abdomen, as well as distention, nausea, vomiting, constipation or diarrhea, chills, and fever. Diverticular diseases are rare in societies in which high-fiber and low red meat diets are consumed (Aldoori et al., 1994). A diet high in total dietary fiber decreases risk of diverticular disease, regardless of technique used to assess fiber (Aldoori, 1998). More than half of individuals older than 70 years of age are affected, with sigmoid involvement a common site.

Bowel cancer has been associated with the presence of diverticular disease. Low serum albumin and H&H levels may be indicative of a longer length of stay in diverticular disease (Wunderlich and Tobias, 1992).

Diverticular disease-associated chronic sigmoid colitis has morphologic features traditionally reserved for idiopathic inflammatory bowel disease (Makapugay and Dean, 1996). Medical management is usually sufficient for acute or uncomplicated diverticulitis, but complicated diverticulitis is generally managed promptly with sigmoid resection with a high success rate (Wolff and Devine, 2000).

OBJECTIVES

Diverticulitis (Inflamed State)

- Allow complete bowel rest to prevent perforation.
- Avoid the laxative effect of excess fiber.
- Eliminate food particles that accumulate in sacs. These food particles are capable of causing bacterial contamination.
- Prevent peritonitis and abscess.
- Correct any GI bleeding, hypoalbuminemia, or anemia.

Diverticulosis (Convalescent State)

- Increase stool caliber and volume, mostly from fiber (bran is useful).
- Distend the bowel wall to prevent development of high-pressure segments.
- Relieve intraluminal pressure; decrease the contractions of colonic circular smooth muscle.
- Prevent inflammation.

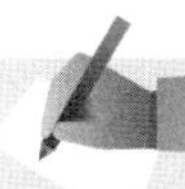

DIETARY AND NUTRITIONAL RECOMMENDATIONS

Diverticulitis (Inflamed State)

- An elemental diet should be used if patient is acutely ill. Progress to clear liquids.
- As treatment progresses, use a soft diet with no excess spices or fiber. Avoid nuts, seeds, popcorn, and fibrous vegetables.
- Ensure adequate intake of protein and iron sources.
- Gradually progress to normal fiber intake as inflammation decreases.
- A low-fat diet also may be beneficial.

Diverticulosis (Convalescent State)

- Diet should include a high intake of fluid.
- Diet should be high in fiber; over 30 g per day is desirable. Begin with 1 teaspoon of bran daily, working up to 2 T. Barley bran flour is 70% total dietary fiber, mostly insoluble (Lupton, Morin, and Robinson, 1993). Whole grains, stewed or dried fruits, potato skins, raw carrots, or celery may also be used. Increase fiber gradually. Popcorn, seeds, and nuts may not be tolerated.
- A low-fat diet may also be indicated to reduce intracolonic pressure.

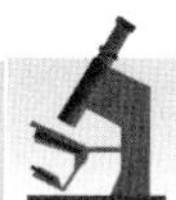

PROFILE

Clinical/History	Lab Work	
Height	H&H, Serum Fe	Alb, prealbumin
Weight	Transferrin, TIBC	Na+, K+
BMI	Erythrocyte sedimentation rate (ESR) (increased)	Ca++, Mg++
Stool number, frequency		WBC (may be increased)
BP		Sigmoidoscopy
		Barium enema

Common Drugs Used and Potential Side Effects

- Bulk-forming agents (methylcellulose) may be used to initiate normal colonic function and bowel action.
- Anticholinergics, stool softeners, and antibiotics may be used. Monitor accordingly.

Herbs, Botanicals and Supplements

- Herbs and botanical supplements should not be used without discussing with the physician.

- Flax, wheat, wild yam, slippery elm, and camomile have been recommended for this condition, but no clinical trials have proven efficacy.

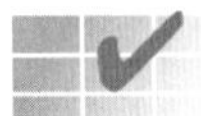

PATIENT EDUCATION

- ✔ Instruct patient concerning dietary fiber. Some ingested plant material is not digested by GI enzymes, including cellulose, pectin, lignin, and hemicelluloses. Some dietary fibers (whole grains) resist intestinal disintegration, whereas others (fruits and vegetables) are more or less disintegrated. In general, increased fiber increases tools volume, frequency, transit rate and decreases intracolonic pressure. Increased stool volume and decreased intracolonic pressure alter transit time.
- ✔ High-fiber foods are not synonymous with foods that are high in residue.
- ✔ Instruct patient to chew slowly.
- ✔ Instruct patient to avoid constipation and straining.
- ✔ Fluid intake should be adequate.
- ✔ If flatulence is a problem, advise the individual that approximately 6 weeks will be needed to allow bacterial flora to adapt to increased fiber intakes.
- ✔ Adequate activity and exercise are beneficial.

PERITONITIS

NUTRITIONAL ACUITY RANKING: LEVEL 2

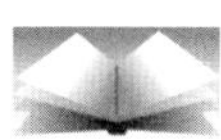

DEFINITIONS AND BACKGROUND

In peritonitis, inflammation of the peritoneal cavity due to infiltration of intestinal contents occurs. Contents from such conditions as ruptured appendix, gastric or intestinal perforation, trauma, fistula, anastomotic leaks, or failure in peritoneal dialysis may initiate the problem.

Spontaneous bacterial peritonitis is a common illness in patients with cirrhosis and ascites that occurs related to bacterial translocation; the gut is a major source of this bacteria (Ramachandran and Balasubramanian, 2001).

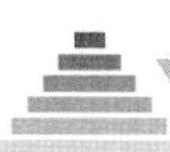

OBJECTIVES

- ▲ Provide bowel rest and recovery.
- ▲ Improve anorectic state; correct ileus if present.
- ▲ Correct dehydration and fluid/electrolyte imbalances where present.
- ▲ Improve nutritional status, especially if patient has been malnourished over a period of time.

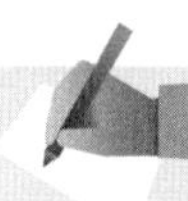

DIETARY AND NUTRITIONAL RECOMMENDATIONS

- Patient generally is NPO with intravenous feedings for at least 24 hours.
- Progress to an increased liquid diet as tolerated such as a diet including Ensure Plus HN or other supplemental feeding.
- Progress as tolerated to a soft or general diet appropriate for the condition that caused the peritonitis originally.
- Increase protein intake to correct catabolic state. Increase calories because BEE is generally elevated by 10–17%.

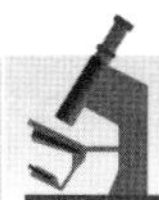

PROFILE

Clinical/History	I & O	Gluc
Height	**Lab Work**	Alb, prealbumin
Weight	H&H, Serum Fe	Na+, K+
BMI	WBC	TLC
Temperature	BUN, Creat	X-rays
BP		Laparoscopy

Common Drugs Used and Potential Side Effects

- Ciprofloxacin is effective in the treatment of serious, nonself-limiting intra-abdominal infections and peritonitis from continuous ambulatory peritoneal dialysis (CAPD) (Finch, 2001).
- Other antibiotics are used for bacterial peritonitis. Monitor for specific side effects.

Herbs, Botanicals and Supplements

- Herbs and botanical supplements should not be used without discussing with the physician.

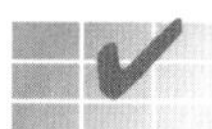

PATIENT EDUCATION

- ✓ With patients on CAPD, diet may need to be limited to 1.2–1.5 g protein/kg + 35 kcal/kg as is typical for renal patients.
- ✓ Discuss diet appropriate for the illness of origin (such as diabetes, hypertension, toxemia, or renal disease.)

CARCINOID SYNDROME

NUTRITIONAL ACUITY RANKING: LEVEL 2

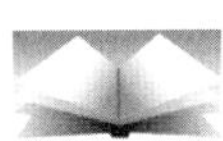

DEFINITIONS AND BACKGROUND

A rare growth that develops in the wall of the intestine, carcinoid syndrome (CS) is usually discovered in x-rays performed for other reasons. The growth can become so large as to cause intestinal obstruction; 10% of these growths metastasize to the liver, producing hormone-producing tumors that have signs that include flushing of the head and neck (usually triggered by alcohol or exercise). The symptoms can last for several hours. In addition, the patient may have swollen and watery eyes, explosive diarrhea and abdominal cramps, wheezing as in asthma, breathlessness, and symptoms similar to heart failure; 35% of patients will get heart disease from fibrosis of the endocardium. Survival is 3–20 years.

Diversion of tryptophan to 5-hydroxytryptamine (5-HT) synthesis occurs, resulting in less tryptophan for protein and nicotinamide synthesis. 5-Hydroxyindole acetic acid (5HIAA) testing requires several days of a diet free from intake of avocados, pineapple, bananas, kiwi fruit, plums, eggplant, walnuts, hickory nuts, and pecans.

Cardiac valvular lesions are seen in the majority of patients with CS and represent the most clinically significant consequence of CS. Tricuspid valvular disease is especially common, and advanced valvular involvement is associated with poor long-term survival. Active surgical and medical therapy of the tumor disease reduces the hormonal secretion and makes right ventricular heart failure a rare cause of death in these patients (Westberg et al., 2001).

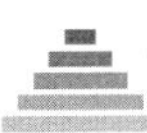

OBJECTIVES

- Ease symptoms and reduce any pain.
- Control secretory diarrhea and wheezing.
- Slow progression of the disease, which is not curable through surgery.
- Control side effects of medications.
- Replenish electrolyte and fluid losses.
- Correct pellagra-like rash.

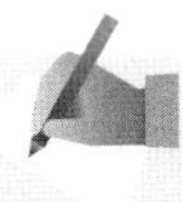

DIETARY AND NUTRITIONAL RECOMMENDATIONS

- Decrease fiber intake during acute stages of diarrhea. Add pectin and ensure adequate fluid intake during those periods.
- Use a diet controlled in protein and carbohydrate with use of bronchodilators.
- Avoid alcoholic beverages. Limit caffeine intake to a controlled amount.

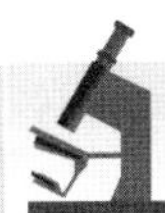

PROFILE

Clinical/History

Height
Weight
BMI
Wheezing
Explosive diarrhea
Number of stools, consistency

Lab Work

Alb, prealbumin
Transferrin
5HIAA test
K+
TLC
H&H, Serum Fe
Na+
Biopsy
Endoscopy
X-rays of GI tract

Common Drugs Used and Potential Side Effects

- The standard treatment used to control the symptoms of CS involves subcutaneous injections of the somatostatin analogue octreotide; this is expensive and treatment may be for many years. Some other vasoconstricting drugs may be used to control side effects.
- Kaolin (Kaopectate) and other medications may be used to control diarrhea. Constipation is a possible side effect.
- Bronchodilators may be used to control wheezing. Check the specific type of drug to evaluate potential side effects.
- Cytotoxic drugs may be used in severe cases.
- Prednisone helps to reduce flushing. Chronic use may decrease nitrogen and calcium absorption.

Herbs, Botanicals and Supplements

- Herbs and botanical supplements should not be used without discussing with the physician.

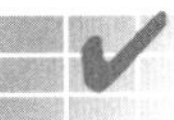

PATIENT EDUCATION

- Discuss measures specifically designed for the patient's status and tolerance levels.
- Suggest ways to make meals more appetizing if appetite is poor.

CROHN'S DISEASE (REGIONAL ENTERITIS)

NUTRITIONAL ACUITY RANKING: LEVEL 4

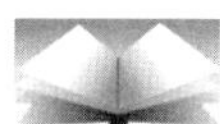

DEFINITIONS AND BACKGROUND

Crohn's disease is a chronic granulomatous IBD with cobblestone effect (usually of the terminal ileum and cecum, less often of the colon). Crohn's disease is believed to be hereditary, although recent studies suggest that high intakes of animal protein and polyunsaturated fatty acids (PUFAs) and low intake of omega-3 fatty acids may contribute to its development (Shoda et al., 1996). Onset is generally between 15 and 30 years of age. Crohn's disease differs from ulcerative colitis (UC) by affecting the GI tract from oral cavity to rectum; UC involves the mucosal tissue of the colon and rectum. At the time of diagnosis, many patients with IBD already show signs of malnutrition (Geerling et al., 2000).

In Crohn's disease, the intestinal lumen decreases; peristalsis from food intake causes cramping pain, especially in the right lower quadrant. Other symptoms include fever, weight loss, debility, bowel narrowing, nausea, mouth sores, anal fissures, vomiting, abdominal pain, intestinal bleeding, and sporadic flare-ups. Chronic watery diarrhea results from edema, bile salt malabsorption, bacterial overgrowth, and ulceration. Stricture may precipitate bowel obstruction. Arthritis, iritis or uveitis, conjunctivitis, jaundice, or pruritus may also be present (Jackson and Eastwood, 1991). Approximately one-third of children present with growth failure; their symptoms may not be of GI origin but may include inflammation, fever, and anemia. Malnutrition and pallor are also common findings.

One million people suffer from this disorder. In one-third of cases, only the ileum is involved; in 45%, both the ileum and the large intestine are affected. Only 25% of cases ever go into remission. Fish oil has been proposed as adjunct therapy to prevent relapses (Belluzzi et al., 1996). Persons with Crohn's disease are at increased risk for colon cancer, obstruction, anorectal fistulas, and abscesses.

Nutritional therapy is an important adjunctive treatment. Elemental diets seem to be effective in reducing whole-body protein losses. In other cases in which only a small amount of intestine remains, TPN may be essential. Vitamin E is among the antioxidant nutrients that inhibit lipoxidase enzymes and may play a part in attenuating disease activity (Coulston and Rock, 1993). Despite statistical advantage of steroids in treating active Crohn's disease, nutrition may be the preferred therapy for children with specific needs and problems; the ideal candidate is an adolescent with newly diagnosed Crohn's disease and terminal ileitis complicated by growth failure and delayed maturation (Ruemmele et al., 2000). Research now suggests that colostrum and milk-derived peptide growth factors may be useful in treatment of GI disorders, including IBD (Playford et al., 2000).

Figure 7–2 shows possible consequences of malnutrition in IBD.

- Replace fluid and electrolytes lost through diarrhea and vomiting. Lessen mechanical irritation and promote rest, especially with diarrhea.
- Replenish nutrient reserves; correct malabsorption or anemia. Wasting in patients with Crohn's disease is a consequence of malnutrition but not of hypermetabolism (Schneeweiss et al., 1999).
- Monitor intolerances (lactose, gluten, etc.).
- Promote healing; rest bowel from offending agents but feed to prevent loss of critical protein mass. Provide foods, which contain short-chain fatty acids and glutamine to promote healing.
- Prevent peritonitis, obstruction, renal calculi, or fistulas.
- Promote weight gain or prevent losses from exudates or inadequate intake. Elevated metabolic rate is not common (Rigaud et al., 1994). Diet-induced thermogenesis (DIT) and lipid peroxidation rate are significantly higher in people with Crohn's disease than in healthy people.
- Prepare for surgery if necessary (perhaps from failed medical management, obstruction, fistula, or peritonitis). A total colectomy or a right-sided ileocolectomy may be necessary. Enteral nutrition with elemental products seems to be sufficient to prepare patients for the surgery (Steffes and Fromm, 1992).
- In a child, promote growth. Growth spurts follow sustained weight gain.
- When controlled, higher fiber and fish oil intakes may reduce severity of symptoms.
- Monitor mineral and trace element levels carefully to ensure adequacy.
- Prevent or correct metabolic bone disease (e.g., osteopenia, arthropathies) from the disease itself, from nutrient malabsorption, side effects of medications, and lifestyle factors.
- Patients with Crohn's disease have altered plasma levels of several antioxidants and decreased total radical trapping antioxidant potential (Genser et al., 1999). Antioxidant intake should be increased

DIETARY AND NUTRITIONAL RECOMMENDATIONS

- With strictures or fistulas, use a low-residue (elemental) or low-fiber diet that is high in calories with a high protein content of 1–1.5 g/kg (especially high biologic value [HBV] proteins). Use TPN if needed, usually for 2 weeks or longer. For some, tube feeding with added glutamine may be useful.

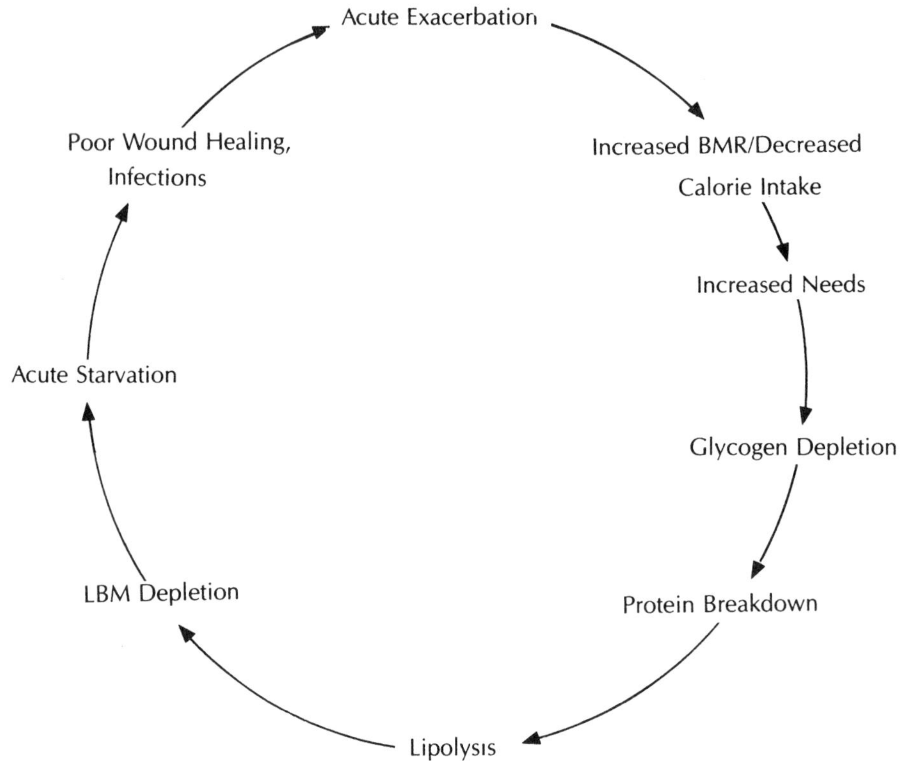

Figure 7–2 Nutritional depletion in IBD. (Adapted from Newman, McCorkle, Turner. In: Lang C, ed. *Nutritional support in critical care.* Aspen Publishers: Rockville, MD, 1987.)

- BEE × 1.5 may be calculated. For infants, use 120 kcal/kg; for children, use 80–100 kcal/kg; for teens, use 60–80 kcal/kg.
- A diet relatively high in fat may improve energy balance (Mingrone et al., 1999). Limit fat intake only if steatorrhea is present. MCTs may be better tolerated. Use of omega-3 fatty acids may be indicated.
- Reduce lactose intake if not tolerated. Check for wheat and gluten tolerances.
- Antioxidant therapy is likely to be beneficial. Supplement diet with adequate amounts of vitamins C, E, and B12, iron, zinc, vitamin B6, copper, calcium, potassium, folate, vitamin D, and magnesium. Vitamins A and K should be given every other day.
- Monitor progress carefully; patients may be finicky.
- Small, frequent meals may be better tolerated.
- With resection greater than 200 cm, selenium may become deficient; monitor carefully.

PROFILE

Clinical/History

Height
Weight
BMI
BP
Temperature
Number of bowel movements, frequency

Lab Work

H&H, Serum Fe (decreased)
K+
Alb, prealbumin (low)
RBP
Transferrin, TIBC
Serum folate
N balance
Schilling test (for B12)
Ca++
Serum B12
Total protein
BUN, Creat
Serum carotene
Serum zinc (decreased)
TLC
Serum Cu
WBC, ESR (increased)
Breath hydrogen test
Crohn's Disease Activity Factor (CDAI)
Sigmoidoscopy
X-rays, endoscopy
Barium enema, barium swallows
Fecal fat analysis

Common Drugs Used and Potential Side Effects

- Human growth hormone (GH) and a high-protein diet can offer remission in some cases. Infliximab infusions seem to provide relief for some who suffer from Crohn's disease and have not found help from standard therapies. Infliximab blocks tumor necrosis factor alpha and reduces its resulting inflammation.
- Corticosteroids. Use of corticosteroids commonly causes electrolyte imbalance; they are more effective for colon involvement. The patient may then need a diet that provides sodium restriction, with extra protein, calcium, and potassium for increased losses. Whole protein enteral nutrition is effective for many patients, but active Crohn's disease usually requires some steroid therapy (Griffiths et al., 1995). Cumulative corticosteroid dose is a significant predictor of reduced bone mineral density (BMD) in IBD (Gokhale et al., 1998).
- Methotrexate may be useful in reducing the need for steroids and for improving symptoms (Feagan, 1995). Stomatitis, gingivitis, nausea, or diarrhea may occur.
- Antidiarrheal agents. Diet should include 2 L of water daily. Sulfasalazine (Azulfidine) decreases inflammation but also decreases folate levels; the patient may need folate supplements. Fever, hair loss, bone marrow suppression, or nephrotoxicity can occur.
- Antibiotics work well for fistulas; vitamin K may be needed. Metronidazole may be used when there is anal involvement; nausea, vomiting, anorexia, or diarrhea may occur. Mesalamine or olsalazine may be used if sulfasalazine causes allergic reactions; nausea or vomiting may occur.
- Antacids, analgesics, and antispasmodics may be used.
- Psyllium laxatives (Metamucil) can help with constipation and diarrhea. Long-term use alters electrolytes. Flatulence or steatorrhea may occur.

Herbs, Botanicals and Supplements

- Onion, valerian, and tea have been recommended for this condition, but no clinical trials have proven efficacy.
- Few data are available, but patients who do not tolerate aminosalicylic acid may benefit from supplemental omega-3 fatty acids.

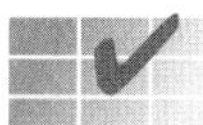

PATIENT EDUCATION

- ✔ Encourage patient to eat. Alleviate fears associated with mealtimes.
- ✔ Tell patient to avoid seasonings if they are poorly tolerated.
- ✔ Ensure that sources of potassium are increased during periods of diarrhea.
- ✔ Help patient evaluate tolerance of chilled foods. Instruct patient to chew foods well and avoid swallowing air.
- ✔ Discuss the roles of fiber, supplements, and fluid intake.
- ✔ Highlight calcium and vitamin D in their roles in bone mineralization; discuss alternate sources when milk cannot be used. Bone density should be monitored yearly.
- ✔ Periodic assistance or reevaluation by a dietitian may be helpful regarding dietary intake.
- ✔ No definite role for sugar or food processing has been documented.
- ✔ Nocturnal tube feedings have been useful to regain weight or for growth.

For More Information

- ✦ Crohn's and Colitis Foundation of America, Inc. (CCFA)
  386 Park Ave. S., 17th Floor
  New York, NY 10016-8804
  212-685-3400
  1-800-932-2423
  http://www.ccfa.org/
- ✦ Healingwell Crohn's Disease Resource Center
  http://www.healingwell.com/ibd/

ULCERATIVE COLITIS

NUTRITIONAL ACUITY RANKING: LEVEL 4

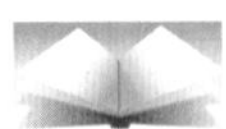

DEFINITIONS AND BACKGROUND

An ulceration of the surface mucosa of the large bowel, ulcerative colitis (an IBD) causes crampy abdominal pain, fever, violent and bloody diarrhea, pus or mucus discharged between stools, anemia, pyoderma, endocarditis, cirrhosis, splenomegaly, and stomatitis. Approximately 14% of children who present with it have growth failure.

The condition is usually one relentless, continuous lesion of the colon with some involvement of the terminal ileum. It does not affect full thickness of the intestine and never affects the small intestine. Ulcerative colitis usually begins in the rectum or sigmoid colon.

It may be acute, mild, or chronic. There are four theories of its cause: autoimmunity, bacteria, allergy, or milk intolerance. Onset is usually between 15 and 35 years of age, often in women. There is a second, lesser peak of onset at ages 50–70. Flares often involve non-GI symptoms such as arthritis, uveitis, and ankylosing spondylitis.

Surgery to remove the large intestine and rectum is potentially curative. The ileocecal valve should be preserved, if possible. Increased risk of colon cancer exists, especially with duration of 10+ years. The risk of cancer is greater than that for Crohn's disease (Coulston and Rock, 1993). Research now suggests that colostrums and milk-derived peptide growth factors may be useful in treatment of GI disorders, such as IBD (Playford et al., 2000).

OBJECTIVES

- ▲ Correct fluid and electrolyte imbalance.
- ▲ Replenish depleted stores and correct poor nutritional status, anemia, negative nitrogen balance, etc.
- ▲ Avoid further irritation and inflammation of the bowel by decreasing fiber—large fecal volume distends the bowel. Be careful not to create obstructions.
- ▲ Correct for diarrhea, steatorrhea, obstruction, and anemia.
- ▲ In acute stages, allow the bowel to heal and use products, which contain short-chain fatty acids and glutamine to prevent a decline in nutritional status.
- ▲ Provide antioxidants such as vitamin E, as well as omega-3 fatty acids (EPA), which play a role in inflammatory processes.
- ▲ Prolonged use of corticosteroids, calcium and vitamin D deficiency, and a low BMI are some of the possible contributing factors to bone disease in patients with IBD (Lopez and Buchman, 2000).

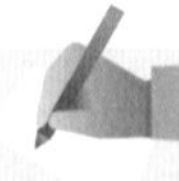

DIETARY AND NUTRITIONAL RECOMMENDATIONS

- To treat the condition in its acute state, an elemental diet is needed to minimize fecal volume. A tube feeding that contains glutamine is often useful. See Table 7–14 for preoperative and postoperative diets.
- TPN is useful if needed, often for 2 weeks in the acute stage, or long-term when surgical intervention has left a small amount of functioning gut remaining.
- As the patient progresses, a high-protein (1–1.5 g/kg), high-calorie diet, given in six small feedings, should be used. This is especially important for infants.
- Diet should exclude nuts, seeds, legumes, and coarse whole grains. Fresh fruits and vegetables may not be tolerated if they are highly fibrous; monitor carefully.
- If needed, a low-residue diet should be used. Intake of fiber and milk should be controlled. Persons with this condition often have lactose, wheat, or gluten intolerance.
- Supplement the diet with multivitamins and minerals, especially thiamine, folacin, vitamin E, zinc, calcium, and iron. Vitamin D may also be needed if bone disease is present.
- MCTs may be helpful. Use more omega-3 fatty acid sources, such as mackerel and tuna; supplements also may be indicated.

TABLE 7–14 Nutritional Guidelines for Colectomy and Ileostomy

Preoperative diet. A low-residue diet leading to a clear liquid diet or use of an elemental tube feeding is recommended.

Postoperative diet. Intravenous feeding should continue for 1–2 days. Diet should progress slowly from clear to full liquids and then a low-fiber, high-protein regimen with high calories (especially carbohydrates). Diet also should provide a high intake of vitamins and minerals. The patient will need vitamin B12 injections and adequate intake of sodium and potassium and fluids. TPN may be ordered. In a liberalized diet, foods (those least likely to cause problems) are added one at a time. Avoid gas-forming or acidic foods (the latter may cause increased peristalsis); products such as Bean-O may help reduce flatulence.

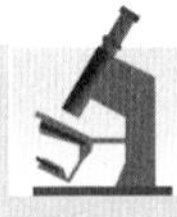

PROFILE

Clinical/History		
Height	Alb, RBP	H&H, Serum Fe
Weight	Ca++	Serum folate
BMI	Mg++	Gluc
Temperature	Serum phosphorus, Alk Phos	Complete blood count (CBC), ESR
Stool sample	PT	WBC
Lab Work	Cl−	Breath hydrogen test
Bilirubin	Transferrin, TIBC	Biopsy
Chol, Trig	N balance	Sigmoidoscopy
K+	Schilling test (B12) Serum B12	Colonoscopy
BUN, Creat		Fecal fat study

Common Drugs Used and Potential Side Effects

- Sulfasalazine (Azulfidine) requires the patient to drink 8–10 glasses of fluid daily to avoid renal stones. Anorexia, nausea, vomiting, and GI distress may occur. Folic acid supplements also may be required.
- Corticosteroids may require restriction of sodium intake. Adrenocorticotropic hormone (ACTH) is usually more effective than hydrocortisone sodium succinate (Solu-Cortef). Negative nitrogen and calcium balances may result. Monitor the need for extra vitamins and minerals. Cumulative corticosteroid dose is a significant predictor of reduced BMD in IBD (Gokhale et al., 1998).
- Use of methotrexate is being studied. Monitor for nausea, vomiting, diarrhea, gingivitis, and stomatitis.
- Antispasmodics or antidiarrheals are often used.
- With antibiotic therapy, diarrhea can be aggravated and vitamin K may be lost.
- Olsalazine (Dipentum) is used for persons who cannot tolerate Azulfidine. Beware of renal toxicity, cramping, rectal bleeding, and indigestion.
- Psyllium laxatives (Metamucil) can help with constipation and diarrhea. Long-term use alters electrolytes. Flatulence or steatorrhea may occur.

Herbs, Botanicals and Supplements

- Herbs and botanical supplements should not be used without discussing with the physician.
- Onion, valerian, and tea have been recommended for this condition, but no clinical trials have proven efficacy.

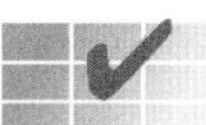

PATIENT EDUCATION

- ✔ Ensure that the patient avoids foods that are known to cause diarrhea. Avoid extremes in food or beverage temperatures.
- ✔ Explain that pleasant mealtimes are an important part of treatment.
- ✔ Indicate that frequent, small meals may increase the patient's total nutritional intake.
- ✔ Avoid iced or carbonated beverages, which may stimulate peristalsis in times of discomfort.
- ✔ Instruct the patient to eat slowly and chew foods well.
- ✔ Discuss fears related to eating.
- ✔ Frequent counseling by a dietitian may be helpful.
- ✔ Stop eating 2–3 hours before bedtime.

INTESTINAL FISTULA

NUTRITIONAL ACUITY RANKING: LEVEL 4

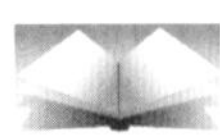

DEFINITIONS AND BACKGROUND

An intestinal fistula is an unwanted pathway from intestines to other organs, e.g., the bladder. External fistulas are between the small intestine and the outside (e.g., skin). Internal fistulas are between two internal organs. They may occur from Crohn's disease, intestinal cancer, trauma, or after surgery. Weight loss and hypoalbuminemia will affect mortality. Hyperbaric oxygen therapy may be considered for patients with poorly healing fistulas. Persistent perineal sinus is a common and serious cause of morbidity after proctectomy for Crohn's disease; omentoplasty may be an effective procedure for the treatment of this condition (Yamamoto et al., 2001).

OBJECTIVES

- Promote rest and healing; minimize drainage from fistula.
- Monitor the type of dietary regimen according to the location of the fistula and surgical or medical treatment. Surgery may be performed to drain infection, to establish a stoma, or to remove the fistula if possible.
- Replace fluid and electrolyte losses.
- Decrease malnutrition and infections through aggressive nutritional support.
- Promote positive nitrogen balance.
- Prevent organ damage and death.

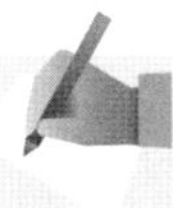

DIETARY AND NUTRITIONAL RECOMMENDATIONS

- Use TPN or elemental diet at first, especially TPN for jejunal fistulas. A jejunostomy may help a duodenal fistula. A higher protein intake than usual may be needed.
- Use of an elemental formula diet also may be beneficial for an extended period of time to support GI tract recovery.
- Progress to a low-residue, soft or normal diet as tolerated.

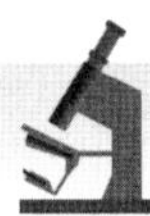

PROFILE

Clinical/History	I & O	Alb, prealbumin
Height	**Lab Work**	RBP
Weight		BUN, Creat
BMI	H&H, Serum Fe	K+, Na+
Weight loss	Serum folate	Cl−
Temperature	N balance	Transferrin

Common Drugs Used and Potential Side Effects

- Antibiotics commonly are used.
- Octreotide (somatostatin analog) inhibits endocrine/exocrine secretions and excessive GI motility. It is only used parenterally and can cause nausea, vomiting, abdominal pain, diarrhea, or flatulence.

Herbs, Botanicals and Supplements

- Herbs and botanical supplements should not be used without discussing with the physician.

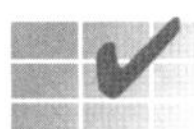

PATIENT EDUCATION

- Defined formula diets can help support spontaneous closure in approximately 4–6 weeks. If closure has not occurred, surgery is aided by better nutritional status.
- Instruct the patient regarding the fiber content of foods. Discuss how much to include during periods of flare-up and how to gradually increase fiber to achieve the goal set individually for that person.

ILEOSTOMY

NUTRITIONAL ACUITY RANKING: LEVEL 3

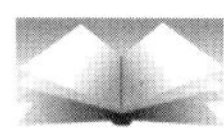

DEFINITIONS AND BACKGROUND

Used to treat intractable cases of ulcerative disease, Crohn's disease, polyposis, and colon cancer, an ileostomy is a surgical procedure (stoma/opening formation) that brings the ileum through the abdominal wall. It may be temporary or permanent. This procedure causes a decrease in fat, bile acid, and vitamin B12 absorption, as well as greater losses of sodium and potassium. Patients will be incontinent of gas and stool. Ideally, ileocecal valve can be kept to decrease bacterial influx into the small intestine. Of these patients, 50–70% will have recurrent disease.

Ileoanal anastomosis is now the most common alternative to conventional ileostomy. Technically, it is not an ostomy because there is no stoma. Most of the rectum is surgically removed; an internal pouch is formed out of the terminal ileum. It is called a J-pouch or pelvic pouch. Opening at the bottom of this pouch is attached to the anus to provide continence. It is used for patients with ulcerative colitis or familial polyposis who have not lost their rectum or anus previously.

Another alternative involves ileal reservoir after proctocolectomy. The colon is the primary site for sodium, potassium, and water absorption and for formation and absorption of vitamin K. This procedure allows fairly normal resumption of colonic functions. No problems with vitamins B12 or K or bile salt absorption have been noted. A high-fiber diet is recommended to normalize elimination. Fluids may be given between meals, with consideration for sodium and potassium needs. Caffeine should be controlled to decrease diarrhea; concentrated sweets should be avoided to prevent osmotic diarrhea; and specific intolerances should be omitted.

A continent ileostomy is also called a Kock pouch. A reservoir pouch is created inside the abdomen with a portion of the terminal ileum. A valve is constructed in the pouch, which is brought through the abdominal wall. A catheter or tube is inserted into the pouch several times a day to drain feces from the reservoir. This procedure has generally been replaced in popularity by the ileoanal pouch, which has demonstrated good results (Regimbeau, 2001). A modified version of this procedure called the Barnett Continent Ileal Reservoir is practiced at a limited number of facilities.

OBJECTIVES

- Modify the diet to counteract malabsorption of nutrients secondary to diarrhea, protein and fluid losses, negative nitrogen balance from nutrient loss, and anorexia.
- Correct anemia caused by inadequate intake or blood losses.
- Counteract weakness and muscle cramping from potassium losses.
- Counteract increased basal metabolic needs in the presence of fever and infection.
- Replenish calcium to reverse arthritic joint involvement caused by steatorrhea and the side effects of steroid therapy.
- Prevent gallstones, renal oxalate stones, bacterial overgrowth, and fatty acid malabsorption.

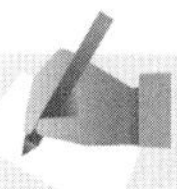

DIETARY AND NUTRITIONAL RECOMMENDATIONS

- If needed, provide a high-calorie, high-protein diet that is low in excess insoluble fiber. Pectin in apples and oligosaccharides in oatmeal may be beneficial.
- Use dairy products cautiously for preoperative patients, because some may have lactose intolerances. Be careful of nuts, legumes, whole grains, and leafy greens for the preoperative patient because of their high residue content with resultant bowel stimulation.
- Diet should provide an adequate amount of fluids, especially in hot weather.
- Postoperatively, spinach or parsley may be used as a natural intestinal deodorizer, but beware of excesses of oxalate-rich foods.
- The patient needs an adequate intake of protein (provided by low-fat sources such as lean meats and egg white), vitamin B12 (provided by liver, fish, and eggs), folacin, calcium, magnesium, iron, sodium, vitamin C, and potassium. Add salt as needed to the diet.

Common Drugs Used and Potential Side Effects

- Prednisone. Restrict excessive sodium intake. Monitor nitrogen and calcium losses.
- Lomotil. This drug is a stool thickener and deodorizer. Plenty of fluids should be used.
- Psyllium (Metamucil) is used as a bulk-forming agent. Increased peristalsis will occur.

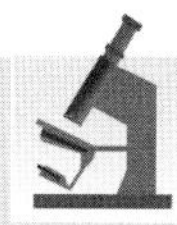

PROFILE

Clinical/History	Lab Work	
Height	H&H, Serum Fe	TIBC
Weight	BUN, Creat	Gluc
BMI	K+, Na+	WBC
Stool (occult blood)	Alb, prealbumin	Ca++
BP	Transferrin	Mg++
		Serum B12
		Schilling test if needed

Herbs, Botanicals and Supplements

- Herbs and botanical supplements should not be used without discussing with the physician.

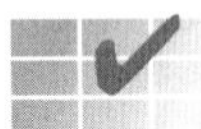

PATIENT EDUCATION

- ✓ Explain which foods are common sources of the needed nutrients in a diet or suggest supplementation with multivitamins and minerals.
- ✓ Monitor individual tolerance to offending foods such as gas-forming or fried foods, highly seasoned foods, nuts, raisins, and pineapple. Patients may try a product such as Bean-O to reduce flatulence; positive results are not guaranteed.
- ✓ An enterostomal therapist may be of assistance.
- ✓ Discuss the role of fluid and sodium during hot weather.
- ✓ The patient should avoid obesity.
- ✓ Eating before bedtime should be avoided.

For More Information

- United Ostomy Association (UOA)
  19772 MacArthur Blvd., Suite 200
  Irvine, CA 92612-2405
  1-800-826-0826
  http://www.uoa.org/

COLOSTOMY

NUTRITIONAL ACUITY RANKING: LEVEL 3

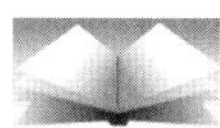

DEFINITIONS AND BACKGROUND

The colon functions primarily to absorb water and sodium and to excrete potassium and bicarbonate. A colostomy is an artificial outlet for intestinal wastes created surgically by bringing a portion of the colon through the abdominal wall, resulting in a stoma. Colostomy can be permanent or temporary. It may be indicated for intestinal cancer, diverticulitis, perforated bowel, radiation enteritis, obstruction, and Hirschsprung's disease. Constipation and fecal incontinence are common symptoms in neurological patients; sacral nerve stimulation is an experimental therapy that should precede surgery.

Colostomy output is generally more formed than ileostomy output. A sigmoid or descending colostomy is the most common type, usually located on the lower left side of the abdomen. A transverse colostomy may result in one or two openings; it is located in the upper abdomen and can be right or left sided. A loop colostomy is usually created in the transverse colon; it is one stoma with two openings. An ascending colostomy is relatively rare and is located on the right side of the abdomen.

Some colostomates can "irrigate," using a procedure similar to an enema to clean stool directly out of the colon through the stoma. This requires special irrigation appliances: an irrigation bag and a connecting tube (or catheter), a stoma cone, and an irrigation sleeve. A special lubricant is sometimes used on the stoma in preparation for irrigation. Following irrigation, some colostomates can use a stoma cap, a one- or two-piece system which simply covers and protects the stoma. This procedure is usually done to avoid the need to wear an appliance.

To avoid major problems of blockage, increased flatulence, and problems with certain foods, preoperative teaching and postoperative follow-up must include anticipatory guidance on food selection (Floruta, 2001).

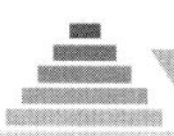

OBJECTIVES

- Speed wound healing and recovery.
- Prevent weight loss. Correct malnutrition from GI blood loss, anemia, protein malabsorption, and steatorrhea.
- Prevent blockage.
- Prevent watery or unscheduled bowel movements. Correct or prevent dehydration.
- Individualize the diet: Eat regularly, avoid odor-causing foods, and monitor food preferences.
- Normalize the patient's lifestyle as much as possible.
- Avoid infection and skin irritants.

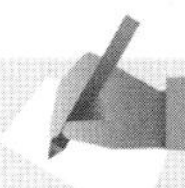

DIETARY AND NUTRITIONAL RECOMMENDATIONS

- Initially, after the operation, use liquids. As the patient progresses, use a low-residue diet to reduce stoma discharge and irritation. To speed healing, diet should also be high in protein and calories. Gradually introduce new foods; if done slowly, offending foods can be identified and obstruction can be controlled or prevented. Foods most often avoided because of an ostomy include fresh fruits, nuts, coconut, and vegetables such as corn, popcorn, cabbage, beans, and onions (Floruta, 2001).
- Diet should provide normal or increased salt intake. One to two quarts of fluid, taken between meals, should be ingested daily.
- Beware of highly spiced foods and excessive raw fruits and vegetables, if these foods cause diarrhea. Prune juice may also be a problem for some patients.
- Odor-causing foods may include alcohol (beer), beans, onions, green peppers, cabbage, turnips, beets, Brussels sprouts, radishes, cucumbers, fish, eggs, and garlic. Fresh parsley is a natural deodorizer.
- Gas-forming vegetables such as corn, broccoli, and cauliflower may cause discomfort; omit if necessary. Bean-O is a product that is helpful in reducing flatulence.
- Regular meals and "constipating foods" like boiled milk, rice, or peanut butter help to normalize evacuation times.
- Progress to a high-fiber diet with short-fibered foods—no whole-kernel corn, celery, nuts, pineapple, popcorn, coleslaw, apple skins, seeds, or coconut.
- If diarrhea results from the colostomy, try strained bananas, applesauce, boiled rice, boiled milk, and peanut butter.
- If calcium oxalate stones develop after the colostomy, diet should provide a high fluid intake. Restrict intake of oxalates from spinach, rhubarb, wild greens, coffee and tea, and chocolate.

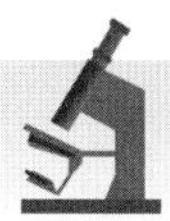

PROFILE

Clinical/History	Lab Work	
Height	H&H, Serum Fe	Ca++, Mg++
Weight	K+, Na+	Chol, Trig
BMI	Gluc	Transferrin, TIBC
I & O; hydration status	Alb, prealbumin	Serum B12
		Serum folate
		PT

Common Drugs Used and Potential Side Effects

- Prednisone. Restrict excessive sodium intake. Monitor nitrogen, calcium, and potassium losses when used over a long period of time.
- Lomotil is a stool thickener and deodorizer; use plenty of fluids.
- Bulk-forming agents such Psyllium (Metamucil) may be useful. Increased peristalsis occurs.

Herbs, Botanicals and Supplements

- Herbs and botanical supplements should not be used without discussing with the physician.

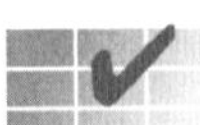

PATIENT EDUCATION

✔ Approximately 6 weeks are required to acclimate the bowel to new procedures of irrigation. Enemas are used to wash the bowel up to the ileocecal valve (with 1,000 mL of tap water). Constipation can occur with dehydration; therefore, adequate intake of fluid and fiber is important.

✔ Use of a commercial deodorant in the colostomy bag is preferred to eliminating highly flavored or nutrient-dense foods.

✔ Instruct the patient to eat slowly, chew foods well, and avoid swallowing air.

✔ Irrigations should not be performed when there is vomiting or diarrhea.

✔ Regular mealtimes should be encouraged.

✔ Enterostomal therapy can be helpful.

✔ Reassurance is needed, without misleading the patient.

✔ Patients should limit intake of aspirin, NSAIDs, red meat, poultry, fish, some raw vegetables, and vitamin C prior to lab testing (American College of Physicians, 1997).

For More Information

✦ United Ostomy Association (UOA)
19772 MacArthur Blvd., Suite 200
Irvine, CA 92612-2405
1-800-826-0826
http://www.uoa.org/

SHORT BOWEL SYNDROME

NUTRITIONAL ACUITY RANKING: LEVEL 4

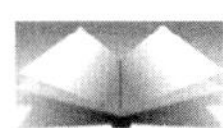

DEFINITIONS AND BACKGROUND

Short bowel syndrome (SBS) usually involves surgical resection of a portion of the small bowel, compromising the absorptive surface and resulting in malabsorption (especially if more than 50% of the small intestine has been removed). Malnutrition from maldigestion, malabsorption diarrhea, and steatorrhea may result. A bowel resection that may result in SBS may be necessary in Crohn's disease, intestinal cancer, scleroderma, or fistula. Necrotizing enterocolitis is the major cause of SBS in infants; another problem may be intestinal atresia or mesentery artery occlusion.

The small bowel is presented with 7–9 L of nutrient-containing fluid each day; the intestinal mucosa is so efficient that only 100–200 mL of stool is excreted in a normal person without SBS (Purdum and Kirby, 1991). If only 30% of the SI remains in an adult (or less than 30 cm in infants), the resulting malabsorption may be life threatening. Problems are significant when more than 70% of the bowel is resected, unless terminal ileum and ileocecal valve remain. Every attempt should be made to keep the ileocecal valve to prevent contamination of the small intestine.

SBS generally leaves less than 150 cm of small intestine; 100 cm is necessary to completely absorb bile salts; 50–70 cm of jejunum-ileum maintains minimal intestinal autonomy. The minimal length of functional bowel needed for enteral feeding is over 100 cm in the absence of an intact colon and over 60 cm in continuity with the colon (Johnson, 2000). Length of small intestine remaining after resection is the best predictor of final success in terminating PN in children with SBS; PN is required longer when there is bacterial overgrowth and associated enteritis (Kaufman et al., 1997). Home PN may cost between \$250–\$400/day, and most insurance companies cover up to \$1 million, or about 10 years of reimbursement.

Effects of SBS include dehydration, electrolyte losses, hypokalemia, deficiencies of calcium, magnesium, and zinc, carbohydrate and lactose malabsorption, protein malabsorption, renal oxalate stone formation, cholesterol biliary stones, gastric acid hypersecretion, vitamin B12 or iron deficiency, fat-soluble vitamin deficiency, and diarrhea. See Table 7–15 regarding the implications of bowel resections and Table 7–16 for malabsorption concerns. Early and aggressive nutritional intervention is necessary for resolution of nutritional deficits and recovery of health. Early oral feeding after colorectal surgery is safe (Hartsell et al., 1997). Postresection phases are in 3 stages (Johnson, 2000). Bowel adaptation takes about 1 year; use of growth hormone, insulin-like growth factor-1 (IGF-1) and glutamine may help enhance this process.

Transplantation of the small bowel restores quality of life for recipients who have functioning grafts (DiMartini et al., 1998). Advances in transplantation hold promise as an alternative to intestinal failure and chronic dependence on TPN (Silver et al., 2000). Surgery and high-dose immunosuppression are a problem. Recovery of normal motility and absorptive capacity are the goals. Diarrhea and high stomal output are common problems and can lead to nutrient deficits, especially electrolytes.

TABLE 7–15 Implications of Bowel Resections

Loss of jejunum. Ileum undergoes hyperplasia; length and absorption per cm increases.

Loss of ileum. This is more serious than loss of jejunum because vitamin B12 and bile salts will be reabsorbed poorly as a result. The ileocecal valve keeps colonic bacteria out of the small intestine and regulates chyme flow. Some colonic adaptation occurs during the next 2–5 years.

Loss of colon. Overall, with removal of the colon versus the small intestine, fewer malabsorption problems occur. Loss of electrolyte and water-absorbing capacity occurs, as well as loss of salvage absorption of CHO and other nutrients. Most oxalate absorption occurs here.

In SBS, short-chain triglycerides have a precursor in pectin; oligosaccharides increase O2 uptake in the colon, thereby maintaining gut integrity. Early refeeding (i.e., free fatty acids, sugars, proteins) stimulates mucosal growth. Hyperphagia can increase enterocyte production. Adaptation requires adequate nutrition, intraluminal nutrients, and bile and pancreatic secretions. Enhancers of the adaptive process seem to include gastrin, glutamine, growth hormone, insulin, short-chain fatty acids, fats, some dietary fibers, cholecystokinin (CCK), glucagon, IGF-1, neurotensin, and glucose.

OBJECTIVES

- Prevent and correct fluid and electrolyte imbalances and dehydration. Oral intake could aggravate already massive losses of fluid (3–10 L/day is common).
- Use remaining bowel surface and maximize efficacy. Prevent atrophy of small bowel mucosa from long-term TPN use.
- Correct symptoms of deficiency and malabsorption, when possible, for trace minerals and for vitamins B12, A, D, E, and K.
- Decrease weight loss (approximately 10 lb monthly until adaptation occurs).
- Omit lactose if not tolerated; provide adequate calcium replacements.

TABLE 7–16 Malabsorption Concerns in Short Bowel Syndrome

Decreased bile acid concentration (with loss of ileum and bacterial overgrowth)

Decreased surface area and lessened fluid reabsorption

Maladaptive remaining small bowel, especially from original bowel disease, lactase deficiency

Dumping syndrome from rapid transit and reduced bowel length

Bacterial overgrowth, if ileocecal valve is absent

Gastric acid over secretion with resulting damage to duodenal cells and altered pH, thus affecting pancreatic enzyme and bile activity

Decreased pancreatic enzyme activity in duodenum, with malnutrition

- Decrease oxalate from the diet to reduce renal stone formation. Excess bile in the colon from decreased ileal absorption enhances absorption of free oxalate (normally only 10–15% is absorbed).
- Control or prevent gallstone formation (increased risk of 2–3 times normal), anemia, protein-losing enteropathy, peptic ulcer from increased gastric acid secretion, and liver disease (often in home TPN).
- Allow remaining intestine to compensate over time by hypertrophy of villi and increased diameter. Less than 100 cm yields more severe problems; less than 60 cm remaining intestine may require long-term PN. Home TPN is expensive but can be lifesaving for months to years. Transitional feedings may be needed over several months from PN to oral diet.
- Provide nutrient replacements, dependent on area of resection (proximal jejunum—calcium, iron, magnesium, protein, CHO, and fat absorbed here; terminal ileum—bile acids and intrinsic factor-bound vitamin B12 absorbed here).
- For care of colostomy or ileostomy, see appropriate entries.
- Reduce symptoms of dumping syndrome from CHO intolerance.

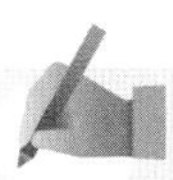

DIETARY AND NUTRITIONAL RECOMMENDATIONS

- IVs or TPN may be appropriate immediately before and approximately 5 days after surgery to allow rest. Determine whether the patient has problems with bloating, etc. TPN should continue until adaptive processes are established. Glutamine-enriched solutions may be beneficial against intestinal atrophy during TPN (Purdum and Kirby, 1991).
- The first phase (1–3 weeks) involves extensive diarrhea greater than 2 liters daily; TPN is used, advancing slowly to avoid refeeding syndrome. If diarrhea continues, at the end of this time, to be greater than 2 liters, TPN may be lifelong.
- In the second phase (3 weeks to 2 months), diarrhea is lessened and intestinal adaptation begins; TPN may be slowly reduced and TF started at a slow, continuous rate according to stomal output or stool output. Need 40–60 kcals/kg and 1.2–1.5 g protein/Kg. If weight loss is greater than 1 kg/week or if diarrhea is greater than 600 g/day, TPN may need to be restarted (Johnson, 2000). When TF is used, polymeric solutions may be beneficial. Glutamine is the major fuel for the GI tract; include with either TF or TPN use. Consider nocturnal TF if patient does not do well with weight gain.
- In the third stage, complete bowel adaptation begins as TF is tolerated and oral diet is slowly resumed (from 2 months to 1 year.) Six small feedings that are high CHO and low fat may be tolerated (60% CHO, 20% protein, 20% fat with limit in MCT of 40 g/day). With no colon, the diet may need to be 30–40% fat, 20% protein, and 40–50% CHO; jejunostomy feedings may be needed, and oxalates need not be restricted (Johnson, 2000).
- Suggestions to increase the transit time of ingested foods are included in a special "SBS diet" plan (Clark Lykins and Stockwell, 1998). Patients are taught after surgery and have bimonthly contact with the dietitian after leaving the hospital.
- Adequate zinc, potassium, liquid magnesium, oral calcium (600–1000 mg), manganese, iron, vitamin C, selenium, B-complex (especially folic acid), and other nutrients may be needed as supplements—determine needs based on site of resection and signs of malnutrition. With antibiotic use, will need extra vitamin K. Monitor for needs for vitamins A, E, and D. Water-miscible forms of the fat-soluble vitamins may be useful.
- Lactose-restricted and oxalate-restricted diets may be needed for an extended period of time. Rhubarb, spinach, beets, cocoa and chocolate, sweet potatoes, strawberries, celery, and peanuts are high-oxalate foods; nuts and nut butters, berries, Concord grapes, sweet potatoes and potatoes, and most vegetables have smaller amounts.
- Omit alcoholic beverages and caffeine unless physician permits small quantities.
- Taking fluids between instead of with meals may be helpful in reducing dumping. Restrict at first to 1,500 mL; progress as tolerated.
- With osmotic diarrhea, a reduction in simple carbohydrates and an increase in complex carbohydrates may be needed. Sorbitol, mannitol, and xylitol are usually poorly absorbed.
- Restricted foods such as lactose may be attempted and added back to the diet if they are tolerated. Bowel adaptation occurs over time and may eventually lead the patient back to an unrestricted diet.

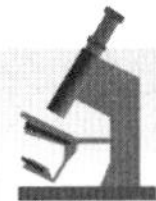

PROFILE

Clinical/History		
Height	Serum gastrin (increased)	RBP
Weight	Ca++	N balance
BMI	25 Hydroxy-vitamin D level	Serum oxalate
Weight changes	Alk Phos	Alb, prealbumin
I & O	Mg++	Schilling test
Steatorrhea	Na+ (serum, urine, stool)	Serum B12
Lab Work	K+ (serum, urine, stool)	Serum amylase, lipase
H&H, Serum Fe	Fecal nitrogen	Bile acid breath test
Transferrin	GTT	Lactose tolerance test
D-xylose absorption	Gluc	Hydrogen breath test
		Fecal fat test

Common Drugs Used and Potential Side Effects

Note–most oral medications are poorly tolerated in this condition!

- Cholestyramine may be used for choleraic diarrhea when less than 100 cm is resected and when the colon is in continuity; prevent excessive use. Take before meals. Nausea, vomiting, or constipation may occur.
- Pancrelipase may improve fat and protein absorption after jejunal resection; results are variable.
- Cimetidine and omeprazole may be needed to decrease gastric hypersecretion. Serum gastrin levels should be monitored. A dose 2–3 times higher than normal may be needed. Vitamin B12 absorption decreases.
- Oral calcium supplements (OsCal or Tums four times daily) often are used to bind oxalate excesses and to decrease diarrhea. Do not take with a bulk-forming laxative or with an iron supplement. Increase water intake.
- Antibiotics may be needed, such as Tetracycline, Flagyl, Septra, or Cipro, for bacterial overgrowth. Monitor hydrogen breath tests (especially with blind loop).
- Vitamins that are chewable or in liquid form may be better tolerated. Parenteral vitamin B12 may be necessary. Add extra fat-soluble vitamins A, E, D, and K if deficiency occurs. Do not use vitamin C in excessively large quantities; some links with oxalate stones have been noted in the literature.
- Minerals such as liquid potassium and intravenous or intramuscular magnesium may be needed.
- Growth hormone increases water/sodium transport. It is often useful when used in combination with glutamine and a modified diet (Byrne et al., 1995).
- Antidiarrheals such as Lomotil, Imodium, and Codeine are useful. Liquid preparations often are better tolerated. If dehydration occurs, use oral rehydration therapy but not sports drinks, which do not have the adequate electrolyte replacements.

Herbs, Botanicals and Supplements

- Herbs and botanical supplements should not be used without discussing with the physician.
- Probiotics such as yogurt are a useful aid in bowel adaptation phases.

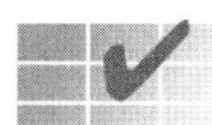

PATIENT EDUCATION

- ✓ Importance of adequate nutrition and supplementation must be discussed to prevent or correct malnutrition and malabsorption. After adaptation, some people will require up to three times their resting energy expenditure (REE) levels to achieve weight maintenance.
- ✓ A supportive attitude from family and caregivers is essential.
- ✓ Recipes and food preparation tips will be needed to support the specific dietary regimen and to evaluate tolerances over time.
- ✓ Progression in diet is allowed when the small intestine hypertrophies over several weeks or months.
- ✓ Discuss the need for free water.

INTESTINAL LYMPHANGIECTASIA

NUTRITIONAL ACUITY RANKING: LEVEL 3

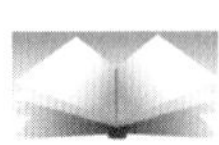

DEFINITIONS AND BACKGROUND

Intestinal lymphangiectasia (idiopathic hypoproteinemia) is a generalized disorder of intestinal lymphatics that results in a protein-losing enteropathy; it can be congenital or secondary to a disease that blocks intestinal lymph drainage (Salvia et al., 2001).

Increased intestinal lymphatic pressure with vessel dilatation occurs, discharging fluid into the bowel lumen. The fluid is then digested by intestinal enzymes and is reabsorbed. Massive fluid retention occurs from obstructed lymph vessels, especially in the abdomen and pleural cavities. While malabsorption and protein-losing enteropathy occur, only marginal loss of protein occurs in most cases. Nausea, vomiting, diarrhea, and abdominal pain result.

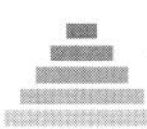

OBJECTIVES

- Identify and correct the cause (e.g., constrictive pericarditis).
- Decrease symptoms and promote recovery.
- Decrease ingested fat because it stimulates lymphatic flow into the gut.
- Meet all nutritional needs for age and sex.
- Monitor absorption of fat-soluble vitamins; ensure adequacy from dietary or supplemental sources.

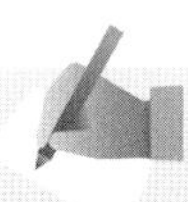

DIETARY AND NUTRITIONAL RECOMMENDATIONS

- A formula or low-fat diet using a high concentration of MCT is useful (Alfano et al., 2000).
- Adequate protein and calories are needed, appropriate to the individual's needs.
- Fat-soluble vitamins may be required in water-miscible form for adequate absorption.

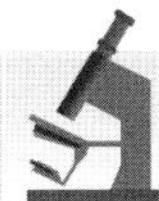

PROFILE

Clinical/History

Height
Weight
BMI
Steatorrhea
Peripheral edema

Lab Work

BUN, Creat
Serum alb, prealbumin (decreased)
RBP
Chol, Trig
Triceps skinfold (TSF), midarm circumference (MAC), midarm muscle circumference (MAMC)
H&H, Serum Fe
Transferrin (decreased)
TLC
Gluc
Fecal concentration of alpha (1)-antitrypsin
Jejunal biopsy (dilated lymphatic lacteal vessels)

Common Drugs Used and Potential Side Effects

- Octreotide may be used with positive results.

Herbs, Botanicals and Supplements

- Herbs and botanical supplements should not be used without discussing with the physician.

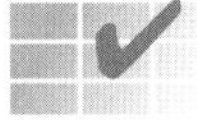

PATIENT EDUCATION

- Discuss the role of fat in digestion, along with the need for MCT oils in the daily diet.
- Discuss fat-soluble vitamins and their sources in the diet.

INTESTINAL LIPODYSTROPHY (WHIPPLE'S DISEASE)

NUTRITIONAL ACUITY RANKING: LEVEL 4

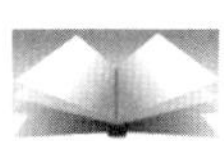

DEFINITIONS AND BACKGROUND

An uncommon systemic disease, Whipple's disease involves infiltration of the small intestine with glycoprotein-laden macrophages and some rod-shaped bacilli (*Tropheryma whippleii*) in varying body tissues. Whipple's disease is noncontagious, occurs mainly in middle-aged white males (ages 30–60 years), and displays many, but not all, of the complications of hereditary hemochromatosis; one hypothesis is that host susceptibility may be exacerbated by iron loading, which impairs microbial iron acquisition ability (Weinberg, 2001). Consideration should be given to have patients evaluated for levels of interferon-gamma and interleukin-4 as well as for serum ferritin and transferrin iron saturation (Weinberg, 2001).

Endocarditis and heart murmur are common. The Whipple bacillus is related to coronary disease and all aspects of atherosclerosis (James, 2001). Patients may have arthralgias for years before diarrhea occurs (Dobbins, 1995). Other signs and symptoms include malabsorption and cholestasis, fever of unknown origin, anemia, hypoproteinemia, gray-to-brown skin pigmentation, CNS involvement, lymphadenopathy, edema, wasting, and sarcoidosis-like illness. The disease is usually fatal if left untreated.

OBJECTIVES

- Reduce fever and inflammatory processes.
- Correct malnutrition and malabsorption.
- Prevent or correct weight loss.
- Correct anemia, iron overloading, or hypoproteinemia where present.
- Prevent or correct dehydration and electrolyte imbalances.

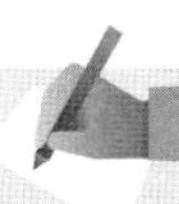

DIETARY AND NUTRITIONAL RECOMMENDATIONS

- Use a high-protein/high-calorie diet appropriate for the patient's age and sex.
- Ensure that diet includes sufficient vitamins and minerals, especially for vitamin D and calcium, when steatorrhea is a problem. Vitamins A, B-complex, and K may also be needed.
- Provide adequate fluid intake to reduce fever and replenish tissues. If edema is a problem, control excess sodium.

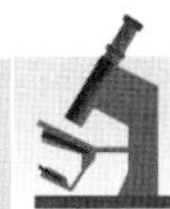

PROFILE

Clinical/History	Lab Work	
Height	Serum Ca++	Serum Fe, serum ferritin
Weight	Alk Phos	Transferrin
BMI	Na+	K+
Temperature	Mg++	RBP
I & O	Alb (decreased)	PT
	H&H (decreased)	Macrophages

Common Drugs Used and Potential Side Effects

- Tetracycline—Do not take with calcium antacids or with dairy products.
- Penicillin also may be used to reduce bacterial overgrowth. Nausea, vomiting, GI distress, or diarrhea may occur.
- Sulfasalazine (Azulfidine) requires the patient to drink 8–10 glasses of fluid daily to avoid renal stones. Anorexia, nausea, vomiting, and GI distress may occur. Folic acid supplements may also be required.
- Trimethoprim-sulfamethoxazole combinations and other drugs may also be used with numerous side effects; monitor closely.

Herbs, Botanicals and Supplements

- Herbs and botanical supplements should not be used without discussing with the physician.

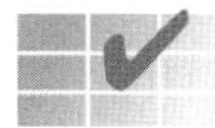

PATIENT EDUCATION

- ✔ Discuss inclusion of high-quality proteins in the diet. Frequent snacks may be beneficial if large meals are not tolerated.
- ✔ Provide lists for nutrient-dense foods rich in specific and needed nutrients (e.g., iron, calcium, etc.).

INTESTINAL TRANSPLANTATION

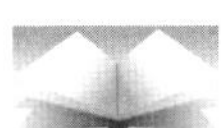

DEFINITIONS AND BACKGROUND

PN is standard therapy for children with SBS and other causes of intestinal failure (Kaufman et al., 2001). Intestinal transplantation (Tx) can now be recommended for a select group of patients for whom morbidity continues to be severe. Life-threatening complications warranting consideration of intestinal transplantation include parenteral nutrition-associated liver disease, recurrent sepsis, and threatened loss of central venous access (Kaufman et al., 2001). SBS, cancers, and other major intestinal diseases may also warrant intestinal transplantation. A critical shortage of donor organs exists, and waiting time is often extensive.

Transplantation of the small bowel restores quality of life for recipients who have functioning grafts (DiMartini et al., 1998). Advances in transplantation hold promise as an alternative to intestinal failure and chronic dependence on TPN (Silver et al., 2000). Morbidity and mortality following intestinal transplant are greater than that following liver or kidney transplant, but long-term survival is now at least 50–60%; outcomes will improve with continued refinements in operative technique and postoperative management, including immunosuppression (Kaufman, 2001). Surgery and high-dose immunosuppression must be managed. Radiation to the small bowel before transplanting the organ, then administration of donor's bone marrow stem cells seems to reduce organ rejection.

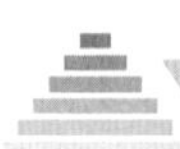

OBJECTIVES

- ▲ Timely nutrition assessment and intervention may improve outcomes; a pretransplant nutrition assessment should be very thorough (Hasse, 2001).
- ▲ Recovery of normal motility and absorptive capacity are the goals.
- ▲ Prevent infection and promote wound healing.
- ▲ Replenish lost nutrient stores. Malnutrition compromises posttransplant survival; prolonged waiting times worsen outcomes when patients are already malnourished (Hasse, 2001).
- ▲ Meet metabolic demands and support recovery.
- ▲ Control complications. Diarrhea and high stomal output are common problems and can lead to nutrient deficits, especially electrolytes.

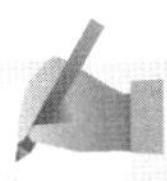

DIETARY AND NUTRITIONAL RECOMMENDATIONS

- PN is rarely needed pretransplant except in cases of intestinal failure (Hasse, 2001).
- Posttransplant, progress from clear liquids to solids as quickly as possibly postoperatively. Monitor fluid status and adjust as needed.
- Daily intake of protein should be appropriate for RDAs (age, sex); 1.5 g-kg while on steroids may be recommended. Calories should be calculated as 30–35 kcal/kg or 1.3–1.5 BEE.
- Daily intake of sodium should be 2–4 g until the drug regimen is reduced. Adjust potassium levels as needed.
- Daily intake of calcium should be 1–1.5 times the RDA to offset poor absorption. Children especially need adequate calcium for growth. Daily intake of phosphorus should be equal to calcium intake.
- Supplement diet with vitamin D, magnesium, and thiamine if needed.
- Control CHO intake with hyperglycemia (50% total kcal) and limit concentrated sweets. Encourage complex CHOs.
- Plan fats at 30–35% of total kcal (encourage monounsaturated fats and omega-3 fatty acids.) Low saturated fats and cholesterol may be needed. A low-fat regimen is recommended for prevention and treatment of hyperlipidemia.
- Reduce gastric irritants as necessary, if GI distress or reflux occurs.
- The special diet may be discontinued when drug therapy is reduced to maintenance levels. Encourage exercise and a weight control plan thereafter.

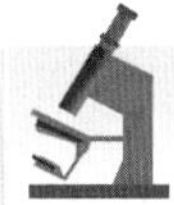

PROFILE

Clinical/History	Lab Work	
Height	Alb, prealbumin	WBC, TLC
Dry weight, present weight	Ca++	Gluc
BMI	K+, Na+	Chol, Trig
BP	H&H, Serum Fe	N balance
I & O	Serum folacin	Glomerular filtration rate (GFR)
Temperature	BUN, Creat	Alk phos, phosphorus
	Mg++	AST, ALT
	TSF, MAC, MAMC	Bilirubin

Common Drugs Used and Potential Side Effects

- Corticosteroids (such as Prednisone, Solu-Cortef) are used for immunosuppression. Side effects include increased catabolism of proteins, negative nitrogen balance, hyperphagia, ulcers, decreased glucose tolerance, sodium retention, fluid retention, and impaired calcium absorption and osteoporosis. Cushing's syndrome, obesity, muscle wasting, and increased gastric secretion may result. A higher protein intake and lower intake of simple CHOs may be needed.
- Cyclosporine does not retain sodium as much as corticosteroids do. Intravenous doses are more effective

than oral doses. Nausea, vomiting, and diarrhea are common side effects. Hyperlipidemia, HPN, and hyperkalemia may also occur; decrease sodium and potassium as necessary. Elevated glucose and lipids may occur. The drug also is nephrotoxic; a controlled renal diet may be beneficial.

- Immunosuppressants such as Muromonab or Orthoclone (OKT3) and antithymocyte globulin (ATG) are less nephrotoxic than cyclosporine but can cause nausea, anorexia, diarrhea, and vomiting. Monitor carefully. Fever and stomatitis also may occur; alter diet as needed.
- Azathioprine (Imuran) may cause leukopenia, thrombocytopenia, oral and esophageal sores, macrocytic anemia, pancreatitis, vomiting, diarrhea, and other side effects that are complex. Folate supplementation and other dietary modifications (liquid or soft diet, use of oral supplements) may be needed. The drug works by lowering the number of T cells; it often is prescribed along with prednisone for conventional immunosuppression.
- Tacrolimus (Prograf, FK506) suppresses T-cell immunity; it is 100 times more potent than cyclosporine, thus requiring smaller doses. Side effects include GI distress, nausea, vomiting, hyperkalemia, and hyperglycemia.
- Diuretics such as Lasix may cause hypokalemia. Aldactone actually spares potassium; monitor drug changes closely.
- Analgesics are also used to reduce pain. Long-term use may affect such nutrients as vitamin C and folacin; monitor carefully for each specific medication.
- Antihypertensive, antilipemics, diuretics, and potassium supplements may be used. Monitor side effects accordingly.
- Grapefruit juice decreases drug metabolism in the gut (via P450-CYP3A4 inhibition.) One glass can affect medications up to 24 hours later. Avoid taking with alprazolam, buspirone, cisapride, cyclosporine, statins, tacrolimus, and many others.

Herbs, Botanicals and Supplements

- Herbs and botanical supplements should not be used without discussing with the physician.

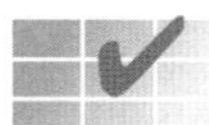

PATIENT EDUCATION

- ✔ Indicate which foods are sources of protein, calcium, and other key nutrients in the diet.
- ✔ If the patient does not prefer milk, show how other sources of calcium may be used in the diet.
- ✔ Alcohol should be avoided unless permitted by the doctor.
- ✔ Discuss control of hyperglycemia when appropriate.
- ✔ Patients should learn appropriate self-medication and when to seek medical attention.
- ✔ Discuss problems with long-term obesity and hypercholesterolemia.
- ✔ Encourage moderation in diet; promote adequate exercise.

For More Information

- ✦ American Council on Transplantation
  700 North Fairfax Street, Suite 505
  Alexandria, VA 22314
  (703) 836-4301

HEMORRHOIDS AND HEMORRHOIDECTOMY

NUTRITIONAL ACUITY RANKING: LEVEL 1

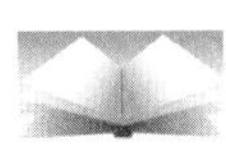

DEFINITIONS AND BACKGROUND

Chronic constipation is believed to be the main cause of hemorrhoids. The disorder is common in Americans (50% of Americans older than 50 years of age will have suffered at least once, especially if obese). Causes include increased abdominal pressure secondary to straining during bowel movements, heavy lifting, childbirth, and benign prostatic hypertrophy.

The theory of a sliding anal canal lining and the knowledge that hemorrhoidal cushions are a normal part of the anal anatomy should encourage symptom control rather than radical removal of tissue (Hulme-Moir, Bartolo, 2001). Internal hemorrhoids are normal anatomical structures and rarely are painful (they may only bleed). External hemorrhoids are usually from excessive diarrhea or from constipation; they are tender, painful, bluish, localized swellings of varicose veins at the anal margin. Bright red bleeding with stool is common.

Techniques that fix the cushions back in position can be performed in outpatients with reasonable success rates. If required, surgery should be aimed at symptomatic hemorrhoids; sutureless closed hemorrhoidectomy is a new procedure that has been well received (Sayfan et al., 2001).

It is hoped that new developments such as circular stapling and better pain management will promote increased day surgery, better pain control, and less time off work for patients (Hulme-Moir, Bartolo, 2001).

OBJECTIVES

Hemorrhoids

- Provide comfort. Prevent prolapse and thrombosis.
- Avoid constipation, infection, and anemia.
- Reduce possible irritation from too much roughage.
- Avoid irritants such as laxatives.

Hemorrhoidectomy

- Reduce irritation while patient heals.
- Promote rapid healing. Prevent future recurrence.

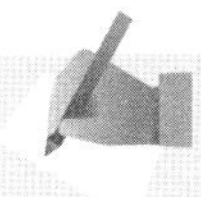

DIETARY AND NUTRITIONAL RECOMMENDATIONS

Hemorrhoids

- Diet should be low in fiber only when the patient is in pain. Otherwise, a high-fiber (25–35 g) diet should be used.
- Fluids should be increased to 8–10 glasses daily.
- Exclude highly seasoned foods or relishes.

Hemorrhoidectomy

- Begin with clear liquids and progress to full liquids.
- A low-fiber/soft diet should be used until full recovery occurs.
- Eventually, adequate to high fiber (25–35 g) should be taken.
- Omit lactose only if necessary.

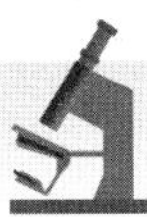

PROFILE

Clinical/History		
Height	History of diarrhea	BUN
Weight	Constipation	Transferrin, TIBC
BMI		PT
I & O	**Lab Work**	Alb, prealbumin
BP	H&H, Serum Fe	Stool (occult blood)

Common Drugs Used and Potential Side Effects

- Laxatives and enemas may have caused faulty bowel function. Avoid use unless prescribed by the doctor.
- Troxerutin and carbazochrome are new medications often used as combination therapy. Monitor for any untoward side effects.
- Preparation H contains vitamin A from shark oil, as well as yeast derivatives; shrinkage is not always guaranteed.
- Lubrication with glycerin suppositories may help to reduce symptoms.
- Medicated suppositories such as Anusol HC (contains hydrocortisone) may help to decrease inflammation. Limit steroid-containing medications to less than 2 weeks of continuous use to avoid atrophy of anal tissues.
- Psyllium laxatives (Metamucil) can help with constipation; long-term use alters electrolytes. Flatulence or steatorrhea may occur.

Herbs, Botanicals and Supplements

- Herbs and botanical supplements should not be used without discussing with the physician.
- Comfrey, plantain, butcher's broom, horse chestnut, and witch hazel have been recommended for this condition, but no clinical trials have proven efficacy.

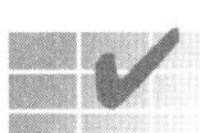

PATIENT EDUCATION

- ✓ Ensure that the patient adequately exercises, rests, and maintains regular bowel habits.
- ✓ Teach the patient about the role of fiber in the diet.
- ✓ Persistent or recurrent bleeding requires medical attention, especially to monitor vitamin K, iron, and B-complex levels and to prevent additional losses.
- ✓ It is important to keep the anal skin area dry.
- ✓ Over-the-counter products may aggravate an allergic response.
- ✓ Warm sitz baths may help to reduce symptoms.

REFERENCES

Cited References

Abell T, Werkman R. Gastrointestinal motility disorders. *Am Fam Phys*. 1996;53:895.

Abdulkarim A, Murray J. Celiac disease. *Curr Treat Options Gastroenterol*. 2002;5:27.

Abraczinskas D, et al. Propranolol for the prevention of first esophageal variceal hemorrhage: a lifetime commitment? *Hepatology*. 2001;34:1096.

Aldoori W, et al. A prospective study of dietary fiber types and symptomatic diverticular disease in men. *J Nutri*. 1998;128:714.

Aldoori W, et al. A prospective study of diet and the risk of symptomatic diverticular disease in men. *Am J Clin Nutri*. 1994;60:757.

Aldoori W, et al. Prospective study of diet and risk of duodenal ulcer in men. *Am J Epid*. 1997;145:42.

Alfano V, et al. Stable reversal of pathologic signs of primitive intestinal lymphangiectasia with a hypolipidic, MCT-enriched diet. *Nutrition*. 2000;16:303.

Altuntas B, et al. Etiology of chronic diarrhea. *Indian J Pediatr*. 1999; 66:657.

American College of Physicians. Clinical guideline: Part 1. Suggested technique for fecal occult blood testing and interpretation in colorectal cancer screening. *Ann Int Med*. 1997;126:808.

American Gastroenterology Association. Medical position statement: Celiac sprue. *Gastroenterology*. 2001;120:1522.

American Gastroenterology Association. Medical position statement: guidelines for the evaluation and management of chronic diarrhea. Clinical Practice and Practice Economics Committee. *Gastroenterology*. 1999;116:1461.

American Gastroenterology Association. Medical position statement: role of nutrition support in GI function. *Gastroenterology*. 1995; 108:1280.

Arranz E, Ferguson A. Intestinal antibody pattern of celiac disease: occurrence in patients with normal jejunal biopsy history. *Gastroenterology*. 1993;104:1263.

Balasekaran R, et al. Positive results on tests for steatorrhea in persons consuming olestra potato chips. *Ann Int Med*. 2000;132:279.

Banerjee S, et al. Effect of Helicobacter pylori and its eradication on gastric juice ascorbic acid. *Gut*. 1994;35:317.

Bardella M, et al. Increased prevalence of celiac disease in patients with dyspepsia. *Arch Int Med*. 2000;160:1489.

Barera G, et al. Body composition in children with celiac disease and the effects of a gluten-free diet: a prospective, case-control study. *Am J Clin Nutri*. 2000;72:71.

Belluzzi A, et al. Effect of an enteric-coated fish-oil preparation on relapses in Crohn's disease. *N Engl J Med*. 1996;334:1557.

Beyer P. Role of the dietitian in gastrointestinal disorders. *J Am Diet Assoc*. 1998;98:108.

Booth I. Dietary management of acute diarrhea in childhood (commentary). *Lancet*. 1993;341:996.

Bozymski E, Isaacs K. Special diagnostic and therapeutic considerations in elderly patients with upper gastrointestinal disease. *J Clin Gastroenterol*. 1991;13:S65.

Brown T, et al. The effect of liquid fibre on gastric emptying in the rat and humans and the distribution of small intestinal contents in the rat. *Gut*. 1993;34:1177.

Bruce B, et al. Diet high in whole and unrefined foods favorably alters lipids, antioxidant defenses, and colon function. *J Am Col Nutri*. 2000;19:61.

Carroccio A, et al. Role of pancreatic impairment in growth recovery during gluten-free diet in childhood celiac disease. *Gastroenterology*. 1997;112:1839.

Cassidy A, et al. Starch intake and colorectal cancer risk: an international comparison. *Br J Cancer*. 1994;69:937.

Cheskin L, et al. Mechanisms of constipation in older persons and effects of fiber compared with placebo. *J Am Geriatr Soc*. 1995; 43:666.

Chovet M. Gastrointestinal functional bowel disorders: new therapies. *Curr Opin Chem Biol*. 2000;4:428.

Clark-Lykins T, Stockwell J. Comprehensive modified diet simplifies nutrition management of adults with short-bowel syndrome. *J Am Diet Assoc*. 1998;98:309.

Colston K, et al. Localization of vitamin D receptor in normal human duodenum and in patients with celiac disease. *Gut*. 1994; 35:1215.

Coulston A, Rock C. *A summary of the current state of knowledge in clinical nutrition and dietetic practice: suggestions for future research in dietetic practice and implications for health care*. Chicago: The American Dietetic Association, 1993.

Corazza G, et al. Bone mass and metabolism in patients with celiac disease. *Gastroenterology*. 1995;109:122.

DeVault K, Castell D. Guidelines for the diagnosis and treatment of gastroesophageal reflux disease. *Arch Intern Med*. 1995;155: 2165.

DiMartini A, et al. Quality of life after small intestine transplantation and among home parenteral nutrition patients *Parenter Enter Nutri*. 1998;22:357.

Dobbins W. The diagnosis of Whipple's disease. *N Engl J Med*. 1995; 332:390.

Drossman D, et al. American Gastroenterological Association Medical Position Statement: Irritable Bowel Syndrome. *Gastroenterology*. 1997;112:2118.

Elta, G. Acute nonvariceal upper gastrointestinal hemorrhage. *Curr Treat Options Gastroenterol* 2002;5:147

Emery E, et al. Banana flakes control diarrhea in enterally fed patients. *Nutr Clin Pract*. 1997;12:72.

Farrell R, Kelly C. Celiac sprue. *N Engl J Med*. 2002;346:180.

Feagan B, et al. Methotrexate for the treatment of Crohn's disease. *N Engl J Med*. 1995;332:92.

Feldman M, Barnett C. Relationships between acidity and osmolality of popular beverages and reported postprandial heartburn. *Gastroenterology*. 1995;108:125.

Finch R. Ciprofloxacin: efficacy and indications. *J Chemother*. 2000; 12:5S.

Fine K, et al. The prevalence and causes of chronic diarrhea in patients with celiac sprue treated with a gluten free diet. *Gastroenterology*. 1997;112:1830.

Flourie B, et al. Can diarrhea induced by lactulose be reduced by prolonged ingestion of lactulose? *Am J Clin Nutri*. 1993;58: 369.

Floruta C. Dietary choices of people with ostomies. *J Wound Ostomy Continence Nurs*. 2001;28:28.

Francis C, Whorwell P. Bran and irritable bowel syndrome: time for reappraisal. *Lancet.* 1994;344:39.

Fraser A, Woollard G. Gastric juice ascorbic acid is related to Helicobacter pylori infection but not ethnicity. *J Gastroenterol Hepatol.* 1999;14:1070.

Ganiats T, et al. Does Bean-O prevent gas? A double-blind crossover study of oral a-galactosidase to treat dietary oligosaccharide intolerance. *J Fam Pract.* 1994;39:441.

Geerling B, et al. Comprehensive nutritional status in recently diagnosed patients with inflammatory bowel disease compared with population controls. *Euro J Clin Nutri.* 2000;54:514.

Genser D, et al. Status of lipid-soluble antioxidants and TRAP in patients with Crohn's disease and healthy controls. *Euro J Clin Nutri.* 1999;53:675.

Goepp J, Katz S. Oral rehydration therapy. *Am Fam Physician.* 1993;47:843.

Gokhale R, et al. Bone mineral density assessment in children with inflammatory bowel disease. *Gastroenterol.* 1998;114:902.

Goldstein R, et al. Carbohydrate malabsorption and the effect of dietary restriction on symptoms of irritable bowel syndrome and functional bowel complaints. *Isr Med Assoc.* 2000;2:583.

Gorman M, Bowman C. Position of the American Dietetic Association: health implications of dietary fiber. *J Am Diet Assoc.* 1993;93:1446.

Graczyk T, Schwab K. Foodborne infections vectored by molluscan shellfish. *Current Gastroenterol Reports.* 2000;2:305.

Gray G. Intestinal lactase: what defines the decline? (editorial). *Gastroenterol.* 1993;105:931.

Green K, et al. A predominant role for Norwalk-like viruses as agents of epidemic gastroenteritis in Maryland nursing homes for the elderly. *J Infect Dis.* 2002;185:133.

Griffiths A, et al. Meta-analysis of enteral nutrition as a primary treatment of active Crohn's disease. *Gastroenterol.* 1995;108:1056.

Guerrant R, et al. Micronutrients and infection: interactions and implications with enteric and other infections and future priorities. *J Infect Dis.* 2000;182:S134.

Hakanen M, Clinical and subclinical autoimmune thyroid disease in adult celiac disease. *Dig Dis Sci.* 2001;46:2631.

Hasse J. Nutrition assessment and support of organ transplant recipients. *J Parenter Enteral Nutri.* 2001;25:120.

Hartsell P, et al. Early postoperative feeding after elective colorectal surgery. *Arch Surg.* 1997;132:518.

Hill I, et al. The prevalence of celiac disease in at-risk groups of children in the United States. *J Pediatr.* 2000;136:86.

Hulme-Moir M, Bartolo D. Hemorrhoids. *Gastroenterol Clin North Am.* 2001;30:183.

Kopp-Hoolihan L. Prophylactic and therapeutic uses of probiotics: A review. *J Am Diet Assoc.* 2001;101:229.

Jackson J, et al. Treatment of functional gastrointestinal disorders with antidepressant medications: a meta-analysis. *Am J Med.* 2000;108:65.

Jackson M, Eastwood G. Diagnosis: Crohn's disease. *Hosp Med.* 1991;142:121.

James T. The protean nature of Whipple's disease includes multiorgan arteriopathy. Trans *Am Clin Climatol Assoc.* 2001;112: 196.

Johnson M. Management of short bowel syndrome—a review. *Support Line.* 2000;22:11.

Juckett G. Intestinal protozoa. *Am Fam Physician.* 1996;53:2507.

Juckett G. Prevention and treatment of traveler's diarrhea. *Am Fam Phys.* 1999;60:119.

Jung A. Gastroesophageal reflux in infants and children. *Am Fam Physician.* 2001;64:1853.

Kaptan K, et al. *Helicobacter pylori*—is it a novel causative agent in Vitamin B12 deficiency? *Arch Intern Med.* 2000;160:1349.

Kaufman S, et al. Indications for pediatric intestinal transplantation: a position paper of the American Society of Transplantation. *Pediatr Transplant.* 2001;5:80.

Kaufman S, et al. Influence of bacterial overgrowth and intestinal inflammation on duration of parenteral nutrition in children with short bowel syndrome. *J Pediatrics.* 1997;131:356.

Kilgore P, et al. Trends of diarrheal disease-associated mortality in U.S. children, 1968 through 1991. *JAMA.* 1995;274:1143.

King T, et al. Abnormal colonic fermentation in irritable bowel syndrome. *Lancet.* 1998;352:1187.

Klinkenberg-Knol E, et al. Long-term treatment with omeprazole for refractory reflux esophagitis: efficacy and safety. *Ann Intern Med.* 1994;121:161.

Kowdley K, et al. Vitamin E deficiency and impaired cellular immunity related to intestinal fat malabsorption. *Gastroenterol.* 1992; 102:2139.

Lebenthal E, et al. Thermophilic amylase-digested rice-electrolyte solution in the treatment of acute diarrhea in children. *Pediatrics.* 1995;95:198.

Ligumsky M, et al. Effect of long-term, continuous versus alternate-day omeprazole therapy on serum gastrin in patients treated for reflux esophagitis. *J Clin Gastroenterol.* 2001;33:32.

Lima-Dutra S, et al. Whole-body protein metabolism assessed by leucine and glutamine kinetics in adults patients with active celiac disease. *Metab: Clin and Experimental.* 1999;47:1429.

Locke G, et al. Familial association in adults with functional gastrointestinal disorders. *Mayo Clin Proc.* 2000;75:907.

Lopez I, Buchman A. Metabolic bone disease in IBD. *Gastroenterol.* 2000;2:317.

Lupton J, Morin J, Robinson M. Barley bran flour accelerates gastrointestinal transit time. *J Am Diet Assoc.* 1993;93:881.

MacDonald W, Owen D. Gastric carcinoma after surgical treatment of peptic ulcer: an analysis of morphologic features and a comparison with cancer in the nonoperated stomach. *Cancer.* 2001; 91:1732.

Madhotra R, et al. Prediction of esophageal varices in patients with cirrhosis. *J Clin Gastroenterol.* 2002;34:81.

Madsen L, et al. Menetrier's disease. Another *Helicobacter pylori* associated disease. *Ugeskr Laeger.* 2000;162:4250.

Makapugay L, Dean P. Diverticular disease-associated chronic colitis. *Am J Surg Pathol.* 1996;20:94.

Marsh M. Gluten sensitivity and latency: can patterns of intestinal antibody secretion define the great "silent majority?" *Gastroenterology.* 1993;104:1550.

McClung H, et al. Is combination therapy for encopresis nutritionally safe? *Pediatrics.* 1993;91:591.

Mendez L, et al. Swallowing disorders of the elderly. *Clin Geriatr Med.* 1991;7:215.

Meyers A. Oral rehydration therapy: what are we waiting for? (editorial). *Am Fam Physician.* 1993;47:740.

Mingrone G, et al. Elevated diet-induced thermogenesis and lipid oxidation rate in Crohn's disease. *Am J Clin Nutri.* 1999;69: 325.

Misciagna G, et al. Diet and duodenal ulcer. *Dig Liver Dis.* 2000; 32:468.

Mistiaen W, et al. Gastric emptying rate for solid and for liquid test meals in patients with dyspeptic symptoms after partial gastrectomy and after vagotomy followed by partial gastrectomy. *Hepatogastroenterology*. 2001;48:299.

Montes R, Perman J. Lactose intolerance: pinpointing the source of nonspecific gastrointestinal symptoms. *Postgrad Med*. 1989;89: 175.

Mora S, et al. Reversal of low bone mineral density with a gluten-free diet in children and adolescents with celiac disease. *Am J Clin Nutri*. 1998;67:459.

Morales M, et al. Exocrine pancreatic insufficiency in tropical sprue. *Digestion*. 2001;63:30.

Murphy O. Nonpolyol low-digestible carbohydrates: food applications and functional benefits. *Br J Nutri*. 2001;85:47S.

Olden K, Drossman D. Psychologic and psychiatric aspects of gastrointestinal disease. *Med Clin North Am*. 2000;84:131.

Playford R, et al. Colostrum and milk-derived peptide growth factors for the treatment of gastrointestinal disorders. *Am J Clin Nutri*. 2000;72:5.

Pribela B, et al. Improved lactose digestion and intolerance among African-American adolescent girls fed a dairy-rich diet. *J Am Diet Assoc*. 2000;100:524.

Probert C, et al. Evidence for the ambiguity of the term constipation: the role of irritable bowel syndrome. *Gut*. 1994;35:1455.

Purdum P, Kirby D. Short-bowel syndrome: a review of the role of nutrition support. *J Parenter Enteral Nutri*. 1991;15:93.

Ramachandran A, Balasubramanian K. Intestinal dysfunction in liver cirrhosis: Its role in spontaneous bacterial peritonitis. *J Gastroenterol Hepatol*. 2001;16:607.

Ramakrishna B, et al. Amylase-resistant starch plus oral rehydration solution for cholera. *N Engl J Med*. 2000;343:308.

Ramirez F, et al. All lactase preparations are not the same: results of a prospective, randomized placebo-controlled trial. *Am J Gastroenterol*. 1994;89:566.

Regimbeau J, et al. Long-term results of ileal pouch-anal anastomosis for colorectal Crohn's disease. *Dis Colon Rectum*. 2001;44:769.

Rhee P, et al. Evaluation of individual symptoms cannot predict presence of gastric hypersensitivity in functional dyspepsia. *Dig Dis Sci*. 2000;45:1680.

Rigaud D, et al. Effect of psyllium on gastric emptying, hunger feeling, and food intake in normal volunteers: a double blind study. *Euro J Clin Nutri*. 1998;52:239.

Rigaud D, et al. Mechanisms of decreased food intake during weight loss in adult Crohn's disease patients without obvious malabsorption. *Am J Clin Nutri*. 1994;60:775.

Ruemmele F, et al. Nutrition as primary therapy in pediatric Crohn's disease: fact or fantasy? *J Pediatr*. 2000;136:285.

Sayfan J, et al. Sutureless closed hemorrhoidectomy: a new technique. *Ann Surg*. 2001;234:21.

Scarinci I, et al. Altered pain perception and psychosocial features among women with gastrointestinal disorders and history of abuse. *Am J Med*. 1994;97:108.

Schneeweiss B, et al. Energy and substrate metabolism in patients with active Crohn's disease. *J Nutri*. 1999;129:844.

Schwarz S, et al. Diagnosis and treatment of feeding disorders in children with developmental disabilities. *Pediatrics*. 2001;108: 671.

Shah V, et al. All that scallops is not celiac disease. *Gastrointest Endosc*. 2000;51:717.

Shaker J, et al. Hypoglycemia and skeletal disease as presenting features of celiac disease. *Arch Int Med*. 1997;157:1013.

Shamburek R, Farrar J. Disorders of the digestive system in the elderly. *N Engl J Med*. 1990;322:438.

Shermak M, et al. Effect of yogurt on symptoms and kinetics of hydrogen production in lactose-malabsorbing children. *Am J Clin Nutri*. 1995;62:1003.

Shoda R, et al. Epidemiologic analysis of Crohn's disease in Japan: increased dietary intake of n-6 polyunsaturated fatty acids and animal protein relates to increased incidence of Crohn's disease in Japan. *Am J Clin Nutri*. 1996;63:741.

Silver H, et al. Nutritional complications and management of intestinal transplant. *J Am Diet Assoc*. 2000;100:680.

Soll A. Medical treatment of peptic ulcer disease. *JAMA*. 1996;275: 622.

Spellett G. Nutritional management of common gastrointestinal problems. *Nurse Pract Forum*. 1994;5:24.

Steffes C, Fromm D. Is preoperative parenteral nutrition necessary for patients with predominantly ileal Crohn's disease? *Arch Surg*. 1992;127:1210.

Suarez F, et al. Lactose maldigestion is not an impediment to the intake of 1500 mg calcium daily as dairy products. *Am J Clin Nutri*. 1998;68:1118.

Suarez F, Saviano, D. Diet, genetics, and lactose intolerance. *Food Technology*. 1997;51:74.

Su Y, et al. The association between *Helicobacter pylori* infection and functional dyspepsia in patients with irritable bowel syndrome. *Am J Gastroenterol*. 2000;95:1900.

Suter W, et al. Cytomegalovirus-induced transient protein-losing hypertrophic gastropathy in an immunocompetent adult. *Digestion*. 2000;62:276.

Thaler E, et al. Feasibility and outcome of endoscopic staple-assisted esophagodiverticulostomy for Zenker's diverticulum. *Laryngoscope*. 2001;111:1506.

Thompson T. Do oats belong in a gluten-free diet? *J Am Diet Assoc*. 1997;97:1413.

Thompson T. Folate, iron, and dietary fiber contents of the gluten-free diet. *J Am Diet Assoc*. 2000;100:1389.

Thomson A. Gastro-Oesophageal reflux in the elderly: role of drug therapy in management. *Drugs Aging*. 2001;18:409.

Vandenplas Y. Diagnosis and treatment of gastroesophageal reflux disease in infants and children. *Can J Gastroenterol*. 2000;14:26D.

Vieira M, et al. Preoperative assessment in cases of adult megacolon suffering from moderate malnutrition. *Nutrition*. 1996;12:491.

von Holstein C. Long-term prognosis after partial gastrectomy for gastroduodenal ulcer. *World J Surg*. 2000;24:307.

Weinberg E. Iron loading: a risk factor for Whipple's disease? *Med Hypotheses*. 2001;57:59–60.

Wenzl H, et al. Determinants of decreased fecal consistency in patients with diarrhea. *Gastroenterol*. 1995;108:1729.

Westberg G, et al. Prediction of prognosis by echocardiography in patients with midgut carcinoid syndrome. *Br J Surg*. 2001;88:865.

Willetts I, et al. Cow's milk enteropathy: surgical pitfalls. *J Pediatr Surg*. 1999;34:1486.

Williams M, et al. Diarrhea management in enterally fed patients. *Nutr in Clinical Practice*. 1998;13:225.

Wolff B, Devine R. Surgical management of diverticulitis. *Am Surg*. 2000;66:153.

Wunderlich S, Tobias A. Relationship between nutritional status indicators and length of hospital stay for patients with diverticular disease. *J Am Diet Assoc*. 1992;92:430.

Yamamoto T, et al. Omentoplasty for persistent perineal sinus after proctectomy for Crohn's disease. *Am J Surg*. 2001;181:265.

Yip R, et al. Pervasive occult gastrointestinal bleeding in an Alaska Native population with prevalent iron deficiency: Role of *Helicobacter pylori* gastritis. *J Am Med Assoc*. 1997;277:1135.

Zaman A, et al. Risk factors for the presence of varices in cirrhotic patients without a history of variceal hemorrhage. *Arch Intern Med.* 2001;26:2564.

Suggested Readings

American Gastroenterology Association medical position statement: Irritable bowel syndrome. *Gastroenterology.* 1997;112:2118.

American Gastrointestinal Association medical position statement on management of oropharyngeal dysphagia. *Gastroenterol.* 1999; 116:452.

Angtuaco T, et al. The utility of urgent colonoscopy in the evaluation of acute lower gastrointestinal tract bleeding: a 2-year experience from a single center. *Am J Gastroenterol.* 2001;96: 1782.

Beyer P. Digestion. In: Mahan K, Escott-Stump S, eds. *Krause's food, nutrition, and diet therapy.* 10th ed. Philadelphia: WB Saunders, 2000.

Beyer P. Nutritional care and the lower GI system. In: Mahan K, Escott-Stump S, eds. *Krause's food, nutrition, and diet therapy.* 10th ed. Philadelphia: WB Saunders, 2000.

Beyer P. Nutritional care and the upper GI system. In: Mahan K, Escott-Stump S, eds. *Krause's food, nutrition, and diet therapy.* 10th ed. Philadelphia: WB Saunders, 2000.

Brody R, et al. Role of registered dietitians in dysphagia screening. *J Am Diet Assoc.* 2000;100:1029.

Buchholz A. Weaning patients with dysphagia from tube feeding to oral nutrition: A proposed algorithm. *Can J Diet Pract Res.* 1998;59:208.

Collin P, et al. Clinical features of celiac disease today. *Dig Dis.* 1999; 17:100.

Dua K, et al. Coordination of deglutitive glottal function and pharyngeal bolus transit during normal eating. *Gastroenterol.* 1997; 112:73.

Iacomo G, et al. Intolerance to cow's milk and chronic constipation in children. *N Engl J Med.* 1998;339:1100.

Inman-Felton A. Overview of gluten-sensitive enteropathy (celiac sprue). *J Am Diet Assoc.* 1999;99:352.

Inman-Felton A. Overview of lactose maldigestion (lactose nonpersistence). *J Am Diet Assoc.* 1999;99:481.

Khan S, et al. Surgical treatment of hemorrhoids: prospective, randomized trial comparing closed excisional hemorrhoidectomy and the harmonic scalpel technique of excisional hemorrhoidectomy. *Dis Colon Rectum.* 2001;44:845.

Lagares-Garcia J, et al. Colonoscopy in octogenarians and older patients. *Surg Endosc.* 2001;15:262.

Lee A. The *Helicobacter pylori* genome—New insights into pathogenesis and therapeutics. *N Engl J Med.* 1998;338:832.

McBean L, Miller G. Allaying fears and fallacies about lactose intolerance. *J Am Diet Assoc.* 1998;98:671.

Sandler R, et al. Gastrointestinal symptoms in 3181 volunteers ingesting snack foods containing olestra or triglycerides: A 6-week randomized, placebo-controlled trial. *Ann Int Med.* 1999;130:253.

Savilahti E. Food-induced malabsorption syndromes. *J Pediatr Gastroenterol Nutri.* 2000;30:S61.

Schwesinger W, et al. Jejunoileal causes of overt gastrointestinal bleeding: diagnosis, management, and outcome. *Am Surg.* 2001; 67:383.

Stollman N, et al. Diagnosis and management of diverticular disease of the colon in adults. *Am J Gastroenterology.* 1999;94:3110.

Tomb J, et al. The complete genome sequence of the gastric pathogen *Helicobacter pylori. Nature.* 1997;388:539.

Wasserman T, et al. Management of swallowing in supraglottic and extended supraglottic laryngectomy patients. *Head Neck.* 2001; 23:1043.

S E C T I O N

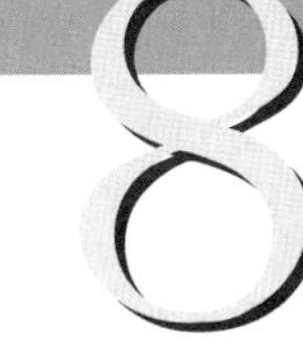

Hepatic, Pancreatic, and Biliary Disorders

CHIEF ASSESSMENT FACTORS

CLINICAL FACTORS

- MALNUTRITION, SUBJECTIVE GLOBAL ASSESSMENT (SGA)
- ABDOMINAL OR RADIATING PAIN
- HEPATOMEGALY OR SHRUNKEN LIVER (IN CIRRHOSIS)
- ASCITES, LARGE ABDOMINAL GIRTH, EDEMA
- ABNORMAL LIVER MRI, ULTRASOUND OR BIOPSY
- VARICES, GASTROINTESTINAL (GI) BLEEDING, ENCEPHALOPATHY?
- DIARRHEA, STEATORRHEA
- VOMITING, NAUSEA
- ANOREXIA, MALAISE, FATIGUE
- DIABETES, HYPERGLYCEMIA, HYPOGLYCEMIA
- JAUNDICE

LABORATORY ASSESSMENT

- ALTERED SERUM BILIRUBIN (TOTAL OR INDIRECT)
- ABNORMAL LIVER ENZYMES: ALANINE AMINOTRANSFERASE (ALT), ASPARTATE AMINOTRANSAMINASE (AST), LACTIC ACID DEHYDROGENASE (LDH)
- ABNORMAL CHOLESTASIS TESTS: SERUM ALKALINE PHOSPHATASE (ALK PHOS), GAMMA GLUTAMYLTRANSFERASE (GGT)
- MARKERS OF SPECIFIC LIVER DISEASE: SERUM FERRITIN, CERULOPLASMIN, ALPHA-FETOPROTEIN, ALPHA-1-ANTITRYPSIN
- SPECIFIC VIRAL HEPATITIS TESTS
- ALTERED SERUM PROTEINS: PRO TIME (PT), INTERNATIONAL NORMALIZED RATIO (INR), PROTHROMBIN TIME (PTT), ALBUMIN, GLOBULIN, MITOCHONDRIAL ANTIBODIES, ANTINUCLEAR AND SMOOTH MUSCLE ANTIBODIES
- ELEVATED SERUM AMMONIA
- ALTERED PANCREATIC ENZYME LEVELS
- ALTERED BLEEDING/CLOTTING TIMES

LIVER FACTS

Nutrition and the liver are interrelated in many ways. Everything that we eat, breathe, and absorb through our skin must be refined and detoxified by the liver. In a number of different kinds of liver disease, nutrition takes on considerably more importance. The liver is the largest organ in the body, and it plays a vital role, performing many complex functions, which are essential for life (Table 8–1); it is the body's internal chemical power plant. It is impossible to live without a liver, and the health of the liver is a major factor in the quality of one's life (source:www. liverfoundation.org). (Fig. 8–1)

For More Information

- American Association for the Study of Liver Diseases
  http://www.aasld.org/
- American Liver Foundation
  75 Maiden Lane, Suite 603
  New York, NY 10038
  1-800-GOLIVER
  http://www.liverfoundation.org/
- National Digestive Diseases Information Clearinghouse
  2 Information Way
  Bethesda, MD 20892-3570
  http://www.niddk.nih.gov/health/digest/nddic.htm
- National Institute of Diabetes & Digestive & Kidney Diseases
  http://www.niddk.nih.gov/

TABLE 8–1 Liver, Gallbladder, and Pancreatic Functions

LIVER:
The largest single organ of the body; it is the central biochemical organ of the body. Functionally, it:

1. Converts galactose and fructose to glucose; makes glycogen; degrades glycogen upon demand.
2. Converts proteins into glucose; synthesizes albumin, globulin, fibrinogen, prothrombin, and transferrin; removes nitrogenous wastes (ammonia); provides transamination; synthesizes purines and pyrimidines; forms amines by decarboxylation.
3. Synthesizes triglycerides; forms very low density lipoproteins (VLDLs); oxidizes fatty acids for energy and ketones.
4. Synthesizes cholesterol from acetate; makes high-density lipoproteins (HDLs).
5. Stores vitamins A, D, E, and K and some vitamin B12 and C.
6. Hydroxylates vitamin D for renal activation; activates folic acid to tetrahydrofolic acid (THFA).
7. Stores minerals (e.g., iron, copper, zinc, magnesium).
8. Detoxifies drugs.
9. Produces bile.

GALLBLADDER:
Stores bile, which helps counteract stomach acidity and aids in fat digestion through emulsification

PANCREAS:

1. The pancreas produces pancreatic juice when stimulated by secretin. Pancreatic juice contains bicarbonate, which helps neutralize acid chyme.
2. The pancreas also secretes insulin and glucagon hormones.
3. The pancreas secretes digestive enzymes (trypsin, lipase, and amylase) into the collecting duct as stimulated by cholecystokinin (also called pancreozymin), which is produced by the duodenum.
4. The pancreas secretes metabolic/digestive enzymes involved in protein, carbohydrate, and fat metabolism. Pancreatic secretion has gastric, cephalic, and intestinal phases. The islets secrete insulin (β) and glucagon (α). The acini secrete lipase, amylase, trypsin, chymotrypsin, ribonuclease, and carboxypolypeptidase.

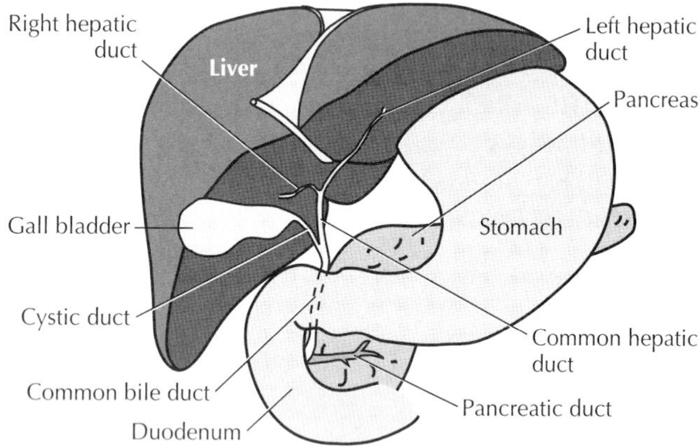

Figure 8–1 Liver and biliary system.

ALCOHOLIC LIVER DISEASE

NUTRITIONAL ACUITY RANKING: LEVEL 3

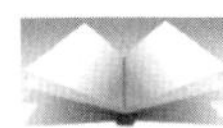

DEFINITIONS AND BACKGROUND

Alcohol may increase resting energy expenditure, nitrogen excretion, and appetite and can lead to cirrhosis of the liver; it affects most organs (Falck-Ytter & McCullough, 2000). Alcohol cannot be stored and is used preferentially over other energy fuels. Alcoholics may replace as much as 30% of their daily kilocalories with alcohol; alcoholic beverages account for about 6% of total kilocalories consumed in the United States.

Alcoholism affects approximately 14 million people in the United States or 10% of the population. Alcohol is a hepatotoxin and is also ulcerogenic, especially to the esophagus. Moderate alcohol use contributes to the risk of specific types of infertility, including endometriosis (Grodstein et al., 1994). Classic nervous system effects include Wernicke's encephalopathy and Korsakoff's psychosis. There is a high incidence of muscle wasting, weight loss, and malnutrition with alcoholic liver disease.

Alcohol abuse may cause deficiencies of protein, folic acid, thiamin, vitamin A, and zinc (Lieber, 1992). Alcohol dehydrogenase is made with zinc. Ethanol alters both the activation and degradation of key nutrients, and nutritional factors have a striking effect on detoxification (Lieber, 1993). Alcohol decreases absorption of fats, fat-soluble vitamins, thiamine, folic acid, and vitamin B12. Nicotine-adenine dinucleotide (NAD) is the rate-limiting factor in the metabolism of alcohol. Metabolism of alcohol is slower during the deprivation of calories. Oxidative balance is restored by use of nicotinamide; effects of wine on plasma rate of lactate to pyruvate are reduced by the addition of this substance (Volpi, 1997).

The hepatotoxicity of alcohol generates oxidative stress despite an adequate diet through microsomal cytochrome P4502E1 (Lieber, 2000). Methionine metabolism, which needs to be activated to S-adenosylmethionine (SAMe), is also impaired in liver disease. Acute liver diseases such as alcoholic hepatitis are considered hypercatabolic diseases and thus require prompt nutritional intervention with a high-calorie enteral or parenteral formula (Teran, 1999).

Women have greater clearance of alcohol per unit of lean body mass (LBM) than do men, even with approximately the same liver volume as men. This explains the equivalent alcohol elimination rates seen when men and women are compared on the basis of liver size; mean LBM is 42% greater in men than in women (Kwo et al., 1998). Intake of 1–2 alcoholic beverages daily for men and less than 1 drink for women is associated with lowest mortality (Liao et al., 2000).

Alcohol adversely affects skeletal muscle. In addition to the mechanical changes to muscle, there are important metabolic consequences; skeletal muscle is 40% of body mass and an important contributor to whole-body protein turnover (Preedy et al., 2001).

Although recalled alcohol intake is a better predictor of past intake than are reports of current intake, current drinking habits may influence recall of alcohol intake in the distant past. Current heavier drinkers tend to underestimate their past alcohol intakes (Liu et al., 1996). Detoxification takes 5–7 days; most program rehabilitation takes 3–6 weeks; and convalescence takes 6–12 months. True recovery takes months to years. Symptoms and signs of alcoholism include restlessness, agitation, spider angiomas on the face, insomnia, anorexia, weight loss, GI cramps, malnutrition, delirium tremens, and hand tremors. Counselors must understand addiction; see also Substance Abuse in section 4. Women and young persons are especially vulnerable to higher mortality risks from heavy alcohol use (Klatsky et al., 1992). (See Table 8–2.)

OBJECTIVES

- ▲ Remove alcohol.
- ▲ Allow the disabled liver to function more effectively while protecting it from metabolic stress.
- ▲ Prevent hypoglycemia from blocked gluconeogenesis. Correct alternate states of hyperglycemia, especially with hypertriglyceridemia.
- ▲ Repair hepatic damage from fatty liver and diminished bile salt synthesis.
- ▲ Repair neural damage from malnutrition and malabsorption.
- ▲ Help liver tissue regenerate and replenish plasma proteins that are lost from increased nitrogen excretion.
- ▲ Correct fluid and electrolyte imbalances, nutritional deficits (such as iron deficiency anemia from chronic blood loss in varices, ulcers, etc.), and vomiting. Scurvy may occur from inadequate consumption of sources of vitamin C; fatigue is the earliest symptom, then cutaneous and gum abnormalities follow (Hirschmann and Raugi, 1999).
- ▲ Improve skeletal muscle synthesis.
- ▲ Improve health of liver so it can synthesize albumin and other serum proteins.
- ▲ Be honest and direct in approach. Confront conflicting information when stated by the patient.

TABLE 8–2 Stages of Alcoholism-Related Effects

I. Obesity, hyperlipidemia, hypertension, and diabetes mellitus
II. Hepatomegaly, hypertriglyceridemia, and hypoalbuminemia
III. Chronic hepatitis and pancreatitis
IV. Cirrhosis
V. Encephalopathy (note that not all patients with cirrhosis become encephalopathic)
VI. Coma and death, if untreated

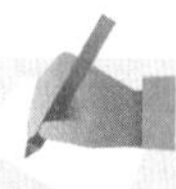

DIETARY AND NUTRITIONAL RECOMMENDATIONS

- Diet should provide adequate protein (1.5 g/kg body weight if malnourished, less if not malnourished). Plan adequate amounts of carbohydrates and fat to spare protein. Monitor carbohydrate (CHO) and fat intake carefully in hyperglycemia and type IV hyperlipoproteinemia.
- Diet should provide adequate intake of potassium.
- Supplement the diet with B-complex vitamins. Synthetic folacin is also needed, because the patient is less able to use what is provided by the diet. Diet should provide adequate amounts of vitamins A, D, E, and K, as well as thiamin, phosphorus, selenium, folate, magnesium, zinc, and calcium. Include fruits and vegetables or supplement vitamin C if dietary intake is low.
- Make meals appetizing to stimulate the appetite.
- Use no alcohol in any form.
- If tube feeding (TF) or total parenteral nutrition (TPN) is needed, do not use a glutamine-enriched formula, which may increase ammonia levels.

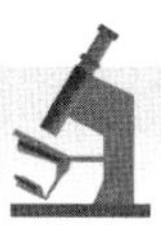

PROFILE

Clinical/History	Lab Work	
Height Weight Body mass index (BMI) Blood pressure (BP) Intake and output (I & O) Ascites Signs of scurvy—large ecchymoses, hemorrhagic gingivitis, corkscrew hairs, perifollicular hemorrhages, leg edema, and poor wound healing	Glucose (gluc) (increased or decreased) Serum ammonia Cholesterol (chol) Blood urea nitrogen (BUN) (may be low) Albumin (alb), prealbumin Triglycerides (Trig) (increased) PT White blood cell count (WBC) Serum B12 Serum folate ALT AST (increased) GGT Bilirubin	Na+ (hyponatremia may occur) K+ Hemoglobin and hematocrit (H&H) (decreased) Uric acid (increased) Globulin Alk phos (increased) Transferrin Total iron-binding capacity (TIBC) Mg++(decreased) Ca++ Serum phosphorus (decreased) DEXA bone scan

Common Drugs Used and Potential Side Effects

- Antabuse (Disulfiram) is given with patient's consent. It causes the patient to vomit after ingesting alcohol and can be dangerous. Avoid alcohol in vinegar, sauces, and cough syrup.
- Insulin may be necessary. Do not mix with alcohol. Alcohol creates decreased insulin sensitivity but also hypersecretion of insulin postprandially, with relatively stable plasma glucose levels as a result (Knip et al., 1995).
- Avoid excesses of supplemental vitamins A and D, which may not be well tolerated by the liver.
- Methylprednisolone may be used in alcoholic hepatitis, with improved ability to produce albumin and to normalize PT and bilirubin levels. As a steroid, there are many possible side effects (i.e., negative nitrogen or calcium balance, hyperglycemia, etc.).
- Supplements of vitamin C may be needed if deficiency is evident. Initial dose of 1–2 g/day for 2 days, followed by a 500-mg dose daily for a week (Oeffinger, 1993).
- Beta-blockers (propanolol, nadolol, etc.) may be used to treat portal hypertension if varices occur.
- Metformin should be avoided with liver disease.

Herbs, Botanicals and Supplements

- Herbs and botanical supplements should not be used without discussing with the physician, even if herbalists and indigenous healers worldwide have traditionally used them (Luper, 1998).
- Chaparral is an herbal product used for antioxidant properties; severe hepatitis or liver failure may result (Gordon et al., 1995). Avoid, especially while drinking alcohol.
- Milk thistle (silybum marianum) may have some therapeutic effect in liver disease, but controlled trials are necessary before patients with alcoholic liver disease are advised to use it (Luper, 1998; Bass, 1999).
- Curcuma longa (turmeric), Camellia sinensis (green tea), and Glycyrrhiza glabra (licorice) have also been studied for their potential effects (Luper 1999; Luper 1998).

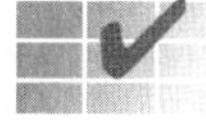

PATIENT EDUCATION

- ✓ Help patient in the preparation of appetizing, nutrient-dense meals.
- ✓ Instruct patient in the sources of necessary nutrients in the diet and use of the prescribed multivitamins.
- ✓ Explain that alcohol is the preferred fuel by the liver but cannot be used for muscular activity.
- ✓ Zinc supplementation may improve a poor appetite.
- ✓ Discuss chemical addiction as a disease. Self-help programs and follow-up can reduce dependency.
- ✓ Obesity, diabetes, and hyperinsulinemia play a role in the development of hepatic steatosis; weight loss remains a critical part of protecting the liver against damage (Neuschwander-Tetri, 2001).
- ✓ Identify sources of assistance for persons who need help with meal preparation or with access to meals.

For More Information

- ✦ Alcoholics Anonymous (AA) World Services
  475 Riverside Drive, 11th Floor
  New York, NY 10115
  http://www.alcoholics-anonymous.org/

- International Society for Biomedical Research on Alcoholism
  http://www.isbra.com/
- National Council on Alcoholism and Drug Dependence
  12 W. 21 St.
  New York, NY 10010
  212-206-6770
  Hopeline: 1-800-NCA-CALL
  http://www.ncadd.org/
- National Institute on Alcohol Abuse and Alcoholism (NIAAA)
  6000 Executive Boulevard--Willco Building
  Bethesda, Maryland 20892-7003
  http://www.niaaa.nih.gov/
- Research Society on Alcoholism
  http://www.rsoa.org/
- Substance Abuse & Mental Health Administration (DHHS)
  http://www.isbra.com/

ASCITES

NUTRITIONAL ACUITY RANKING: LEVEL 3

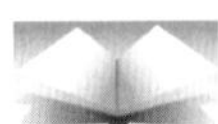

DEFINITIONS AND BACKGROUND

Ascites is defined as pathological fluid in the peritoneal cavity caused by portal hypertension. Low serum proteins or sodium retention may contribute also in cases of liver failure or portal hypertension. It is seen in patients with hepatic cirrhosis, cardiac failure, or renal insufficiency and may result from fluid loss from cells because of osmolar or nutrient imbalances. A distended abdomen results.

Although weight is not used for nutritional assessment here, it does help determine fluid balance. Goal of diuretic therapy is to promote weight loss of 1–3 kg/day with ascites and up to 4–7 kg if both edema and ascites are present (Hasse et al., 1997). With hyponatremia from protein losses in paracentesis, diuretics, and excessive dietary restriction, IV albumin may be useful or fluid restriction will be needed.

Sodium restriction is needed with ascites—2–4 g per day is best tolerated and accepted (Crippin, 1997). Hyponatremia may be a side effect, and fluid restriction is common. Renal compromise may also occur with aggressive diuretic therapy. Paracentesis can complement diuretic therapy; IV albumin often follows this procedure. Spontaneous bacterial peritonitis (SBP) occurs in 10–20% of patients with ascites (Crippin, 1997). Prognosis is poor for patients with ascites; a 2-year survival rate is common after onset (Runyon, 1994).

Hepatic hydrothorax occurs when ascitic fluid in the pleural space accumulates and requires treatment including salt restriction, diuretics, and thoracentesis (Xiol and Guardiola, 1998).

Chylous ascites is a rare form of ascites. This condition results from increased hydrostatic pressure and lymphatic blockade, with accumulation of LCT-dense chyle in the peritoneum. Chylous ascites may result from trauma, cancer, or fistula. Chylous ascites is sometimes associated with a poor outcome when it is secondary to neoplasms (Laterre et al., 2000). Any source of large fluid volume losses, lymph vessels obstruction, or leakage may cause these chylous effusions in the peritoneal cavities. A vast majority of chylous effusions heal spontaneously, but early and full treatment has to be initiated in order to reduce morbidity and mortality associated with this condition (Laterre et al., 2000). Nutrient depletion can occur if left untreated; fat, proteins, fat-soluble vitamins, and electrolytes may be lost (Cardillo, 2001). Paracentesis improves patient comfort, reduces intra-abdominal pressure, and secondary renal dysfunction; it also carries risk for peritonitis.

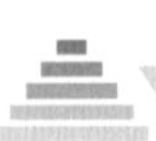

OBJECTIVES

- Reduce fluid retention, usually by diuretics.
- Prevent electrolyte imbalances.
- Prevent further pain, dyspnea, fatigue, loss of LBM, and anorexia.
- If possible, prevent hepatorenal syndrome, which can occur in patients with severe liver disease. If severe, it may require transplantation.
- Individualize diet as needs change.
- For chylous ascites, treatment of the underlying cause will be essential. Malnutrition is a common result if left untreated; essential fatty acid deficiency must be avoided.

DIETARY AND NUTRITIONAL RECOMMENDATIONS

- Restrict patient's intake of sodium (usually to 2–4 g).
- Fluid restriction may be necessary (1–1.5 L/day), two-thirds with meals and one-third for thirst/medicines. Caffeine may be limited if necessary.
- Diet should be altered in potassium if serum levels so indicate. Often, patients take Aldactone or have renal insufficiency, which may increase potassium retention. Other diuretics may cause potassium losses.
- Energy needs are often as high as 1.5 times normal. Protein needs are often 1.25–1.75 g/kg of body weight after paracentesis.
- If TF or TPN is needed, a nutrient-dense formula may help. No glutamine-enriched formulas should be used, because they may increase ammonia production.
- Ensure intake of vitamins and minerals is adequate. Check for physical signs of malnutrition.
- For **chylous ascites,** a low-fat diet or enteral feeding is needed with medium-chain triglycerides (MCT) the preferred fat source; the addition of essential fatty acids (EFAs) will be needed. Adequate protein and calories are needed. If oral diet fails, TPN may be needed, with extra water-miscible forms of fat-soluble vitamins.

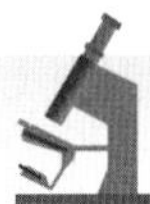

PROFILE

Clinical/History

Height
Weight
BMI
BP
I & O
Temperature
Abdominal girth

Lab Work

Ultrasonography
Serum ascites-albumin gradient (more than 1.1 g/dL = portal hypertension)
Alb (decreased)
Prealbumin
Na+
K+
BUN, creatinine (creat)
ALT
AST
H&H, serum ferritin
TIBC, % saturation
Globulin
Somatomedin C
Transferrin
Gluc
Total lymphocyte count (TLC) (decreased)
Chol, Trig
Triceps skinfold (TSF), mid-arm circumference (MAC)

Common Drugs Used and Potential Side Effects

- Somatostatin analogues have been demonstrated to be effective in reducing lymphorrhagia and may be proposed prior to surgery (Laterre et al., 2000).
- Diuretics. Check whether the specific drug retains or spares potassium; if furosemide (Lasix) is used, added potassium is needed. Spironolactone and Lasix are commonly administered. Use of spironolactone must require monitoring of serum K+ levels closely, because it spares potassium.
- Albumin replacement may help maintain oncotic pressure. It is expensive.
- For bacterial peritonitis, antibiotic therapy is needed, e.g., norfloxacin or trimethoprim.

Herbs, Botanicals and Supplements

- Herbs and botanical supplements should not be used without discussing with physician.
- Milk thistle may have some therapeutic effects in liver disease, but no controlled trials have shown efficacy for ascites at this time.

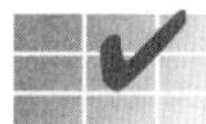

PATIENT EDUCATION

- ✓ Instruct patient concerning good sources of potassium.
- ✓ Ensure that the patient follows a low-sodium diet. Explain which foods have hidden sources of sodium.
- ✓ Salt substitutes (e.g., KCl) can lower pH of the ileum, making vitamin B12 absorption less effective. They may be discouraged when Aldactone is used. Otherwise, use judiciously, if at all.

JAUNDICE

NUTRITIONAL ACUITY RANKING LEVEL 1 OR 2

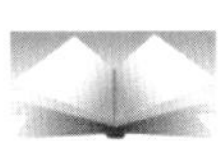

DEFINITIONS AND BACKGROUND

A yellowish discoloration of the skin, mucous membranes, and some body fluids, jaundice results from accumulation of bile or bilirubin. It is a sign, not a disease. Causes of jaundice include excessive red blood cell count (RBC) destruction, liver cell infection, and bile obstruction from gallstones, tumors, or parasites. Jaundice is classified as hemolytic (from excess bilirubin production), hepatic (from an immature liver or from damage), or obstructive (from obstructed biliary ducts).

In the obstructive type, no bile pigment gets to the stool and the stool becomes pale and clay colored, indicating fat maldigestion or malabsorption. Anorexia is a frequent finding in patients with biliary obstruction (BO). Decreased food intake may be related to the degree of obstruction and increases in cholecystokinin levels; biliary drainage improves biochemical and food intake (Padillo et al., 2001).

In neonatal jaundice, there is a somewhat normal pattern of hyperbilirubinemia that is not detrimental. The challenge to clinicians is to distinguish the features of normalcy from abnormal conditions that place the infant into a risk category (Gartner and Herschel, 2001).

OBJECTIVES

- Correct underlying cause of jaundice.
- Correct inadequate fat absorption.
- Prevent osteopenia.
- Correct anorexia and poor intake.

DIETARY AND NUTRITIONAL RECOMMENDATIONS

- Use a high-calorie, high-protein diet.
- Include rich dietary sources of calcium, vitamin K, and other nutrients. Check the need for vitamin D.
- Exclude alcoholic beverages from the diet.
- Monitor protein intake according to clinical status.

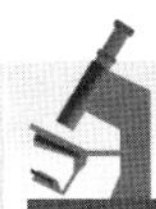

PROFILE

Clinical/History

Height
Weight
BMI

Lab Work

ALT
AST
GGT
Serum lipase
Chol (increased if obstructive)
Alb
BUN
Bilirubin
Amylase
Trig
Alk phos
Ca++
H&H
Carotenoids (increased/decreased)
Gluc

Common Drugs Used and Potential Side Effects

- Bile salts (Festal) may be used to correct faulty fat absorption if that is related.
- Avoid excesses of vitamins A and D, because liver function is abnormal and toxicity may occur.

Herbs, Botanicals and Supplements

- Herbs and botanical supplements should not be used without discussing with physician.
- While milk thistle may have some role in liver disease, it has not been proven efficacious in jaundice through controlled clinical trials.

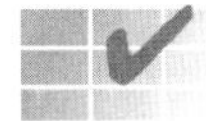

PATIENT EDUCATION

- ✔ Show the patient how to make meals that are appetizing and balanced in all key nutrients.
- ✔ Discuss the role of organs in digestion and absorption. Jaundice does not always involve fat malabsorption, although this may occur in the obstructive form.

HEPATITIS

NUTRITIONAL ACUITY RANKING: LEVEL 2

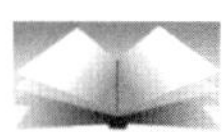

DEFINITIONS AND BACKGROUND

Hepatitis is defined as liver inflammation resulting from alcohol use, toxic materials (carbon tetrachloride), or viral infection (transmitted in food, liquids, or blood transfusions). There is also an autoimmune hepatitis and a nonalcoholic steatohepatitis (NASH). Hepatitis causes nausea, fever, liver tenderness and enlargement, jaundice, pale stools, and anorexia. Fifty percent of hepatitis cases are due to hepatitis A; hepatitis B is considered a sexually transmitted disease; hepatitis D is an incomplete virus found accompanying hepatitis B.

The first stage of viral hepatitis is preicteric/prodromal (with flu-like symptoms); the second stage is icteric (with jaundice, dark urine, light stools); and the third stage is posticteric/convalescent With chronic active hepatitis, inflamed liver cells continue for years. It usually is an autoimmune response after type B or C hepatitis. Of persons with type B, 20% develop some form of chronic liver disease; 50–70% with type C develop chronic disease. Nearly 20% of Americans test positive for hepatitis C antibody; most are adults aged 30–49, higher among minority populations. A higher risk of liver cancer occurs with hepatitis C; it often leads to cirrhosis and liver failure.

See Table 8–3 for various types and symptoms or treatments for the many forms of hepatitis.

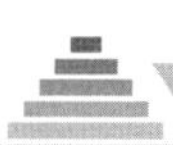

OBJECTIVES

- ▲ Promote liver regeneration. Prevent further injury. Promote rest.
- ▲ Prevent or correct weight loss, which often results from a poor appetite, nausea, and vomiting.
- ▲ Spare protein by providing a diet high in carbohydrates.
- ▲ Force fluids to prevent dehydration, unless contraindicated.
- ▲ Prevent the spread to others.

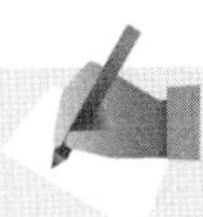

DIETARY AND NUTRITIONAL RECOMMENDATIONS

- For patients with acute hepatitis, provide a balanced diet. If nutritional support is necessary, consider tube feeding.
- As the patient progresses, use a liquid diet and then a diet of small, frequent feedings of regular or soft foods. TPN only if necessary. Avoid glutamine.
- Diet should be high in calories (30–35 kcal/kg body weight). Intake of carbohydrates should be between 50 and 55% of energy.
- Intake of protein should be 1–1.2 g/kg body weight. Well-nourished or chronic active hepatitis patients may need less.
- Fat intake should be moderate to liberal (150 g), depending on tolerance.
- Supplement diet with vitamin B complex (especially thiamine, folate, and vitamin B12), vitamin K (to normalize bleeding tendency), vitamin C, and zinc for impoverished appetite and to improve encephalopathy.
- Extra fluid should be encouraged, unless contraindicated.

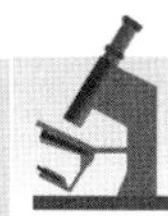

PROFILE

Clinical/History		
Height	AST (increased)	PT
Weight	ALT	Gluc
BMI	Alk phos (increased)	Transferrin (increased in acute stage)
Joint pain	Chol	H&H
Upper GI pain	LDH (increased)	I & O
Jaundice	Alb	WBC
Lab Work	BUN	GGT
Globulin	Serum ammonia	Antigen and antibody tests
Bilirubin (increased)	Lipase	
	Amylase (increased)	

Common Drugs Used and Potential Side Effects

- ■ Analgesics are used for pain. Monitor for vitamin C depletion.
- ■ Steroids may cause side effects (i.e., sodium retention, nitrogen depletion, or hyperglycemia).
- ■ Avoid excessive fat-soluble vitamin intake (vitamins A and D). Vitamin A toxicity is possible in compromised liver function; monitor all supplements carefully. B-carotene is much less toxic (Hathcock et al., 1990).
- ■ Interferon a-2b (Intron-A) shows promise for HBV and HCV. Dry mouth, stomatitis, nausea, vomiting, and calcium depletion can occur.
- ■ Niacin-induced hepatitis has been noted after long years of use, especially with time-released capsules (Reimund and Ramos, 1994). Investigate megavitamin use for all patients; discourage long-term use of niacin, especially with high doses.
- ■ Ribavirin and interferon work on only about 40% of patients. There are also hemolytic side effects, possible depression, and weight and lipid changes.

TABLE 8–3 Hepatitis Symptoms, Transmission, and Treatment

Type	*Incubation*	*Symptoms*	*Transmission*	*Treatment*
Hepatitis A Infectious HAV	30 days	Flu-like illness, jaundice, nausea, fatigue, abdominal pain, anorexia, diarrhea, fever.	Ingestion of items contaminated with infected feces, drinking water or ice contaminated with raw sewage, eating fruits, vegetables, or uncooked food contaminated during handling. Risk factors: overseas travel, anal sex, IV drug use, living in poor sanitation.	Immune globulin 2–3 months before or 2 weeks after exposure. Vaccine is available.
Hepatitis B Serum HBV	Can survive 7 days outside of the body	Flu-like illness, jaundice, nausea, fatigue, vomiting, fever, often no symptoms	Contact with contaminated body fluids, exposure to sharp instruments that contain contaminated blood, human bites, blood transfusion before 1975. Risk factors: IV drug use, multiple sex partners, travel or work in developing countries, transfusion before 1975.	Interferon alfa and lamivudine. Hepatitis-B immune globulin (HBIG) within 14 days of exposure. There are safe and effective vaccines. Ribavirin is under study.
Hepatitis C HCV	Average 7–9 weeks; can live 28 weeks	Often no symptoms until liver damage occurs, flu-like illness, fatigue, nausea, headaches, abdominal pain.	Blood-to-blood contact, especially IV drug use and shared needles. Exposure to items with contaminated blood, such needles (tattoo, body piercing, acupuncture), razors, nail files, toothbrushes, scissors, tampons. Sexually transmitted disease with rashes or sores. Blood transfusions before July 1992. At risk: IV drug use, had a blood transfusion or organ transplant before July 1992, snorts cocaine. Widespread—affects 4 million people. Silent. Leading cause Of cirrhosis in the U.S.	Interferon or combination drug treatments. Liver transplant for end-stage. There are no vaccines. Treatment takes minimum of 1 year. Ribavirin is under study.
Hepatitis D	Occurs only with Hepatitis B infection, cannot survive on own	Flu-like illness, jaundice, nausea, fatigue, vomiting, fever, often no symptoms.	Sexual contact with HBV-infected person. Exposure to sharp instruments contaminated with HBV. At risk: IV drug use.	Interferon alpha for chronic cases. Vaccination against HBD provides protection against type D.
Hepatitis E HEV	2–9 weeks	Malaise, loss of appetite, abdominal pain, joint pain, fever.	Fecal transmission, often through contaminated water. At risk: pregnant women, those who travel in developing countries.	No specific treatment.
Hepatitis G	Average 7–9 weeks; can live up to 28 weeks	Often no symptoms until liver damage occurs. Flu-like illness, fatigue, nausea, headaches, abdominal pain.	Transmitted through blood.	No proven treatment.

Herbs, Botanicals and Supplements

- Herbs and botanical supplements should not be used without discussing with the physician.
- Chaparral is an herbal product used for antioxidant properties; severe hepatitis or liver failure may result (Gordon et al., 1995).
- Carrot, schisandra, dandelion, Indian almond, and licorice have been recommended for this condition but without clinical trials to prove efficacy.
- Silybum marianum (milk thistle) has been shown to have clinical applications in the treatment of toxic hepatitis and viral hepatitis via its antioxidative, antilipid peroxidative, antifibrotic, anti-inflammatory, immunomodulating, and liver-regenerating effects (Luper, 1998). Further studies are under way.

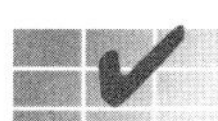

PATIENT EDUCATION

- ✓ Ensure patient abstains from alcohol.
- ✓ Help patient make attractive, appetizing meals. Encourage frequent, small meals.
- ✓ Teach safe personal hygiene in regard to handwashing and disinfectants.
- ✓ Educate patient about how to increase calorie, protein, and vitamin intakes. Discuss pros and cons of supplemental products.

For More Information

- CDC Information
  http://www.cdc.gov/ncidod/diseases/hepatitis/
- Hepatitis Information Network
  http://www.hepnet.com/
- Hepatitis Information
  http://www.hepatitis.org
- Hepatitis B Foundation
  http://www.hepb.org/
- Hepatitis C Central
  http://www.hepatitis-central.com/
- Hepatitis D Info Center
  http://www.hepnet.com/hepd.html
- Hepatitis G Info Center
  http://www.hepnet.com/hepg.html

HEPATIC CIRRHOSIS

NUTRITIONAL ACUITY RANKING: LEVEL 3–4

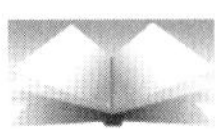

DEFINITIONS AND BACKGROUND

Hepatic cirrhosis is caused by chronic degeneration of the parenchymal liver cells and thickening of the surrounding tissue. Symptoms and signs may include fatigue, weight loss, lowered immune resistance, jaundice, and GI disturbances. It may result from alcohol use, viral hepatitis, cystic fibrosis, biliary stenosis, or other diseases; alcohol use is the most common cause of cirrhosis.

In the United States, cirrhosis is the ninth leading cause of death, causing about 25,000 deaths annually. Alcoholic cirrhosis, also called Laennec's cirrhosis, is the fourth leading cause of death after 40 years of age (see Fig. 8–1). Whereas light-to-moderate drinking may lower cardiac mortality rates among women, heavier drinking is associated with breast cancer and cirrhosis (Fuchs et al., 1995). Nonalcoholic steatohepatitis (NASH) is common in women who are overweight and have type 2 diabetes.

The pathogenesis of protein-energy malnutrition in cirrhosis involves many factors, including poor oral intake, malabsorption, and metabolic abnormalities similar to stress (Teran, 1999). Cirrhosis is a disease of accelerated use of alternative fuels (e.g., fat). Approximately 50–60% of kilocalories as CHO should be consumed to minimize use of fat and protein for energy. Glucose intolerance occurs in one third of patients with cirrhosis, mainly from insulin resistance or higher circulating glucagon (Hasse et al., 1997). In patients with chronic liver disease, early satiety and hypophagia may be caused by hyperinsulinemia; those with cirrhosis are found to be especially nutritionally depleted (Richardson et al., 1999).

Plasma aromatic amino acids concentrations (AAAs—phenylalanine, tyrosine, tryptophan) tend to increase from rapid muscle proteolysis, decreased synthesis of proteins, and decreased liver clearance (Hasse et al., 1997). Branched chain amino acid (BCAA) levels increase. The imbalance in BCAA:AAA has been suggested as an etiologic factor—when AAAs are high, BCAAs are limited in cerebral uptake. A higher BCAA intake is hypothesized to improve this status; this therapy is suggested for patients with hepatic encephalopathy who do not tolerate standard proteins and have not responded to lactulose or neomycin therapy.

There is a high incidence of muscle wasting, weight loss, and malnutrition with cirrhosis. Nutrition support improves nutritional status in patients with alcoholic cirrhosis. Daily drinking of oral supplements for 6 months has been shown to improve status by providing about 1,000 additional kilocalories and 35 g additional protein (Hirsch et al., 1999). An accurate diet history will help to determine current intake. Nutritionally depleted patients may need 1.5 g/Kg—as much as possible without inducing encephalopathy (Hasse et al., 1997).

Severe cirrhosis may lead to decreased total cholesterol (TC), HDL, LDL, and VLDL (Hasse et al., 1997). A low respiratory quotient (RQ) indicates reduced glucose and increased lipid oxidation and may be a useful marker for assessment when BMI and anthropometric measurements may suggest use of normal nutrition (Scolapio et al., 2000).

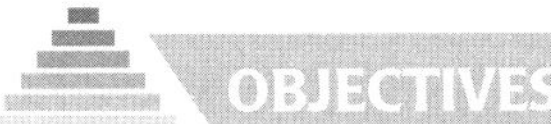

OBJECTIVES

- Support residual liver function.
- Provide supportive treatment for ascites, edema, muscle wasting, weight loss, esophageal varices, and portal hypertension.
- Monitor fat stasis and steatorrhea; offer suggestions for managing.
- Correct nutritional deficiencies. Cirrhotic patients' spontaneous dietary intake is lower than that of controls and recommended intakes; it is unclear whether associated nutrient deficits are metabolically driven and dictated by primary cause (Davidson et al., 1999).
- Drowsiness and disorientation are potential signs of hepatic encephalopathy; monitor closely.
- Provide adequate glucose for brain metabolism but beware of glucose intolerance, especially in alcoholic cirrhosis.

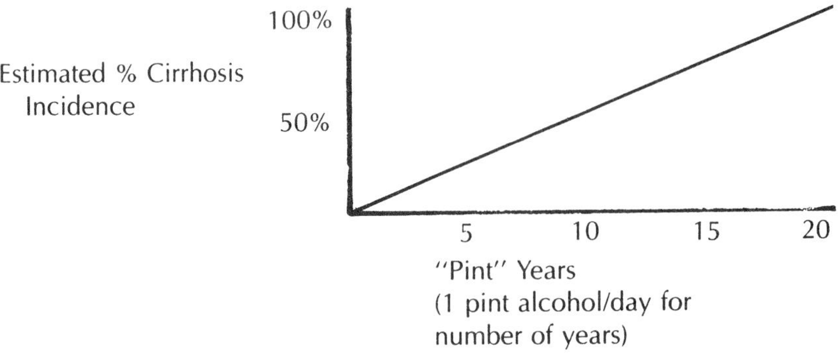

Figure 8–2 Role of alcohol in creating cirrhosis (Lelbach).

- Prevent bone disease, hyper- or hypokalemia, hyponatremia, renal problems, and anemia.

DIETARY AND NUTRITIONAL RECOMMENDATIONS

- Increased energy is needed. Calculate basal energy expenditure (BEE) and use a factor of 1.5–1.75 accordingly, if malabsorption is present or if repletion is desired. Use ideal or estimated dry weight; fat is the preferred fuel in cirrhosis and frequent small meals are needed (Hasse et al., 1997). Diet should provide 1–1.5 g protein/kg body weight (a high percentage should be high biologic value [HBV] proteins). It also should provide adequate carbohydrates to spare protein.
- Ensure that fat intake is sufficient. Ensure adequate EFA intake. In general, 40–50% nonprotein calories should be from fat.
- Malabsorption occurs from diminished lipase output. With steatorrhea, decrease LCTs. Monitor use of MCTs; they may cause diarrhea or acidosis.
- Supplement diet with vitamin B-complex, vitamins C and K, zinc, and magnesium-rich foods or supplements. Monitor need for vitamins A and D.
- Meat has a high level of aromatic amino acids; vegetable proteins have less. Encourage use of vegetable proteins and BCAAs (pasta, vegetables, rice, fruits, and lima beans). Casein is another form of protein that is often better tolerated than meat protein.
- Check use of tube feedings. Tube feeding does not necessarily increase rates of survival in cirrhosis (Borum, 2000).
- Glutamine is not generally recommended in liver disease.
- Avoid alcoholic beverages.

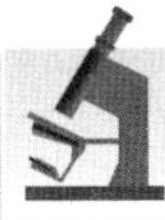

PROFILE

Clinical/History

Height
Weight
BMI
Bowel changes
BP

Lab Work

BUN
TSF
Alb, prealbumin (not valid in cirrhosis)
Retinol-binding protein (RBP)
Globulin
Somatomedin C
Total protein
Uric acid (UA)
Gluc (increased or decreased)
PT (prolonged)
Na+, K+
Ca++
Transferrin
H&H (decreased)
Serum ammonia
ALT
AST (increased)
Bilirubin (increased)
K+
Mg++
Alk phos (increased)
WBC
Trig (increased)
Chol
LDH (increased)
Copper, ceruloplasmin (increased)
Folate
GGT
Liver biopsy
Computed tomography (CT) scan

- Control CHO intake if diabetic.
- Low sodium intake (2–4 g) is recommended with ascites.
- Decrease fluid in hyponatremia.
- Enhance nutrient density of food choices if malnourished.
- Vitamin and mineral supplements may be needed in liquid form for some patients, especially with esophageal varices.

Common Drugs Used and Potential Side Effects

- Neomycin is often used to destroy intestinal bacteria. Chronic antibiotic use (neomycin, metronidazole) requires careful renal and neurological monitoring.
- Albumin replacement may be used. Check tolerance and encephalopathic status.
- Insulin may be needed. Monitor for hypoglycemic episodes.
- Colchicine has been demonstrated to improve survival of some patients with cirrhosis. More studies are being completed at this time. Nausea, vomiting, and diarrhea may result.
- Lactulose (Cephulac) and kristalose (Chronulac) stimulate catharsis to change pH and to bind ammonia. Take with food or milk. Flatulence and cramping are common. Nausea, abdominal pain, bloating, and diarrhea can also occur.
- Other drugs are used for patient-specific symptoms. Antihistamines and cholestyramine are commonly prescribed. Nausea or constipation can result.
- Between 25 and 35% of patients with either alcoholic or nonalcoholic liver disease with known varices will eventually bleed. Beta-blockers are often useful: propanolol, nadolol, metoprolol may be prescribed.
- Megestrol acetate is thought to be useful for anorexia in ESLD by interfering with production of cachectin; oral solutions are usually tolerated (Gurk-Turner, 1997). Diarrhea, flatulence, nausea, and vomiting (N&V) can occur.

Herbs, Botanicals and Supplements

- Herbs and botanical supplements should not be used without discussing with the physician.
- Some herbal tea preparations may be harmful (such as Comfrey tea); check with physician.
- Chaparral is an herbal product used for antioxidant properties; severe hepatitis or liver failure may result (Gordon et al., 1995).
- Silybum marianum (milk thistle) has been shown to have clinical applications in the treatment of cirrhosis through its antioxidative, antilipid peroxidative, antifibrotic, anti-inflammatory, immunomodulating, and liver-regenerating effects (Luper, 1998). Picrorrhiza kurroa is also under study.

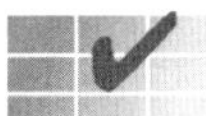

PATIENT EDUCATION

- A better appetite at certain meals may be common. Identify if breakfast or another meal is best tolerated. Some patients sleep late with a sleep reversal pattern.
- Dietary intake must be adjusted according to the changing status of the patient.
- Large meals increase portal pressure. Ensure patient eats smaller meals more frequently.
- Avoid skipping meals. Discuss proper menu planning.
- Avoid high doses of vitamins A and D, which may become toxic in the diseased liver.

For More Information

- American Gastroenterological Association
  http://www.gastro.org/public/cirrhosis.html
- National Institutes of Health—Cirrhosis
  http://www.nlm.nih.gov/medlineplus/cirrhosis.html

PORTACAVAL-SPLENORENAL SHUNT FOR PORTAL HYPERTENSION

NUTRITIONAL ACUITY RANKING: LEVEL 3

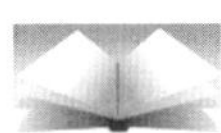

DEFINITIONS AND BACKGROUND

A serious problem for people with cirrhosis is pressure on blood vessels that flow through the liver. Normally, blood from the intestines and spleen is pumped to the liver through the portal vein. However, in cirrhosis, normal flow of blood is slowed, building pressure in the portal vein (portal hypertension). This blocks the normal flow of blood, causing the spleen to enlarge. Blood from the intestines then tries to find a way around the liver through new vessels.

When end-stage liver disease results in portal hypertension with increased collateral flow, it causes varices in any part of the GI tract. Esophageal varices are the most serious complication of cirrhosis. Between 25 and 35% of patients with either alcoholic or nonalcoholic liver disease with known varices will eventually bleed (Crippin, 1997). The pathogenesis of portal-systemic hepatic encephalopathy probably is multifactorial, although the key causative agent appears to be ammonia (Abou-Assi and Vlahcevic, 2001).

Splenorenal shunting is performed when flow is diverted from the liver by anastomosis of the splenic vein to the renal vein (performed when the portal vein is obstructed). The shunt is performed for intrahepatic obstruction. Portacaval blood flow is diverted from the liver by anastomosing the portal vein to the inferior vena cava. A new shunt procedure, the transjugular intrahepatic portosystemic shunt (TIPS) has resulted in the need for fewer surgical shunts; it may, however, cause hepatic encephalopathy in 33% of cases (Crippin, 1997).

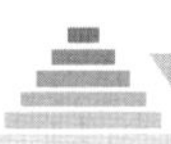

OBJECTIVES

- Decrease hypertension and GI bleeding.
- Support preoperative and postoperative medical care. The liver fares better when adequate glycogen stores are available.
- Correct inadequate intake, which is a common problem.
- Avoid encephalopathy and coma.

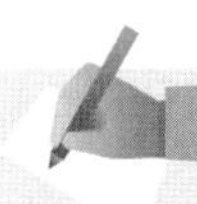

DIETARY AND NUTRITIONAL RECOMMENDATIONS

- Progress, as tolerated, to a diet with regulated protein, adequate-to-high carbohydrate, controlled sodium (lower with ascites), and adequate calories. Limitation of protein in the diet may be useful for short periods but is not recommended for long-term use because of potential worsening of already poor nutrition (Abou-Assi and Vlahcevic, 2001). Generally, 1–1.5 g protein/kg can be tolerated if the patient is not comatose.
- Provide a multivitamin/mineral supplement if needed, especially ensuring that fat-soluble vitamins A, D, E, and K are available in an appropriate form.
- Control fluid intake—prevent dehydration and overhydration.
- No alcoholic beverages should be consumed.
- Provide TPN or TF when needed; increased BCAAs seem to be beneficial. Avoid glutamine-enriched formulas, which can add to ammonia production.

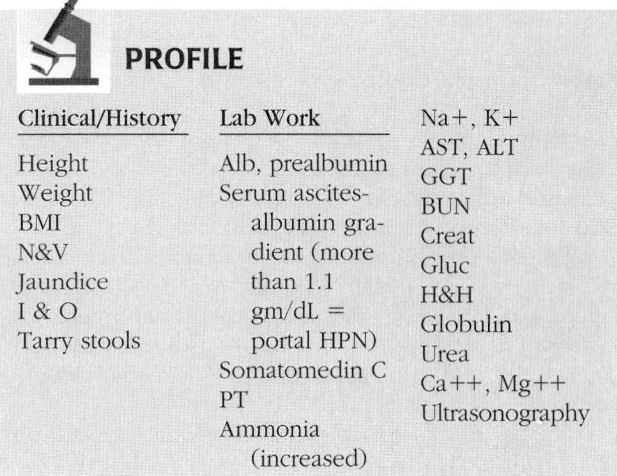

PROFILE

Clinical/History	Lab Work	
Height	Alb, prealbumin	Na+, K+
Weight	Serum ascites-albumin gradient (more than 1.1 gm/dL = portal HPN)	AST, ALT
BMI	Somatomedin C	GGT
N&V	PT	BUN
Jaundice	Ammonia (increased)	Creat
I & O		Gluc
Tarry stools		H&H
		Globulin
		Urea
		Ca++, Mg++
		Ultrasonography

Common Drugs Used and Potential Side Effects

- Lactulose may be used for the underlying encephalopathy.
- Use of oral antibiotics and BCAAs is of some benefit in patients who do not respond to lactulose. Extensive use may deplete vitamin K levels. Evaluate individually for preferred administration (with milk, food, etc.).
- Albumin replacement may be used.

Herbs, Botanicals and Supplements

- Herbs and botanical supplements should not be used without discussing with physician.
- Chaparral is an herbal product used for antioxidant properties; severe hepatitis or liver failure may result (Gordon et al., 1995).
- Milk thistle is under study for this condition.

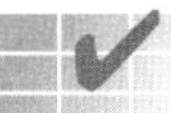

PATIENT EDUCATION

- The importance of dietary regulation should be addressed extensively.
- The patient should be advised to omit alcoholic beverages from the diet, probably permanently.
- The patient should eat slowly and chew well.

HEPATIC ENCEPHALOPATHY, FAILURE, OR COMA

NUTRITIONAL ACUITY RANKING: LEVEL 4

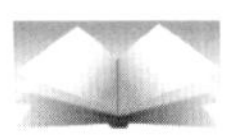

DEFINITIONS AND BACKGROUND

The pathogenesis of portal-systemic hepatic encephalopathy (HE) is multifactorial, although the predominant causative agent appears to be ammonia (Abou-Assi and Vlahcevic, 2001). The basis of neurotoxicity of ammonia or other agents implicated in the condition is not clear. Encephalopathy may complicate cirrhosis but is usually not caused by diet (Teran, 1999). Protein restriction is only necessary in rare patients with refractory encephalopathy.

Hepatic encephalopathy is a recognized clinical complication of chronic liver disease. It can be precipitated by GI bleeding, abnormal electrolytes, renal failure, infection, use of sedatives, and constipation. Decreased dopamine and elevated serotonin can occur, as well as decreased BCAAs and increased aromatic AAs. The use of branched-chain amino-acid solutions is not fully supported by the literature.

There is a possible relationship between manganese neurotoxicity and chronic HE (Krieger et al., 1995). Zinc deficiency may be involved in pathogenesis of encephalopathy because it is a cofactor in ornithine transcarbamylase (OTC) activity and also influences ammonia production from aspartate (Hasse et al., 1997).

The spectrum of HE ranges from minimal cerebral functional deficits, which can only be found by sensitive tests, to coma with signs of decerebration (Gerber and Schomerus, 2000). See Table 8–4 for stages of HE. Therapy includes timely recognition and correction of precipitating factors.

Hepatic coma is a potentially serious complication of advanced liver disease; signs of impending coma are noted in Table 8–5. About 30% of patients with cirrhosis die in hepatic coma (Abou-Assi and Vlahcevic, 2001). These patients have increased intracranial pressure and brain edema with a deleterious clinical course and poor prognosis unless liver transplantation is available.

Hepatic failure is common in critical illnesses. With liver failure, renal insufficiency and hepatorenal syndrome may occur. Creatinine measures are not accurate here; glomerular filtration rate (GFR) is more useful. Hemodialysis may be needed until an appropriate donor is available.

TABLE 8–4 Stages of Hepatic Encephalopathy

Stage 1: Mild confusion, irritability, agitation, sleep disturbance, decreased attention
Stage 2: Lethargy, disorientation, inappropriate behavior, drowsiness
Stage 3: Arousable somnolence, incomprehensible speech, aggression when awake, confusion
Stage 4: Coma

Adapted from: Hasse J, Matarese L. Medical nutrition therapy for liver, biliary system, and exocrine pancreas disorders. In: Mahan L and Escott-Stump S. *Krause's food nutrition and diet therapy*. 10th edition. Philadelphia: WB Saunders Co., 2000.

TABLE 8–5 Signs of Impending Hepatic Coma

1. Irritability, change in mentation.
2. Disorientation to time and place.
3. Asterixis or metabolic flap (involuntary jerky movements, especially of hands).
4. Constructional apraxia (inability to draw simple diagrams).
5. Difficulty in writing.
6. Ascites, edema, and fetor hepaticus (sweet, musty odor of the breath).
7. Bleeding.

OBJECTIVES

According to The Practice Parameters Committee of the American College of Gastroenterology (Beil and Cordoba, 2001):

For acute encephalopathy in cirrhosis, correct the precipitating factor. Withhold oral intake for 24–48 hours and provide intravenous glucose until improvement is noted. Tube feeding can be started if the patient appears unable to eat after this period. Protein intake begins at a dose of 0.5 g/kg/day, with progressive increase to 1–1.5 g/kg/day.

For chronic encephalopathy in cirrhosis, avoid and prevent precipitating factors. Focus protein intake on dairy products and vegetable-based diets. Consider oral branched-chain amino acids for individuals intolerant of all protein.

For problematic encephalopathy (nonresponsive to therapy), consider the combination of lactulose and neomycin, oral zinc, and invasive approaches such as surgical shunts.

In general:

- Avoid skeletal muscle catabolism; decrease ammonia and toxin production. Normalize serum amino acid patterns.
- Avoid hypoglycemia.
- Provide nutrition support because of elevated catabolic hormone levels.
- Promote regeneration of liver tissue.
- Support other systems (respiratory, neurological, GI, circulatory) while the liver regenerates.
- Correct anemia, zinc deficiency, and other nutritional deficits (see Table 8–6).
- Prevent hypokalemia, sepsis, starvation, and acute crises.

TABLE 8–6 Nutrient Relationships in Hepatic Failure and Hepatic Encephalopathy

Decreased protein—Swollen belly (ascites) from decreased albumin production
Decreased niacin—Memory loss
Decreased folacin—Degeneration of spinal cord
Decreased B-complex, iron, and protein—Glossitis, anemias
Decreased vitamins C and K—Hemorrhage, scurvy
Decreased zinc—Poor taste acuity, impaired wound healing
Decreased magnesium, niacin, thiamine—Hallucinations, delirium, beriberi, pellagra
Increased Na+ and fluid—Fluid retention
Decreased thiamine—Amnesia, confabulation, Korsakoff's psychosis
Decreased vitamin A—Increased respiratory infections
Decreased vitamin K—Muscle weakness
Decreased protein and fat with malabsorption—Somnolence, euphoria, asterixis, coma
Decreased magnesium—Marked anxiety, hyperirritability, confusion, seizures, tremor

- Reduce circulating amines and lessen shunting of blood around the liver.
- Control hemorrhage and blood loss into the gut.

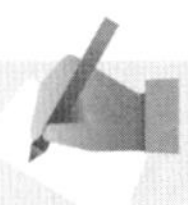

DIETARY AND NUTRITIONAL RECOMMENDATIONS

- Management by protein restriction has been abandoned in recent years. For the patient who is not comatose, diet should provide moderate-to-high levels of protein.
- Glucose is administered to reduce hypoglycemia.
- For the patient with coma, use tube feeding with 0.5–0.6 g protein/kg body weight; advance to 1–1.5 g/kg IBW. It may be useful to ensure higher intake of BCAAs as in Hepatic Aid II, Nutri-Hep, or similar products. HepatAmine is used for parenteral and contains 35% BCAAs; leucine is most essential. Avoid glutamine-enriched products.
- To minimize muscle catabolism, diet should provide 1.3 × resting energy expenditure (REE) per day. Adequate intake of carbohydrates and fats is needed; 25–30 kcal/kg body weight (BW) is common; measure using indirect calorimetry whenever possible. Fats should be 30–35% of kcal, using MCT if needed.
- In parenteral solutions, use up to 50% of energy as non-protein kilocalories.
- Ensure adequate intake of fluids and electrolytes as monitoring determines. Often, sodium is limited to aid diuresis.
- Restrict fluid only with dilutional hyponatremia; usually 1,000–1,500 mL.
- Vitamin–mineral supplements may be needed (vitamins A, D, E, and K, niacin, thiamine, folate, phosphate, and zinc). Calcium or magnesium may be supplemented as needed.
- Monitor fat-soluble vitamin use with damaged liver. Avoid copper and manganese at this time.

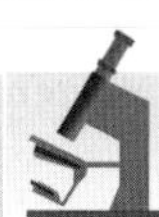

PROFILE

Clinical/History

Height
Weight
BMI
I & O
BP
Subjective global assessment

Lab Work

BUN (decreased)
Bilirubin (increased)
Alk phos (increased)
AST (increased)
ALT
GGT
Mg++
Ca++
H&H (decreased)
K+
Chol, Trig
UA
Ammonia
Alb (decreased)
Prealbumin, RBP
PT
Na+
Transferrin
Nitrogen (N) balance
Gluc (decreased)
Globulin (decreased)
Plasma AAs (isoleucine, leucine, valine, tryptophan, phenylalanine, tyrosine)
Serum insulin, epinephrine, adrenocortical, steroids, thyroxine

Common Drugs Used and Potential Side Effects

- Nonabsorbable antibiotics (aminoglycosides) have adverse effects and are limited to higher grades of HE.
- Intestinal cleansing with Neomycin is used to destroy intestinal bacteria; treatment is started before protein restriction begins. This drug alters the absorption of most nutrients and can cause nausea, vomiting, diarrhea, sore mouth, and elevated BUN/creatinine.
- Administration of disaccharides that are undigested in the small intestine are often used (Abou-Assi and Vlahcevic, 2001). Lactulose (Cephulac) or kristalose (Chronulac) may have side effects including N, abdominal pain, bloating, or diarrhea. It is used to decrease ammonia and aromatic AA formation and to improve protein tolerance. Lactulose, branched chain amino acids, and ornithine aspartate are effective and can be applied for long-term use in patients with lower grades of HE (Gerber and Schomerus, 2000).
- Zinc sulfate or acetate may be needed.
- Megestrol acetate is thought to be useful for anorexia in ESLD by interfering with production of cachectin; oral solutions are usually tolerated (Gurk-Turner, 1997). Diarrhea, flatulence, and N&V can occur.
- Dronabinol works on the central nervous system (CNS) and euphoria can occur, along with slurred speech, lethargy, and postural hypotension.
- For hyperglycemia, glipizide and glyburide are more favorable than first-generation drugs (Gurk-Turner, 1997).
- With renal insufficiency, avoid aspirin and NSAIDs because of their effect on renal insufficiency; cut out any potentially nephrotoxic drugs including diuretics.

- Pruritus is common, and cholestyramine or ursodeoxycholic acid may be useful.
- Osteoporosis can also occur; vitamin D supplements or estrogen may be given.
- Bromocriptine is sometimes used for refractory encephalopathy.
- Silybum marianum (milk thistle) has been shown to have clinical applications in the treatment of liver disease for its antioxidative, antilipid peroxidative, antifibrotic, anti-inflammatory, immunomodulating, and liver-regenerating effects (Luper, 1998). It is not clear yet if it has a therapeutic role in management of liver failure.

Herbs, Botanicals and Supplements

- Herbs and botanical supplements should not be used without discussing with physician.
- Chaparral is an herbal product used for antioxidant properties; severe hepatitis or liver failure may result (Gordon et al., 1995).

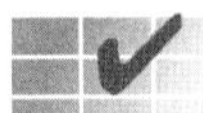

PATIENT EDUCATION

- ✔ Milk and eggs produce less ammonia than meats.
- ✔ Explain that guidelines for hepatic cirrhosis also apply.
- ✔ Discuss the importance of refraining from use of alcoholic beverages.

LIVER TRANSPLANTATION

NUTRITIONAL ACUITY RANKING: LEVEL 4

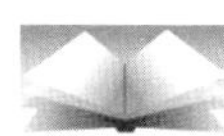

DEFINITIONS AND BACKGROUND

Liver transplantation is now a viable alternative for patients with end-stage hepatic failure due to cirrhosis from alcohol and other causes, viral hepatitis, chronic active liver disease, alpha-1-antitrypsin deficiency, primary sclerosing cirrhosis, cholangiocarcinoma, hemochromatosis, autoimmune hepatitis, Budd-Chiari syndrome, hepatoma, primary biliary cirrhosis, and other diseases.

Obesity is a major risk factor in the development of NASH, a precursor to cirrhosis; diabetes and hyperinsulinism may also play a role in the 1–2% of liver transplants performed because of a pretransplant diagnosis of NASH (Neuschwander-Tetri, 2001). Alcohol is a major contributor to cirrhosis and the need for transplantation; abstinence, along with vitamin supplements and nutritional considerations, will allow better transplant results (Walsh & Alexander, 2000).

Patients are screened carefully for other underlying conditions; many will not be suitable for transplantation. Symptoms and signs leading to the need for transplant include ascites, jaundice, edema, CNS dysfunction, and cachexia. Transplant patients who are not hospitalized when a donor becomes available are more likely to have higher survival rates than patients who are hospitalized before transplantation (Crippin, 1997).

Preoperative and early postoperative nutrition may speed recovery, lessen time in the intensive care unit, and promote fewer infections. Subjective global assessment (SGA) is often the most useful series of tests, because lab work varies so much in liver disease. Subjective global assessment includes physical signs and symptoms, dietary changes and intolerances, medical/surgical history, GI symptoms and complaints, history (hx) of weight loss, and functional capacity (Labbe and Veldee, 1994).

In general, enteral nutrition is as effective as TPN in maintaining nutritional status after transplantation, with potential benefits such as reduced complications and costs (Wicks et al., 1994). Nutritional supplementation after liver transplantation quickly restores protein synthesis in the allograft (Geevarghese et al., 1999).

In patients who have received a transplant because of hepatitis C, it is important to monitor carefully for recurrence of the underlying disorder to prevent allograft rejection (Testa et al., 2000).

OBJECTIVES

Pretransplantation:

- Correct malnutrition; lessen edema, ascites.
- Treat hyponatremia and electrolyte imbalances, depending on medications and renal function.
- Prevent or correct catabolic wasting of muscle mass from increased hormonal levels (insulin, glucagon, epinephrine, and cortisol may be elevated).
- Provide nutritional support in an appropriate mode of feeding (considering nausea, vomiting, etc.) to provide a normalized nitrogen balance and other normalized laboratory values.
- Normalize blood glucose levels and prevent hypoglycemia; diabetes is common.
- Correct fat malabsorption, with or without steatorrhea and diarrhea.
- Correct abnormal amino acid metabolism and neural accumulation of amino acids that are precursors for dopamine, serotonin, and norepinephrine. Normalize serum ammonia.

Posttransplantation:

- Promote normalized protein synthesis in the liver (i.e., albumin, globulins, clotting factors, etc.).
- Prevent or correct hyperglycemia, fasting hypoglycemia, and abnormal glucagon storage. Diabetes is a common complication. Transplant patients are at risk of glucose intolerance from use of prednisone, cyclosporine, and tacrolimus (Hasse et al., 1997).
- Support wound healing.
- Manage long-term hypercholesterolemia, osteopenia, hypertension, and obesity (Blue et al., 1993).

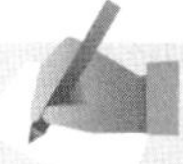

DIETARY AND NUTRITIONAL RECOMMENDATIONS

Pretransplantation:

- Protein requirements may be 1–1.5 g/kg dry weight, unless in encephalopathy.
- Energy should be 35–45 kcals/kg.
- Modify for sodium, potassium, and other electrolytes depending on lab values and renal status.
- If TF, use a low-volume, diluting concentration as needed. Avoid glutamine-enriched solutions if ammonia levels are a concern.
- Beware of excess vitamins and minerals because of liver functioning; use recommended dietary allowance (RDA) levels.

Posttransplantation:

- Use 1–1.2 g protein per kg /dry weight per day. Negative nitrogen balance may persist for several weeks postoperatively. Increase BCAAs and decrease aromatic amino acids (tyrosine, phenylalanine, tryptophan). For patients with encephalopathy, decreasing methionine may also be necessary.
- Adequate calories are needed—30 kcals/kg to maintain. Increase to 35 kcal/kg (1.1–1.3 × BEE) if weight gain is needed. Refeed as early as possible to prevent GI atrophy and bacterial translocation (Hasse et al., 1994).
- For adequate kilocalories, 25–40% of total kilocalories as fat may be needed.
- For hyperglycemia, decrease glucose administration. For oral diets, decrease simple sugars. CHO should be 50–60% of calories.

- Mineral supplementation may be helpful. Use 1,000–1,200 mg calcium. Encourage intake of foods high in magnesium and phosphorus when levels are low; supplement or restrict according to serum levels.
- Alter sodium and potassium intakes according to the profile. Usually, sodium is maintained at a maximum of 2–4 g (3–4 g long-term). In hyponatremia, correct immediately but do not over-treat to avoid brain damage. Hyperkalemia can be a problem with cyclosporine or tacrolimus.
- Adequate vitamin intake will be essential to maintain immunity and to support wound healing.

PROFILE

Clinical/History	Lab Work	
Height	BUN, Creat	Cerebrospinal fluid (CSF)
Weight—usual	Alb, prealbumin	Mg++, Ca++
Present weight	N balance	H&H, Serum Fe
BMI	Amino acid profiles	Transferrin
Edema	Na+, K+	Urea
N&V	Bilirubin	Chol, Trig
I & O	Serum ammonia	Carotenoids
BP		AST, ALT
SGA		GGT
		Gluc

Common Drugs Used and Potential Side Effects

- Corticosteroids (such as Prednisone, Solu-Cortef) are used for immunosuppression. Side effects include increased catabolism of proteins, negative nitrogen balance, hyperphagia, GI ulcers, decreased glucose tolerance, sodium retention, fluid retention, and impaired calcium absorption and osteoporosis. Cushing's syndrome, obesity, muscle wasting, and increased gastric secretion may result. A high protein intake and low intake of simple CHOs may be needed.
- Cyclosporine does not retain sodium as much as corticosteroids do. Intravenous doses are more toxic than oral doses; avoid if possible. Nausea, vomiting, and diarrhea are common side effects. Hyperlipidemia, HPN, and hyperkalemia also may occur; decrease sodium and potassium as necessary. Elevated glucose and lipids may occur. The drug is also nephrotoxic; a controlled renal diet may be beneficial if GFR declines and when trying to slow deterioration or chronic renal failure. Avoid taking with grapefruit and its juice.
- The depletion paradigm enables drugs to bind to lymphocyte cell surface markers, creating cell lysis and/or inactivation; these include polyclonal antithymocyte globulin (ATG) and thymoglobulin, and monoclonal OKT3 antilymphocyte antibodies (Hong and Kahan, 2000). These immunosuppressants such as Muromonab, Orthoclone (OKT3), and ATG are less nephrotoxic than cyclosporine but can cause nausea, anorexia, diarrhea, and vomiting. Monitor carefully. Fever and stomatitis also may occur; alter diet as needed.
- Azathioprine (Imuran) may cause leukopenia, thrombocytopenia, oral and esophageal sores, macrocytic anemia, pancreatitis, vomiting, diarrhea, and other complex side effects. Folate supplementation and other dietary modifications (liquid or soft diet, use of oral supplements) may be needed. The drug works by lowering the number of white blood cells; it is often prescribed along with prednisone for conventional immunosuppression.
- Tacrolimus (Prograf, FK506) suppresses T-cell immunity; it is 100 times more potent than cyclosporine, thus requiring smaller doses. Side effects include GI distress, nausea, vomiting, hyperkalemia, and hyperglycemia. It may be necessary to supplement with magnesium; check lab work. Avoid taking with grapefruit and its juice.
- Insulin may be necessary during periods of hyperglycemia. Monitor for hypoglycemic symptoms during use.
- Furosemide (Lasix) and other diuretics may be needed with edema. Assess each medication's effects.
- Other drugs such as CellCept and sirolimus may be used (Hong and Kahan, 2000; McAlister et al., 2001).

Herbs, Botanicals and Supplements

- Herbs and botanical supplements should not be used without discussing with physician.
- Chaparral is an herbal product used for antioxidant properties; severe hepatitis or liver failure may result (Gordon et al., 1995). Avoid after transplantation.
- Silybum marianum (milk thistle) has been shown to have clinical applications in the treatment of liver disease through its antioxidative, antilipid peroxidative, antifibrotic, anti-inflammatory, immunomodulating, and liver-regenerating effects (Luper, 1998).
- St. John's Wort interferes with the metabolism of cyclosporin-A and should not be used after transplantation (Karliova et al., 2000).

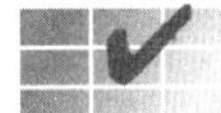

PATIENT EDUCATION (POSTTRANSPLANTATION)

- ✓ Discuss the role of diet in wound healing, graft retention, and improvement in health status.
- ✓ Provide patient or family with recipes for no-added-salt and sugar-free foods as needed.
- ✓ Discuss sources of foods that contain calcium and magnesium, etc. Individualize to patient preferences and needs.
- ✓ Discuss the need for alcohol rehabilitation, family counseling, and other available services. Ethanol/ethyl alcohol (ETOH) abuse affects such key nutrients as niacin, folate, vitamin B12, zinc, phosphorus, and magnesium.
- ✓ Obesity can occur unless energy intakes are controlled.
- ✓ Prevent infections from food-borne illness; patients who have undergone transplantation may be prone to increased risk more than other individuals.

For More Information

- American Council on Transplantation
  700 North Fairfax Street, Suite 505
  Alexandria, VA 22314
  (703) 836-4301
- Biliary Atresia and Liver Transplant Network
  3835 Richmond Ave., Box 190
  Staten Island, New York 10312
  Voice mail and fax: 718-987-6200
  Email: OrganTrans@msn.com

PANCREATITIS, ACUTE

NUTRITIONAL ACUITY RANKING: LEVEL 3

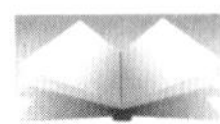

DEFINITIONS AND BACKGROUND

The exocrine pancreas secretes proteolytic, lipolytic, and amylolytic enzymes for nutrient digestion in the intestines. Therefore, pancreatitis allows autodigestion and premature enzyme release to occur. A balance between activated proteases and enzyme inhibitors results in cellular necrosis.

Pancreatitis involves inflammation with edema, fat necrosis, and cellular exudate. Acute pancreatitis (AP) is an acute inflammatory disease in which autodigestion occurs from obstruction of the pancreatic duct. Enzymes become activated in the pancreas instead of the duodenum.

AP is a condition that occurs primarily from alcohol abuse and secondarily from gallstones (cholelithiasis). Gallstones are responsible for about 45% of all cases of AP. Pancreatitis also results from choledocholithiasis, because the pancreatic duct, which carries digestive enzymes, joins the common bile duct right after it enters the intestine and so may be blocked by common duct stones. It is difficult to differentiate between pancreatitis and acute cholecystitis; a correct diagnosis is important because treatment is very different.

Other causes include end-stage renal disease, lupus, biliary tract disease, abdominal trauma, certain hyperlipidemias (especially triglycerides over 1,000 or type IV hyperlipoproteinemia [HLP]), AIDS, or pancreatic cancer. In 20–40% of cases of idiopathic AP, biliary sludge has been found as a possible cause (Lee et al., 1992).

Symptoms include sudden, severe abdominal pain, nausea, vomiting, and diarrhea. Abdominal pain can be constant and disabling, causing some patients to become addicted to pain medications. About 25% of persons with AP go on to have chronic pancreatitis. Surgery for AP may include necrosectomy, pancreaticoduodenectomy, or sphincterotomy.

OBJECTIVES

- Inhibit activity and secretion of pancreatic enzymes to promote rest and reduce pain.
- Avoid pancreatic irritants, especially alcohol and caffeine.
- Correct fluid and electrolyte imbalances and malnutrition; avoid overfeeding. Acid-base imbalance is common with nasogastric (NG) suctioning, fistula losses, renal failure, nausea, and vomiting.
- In acute cases, allow the pancreas to rest; reduce fever; prevent shock and hypovolemia, hypermetabolism, sepsis, and compression of the stomach or colon.
- Avoid or control complications (cardiovascular, pulmonary, hematological, renal, neurological, or metabolic); prevent multiple organ system failure.
- Feed intravenously if necessary to reduce morbidity. Use TPN if abdominal pain is refractory; TPN will promote positive nitrogen balance.
- If TF, monitor for needed increases of pancreatic enzymes, abdominal pain, or discomfort; hold TF for resolution. Minimize pancreatic secretions.

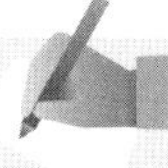

DIETARY AND NUTRITIONAL RECOMMENDATIONS

- For the patient with AP, start nil per os (NPO, not by mouth) with intravenous feedings for 48 hours. Use TPN for excessively slow progression such as ileus or fistula. Remember that TPN can cause or aggravate sepsis.
- Transition to jejunostomy can be considered, using a low-fat elemental formula; the jejunostomy should be distal to the ligament of Treitz (Pisters and Ranson, 1992). Needle catheter jejunostomy may be especially useful. For enteral therapy, Peptamen is good for its MCT content. For short-term, a nasoenteric tube may be placed.
- Check glucose tolerance and progress to clear liquids. Eventually, add amino acids and predigested fats. MCTs may be tolerated as well but may cause some bloating. Progress to a diet given in six daily feedings, used with pancreatic enzymes for all meals and snacks.
- Alcoholic beverages are prohibited. In addition, caffeine, nicotine, and gastric stimulants should be prohibited.
- Adequate calcium and fat-soluble vitamin supplementation should be provided. Magnesium may be needed.
- Diet should include adequate amounts of vitamin C, B-complex, and folate for water-soluble vitamin needs, as well as zinc. Thiamine is especially needed.
- For patients with severe steatorrhea, diet should include an increase of MCTs. Mild cases are not a problem.
- Antioxidant therapy may allow cessation of abdominal pain; glutathione production may be involved.

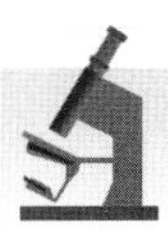

PROFILE (SEE TABLE 8–7):

Clinical/History

Height
Weight
BMI (obese?)
BEE
BP (low)
Left upper quadrant abdominal pain
Vomiting
Temperature
Chvostek's sign
Steatorrhea

Lab Work

Lipase (over 110; more sensitive than amylase)
Amylase (over 250)
K+ (decreased)
Na+ (decreased)
PT
Bilirubin (elevated)
Ca++ (decreased)
Gluc (increased, over 200)
Chol (LDL up, or total decreased)
Trig (increased)
Mg+ (decreased)
LDH (over 700)
ALT (elevated)
AST (over 250)
WBC (over 10,000 cells/mm3)
Alb (low)
RBP
Partial pressure of carbon dioxide (pCO2) (increased)
Partial pressure of oxygen (pO2) (decreased)
BUN
H&H
Serum folate
Alk phos (increased)
CT scan for necrosis
Ultrasound
Fecal fat study

TABLE 8–7 Ranson's Prognostic Criteria for Acute Pancreatitis

Older than 55-years-old
WBC over 16,000
Glucose over 200 mg/dL
Serum LDH over 350 units/mL
Serum AST over 250 units/mL
Low hematocrit (Hct) (below 40% [males]; 37% [females])
BUN elevated (not immediately)
Arterial p02 under 60 mm Hg
Fluid sequestered over 6 L
Base deficit over 4

Source: http://blue.temple.edu/~pathphys/gi/acute_pancreatitis.html#Ranson's Criteria; http://www.thenar.com/Ranson/

Common Drugs Used and Potential Side Effects

- Pancreatic enzymes or 30,000 international units (IU) of lipase per meal may be needed to reduce steatorrhea to less than 20 g/day. Enteric coating is necessary to prevent destruction by enzymes. Capsules or tablets should be swallowed whole. Take enteric-coated enzymes with cimetidine, food, or antacids.
- Antibiotics, antispasmodics, and anticholinergics may be used.
- Diuretics such as acetazolamide (Diamox) may be needed to control fluid retention. Nausea, vomiting, and diarrhea may result.
- Antacids may be helpful; beware of extended use. Side effects on various mineral or nutrient absorption are not always desirable.
- Insulin may be necessary. Monitor for hypoglycemia during use.
- Bile salts or water-miscible forms of fat-soluble vitamins may be needed.
- Medications often associated with AP include: acetaminophen, azathioprine, estrogens, furosemide, methyldopa, nitrofurantoin, steroids, thiazides, cimetidine, erythromycin, salicylates, sulfonamides, and tetracyclines.
- Octreotide may have a beneficial role in the management of AP.

Herbs, Botanicals and Supplements

- Herbs and botanical supplements should not be used without discussing with physician.

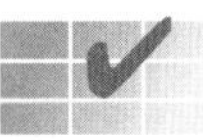

PATIENT EDUCATION

- ✔ Instruct patient to watch for signs and symptoms of diabetes, tetany, peritonitis, fat necrosis, acute respiratory distress syndrome, and pleural effusion.
- ✔ Discuss omission of alcohol from the typical diet.
- ✔ Discuss tips for handling nausea and vomiting (e.g., dry meals, taking liquids a few hours before or after meals, use of ice chips, sipping beverages, asking physician about available antiemetics, etc.).
- ✔ Coffee, tea, and gas-forming foods may need to be omitted.

For More Information

- American Gastroenterological Association
  http://www.gastro.org/public/pancreatitis.html

PANCREATITIS, CHRONIC

NUTRITIONAL ACUITY RANKING: LEVEL 3

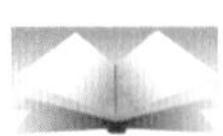

DEFINITIONS AND BACKGROUND

Pancreatitis involves inflammation with edema, fat necrosis, and cellular exudate. Chronic pancreatitis is a fibrotic, necrotic disease state with decreased enzymatic processes with abdominal pain, nausea, vomiting, and distention. Permanent damage to the pancreas occurs.

The most common cause is chronic alcohol abuse (60–70% of cases); other causes include nonalcoholic tropical chronic pancreatitis, pancreatic carcinoma, hypercalcemia, cystic fibrosis, pancreatic fistulae, trypsinogen-enterokinase deficiency, and enzyme deficiencies such as lipase deficiency.

Abdominal pain can be constant and disabling, causing some patients to become addicted to pain medications. Approximately 5% of persons with AP go on to have chronic pancreatitis. Supportive treatments, inhibition of gastric acid secretion, nerve blocks, reduction of oxidative stress, and endoscopic and surgical treatments are all possibilities for treating patients with chronic pancreatitis (American Gastroenterological Association, 1998). Distal pancreatectomy achieves pain relief and good quality of life in a large percentage (80%) of patients (Sakorafas et al., 2001).

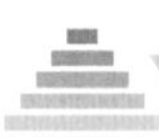

OBJECTIVES

- Provide optimal nutrition support.
- Decrease pain by minimizing stimulation of the exocrine pancreas. Because cholecystokinin (CCK) stimulates secretion from the exocrine pancreas, one approach is to decrease CCK levels through modulation of diet (Shea et al., 2000).
- Avoid pancreatic irritants, especially alcohol and caffeine.
- Correct fluid and electrolyte imbalances and malnutrition; avoid over-feeding. Acid-base imbalance is common with NG suctioning, fistula losses, renal failure, nausea, and vomiting.
- Alleviate steatorrhea and prevent or control secondary tetany, hyperglycemia, protein–calorie malnutrition (PCM), maldigestion, and diarrhea.
- Avoid or control complications (cardiovascular, pulmonary, hematological, renal, neurological, or metabolic); prevent multiple organ failure.
- If postprandial pain is a limiting factor, enteral therapies that minimally stimulate the pancreas may be beneficial (Shea et al., 2000). Aggressive support will minimize pain and decrease complications; TPN may be needed for resistant cases.
- If tube fed, monitor for needed increases of pancreatic enzymes, abdominal pain, or discomfort; hold TF if needed for resolution. Minimize pancreatic secretions.

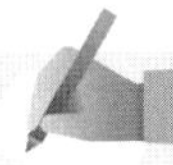

DIETARY AND NUTRITIONAL RECOMMENDATIONS

- Needle catheter jejunostomy may be useful. High calorie, peptide-based semi-elemental feeding is better than PN, although TPN may be needed in complicated cases.
- Use a diet with low-to-moderate fat, moderate protein (1 g for renal or liver failure, 2 g/kg for repletion), and high carbohydrates (no more than 5 mg/kg/minute of glucose); calculate accordingly.
- Diet should be low fiber with six small meals a day. The benefits are not yet known regarding the use of BCAAs and glutamine. If intravenous lipids are used, do not use more than 1.5 g/kg for adults.
- Alcoholic beverages are prohibited. In addition, caffeine or gastric stimulants should be prohibited.
- Adequate calcium and fat-soluble vitamin supplementation should be provided. Magnesium may be needed.
- Diet should include adequate amounts of vitamin C, B-complex, and folic acid for water-soluble vitamin needs, as well as zinc.
- For patients with severe steatorrhea, diet should include an increase of MCTs. Mild cases usually are not a problem.

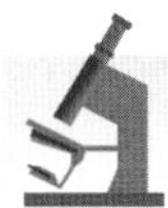

PROFILE

Clinical/History

Height
Weight
BMI
BEE
Left upper quadrant abdominal pain
Vomiting
Steatorrhea
Temperature
I & O
Chvostek's sign

Lab Work

K+ (decreased)
Na+ (decreased)
PT
Bilirubin
Ca++ (decreased)
Gluc (increased)
Lipase (increased)
Chol (LDL up, or total decreased)
Trig (increased)
Mg+ (decreased)
LDH (over 700)
AST (over 250)
WBC (over 200)
Amylase (over 200)
Alb, RBP
BUN
H&H
Serum folate
Alk phos (increased)
CT scan or ultrasound
Fecal fat study
pCO2 (increased)
pO2 (decreased)

Common Drugs Used and Potential Side Effects

- Pancreatic enzymes may be needed to reduce steatorrhea to less than 20 g/day. Enteric coating is necessary to prevent destruction by enzymes. Capsules or tablets should be swallowed whole. Take enteric-coated enzymes with cimetidine, food, or antacids.
- Antibiotics, antispasmodics, and anticholinergics may be used.
- Diuretics such as acetazolamide (Diamox) may be needed to control fluid retention. Nausea, vomiting, and diarrhea may result.
- Antacids may be helpful; beware of extended use. Side effects on various mineral or nutrient absorption are not always desirable.
- Steroids can cause sodium retention, potassium and calcium depletion, and negative nitrogen balance.
- Insulin may be necessary. Monitor for hypoglycemia during use.
- Bile salts or water-miscible forms of fat-soluble vitamins may be needed.
- Histamine and cimetidine may be given to decrease hydrochloric acid (HCl) output. Cimetidine may deplete vitamin B12, especially among the elderly. Histomine H2 receptor antagonists (cimetidine or ranitidine) or proton pump inhibitors can improve fat malabsorption and steatorrhea.

Herbs, Botanicals and Supplements

- Herbs and botanical supplements should not be used without discussing with physician.

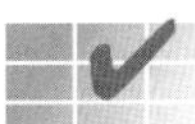

PATIENT EDUCATION

- ✓ Instruct patient to watch for signs and symptoms of diabetes, tetany, peritonitis, fat necrosis, acute respiratory distress syndrome, and pleural effusion.
- ✓ Discuss omission of alcohol from the typical diet.
- ✓ Discuss tips for handling nausea and vomiting (e.g., dry meals, taking liquids a few hours before or after meals, use of ice chips, sipping beverages, asking physician about available antiemetics, etc.).
- ✓ Coffee, tea, and gas-forming foods may need to be omitted.

PANCREATIC INSUFFICIENCY

NUTRITIONAL ACUITY RANKING: LEVEL 3

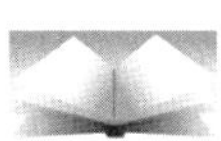

DEFINITIONS AND BACKGROUND

Pancreatic insufficiency is caused by decreased secretion of lipase, often from cystic fibrosis, PCM, congenital problems, pancreatic cancer, or pancreatitis. In cystic fibrosis, there may be recurrent problems with management of fatty acid abnormalities. Arachidonic acid is the pro-inflammatory culprit.

Lipase is the key enzyme for breaking down triglycerides. Patients often have mild-to-moderate fat malabsorption, as well as CHO malabsorption (Ladas et al., 1993).

OBJECTIVES

- Correct fatty acid abnormalities
- Correct states of maldigestion, diarrhea, and steatorrhea.
- Provide adequate caloric intake while lowering intake of fats.
- Provide missing fat-soluble vitamins, if needed, from malabsorption.
- Prevent iron overloading.

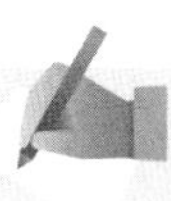

DIETARY AND NUTRITIONAL RECOMMENDATIONS

- Use a moderate-to-low fat diet. MCTs also may be tolerated, because they do not require lipase. They may be taken with simple sugars, jelly, and jams in mixed dishes.
- Use tender meats and low-fiber fruits and vegetables.
- Alcoholic beverages are prohibited.
- Zinc may be needed in supplemental form or from an elemental diet.
- Tube feed in severe cases.
- Correct the ratio of linoleic to arachidonic acid; increase use of omega-3 fatty acids from tuna, mackerel, and salmon.

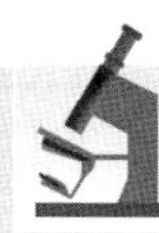

PROFILE

Clinical/History	Lab Work	
Height	K+	Alk phos
Weight	Ca++	Lipase
BMI	Trig	H&H
I & O	PT	Amylase (increased)
Stool weight	Bicarbonate	Serum carotene
Steatorrhea	Gluc	CT scan or ultrasound
	Na+	Fecal fat study
	Chol	

Common Drugs Used and Potential Side Effects

- Pancreatic enzymes (pancreatin or pancrelipase [Cotazym]) should be taken with food. Take enteric-coated tablets with cimetidine or antacids.
- Fat-soluble vitamins should be taken in water-miscible form.

Herbs, Botanicals and Supplements

- Herbs and botanical supplements should not be used without discussing with physician.

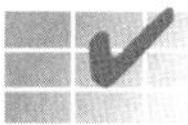

PATIENT EDUCATION

- ✔ Instruct patient in the role of the pancreas in digestion.
- ✔ Discuss appropriate measures for recovery and control.

PANCREATIC TRANSPLANTATION

NUTRITIONAL ACUITY RANKING: LEVEL 4

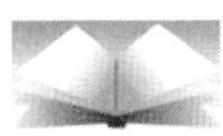

DEFINITIONS AND BACKGROUND

Pancreatic transplantation may be a viable option for type 1 diabetes mellitus. It helps to decrease nephropathy, early or mild retinopathy, and neuropathy; it does not improve gastroparesis. One of four types of surgeries may be completed: combined pancreas-kidney transplant; pancreas-after-kidney transplant; isolated pancreas transplant; islet or isolated beta cell transplant. Most common is anastomosis to the recipient's intestine.

OBJECTIVES

- Preoperatively: Meet nutritional needs; improve visceral protein stores; maintain lean tissue.
- Postoperatively: Support graft survival. Promote wound healing. Improve or maintain nutritional status.
- Long-term: Prevent weight gain. Prevent complications such as gastroparesis, hypertension, hyperlipidemia, hyperglycemia, and osteoporosis.

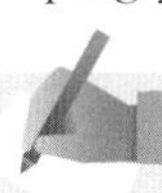

DIETARY AND NUTRITIONAL RECOMMENDATIONS

- Postoperatively, progress to clear liquids and then a high-protein diet to prevent side effects of antirejection medications. Tube feeding may be needed if oral intake is inadequate. Use 1.3–2.0 g protein/kg dry weight. Long-term, use 0.8–1.0 g protein/kg.
- If serum glucose levels are altered, offer an appropriate dietary regimen. If weight is a concern, use low-calorie snacks and meals. Keep CHO at 50% of kilocalories consumed.
- After 3–6 months, decrease saturated fatty acids and keep cholesterol at or below 300 mg/day.
- Increase calcium intake to 1,500 mg/day.
- Use ample fluids (30–40 mL/kg daily).
- Use extra magnesium, calcium, and phosphorus, if depleted. Restrict if levels are elevated.

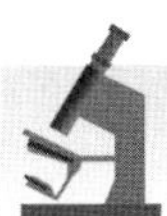

PROFILE

Clinical/History		
Height	BP	Serum amylase
Weight, dry	Temperature	Urinary amylase (only if bladder drained)
BMI	**Lab Work**	K+
Weight changes and goals	Gluc	Na+
I & O	BUN, Creat	Ca++, Mg++
	H&H, Serum Fe	

Common Drugs Used and Potential Side Effects

- Corticosteroids (such as Prednisone, Solu-Cortef) are used for immunosuppression. Side effects include increased catabolism of proteins, negative nitrogen balance, hyperphagia, GI ulcers, decreased glucose tolerance, sodium retention, fluid retention, and impaired calcium absorption and osteoporosis. Cushing's syndrome, obesity, muscle wasting, and increased gastric secretion may result. A higher protein intake and lower intake of simple CHOs may be needed.
- Cyclosporine does not retain sodium as much as corticosteroids do. Nausea, vomiting, and diarrhea are common side effects. Hyperlipidemia, HPN, gum hyperplasia, hypomagnesemia, and hyperkalemia also may occur; decrease sodium and potassium as necessary. Elevated glucose and lipids may occur. Do not use intravenously if possible. The drug is also nephrotoxic; a controlled renal diet may be beneficial if renal failure is imminent. Do not use grapefruit or grapefruit juice.
- The depletion paradigm enables drugs to bind to lymphocyte cell surface markers, creating cell lysis and/or inactivation; these include polyclonal ATG and Thymoglobulin, and monoclonal OKT3 antilymphocyte antibodies (Hong and Kahan, 2000). Immunosuppressants such as Muromonab, OKT3, and ATG are less nephrotoxic than cyclosporine but can cause nausea, anorexia, diarrhea, and vomiting. Monitor carefully. Fever and stomatitis also may occur; alter diet as needed. Do not use grapefruit or its juice.
- Azathioprine (Imuran) may cause leukopenia, thrombocytopenia, oral and esophageal sores, macrocytic anemia, pancreatitis, vomiting, diarrhea, and other complex side effects. Folate supplementation and other dietary modifications (liquid or soft diet, use of oral supplements) may be needed. The drug works by lowering the number of white blood cells; it is often prescribed along with prednisone for conventional immunosuppression.
- Tacrolimus (Prograf, FK506) suppresses T-cell immunity; it is 100 times more potent than cyclosporine, thus requiring smaller doses. Side effects include GI distress, nausea, vomiting, hyperkalemia, hypophosphatemia, hypomagnesemia, and hyperglycemia.
- Antibiotics may be used. Monitor for GI distress and other side effects.
- Pancreatic enzymes may be needed if pancreatitis occurs again after transplant.
- Other drugs such as CellCept and sirolimus may be used (Hong and Kahan, 2000; McAlister et al., 2001).

Herbs, Botanicals and Supplements

- Herbs and botanical supplements should not be used without discussing with physician.
- St. John's Wort interferes with the metabolism of cyclosporin-A and should not be used after transplantation (Karliova et al., 2000).

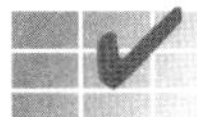

PATIENT EDUCATION

- ✓ Encourage activity to prevent excessive weight gain; 14–30 pounds may be a common gain.
- ✓ Discuss surgical stress. Encourage positive protein balance for short-term to promote anabolism and wound healing.
- ✓ Long-term, follow a low cholesterol and saturated fatty acid dietary plan.
- ✓ Sudden abdominal pain, fever, increased amylase, and glucose can occur and are signs of pancreatitis even after transplant. Report these warning signs immediately to the physician.

ZOLLINGER-ELLISON SYNDROME

NUTRITIONAL ACUITY RANKING: LEVEL 3

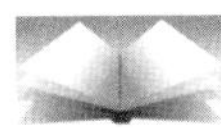

DEFINITIONS AND BACKGROUND

The Zollinger-Ellison syndrome is a severe form of peptic ulcer disease with ulceratogenic tumor (gastrinoma) of the delta cells of the pancreatic islets of Langerhans. It results in hypersecretion of gastric acid and fulminating ulceration of the esophagus, stomach, duodenum, and jejunum. D-cell adenoma may be malignant or benign. Widespread metastasis indicates a poor prognosis.

It frequently is accompanied by secretory diarrhea. Interestingly, insulin production is often increased in the beta cells. Of all cases, 60% occur in males; two-thirds are malignant.

OBJECTIVES

- Overcome malabsorption.
- Decrease steatorrhea with losses of nitrogen, fat, sodium, and potassium.
- Lessen diarrhea.
- Eliminate gastric acid secretion, usually with medications or, less often, surgery (gastrectomy).
- Where existing, lessen problems with dysphagia and reflux.

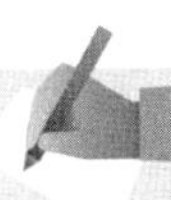

DIETARY AND NUTRITIONAL RECOMMENDATIONS

- Diet should provide low-to-moderate fat (50–70 g).
- According to the patient's stool losses, modify calories, fat, protein, and electrolytes as needed.
- Modify fiber, seasonings, and textures as necessary.
- Alter feeding modality to TF or TPN if needed.

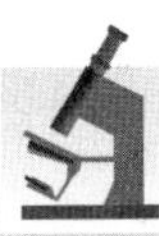

PROFILE

Clinical/History	Lab Work	
Height	N balance	Mg++
Weight	Na+	BUN
BMI	Ca++ (usually increased)	Serum insulin
Steatorrhea	Alb	Serum gastrin
Stool volume	H&H	Trig, Chol
BP	K+ (decreased)	Gluc
I & O		Gastrin radioimmunoassay
		CT scan

Common Drugs Used and Potential Side Effects

- Histamine H2 receptor antagonists (ranitidine or cimetidine) can reduce hypergastric acid secretion. Vitamin B12 may be depleted, especially in elderly persons.
- Omeprazole also can inhibit gastric acid secretion. Take before meals. Iron and vitamin B12 levels may become depleted.
- Pancreatic enzymes may be needed if steatorrhea is excessive.
- Zantac may be used to reduce acid production. Monitor for abdominal distress, nausea, and vomiting.

Herbs, Botanicals and Supplements

- Herbs and botanical supplements should not be used without discussing with physician.

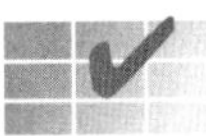

PATIENT EDUCATION

- ✓ Explain which modifications of fiber in the diet are appropriate.
- ✓ Explain how malabsorption compromises nutritional status.
- ✓ Discuss limiting fat intake, as appropriate for the patient.

GALLBLADDER DISEASE

NUTRITIONAL ACUITY RANKING: LEVEL 2

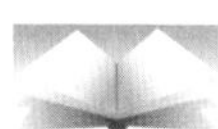

DEFINITIONS AND BACKGROUND

Cholelithiasis is defined as the presence of gallstones; 10% of the general population (especially women) over age 40, and 70% of Native American women over age 30 have gallstones. Incidence increases with aging, diabetes, obesity, pregnancy, and use of estrogens (see Table 8–8). Low intake of vitamin C in both animals and humans can also cause gallstones (Simon, 1993).

A low-energy diet with a relatively high fat content may maintain adequate gallbladder emptying and prevent gallstone formation during rapid weight loss (Festi et al., 1998). Other preventive measures include a controlled weight loss rate, reduction of the length of overnight fast, and maintenance of a small amount of fat in the diet (Erlinger, 2000).

Some gallbladders can concentrate bile normally but cannot acidify it. The result is that calcium may be less soluble in bile and precipitates out. Gallstones contain primarily cholesterol, bilirubin, and calcium salts. There are two forms of stones—cholesterol or pigment stones. Cholesterol precipitates as gallstones whenever cholesterol is greater than bile acids and phospholipids. Cholesterol is the primary component of stones in Western society; thickened mucoprotein with tiny entrapped cholesterol crystals (sludge) tends to precede stone development (Johnston and Kaplan, 1993). Caffeine may actually help prevent gallbladder disease (GBD) by helping to dissolve mineral deposits.

Cholecystitis is inflammation of the gallbladder. Gallstones are almost always the cause of the acute form. Symptoms and signs include abdominal pain (radiating to back), vomiting, nausea, and fever. Surgery is needed unless the condition subsides because of medical therapy. Extracorporeal lithotripsy breaks up gallstones with shock waves and is performed on an outpatient basis. Laparoscopic cholecystectomy reduces the length of hospital stay; lithotripsy is now less common (Festi, 1998).

Chronic GBD (chronic cholecystitis) involves prolonged presence of gallstones and low-grade inflammation. Scarring causes the gallbladder to become stiff and thick; nausea and abdominal discomfort are common. Gallbladder cancer is usually associated with gallstone disease, late diagnosis, unsatisfactory treatment, and poor prognosis.

TABLE 8–8 Hypotheses for Risk Factors in Gallbladder Disease

Risk factors
Advanced age
Sex (female)
Obesity, especially with the highest BMI (Erlinger, 2000)
Hormonal imbalance, use (estrogen, progestin, insulin)
Drugs (oral contraceptives [OCs], clofibrate, cholestyramine)
Enzyme defects
Diabetes
Low intake of vitamin C

OBJECTIVES

- Lose excess weight, if needed. Avoid rapid weight loss, which can lead to gallstone formation.
- Limit foods that cause pain or flatulence.
- For the patient with cholelithiasis, overcome fat malabsorption caused by obstruction and prevent stagnation in a sluggish gallbladder, which may be caused by decreased bile secretion, bile stasis, bacteria, hormones, or fungi. Bacterial overgrowth alters bile acids so that they can no longer emulsify fats.
- Prevent biliary obstruction, cancer, and pancreatitis.
- Provide fat-soluble vitamins, if needed.
- Vitamin C helps break down cholesterol into bile acids. Increase intake from fruits and vegetables; supplement if needed.

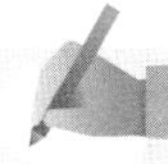

DIETARY AND NUTRITIONAL RECOMMENDATIONS

- Provide a calorie-controlled, balanced diet. Use NPO during an acute attack.
- For the patient with **acute cholecystitis,** use a low-fat diet. Progress to a diet with fewer condiments and gas-forming vegetables, which cause distention, increased peristalsis, and irritation.
- For the patient with **chronic cholecystitis,** use a fat/calorie-controlled diet to promote drainage of the gallbladder without excessive pain. Patient should consume adequate amounts of CHO, especially fiber (such as pectin, which binds excess bile acids).
- For the patient with **cholelithiasis,** encourage a diet that is high in fiber and, when needed, low in calories.
- Fat-soluble vitamins may need to be replaced in water-miscible forms.
- Increase intake of sources of vitamin C such as citrus fruits and juices.

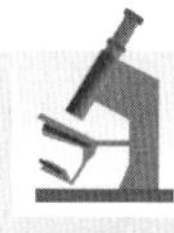

PROFILE

Clinical/History	Lab Work	
Height	Alb, prealbumin	Lipase (often increased)
Weight	Bilirubin (increased)	Amylase
BMI	Trig	Ca++
WBC	AST	Alk phos
Jaundice	PT	GGT (increased)
Nausea	H&H	CT scan or ultrasound
I & O	Chol	Cholecystoscintigraphy
Temperature	LDH	Cholecystography
	K+	
	Na+	

Common Drugs Used and Potential Side Effects

- Ursodeoxycholic acid decreases cholesterol saturation of bile and gallstone incidence during weight loss (Erlinger, 2000). Chenodeoxycholic acid and lithium may be used to dissolve small stones and prevent new formation, if consumed daily for at least 6 months. Chenodiol (Chenix) may cause nausea, vomiting, or diarrhea; take with food or milk.
- Actigall (ursodiol) may dissolve certain small, high-cholesterol gallstones. Metallic taste, abdominal pain, and vomiting may occur.
- Bile salts (Festal) are used to facilitate fat metabolism. They contain protease, lipase, hemicellulose, amylase, and bile constituents.
- Antibiotics may be used to counteract any infection. Evaluate the need to take with food or milk or with other specific liquids.
- OCs and estrogens may increase the risk of GBD, especially after years of use.
- Analgesics (Demerol, meperidine) may be used to relieve pain. Nausea, vomiting, constipation, and GI distress can occur.
- Risk of formation of gallstones during weight loss may actually be lowered with orlistat (Trouillot et al., 2001).

Herbs, Botanicals and Supplements

- Herbs and botanical supplements should not be used without discussing with physician.
- Turmeric, celandine, peppermint, couch grass, and goldenrod have been recommended for this condition but without clinical trials to prove efficacy.

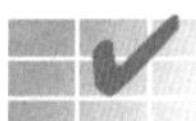

PATIENT EDUCATION

- ✓ After a cholecystectomy, fat intake should be limited for several months to allow the liver to compensate for the gallbladder's absence. Fats should be introduced gradually; excessive amounts of fat or bulky foods at one meal should be avoided.
- ✓ Recommend weight control because stone formation can occur even after cholecystectomy.
- ✓ Avoid fasting and rapid weight loss schemes.
- ✓ People who have had their gallbladders removed should have their cholesterol levels checked periodically, as should every adult.

For More Information

- ✦ Gallbladder Disease Information
  http://www.nlm.nih.gov/medlineplus/gallbladderandbileductdiseases.html

BILIARY CIRRHOSIS

NUTRITIONAL ACUITY RANKING: LEVEL 3

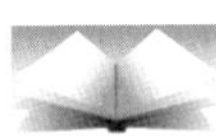

DEFINITIONS AND BACKGROUND

Primary biliary cirrhosis (PBC) is a chronic cholestatic liver disease that predominantly affects middle-aged women. Biliary cirrhosis, also called cholangiolitic hepatitis (obstructive jaundice), causes progressive, segmental necrosis, and destruction of intrahepatic bile ducts. Symptoms include pruritus, jaundice, fatigue, and portal hypertension.

Etiology of PBC remains unknown. Environmental or autoimmune factors may act to trigger the disease in genetically susceptible hosts. Sjögren's syndrome, Raynaud's syndrome, a high rate of urinary tract infection (UTI), and a history of smoking have been reported in cases of PBC (Parikh-Patel et al., 2001).

PBC slowly progresses and may lead to liver failure. In symptomatic patients, advanced age, elevated serum bilirubin levels, decreased serum albumin levels, and cirrhosis each correlate with shortened survival (Nishio et al., 2001). Transplantation is the only effective therapy in the end-stage of the disease.

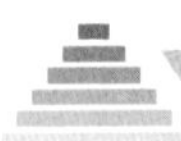

OBJECTIVES

- Correct diarrhea, steatorrhea, malnutrition, and osteomalacia.
- Limit or control symptoms.
- Correct a zinc deficiency if present.

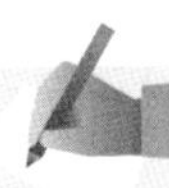

DIETARY AND NUTRITIONAL RECOMMENDATIONS

- Increase vitamin D and calcium intake if osteopenia occurs.
- Increase water-miscible sources of vitamins A, D, E, and K in steatorrhea.
- Reduce cholesterol and saturated fats in hypercholesterolemia.
- Ensure adequate intake of zinc from diet.

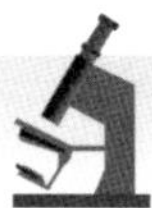

PROFILE

Clinical/History

Height
Weight
BMI
Jaundice
Xanthomas

Lab Work

Alb, prealbumin
Mitochondrial antibodies
PT (decreased)
Transferrin
Globulin
Bilirubin (increased)
Gluc
Alk phos (increased)
Ca++
Chol (increased)
Ceruloplasmin
ALT/AST
GGT

Common Drugs Used and Potential Side Effects

- Prolonged administration of ursodeoxycholic acid (UDCA) in patients with PBC is associated with survival benefit and a delaying of liver transplantation; it might even prevent progression of the histologic stage of PBC (Kumar and Tandon, 2001). Studies with UDCA and immunosuppressants such as prednisone, budesonide, and azathioprine have shown that in selected patients combination therapy may be superior to UDCA monotherapy (Holtmeier and Leuschner, 2001).
- Cholestyramine may be used to decrease bile acids. Belching or constipation may occur.
- Colchicine may cause diarrhea, nausea, vomiting, and stomach pain.

Herbs, Botanicals and Supplements

- Herbs and botanical supplements should not be used without discussing with physician.

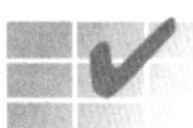

PATIENT EDUCATION

✓ Discuss the role of bile salts in fat and fat-soluble vitamin absorption.

CHOLESTATIC LIVER DISEASE (CHOLESTASIS)

NUTRITIONAL ACUITY RANKING: LEVEL 3

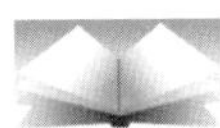

DEFINITIONS AND BACKGROUND

Disturbance of the flow of bile leads to intracellular retention of biliary constituents. In the sequence of events that leads to liver injury, the cytotoxic action of bile salts is pivotal to all forms of cholestasis (Kullak-Ublick and Meier, 2000). Cholestatic liver disease involves any liver disease with bilirubin over 2.0 mg/dL.

Common hepatic causes are viral hepatitis, alcoholic liver disease, hemochromatosis, and autoimmune hepatitis. Biliary causes include primary sclerosing cholangitis (in which the intra and/or extrahepatic bile ducts undergo inflammation and fibrosis), choledocholithiasis, primary biliary cirrhosis, and biliary atresia. Cholestasis and jaundice can occur after hematopoietic cell transplantation and may have multiple causes, including sepsis, hemolysis, cyclosporine administration, drug toxicity, parenteral nutrition, graft-versus-host disease, viral infection, and extrahepatic obstruction (Strasser et al., 1999).

Cholestasis interferes with excretion of the bile salts required for emulsification and absorption of dietary fat. Vitamin and mineral deficiencies and alterations are common, especially with significant cholestasis. Zinc, magnesium, and calcium may be deficient, because they are albumin-bound, and the liver is not working properly. Deficiency of fat-soluble vitamins A, D, E, and K may occur. Of particular concern is vitamin E, which tends to be low in this condition; vitamin E circulates in the blood almost exclusively attached to the lipoprotein fractions. Vitamin E deficiency may cause neurologic degeneration, often leading to wheelchair dependency in this condition, if untreated (Sokol et al., 1993). In chronic cholestasis with biliary obstruction, hyperlipidemia and accumulation of copper result, and manganese can accumulate in the brain; avoid over-feeding with copper or manganese.

Chronic total parenteral nutrition may induce fatty liver and inflammation, especially in patients with short-bowel syndrome. Deficiency of choline in parenteral solutions has been proposed as the mechanism for liver disease. With TPN, cholestatic jaundice may occur from a lack of enteral nutrition and failure of biliary stimulation. In patients receiving home PN, prevalence of liver disease increases with duration of HPN. PN intake of lipid emulsion rich in omega-6 fatty acids should be under 1 g/kg BW (Cavicchi et al., 2000).

Signs and symptoms of cholestasis can include glossitis from B-complex deficiency, protein and iron deficiency, hemorrhagic tendencies due to vitamins C or K inadequacy, and flatulence. Patients with steatorrhea may benefit from a low-fat diet or from use of MCTs. Intrahepatic cholestatic syndromes cause a decrease in bile flow with no overt bile duct obstruction; bile constituents accumulate in the liver and blood. Treatment of extrahepatic manifestations of cholestatic liver disease such as pruritus, fatigue, osteoporosis, and steatorrhea can be problematic and time consuming (Holtmeier and Leuschner, 2001).

The central role of bile salts in the pathogenesis of cholestasis has become evident from the improvement of many cholestatic syndromes with oral bile salt therapy (Kullak-Ublick and Meier, 2000). Ursodeoxycholic acid and adequate nutritional support are the usual treatments (Qureshi, 1999).

OBJECTIVES

- Promote return of normal liver function and bile flow.
- Treat fat malabsorption and deficiency of any nutrients.
- Correct steatorrhea, GI bleeding, and copper overloading where present.
- Prevent or correct for liver failure, osteomalacia, or osteoporosis.
- Correct nutrient excesses, e.g., copper and manganese.
- Prepare for liver transplantation, where selected.

DIETARY AND NUTRITIONAL RECOMMENDATIONS

- In chronic cases, 10–20% added kilocalories may be needed. Infants need more kilocalories, and adults tend to use CHO poorly. In acute stages, use IV glucose to prevent hypoglycemia and protein catabolism.
- In acute stages, infants will need 1.0–1.5 g/kg protein. Children, teens, and adults need 0.5–1.2 g protein/kg; highlight branched chain amino acid sources. In chronic cases, use 3 g protein/day for infants and 1–1.5 g protein/kg in adults.
- Some research suggests the need for adequate taurine in infants, especially if tube fed.
- Supplement with vitamins and minerals, especially fat-soluble vitamins. Vitamin D and calcium will be needed if osteoporosis or osteomalacia is present.
- Small, frequent feedings and snacks may be better tolerated than large meals.
- Use enteral nutrition (where possible), if TPN has caused cholestasis. If TPN is required, early use of cyclic TPN may be useful (Hwang et al., 2000). Avoid excesses of copper and manganese in the solutions.
- Zinc and selenium may be needed.

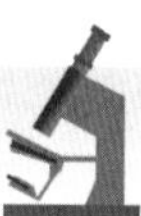

PROFILE

Clinical/History		
Height	PT (prolonged)	Alb, prealbumin
Weight	AST, ALT (increased)	Serum carotene (increased or decreased)
BMI	Bilirubin (increased, more than 2 mg/dL)	Transferrin
Ascites	Somatomedin C	Globulin
Edema	Alk phos (increased)	GGT
I & O	RBP	Amylase, lipase
Nausea	Bun, Creat	Serum manganese
Lab Work	H&H, Serum Fe	Serum zinc
Chol, Trig (increased)		

Common Drugs Used and Potential Side Effects

- Bile salts may be needed with extensive malabsorption. Ursodeoxycholic acid is currently the only established drug for treatment of chronic cholestatic liver diseases. It has cytoprotective, antiapoptotic, membrane-stabilizing, and antioxidative and immunomodulatory effects (Kumar and Tandon, 2001).
- Water-miscible forms of fat-soluble vitamins A, D, E, and K may be needed. Vitamin E may be given intramuscularly if malabsorption is severe. Otherwise, a daily dose of 20–25 IU of *d*-α-tocopherol is useful for most children (Sokol et al., 1993).

Herbs, Botanicals and Supplements

- Herbs and botanical supplements should not be used without discussing with physician.

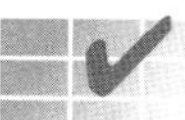

PATIENT EDUCATION

- ✔ Discuss the role of fat in normal metabolic processes; simplify explanation in correlation to absorption of fat-soluble vitamins and other nutrients affected by the liver.
- ✔ Discuss ways to increase satiety from the diet with appetizing recipes.
- ✔ Discuss use of over-the-counter (OTC) vitamin and mineral supplements, especially regarding copper and manganese for possible toxic levels.
- ✔ Liver transplantation works best in a well-nourished patient. Promote good tolerance and intake.

REFERENCES

Cited References

Abou-Assi S, Vlahcevic Z. Hepatic encephalopathy. Metabolic consequence of cirrhosis often is reversible. *Postgrad Med.* 2001;109: 52.

American Gastroenterological Association Medical Position Statement: Treatment of pain in chronic pancreatitis. *Gastroenterology.* 1998;115:763.

Bass N. Is there any use for nontraditional or alternative therapies in patients with chronic liver disease? *Cur Gastroenterol Rep.* 1999;1:50.

Blei A, Cordoba J, et al. Hepatic encephalopathy. *Am J Gastroenterol.* 2001;96:1968.

Blue L, et al. Effect of obesity on clinical outcomes in liver transplantation. *J Am Diet Assoc.* 1993;93S:49A.

Borum M, et al. The effect of nutritional supplementation on survival in seriously ill hospitalized adults: an evaluation of the SUPPORT data. Study to Understand Prognoses and Preferences for Outcomes and Risks of Treatments. *J Am Geriatr Soc.* 2000;48: 33S.

Cardillo K. Nutrition interventions for chylous effusions. *Support Line.* 2001;23:18.

Cavicchi M, et al. Prevalence of liver disease and contributing factors in patients receiving home parenteral nutrition for permanent intestinal failure. *Ann Int Med.* 2000;132:525.

Crippin, J. Medical management of end-stage liver disease: a bridge to transplantation. *Support Line.* 1997;XIX:3.

Davidson H, et al. Macronutrient preference, dietary intake, and substrate oxidation among stable cirrhotic patients. *Hepatology.* 1999;29:1380.

Erlinger S. Gallstones in obesity and weight loss. *Eur J Gastroenterol Hepatol.* 2000;12:1347.

Falck-Ytter Y, McCullough A. Nutritional effects of alcoholism. *Gastroenterology.* 2000;2:331.

Festi D, et al. Gallbladder motility and gallstone formation in obese patients following very low calorie diets. Use it (fat) or lose it (well). *Int J Obesity and Related Metabolic Disorders.* 1998;22: 592.

Fuchs C, et al. Alcohol consumption and mortality among women. *N Engl J Med.* 1995;332:1245.

Gartner L, Herschel M. Jaundice and breastfeeding. *Pediatr Clin North Am.* 2001;48:389.

Geevarghese S, et al. The effect of nutritional and hormonal supplementation on protein synthesis immediately after liver transplantation. *J Surg Res.* 1999;81:196.

Gerber T, Schomerus H. Hepatic encephalopathy in liver cirrhosis: pathogenesis, diagnosis and management. *Drugs.* 2000;60:1353.

Gordon D, et al. Chaparral ingestion: the broadening spectrum of liver injury caused by herbal medications. *JAMA.* 1995;273:489.

Grodstein F, et al. Infertility in women and moderate alcohol use. *Am J Public Health.* 1994;84:1429.

Gurk-Turner C. Management of the metabolic complications of liver disease: an overview of commonly used pharmacologic agents. *Support Line.* 1997;XIX:17.

Hasse J, et al. Early enteral nutrition support in patients undergoing liver transplantation. *J Parenter Enteral Nutri.* 1995;19:437.

Hasse J, et al. Nutrition therapy for end-stage liver disease: a practical approach. *Support Line.* 1997;XIX:8.

Hasse J, Matarese L. Medical nutrition therapy for liver, biliary system and exocrine pancreas disorders. In: Mahan L, Escott-Stump S. *Krause's food nutrition and diet therapy.* 10th edition. Philadelphia: WB Saunders Co., 2000.

Hathcock J, et al. Evaluation of vitamin A toxicity. *Am J Clin Nutri.* 1990;52:183.

Hirsch S, et al. Nutritional support in alcoholic cirrhosis patients improves host defenses. *J Am Col Nutri.* 1999;18:434.

Hirschmann J, Raugi G. Adult scurvy. *J Am Acad Dermatol.* 1999;41: 895.

Holtmeier J, Leuschner U. Medical treatment of primary biliary cirrhosis and primary sclerosing cholangitis. *Digestion.* 2001;64:137.

Hong J, Kahan B. Immunosuppressive agents in organ transplantation: past, present, and future. *Semin Nephrol.* 2000;20:108.

Hwang T, et al. Early use of cyclic TPN prevents further deterioration of liver functions for the TPN patients with impaired liver function. *Hepatogastroenterology.* 2000;47:1347.

Johnston D, Kaplan M. Pathogenesis and treatment of gallstones. *N Engl J Med.* 1993;328:412.

Karliova M, et al. Interaction of Hypericum perforatum (St John's wort) with cyclosporin A metabolism in a patient after liver transplantation. *J Hepatol.* 2000;33:853.

Klatsky A, et al. Alcohol and mortality. *Ann Intern Med.* 1992;117: 646.

Knip M, et al. Ethanol induces a paradoxical simultaneous increase in circulating concentrations of insulin-like growth factor binding protein-1 and insulin. *Metab Clin Exp.* 1995;44:1356.

Krieger D, et al. Manganese and chronic hepatic encephalopathy. *Lancet.* 1995;346:270.

Kullak-Ublick G, Meier P. Mechanisms of cholestasis. *Clin Liver Dis.* 2000;4:357.

Kwo P, et al. Gender differences in alcohol metabolism: relationship to liver volume and effect of adjusting for body mass. *Gastroenterology.* 1998;115:1552.

Kumar D, Tandon R. Use of ursodeoxycholic acid in liver diseases. *J Gastroenterol Hepatol.* 2001;16:3.

Labbe R, Veldee M. Optimizing laboratory services. In: *Report of the 14th Ross Roundtable on Medical Issues: laboratory utilization for nutrition support: current practice, requirements, expectations.* Columbus, OH: Ross Laboratories, 1994:2.

Laterre P, et al. Chylous ascites: diagnosis, causes, and treatment. *Acta Gastroenterol Belg.* 2000;63:260.

Lee S, et al. Biliary sludge as a cause of acute pancreatitis. *N Engl J Med.* 1992;326:589.

Liao Y, et al. Alcohol intake and mortality: findings from the National Health Interview Surveys (1988 and 1990). *Am J Epid.* 2000;151:651.

Lieber C. Alcohol: its metabolism and interaction with nutrients. *Annu Rev Nutri.* 2000;20:395.

Lieber C. Herman Award lecture, 1993: a personal perspective on alcohol, nutrition, and the liver. *Am J Clin Nutri.* 1993;58:430.

Lieber C. *Medical and nutritional complications of alcoholism: mechanism and management.* New York: Plenum Medical Book Co., 1992.

Liu S, et al. Reliability of alcohol intake as recalled from 10 years in the past. *Am J Epid.* 1996;143:177.

Luper S. A review of plants used in the treatment of liver disease: part two. *Altern Med Rev.* 1999;4:178.

Luper S. A review of plants used in the treatment of liver disease: part 1. *Altern Med Rev.* 1998;3:410.

McAlister V, et al. Orthotopic liver transplantation using low-dose tacrolimus and sirolimus. *Liver Transpl.* 2001;7:701.

Neuschwander-Tetri B. Fatty liver and nonalcoholic steatohepatitis. *Clin Cornerstone.* 2001;3:47.

Nishio A, et al. Primary biliary cirrhosis: from induction to destruction. *Semin Gastrointest Dis.* 2001;12:89.

Oeffinger K. Scurvy: more than historical relevance. *Am Fam Physician.* 1993;48:609.

Padillo F, et al. Anorexia and the effect of internal biliary drainage on food intake in patients with obstructive jaundice. *J Am Col Surg.* 2001;192:584.

Parikh-Patel A, et al. Risk factors for primary biliary cirrhosis in a cohort of patients from the United States. *Hepatology.* 2001;33:16.

Pisters P, Ranson J. Nutritional support for acute pancreatitis. *Surg Gynecol Obstet.* 1992;175:275.

Preedy V, et al. Alcoholic skeletal muscle myopathy: definitions, features, contribution of neuropathy, impact, and diagnosis. *Eur J Neurol.* 2001;8:677.

Qureshi W. Intrahepatic cholestatic syndromes: pathogenesis, clinical features, and management. *Dig Dis.* 1999;17:49.

Reimund E, Ramos A. Niacin-induced hepatitis and thrombocytopenia after ten years of niacin use. *J Clin Gastroenterol.* 1994;18:270.

Richardson R, et al. Influence of the metabolic sequelae of liver cirrhosis on nutritional intake. *Am J Clin Nutri.* 1999;69:331.

Sakorafas G, et al. Postobstructive chronic pancreatitis: results with distal resection. *Arch Surg.* 2001;136:643.

Scolapio J, et al. Substrate oxidation in patients with cirrhosis: comparison with other nutritional markers. *J Parenter Enteral Nutri.* 2000;24:150.

Shea J, et al. Advances in nutritional management of chronic pancreatitis. *Cur Gastroenterol Rep.* 2000;2:323.

Simon J. Ascorbic acid and cholesterol gallstones. *Med Hypotheses.* 1993;40:81.

Sokol R, et al. Multicenter trial of d-a-tocopherol polyethylene glycol 1,000 succinate for treatment of vitamin E deficiency in children with chronic cholestasis. *Gastroenterology.* 1993;104:1727.

Strasser S, et al. Cholestasis after hematopoietic cell transplantation. *Clin Liver Dis.* 1999;3:651.

Teran J. Nutrition and liver diseases. *Cur Gastroenterol Rep.* 1999;1:335.

Testa G, et al. Liver transplantation for hepatitis C: recurrence and disease progression in 300 patients. *Liver Transpl.* 2000;6:553.

Trouillot T, et al. Orlistat maintains biliary lipid composition and hepatobiliary function in obese subjects undergoing moderate weight loss. *Am J Gastroenterol.* 2001;96:1888.

Volpi E, et al. Nicotinamide counteracts alcohol-induced impairment of hepatic protein metabolism in humans. *J Nutri.* 1997;127:2199.

Walsh K, Alexander G. Alcoholic liver disease. *Postgrad Med.* 2000;J76:280.

Wicks C, et al. Comparison of enteral feeding and total parenteral nutrition after liver transplantation. *Lancet.* 1994;344:837.

Xiol X, Guardiola J. Hepatic hydrothorax. *Cur Opin Pulm Med.* 1998;4:239.

Suggested Readings

Alexander G, Walsh K. Chronic viral hepatitis. *Int J Clin Pract.* 2000;54:450.

Bulger E, Helton W. Nutrient antioxidants in gastrointestinal diseases. *Gastroenterol Clin North Am.* 1998;27:403.

Cardillo K. Nutrition interventions for chylous effusions. *Support Line.* 2001;23:6.

Curtis A, et al. Alcohol consumption and changes in blood pressure among African Americans: The Pitt County Study. *Am J Epid.* 1997;146:727.

Dufouil C, et al. Sex differences in the association between alcohol consumption and cognitive performance. *Am J Epid.* 1997;146:405.

Habib A, et al. Long-term management of cirrhosis. Appropriate supportive care is both critical and difficult. *Postgrad Med.* 2001;109:101.

Halonen K, et al. Severe acute pancreatitis: prognostic factors in 270 consecutive patients. *Pancreas.* 2000;21:266.

Kaufman S, et al. Indications for pediatric intestinal transplantation: a position paper of the American Society of Transplantation. *Pediatr Transplant.* 2001;5:80.

Kelly D. Liver complications of pediatric parenteral nutrition—epidemiology. *Nutrition.* 1998;14:153.

Loguercio C, et al. Can dietary intake influence plasma levels of amino acids in liver cirrhosis? *Dig Liver Dis.* 2000;32:611.

Richardson R, et al. Influence of the metabolic sequelae of liver cirrhosis on nutritional intake. *Am J Clin Nutri.* 1999;69:331.

Santolaria F, et al. Osteopenia assessed by body composition analysis is related to malnutrition in alcoholic patients. *Alcohol.* 2000;22:147.

Scolapio J, et al. Substrate oxidation in patients with cirrhosis: comparison with other nutritional markers. *J Parenter Enteral Nutri.* 2000;24:150.

Westerterp-Plantenga M, Verwergen C. The appetizing effect of an aperitif in overweight and normal-weight humans. *Am J Clin Nutri.* 1999;69:205.

SECTION 9

Endocrine Disorders

CHIEF ASSESSMENT FACTORS

Diabetes:

- FREQUENT URINATION
- EXCESSIVE THIRST
- UNEXPLAINED WEIGHT LOSS
- EXTREME HUNGER
- SUDDEN VISION CHANGES
- TINGLING OR NUMBNESS IN HANDS OR FEET
- FEELING TIRED MUCH OF THE TIME
- DRY SKIN
- SORES THAT ARE SLOW TO HEAL
- MORE INFECTIONS THAN USUAL

Other Endocrine Conditions:

- NUMBNESS, TINGLING, PARESTHESIA
- BONE PAIN
- HEADACHE, SEIZURES, SYNCOPE
- ANOREXIA, NAUSEA, ABDOMINAL PAIN, MALABSORPTION, GASTROPARESIS
- HYPERGLYCEMIA, HYPOGLYCEMIA
- WEIGHT CHANGES
- SHORTNESS OF BREATH, HOARSENESS
- DECREASED LIBIDO, ERECTILE DYSFUNCTION
- DYSURIA
- PRURITUS, DRYNESS OF SKIN OR HAIR
- ALTERED CONSCIOUSNESS
- HORMONE THERAPY: ANABOLIC HORMONES—GROWTH HORMONES, ANDROGENS, SEX HORMONES; CATABOLIC HORMONES—STRESS HORMONES (CAUSING GLUCONEOGENESIS FROM PROTEIN) SUCH AS CATECHOLAMINES (EPINEPHRINE, NOREPINEPHRINE), GLUCOCORTICOIDS (CORTISONE, CORTISOL), AND GLUCAGON
- GOITER; EXOPHTHALMUS; INTOLERANCE TO HEAT, COLD
- ADULT CHANGES IN SIZE OF HEAD, HANDS, FEET
- POSTURAL HYPOTENSION, WEAKNESS
- DIAGNOSIS OF THYROID DISEASE, ETC.
- HORMONE IMBALANCES (see Table 9–1)

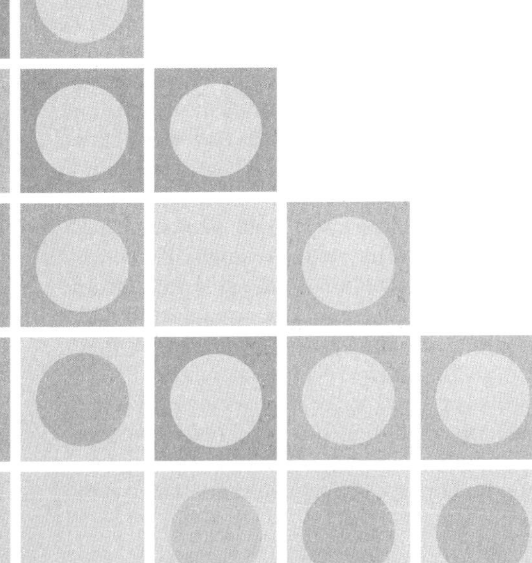

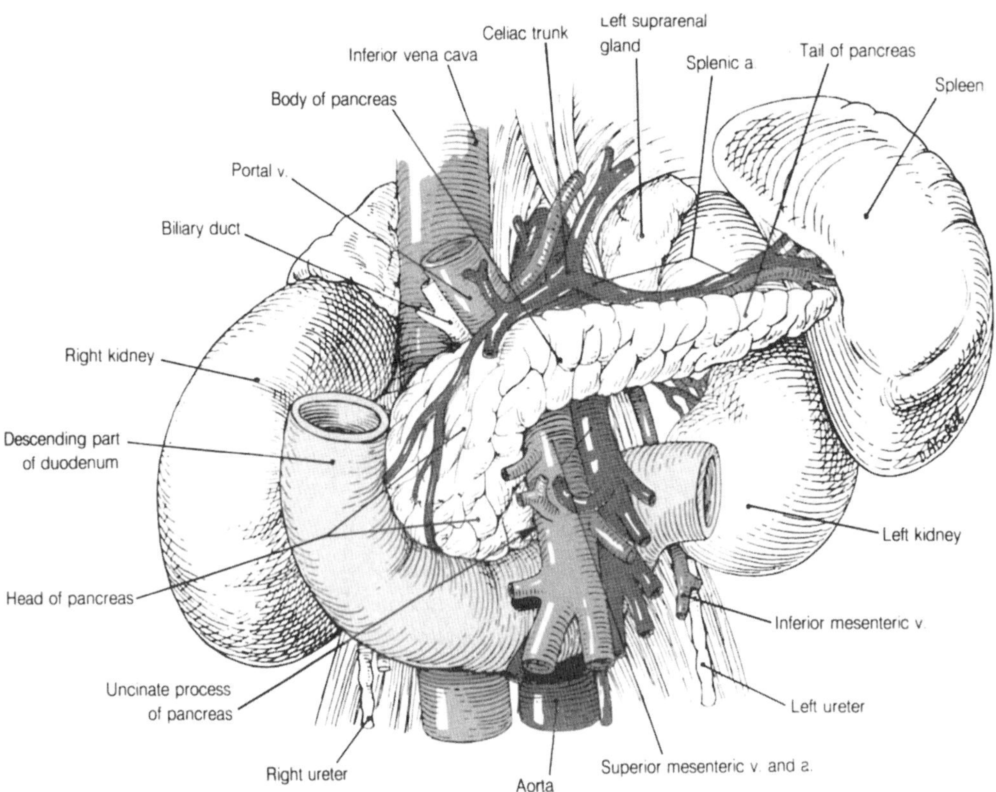

The pancreas and its nearby relationships. (Reprinted with permission from Hall-Craggs, ECB. *Anatomy as a Basis for Clinical Medicine.* 2nd Ed. Baltimore: Urban & Schwartzenberg, 1990.)

OVERVIEW OF DIABETES MELLITUS

Diabetes mellitus is a group of metabolic diseases characterized by hyperglycemia resulting from defects in insulin secretion, insulin action, or both. It affects over 16 million Americans. Hyperglycemia of diabetes is associated with long-term damage, dysfunction, and failure of various organs, especially the eyes, kidneys, nerves, heart, and blood vessels. Diabetes mellitus is divided into distinct types—type 1, type 2, gestational diabetes mellitus (GDM), and other types; see Tables 9–1 and 9–2 Type 2 diabetes, with 90% of cases of the disease, is especially affected by both genetic and environmental factors (Busch and Hegele, 2001).

MEDICAL NUTRITION THERAPY (MNT) replaced "diet therapy," and self-management training replaced "patient education" in diabetes management. Today, there is no one "diabetic" or "ADA" diet. The recommended diet is a nutrition prescription based on assessment and treatment goals and outcomes. MNT for people with diabetes should be individualized, with consideration given to usual eating habits and other lifestyle factors. Large population study findings support the hypothesis that the vast majority of cases of type 2 diabetes could be prevented by the adoption of a healthier lifestyle (Hu et al., 2001).

According to the American Diabetes Association Clinical Practice Guidelines 2001: "Patients beginning treatment with MNT or oral glucose-lowering agents may need to be contacted as often as weekly until reasonable glucose control is achieved and they are competent to conduct the treatment program. Regular visits should be scheduled for all patients with diabetes. Patients should generally be seen at least quarterly until achievement of treatment goals. Thereafter, the frequency of visits may be decreased as long as patients continue to achieve all treatment goals. More frequent contact may also be required if patients are undergoing intensive insulin therapy, not meeting glycemic or blood pressure goals, or have evidence of progression in microvascular or macrovascular complications. Patients must be taught to recognize problems with their glucose control as indicated by their self-monitoring blood glucose (SMBG) records and to promptly report concerns to the health care team to clarify and strengthen their self-management skills. Patients also should be taught to recognize early signs and symptoms of acute and chronic complications and to report these immediately. Severe hypoglycemic reactions requiring the assistance of another person must be reported as soon as possible." (http://www.diabetes.org/clinicalrecommendations/Supplement101/S33.htm)

Goals should be negotiated to be responsive to patient needs (Holler and Pastors, 1997). While the initial sessions will require that the nutrition counselor take a leading role, eventually the patient should set new goals and design new

TABLE 9–1 Etiologic Classification of Diabetes Mellitus

I. Type 1 diabetes* (beta-cell destruction, usually leading to absolute insulin deficiency)
   A. Immune mediated
   B. Idiopathic
II. Type 2 diabetes (may range from predominantly insulin resistance with relative insulin deficiency to a predominantly secretory defect with insulin resistance)
III. Other specific types
   A. Genetic defects of beta-cell function
      1. Chromosome 12, HNF-1alpha (MODY3)
      2. Chromosome 7, glucokinase (MODY2)
      3. Chromosome 20, HNF-4alpha (MODY1)
      4. Mitochondrial DNA
   B. Genetic defects in insulin action
      1. Type A insulin resistance
      2. Leprechaunism
      3. Rabson-Mendenhall syndrome
      4. Lipoatrophic diabetes
   C. Diseases of the exocrine pancreas
      1. Pancreatitis
      2. Trauma/pancreatectomy
      3. Neoplasia
      4. Cystic fibrosis
      5. Hemochromatosis
      6. Fibrocalculous pancreatopathy
   D. Endocrinopathies
      1. Acromegaly
      2. Cushing's syndrome
      3. Glucagonoma
      4. Pheochromocytoma
      5. Hyperthyroidism
      6. Somatostatinoma
      7. Aldosteronoma
   E. Drug- or chemical-induced
      1. Vacor
      2. Pentamidine
      3. Nicotinic acid
      4. Glucocorticoids
      5. Thyroid hormone
      6. Diazoxide
      7. Beta-adrenergic agonists
      8. Thiazides
      9. Dilantin
      10. Alpha-interferon
   F. Infections
      1. Congenital rubella
      2. Cytomegalovirus
   G. Uncommon forms of immune-mediated diabetes
      1. "Stiff-man" syndrome
      2. Anti-insulin receptor antibodies
   H. Other genetic syndromes sometimes associated with diabetes
      1. Down's syndrome
      2. Klinefelter's syndrome
      3. Turner's syndrome
      4. Wolfram's syndrome
      5. Friedreich's ataxia
      6. Huntington's chorea
      7. Laurence-Moon-Biedl syndrome
      8. Myotonic dystrophy
      9. Porphyria
      10. Prader-Willi syndrome
IV. Gestational diabetes mellitus (GDM)

*Patients with any form of diabetes may require insulin treatment at some stage of their disease.
American Diabetes Association Clinical Practice Guidelines 2001. (Copyright © 2001 American Diabetes Association. From Diabetes Care, Vol. 24, Supplement 1, 2001; S5–S20. Reprinted with permission from *The American Diabetes Association*.)

meal plans according to lifestyle changes. Sample questions that can be asked to solicit information about the patient's goals may include (Holler and Pastors, 1997):

"What goals are most likely to help you develop a healthier lifestyle?"

"What behavior would you like to change?"

"What changes can you make in your current lifestyle?

"What obstacles do you see to making these changes?"

"What benefits do you see as a result of these changes?"

"What are you willing to do right now?"

Holler and Pastors (1997) also suggest that medical nutrition therapy be offered in three steps: 1) Basic Nutrition Guidelines (basic principles of nutrition and guidance for selecting a healthy diet—such as using Dietary Guidelines for Americans, Guide to Good Eating; Food Guide Pyramid); 2) Diabetes Nutrition Guidelines (Diabetes Meal Planning and other single topic tools from The American Diabetes Association and The American Dietetic Association); and 3) In-Depth Nutrition Intervention (menu approaches, exchange lists for meal planning, carbohydrate counting, or calorie and fat counting). The timing of introducing each new step will depend on the patient's comprehension and readiness to learn. Many tools are available, and it is not acceptable to simplify medical nutrition therapy into a diet order for "no concentrated sweets." An individual approach is best.

The American Dietetic Association recommends 3–4 MNT visits over the first 3 months of treatment for Type 1 diabetes, then 1–2 annually; for Type 2 diabetes, 4 MNT visits are recommended initially, then 1 every 6–12 months (http://www.knowledgelinc.com/ada/mntguides/). Steps include assessment, goal setting, intervention, and evaluation/problem solving. Nutrition management; evaluation of renal status; monitoring of blood glucose, medications, physical activity, and behavior modification. A new credential has been developed for registered dietitians (RDs), nurses, and pharmacists who have advanced degrees and meet experiential requirements; this credential is cited as BC-ADM (Daly et al., 2001).

TABLE 9–2 Potential Complications of Diabetes

ACUTE:

Signs and Symptoms of Hyperglycemia: Polyphagia, polydipsia, polyuria, dehydration, weight loss, weakness, muscle wasting, recurrent or persistent infections, hypovolemia, ketonuria, glycosuria, blurred or changed vision, fatigue, muscle cramps, and dry mouth. Blood glucose greater than 250 mg/dL should be evaluated; monitor urine ketones to check for diabetic ketoacidosis (DKA). In children, DKA and Nonketotic hyperosmolar syndrome (NKHS) crisis are associated with high morbidity and mortality, and cerebral edema can occur in either circumstance. Early consultation and referral to a diabetologist or endocrinologist should be considered.

Signs and Symptoms of Hypoglycemia: Shakiness, confusion, diplopia, irritability, hunger, weakness, headache, rapid and shallow breathing, numbness of mouth/lips/tongue, pulse normal or abnormal, convulsions, lack of coordination, dizziness, staggering gait, pallor, slurred speech, tingling, diaphoresis, and nausea. Hypoglycemia can cause sweating, tremors, hunger, and nightmares (Boyle et al., 1995). Treat when blood glucose level is below 70 mg/dL with 15 g of pure glucose or other simple carbohydrates (CHO); wait 15 minutes and retest, then treat with another 15 g of CHO if still below 70 mg/dL. Feed a small snack, if mealtime is still several hours away. Continue to monitor until next meal.

The **Somogyi effect** is defined as hormonal rebounding effects of insulin/blood sugar levels. Hypoglycemia or fasting hyperglycemia occurs, with potentially dangerous results. Check blood glucose 4 hours after bedtime.

Acute Illness: The risk for diabetic ketoacidosis is higher during this time; test blood glucose, drink adequate amounts of fluid, ingest CHO if levels are low, and adjust medications to keep glucose in desired range and to prevent starvation ketosis (Franz et al., 2002).

INTERMEDIATE:

For Children with type 1 diabetes: Children's growth and development may be impaired; adequate protein and energy for growth must be provided.

For Children with type 2 diabetes: They are usually overweight or obese and present with glycosuria without ketonuria, absent or mild polyuria and polydipsia, and little or no weight loss. Up to 33% have ketonuria at diagnosis, and some may have ketoacidosis without any associated stress, other illness, or infection. Because DKA and NKHS crisis are associated with high morbidity and mortality in children and cerebral edema can occur in either circumstance, early consultation and referral to pediatric and adolescent diabetologists/endocrinologists should be considered.

For Pregnancy: Infant mortality rates are approximately twice as high for babies born to women with uncontrolled diabetes compared with babies born to women without diabetes. To reduce the risk of fetal malformations and maternal or fetal complications, pregnant women and women planning to become pregnant require excellent blood glucose control. These women need to be seen frequently by a multidisciplinary team. Specialized laboratory and diagnostic tests may be needed; these women must be trained in SMBG. The American Diabetes Association suggests that nutrition recommendations for women with preexisting diabetes be based on a thorough assessment. Monitoring blood glucose levels, urine ketones, appetite, and weight gain is needed to develop an individualized nutrition prescription and to make adjustments to the meal plan. In one study, a higher fiber intake was associated with lower daily insulin requirements during pregnancy (Kalkwarf et al., 2001). For more details, review the specific guidelines available from The American Diabetes Association: Use an extra 300 kcals daily during the second and third trimester; protein calculated as 0.75 g/Kg daily plus an additional 10 g; 400 mcg folic acid (Franz et al., 2002). Added iron and calcium may also be required, depending on the usual and current dietary intake patterns.

For Gestational Diabetes: See appropriate entry.

For Lactation: Extra kilocalories, protein, calcium, and folic acid will be needed. Close monitoring of blood glucose is recommended, but episodes of hypoglycemia should be avoided. Breastfeeding lowers blood glucose and may require women to eat a CHO-containing snack either before or during breastfeeding; overall, an extra 200 kcals or average plan for 1,800 kcals meets the needs of most lactating mothers (Franz et al., 2002).

For Older Adults: There is little research on the aging individual who has diabetes, and therefore typical signs such as unexplained weight loss should be viewed as a symptom of a problem (Franz et al., 2002). A multivitamin–mineral supplement may be beneficial for this population. Strict diets in long-term care are not warranted and may lead to dehydration and malnutrition; specialized diabetic diets are not required, and a balanced diet with consistent timing of CHO is to be recommended (Franz et al., 2002). Modify medications, rather than diet, as needed.

(continued)

TABLE 9–2 Potential Complications of Diabetes (*Continued*)

CHRONIC: Achieve and maintain normal blood glucose and lipids. Intensive therapy (IT) helps reduce onset or progression of vascular problems.
Microvascular: Diabetic retinopathy and ocular abnormalities, nephropathy, neuropathy (sensory or motor conditions, which may lead to ulceration or even limb amputation, orthostatic hypotension, intractable nausea and vomiting, diabetic gastroenteropathy), diabetic cystopathy, and diabetic diarrhea.

Retinopathy accounts for 12,000–24,000 cases of blindness each year.

Nephropathy is preceded by microalbuminemia over 300 mg albumin/day for several years. For diabetic nephropathy, liberalize CHO intake and control insulin levels accordingly. Prevent loss of lean body mass to slow the progression of end-stage renal disease (ESRD). There is some evidence that controlled protein intake will slow down progression of nephropathy. Adults need 0.8–1 g protein/kg daily. Protein restriction before evidence of nephropathy is not currently recommended. Inclusion of plant protein may be suggested, but there is no clear evidence yet about the importance of this change (Franz et al., 2002). Phosphorus should be controlled at 8–12 mg/kg per day; some people may need phosphate binders and calcium supplements. Control of blood pressure (below 125/75) and blood glucose levels is extremely important. In addition, smoking cessation and control of hyperlipidemia are useful for decreasing progression of renal disease. Diabetes is now the leading cause of ESRD, especially among blacks, Mexican Americans, and American Indians. Early signs of nephropathy include hyperfiltration, renal hypertrophy, and microalbuminemia (loss of 30–300 ug/mg creatinine in the urine); protein losses at a rate of over 300 ug/mg creatinine may indicate advancement toward ESRD. The onset of ESRD is 5.7 years after noted renal damage. Diagnosis involves persistently positive urinary albumin over 0.3 g/dL in the absence of other renal diseases.

Neuropathy may be delayed with careful blood glucose management. Lower extremity amputations are painful and disabling; prevention is desirable in all cases. Neuropathy is more common in obese patients; weight loss may be beneficial. About 70% of persons who have diabetes have some degree of neuropathy, including impaired sensation in the hands and feet, slowed digestion, or carpal tunnel syndrome.

Diabetic gastroparesis is a consequence of neuropathy, and is more common in type 2 diabetes.

Macrovascular: Coronary artery disease, stroke, and peripheral vascular disease. Risk factors include insulin resistance, hyperglycemia, hypertension, hyperlipidemia, and smoking.

Hyperlipidemia and coronary heart disease should be addressed. The new National Cholesterol Education Program (NCEP) guidelines promote low density lipoprotein-C (LDL-C) levels of less than 100 mg/dL as optimal for all patients, and increase attention on high triglyceride levels (above 200 mg/dL). Lowering saturated fat intake, monitoring of homocysteine levels, and related actions should be taken. Adequate insulin therapy often returns lipids to normal in type 1 diabetes (Franz et al., 2002). Elevated levels in type 2 DM require use of rigorous management guidelines; limit saturated fat to 7–10% of total kilocalories. See entries for coronary heart disease. The rate of heart disease is about 2–4 times higher in adults who have diabetes; it is the leading cause of diabetes-related deaths.

Hypertension is common (2.5 million people have both hypertension and diabetes). Maintain desirable body mass index (BMI); prevent hypokalemia, which can blunt insulin release; control glucose; omit alcohol and smoking; add exercise. Control of hypertension in diabetes has been linked to reduction in the progression of nephropathy. Use of the DASH diet is very effective because it increases intake of calcium, magnesium, and potassium while lowering alcohol and excess weight (Franz et al., 2002). Stroke risk is 2–4 times higher among persons with diabetes.

Other Complications:

Catabolic Illness changes body compartments, with increased extracellular fluid and shrinkage of body fat and body cell mass (Franz et al., 2002). Monitor unexplained weight losses carefully, especially 10% or more of usual weight. Standard tube feedings are usually well tolerated in persons with diabetes (50% CHO or lower); monitor fluid status, weight, plasma glucose and electrolytes, and acid-base balance (Franz et al., 2002). Overfeeding is to be avoided; start with 25–35 kcals/kg of body weight. Protein needs may be 1 g/kg up to 1.5 g/kg in stressed individuals.

OTHER ENDOCRINE CONDITIONS

There are many other disorders of endocrine function that require some level of nutritional intervention. Listed below are some of the essential functions of the endocrine glands.

Gland	*Hormones*	*Functions*
Pituitary (anterior)	Adrenocorticotropic hormone (ACTH), growth hormone (corticotropin), gonadotropins (FSH, LH)	Growth, lactation, control of other endocrine glands
Pituitary (posterior)–Hypothalamus	Oxytocin, pitocin, vasopressin, corticotropin-releasing factor	Body temperature regulation, sleep, behavior, appetite, emotional response
Thyroid	Thyroxine Triiodothyronine	Growth and development, metabolism
Pancreas	Glucagon (A cells) Insulin (B cells) Gastrin (D cells)	Control of many metabolic functions, blood glucose control
Pineal gland	Melatonin	Skin blanching
Thymus	Thymosin	Immunity/T cells/lymphocytes
Gonads	Estrogen, progesterone, androgens	Reproduction
Adrenal glands	Mineralocorticoids, glucocorticoids, androgens (adrenal cortex) Epinephrine and norepinephrine (adrenal medulla)	Control of many hormones (28)
Parathyroids	Parathormone, calcitonin	Regulation of calcium and phosphorus

For More Information About Diabetes Mellitus

- American Association of Diabetes Educators
  http://www.aadenet.org/
- American Diabetes Association
  1701 North Beauregard Street
  Alexandria, VA 22311
  1-800-232-3472
  http://www.diabetes.org/
- American Dietetic Association
  Type 1 Diabetes protocols (initial, continuing, intensive)
  www.eatright.org
- Canadian Diabetes Association
  http://www.diabetes.ca/
- Canadian guidelines for diabetes management
  http://www.diabetes.ca/prof/nutritional_guide_eng.pdf
- CDC Division of Diabetes
  http://www.cdc.gov/diabetes
- Children with Diabetes
  http://www.childrenwithdiabetes.com/index_cwd.htm
- Diabetic Gourmet Magazine
  http://diabeticgourmet.com/dgarchiv2.shtml
- Diabetic Recipes (Berkley)
  http://soar.berkeley.edu/recipes/diabetic/
- Diabetes Research Institute Foundation
  http://www.drinet.org/
- Joslin Diabetes Center
  One Joslin Place
  Boston, MA 02215
  http://www.joslin.org/
- National Institutes of Diabetes and Digestive and Kidney Diseases (NIDDK)
  Office of Communications and Public Liaison
  NIDDK, NIH, 31 Center Dr., MSC 2560
  Bethesda, MD 20892-2560
  http://www.niddk.nih.gov/
  http://www.niddk.nih.gov/health/diabetes/pubs/nutritn/index.htm
- National Diabetes Information Clearinghouse
  http://www.niddk.nih.gov/health/diabetes/ndic.htm
- National Diabetes Education Program
  http://ndep.nih.gov/
- Practice Guidelines
  http://www.diabetes.org/clinicalrecommendations/Care-Sup1Jan01.htm

For More Information on Other Endocrine Conditions

- American Association of Clinical Endocrinologists
  http://www.aace.com/
- Endocrine Society
  http://www.aace.com/
- The Hormone Foundation
  http://www.hormone.org/

TYPE 1 DIABETES MELLITUS

NUTRITIONAL ACUITY RANKING: LEVEL 3

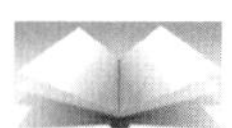

DEFINITIONS AND BACKGROUND

Type 1 diabetes mellitus (DM) is absolute insulin deficiency with total failure to produce it. Resulting from a defect in the pancreatic beta cells (the islets of Langerhans), type 1 may be related to the adrenal cortex, thyroid, anterior pituitary gland, or other organs. The immune-mediated form usually starts in children or young adults but can arise at any age. Idiopathic type 1 is a rare form with no known cause. The extent of beta-cell damage differs between patients diagnosed with type 1 diabetes before and after puberty. The process is more damaging in children less than 7 years of age because residual beta-cell function is not affected by the presence or absence of islet cell-related antibodies (Pozzili et al., 1998). Type 1 accounts for 10% of all cases of DM.

Previously used terms include "type I," "insulin-dependent diabetes mellitus or IDDM," "juvenile," "brittle," or "ketosis-prone" diabetes. Onset often follows viral infection such as mumps. Studies have implicated exposure to bovine serum albumin as related to type 1 DM, but this has not been further documented. In an ethnically homogeneous population at high risk for type 1 diabetes, early exposure to cow's milk and dairy products did not increase the risk for developing it (Meloni et al., 1997).

Diagnosis finds greater than 126 mg/dl glucose on fasting, repeated on a different day. Casual plasma glucose taken any time of day with results over 200 mg/dl with increased urination, increased thirst, and unexplained weight loss can be another diagnostic test. Another test is the oral glucose tolerance test (OGTT) over 200 mg/dL in a 2-hour sample—this is least effective and more costly. Hemoglobin A1c test (HbA1c) is NOT recommended for diagnosis; finger-prick tests are also not valid. The upper limit of normal blood glucose is 110 mg/dl.

DM is the number 4 killer in the United States, usually related to coronary heart disease (CHD) or stroke. Increased postprandial levels of potentially atherogenic oxidized lipids may contribute to the accelerated atherosclerotic heart disease (ASHD) associated with diabetes (Staprans et al., 1999). Diabetes is the chief cause of blindness, renal failure, and amputations and is a leading cause of birth defects. Serious complications begin earlier than thought previously. Glucose control really matters, as proven by the results of the Diabetes Control and Complications Trial (DCCT).

Intensive therapy to achieve near normal glucose levels gives lower onset and progression of complications. Caution is needed to prevent hypoglycemia, especially in the very young, elderly, persons with ESRD, and those with vision loss. An electroencephalogram (EEG) performed shortly after diagnosis of type 1 may be helpful in identifying those at risk for symptoms of severe hypoglycemia (Rajantie et al., 1998).

Signs and symptoms of diabetes include polyuria (frequent urination, including frequent bedwetting in otherwise trained children), polydipsia (excessive thirst), polyphagia (extreme hunger), weakness, fatigue, irritability, and sudden weight loss. The prevalence of overweight is lower in type 1 diabetes than in the general population (Williams et al., 1999).

Protein and nutrient metabolism are affected by insulin availability. The long-term effects of diets high in protein and low in CHO are unknown at this time (Franz et al., 2002). Studies have evaluated use of daily vitamin E (100 IU) and vitamin C (200–600 mg) supplementation to improve glycemic control by enhancing insulin action (Cunningham, 1998). Studies have also suggested that vitamin D supplementation may reduce the risk of type 1 diabetes (Hypponen et al., 2001), but further studies are needed regarding specific amino acids and nutrient supplementation.

The pancreatic b-cell hormone amylin is secreted with insulin after a meal and appears to suppress secretion of glucagon (which reduces hepatic glucose production) and to slow gastric emptying (which slows absorption of ingested glucose). In diabetes, deficient secretion of amylin parallels deficient secretion of insulin, contributing to elevated blood glucose levels after meals (Kruger et al., 1999).

Over a lifetime, intensive diabetes therapy can be expected to increase length of life and to improve quality of life by having less renal disease and fewer complications (DCCT Research Group, 1996). Clearly cost-saving interventions included nephropathy prevention in type 1 DM and improved glycemic control (Klonoff and Schwartz, 2000). Possible cost-effective interventions include self-management training. MEDEM is a mnemonic to support the importance of Monitoring, Education, Diet, Exercise, and Medication as steps of diabetes management (Department of Medicine, 2001).

Medical costs for patients with diabetes accounts for a significant percentage of all health care costs. MNT implemented according to the field-tested nutrition practice guidelines results in significantly greater reductions in HbA1c at 3 months than usual care; dietitians who use practice guidelines pay closer attention to the control goals on the first visit and spend more time with the patient (Delahanty, 1998). According to a study of 55 midwestern community health centers, the charts of 2,865 diabetic adults were evaluated for American Diabetes Association measures of quality; practice guidelines were independently associated with higher quality of care (Chin et al., 2000).

National Standards for Diabetes Self-Management (American Diabetes Association, 2001) have been written to support a team approach to patient care; they include the RD as an essential team member. Ongoing nutrition self-management education includes assessment, care plans, treatment goals, desired outcomes, and monitoring metabolic parameters such as blood glucose, lipids, HbA1c, etc. Multidisciplinary team interventions reveal improved HbA1c levels, fewer diabetes complications, fewer hospital readmissions, shorter hospital stays, improved quality of life, improved coping skills, and more frequent blood glucose monitoring (American Diabetes Association, 2001). The American Dietetic Association recommends 3–4 MNT visits over the first 3 months of treatment for Type 1 diabetes, then a minimum of 1–2 annually (http://www.knowledgelinc.com/ada/mntguides/).

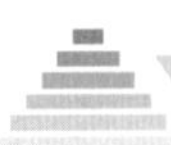

OBJECTIVES

(Derived from American Diabetes Association, 2001; Franz et al., 2002)

Goal-directed therapy with the patient's goals having greater importance than benchmark clinical goals is the most important objective!

- Attain and maintain optimal metabolic outcomes, including near-normal blood glucose levels as possible by balancing food intake with insulin (either endogenous or exogenous) or oral glucose-lowering medications and activity levels. Maintain HbA1c levels less than 7% and fasting blood sugar (FBS) levels between 80–120 mg/dL fasting and between 100–140 mg/dL at bedtime. A normal range for the patient may vary by age and by underlying disorders. Use of the HbA1c test is convenient.
- Achieve optimal serum lipid levels to reduce the risk for macrovascular disease; maintain blood pressure levels that reduce the risk for vascular disease.
- Provide adequate calories for maintaining or attaining reasonable weights for adults, normal growth and development rates in children and adolescents, increased metabolic needs during pregnancy and lactation, or recovery from catabolic illnesses. Reasonable weight is defined as the weight an individual and health care provider acknowledge as achievable and maintainable, both short- and long-term. This may not be the same as the traditionally defined desirable or ideal body weight.
- Prevent and treat acute complications in insulin-treated diabetes such as hypoglycemia, short-term illnesses, and exercise-related problems and the long-term complications of diabetes such as renal disease, autonomic neuropathy, hypertension, and cardiovascular disease (see Table 9–2).
- Improve overall health through optimal nutrition and physical activity. Dietary Guidelines for Americans and the Food Guide Pyramid summarize and illustrate nutritional guidelines and nutrient needs for all healthy Americans and can be used by people with diabetes and their family members. Encourage regular mealtimes. If necessary, make two plans—one for weekdays and one for weekends. A specific diabetes pyramid is available at http://www.diabetes.org/nutrition/article031799.asp.
- Address individual needs according to culture, ethnicity, and lifestyle, while respecting willingness to change. For older adults, provide for nutritional and psychosocial needs. For youth, provide adequate energy for growth and development and integrate insulin regimen according to meal pattern and lifestyle. For pregnant or lactating women, provide adequate energy and nutrients for optimal outcomes.

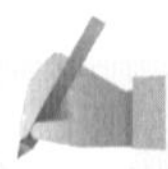

DIETARY AND NUTRITIONAL RECOMMENDATIONS

- A meal plan based on the individual's usual food intake should be used as the basis for integrating insulin therapy into the usual eating and exercise patterns (American Diabetes Association, 2001). Individuals using insulin therapy should eat at consistent times synchronized with the time-action of the insulin preparation used, monitor their blood glucose levels, and adjust their insulin doses for the amount of food usually eaten. Premeal insulin doses should be adjusted for the CHO content of the meal. Meal skipping should be discouraged.
- Intensified therapy, including multiple daily injections, continuous subcutaneous insulin infusion (CSII) using an insulin pump, and rapid-acting insulin, allows for more flexibility in the timing of meals and snacks, as well as in the amount of food eaten. Individuals on intensified insulin regimens can make adjustments in rapid- or short-acting insulin to cover the CHO content of their meals and, possibly, snacks and for deviations from usual eating and exercise habits (American Diabetes Association, 2001).
- Plan meals and snacks according to patient's preferences. Overall intake should be 10–20% protein, 60–70% monounsaturated fatty acids (MUFA) + CHO (Franz et al., 2002). Maintain kilocalories at 10% saturated fats; include omega-3 fatty acids regularly. Consensus about protein currently suggests maintaining recommended dietary allowance (RDA) levels (0.8 g–1g/kg in adults) and lowering to 0.6 g/kg with early signs of nephropathy. The dietitian should determine fat and CHO levels according to patient history (i.e., obesity, FBS levels, elevated lipid levels, etc.).
- Determine appropriate calorie level for age, with conditions of pregnancy or growth receiving more. Sedentary = 25 kcal/kg; normal = 30 kcal/kg; undernourished or active = 45–50 kcal/kg. Reassess as activity changes. Prevent ketosis by including at least 40–45% kilocalories as CHO daily. It is acceptable to use artificial sweeteners to enhance flavors. The Food and Drug Administration (FDA) has approved use of saccharin, aspartame, acesulfame potassium, and sucralose; see Table 9–3.
- Teach the food pyramid principles, use of exchanges (only if needed), and/or carbohydrate counting (see Table 9–4).
- Assess dietary history, physical exercise, and activity patterns.
- Discuss use of alcohol. To avoid hypoglycemia, alcohol should be consumed with food and limited to one drink daily for women and two for men (Franz et al., 2002). Alcohol calories = 0.8 3 proof 3 number of ounces. Abstention from alcohol is recommended for pregnant women, and for those persons who have pancreatitis, advanced neuropathy, elevated triglycerides, or a history of alcohol abuse (Franz et al., 2002).
- Use of a sports drink before and during exercise may be beneficial to prevent hypoglycemia for up to 1 hour after exercise; it does not seem to cause hyperglycemia (Tamis-Jortberg et al., 1996). Late-onset postexercise hypoglycemia can be avoided by consuming whole milk or sports drinks during exercise (Hernandez et al., 2000).
- Increase intake of fiber from rice, beans, vegetables, barley, oat bran, fruits, and vegetables. Whole grains are good sources of vitamin E, fiber, and magnesium—all of which affect insulin metabolism.
- Encourage control or reduction in total sodium, cholesterol, and saturated fat intake. Cut down or eliminate fried or creamed foods. Inclusion of omega-3 fatty acids (as from salmon, mackerel, tuna), garlic, and amylose are sug-

TABLE 9–3 Sugar and Sweeteners: Some Facts (used with permission American Diabetes Association, 2001)

The percent of calories from carbohydrate in the diet for diabetes will vary; it is individualized based on eating habits and glucose and lipid goals. For most of the 20th century, the most widely held belief about the nutritional treatment of diabetes had been that simple sugars should be avoided and replaced with starches. This belief was based on the assumption that sugars are more rapidly digested and absorbed than are starches and thereby aggravate hyperglycemia to a greater degree; there is little scientific evidence that supports this assumption. Fruits and milk have been shown to have a lower glycemic response than most starches, and sucrose produces a glycemic response similar to that of bread, rice, and potatoes. Although various starches do have different glycemic responses, from a clinical perspective, first priority should be given to the total amount of CHO consumed rather than the source of the carbohydrate.

Sucrose: Scientific evidence has shown that the use of sucrose as part of total CHO of the diet does not impair blood glucose control in individuals with type 1 or type 2 diabetes. Sucrose and sucrose-containing foods must be substituted for other carbohydrates gram for gram and not simply added to the meal plan. The nutrient content of concentrated sweets and sucrose-containing foods, as well as the presence of other nutrients such as fat, must be considered.

Fructose: Dietary fructose produces a smaller rise in plasma glucose than isocaloric amounts of sucrose and most starches. In that regard, fructose may offer an advantage as a sweetening agent in the diabetic diet. However, because of the potential adverse effects of large amounts of fructose (i.e., double the usual intake [20% of calories]) on serum cholesterol and LDL cholesterol, fructose may have no overall advantage as a sweetening agent in the diabetic diet. Although people with dyslipidemia should avoid consuming large amounts of fructose, there is no reason to recommend that people with diabetes avoid consumption of fruits and vegetables, in which fructose occurs naturally, or moderate consumption of fructose-sweetened foods.

Other nutritive sweeteners: This group includes corn sweeteners such as corn syrup, fruit juice or fruit juice concentrate, honey, molasses, dextrose, and maltose. There is no evidence that foods sweetened with these sweeteners have any significant advantage or disadvantage over foods sweetened with sucrose in decreasing total calories or CHO content of the diet or in improving overall diabetes control. Sorbitol, mannitol, and xylitol are common sugar alcohols (polyols) that produce a lower glycemic response than sucrose and other carbohydrates. Starch hydrolysates are formed by the partial hydrolysis and hydrogenation of edible starches, thus becoming polyols. Although the exact caloric value of sugar alcohols varies, they average ~2 kcal/g compared with the 4 kcal/g from other carbohydrates. Evidence is limited to suggest that this can be expected to contribute to a major reduction in total calories or in the total CHO content of the daily diet. Furthermore, excessive amounts of polyols may have a laxative effect. The calories and CHO content from all nutritive sweeteners must be accounted for in the meal plan and have the potential to affect blood glucose levels.

Nonnutritive sweeteners: the FDA approves saccharin, aspartame, acesulfame K, and sucralose for use in the U.S. For all food additives, including nonnutritive sweeteners, the FDA determines an acceptable daily intake (ADI), which is defined as the amount of a food additive that can be safely consumed on a daily basis over a person's lifetime without any adverse effects and includes a 100-fold safety factor. Actual intake by individuals with diabetes for all nonnutritive sweeteners is well below the ADI.

Sugar (sucrose)	16 kcal/t (4 g CHO)
Saccharin	300–400 × sweeter than sugar
Cyclamate	30 times sweeter than sugar; banned in 1970; revisited
Acesulfame-K (Sunette)	200 times sweeter than sugar and suited for baking
Fructose	11 kcal/t (3 g CHO)
Sorbitol	50% as sweet as sucrose; a sugar alcohol
Xylitol	16 kcal/t (4 g CHO)
Aspartame	180 times sweeter than sugar; 4 kcal/t
Stieva (an herb; not FDA approved)	300 times sweeter than sugar
Trehalose (naturally occurring sugar; reviewed for "Generally Recognized As Safe" List [GRAS])	45% as sweet as sugar
Alitame	2,000 times sweeter than sugar
Tagatose (noncaloric, D-sugar); testing for GRAS	Taste, bulk, and browning ability of sugar
Neotame (developed by Nutra Sweet; FDA pending)	6,000 times sweeter than sugar

gested for control of blood lipids and glucose. Consumption of fat-modified foods by individuals with DM may help decrease intake of fat, cholesterol, and saturated fatty acid (SFA) (Rodriguez and Castelanos, 2000).

- For minerals: assess for adequacy of intake. Routine supplementation is not advised at this time (Franz et al., 2002). Studies are investigating use of chromium supplements, which may prove useful in improving glucose tolerance (Anderson, 2000). Replenish potassium and magnesium, if needed. Adequate calcium is needed, especially in older persons; 1,000–1,500 mg should be attained daily (Franz et al., 2002).
- For vitamins: Assess for adequate intake. Glucose and vitamin C compete for uptake; plasma vitamin C may be inversely associated with glycated hemoglobin levels (Sargeant et al., 2000). Routine supplementation of antioxidants is not advised at this time (Franz et al., 2002).
- With tube feeding, consider products with increased fiber. There are several formulas on the market that are low in CHO and higher than usual in MUFA that are useful for

TABLE 9–4 Carbohydrate Counting

1. Focus on CHOs more than total kilocalories
2. Provide consistent CHOs at each meal and snack
3. Determine CHO/insulin ratio for patient (e.g., use .5–1 unit insulin for 10–15 g CHO)
4. One CHO exchange = 12–15 g of CHO. Starch (15 g); fruit (15 g); milk group (12 g)

some patients whose blood glucose levels are difficult to maintain within desired limits.

- In total parenteral nutrition (TPN), it may be useful to plan 30% kilocalories as fat, 50% CHO, and 20% protein unless additional disease states indicate otherwise.

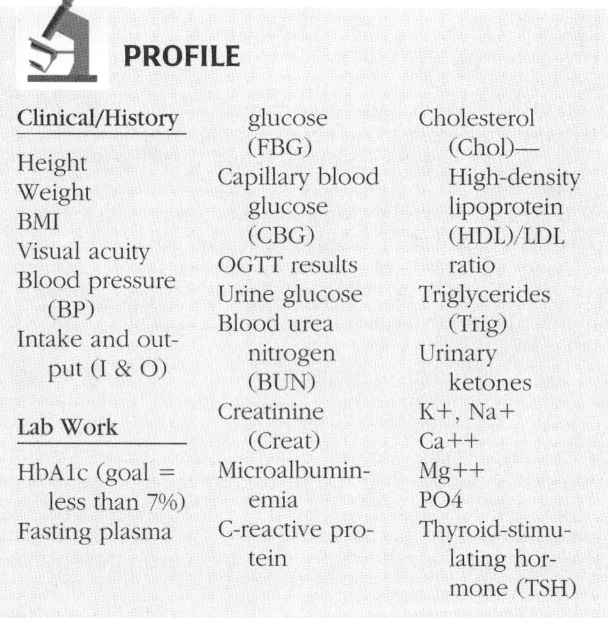

PROFILE

Clinical/History

Height
Weight
BMI
Visual acuity
Blood pressure (BP)
Intake and output (I & O)

Lab Work

HbA1c (goal = less than 7%)
Fasting plasma glucose (FBG)
Capillary blood glucose (CBG)
OGTT results
Urine glucose
Blood urea nitrogen (BUN)
Creatinine (Creat)
Microalbuminemia
C-reactive protein
Cholesterol (Chol)—High-density lipoprotein (HDL)/LDL ratio
Triglycerides (Trig)
Urinary ketones
K+, Na+
Ca++
Mg++
PO4
Thyroid-stimulating hormone (TSH)

Common Drugs Used and Potential Side Effects

- Insulin/diet correlation is essential. Persons with type 1 diabetes are dependent on insulin for life. The primary potential effect is hypoglycemia. Sources of insulin must be noted because they affect the speed of absorption, peak times of effect, and duration of effect (Table 9–5). Human insulin is produced synthetically and tends to produce fewer antibodies than that from animals.
- CSII may be good to maintain glucose levels. A pump is used; meal schedules are not as strict but should not be abused. With multiple daily insulin injections (MDII), test FBS 30 minutes before injections. There are now insulin pens available that are convenient.
- Vitamin C in high doses can give false-positive urinary glucose results; check use of supplements (Branch 1999).
- Check drugs for content of sugars and alcohol.
- In people with mild-to-moderate peripheral neuropathy, pharmacologic doses of vitamin E may improve defective nerve conduction (Tutuncu et al., 1998). This is not currently common practice.
- Low-dose aspirin is sometimes recommended to protect against cardiovascular events in persons with diabetes who are at high risk.

Herbs, Botanicals and Supplements (Clairmont, 2000)

- Herbs and botanical supplements should not be used without discussing with the physician—beans, peanut, onion, garlic, and bitter gourd have been recommended, but no clinical trials prove efficacy.
- Alpha-lipoic acid (thioctic acid) may have some potential benefits. It is found in the mitochondria and seems to have antioxidant properties that protect vitamin C, vitamin E, and glutathione. Natural sources include red meat, yeast, potatoes, and spinach. Supplementation may provide protection against cataracts and neuropathy in diabetes; it may also improve glucose uptake by the heart, although these studies are inconclusive at this time.
- Bilberry contains anthocyanosides that counteract cellular damage to the retina. Mild drowsiness and skin rashes have been noted.
- Chromium enhances use of insulin. Skin allergies, renal toxicity, and altered iron and zinc absorption can occur. Use only with noted deficiency levels, because there are no proven benefits if a patient is not deficient.
- Evening primrose oil may prevent or limit neuropathy due to gamma linoleic acid, an essential fatty acid. It can cause headache and gastrointestinal (GI) distress in susceptible individuals.
- Fenugreek may lower glucose levels due to psyllium content. It is part of the peanut family and may cause allergic reactions. Do not take with monoamine oxidase (MAO) inhibitors for depression. It has the potential for drug interactions with other medications as well.
- Garlic may lower blood glucose levels if used in large amounts
- Gingko biloba may help control neuropathy by maintaining integrity of blood vessels and reducing stickiness of blood and clotting. It has some antioxidant properties. Avoid taking with warfarin, aspirin, and other anticoagulant drugs, because it functions as a blood thinner. Headache and interactions with other drugs can occur.
- Ginseng may lower blood glucose levels. It increases energy and activity levels, which may lead to better glucose control. Do not take with warfarin, aspirin, MAO inhibitors, caffeine, antipsychotics, insulin, and oral hypoglycemics because of fluctuations in blood glucose levels, bleeding and platelet functioning, and changes in blood pressure and heart rate. Avoid taking with steroids because it functions as a steroidal herb. Headache, insomnia, nausea, and occasional menstrual difficulties can occur. Take with a meal.
- Gymnemna sylvestre is a hypoglycemic herb. It is highly potent and should be used only under doctor's supervision, because it may change insulin requirements.
- Vanadium acts like insulin to lower glucose levels. It has been associated with cancer cell growth and can be toxic at therapeutic levels.
- Zinc should not be used with immunosuppressants, tetracycline, ciprofloxacin, or levofloxacin because of potential antagonist effects.

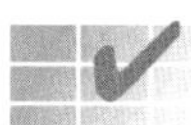

PATIENT EDUCATION

Note: Table 9–6 provides a detailed list of roles of various levels of dietetics professionals in diabetes self-management.

TABLE 9–5 Insulin Onset, Peaks, and Duration

Note: Physiologic insulin has immediate onset, peaks in ½–1 hour and lasts 2–3 hours.
Most insulins today now contain 100 units/mL (U-100). Mixtures–Rapid-acting insulins (regular and lispro) can be mixed with intermediate acting (NPH or lente- or long-acting (ultralente) insulins in the same syringe to increase convenience. Examples include 70/30 (NPH/Reg), 75/25 (NPL/LIS.)

Insulin type	Onset of action	Peak effect	Duration of activity
Rapid-acting			
Lispro	15–30 minutes	30–90 minutes	3–5 hours
Regular	30–60 minutes	2–4 hours	6–8 hours
Aspartate (Novolog)	5 minutes	15 minutes	3–4 hours
Intermediate-acting			
NPH (isophane)	1–2 hours	6–12 hours	18–24 hours
Lente (zinc)	1–3 hours	6–12 hours	18–26 hours
Humulin L, Novolin L	1–2.5 hours	6–12 hours	18–24 hours
Long-acting			
Ultralente	4–6 hours	10–16 hours	24–48 hours
PZI (protamine zinc insulin)	3–8 hours	14–24 hours	24–40 hours
Extra long-acting			
Glargine (Lantus)	4–6 hours	6–24 hours	Over 24 hours

Adapted from: Department of Medicine. *Washington Manual of Medical Therapeutics*. 30th ed. St. Louis, MO: Washington University School of Medicine, 2001.

- ✔ Teach patient about the importance of careful control, self-care, and optimal functioning, and the role of exercise and planned snacks in maintaining dietary control.
- ✔ Identify potential or real obstacles and discuss options, e.g., negative emotions, resisting temptations, dining away from home, feeling deprived, time pressures, temptations to relapse, planning, competing priorities, social events, family support, food refusal, and lack of friends' support (Schlundt et al., 1994).
- ✔ Encourage regular mealtimes and snacks. Children and teens in particular may need planned snacks.
- ✔ Discuss typical downfalls—restaurants, food offers from others. Reduced-fat foods often contain extra sugars—this must be monitored carefully.
- ✔ Discuss visual assessment of portions. Practice with scales if necessary. Read labels.
- ✔ Empowerment is important—help patients to gain mastery over their affairs and to effect change. Personal strengths, self-selected learning, self-generated problems and solutions, and internal reinforcement are key steps (Funnell et al., 1991). Discuss emotional eating—from boredom, anger, frustration, loneliness, and depression. Alternative choices should be recommended.
- ✔ Discuss the possibility of weight gain that occurs with intensive therapy and improved glucose control.
- ✔ A "Non-Diet" approach to diabetes management encourages regular eating according to actual hunger; listening to own signals and stopping eating when full; making gradual change to healthier eating; integrating activity into lifestyle; monitoring blood glucose in relationship to different meals or times; and making small changes gradually (Diabetes Care and Education, 2001).
- ✔ For sick days: Patients may require more insulin when ill. Liquid diets should provide 200 g CHO in equally divided amounts at mealtime and snacks; liquids should not be sugar-free (American Diabetes Association, 2001).
- ✔ For surgery: Blood glucose should be 100–200 mg/dL and perioperative hyperglycemia can be managed with doses of short-acting insulin. Correct abnormalities before surgery when possible.
- ✔ Eating disorders occur in young women with diabetes; refer for therapy (Rydall, 1997).
- ✔ Discuss the glycemic index—see Table 9–7. Current recommendations do not support its use in meal planning for diabetes (Franz et al., 2002).
- ✔ Guidelines for exercise are found in Table 9–8.

For More Information

- ✦ American Dietetic Association
  Type 1 Diabetes protocols (initial, continuing, intensive)
  www.eatright.org

TABLE 9–6 Roles for Dietetics Professionals in Diabetes Self-Management (Based on data from Diabetes Care and Education Practice Group, 2000)

Dietetic Technician (DTR) Roles:
Complete nutrition screening
Provide basic diabetes nutrition information
Explain restaurant dining and alcohol use guidelines
Provide label-reading guidelines
Recommend use of modified foods, as appropriate
Collaborate and communicate with health care providers (example: physician, nurse, RD, RD/CDE)

Registered Dietitian Roles:
The RD may perform all of the duties mentioned above for the DTR plus the following:
Nutrition assessments
Interpret appropriate laboratory results and recommend changes in therapy
Consider patient's readiness to change and negotiate goals appropriately or postpone education for a later time
Provide information on the pathophysiology of diabetes and an overview of diabetes management
Provide individualized nutrition prescription utilizing the appropriate meal planning approach, including but not limited to exchanges, carbohydrate counting, Food Guide Pyramid, calorie, and/or fat-gram counting
Use a variety of nutrition intervention and behavior management approaches
Coordinate exercise and nutrition management strategies
Depending on the setting, teach use of blood glucose meters, how to interpret results and make adjustments in food, medication, or physical activity
Review the effect of insulin or oral diabetes medication on blood glucose levels
Explain management of hypoglycemia and hyperglycemia
Provide sick-day guidelines for food intake
Recommend and implement modifications to the eating plan to address complications of diabetes and other comorbid conditions as needed
Guide clients to establish problem-solving skills
Develop/maintain educational resources appropriate to practice needs
Evaluate and adjust a client's meal plan and goals based on blood glucose levels
Monitor outcomes of MNT; revise therapy as needed
Refer clients to other health professionals, as needed
Participate as a member of the multidisciplinary diabetes care team
Document outcomes
Monitor and collect data on referral patterns and reimbursement practices
Become involved with legislative efforts to improve diabetes care, which includes MNT, at the local and national level

Registered Dietitian/Certified Diabetes Educator Roles:
The RD/CDE may perform all of the duties described for the DTR and the RD, plus the following:
Provide in-depth information on the pathophysiology of diabetes and an overview of diabetes management
Provide sick-day management guidelines, beyond those relative to food intake
Interpret blood glucose results and discuss adjustments in food, insulin, or medication; RD/CDE uses this in more depth for recommending treatment changes
Review the effect of insulin or oral hypoglycemic agents on blood glucose levels and recommend changes in therapy
Teach insulin administration skills/techniques, depending on the practice setting
Help select clients as candidates for intensive therapy and develop protocols to ensure quality diabetes care
Recommend and develop protocols and clinical pathways to ensure quality diabetes care
Refer clients to other team members, as appropriate
Provide professional expertise to other members of the diabetes care team and the community
Develop, coordinate, and/or manage diabetes education programs
Market diabetes management services to the medical community and the community at large
Provide case management services in inpatient and outpatient settings

TABLE 9–7 Glycemic Index

Glycemic index (GI) is a measure of serum glucose response to a food relative to a reference food that contains equal amounts of CHO (Salmeron et al., 1997). Because the index is a ratio, it does not refer directly to quantified food exchanges. A mixed diet yields varying results on blood glucose levels. A diet with lower GI results in lower plasma glucose and insulin levels throughout the day and a more favorable lipid profile and capacity for fibrinolysis than does a diet with a high GI (Jarvi et al., 1999). The same quantity of available CHO in different foods can induce very different glycemic responses.

Glycemic index yields:

½ cup instant potatoes @ an index of 86
1 slice of white bread @ 70
1 apple @ 53
½ cup canned corn @ 55
½ cup oat bran cereal @ 50
½ cup sucrose @ 86
1 cup watermelon @ 72
1 cup milk @ 49
1 cup of green grapes @ 46

The method of food preparation and the characteristics of each food are important predictors of glycemic response to food. Relative glycemic potency (RGP) and GI adjusted exchange value (EVG) are useful tools to derive common standard quantities to allow food exchange (Monro, 1999). More recently, use of the term glycemic load has been proposed, using calculation of the product of a food's CHO content and its GI as equivalent to 1 g of CHO from white bread (Liu et al., 2001). Type 1 diabetes management has been positively impacted in some studies by use of GI to evaluate dietary intakes against outcomes such as glycated hemoglobin and lipid levels (Buyken et al., 2001). However, use of the GI remains controversial in diabetes management (Franz et al., 2002). Further controlled research studies are recommended.

TABLE 9–8 American Diabetes Association General Guidelines for Regulating Glycemic Response to Exercise

1. **Metabolic control before exercise**
   - Avoid exercise if fasting glucose levels are >250 mg/dl and ketosis is present, and use caution if glucose levels are >300 mg/dl and no ketosis is present.
   - Ingest added carbohydrate if glucose levels are <100 mg/dl.
2. **Blood glucose monitoring before and after exercise**
   - Identify when changes in insulin or food intake are necessary.
   - Learn the glycemic response to different exercise conditions.
3. **Food intake**
   - Consume added CHO, as needed, to avoid hypoglycemia.
   - CHO-based foods should be readily available during and after exercise.

The Surgeon General's Report on Physical Activity and Health (U.S. Department of Health and Human Services, 1996) discusses the pivotal role physical activity plays in health promotion and disease prevention. It recommends that individuals accumulate 30 minutes of moderate physical activity on most days of the week. In the context of diabetes, it is becoming increasingly clear that the epidemic of type 2 diabetes is associated with decreasing levels of activity and an increasing prevalence of obesity. Exercise is a vital component of the prevention, as well as management of type 2 diabetes. Exercise improves the metabolic abnormalities of type 2 diabetes, especially when used early in the progression from insulin resistance, to impaired glucose tolerance (IGT), to overt hyperglycemia.

ISLET CELL TRANSPLANTATION

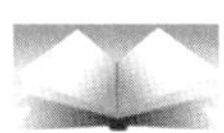

DEFINITIONS AND BACKGROUND

Islet cell transplantation is moving toward widespread clinical use. Knowing that there are not enough donated pancreases to allow for more organ donations, the Diabetes Research Institute Foundation has developed a stem cell developmental laboratory in Sweden to define the path that young cells take to become islets so that investigators can mimic these conditions (http://www.drinet.org/html/dri_stem_cell_program.htm).

Islet cell transplantation in type 1 diabetes can lead to insulin independence with excellent metabolic control when glucocorticoid-free immunosuppression is used (Shapiro et al, 2000). Transplantation is not always successful and is not common.

High doses of glucocorticoid drugs are needed to prevent rejection. The acute posttransplantation phase lasts up to 2 months; the chronic phase starts after 2 months. Complications sometimes include osteoporosis and hyperlipidemia.

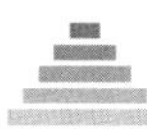

OBJECTIVES

- Prevent infection and promote healing.
- Normalize diet to meet specific needs of patient and modify diet according to drug therapy to enhance outcome.
- Monitor for abnormal electrolyte levels (Na+, K+).
- Monitor CHO intolerance but make sure that diet provides enough CHO to spare proteins.
- Alleviate rejection episodes. Control infections, especially during the acute phase. Support serum albumin levels to prevent additional infections.
- Force fluids unless contraindicated, as in retention. Match fluid output.
- Help patient adjust to a lifelong medical regimen during chronic phase. Improve survival rate by supporting immune response.
- Correct or manage complications that occur.
- Control weight gain in the first year after transplantation.

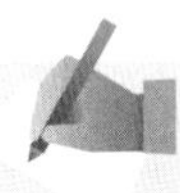

DIETARY AND NUTRITIONAL RECOMMENDATIONS

- Progress from clear liquids to solids as quickly as possibly postoperatively. Monitor fluid status and adjust as needed.
- Daily intake of protein should be appropriate for RDAs (age, sex); 1.5 g/kg while on steroids may be recommended. Calories should be calculated as 30–35 kcal/kg or 1.3–1.5 basal energy expenditure (BEE).
- Daily intake of sodium should be 2–4 g until the drug regimen is reduced. Adjust potassium levels as needed.
- Daily intake of calcium should be 1–1.5 times the RDA to offset poor absorption. Children especially need adequate calcium for growth. Daily intake of phosphorus should be equal to calcium intake.
- Supplement diet with vitamin D, magnesium, and thiamine as needed.
- Control CHO intake with hyperglycemia (50% total kilocalories) and limit sugars; encourage starch and fiber sources. Transplant patients are at risk of further glucose intolerance from use of prednisone, cyclosporine, and tacrolimus (Hasse et al., 1997).
- Plan fats at 30–35% of total kilocalories (encourage monounsaturated fats and omega-3 fatty acids). Low saturated fats and cholesterol may be needed. A low-fat regimen is recommended for prevention and treatment of hyperlipidemia.
- Reduce gastric irritants as necessary, if GI distress or reflux occurs.
- Monitor electrolytes carefully; hyperkalemia is common with cyclosporine or tacrolimus.
- Adequate vitamin intake will be essential to maintain immunity and to support wound healing.
- The special diet may be discontinued when drug therapy is reduced to maintenance levels. Encourage exercise and a weight control plan thereafter.

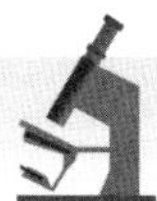

PROFILE

Clinical/History

Height
Dry weight, present weight
BMI
I & O
BP
Temperature

Lab Work

Alb, prealbumin
Ca++
Phosphorus
K+
Na+
H&H, Serum Fe
Serum folacin
BUN, Creat
Mg++
Triceps skinfold (TSF), mid-arm circumference (MAC), mid-arm muscle circumference (MAMC)
White blood cell count (WBC), total lymphocyte count (TLC)
Glucose (gluc)
Chol, Trig
C-reactive protein
Nitrogen (N) balance
Glomerular filtration rate (GFR)
Alk phos
Aspartate aminotransaminase (AST), alanine aminotransferase (ALT)
Bilirubin

Common Drugs Used and Potential Side Effects

- Tacrolimus (Prograf, FK506) suppresses T-cell immunity; it is 100 times more potent than cyclosporine, thus requiring smaller doses. Side effects include GI distress, nausea, vomiting, hyperkalemia, and hyperglycemia; there is also an increased risk of atherosclerosis. It may be necessary to supplement with magnesium; check lab work. Avoid taking with grapefruit and its juice.
- Corticosteroids (such as Prednisone, Solu-Cortef) are not as successful for immunosuppression. Side effects include increased catabolism of proteins, negative nitrogen balance, hyperphagia, ulcers, decreased glucose tolerance, sodium retention, fluid retention, and impaired calcium absorption and osteoporosis. Cushing's syndrome, obesity, muscle wasting, and increased gastric secretion may result. A higher protein intake and lower intake of simple CHOs may be needed.
- Cyclosporine does not retain sodium as much as corticosteroids do. Intravenous doses are not recommended. Nausea, vomiting, and diarrhea are common side effects. Hyperlipidemia, hypertension, and hyperkalemia also may occur; decrease sodium and potassium as necessary. Elevated glucose and lipids may occur. The drug is also nephrotoxic; therefore, adjustment of medications may be needed.
- Depletion paradigm enables drugs to bind to lymphocyte cell surface markers, creating cell lysis and/or inactivation; these include thymoglobulin and monoclonal OKT3 antilymphocyte antibodies (Hong and Kahan, 2000). Immunosuppressants such as Muromonab, OKT3, and antithymocyte globulin (ATG) are less nephrotoxic than cyclosporine but can cause nausea, anorexia, diarrhea, and vomiting. Monitor carefully. Fever and stomatitis also may occur.
- Azathioprine (Imuran) may cause leukopenia, thrombocytopenia, oral and esophageal sores, macrocytic anemia, vomiting, diarrhea, and other complex side effects. Folate supplementation and other dietary modifications may be needed such as liquid or soft diet for sore mouth. The drug works by lowering the number of T cells; it often is prescribed along with prednisone for conventional immunosuppression.
- Other drugs such as CellCept and sirolimus may be used (Hong and Kahan, 2000; McAlister et al., 2001).

Herbs, Botanicals and Supplements

- Herbs and botanical supplements should not be used without discussing with physician.
- Chaparral is an herbal product used for antioxidant properties; severe hepatitis or liver failure may result (Gordon et al., 1995). Avoid after transplantation.
- Silybum marianum (milk thistle) has been shown to have clinical applications in the treatment of liver disease through its antioxidative, antilipid peroxidative, antifibrotic, anti-inflammatory, immunomodulating, and liver-regenerating effects (Luper, 1998). Its role in pancreatic disease has not been proven.
- St. John's Wort interferes with the metabolism of cyclosporin-A and should not be used after transplantation (Karliova et al., 2000).

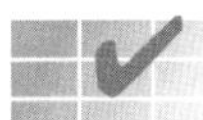

PATIENT EDUCATION

✔ Indicate which foods are sources of key nutrients such as protein in the diet. If patient does not prefer milk, show how other sources of calcium may be used in the diet.
✔ Alcohol should be avoided unless permitted by the doctor.
✔ Patients should know when to seek medical attention.
✔ Discuss problems with long-term obesity and hypercholesterolemia.
✔ Encourage moderation in diet; promote adequate exercise.

For More Information

- American Council on Transplantation
  700 North Fairfax Street, Suite 505
  Alexandria, VA 22314
  (703) 836-4301
- Joslin Diabetes Center–Islet Transplantation
  http://www.joslin.org/news/islet_transplant_july.html
- Immune Tolerance Network (ITN)
  http://www.immunetolerance.org

TYPE 2 DIABETES MELLITUS

NUTRITIONAL ACUITY RANKING: LEVEL 3

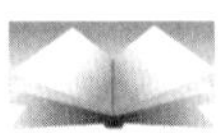

DEFINITIONS AND BACKGROUND

Type 2 DM arises because of insulin resistance, where there is failure to use insulin properly, combined with relative insulin deficiency. Individuals are usually overweight and sedentary with a family history of diabetes. There are 16 million Americans with type 2; they account for 90% of all persons with diabetes. Previous names for type 2 diabetes include "noninsulin-dependent diabetes or NIDDM," "Adult-Onset," "Type II," "Maturity-Onset," or "Ketosis-Resistant" diabetes. Risk factors include genetics, obesity, and age.

Genetics of type 2 have been reported in the GENNID (Genetics of NIDDM) Study of The American Diabetes Association. These resources are ideally suited for genetic linkage because Caucasian, Hispanic, African-American, and Japanese-American populations have been included. Rates of type 2 DM are high among Native Americans (almost 50%), non-Hispanic blacks (almost 20%), and Mexican-Americans and Hispanics (almost 25%). Tailoring of diets according to preferred foods and lifestyles is important. DM risk is greater for black vs. white Americans at low BMI and equivalent for both groups at high BMI (Resnick et al., 1998). There is a general lack of data on the incidence of obesity and type 2 diabetes among Asian Americans (Crawford et al., 2001); however, risk is higher because of greater central adiposity (McNeely et al., 2001).

The United Kingdom Prospective Diabetes Study (UKPDS) was a multicenter, prospective study of type 2 diabetes with 5,000+ individuals studied over a decade. The UKPDS conclusively demonstrated that improved blood glucose control in these patients reduces the risk of developing retinopathy, nephropathy, and possibly neuropathy (American Diabetes Association, Clinical Practice Recommendations 2001). Overall, the microvascular complications rate was decreased by 25% in patients receiving intensive therapy vs. conventional therapy; for every percentage point decrease in HbA1c (e.g., 9–8%) there was a 35% reduction in the risk of microvascular complications. The UKPDS also showed that aggressive control of BP, consistent with American Diabetes Association recommendations, significantly reduces strokes, diabetes-related deaths, heart failure, microvascular complications, and visual loss. Initial dietary therapy in patients with newly diagnosed Type 2 diabetes substantially reduces plasma triglyceride, improves total cholesterol and subfractions and results in a potentially less atherogenic profile; this does not eliminate the excess cardiovascular risk in patients with Type 2 diabetes (Manley et al., 2000).

Progressive deterioration of beta cells occurs in type 2 DM (Grill and Bjorklund, 2001). Patients with type 2 diabetes also have insulin resistance in liver and peripheral tissues (muscle, fat). Hyperinsulinism decreases insulin receptors (down regulation). Being obese (BMI over 25) for 10+ years is an important factor (Sakurai et al., 1999).

Impaired glucose metabolism is a risk factor for future diabetes and coronary heart disease. Pre-diabetes affects about 21 million Americans, and many convert to type 2 DM. Impaired Fasting Glucose (IFG) is a fasting level greater than or equal to 110 but less than 126 mg/dL. IGT is a 2-hour blood glucose value between 140 and 200 mg/dL on an oral glucose tolerance test (OGTT). Testing should be done in a health care setting on people who are over age 45 or earlier if the patient has risks for diabetes. Risks include obesity (BMI over 27); having a first-degree relative with DM; high-risk ethnic group; history of gestational diabetes mellitus (GDM) or baby born over 9 lbs; being hypertensive (140/90 or higher); having HDL of 35 or lower; having triglycerides (TG) of 250 or higher; previous test results of IFG or IGT; or hx of polycystic ovary syndrome.

Undiagnosed type 2 DM is common in older persons with essential hypertension (HPN) (Johnson et al., 1997). Odds of developing insulin resistance syndrome (hyperlipidemia, hyperinsulinemia, and dyslipidemia) by middle adulthood are related to weight gain over the preceding 30 years (Everson et al., 1998). Upper body (android) obesity is more strongly associated with type 2 diabetes than lower body (gynoid) obesity. High risk for nephropathy in type 2 DM seems to be: moderately elevated BP, total cholesterol, HbA1c, and high BMI (Ravid et al., 1998).

Studies are currently evaluating the role of proteins on inflammation and apo-A (Quilliot et al., 2001). There is also research on the kinase that is responsible for protein synthesis when under stress. Loss of a specific kinase results in destruction of insulin-producing b cells in the pancreas and dysregulation of glucose homeostasis (Sonenberg and Newgard, 2001). These studies promote interesting speculation on the role of proteins in diabetes.

High serum levels of carotenoids may play a protective role in the pathogenesis of insulin resistance and diabetes (Ford et al., 1999). Daily vitamin E and C supplementation does not seem to improve glycemic control in type 2 diabetes, but more studies are suggested (Konen et al., 2000).

Healthy men who drink light or moderate amounts of alcohol have a lower risk of developing type 2 diabetes than men who drink no alcohol (Ajani et al., 2000) or large amounts (Wei et al., 2000). Diabetes and liver injury appear to be related; BMI, heavy alcohol consumption, and male gender are associated with increased likelihood of elevated serum ALT over 43 international units (IU)/L, a sign of liver disease (Meltzer and Everhart, 1997). There also seems to be a large number of persons with type 2 DM who have fatty liver, regardless of alcohol intake (Marchesini et al., 2001).

It may be cost effective to screen young adults for type 2 or pre-diabetes (CDC Diabetes Cost Effectiveness Study Group, 1999). Benefits of early detection and treatment accrue from prevention of complications and resulting improvement in quality of life. Day-to-day quality of life in patients with type 2 diabetes can be improved with better blood glucose control and should be considered when implementing disease management programs, evaluating health outcomes, and estimating costs and benefits of therapeutic or prevention programs (Testa and Simonson, 1999). The care plan needs modification when HgA1c exceeds 8% (McFarland, 1997). Careful drug management will be needed.

Type 2 diabetes increases with age and affects more than 10% of U.S. population over age 65. Dietary intake of grains, especially whole grains, cereal fiber, and magnesium, is inversely related to development of type 2 DM in older adult women; total CHO, refined grains, fruit and vegetable intakes, soluble fiber, and glycemic index of the diet are unrelated to diabetes risk (Meyer et al., 2000; Nicholson et al., 1999; Liu et al., 2000).

Diagnosis of children with type 2 diabetes is increasing. They are usually diagnosed over the age of 10 years, in middle to late puberty. As children become increasingly overweight, type 2 diabetes may be expected to occur in younger children. Obesity is increasing not only in the U.S. but in many places throughout the world, and the incidence of type 2 diabetes increases as well. Physical inactivity, family history of type 2 diabetes, increased energy, and fat intake from the diet are important factors. Puberty seems to play a role in the onset of type 2 diabetes in children, when there is increased resistance to insulin action as related to a natural surge of growth hormone. The American Diabetes Association recommends that children be tested for type 2 diabetes if they have a family history of type 2 diabetes in first- and second-degree relatives; belong to a certain race/ethnic group (American Indians, African Americans, Hispanic Americans, Asians/ South Pacific Islanders); or have signs of insulin resistance or conditions associated with insulin resistance (acanthosis nigricans, hypertension, dyslipidemia, polycystic ovary syndrome [PCOS]).

Hypertensive patients with type 2 diabetes are at greater risk of cardiovascular complications, renal disease and, ultimately, renal failure. Prospective morbidity and mortality trials have demonstrated that tight blood pressure control improves cardiovascular prognosis and provides target organ protection (Weber and Weir, 2001). Current treatment guidelines recommend a target blood pressure of less than 130/85 mm Hg for patients with hypertension and diabetes.

Controversy exists about relations between the amount and types of dietary fat and carbohydrate and the risk of diabetes. In a study by Hu, van Dam, and Liu (2001), findings indicate that a higher intake of polyunsaturated fat and possibly long-chain omega-3 fatty acids could be beneficial, whereas a higher intake of saturated fat and trans-fat adversely affect glucose metabolism and insulin resistance. In addition, higher amounts of fiber and minimally processed whole grain products reduce glycemic and insulinemic responses and lower the risk for type 2 diabetes. Dietary recommendations to prevent type 2 diabetes should focus on the quality of fat and carbohydrate in the diet, in addition to balancing total energy intake to avoid overweight and obesity (Hu, van Dam, and Liu, 2001).

A large NIH-sponsored clinical trial found that eating less fat, exercising 2½ hours per week, and losing moderate amounts of weight cuts the incidence of type 2 DM by more than half among those most at risk. The study included 3,234 participants at 27 medical centers; they had impaired glucose tolerance and most were either overweight or had a family history of diabetes. The study showed that diabetes can be prevented in those at risk by using these behavioral changes (http://www.niddk.nih.gov/welcome/releases/8_8_01.htm).

MNT results in significant improvements in medical and clinical outcomes in type 2 diabetes (Franz et al., 1995); MNT interventions may result in minimum savings of $2,178 annually per patient case. See Tables 9–9 and 9–10 for further guidance. Table 9–11 provides background for handling MODY. Dietitians need to focus on lifestyle strategies that will improve blood glucose, BP, and lipids. The American Dietetic Association recommends 4 MNT visits initially, then 1 visit for every 6–12 months for Type 2 diabetes (http://www.knowledgeinc.com/ada/mntguides/).

TABLE 9–9 Diabetes Care Guidelines (American Diabetes Association, 2001)

1) MNT is integral to total diabetes care and management. Although adherence to nutrition and meal planning principles is one of the most challenging aspects of diabetes care, nutrition therapy is an essential component of successful diabetes management. Achieving nutrition-related goals requires a coordinated team effort that includes the person with diabetes. Because of the complexity of nutrition issues, it is recommended that a registered dietitian, knowledgeable and skilled in implementing diabetes MNT, be the team member providing nutrition care and education.

2) Effective nutrition self-management training requires an individualized approach appropriate for the personal lifestyle and diabetes management goals of the individual with diabetes.

3) Monitoring of glucose and glycated hemoglobin, lipids, blood pressure, and renal status is essential to evaluate nutrition-related outcomes. If goals are not met, changes must be made in the overall diabetes care and management plan. A nutrition assessment is used to determine the nutrition prescription, which is based on treatment goals, and what the individual with diabetes is able and willing to do.

4) To facilitate adherence, sensitivity to cultural, ethnic, and financial considerations is of prime importance.

TABLE 9–10 National Diabetes Education Program

The National Diabetes Education Program (NDEP) is designed to positively impact the health and outcomes of persons with diabetes. Most Americans do not consider diabetes to be a serious disease, or at least not as serious as cancer, AIDS, or heart disease; yet type 2 DM affects more than 7% of the adult population. The NDEP is to increase public awareness that diabetes is costly, common, and serious. Self-management among patients with diabetes is promoted. The goal of normoglycemia is recommended. An integrated approach to health care is suggested, and access to quality health care is needed. Website information is found at: http://ndep.nih.gov/.

TABLE 9–11 Maturity Onset Diabetes of the Young (MODY)

MODY is a relatively rare type of type 2 diabetes that is characterized by an early age of onset (age 9–25) and autosomal dominant inheritance. Unlike type 2 diabetes, often associated with insulin resistance, MODY is caused by a primary defect in pancreatic beta cell function resulting in decreased insulin secretion. Patients with MODY are not usually obese. Environmental stressors such as illness or puberty may unmask the genetically limited insulin secretory reserve of patients with undiagnosed MODY. Unlike type 1, MODY does not cause polyuria, thirst, or extreme hunger and may be undiagnosed until later in life. The primary goal is euglycemia (Cabanas, 1998).

MODY presentation is broad, ranging from asymptomatic hyperglycemia to a severe acute presentation. MODY has been reported in all races/ethnicities. Individuals with type 2 diabetes do not generally have autoantibodies to *b*-cell proteins; fasting insulin and C-peptide levels are usually normal or elevated, although not as elevated as might be expected for the degree of hyperglycemia. These gene abnormalities are thought to be rare, and molecular diagnostic testing, currently only available in research laboratories, is required for specific classification. Until such testing becomes commonplace, children with MODY should be classified as having the type of diabetes that best fits their clinical picture.

OBJECTIVES

(Derived from American Diabetes Association, 2001)

Goal-directed therapy with the patient's goals having greater importance than benchmark clinical goals is the most important objective!

- Maintain as near-normal blood glucose levels as possible by balancing food intake with insulin (either endogenous or exogenous) or oral glucose-lowering medications and activity levels. Maintain glycosylated HbA1c levels less than 7% and FBS levels between 80 and 120 mg/dL fasting and between 100 and 140 mg/dL at bedtime. A normal range for the patient may vary by age and underlying disorders. Protect beta cell function by controlling hyperglycemia. Use of the HbA1c test is convenient.
- Achievement of optimal serum lipid levels to reduce the risk for macrovascular disease. Dyslipidemia is a central component of insulin resistance in all ethnic groups (Howard et al., 1998).
- Provide adequate calories for maintaining or attaining reasonable weights for adults, normal growth and development rates in children and adolescents, increased metabolic needs during pregnancy and lactation, or recovery from catabolic illnesses. Reasonable weight is defined as the weight an individual and health care provider acknowledge as achievable and maintainable, both short- and long-term, not the traditionally defined desirable or ideal body weight. Calculate 30 kcal/kg for a person at normal weight, 25 kcal/kg to lose weight, and 35 kcal/kg to gain weight.
- Prevent and treat the acute complications of insulin-treated diabetes such as hypoglycemia, short-term illnesses, and exercise-related problems and of the long-term complications of diabetes such as renal disease, autonomic neuropathy, hypertension, and cardiovascular disease (see Table 9–2). Consensus about protein currently suggests maintaining RDA levels (0.8 g/kg in adults) and lowering to 0.6 g/Kg with early signs of nephropathy.
- Improvement of overall health through optimal nutrition and physical activity. Dietary Guidelines for Americans and the Food Guide Pyramid summarize and illustrate nutritional guidelines and nutrient needs for all healthy Americans and can be used by people with diabetes and their family members. Encourage regular mealtimes. If necessary, make two plans—one for weekdays and one for weekends. Maintain the diet through behavior modification, education, and problem solving strategies. A specific diabetes pyramid is available at http://www.diabetes.org/nutrition/article031799.asp.
- Address individual needs according to culture, ethnicity, and lifestyle, while respecting willingness to change. For older adults, provide for nutritional and psychosocial needs. For pregnant or lactating women, provide adequate energy and nutrients for optimal outcomes. Regulate patient's individual medication plan according to meal pattern and lifestyle.
- Maintain BP levels that reduce risk for vascular disease. Elevated BP has a major impact on renal function.
- Manage problems related to compulsive or binge eating. Patients often report deliberate omission of insulin or oral hypoglycemic agents (OHA) to lose weight (Herpertz et al., 1998).

DIETARY AND NUTRITIONAL RECOMMENDATIONS

- Weight control is important. A moderate caloric restriction (250–500 calories less than average daily intake as calculated from a food history) and a nutritionally adequate meal plan with a reduction of total fat, especially saturated fat, accompanied by an increase in physical activity should be recommended (American Diabetes Association, 2001). Moderate weight loss in an obese patient (5–9 kg or 10–20 lbs), irrespective of starting weight, may reduce hyperglycemia, dyslipidemia, and hypertension. For teen boys over age 15, it may be useful to calculate as 18 kcal/lb for usual activity and 16 kcal/lb if sedentary; teen girls over age 15 have needs estimated the same as an adult. Extremely low calorie diets for adults should be performed only in a hospital setting. In morbidly obese patients, gastric bypass surgery has sometimes been used with favorable results (Pories and Albrecht, 2001).
- Spacing of meals (spreading nutrient intake, particularly carbohydrate, throughout the day) is important. Meal skipping should be discouraged. Individualize meal plan according to patient preferences.
- The dietitian should calculate CHO and fat requirements individually according to lipid and glucose levels. Assess dietary history, physical exercise, and activity patterns. A diet that emphasizes fruits, nonstarchy vegetables, and dairy products may benefit patients with type 2 diabetes (Gannon et al., 1998).
- Evidence regarding the role of controlled protein in reduction of progression of nephropathy has not been clearly proven. Use RDA levels for age and sex.

- Use the Food Guide Pyramid principles, current guidelines for lipid management, and proper energy intake. Teach food exchanges only at the request of a highly motivated patient. For Carbohydrate Counting: See Table 9–4.
- Although selected soluble fibers are capable of inhibiting absorption of glucose from the small intestine in the amounts likely to be consumed from foods, the clinical significance of this effect on blood glucose levels is probably insignificant (American Diabetes Association, 2001). Recommendations for people with diabetes are the same as for the general population related to fiber and a healthful diet: 25 g dietary fiber per 1,000 kilocalories from both soluble and insoluble fibers with a wide variety of food sources is recommended. Use more rice, beans, vegetables, oat bran, legumes, barley, produce with skins, apples, etc.
- Use of MUFAs has some positive effects (Garg et al., 1994). Limit intake of cholesterol to less than 300 mg daily; ensure that only 10% of total fat intake is saturated (Franz et al., 2002).
- As a healthy lifestyle, teach the principles of the DASH diet. For people with mild-to-moderate hypertension, <2,400 mg/day of sodium is recommended; for people with hypertension and nephropathy, <2,000 mg/day of sodium is recommended (American Diabetes Association, 2001).
- For vitamins and minerals, ensure that patient has adequate dietary intakes. Higher levels of magnesium, chromium, and potassium have been recommended when serum levels are low. There is not a clear need for daily supplementation at this time (Franz et al., 2002).
- Assess dietary history, physical exercise, and activity patterns. Discuss use of artificial sweeteners and food diaries.
- Discuss use of alcohol. To avoid hypoglycemia, alcohol should be consumed with food and limited to one drink daily for women and two for men (Franz et al., 2002). Alcohol calories = 0.8 × proof × number of ounces. Abstention from alcohol is recommended for pregnant women and for those persons who have pancreatitis, advanced neuropathy, elevated triglycerides, or a history of alcohol abuse (Franz et al., 2002). When calories from alcohol need to be calculated as part of the total caloric intake, alcohol is best substituted for fat exchanges (1 alcoholic beverage = 2 fat exchanges) or fat calories.

PROFILE

Clinical/History	Lab Work	
Height	HbA1c	Alk Phos, PO4
Weight	Fasting gluc	Lipid Panel—Chol (usually low HDL/high LDL)
BMI and waist measurement	Urinary glucose or ketones	Trig (increased)
BP (often increased)	BUN, Creat	Ca++
	K+, Na+	Mg++
	ALT, AST	Microalbuminemia
	Lactic acid dehydrogenase (LDH)	

Common Drugs Used and Potential Side Effects

- Insulin may be needed for refractory hyperglycemia, DKA, stress, infection, or pregnancy. If monotherapy does not achieve normoglycemia, combined oral therapies (drugs from two classes) can be initiated (Table 9–12). If combination oral therapy does not work, then insulin may be needed. Insulin is often given twice daily (McFarland, 1997).
- Steroids, beta-blockers, and diuretics may cause hyperglycemia. Angiotensin-converting enzyme (ACE) inhibitors are better to keep blood glucose levels within normal limits.
- Xenical (fat blocker) may help cut heart risk in patients with type 2 diabetes.
- Vitamin E supplementation may help reduce oxidative stress in patients with diabetes (Sharma et al., 2000). Large doses of vitamin C can cause false-positive urinary glucose levels; but studies show that plasma vitamin C is inversely associated with glycated hemoglobin levels (Sargeant et al., 2000). Further studies are needed on the role of these vitamins in diabetes management.
- Oral 5-hydroxy-tryptophan (5-HTP) the precursor of serotonin stimulates the serotonergic system in the brain, causing decreased CHO intake and weight loss. Type 2 DM is associated with decreased levels of serotonin, hyperphagia, and CHO cravings. Eventually, oral 5-HTP may help patients with type 2 DM adhere to dietary prescriptions (Cangiano et al., 1998).
- When used, H2 receptor antagonists such as cimetidine can positively impact diabetes control, decrease appetite, and decrease body weight in individuals with type 2 diabetes (Stoa-Birketvedt et al., 1998).
- High blood pressure is often managed with ACE inhibitors or beta-blockers.
- Adding psyllium to a diabetic diet may improve glycemic and lipid control in men with type 2 diabetes and hypercholesterolemia (Anderson et al., 1999; Chandalia et al., 2000).
- Low dose aspirin is sometimes recommended to protect against cardiovascular events in persons with diabetes, who are at high risk.
- Metformin may have some role in improving insulin sensitivity in patients with IGT because of the reversal of the glucose fatty acid cycle. This Finnish study should be replicated in other centers to identify if these effects can prevent progression of type 2 diabetes and cardiovascular morbidity and mortality (Lehtovirta et al. 2001).

Herbs, Botanicals and Supplements (Clairmont, 2000)

- Herbs and botanical supplements should not be used without discussing with physician.
- Bilberry contains anthocyanosides that counteract cellular damage to the retina. Mild drowsiness and skin rashes have been noted.

TABLE 9–12 Drugs Used For Type 2 Diabetes

Drugs	*Action*	*How Taken*	*Potential Effects*	*Other*
Secretagogues				
Sulfonylureas	Lower blood glucose by augmenting insulin secretion	30–60 minutes before eating	Weight gain and hypoglycemia can occur.	Never give to a patient who is fasting for any reason. Avoid taking with alcohol to avoid flushing, altered heart rate.
First-generation: Tolazamide (Tolinase); Tolbutamide (Orinase); Acetohexamide (Dymelor); chlorpropamide (Diabinese)			Diarrhea, GI distress, nausea, vomiting, and metallic taste also may occur.	
Long-acting: Glyburide (DiaBeta, Micronase); Glipizide (Glucotrol); Glimepiride (Amaryl)		Take with breakfast or a main meal.	Nausea, GI distress, diarrhea, and heartburn may occur. With Amaryl, elevated liver enzymes may occur; hypoalbuminemia can increase effects.	
Short-acting: Repaglinide (Prandin); Senaglinide (Starlix)	Action on insulin secretion is more rapid and shorter than that of sulphonylureas. Offers better control of post-prandial hyperglycemia and is associated with a lower risk of delayed hypoglycemic episodes.	Take within 30 minutes before meals		
Sensitizers	Inhibit glucose release by the liver.	Take with the first bite of each meal.		
Metformin HCL (Glucophage), Acarbose (Precose), Glyset (Miglitol)	Hepatic glucose output is inhibited; peripheral glucose uptake is enhanced.	Take with food; increase dose slowly over 1–2 weeks until optimal glycemic effect is seen.	Diarrhea, abdominal pain, and flatulence	Persons with high serum creatinine or low GFR, cirrhosis, IBD, colonic ulceration, partial intestinal obstruction, or diabetic ketoacidosis should not receive these medications. Hypoglycemia and weight gain may occur.
Thiazolidinediones: Rosiglitazone (Avandia); and Pioglitazone (Actos)	Increase tissue glucose utilization, mostly in peripheral tissue such as muscle.	Take with or without food.		Should not take with significant heart disease because of potential fluid retention or congestive heart failure (CHF). May be hepatotoxic.
Enzyme Inhibitors				
Acarbose (Precose); Miglitol (Glyset)	Starch blockers that delay intestinal glucose absorption.	Take with food.	GI intolerance may occur.	Exercise enhances effectiveness. Not usually given alone.

- Chromium enhances use of insulin. Skin allergies, renal toxicity, and altered iron and zinc absorption can occur. Use only with noted deficiency levels because there are no proven benefits if patient is not deficient.
- Evening primrose oil may prevent or limit neuropathy due to gamma linoleic acid, an essential fatty acid. It can cause headache and GI distress in susceptible individuals.
- Fenugreek may lower glucose levels due to psyllium content. It is part of the peanut family and may cause allergic reactions. Do not take with MAO inhibitors for depression. It has the potential for drug interactions with other medications as well.
- Garlic may lower blood glucose levels if used in large amounts
- Gingko biloba may help control neuropathy by maintaining integrity of blood vessels and reducing stickiness of blood and clotting. It has some antioxidant proper-

ties. Avoid taking with warfarin, aspirin, and other anticoagulant drugs, because it functions as a blood thinner. Headache and interactions with other drugs can occur

- Ginseng may lower blood glucose levels. It increases energy and activity levels, which may lead to better glucose control. Do not take with warfarin, aspirin, MAO inhibitors, caffeine, antipsychotics, insulin, and oral hypoglycemics because of fluctuations in blood glucose levels, bleeding and platelet functioning, or changes in blood pressure and heart rate. Avoid taking with steroids, because it functions as a steroidal herb. Headache, insomnia, nausea, and occasional menstrual difficulties can occur. Take with a meal.
- Gymnemna sylvestre is a hypoglycemic herb. It is highly potent and should be used only under doctor's supervision, because it may change insulin requirements.
- Vanadium acts like insulin to lower glucose levels. It has been associated with cancer cell growth and can be toxic at therapeutic levels.
- Zinc should not be used with immunosuppressants, tetracycline, ciprofloxacin, or levofloxacin because of potential antagonist effects.

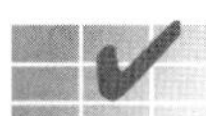

PATIENT EDUCATION

See Table 9–6 for specific tips on diabetes self-management.

- ✔ Emphasize the importance of regular mealtimes, use of medications, and balanced activity.
- ✔ Emphasize the importance of self-care and optimal functioning. Include instructions on how to handle illness, stress, dining out, exercise, label reading, and how to use sucrose or fructose and sugar alcohols.
- ✔ Identify potential or real obstacles and discuss options—e.g., negative emotions, resisting temptations, dining away from home, feeling deprived, time pressures, temptations to relapse, planning, competing priorities, social events, family support, food refusal, and lack of friends' support (Schlundt et al., 1994).
- ✔ Differentiate between "dietetic" and "diabetic" in food labeling; these are not equivalent terms. More education about the food label is important (Miller et al., 1999).
- ✔ Discuss handling parties and food offers from others.
- ✔ Encourage group support, behavior modification, and nutritional counseling for overweight persons. Small-step changes lead to greater self-esteem than continued failures at change. Sequential rather than simultaneous dietary manipulations work better for most people.
- ✔ Doctors should be encouraged to refer newly diagnosed patients to a dietitian. The dietitian should regularly reassess patients who have had diabetes for a while for modification of insulin or other medications to match dietary intakes.
- ✔ Before surgery, blood glucose should be maintained in a range between 100–200 mg/dL. Perioperative hyperglycemia may be managed with doses of short-acting insulin. Correct abnormalities before surgery, when possible.
- ✔ Table 9–8 provides suggested guidelines for exercise.

For More Information

- ✦ American Diabetes Association
  GENNID Resource
  Fax: (703) 549-1715
  http://www.diabetes.org/
- ✦ American Dietetic Association: Type 2 Diabetes protocol
  www.eatright.org

GESTATIONAL DIABETES

NUTRITIONAL ACUITY RANKING: LEVEL 3

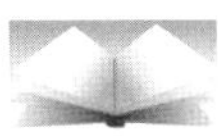

DEFINITIONS AND BACKGROUND

Pregnancy is a metabolic stress test for all women; some, but not all, women acquire gestational diabetes (GDM). In any pregnancy, increased insulin resistance occurs because gestational hormones counteract insulin action. Glycosuria can occur in the presence of normal blood sugars from decreased renal glucose thresholds. During the first half of pregnancy, transfer of maternal glucose to fetus occurs; during the second half of pregnancy, diabetogenic action of placental hormones outweighs glucose transfer (average insulin requirement increases by 67%).

GDM occurs in 1–6% of all pregnancies, with hyperglycemia (over 130 mg/dL) and glycosuria first recognized during pregnancy. Selective screening at 24–28 weeks of pregnancy is generally recommended, with a glucose challenge test and 1-hour assessment (Jovanovich, 2000; Wen et al., 2000). American Diabetes Association criteria for GDM require two plasma glucose values > or = 95 mg/dL (fasting), > or = 180 mg/dL (1 hour), and > or = 155 mg/dL (2 hours) after a 100-g glucose load; World Health Organization (WHO) criteria require a plasma glucose > or = 7.0 mmol/l (fasting) or > or = 7.8 mmol/l (2 hours) (Schmidt et al., 2001). See Table 9–13 for details about risk assessment.

Women at risk for GDM may be obese, hyperglycemic, and insulin-resistant; others may be normal in weight and insulin-deficient. In general, these mothers tend to be older. Central body fat distribution during pregnancy is an independent predictor of GDM (Branchtein, 1997). Saturated fat intake has an independent role in the development of gestational glucose abnormalities (Bo et al., 2001), and PUFA intake may be more protective against GDM (Wang et al., 2000).

Infants born to mothers with GDM who are overweight before pregnancy, gain excess weight during pregnancy, and have elevated blood glucose levels during pregnancy, are at greater risk for macrosomia and elevated blood lipids (Vohr et al., 1995). Glycemic control before conception and during the first trimester may actually influence weight gain more than glycemic control during the later weeks of pregnancy (Gold et al., 1998). Further studies are needed.

Symptoms and signs of GDM include a large weight gain, hypoglycemia, DKA, pregnancy-induced hypertension, and anxiety. This condition yields an abnormally high risk for perinatal complications. Infants may be large for gestational age (LGA) with macrosomatia, hypoglycemia, respiratory distress, hypocalcemia, or hyperbilirubinemia. The condition may lead to diabetes for the mother postnatally. Recurrence of GDM is associated with shortened interval and large weight gain between pregnancies (DeVeciana et al., 1998). Women with GDM are at increased risk for preeclampsia (Catalano et al., 1998).

In spite of the potential for increased morbidity in GDM, the corrected perinatal outcomes are usually quite good (Lucas, 2001). Use of family planning, early screening for fetal abnormalities, delivery early in term, improved compliance, better glycemic control during pregnancy, and improved neonatal care all make the difference.

All women with GDM should receive nutritional counseling by a registered dietitian when possible, as stated by The American Diabetes Association (2001). Individualized MNT relates to maternal weight and height. MNT should include the provision of adequate calories and nutrients to meet the needs of pregnancy and should be consistent with the maternal blood glucose goals that have been established. Nutrition recommendations for women with GDM should be based on a

TABLE 9–13 Risk Assessment for GDM (American Diabetes Association, Clinical Practice Recommendations 2001)

Risk assessment for GDM should be undertaken at the first prenatal visit; women with a high risk of GDM (i.e., marked obesity, personal history of GDM, glycosuria, or a strong family history of diabetes) should undergo glucose testing. If they are found not to have GDM at that initial screening, they should be retested between 24 and 28 weeks of gestation. Women of average risk should have testing undertaken at 24–28 weeks of gestation. A fasting plasma glucose level >126 mg/dl (7.0 mmol/l) or a casual plasma glucose >200 mg/dl (11.1 mmol/l) meets the threshold for the diagnosis of diabetes, if confirmed on a subsequent day, and precludes the need for any glucose challenge.

In the absence of this degree of hyperglycemia, evaluation for GDM in women with average or high-risk characteristics should follow one of two approaches:

One-step approach: Perform a diagnostic OGTT without prior plasma or serum glucose screening. The one-step approach may be cost-effective in high-risk patients or populations (e.g., some Native-American groups).

Two-step approach: Perform an initial screening by measuring the plasma or serum glucose concentration 1 hour after a 50-g oral glucose load (glucose challenge test [GCT]) and perform a diagnostic OGTT on that subset of women exceeding the glucose threshold value on the GCT. When the two-step approach is employed, a glucose threshold value >140 mg/dl (7.8 mmol/l) identifies approximately 80% of women with GDM, and the yield is further increased to 90% by using a cutoff of >130 mg/dl (7.2 mmol/l).

thorough nutrition assessment. Monitoring blood glucose levels, urine ketones, appetite, and weight gain guides the individualized nutrition prescription and meal plan. Adjustments should be made to the meal plan throughout pregnancy to ensure desired outcomes (American Diabetes Association, 2001).

According to the American Dietetic Association, cost-effectiveness of nutritional interventions in GDM saves about $10,538 annually per case. Multidisciplinary prenatal care must include nutritional education, counseling, and support. The American Dietetic Association recommends three MNT visits over the first few months, then every 2–3 weeks during treatment for gestational diabetes (http://www.knowledgelinc.com/ada/mntguides/).

OBJECTIVES

- Optimize growth and development of the fetus. Prevent both low birthweight and macrosomia.
- Prevent complications of diabetes and fetal problems, including infections. Minimize morbidity and prevent death of mother or infant.
- Control blood pressure.
- Normalize blood sugars; maintain normoglycemia. Monitor starvation ketosis (glucose is needed) versus diabetic acidosis (where insulin and potassium are needed). Performance of both preprandial and postprandial self-monitoring of blood glucose levels helps to prevent pronounced postprandial glucose excursions and minimize the risk of neonatal macrosomia.
- Utilize insulin when necessary, based on measures of maternal glycemia with or without assessment of fetal growth. Insulin therapy is recommended when MNT fails to maintain fasting whole blood glucose levels ≤ 95 mg/dl or 2-hour postprandial whole blood glucose levels ≤ 120 mg/dl (6.7 mmol/l).
- Prevent hypoglycemic episodes, urinary tract infections, and candidiasis.
- Achieve an approximate total weight gain of 20–30 lb. Prevent weight loss; avoid excessive weight gain in obese women.
- Monitor development of type 2 diabetes in women with a high prevalence of b-cell dysfunction; risks increase with every 10 lb of weight gained during follow-up years after pregnancy (Peters et al., 1996).

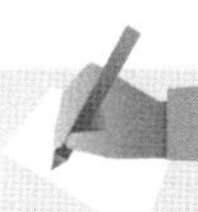

DIETARY AND NUTRITIONAL RECOMMENDATIONS

- Diet should match age needs and weight goals. The typical diet may include 30–35 kcal/kg, 20–25% total calories as protein (1.3+ g/kg), 35–40% CHO (especially from starches and fiber sources), and 35–40% total fat. Restriction of CHOs to 35–40% of calories has been shown to decrease maternal glucose levels and improve maternal and fetal outcomes (http://www.diabetes.org/clinicalrecommendations/Supplement101/S3.htm.) While sufficient CHO intake (at least 250 g/day) is needed to prevent hypoglycemia (Romon et al., 2001), avoidance of excessive sugars is also recommended. Maintain an adequate intake of polyunsaturated fats; keep saturated fats to 10% of total fat or less.
- For obese women with BMI over 30, reduce kilocalories by about 1/3. This translates for many to an energy intake around 1,800 kcals.
- DASH diet principles may be helpful if BP is elevated.
- Ensure intake of prenatal vitamin–mineral supplement (especially for folic acid, vitamin C, 30–60 mg iron, adequate calcium). Include adequate chromium intake from dietary sources (Anderson, 2000).
- Carefully spaced meals and snacks, especially before bedtime, are needed. Four to six small meals may be helpful, and a snack upon arising may be important to prevent hypoglycemia.
- No meals should be skipped.
- Tube feeding with CHO-controlled specialty products may be useful in patients who cannot be fed orally.

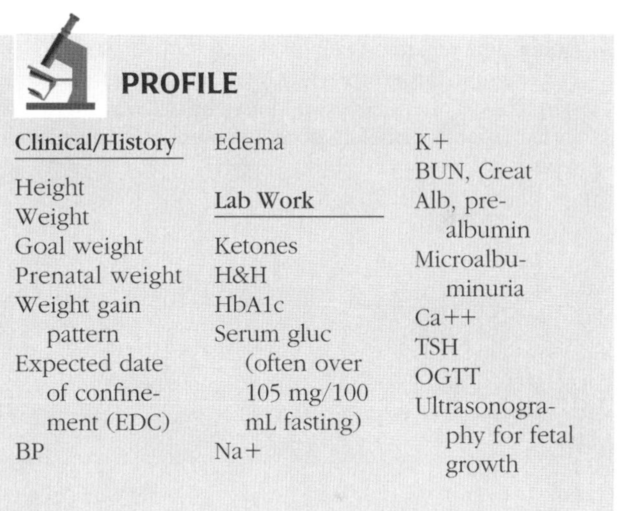

PROFILE

Clinical/History		
Height	Edema	K+
Weight	**Lab Work**	BUN, Creat
Goal weight	Ketones	Alb, pre-albumin
Prenatal weight	H&H	Microalbuminuria
Weight gain pattern	HbA1c	Ca++
Expected date of confinement (EDC)	Serum gluc (often over 105 mg/100 mL fasting)	TSH
BP	Na+	OGTT
		Ultrasonography for fetal growth

Common Drugs Used and Potential Side Effects

- Insulin may be required to control blood glucose, if diet and exercise do not help. Careful physician monitoring will be needed. Self-monitoring may be important for glucose/insulin control. Insulin lispro is associated with fewer hypoglycemic events and attenuates the postprandial response greater than does regular human insulin (Jovanovich, 2000).
- Prenatal vitamin–mineral supplements should be used as prescribed. Be aware that excessive doses of vitamin C may show false-positive urinary glucose levels; more than 200 mg daily probably is not needed.
- Oral glucose-lowering agents are not recommended during pregnancy.
- Low-dose estrogen-progestogen oral contraceptives may be used after GDM, if no medical contraindications exist. However, medications that worsen insulin resistance (e.g., glucocorticoids, nicotinic acid) should be avoided if possible.

Herbs, Botanicals and Supplements

- In general, pregnant women should not take any herbs and botanical products. They should discuss any previous use with their physician.

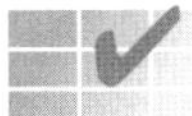

PATIENT EDUCATION

- ✔ Communicate the importance of meal spacing, timing, adequacy, and consistency (i.e., patient should not skip meals).
- ✔ Careful instructions on what to eat and what to avoid will be important.
- ✔ Carrying a snack at all times is helpful (e.g., fruit, milk, crackers).
- ✔ Regular aerobic exercise may be beneficial (Franz et al., 2002). Exercise after meals may help to control blood sugar; walking is often recommended. Upper body exercises are also beneficial.
- ✔ Encourage breastfeeding (Franz et al., 2002).
- ✔ Counseling regarding risk for diabetes should be provided. For example, a person with GDM may continue to be hyperglycemic after delivery and may be determined to have, in fact, type 1 diabetes; obese women may later develop type 2 diabetes.
- ✔ According to The American Diabetes Association, if glucose levels are normal postpartum, reassessment of glycemia should be undertaken at a minimum of 3-year intervals, more frequently for women with IFG or IGT in the postpartum period. Long-term lifestyle modifications that lessen insulin resistance, including maintenance of normal body weight through MNT and physical activity, should be discussed.
- ✔ The need for family planning exists to ensure optimal glucose regulation from the start of subsequent pregnancies.
- ✔ Discuss the potential impact on offspring, who are at increased risk of obesity, glucose intolerance, and diabetes in late adolescence or adulthood.

For More Information

- ✦ American Dietetic Association
  Gestational Diabetes protocol
  www.eatright.org
- ✦ Diabetes care
  Clinical Practice Recommendations
  http://journal.diabetes.org/FullText/Supplements/DiabetesCare/Supplement100/s77.htm
- ✦ March of Dimes
  http://www.modimes.org/

DIABETIC GASTROPARESIS

NUTRITIONAL ACUITY RANKING: LEVEL 3

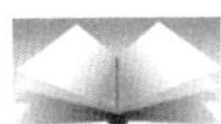

DEFINITIONS AND BACKGROUND

Gastroparesis is a condition in which stomach emptying is prolonged because the nerves are damaged or have stopped working. Gastroparesis occurs in approximately 50% of all cases of diabetes (Goldberg et al., 1997), with delayed gastric emptying in the absence of mechanical obstruction. Problems occur more often in type 1 than in type 2 DM.

Phases of normal digestion include: phase I (45–60 minutes of inactivity); phase II (30–45 minutes of intermittent peristaltic contractions); phase III (10 minutes of intense, regular contractions); and phase IV (brief transition between cycles). In gastroparesis, any of these phases may be prolonged.

The condition occurs as a result of vagal autonomic neuropathy, scleroderma, Parkinson's disease, hypothyroidism, postviral syndromes, surgery on the stomach or the vagus nerve, prolonged hyperglycemia, or vascular insufficiencies. Assessment of patients for possible diabetic gastroparesis includes asking questions about recent changes in appetite; heartburn, abdominal pain, or nausea after eating; early fullness after eating small amounts of food; poor blood glucose control; or weight fluctuations.

Signs and symptoms of gastroparesis include heartburn, nausea, abdominal pain, vomiting, early satiety, weight loss, belching, bloating, gastroesophageal reflux, and constipation. Bezoar formation can occur, which entails formation of food into solid masses that further obstruct the flow from the stomach to the small intestine.

OBJECTIVES

- ▲ Correct dehydration and electrolyte abnormalities.
- ▲ Reduce or control pain, diarrhea, and constipation.
- ▲ Ensure adequate intake of diet as prescribed to prevent weight loss and control malnutrition.
- ▲ Prevent further symptoms and problems such as the need for surgery.
- ▲ Differentiate from ketoacidosis, which has similar symptoms of nausea and vomiting.
- ▲ Prevent bezoar formation of indigestible solids.
- ▲ Pernicious vomiting may occur; distinguish from bulimia.

DIETARY AND NUTRITIONAL RECOMMENDATIONS

- Monitor intake carefully for tolerated foods. Blood sugar delays its return to normal in gastroparesis.
- Soft-to-liquid diet lower in fat may be useful to prevent delay in gastric emptying. Isotonic liquids empty more quickly than hypertonic liquids. Six small meals may be better tolerated than large meals.
- Alter fiber intake according to needs (diarrhea, constipation, etc.).
- If patient complains of dry mouth, add extra fluids and moisten foods with broth or allowed sauces or gravies.
- In severe problems, a jejunostomy tube feeding with an elemental diet may be indicated. It can be used temporarily if needed to correct malnutrition. In rare cases, parenteral nutrition may be needed.

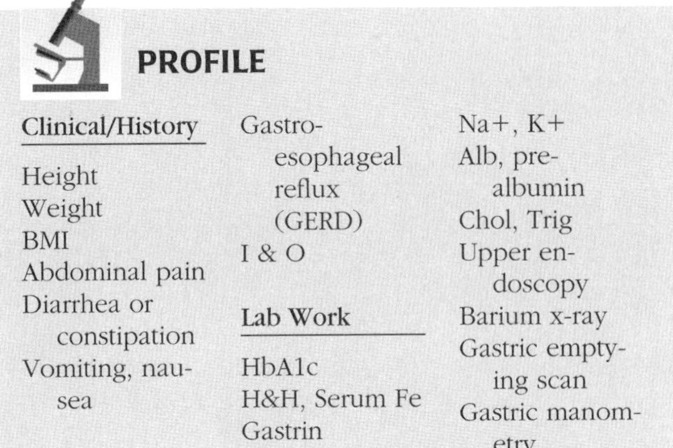

PROFILE

Clinical/History

Height
Weight
BMI
Abdominal pain
Diarrhea or constipation
Vomiting, nausea
Gastroesophageal reflux (GERD)
I & O

Lab Work

HbA1c
H&H, Serum Fe
Gastrin
Gluc
Na+, K+
Alb, prealbumin
Chol, Trig
Upper endoscopy
Barium x-ray
Gastric emptying scan
Gastric manometry

Common Drugs Used and Potential Side Effects

- Metoclopramide (Reglan) may be given 30 minutes before meals to increase gastric contractions and to relax pyloric sphincter. Dry mouth, sleepiness, anxiety, or nausea can be side effects. Emitasol is a nasal spray form of this medication, which is in final trials for effectiveness.
- Rapid-acting insulin should be injected with or after meals. Use SMBG to monitor delayed absorption and glucose changes. Humalog is quite effective, because it starts working within 5–15 minutes after injection. To control blood glucose, it may be necessary to take insulin more often, after eating instead of before, and check blood glucose often after eating (http://www.niddk.nih.gov/health/digest/pubs/gastro/gastro.htm).
- Antiemetics may be used for vomiting. Monitor for specific side effects.
- Erythromycin improves gastric emptying but can cause nausea, vomiting, and cramping.
- Domperidone (Motilium) stimulates peristalsis and has few central nervous system (CNS) side effects; it may be available in Canada but currently not in the U.S.

Herbs, Botanicals and Supplements

- Herbs and botanical supplements should not be used without discussing with physician.

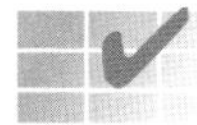

PATIENT EDUCATION

- ✓ Discuss delayed digestion and absorption of food.
- ✓ Discuss role of diet in maintaining weight and controlling pain. Emphasize nutrient-dense foods if intake has been poor.
- ✓ Bezoar formation may occur after eating oranges, coconuts, green beans, apples, figs, potato skins, Brussels sprouts, broccoli, and sauerkraut.

For More Information

- Diabetic gastroparesis
  http://www.niddk.nih.gov/health/digest/pubs/gastro/gastro.htm

DIABETIC KETOACIDOSIS OR DIABETIC COMA

NUTRITIONAL ACUITY RANKING: LEVEL 3

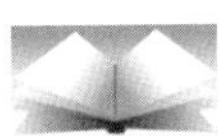

DEFINITIONS AND BACKGROUND

Diabetic ketoacidosis (DKA) is a medical emergency that accounts for over 10% of hospital admissions, with mortality about 2% per episode. Alkaline reserves may be depleted by infection, too little insulin, fever, pregnancy, stress, trauma, or myocardial infarction (MI). Stress and activation of counter regulatory hormones (glucagons, catecholamines) are often precipitating factors. Preceding diabetic coma, symptoms and signs include intense thirst, nausea and vomiting, dim vision, labored breathing, sweet acetone breath, pruritus, polyuria, hot/dry and flushed skin, cramping, seizures, and drowsiness. Hyperketonemia from DKA results in classic metabolic acidosis.

DKA is seen primarily in patients with type 1 diabetes, with about 3% of type 1 diabetic patients initially presenting with DKA. It can occur in type 2 diabetic patients, usually from urinary tract infections, trauma, stress, pregnancy, MI, surgery, or other causes.

OBJECTIVES

- Decrease hyperglycemia; provide insulin. Frequent monitoring is necessary.
- Correct electrolytes and hypovolemia or fluid imbalances. Optimal fluid management for DKA in children is uncertain (Felner and White, 2001).
- Promote return to wellness; patient most likely has been in poor health for several days preceding acidosis.
- Monitor for precipitating factors such as surgery, MI, or trauma.
- Prevent complications such as shock, arterial thrombosis, and cerebral edema.
- For chronically high fasting glucose levels, adjust evening intermediate or long-acting insulin doses or timing. Lose weight to reduce insulin resistance, if obese.

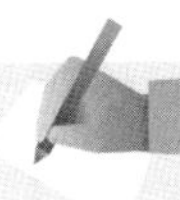

DIETARY AND NUTRITIONAL RECOMMENDATIONS

- If patient is in a coma, intravenous insulin, electrolytes, and fluids are used. A nasogastric tube may be placed to prevent aspiration during feeding.
- As treatment progresses, a 5% glucose solution is usually given as glucosuria and hyperglycemia subside. If glucosuria and hyperglycemia do not decrease, try tea and salty broth. Later, fruit juices and liquids high in potassium may be given.
- Eventually, return to usual diet. Monitor closely.
- A weight loss plan may be needed in obesity.

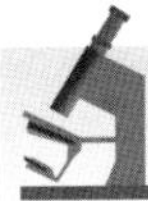

PROFILE

Clinical/History

Height
Weight
BMI
Nausea
Vomiting
BP (often low)
Tachycardia
Flushed face
Temperature
I & O
Diarrhea

Lab Work

Blood pH
BUN (increased)
Creat
K+, Na+ (decreased)
Cl− (decreased)
HbA1c
Amylase (increased)
Gluc (350–750 mg/dL; but may be as low as 250)
WBC (elevated with infections)
pCO2 (decreased); pO2
Acetone (increased)
Uric acid (increased)
Trig
AST (decreased)
ALT, LDH, creatine kinase (CK) (increased)
Bicarbonate < 15 mmol/L
Phosphate (decreased)
Chol (increased)
C-reactive protein
Mg++
pH below 7.3

Common Drugs Used and Potential Side Effects

- Insulin is usually given as an intravenous (IV) bolus. The goal is to decrease blood glucose by 50–75 mg/dL per hour.
- Dextrose in saline is often given once plasma glucose decreases to prevent accidental hypoglycemia.
- Potassium deficit is common, as are deficits of phosphate and magnesium.
- Intravenous antibiotic therapy will be needed for sepsis.

Herbs, Botanicals and Supplements

- Herbs and botanical supplements should not be used without discussing with physician.

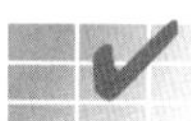

PATIENT EDUCATION

- ✓ Explain role of food and insulin during illness and infection. Discuss how timing, snacks, overconsumption at mealtimes, high-fat meals, insulin regimens, and stress may cause hyperglycemia.
- ✓ Explain role of exercise in lowering blood glucose levels.
- ✓ Discuss the Somogyi effect; discuss how rebounding occurs and how it is treated.
- ✓ Because every episode of DKA implies breakdown in clinical communication, appropriate diabetes education should be reinforced. Self-management skills during sick days, self-testing of urinary ketones, and timely contact with the medical advisor should be addressed.

NONKETOTIC HYPEROSMOLAR SYNDROME

NUTRITIONAL ACUITY RANKING: LEVEL 3

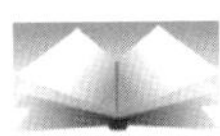

DEFINITIONS AND BACKGROUND

Nonketotic hyperosmolar syndrome (NKHS) is a metabolic disorder that leads to increased serum osmolality and dehydration. Blood glucose is extremely elevated, but ketosis is absent. The condition occurs in elderly patients with type 2 DM. Signs and symptoms include polydipsia, polyuria, nausea and vomiting, diarrhea, fever, respirations that are normal, profound dehydration, lethargy, confusion, grand mal seizures, tachycardia, hypotension, and oliguria.

Predisposing factors for NKHS include long-term uncontrolled hyperglycemia, pancreatic disease, infections or sepsis, stroke, surgery, extensive burns, renal or cardiovascular disease, cortisol steroid use, diuretics, TPN, dialysis, and excessive tube feeding.

OBJECTIVES

- Prevent or correct dehydrated state, shock, cardiac arrhythmias, and death.
- Monitor fluid status and replace deficits, which may be 10–20% of total body weight.
- Reduce elevated blood glucose levels, generally, with isotonic saline and then hypotonic saline.
- Prevent future crises by appropriate diabetes self-management education.
- Acute renal failure may result from prolonged hypovolemia.

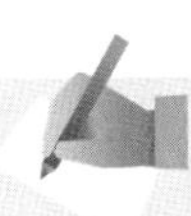

DIETARY AND NUTRITIONAL RECOMMENDATIONS

- Offer fluid replacement; often 1L per hour until volume is restored; 10–12 L may be needed.
- Patient is likely to be nil per os (nothing by mouth, NPO) during a crisis or perhaps tube fed during a comatose state.
- As appropriate, intake may be progressed gradually to a balanced diet, controlling calories as needed.
- Correct electrolyte deficits. Potassium may be needed.
- A renal diet plan may be needed if renal failure is identified.

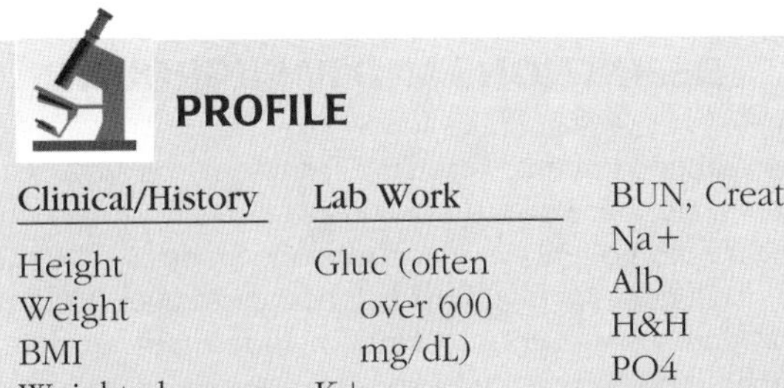

PROFILE

Clinical/History	Lab Work	
Height	Gluc (often over 600 mg/dL)	BUN, Creat
Weight	K+	Na+
BMI	Bicarbonate	Alb
Weight changes	Hyperosmolality (usually over 320mOsm)	H&H
I & O		PO4
Absence of ketonemia		Chol
BP		Trig
		C-reactive protein

Common Drugs Used and Potential Side Effects

- Insulin is needed to normalize blood glucose levels. Infusions will be needed until full rehydration is complete. Potassium replacements may be needed. Monitor carefully.
- Antibiotic therapy may be needed in cases of sepsis.

Herbs, Botanicals and Supplements

- Herbs and botanical supplements should not be used without discussing with physician.

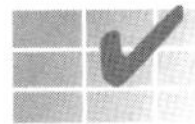

PATIENT EDUCATION

- ✓ Discuss, where possible, predisposing factors, how to avoid future incidents, etc.
- ✓ Calorie-controlled diets may be beneficial if patient can comprehend. Family intervention may be required.

HYPOGLYCEMIA

NUTRITIONAL ACUITY RANKING: LEVEL 2–3

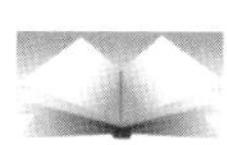

DEFINITIONS AND BACKGROUND

Except in diabetic patients receiving insulin or sulfonylureas, hypoglycemia is a rare disorder. Sources of bodily glucose are dietary intake, glycogenolysis, and gluconeogenesis. The metabolism of glucose involves oxidation and storage as glycogen or fat. Causes of hypoglycemia include medications or toxins capable of decreasing blood glucose, disorders associated with fasting hypoglycemia, and postprandial hypoglycemic disorders (Pourmotabbed and Kitabchi, 2001). Many different causes can stimulate hypoglycemia, and treatments through dietary means will differ accordingly. The most common type of hypoglycemia is insulin-induced hypoglycemia in diabetics. Insulinoma is rare; however, it is the most common hormone-secreting islet cell tumor; it is treated by surgical resection. See Spontaneous Hypoglycemia entry.

True low blood sugar (40 mg/100 mL or lower) releases hormones such as catecholamines, which produce hunger, trembling, headache, dizziness, weakness, and palpitations. Other factors also include skipped or insufficient meals, alcohol consumption, or extra physical exertion (Department of Medicine, 2001).

The body makes great effort to supply glucose for the CNS and red blood cells. Adrenergic stimulation of glucose output by the kidney, a defense mechanism against hypoglycemia in normal subjects, is impaired in patients with type 1 DM and contributes to defective glucose counter regulation (Cersosimo et al., 2001).

OBJECTIVES

- Normalize blood glucose levels. If the problem is recurrent, stabilize blood glucose levels through normal mealtimes, meal and CHO consistency, and blood glucose self-monitoring.
- Minimize length of time between meals.
- Prevent seizures and coma in true hypoglycemia (i.e., neuroglycopenia with confusion, light headaches, aberrant behavior, seizures, and frank coma). Under certain circumstances, ketones and lactate may substitute for glucose as a fuel for the brain, but this is not a predictable response (Veneman et al., 1994).
- Determine frequency, symptoms of hypoglycemia, activity levels, and exercise for the individual.

DIETARY AND NUTRITIONAL RECOMMENDATIONS

- For insulin-induced hypoglycemia, use a normal diet with adequate to high levels of CHOs. Have patient ingest fruit juice or carry candy as needed. Quick sources of glucose may be found in Table 9–14. Fat is not as effective as CHO in normalizing blood glucose.
- Frequent feedings may be beneficial.
- Ingestion of moderate amounts of caffeine may enhance the intensity of hypoglycemia warning symptoms in patients with type 1 DM (Watson et al., 2000). Use cautiously.
- In most cases, mild hypoglycemia can be handled with use of readily available CHOs, including cheese, milk, fruit, and crackers. Balanced, regular mealtimes are also useful.
- For hypoglycemia at night that is caused by excessive insulin or insufficient dinner meal or evening snack, evening and bedtime doses of insulin should be adjusted. A lightly larger dinner or snack containing CHO may be needed as well.

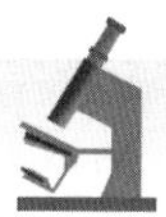

PROFILE

Clinical/History		
Height	Dizziness, weakness	Serum insulin
Weight	Palpitations	Acetone
BMI	Seizures or coma	Na+
I & O	**Lab Work**	K+
Temperature	Serum gluc	Chol, Trig
BP	HbA1c	Ca++, Mg++
Trembling		OGTT results using 1 g gluc/kg
Headache		

TABLE 9–14 Quick Sources of Glucose

1 cup skim milk (12 g CHO)
4 oz orange, apple, pineapple, or grapefruit juice (12–15 g CHO)
4 oz grape, cranberry, or prune juice (19 g CHO)
4 oz ginger ale or cola (13 g CHO)
1 T sugar (13 g CHO)
1 T corn syrup (15 g CHO)
5 lifesavers candies (15 g CHO)
6 oz ginger ale (16 g CHO)
1 T honey (17 g CHO)
½ cup sweetened gelatin (17 g CHO)
3 glucose tablets (15 g CHO)

Common Drugs Used and Potential Side Effects

- IV dextrose is indicated. In rare cases, intramuscular glucagon may be needed; vomiting is one side effect.
- Insulin and other glucose-lowering medications must be carefully prescribed and monitored.
- Chemotherapy (streptozocin, 5-fluorouracil) can be nephrotoxic; these drugs are often used for insulinomas. Monitor GI side effects.
- Glucose tablets (Becton Dickinson) have 15 g of CHO per tablet. Patients should receive instructions regarding their use (quantity, when to use, etc.).

Herbs, Botanicals and Supplements

- Herbs and botanical supplements should not be used without discussing with physician.

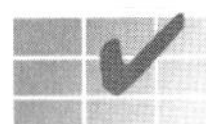

PATIENT EDUCATION

- ✔ Explain which foods are appropriate for between-meal snacks. Beware of the use of "dietetic" items when blood sugar levels need to be controlled more carefully.
- ✔ Discuss appropriate snacking patterns.
- ✔ Discuss observations that require medical attention.
- ✔ Promote regular mealtimes, meal spacing, and planned exercise.
- ✔ Discuss use of alcoholic beverages and potential effects.

SPONTANEOUS HYPOGLYCEMIA AND HYPERINSULINISM

NUTRITIONAL ACUITY RANKING: LEVEL 3

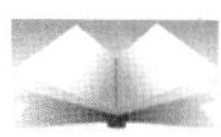

DEFINITIONS AND BACKGROUND

Spontaneous hypoglycemia is unrelated to diabetes. Fasting and postprandial hypoglycemia are categorized as spontaneous forms.

Fasting hypoglycemia may occur from an insulinoma such as an islet cell tumor. Tumor-induced hypoglycemia is secondary to inappropriate insulin secretion by a beta-cell pancreatic tumor (insulinoma) or, more rarely, to an extrapancreatic mesenchymal large tumor secreting IGF-II (Virally and Guillausseau, 1999). Congenital hyperinsulinism (CHI) is characterized by profound hypoglycemia because of excessive insulin secretion; one form, from a beta cell tumor, may be cured by partial pancreatectomy (Fournet et al., 2001).

In postprandial or alimentary hypoglycemia, excessive amounts of insulin are secreted 1.5–5 hours in response to CHO-rich foods. Postprandial hypoglycemia occurs in response to feeding and is generally caused by excessive insulin effect, often after gastric surgery and rarely in early diabetes mellitus (Pourmotabbed and Kitabchi, 2001). Symptoms resemble those of the dumping syndrome: weakness and agitation 2–4 hours after meals, perspiration, nervousness, and mental confusion. Postprandial reactive hypoglycemia (PRH) can be diagnosed if sympathetic and neuroglucopenic symptoms develop concurrently with low blood sugar (Brun et al., 2000). Neither the OGTT nor mixed meals are suitable for this diagnosis due to respectively false-positive and false-negative results. They should be replaced by ambulatory glycemic control or, as recently proposed, a hyperglycemic breakfast test. PRH patients often suffer from an associated adrenergic hormone postprandial syndrome, with consequences such as cardiac arrhythmia.

According to Brun et al. (2000), PRH could result from a) an exaggerated insulin response, either related to insulin resistance or to increased glucagon-like-peptide 1, b) renal glycosuria, c) defects in glucagon response, or d) high insulin sensitivity, probably the most frequent cause (50–70%), which is not adequately compensated by hypoinsulinemia and thus cannot be measured by indices of insulin sensitivity such as the homeostatic model assessment. Such situations are frequent in very lean people, after massive weight reduction, or in women with moderate lower body overweight. PRH is influenced by patient's alimentary habits (high-carbohydrate-low-fat diet, alcohol intake). Thus, diet remains the main treatment, although alpha-glucosidase inhibitors and some other drugs may be helpful. Exercise decreases insulin resistance and may have some effect on hypoglycemia but is not significant.

OBJECTIVES

- Reduce intake of concentrated CHO to a level that does not overstimulate the pancreas to secrete inappropriately large amounts of insulin, which may cause blood sugar to drop to 40 mg/dL or lower.
- Monitor patient carefully, because this condition can precede diabetes or can be related to mild overt diabetes.
- If required, ensure that patient loses weight, gradually.
- Reduce counter regulatory hormone responses to excessive insulin.

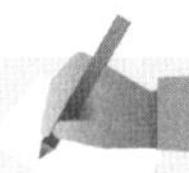

DIETARY AND NUTRITIONAL RECOMMENDATIONS

- Limit CHO intake to 35–40% of calories daily. Use more soluble-fiber foods such as fruits and vegetables. Reduce excess starches. Simple sugars and dried fruits are allowed in limited amounts.
- Maintain protein intake at RDA levels, because protein may stimulate insulin secretion. Fat furnishes the remainder of calories.
- Diet should include frequent small meals and at least a well-balanced diet.

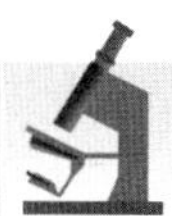

PROFILE

Clinical/History

Height
Weight
BMI
Recent weight losses
BP
Seizures, confusion
Palpitations

Lab Work

Gluc (decreased)
Serum insulin
Serum glucagon
Chol
Trig
K+, Na+
Trig
HgA1c
Ca++, Mg++
Acetone
PO4
C-reactive protein

Common Drugs Used and Potential Side Effects

- Alpha-glucosidase inhibitors may be useful for postprandial hypoglycemia, but this requires further study.
- Monitor all medications for their potential hypoglycemic effects.

Herbs, Botanicals and Supplements

- Herbs and botanical supplements should not be used without discussing with physician.

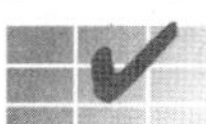

PATIENT EDUCATION

- ✔ Explain that alcohol blocks gluconeogenesis and should be avoided.
- ✔ Ensure that patient keeps snacks available such as cheese and crackers.
- ✔ Emphasize that meals should not be skipped and that large meals should not be taken. Meals should be eaten on time.
- ✔ Avoid any one meal that is unbalanced or especially high in carbohydrates.
- ✔ Control caffeine intake and use of other stimulants, which may aggravate condition.

INSULIN RESISTANCE SYNDROME (METABOLIC SYNDROME)

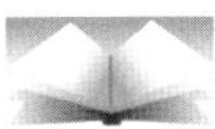

DEFINITIONS AND BACKGROUND

Insulin Resistance Syndrome or Metabolic Syndrome (formerly Syndrome X) has simultaneous insulin resistance, hypertension, dyslipidemia, and an abnormal glucose tolerance test. The syndrome was first labeled in 1988. Persons with insulin resistance often have multiple disturbances that can lead to coronary heart disease and diabetes; this condition may affect as many as 25% of young adults and over half of those persons aged 55 and above (Maki and Kurlandsky, 2001).

In postmenopausal women, the combination of low birth weight (LBW) and adult obesity is a strong determinant of metabolic syndrome (Yarbrough et al., 1998). Genes that increase birth weight also worsen the metabolic syndrome including abdominal obesity, insulin resistance, hyperinsulinemia, glucose intolerance, dyslipidemia, and hypertension (Stern et al., 2000). Whether this syndrome is purely genetic is not known at this time. A stress-related hormone may hold the key; known as HSD-1, this hormone has been studied for its Cushing's syndrome-like effects. Excessive calorie consumption, physical inactivity, excess weight, and smoking may also contribute. Individuals who are obese and insulin resistant are particularly prone to the adverse effects of a high dietary glycemic load (Liu and Manson, 2001).

An "apple-shaped" figure is risky because fat cells located in the abdomen release fat into the blood more easily than fat cells found elsewhere. Release of fat begins 3–4 hours after the last meal compared to many more hours for other fat cells, leading to higher TG and free fatty acid levels. Free fatty acids themselves cause insulin resistance. Obesity should be addressed, especially for those persons with the apple-shaped figure.

Low HDL levels are common, as are elevated triglycerides, hemostatic disturbances, microvascular angina, and central obesity, although not all individuals with this syndrome are obese. Uric acid levels may also be elevated and abnormal blood clotting activity due to increased plasminogen-activating inhibitor-1 may also persist.

More hypertension, coronary heart disease, and age-related disorders seem to occur in this insulin-resistant population (Facchini et al., 2001). It is estimated that 5–10% of individuals with this syndrome will go on to develop type 2 diabetes. Table 9–15 provides clinical identifiers that are used to diagnose the metabolic syndrome.

TABLE 9–15 Clinical Identifiers for Metabolic Syndrome

Abdominal obesity—Waist circumference, men over 40 inches; women over 35 inches
Triglycerides—Over 150 mg/dL
HDL cholesterol below 40 in men; below 50 in women
Blood pressure equal to or over 130/85
Fasting glucose equal to or greater than 110 mg/dL

http://www.nhlbi.nih.gov/guidelines/cholesterol/atp3xsum.pdf

OBJECTIVES

- Reduce underlying causes (i.e., obesity, physical inactivity).
- Reduce lipid risk factors. To match the new Adult Treatment Panel III guidelines for managing the metabolic syndrome, lower elevated blood lipids. The goal for LDL is less than 100; total cholesterol below 200; and HDL at least 40 but preferably 60 or higher. Lower elevated triglycerides to levels below 150 mg/dL.
- Achieve improved body weight; maintain it to lessen abdominal obesity in particular.
- Achieve and maintain blood glucose levels less than 110 mg/dL.
- Lower elevated blood pressure; goal less than 130/85.
- Prevent complications such as type 2 diabetes and atherothrombotic cardiovascular disease (Cohn et al., 2001).

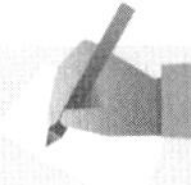

DIETARY AND NUTRITIONAL RECOMMENDATIONS

- To lower LDL cholesterol and lipid levels, control saturated and trans-fatty acid intake; 35–40% kilocalories from total fat is acceptable. Increase use of omega-3 and omega-6 fatty acids (30–35% of kilocalories) and keep SFA down to 5–10%. The Mediterranean diet plan has been somewhat useful (Maki and Kurlandsky, 2001).
- Plan a diet using more fiber and starches, especially whole grains, raw fruits, and vegetables (Liu and Manson, 2001). A diet with 45–50% CHO levels has been suggested; monitor blood glucose levels accordingly.

- Protein should be maintained at 15% kilocalories. Encourage soy protein as a meat substitute several times a week.
- Ensure adequate intake of vitamins such as folate, vitamins B6, B12, C, and E.
- Follow a 3–4 g sodium diet; include good sources of potassium.
- There may be advantages to spreading nutrient load by eating smaller meals or foods with lower glycemic index (Maki and Kurlandsky, 2001).

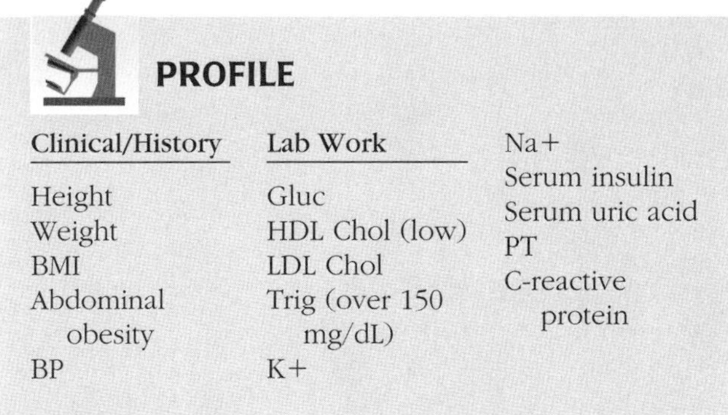

PROFILE

Clinical/History	Lab Work	
Height	Gluc	Na+
Weight	HDL Chol (low)	Serum insulin
BMI	LDL Chol	Serum uric acid
Abdominal obesity	Trig (over 150 mg/dL)	PT
BP	K+	C-reactive protein

Common Drugs Used and Potential Side Effects

- Glucose-lowering medications must be carefully prescribed and monitored. Metformin may be indicated
- Blood pressure medications may be prescribed; monitor for necessary restrictions of sodium and/or higher need for potassium.
- Medications that diminish insulin resistance and directly alter lipoproteins are also necessary; combination therapy is often required to optimize attainment of treatment goals (Cohn et al., 2001).

Herbs, Botanicals and Supplements

- Herbs and botanical supplements should not be used without discussing with physician.

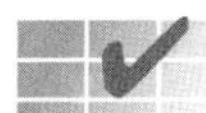

PATIENT EDUCATION

✔ Discuss role of nutrition and weight control in managing or controlling this syndrome.

✔ Exercise daily. Aerobic and strength training exercises are helpful.

✔ Smoking cessation measures should be taken where needed.

✔ Reduce consumption of alcoholic beverages, which may elevate triglycerides.

POLYCYSTIC OVARIAN SYNDROME

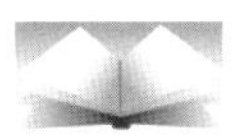

DEFINITIONS AND BACKGROUND

Polycystic ovary syndrome (PCOS) is an endocrine disorder characterized by hyperandrogenism, bilaterally enlarged polycystic ovaries and insulin resistance. This syndrome affects about 6–10% of women of childbearing age; it is a leading cause of infertility (Barbieri, 2000).

The syndrome of hyperandrogenism, insulin resistance, and acanthosis nigricans (HAIR-AN syndrome) is one presentation of the insulin-resistant subset of polycystic ovary syndrome (Barbieri, 2000). Insulin resistance and hyperandrogenism are caused by genetic and environmental factors. Acanthosis nigricans is a dark, velvety patch of skin that indicates insulin resistance (Scalzo and McKittrick, 2000). Women of Caribbean-Hispanic or African-American descent seem to be more prone to this condition.

Women with PCOS may have had a history of GDM. Many adolescents present with hirsutism and irregular menses. In PCOS, elevated luteinizing hormone (LH):follicle-stimulating hormone (FSH) ratio, hirsutism, acne, oily skin, male pattern baldness, menstrual irregularity, oligomenorrhea, and obesity can occur. Abnormally elevated levels of testosterone and LH disrupt the normal maturation process for ovulation. Immature cysts remain on the ovaries, giving the appearance of a "string of pearls." Biochemical abnormalities include hyperandrogenism, acyclic estrogen production, LH hypersecretion, decreased levels of steroid hormone-binding globulin (SHBG), and hyperinsulinemia. Infertility, hypertension, uterine cancer, diabetes, coronary heart disease, and endometrial carcinoma often follow (Legro, 2001; Kahn and Gordon, 1999).

OBJECTIVES

- Lose weight or maintain a normal weight for height; obesity is common in 50% of this population.
- Prevent coronary heart problems, including dyslipidemia and hypertension.
- Reduce serum androgens and improve reproductive function.
- Decrease risk for endometrial cancer.
- Alleviate glucose intolerance and insulin resistance.

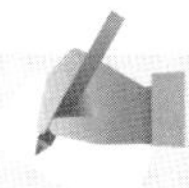

DIETARY AND NUTRITIONAL RECOMMENDATIONS

- Offer a weight control and exercise plan to meet weight goals. Loss of 5–10& may reduce symptoms.
- Lower elevated blood glucose, lipids.
- The DASH diet may be helpful to lower blood pressure. Avoid low fat-high CHO diets, which promote extra insulin secretion (McKittrick, 2002). A diet of 30–40% fat may be needed.

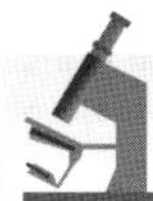

PROFILE

Clinical/History

Height
Weight
BMI
Weight gain pattern
Hx GDM
Irregular menses
Amenorrhea
Hirsutism
Infertility
Acne
Male pattern baldness
Acanthosis nigricans (dark, velvety patches on skin)

Lab Work

Glucose
C-reactive protein
Trig
Serum insulin
Serum estrogen
Serum testosterone
LH
LH:FSH ratio (elevated)
H&H
Alb
BUN/Creat
ALT
BP (elevated)

Common Drugs Used and Potential Side Effects

- Oral contraceptives and other antiandrogens are useful.
- Insulin-sensitizing drugs such as Troglitazone improve ovulation and hirsutism in PCOS (Azziz et al., 2001). Metformin allows for improved insulin sensitivity, reduced LH and testosterone. Do not use with CHF, chronic obstructive pulmonary disease (COPD), or chronic renal failure. Take with food; monitor for GI side effects such as nausea, diarrhea, and flatulence.
- While not FDA approved for this indication, Avandia and Actos may be used for improving serum glucose levels. Monitor for hepatic toxicity.

Herbs, Botanicals and Supplements

- Herbs and botanical supplements should not be used without discussing with physician.

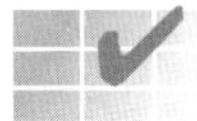

PATIENT EDUCATION

- Counsel about weight loss and nutrition. Regular mealtimes and snacks may help control cravings and overeating.
- Encourage regular exercise.
- Explain relationship of insulin resistance and increased risk for type 2 diabetes.

For More Information

- Polycystic Ovarian Syndrome Association, Inc
  P.O. Box 7007
  Rosemont, IL 60018-7007
  http://www.pcosupport.org

PREGNANCY-INDUCED HYPERTENSION

NUTRITIONAL ACUITY RANKING: LEVEL 3

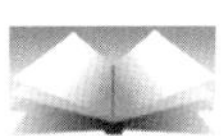

DEFINITIONS AND BACKGROUND

Pregnancy-induced hypertension (PIH) is a syndrome of edema, proteinuria, and hypertension (EPH-gestosis) that occurs during the second half of pregnancy (usually after week 20), more often in primigravidas, multiple gestation, malnutrition, hydatidiform mole, positive family history of PIH, and underlying vascular disease. The condition occurs in approximately 10% of all pregnancies. Early sonogram is recommended in high-risk cases.

Preeclampsia is defined as the presence of hypertension or PIH accompanied by proteinuria, edema, or both. Preeclampsia is divided into mild and severe forms. Criteria for mild preeclampsia include hypertension as defined at 140/90 to 159/109; proteinuria >300 mg/24 hours; mild edema with weight gain >2 lb/week or >6 lb/month; urine output >500 ml/24 hours. Preeclampsia is associated with high body mass index, insulin resistance, and hypertriglyceridemia. One study suggests that high intakes of energy, sucrose, and polyunsaturated fatty acids independently increase the risk for preeclampsia (Clausen et al., 2001).

Criteria for severe preeclampsia include: BP >160/110 on 2 occasions with patient on bed rest; systolic BP rise >60 mm Hg over baseline; diastolic BP rise >30 mm Hg over baseline; proteinuria >5 g/24 hours or 3+ or 4+ on urine dipstick; massive edema; oliguria <400 ml/24 hours; symptoms including pulmonary edema, headaches, visual changes, right upper quadrant pain, elevated liver enzymes, or thrombocytopenia.

Signs and symptoms include increased blood pressure, proteinuria, facial edema, pretibial pitting edema, irritability, nausea and vomiting, nervousness, severe headache, altered states of consciousness, epigastric pain, and oliguria. In eclampsia, there is an occurrence of a seizure. Eclamptic seizures, (hemolysis, elevated liver function tests, low platelet count (HELLP) syndrome, hepatic rupture, pulmonary edema, acute renal failure, placental abruption, intrauterine fetal demise (IUFD), cerebral hemorrhage, cortical blindness, and retinal detachment are all potential risks in the severe state. Home bed rest is usually required.

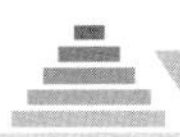

OBJECTIVES

- Normalize abnormal blood pressures to prevent eclamptic seizures and death.
- Prevent, if possible, chronic hypertension after delivery.
- Lessen any edema that is present.
- Correct any underlying protein–calorie malnutrition.
- Monitor any sudden weight gains (more than 1 kg/week) that are unexplained by food intake.

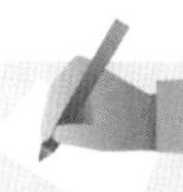

DIETARY AND NUTRITIONAL RECOMMENDATIONS

- Maintain diet as ordered for age and pregnancy stage (generally 300 kcal more than prepregnancy diet). Use extra fruits and vegetables, less sucrose.
- A multivitamin–mineral supplement may be needed, because inadequate intakes of vitamins C and B6 have been implicated by some studies.
- Adequate calcium, protein, calories, and potassium will be necessary.
- Sodium intake may need to be controlled to 1–2 g/day.
- Linoleic and arachidonic acids have been used to serve as vasodilators in some cases. This should be done under careful medical supervision.

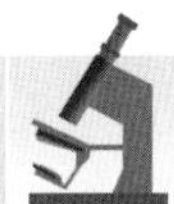

PROFILE

Clinical/History

Height
Weight
BMI
Weight gain pattern
Edema
BP (severe is higher than 160/110)

Lab Work

GFR
Ca++
Alb, prealbumin (often low)
Proteinuria (more than 0.3 g/L/day is mild; more than 5 g/L/day may be severe)
H&H, Serum Fe
Gluc
Mg++
K+, Na+
Uric acid (may be elevated)
BUN, Creat
Coagulation series (PT, prothrombin time [PTT], fibrinogen degradation)
HELLP syndrome
Liver function tests (AST, ALT, LDH)

Common Drugs Used and Potential Side Effects

- Thiazide diuretics can cause electrolyte imbalances, hyperglycemia, hyperuricemia, and pancreatitis. They usually are not beneficial in treatment and may harm the fetus. They are used only in rare cases of congestive heart failure and severe chronic hypertension during pregnancy.
- Magnesium sulfate is often used to control seizures. Excess may cause drowsiness or postpartum hemorrhage.
- Some studies suggest that calcium supplementation may reduce PIH. More studies are needed.

- During pregnancy, ACE inhibitors, diuretics, and many other cardiac drugs are not to be used.
- Monitor side effects of other medications being used for chronic illnesses; some may be high in sodium.

Herbs, Botanicals and Supplements

- Herbs and botanical supplements should not be used without discussing with physician.

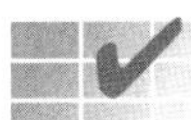

PATIENT EDUCATION

- ✓ Rest is essential during this time. Biofeedback and other forms of stress reduction are often beneficial.
- ✓ Meal skipping should be avoided at all costs.
- ✓ Discuss adequate sources of calcium from the diet, especially if dairy products are not tolerated or preferred.
- ✓ Good sources of potassium include many fruits and vegetables.

OTHER ENDOCRINE DISORDERS

ADRENOCORTICAL INSUFFICIENCY AND ADDISON'S DISEASE

NUTRITIONAL ACUITY RANKING: LEVEL 3

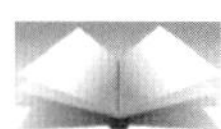

DEFINITIONS AND BACKGROUND

In adrenocortical insufficiency, the adrenal cortex atrophies with loss of hormones (aldosterone, cortisol, and androgens). The condition often results from tuberculosis, cancer, or surgery. Of patients with adrenocortical insufficiency, 33% also have diabetes. Signs and symptoms include abdominal pain, vomiting, weakness, fatigue, weight loss, dehydration, nausea, diarrhea, hyperpigmented (tan or bronze) skin, and hypotension.

Acute adrenal insufficiency involves low blood pressure, low serum sodium, high serum potassium, and low corticosteroid levels. It may be temporary or may become a chronic insufficiency. Addison's disease is a strict insufficiency state. An Addisonian crisis can be precipitated by acute infection, trauma, surgery, or excessive body salt loss.

Note that aldosterone functions to conserve sodium and excrete potassium. When aldosterone is no longer secreted normally, the following events occur: Excretion of sodium takes place; the body's store of water decreases, leading to dehydration, hypotension, and decreased cardiac output. The heart becomes slower due to reduced workload. Increased serum potassium can lead to arrhythmias, arrest, and even death.

Adrenalectomy may require steroid replacement therapy and a 2-g Na+ diet; hyperglycemia may result.

OBJECTIVES

- ▲ Replace lost hormones with synthetic hormones.
- ▲ Prevent hypoglycemia; avoid fasting.
- ▲ Prevent weight loss. Improve appetite and strength.
- ▲ Modify sodium according to drug therapy. Prevent hyponatremia, especially in warm weather when sodium losses from perspiration are higher than usual.
- ▲ Prevent dehydration and shock.
- ▲ Correct diarrhea, hyperkalemia, nausea, and drug overdosage.

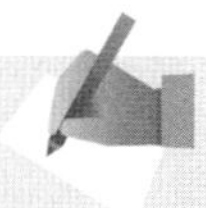

DIETARY AND NUTRITIONAL RECOMMENDATIONS

- Use a high-protein, moderate-carbohydrate diet. Snacks may be needed.
- Ensure intake of sodium is high, unless drugs are used to retain sodium.
- Restrict refined CHO to prevent overstimulation of insulin (with resulting hypoglycemia).
- Supplement diet with vitamins B-complex and C for increased metabolic requirements.
- Beware of foods that are high in potassium, unless drugs are used to control potassium.
- Force fluids—2–3 L if allowed.

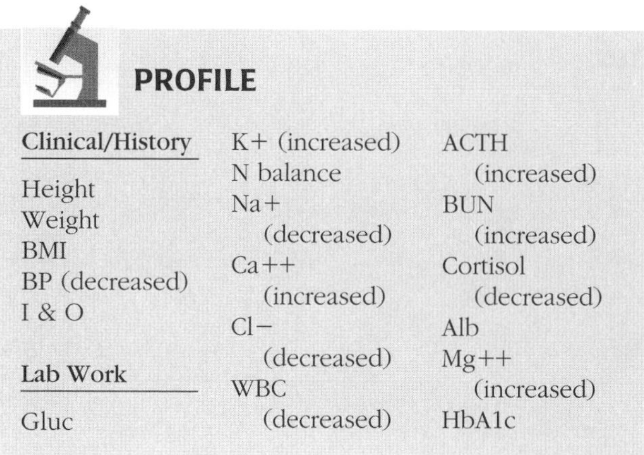

PROFILE

Clinical/History

Height
Weight
BMI
BP (decreased)
I & O

Lab Work

Gluc
K+ (increased)
N balance
Na+ (decreased)
Ca++ (increased)
Cl− (decreased)
WBC (decreased)
ACTH (increased)
BUN (increased)
Cortisol (decreased)
Alb
Mg++ (increased)
HbA1c

Common Drugs Used and Potential Side Effects

- Cortisone (20–30 mg common). Extra dietary salt may be needed.
- Fludrocortisone (Florinef) is a sodium-retaining hormone. Fludrocortisone does not demand an increase in dietary sodium. Be wary about overdosing. Side effects include HPN and ankle edema or postural hypotension with a low dose.

Herbs, Botanicals and Supplements

- Herbs and botanical supplements should not be used without discussing with physician.

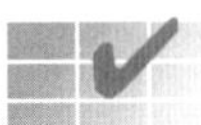

PATIENT EDUCATION

- Help patient individualize diet according to symptoms.
- To decrease gastric irritation, ensure patient takes hormone with milk or antacid.
- Ensure patient does not skip meals. Instruct patient to carry cheese or cracker snack to prevent hypoglycemia.
- Discuss simple meal preparation to lessen fatigue.
- Use of Medic-Alert identification is recommended.
- Pregnancy is possible but must be managed with additional replacement medication.

For More Information

- National Adrenal Diseases Foundation
  505 Northern Blvd.
  Great Neck, NY 11021
  (516) 487-4992
  http://www.medhelp.org/nadf/

CUSHING'S SYNDROME

NUTRITIONAL ACUITY RANKING: LEVEL 2

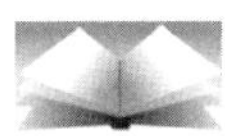

DEFINITIONS AND BACKGROUND

Cushing's Syndrome is a disease caused by an excess of cortisol production or excess use of cortisol or other similar steroid (glucocorticoid) hormones. It can be caused by extrinsic and excessive hormonal stimulation of the adrenal cortex by tumor of the anterior pituitary gland, adrenal hyperplasia, or exogenous cortisol use. Excess ACTH is secreted.

Pituitary Cushing's disease occurs after puberty with equal frequency in boys and girls. In adults, it has a greater frequency in women than men, with most found at ages 25–45. The total incidence is about 5–25 cases per million people per year (http://www.medhelp.org/nadf/nadf4.htm). It is a disorder characterized by virilism, obesity, hyperglycemia, glucosuria, hypertension, moon face, emotional lability, buffalo hump, purple striae over obese areas, and pitting ankle edema. In some cases, massive osteoporosis may also be present.

Treatment varies by cause: ACTH dependent (pituitary or ectopic) or independent (an adrenal tumor) or iatrogenic (from excessive steroid hormone use). If iatrogenic, removal of steroid hormones will be needed. If pituitary, the gland may need to be removed. If from an adrenal tumor, radiation, chemotherapy, or surgery may be needed.

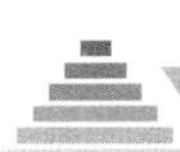

OBJECTIVES

- Control symptoms of elevated blood glucose.
- Promote weight loss if needed. Control patient's weight while increasing lean body mass.
- Control symptoms of hypertension.
- Prevent vertebral collapse and other side effects such as congestive heart failure, bone demineralization, osteoporosis, and hypokalemia.
- Control side effects of corticosteroid therapy.

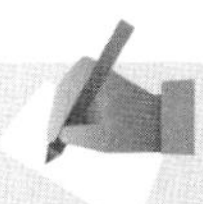

DIETARY AND NUTRITIONAL RECOMMENDATIONS

- Restrict sodium if steroids are used.
- Use a calorie-controlled diet, if needed. Calculate diet according to patient's desirable body weight. Control glucose levels, if required.
- Ensure adequate intake of calcium and potassium.
- Ensure adequate intake of protein, if losses are excessive, e.g., 1 g protein/kg or more.

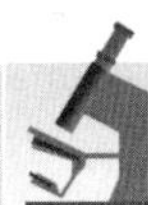

PROFILE

Clinical/History

Height
Weight
BMI
BP (increased)
Edema

Lab Work

ACTH levels (elevated)
Urinary gluc (increased)
Urinary Ca+
Alb
Gluc (increased)
Serum Ca++
Chol
K+ (decreased)
N balance
Na+ (increased)
pCO2 (increased); pO2
WBC, TLC (decreased)
Urinary and plasma cortisol (increased)
Glucose tolerance test (GTT)
HbA1c
CT scan
DEXA scan

Common Drugs Used and Potential Side Effects

- Glucocorticoid therapy. Osteoporosis and hypercalciuria are common side effects of these drugs.
- Large doses of Vitamin D may be necessary; do not use for extended periods of time because toxicity may occur.

Herbs, Botanicals and Supplements

- Herbs and botanical supplements should not be used without discussing with physician.

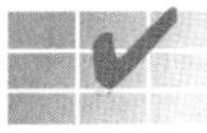

PATIENT EDUCATION

- Help patient control weight as needed.
- Explain which foods are good sources of calcium in the diet.
- Explain how to control elevated blood sugars through balanced dietary intake.

For More Information

- Cushing's Support and Research Foundation
  http://www.world.std.com/~csrf/

ACROMEGALY

NUTRITIONAL ACUITY RANKING: LEVEL 2

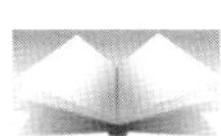

DEFINITIONS AND BACKGROUND

Acromegaly is caused by overproduction of growth hormone (GH). Incidence is rare, with 50–70 cases per million in the U.S. population. Diagnosis commonly is made about a decade after over-secretion of GH begins.

GH (somatotropin) affects the growth of almost all cells and tissues and has direct and indirect effects. Direct effects of GH include hyperinsulinism, lipolysis, insulin resistance in peripheral tissues, ketogenesis, hyperglycemia, and sodium and water retention. Elevated insulin-like growth factor (IGF-1) also occurs in acromegaly; induction of greater protein synthesis, amino acid transportation, muscle and bone growth, DNA and RNA synthesis, and cell proliferation.

Symptoms and signs of acromegaly include disproportionate growth (facial features, tongue, hands, and feet), increase in coarse body hair, coarse and leathery skin, excessive diaphoresis and skin oiliness, visual impairment, premature osteoarthritis, carpal tunnel syndrome, headaches, moderate weight gain, heart failure, and diabetes in 25–30%. Surgical removal of the pituitary gland may help.

OBJECTIVES

- Control weight and metabolic rate, which may be increased.
- Control diabetes and heart disease when involved.
- Alter phosphorus intake when needed (because tubular reabsorption of phosphate may be increased).
- Prevent osteoporosis with calcium balance (often negative in acromegaly).
- Monitor for complications such as colon polyps, which may lead to cancer.

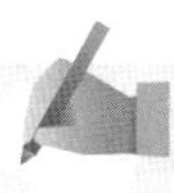

DIETARY AND NUTRITIONAL RECOMMENDATIONS

- A diet with controlled calories (higher or lower) may be needed to control weight.
- Extra fluid intake may be needed, often 2–3 L daily.
- Adequate Ca:P ratio is needed, at least 1:1.
- Control sodium as needed for heart failure.

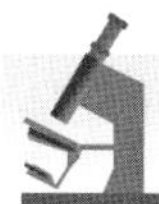

PROFILE

Clinical/History	Lab Work	
Height	N balance	Gluc, HbA1c
Weight	Phosphorus (P) (increased)	Ca++ (decreased)
BMI	BUN	Alb
BP (increased)	Serum Creat (increased)	GH
I & O	Urine sugar	GTT
		K+
		H&H

Common Drugs Used and Potential Side Effects

- Sandostatin (octreotide) injection may be used. Side effects include diarrhea, nausea, gallstones, and loose stools.
- Insulin may be needed if diabetes is also present. Be wary of excess dosages; hypoglycemia is a dangerous side effect.
- Cardiac medications may be needed with heart failure; monitor for specific side effects accordingly.
- Physicians must be aware of the risks of the use of GH in other medical conditions, especially if used for prolonged periods of time or in large doses.

Herbs, Botanicals and Supplements

- Herbs and botanical supplements should not be used without discussing with physician.

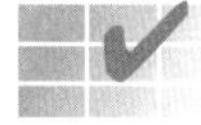

PATIENT EDUCATION

- ✓ Discuss body changes and self-image alterations.
- ✓ Teach patient about control of diabetes, where present.

HYPERALDOSTERONISM

NUTRITIONAL ACUITY RANKING: LEVEL 2

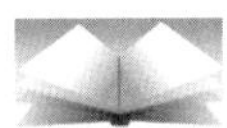

DEFINITIONS AND BACKGROUND

An increased production of aldosterone by the adrenal cortex, hyperaldosteronism may be primary (usually from adenoma) or secondary (cancer, CHF, hyperplasia, malignant hypertension, pregnancy, estrogen use, or cirrhosis). Conn's syndrome is a benign tumor in one adrenal gland that can cause this condition. Signs and symptoms include hypertension, headache, cardiomegaly, hypokalemia, paresthesia, polyuria, polydipsia, azotemia, muscle spasms in hands and feet, and tetany.

OBJECTIVES

- ▲ Hydrate adequately.
- ▲ Alter diet as needed for testing (sodium, potassium).
- ▲ Correct hypokalemia and other altered electrolytes.
- ▲ Prepare for surgery if a tumor is involved.

DIETARY AND NUTRITIONAL RECOMMENDATIONS

- Provide adequate fluid intake (unless contraindicated for other reasons).
- Use a high or low sodium intake for testing (6 g Na+ load is common).
- A high potassium intake may be required.
- Small, frequent feedings may be needed.

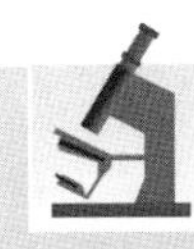

PROFILE

Clinical/History		
Height	BP	Aldosterone levels
Weight	**Lab Work**	K+, Na+
BMI	Urine sugar	H&H, Serum Fe
I & O	Plasma renin	

Common Drugs Used and Potential Side Effects

- Antihypertensives may be used; monitor side effects specifically for the medications prescribed. Spironolactone may be used if surgery is not indicated.
- Digitalis is often used. Avoid herbal teas, high fiber intakes, and excessive amounts of vitamin D. Include adequate amounts of potassium. Take the drug 30 minutes before meals.

Herbs, Botanicals and Supplements

- Herbs and botanical supplements should not be used without discussing with physician.

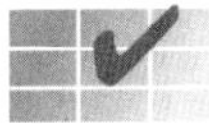

PATIENT EDUCATION

- ✓ Explain altered sodium and potassium requirements, as appropriate.
- ✓ Have patient avoid fasting, skipping meals, and fad dieting.
- ✓ Provide recipe suggestions.

HYPOPITUITARISM

NUTRITIONAL ACUITY RANKING: LEVEL 2

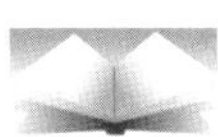

DEFINITIONS AND BACKGROUND

A deficiency in production of pituitary hormones, hypopituitarism may be caused by tumor, aneurysm, infarction, or surgery. The condition is relatively rare. In children, short stature results (10% of all dwarfism). Skinfold thickness greater than 50% for age shows greater subcutaneous fat deposition with decreased muscle mass. Symptoms and signs include sexual dysfunction, weakness, easy fatigue, and lack of resistance to cold and stress. Vascular abnormalities are common (Kearney et al., 2001).

OBJECTIVES

- Replenish stores.
- Prevent dehydration and hypoglycemia.
- Improve lean muscle mass stores.
- Monitor serum levels of cholesterol and triglycerides; prevent side effects of elevated levels.

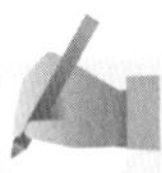

DIETARY AND NUTRITIONAL RECOMMENDATIONS

- High-calorie/high-protein diet with a moderate-to-high salt intake may be needed. A modified fat, cholesterol, and CHO intake should be planned.
- Six small feedings may be better tolerated.
- Increase fluids unless contraindicated.
- Ensure adequate intake of all vitamins and minerals.

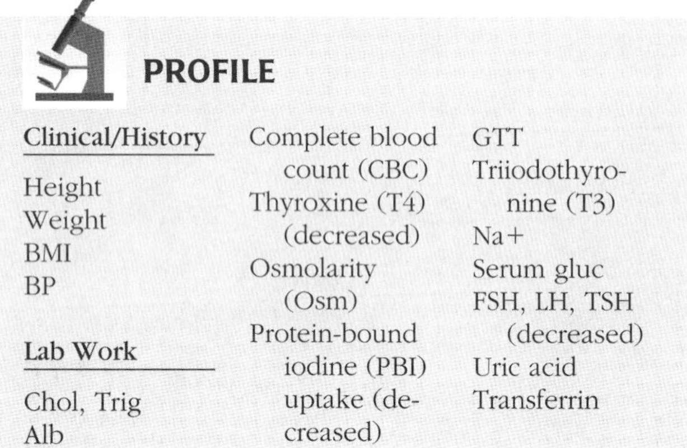

PROFILE

Clinical/History

Height
Weight
BMI
BP

Lab Work

Chol, Trig
Alb
Complete blood count (CBC)
Thyroxine (T4) (decreased)
Osmolarity (Osm)
Protein-bound iodine (PBI) uptake (decreased)
GTT
Triiodothyronine (T3)
Na+
Serum gluc
FSH, LH, TSH (decreased)
Uric acid
Transferrin

Common Drugs Used and Potential Side Effects

- Corticosteroids (hydrocortisone [Cortef], cortisol) are often used and can alter glucose, calcium, and phosphate tolerance. K+ and folacin must be increased and sodium must be decreased. Monitor for signs of diabetes.
- Thyroid preparations may be needed.
- GH, when given, requires no specific dietary interventions. It may help alleviate elevated triglycerides.

Herbs, Botanicals and Supplements

- Herbs and botanical supplements should not be used without discussing with physician.

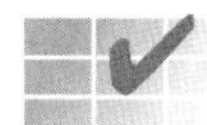

PATIENT EDUCATION

- Have patient avoid fasting and stress.
- Discuss the need to use small, frequent meals instead of large meals.
- Discuss the possibility of hyperglycemia and how to manage.

PHEOCHROMOCYTOMA

NUTRITIONAL ACUITY RANKING: LEVEL 2

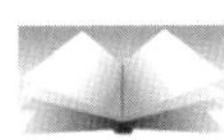

DEFINITIONS AND BACKGROUND

Pheochromocytoma is a rare tumor of the chromaffin cells most commonly arising from the adrenal medulla, resulting in increased secretion of the hormones epinephrine and norepinephrine. It is slightly more common in males and may be transmitted as an autosomal dominant trait.

Symptoms and signs include very high blood pressure, headache, excessive diaphoresis, and palpitations. Less common are symptoms of syncope, pallor or flushing of skin, weight loss, nausea, anorexia, nervousness, and hypermetabolism with normal T4. About 10% of these tumors are malignant.

Diagnosis often involves measurement of urinary catecholamines or their metabolites, vanillylmandelic acid, and total metanephrines; the urinary metanephrines provide a more sensitive clue to the presence of pheochromocytoma. Treatment usually involves surgical removal of the tumor.

OBJECTIVES

- Avoid over-stimulation (even slight exercise, cold stress, or emotional upsets).
- Correct nausea, vomiting, and anorexia.
- Prepare for surgery to remove tumor, if feasible.
- Prevent hypertensive crisis (which could cause sudden blindness or cerebrovascular accidents [CVAs]).

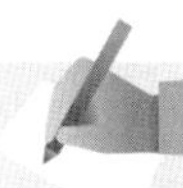

DIETARY AND NUTRITIONAL RECOMMENDATIONS

- Increase fluids but avoid caffeinated beverages.
- Six small feedings may be better tolerated than large meals.
- For testing, a vanillylmandelic acid (VMA)-restricted diet may be required for lab results (i.e., omit chocolate, vanilla extract, and citrus). Check with diagnostic personnel.
- Increase protein and calories if patient will have surgery. Postoperatively, provide adequate vitamins and minerals for wound healing.
- Reexpansion of plasma volume may be accomplished by liberal salt or fluid intake with use of alpha-1 adrenergic receptor antagonists.
- In recurrent cases, long-term drug therapy will be needed. Monitor for specific dietary changes and side effects.

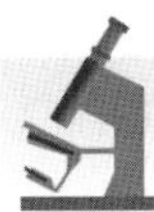

PROFILE

Clinical/History	Lab Work	
Height Weight BMI BP (very elevated) Orthostatic hypotension	Gluc T3, T4 Urinary Epinephrine and Norepinephrine (increased) Urinary catecholamine metabolites (VMA and Metanephrines)	Alb H&H Glucagon test (positive) CT scan

Common Drugs Used and Potential Side Effects

- Pharmacologic treatment of catecholamine excess is mandatory.
- Phenoxybenzamine (or alpha-1 adrenergic receptor antagonists such as prazosin) is needed to block alpha-adrenergic activity. Diuretics should not be used.
- Low doses of a beta-blocker such as propranolol are used to control blood pressure and cardiac tachyarrhythmias, but only after alpha blockade is established.
- Labetalol, an alpha- and beta-adrenergic blocker, has also been shown to be effective in the control of blood pressure and symptoms of pheochromocytoma.

Herbs, Botanicals and Supplements

- Herbs and botanical supplements should not be used without discussing with physician.

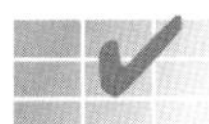

PATIENT EDUCATION

- ✓ Discuss avoidance of caffeinated foods and beverages (e.g., coffee, tea, and chocolate).
- ✓ Maintain a calm atmosphere for patient; prevent undue stress.

HYPERTHYROIDISM

NUTRITIONAL ACUITY RANKING: LEVEL 2

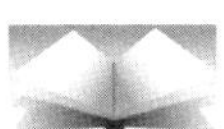

DEFINITIONS AND BACKGROUND

Hyperthyroidism results from over secretion of the thyroid hormones, thyroxine, and/or triiodothyronine. Most often, the entire gland is overproducing thyroid hormone; rarely, a single nodule is responsible for the excess hormone secretion.

An elevated metabolic rate, tissue wasting, diaphoresis, tremor, tachycardia, heat intolerance, cold insensitivity, tremor, nervousness, increased appetite, exophthalmos, and loss of glycogen stores may result. Thyrotoxicosis and Graves' disease (toxic goiter) are the more severe forms. Fifty percent of persons suffering from Graves' disease have had relatives with altered thyroid functioning. Some underlying hereditary condition may exist. Hyperthyroidism is eight times more common in women.

Thyroidectomy may be needed. With thyroidectomy, often subtotal (up to 90%), the patient may require a high-calorie, high-protein diet preoperatively. Antithyroid agents and iodine are often given 4–6 weeks before surgery to minimize risk of thyroid crisis. Evaluate needs postoperatively with the doctor's care plan.

OBJECTIVES

- Prevent or treat complications accompanying high metabolic rate, including bone demineralization.
- Replenish glycogen stores. Replace lost weight (usually 10–20 lb).
- Correct negative nitrogen balance.
- Replace fluid losses from diarrhea, diaphoresis, and increased respirations.
- Exophthalmos, which is caused by increased accumulation of extracellular fluid in the eyes, may require fluid and salt restriction.
- Monitor for fat intolerance and steatorrhea.

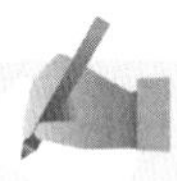

DIETARY AND NUTRITIONAL RECOMMENDATIONS

- Use a high-calorie diet (40 kcal/Kg). The patient's caloric needs may be increased by 50–60% in this condition (or 10–30% in mild cases). Ensure high intake of carbohydrates; use protein in the range of 1–1.75 g/kg body weight.
- Fluid intake should be 3–4 L per day, unless contraindicated by renal or cardiac problems.
- Diet should include 1 quart of milk daily to supply adequate calcium, phosphorus, and vitamin D; equivalent sources will be needed if patient does not consume dairy products.
- Caffeine stimulants should be excluded from diet.
- Supplement diet with vitamins A and C, as well as the B-complex vitamins, especially thiamine, riboflavin, B6, and B12. A general multivitamin–mineral supplement may be beneficial.
- Be cautious regarding use of natural goitrogens (i.e., cabbage, Brussels sprouts, kale, cauliflower, soybeans, peanuts, etc.) concomitant with antithyroid medications. These substances can increase side effects of the drugs; cooking reduces this effect.

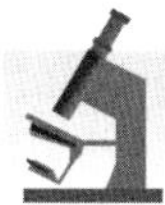

PROFILE

Clinical/History		
Height	T3, increased	Na+
Weight	T4, increased	H&H
BMI	TSH (normal or low)	Chol, Trig (decreased)
Temperature	PBI	Mg++ (decreased)
BP	Gluc (increased)	P
I & O	Alb, prealbumin	N balance
Lab Work	Ca++	Alk phos (increased)
Thyroid scan	K+	

Common Drugs Used and Potential Side Effects

- The goal with this form of drug therapy is to prevent the thyroid from producing hormones. Antithyroid drugs (methimazole [Tapazole], propylthiouracil [PTU]) can cause nausea, vomiting, altered taste sensation, and GI distress; take with food. Watch use of natural goitrogens with these drugs, which can increase effects of the drug; cook these foods rather than using in raw form
- Radioactive iodine may be used to damage or destroy some of the thyroid cells. It can cause a temporary burning sensation in the throat.
- For mild or temporary cases, use of beta-blockers may be beneficial.

Herbs, Botanicals and Supplements

- Herbs and botanical supplements should not be used without discussing with physician.
- Bugleweed, verbena, lemon balm, kelp, and broccoli have been recommended, but no clinical trials prove efficacy.

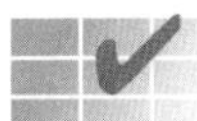

PATIENT ED396UCATION

- ✔ Encourage quiet, pleasant mealtimes.
- ✔ Exclude use of alcohol, which may cause a hypoglycemic state.
- ✔ To avoid obesity, adjust patient's diet as condition corrects itself.
- ✔ Beware of hyperglycemia after carbohydrate-rich meals.
- ✔ Frequent snacks may be needed.

For More Information

- American Thyroid Association
  Townhouse Office Park
  55 Old Nyack Turnpike, Suite 611
  Nanuet, NY 10954
  http://www.thyroid.org/
- European Thyroid Society
  http://www.eurothyroid.com/
- Gland Central–Thyroid health
  http://www.glandcentral.com/home/
- Latin American Thyroid Society
  http://www.lats.org/
- Merck Thyro-Link
  http://www.thyrolink.com/
- National Graves Disease Foundation
  http://www.ngdf.org/
- The Thyroid Foundation
  http://www.tsh.org/
- The Thyroid Society
  http://the-thyroid-society.org/

HYPOTHYROIDISM

NUTRITIONAL ACUITY RANKING: LEVEL 2

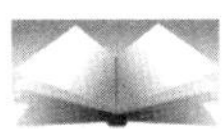

DEFINITIONS AND BACKGROUND

Hypothyroidism, the underfunctioning of the thyroid gland (from surgery, autoimmune disease, or hypofunctioning of the pituitary gland), may show with such signs and symptoms as dry skin, hand and face puffiness, fatigue, weight gain, slow speech, mental apathy, constipation, hearing loss, memory impairment, decreased perspiration, cold intolerance, and brittle nails. Women may experience menstrual irregularities or difficulty conceiving. T3 and T4 are elevated with pregnancy, oral contraceptive, and estrogen use. Hypothyroidism is common among middle-aged and older women. Physicians must treat to avoid long-term complications.

Endemic goiter, enlargement of the thyroid gland with swelling in front of the neck, results from iodine deficiency due to inadequate dietary intake or drug effects. Simple and nodular goiters are unrelated to the presence of iodine. Cretinism is endemic goiter in a child, with dwarfism or short stature, deafness, retardation, and large tongue. It is rare at birth. Myxedema is an endemic goiter in an adult. In myxedema coma, severe unconsciousness can occur with stress. Vitamin A may be poorly converted from carotene. Calcium may be retained.

OBJECTIVES

- ▲ Control weight gain that results from a 15–40% slower metabolic rate, especially in the untreated patient. Measure weight frequently to detect losses or fluid retention.
- ▲ Correct reasons for imbalance, which can be due to inadequate intake of iodine, increased intake of goitrogens, or congenital imbalance.
- ▲ Correct vitamin B12 or iron deficiency anemias, if present.
- ▲ Improve energy levels; reduce fatigue.

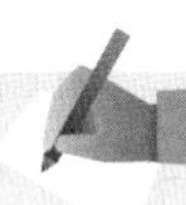

DIETARY AND NUTRITIONAL RECOMMENDATIONS

- Use a calorie-controlled diet adjusted for age, sex, and height.
- Ensure an adequate supply of fiber and laxative foods.
- In diets for pregnant women or children, check to make sure that adequate amounts of iodine are provided.
- Natural goitrogens may be used in moderation or cooked. Goitrogens in cabbage, turnips, rapeseeds, peanuts, cassava, cauliflower, broccoli, and soybeans may block uptake of iodine by body cells; they are inactivated by heating and cooking.
- Soy can interfere with thyroid function and can block absorption of thyroid medications; use with caution.
- To make the thyroid function properly, zinc, copper, and tyrosine are needed.

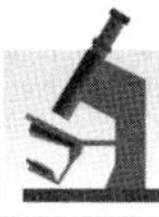

PROFILE

Clinical/History

Height
Weight
BMI
Temperature

Lab Work

T4 (decreased)
T3 (decreased)
TSH (elevated)
PBI
Ca++
H&H (decreased—less O2 needed)
Chol, Trig (increased)
Gluc
Alk phos (decreased)
Copper (Cu) (decreased)
Na+ (decreased)
K+ (decreased)
Serum B12
Serum Fe, ferritin
Creatine phosphokinase (CPK)
Thyrotropin
Somatomedin C (increased)
Uric acid (increased)
Mg++ (increased)
Carotenoids (increased)

Common Drugs Used and Potential Side Effects

- Thyroid hormones (Liotrix, sodium levothyroxine, or Synthroid). Monitor diabetics carefully. Use caution with long-term use of soy protein products and the Brassica family. Changes in appetite and decreased weight can occur. Thyroid hormones elevate glucose and decrease cholesterol.
- Amultivitamin–mineral supplement formula may be beneficial.

Herbs, Botanicals and Supplements

- Herbs and botanical supplements should not be used without discussing with physician.
- Avoid kelp tablets and “thyroid support” supplements.
- Kelp, gentian, walnut, mustard, radish, and St. John’s wort have been recommended, but no clinical trials have proven efficacy.

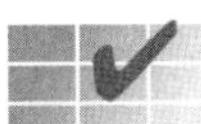

PATIENT EDUCATION

- ✔ Provide a list of the foods that contain progoitrin, an antithyroid agent. Goitrogens in cabbage and Brassica vegetables, turnips, rapeseeds, peanuts, cassava, and soybeans may block uptake of iodine by body cells; they are inactivated by heating and cooking.
- ✔ Urge cooking of vegetables.
- ✔ Encourage use of iodized salt, as permitted.
- ✔ Encourage adequate fluid intake.
- ✔ Be careful not to self-medicate with iodine.

For More Information

- ✦ American Thyroid Association
  Townhouse Office Park
  55 Old Nyack Turnpike, Suite 611
  Nanuet, NY 10954
  http://www.thyroid.org/
- ✦ Synthroid Information
  http://www.synthroid.com/

See Hyperthyroidism for other sites on thyroid health.

DIABETES INSIPIDUS

NUTRITIONAL ACUITY RANKING: LEVEL 2–3 DEFINITIONS AND

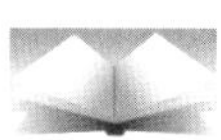

DEFINITIONS AND BACKGROUND

Diabetes insipidus (DI) results from primary (inherited) or secondary (resulting from trauma, tumor, or infection) deficiency of the pituitary gland hormone (vasopressin or antidiuretic hormone [ADH]) and is marked by excessive thirst, drinking, and urination, dry skin, and weakness. Urine output may be 5–10 L/24 hours. The disease is more common in young individuals, especially in males. Children with DI may be irritable or listless and may have problems with bedwetting, fever, vomiting, or diarrhea.

Nephrogenic DI may be an inherited disorder of defective kidney tubules, or it may be acquired. The kidneys' ability to respond to ADH can be impaired by drugs (like lithium) and by chronic disorders including polycystic kidney disease, sickle cell disease, kidney failure, partial blockage of the ureters, and inherited genetic disorders. Sometimes, the cause of nephrogenic DI is not known.

Very rare forms occur because of a defect in the thirst mechanism (dipsogenic DI) or during pregnancy (gestational DI). A medical specialist should determine which form of DI exists before treatment is administered.

OBJECTIVES

- Prevent dehydration and hypovolemic shock from excretion of large amounts of dilute urine. Prolonged dehydration may cause slight brain damage.
- Check patient's weight three times weekly to determine fluid retention and effectiveness of drug therapy.
- Reduce excess workload for the kidney.

DIETARY AND NUTRITIONAL RECOMMENDATIONS

- Ensure increased fluid intake to compensate for losses. Up to 20 L may be needed!
- Ensure potassium intake is adequate.
- If a patient has the nephrogenic form, limit protein intake to RDA levels and liberalize regimen as patient (usually a child) learns to satisfy fluid needs. A low-sodium diet, adequate fluid intake, and diuretics may also be needed to minimize workload of the kidney.

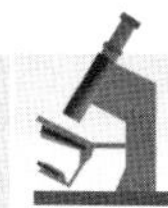

PROFILE

Clinical/History	Lab Work	
Height Weight BMI BP Excessive thirst and urination I & O	Vasopressin (ADH) in serum, urine K+ BUN Osmolality below 300 mOsm/Kg Na+ (increased)	Alb Urinary specific gravity (decreased) Uric acid (increased in adults) Fluid deprivation test Brain MRI

Common Drugs Used and Potential Side Effects

- Vasopressin tannate (Pitressin) or benzothiazide diuretics will reduce volume by 50% for this type of pituitary disorder. Supplements of potassium may be needed. Angina or intestinal cramping can occur. Vasopressin is not effective for the nephrogenic type.
- DDAVP (desmopressin acetate) may cause abdominal pain, headaches, GI distress, and weakness. It is administered parenterally, by pill, or by nasal spray. Patients should drink fluids or water only when thirsty.
- For nephrogenic DI, hydrochlorothiazide (also called HCTZ) or indomethacin, may be used. HCTZ is sometimes combined with amiloride. Patients should drink fluids or water only when thirsty.

Herbs, Botanicals and Supplements

- Herbs and botanical supplements should not be used without discussing with physician.

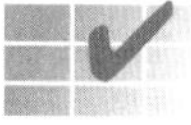

PATIENT EDUCATION

- ✓ Caution patient not to limit fluid intake in an effort to lessen urine output. Cold water may be preferred.
- ✓ Select low-calorie beverages to prevent excessive weight gain.
- ✓ Avoid stimulant/diuretic-type beverages (e.g., coffee, tea, alcohol).

For More Information

- The Diabetes Insipidus Foundation, Inc.
  4533 Ridge Drive
  Baltimore, MD 21229
  (410) 247-3953
  http://diabetesinsipidus.maxinter.net/toc.htm
- The Diabetes Insipidus and Related Disorders Network
  535 Echo Court
  Saline, MI 48176-1270
  (734) 944-0078
  http://hometown.aol.com/ruudh/dipage1.htm
- Nephrogenic Diabetes Insipidus Foundation
  Main Street, P.O. Box 1390
  Eastsound, WA 98245
  1-888-376-6343
  http://www.ndif.org/

SYNDROME OF INAPPROPRIATE ANTIDIURETIC HORMONE

NUTRITIONAL ACUITY RANKING: LEVEL 3

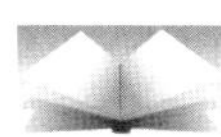

DEFINITIONS AND BACKGROUND

Syndrome of inappropriate antidiuretic hormone (SIADH) involves water intoxication with hyponatremia and hyperosmolarity of urine. Normal renal and adrenal functioning with abnormal elevation of plasma vasopressin occurs (inappropriate for serum osmolality). The condition may occur as a result of oat cell bronchial cancer, pulmonary tuberculosis, acute MI, myxedema, CNS disorders, acute leukemia, stroke, meningitis, or craniotomy. Symptoms and signs include irritability, lethargy, seizures, or confusion.

OBJECTIVES

- Restrict water intake.
- Replace electrolytes as appropriate.
- Normalize ADH secretion.

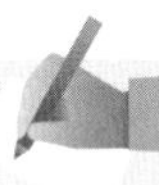

DIETARY AND NUTRITIONAL RECOMMENDATIONS

- Restrict fluid intake.
- Alter dietary sodium and potassium, as deemed appropriate for the condition.
- When enteral feeding is needed, select a formula that is fluid-restricted such as those that are 2 calories/mL. Monitor carefully for signs of dehydration. Check content of formula for Na+ and K1; select according to patient status and needs.

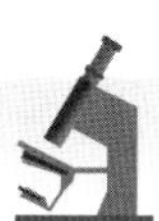

PROFILE

Clinical/History

Height
Current weight
Edema-free weight
BMI
I & O
Temperature
Edema
Irritability
Lethargy, confusion

Lab Work

BUN
Vasopressin (ADH) levels
Creatinine
Na+ (decreased)
Osmolality (decreased)
K+

Common Drugs Used and Potential Side Effects

- Lithium carbonate (Lithane, Lithobid, Lithotabs) may be used. Consistency of sodium intake is required. Weight gain, metallic taste, nausea, vomiting, and other side effects may occur. Limit caffeine intake.
- Demeclocycline (Declomycin) may be used with side effects like those of tetracycline. Avoid taking with calcium or dairy products.

Herbs, Botanicals and Supplements

- Herbs and botanical supplements should not be used without discussing with physician.

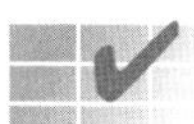

PATIENT EDUCATION

- Provide counseling regarding water restrictions and fluid intake, as ordered.
- Discuss any underlying conditions that may have caused the syndrome; highlight needed dietary alterations.

PARATHYROID DISORDERS AND ALTERED CALCIUM METABOLISM

NUTRITIONAL ACUITY RANKING: LEVEL 3

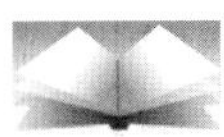

DEFINITIONS AND BACKGROUND

Serum Ca++ levels regulate parathyroid hormone (PTH). PTH affects calcium, phosphorus, and vitamin D metabolism by removing calcium from bone to raise serum levels; it promotes hydroxylation of vitamin D to 1,25 (OH)2-D. Calcitonin, in contrast to PTH, decreases serum calcium levels. Calcitonin is from the thyroid.

Hyperparathyroidism results from adenoma, renal failure, hyperplasia of the parathyroid glands, or from a hypocalcemic state. Signs and symptoms include weakness, fatigue, anorexia, constipation, weight loss, hypercalcemia and hypercalciuria, and elevated PTH. (See also Paget's Disease.) Elevated levels of parathyroid hormone or renal failure cause hyperparathyroidism. Increased serum Ca++, decreased serum P, and dehydration are common. About 28/100,000 people have this condition in the United States. Frequency increases with age, and women tend to have the condition more than men.

Hypoparathyroidism results from a deficiency of PTH from biologically ineffective hormones, damage or accidental removal of the glands, or impaired skeletal or renal response. Vitamin D may be deficient. Signs and symptoms include tetany, thinning hair, coarse skin, cataracts, dental hypoplasia, chronic cutaneous moniliasis, hypocalcemia, hyperphosphatemia, and low PTH. Hypoparathyroidism/hypocalcemia is one of the most common results of damage to parathyroid glands during surgery. Other causes include magnesium deficiency, neonatal immaturity, and defects. In states of permanent hypoparathyroidism, requirements are large for calcium (1–2 g) and vitamin D (25,000/day) to maintain normal calcium.

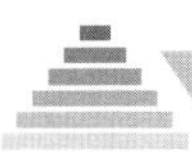

OBJECTIVES

Hypercalcemia/Hyperparathyroidism:

- Lower elevated serum calcium and urinary calcium.
- Normalize serum and urinary phosphate; 80% of phosphorus is usually absorbed from diet. Parathyroidectomy may be necessary.

Hypocalcemia/Hypoparathyroidism:

- Normalize serum and urinary levels of calcium, phosphorus, and vitamin D.
- Prevent long-term bone disease complications.

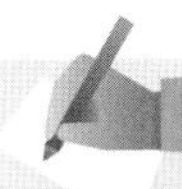

DIETARY AND NUTRITIONAL RECOMMENDATIONS

Hypercalcemia/Hyperparathyroidism:

- Use a low-calcium diet; fewer dairy products, nuts, salmon, peanut butter, and green leafy vegetables.
- Low calcium tube feedings such as Compleat, which is also high in phosphorus, can be used.
- Drink lots of fluid to prevent dehydration, which can elevate serum calcium.

Hypocalcemia/Hypoparathyroidism:

- Use a high-calcium diet; increase dairy products, nuts, salmon, peanut butter, and green leafy vegetables.
- Oral supplements high in calcium may be used.
- Supplements such as calcium carbonate may be needed.
- Reduce excess use of meats, phytates (whole grains), and oxalic acid (spinach, chard, etc.).
- If tolerated, lactose should be included in diet.
- Intake of vitamin D and protein should be adequate, at least meeting RDA levels.

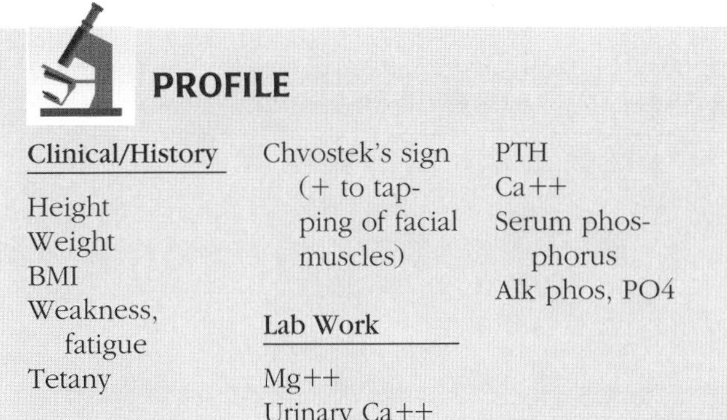

PROFILE

Clinical/History		
Height	Chvostek's sign (+ to tapping of facial muscles)	PTH
Weight	**Lab Work**	Ca++
BMI	Mg++	Serum phosphorus
Weakness, fatigue	Urinary Ca++	Alk phos, PO4
Tetany		

Common Drugs Used and Potential Side Effects

- Overuse of steroids may cause hypocalcemia, with resulting severe muscle spasms and convulsions.
- Beware of hypervitaminosis A or D—either may aggravate or cause hypercalcemia (e.g., 10,000 of vitamin A or 50,000 of vitamin D). It takes 12–36 hours to show changes in serum Ca++ levels.

- Use of antacids and excessive amounts of iron lower phosphorus absorption. Be careful! Antacids also may contain high levels of calcium.
- Calcium lactate (8–12 g) may be used in hypoparathyroidism.
- Ergocalciferol (calciferol) is a vitamin D analog that is used with calcium supplements for hypoparathyroidism. Beware of toxic effects with long-term use. Calcitriol (Rocaltrol) also may be useful.

Herbs, Botanicals and Supplements

- Herbs and botanical supplements should not be used without discussing with physician.

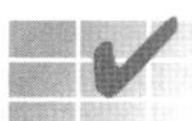

PATIENT EDUCATION

✔ Indicate which foods are sources of calcium, phosphorus, and vitamin D.
✔ Indicate which foods are sources of phytates and oxalates.
✔ Discuss role of sunlight in vitamin D formation.

For More Information

- American Society for Bone and Mineral Research
  2025 M Street, NW, Suite 800
  Washington, DC 20036
  202-367-1161
- National Institutes of Health–Osteoporosis and Related Bone Diseases
  http://www.osteo.org/pdisbone.html
- The Paget Foundation
  120 Wall Street, Suite 1602
  New York, NY 10005
  1-800-23-PAGET

REFERENCES

Cited References

Ajani U, et al. Alcohol consumption and risk of type 2 diabetes mellitus among U.S. male physicians. *Arch Int Med.* 2000;160:1025.

American Diabetes Association. *Maximizing the role of nutrition in diabetes management.* Alexandria, VA: The American Diabetes Association, 2000.

American Diabetes Association. Position statement: Nutrition recommendations and principles for people with diabetes mellitus. *Diabetes Care.* 2000;23:43S.

American Diabetes Association. Position statement: Translation of the diabetes nutrition recommendations for health care institutions. *Diabetes Care.* 2001;24:S48–S50. http://journal.diabetes.org/FullText/Supplements/DiabetesCare/Supplement101/S44.htm.

American Diabetes Association. Clinical Practice Recommendations 2001. http://www.diabetes.org/clinicalrecommendations/Supplement101/S5.htm.

Anderson R. Chromium in the prevention and control of diabetes. *Diabetes Metab.* 2000;26:22.

Anderson J, et al. Effects of psyllium on glucose and serum lipid responses in men with type 2 diabetes and hypercholesterolemia. *Am J Clin Nutri.* 1999;70:466.

Azziz R, et al. Troglitazone improves ovulation and hirsutism in the polycystic ovary syndrome: a multicenter, double blind, and placebo-controlled trial. *J Clin Endocrinol Metab.* 2001;86:1626.

Barbieri R. Induction of ovulation in infertile women with hyperandrogenism and insulin resistance. *Am J Obstet Gynecol.* 2000; 183:1412.

Boyle P, et al. Brain glucose uptake and unawareness of hypoglycemia in patients with insulin-dependent diabetes mellitus. *N Engl J Med.* 1995;333:1726.

Branch D. High-dose vitamin C supplementation increases plasma glucose. *Diab Care.* 1999;22:1218.

Branchtein L, et al. Waist circumference and waist-to-hip ratio are related to gestational glucose tolerance. *Diabetes Care.* 1997;20:509.

Brun J, et al. Postprandial reactive hypoglycemia. *Diabetes Metab.* 2000;26:337.

Busch C, Hegele R. Genetic determinants of type 2 diabetes mellitus. *Clin Genet.* 2001;60:243.

Buyken A, et al. Glycemic index in the diet of European outpatients with type 1 diabetes: relations to glycated hemoglobin and serum lipids. *Am J Clin Nutri.* 2001;73:574.

Cabanas E. Maturity onset diabetes of the young: Recent findings indicate insulin resistance/obesity are not factors. *Diab Educator.* 1998;24:477.

Cangiano C, et al. Effects of oral 5-hydroxy-tryptophan on energy intake and macronutrient selection in non-insulin dependent diabetic patients. *Int J Obesity and Related Disorders.* 1998;22:648.

Catalano P, et al. The relationship between abnormal glucose tolerance and hypertensive disorders of pregnancy in healthy nulliparous women. *Am J Obstet Gynecol.* 1998;98:179.

CD Diabetes Cost Effectiveness Study Group. The cost effectiveness of screening for type 2 diabetes. *J Am Med Assoc.* 1999;280:1757.

Cersosimo E, et al. Abnormal glucose handling by the kidney in response to hypoglycemia in type 1 diabetes. *Diabetes.* 2001;50: 2087.

Chandalia M, et al. Beneficial effects of high dietary fiber intake in patients with type 2 diabetes mellitus. *N Engl J Med.* 2000;342:1392.

Chiasson R, et al. The effect of acarbose on insulin sensitivity in subjects with impaired glucose tolerance. *Diabetes Care.* 1996;19: 1190.

Chin M, et al. Quality of diabetes care in community health centers. *Am J Public Health.* 2000;90:431.

Clairmont M. Diabetes and alternative nutrition. *Today's Dietitian.* 2000;11:43.

Clausen T, et al. High intake of energy, sucrose, and polyunsaturated fatty acids is associated with increased risk of preeclampsia. *Am J Obstet Gynecol.* 2001;185:451.

Cohn G, et al. Pathophysiology and treatment of the dyslipidemia of insulin resistance. *Curr Cardiol Rep.* 2001;3:416.

Crawford P, et al. Ethnic issues in the epidemiology of childhood obesity. *Pediatr Clin North Am.* 2001;48:855.

Cunningham J. Micronutrients as nutriceutical interventions in diabetes mellitus. *J Am Col Nutri.* 1998;17:7.

Daly A, et al. The new credential: Advanced Diabetes Management. *J Am Diet Assoc.* 2001;101:940.

DCCT Research Group. Nutrition interventions for intensive therapy in the Diabetes Control and Complications Trial. *J Am Diet Assoc.* 1993;93:768.

DCCT Research Group. Lifetime benefits and costs of intensive therapy as practiced in the Diabetes Control and Complications Trial. *JAMA.* 1996;276:1409.

Department of Medicine. *Washington manual of medical therapeutics.* 30th ed. St Louis, MO: Washington University School of Medicine, 2001.

De Veciana M, et al. Postprandial versus preprandial blood glucose monitoring in women with gestational diabetes mellitus requiring insulin therapy. *N Engl J Med.* 1995;333:1237.

Diabetes Care and Education Practice Group. Scope of practice for qualified dietetics professionals in diabetes care and education. *J Am Diet Assoc.* 2000;100:1205.

Diabetes Care and Education Practice Group newsletter, *On the Cutting Edge.* 2001;22:23.

Everson S, et al. Weight gain and the risk of developing insulin resistance syndrome. *Diab Care.* 1998;21:1637.

Facchini F, et al. Insulin resistance as a predictor of age-related diseases. *J Clin Endocrinol Metab.* 2001;86:3574.

Felner E, White P. Improving management of diabetic ketoacidosis in children. *Pediatrics.* 2001;108:735.

Ford E, et al. Diabetes mellitus and serum carotenoids: findings from the third National Health and Nutrition Examination Survey. *Am J Epid.* 1999;149:168.

Fournet J, et al. Unbalanced expression of 11p15 imprinted genes in focal forms of congenital hyperinsulinism: association with a reduction to homozygosity of a mutation in ABCC8 or KCNJ11. *Am J Pathol.* 2001;158:2177.

Franz M, et al. American Diabetes Association Position Statement: Evidence-based nutrition principles and recommendations for the treatment and prevention of diabetes and related conditions. *J Am Diet Assoc*. 2002;102:109.

Franz M, et al. Effectiveness of medical nutrition therapy provided by dietitians in the management of noninsulin-dependent diabetes mellitus: a randomized, controlled clinical trial. *J Am Diet Assoc*. 1995;95:1009.

Franz M, et al. *Maximizing the role of nutrition in diabetes management*. Alexandria, VA: American Diabetes Association, 2000.

Funnell M, et al. Empowerment: an idea whose time has come in diabetes education. *Diabetes Ed*. 1991;17:37.

Gannon M, et al. Acute metabolic response of high-CHO, high-starch meals compared with moderate-CHO, low-starch meals in subjects with type 2 diabetes. *Diab Care*. 1998;21:1619.

Gold A, et al. The effect of glycemic control in the preconception period and early pregnancy on birth weight in women with IDDM. *Diab Care*. 1998;21:535.

Goldberg K, et al. Dietary adequacy in patients with diabetic gastroparesis. *J Am Diet Assoc*. 1997;97:420.

Grill V, Bjorklund A. Overstimulation and beta-cell function. *Diabetes*. 2001;5050:S122.

Hernandez J, et al. Fluid snacks to help persons with type 1 diabetes avoid late onset postexercise hypoglycemia. *Med & Sci in Sports & Exercise*. 2000;32:904.

Herpertz S, et al. Comorbidity of diabetes and eating disorders: Does diabetes control reflect disturbed eating behavior? *Diab Care*. 1998;21:1110.

Holler H, Pastors J. *Diabetes medical nutrition therapy*. Chicago: The American Dietetic Association, 1997.

Howard B, et al. Relationship between insulin resistance and lipoproteins in nondiabetic African Americans, Hispanics, and nonHispanic whites: The Insulin Resistance Atherosclerosis Study. *Metabolism*. 1998;47:1174.

Hu F, et al. Diet, lifestyle, and the risk of type 2 diabetes mellitus in women. *N Engl J Med*. 2001;345:790.

Hu F, van Dam R, Liu S. Diet and risk of Type II diabetes: the role of types of fat and carbohydrate. *Diabetologia*. 2001;44:805.

Hypponen E, et al. Intake of vitamin D and risk of type 1 diabetes: a birth-cohort study. *Lancet*. 2001;358:1500.

Jain S, et al. Effect of modest vitamin E supplementation on blood glycated hemoglobin and triglyceride levels and red cell indices in type I diabetic patients. *J Am Col Nutri*. 1996;15:458.

Jarvi A, et al. Improved glycemic control and lipid profile and normalized fibrinolytic activity on a low-glycemic index diet in type 2 diabetic patients. *Diab Care*. 1999;22:10.

Johnson K, et al. Prevalence of undiagnosed noninsulin-dependent diabetes mellitus and impaired glucose tolerance in a cohort of older persons with hypertension. *J Am Geriatr Soc*. 1997;45:695.

Jovanovic L. Optimization of insulin therapy in patients with gestational diabetes. *Endocr Pract*. 2000;6:98.

Kahn J, Gordon C. Polycystic ovary syndrome. *Adolesc Med*. 1999; 10:321.

Kearney T, et al. Hypopituitarism is associated with triglyceride enrichment of very low-density lipoprotein. *J Clin Endocrinol Metab*. 2001;86:3900.

Klonoff D, Schwartz D. An economic analysis of interventions for diabetes. *Diab Care*. 2000;23:390.

Konen J, et al. Measurement feasibility of advanced glycated end-products from skin samples after antioxidant vitamin supplementation in patients with type 2 diabetes. *J Nutr Health Aging*. 2000;4:81.

Kruger D, et al. Clinical implications of amylin and amylin deficiency. *Diab Educator*. 1999;25:389.

Kwalkorf H, et al. Dietary fiber intakes and insulin requirements in pregnant women with type 1 diabetes. *J Am Diet Assoc*. 2001;101: 305.

Legro R. Diabetes prevalence and risk factors in polycystic ovary syndrome. *Obstet Gynecol Clin North Am*. 2001;28:99.

Lehtovirta M, et al. Metabolic effects of metformin in patients with impaired glucose tolerance. *Diabet Med*. 2001;18:578.

Leontos C, et al. National Diabetes Education program: opportunities and challenges. *J Am Diet Assoc*. 1998;98:73.

Liu S, et al. A prospective study of whole-grain intake and risk of type 2 diabetes mellitus in U.S. women. *Am J Pub Health*. 2000; 90:1409.

Liu S, et al. Dietary glycemic load assessed by food-frequency questionnaire in relation to plasma high-density lipoprotein cholesterol and fasting plasma triacylglycerols in postmenopausal women. *Am J Clin Nutri*. 2001;73:560.

Liu S, Manson J. Dietary carbohydrates, physical inactivity, obesity, and the 'metabolic syndrome' as predictors of coronary heart disease. *Curr Opin Lipidol*. 2001;12:395.

Lucas M. Diabetes complicating pregnancy. *Obstet Gynecol Clin North Am*. 2001;28:513.

Maki K, Kurlandsky S. Syndrome X: A tangled web of risk factors for coronary heart disease and diabetes mellitus. *Top Clin Nutri*. 2001; 16:32.

Manley S, et al. Effects of three months' diet after diagnosis of Type 2 diabetes on plasma lipids and lipoproteins (UKPDS 45). UK Prospective Diabetes Study Group. *Diabet Med*. 2000;17:518.

Marchesini G, et al. Nonalcoholic fatty liver disease: a feature of the metabolic syndrome. *Diabetes*. 2001;50:1844.

McFarland K. Type 2 diabetes: stepped-care approach to patient management. *Geriatrics*. 1997;52:22.

McKittrick M. Diet and polycystic syndrome. *Nutrition Today*. 2002; 37:63.

McNeely M, et al. Standard definitions of overweight and central adiposity for determining diabetes risk in Japanese Americans. *Am J Clin Nutri*. 2001;74:101.

Meloni T, et al. IDDM and early infant feeding: Sardinian case-control study. *Diabetes Care*. 1997;20:340.

Meltzer A, Everhart J. Association between diabetes and elevated serum alanine aminotransferase activity among Mexican Americans. *Am J Epid*. 1997;146:565.

Meyer K, et al. Carbohydrates, dietary fiber, and incident type 2 diabetes in older women. *Am J Clin Nutri*. 2000;71:921.

Miller C, et al. Evaluation of a food label nutrition intervention for women with type 2 diabetes mellitus. *J Am Diet Assoc*. 1999;99: 323.

Monro J. Available carbohydrate and glycemic index combined in new data sets for managing glycemia and diabetes. *J Food Comp and Analysis*. 1999;12:71.

Nicholson A, et al. Toward improved management of type 2 DM: a randomized, controlled pilot intervention using a lowfat, vegetarian diet. *Preventive Med*. 1999;29:87.

Pories W, Albrecht R. Etiology of type II diabetes mellitus: role of the foregut. *World J Surg*. 2001;25:527.

Pourmotabbed G, Kitabchi A. Hypoglycemia. *Obstet Gynecol Clin North Am*. 2001;28:383.

Pozzili P, et al. Metabolic and immune parameters at clinical onset of insulin-dependent diabetes in a population-based study. *Metabolism*. 1998;47:12005.

Quilliot D, et al. Effect of the inflammation, chronic hyperglycemia, or malabsorption on the apolipoprotein A-IV concentration in type 1 diabetes mellitus and in diabetes secondary to chronic pancreatitis. *Metabolism*. 2001;50:1019.

Rajantie J, et al. Abnormal electroencephalogram at diagnosis of insulin-dependent diabetes mellitus may predict severe symptoms of hypoglycemia in children. *J Pediatr*. 1998;133:792.

Ravid M, et al. Main risk factors for nephropathy in type 2 diabetes mellitus are plasma cholesterol levels, mean blood pressure, and hyperglycemia. *Arch Int Med*. 1998;158:998.

Reiter S, et al. Blood glucose laboratory for first-year medical students: An interdisciplinary model for nutrition-focused diabetes management. *J Am Diet Assoc*. 2000;100:570.

Resnick H, et al. Differential effects of BMI on diabetes risk among black and white Americans. *Diab Care*. 1998;21:1828.

Rodriguez L, Castelanos V. Use of low-fat foods by people with diabetes decreases fat, saturated fat, and cholesterol intakes. *J Am Diet Assoc*. 2000;100:531.

Romon M, et al. Higher carbohydrate intake is associated with decreased incidence of newborn macrosomia in women with gestational diabetes. *J Am Diet Assoc*. 2001;101:897.

Rydall A, et al. Disordered eating behavior and microvascular complications in young women with insulin-dependent diabetes mellitus. *N Engl J Med*. 1997;336:1849.

Sakurai Y, et al. Association between duration of obesity and risk of non-insulin-dependent diabetes mellitus: the Sotetsu Study. *Am J Epid*. 1999;149:256.

Salmeron J, et al. Dietary fiber, glycemic load, and risk of NIDDM in men. *Diabetes Care*. 1997;20:545.

Salmeron J, et al. Dietary fiber, glycemic load, and risk of NIDDM in women. *J Am Med Assoc*. 1997;277:472.

Sargeant L, et al. Vitamin C and hyperglycemia in the European Prospective Investigation into Cancer—Norfolk study: a population-based study. *Diab Care*. 2000;23:726.

Scalzo K, McKittrick M. Case problem: dietary recommendations to combat obesity, insulin resistance, and other concerns related to polycystic ovary syndrome. *J Am Diet Assoc*. 2000;100:955.

Schlundt D, et al. Situational obstacles to dietary adherence for adults with diabetes. *J Am Diet Assoc*. 1994;94:874.

Schmidt M, et al. Gestational diabetes mellitus diagnosed with a 2-h 75-g oral glucose tolerance test and adverse pregnancy outcomes. *Diabetes Care*. 2001;24:1151.

Shapiro A, et al. Islet transplantation in seven patients with type 1 diabetes mellitus using a glucocorticoid-free immunosuppressive regimen. *N Engl J Med*. 2000;343:230.

Sharma A, et al. Evaluation of oxidative stress before and after control of glycemia and after vitamin E supplementation in diabetic patients. *Metabolism: Clin & Experimental*. 2000;49:160.

Sonenberg N, Newgard C. Protein synthesis. The perks of balancing glucose. *Science*. 2001;293:818.

Staprans I, et al. Effect of oxidized lipids in the diet on oxidized lipid levels in postprandial serum chylomicrons of diabetic patients. *Diab Care*. 1999;22:300.

Stern M, et al. Birth weight and the metabolic syndrome: thrifty phenotype or thrifty genotype? *Diabetes Metab Res Rev*. 2000;16:88.

Stoa-Birketvedt G, et al. Cimetidine reduces weight and improves metabolic control in overweight patients with type 2 diabetes. *Int J Obes*. 1998;22:1041.

Tamis-Jortberg D, et al. Effects of a glucose polymer sports drink on blood glucose, insulin, and performance in subjects with diabetes. *Diabetes Educator*. 1996;22:471.

Testa M, Simonson D. Health benefits and quality of life during improved glycemic control in patients with type 2 diabetes. A randomized controlled double blind trial. *J Am Med Assoc*. 1999;280:1490.

Tutuncu N, et al. Reversal of defective nerve conduction with vitamin E supplementation in type 2 diabetes: a preliminary study. *Diab Care*. 1998;21:1915.

Upritchard J, et al. Effect of supplementation with tomato juice, vitamin E, and vitamin C on LDL oxidation and products of inflammatory activity in type 2 diabetes. *Diabetes Care*. 2000;23:733.

U.S. Department of Health and Human Services: *Physical Activity and Health: A Report of the Surgeon General*. Washington, D.C.: Centers for Disease Control and Prevention, National Center for Chronic Disease Prevention and Health Promotion, U.S. Govt. Printing Office, 1996.

Veneman T, et al. Effect of hyperketonemia and hyperlacticacidemia on symptoms, cognitive dysfunction, and counter regulatory hormone responses during hypoglycemia in normal humans. *Diabetes*. 1994;43:1311.

Virally M, Guillausseau P. Hypoglycemia in adults. *Diabetes Metab*. 1999;25:477.

Vohr B, et al. Effects of maternal gestational diabetes and adiposity on neonatal adiposity and blood pressure. *Diabetes Care*. 1995;18:467.

Vuksan V, et al. American ginseng (*Panax quinquefolius*) reduces postprandial glycemia in nondiabetic subjects and subjects with type 2 diabetes mellitus. *Arch Int Med*. 2000;160:1009.

Wang Y, et al. Dietary variables and glucose tolerance in pregnancy. *Diab Care*. 2000;23:460.

Weber M, Weir M. Management of high-risk hypertensive patients with diabetes: potential role of angiotensin ii receptor antagonists. *J Clin Hypertens*. 2001;3:225.

Wei M, et al. Alcohol intake and incidence of type 2 diabetes in men. *Diab Care*. 2000;23:18.

Wen S, et al. Impact of prenatal glucose screening on the diagnosis of gestational diabetes and on pregnancy outcomes. *Am J Epidemiol*. 2000;152:1009.

Williams K, et al. Improved glycemic control reduces the impact of weight gain on cardiovascular risk factors in type 1 diabetes: The Epidemiology of Diabetes Complications study. *Diab Care*. 1999;22:1084.

Yang W, et al. Weight reduction increases plasma levels of an adipose-derived anti-inflammatory protein, adiponectin. *J Clin Endocrinol Metab*. 2001;86:3815.

Yarbrough D, et al. Birth weight, adult weight, and girth as predictors of the metabolic syndrome in postmenopausal women: The Rancho Bernardo Study. *Diab Care*. 1998;21:1652.

Suggested Readings

Abusabha R, et al. How to make nutrition education more meaningful through facilitated group discussion. *J Am Diet Assoc*. 1999;99:72.

American Diabetes Association. Type 2 diabetes in children and adolescents. American Diabetes Association Consensus Statement. *Diab Care*. 2000;23:381.

Balkau B, et al. Is there a glycemic threshold for mortality risk? *Diab Care*. 1999;22:696.

Bell S, Forse R. Nutritional management of hypoglycemia. *Diab Educator*. 1999;25:41.

Bjornholt J, et al. Fasting blood glucose: an underestimated risk factor for cardiovascular death. Results from a 22-year follow-up of healthy nondiabetic men. *Diab Care.* 1999;22:45.

Brown S, et al. Motivational strategies used by dietitians to counsel individuals with diabetes. *Diab Educator.* 1998;24:313.

Camelon K, et al. The plate model: a visual method of teaching meal planning. *J Am Diet Assoc.* 1998;98:1155.

Charlton M, et al. Role of hyperglucagonemia in catabolism associated with type 1 diabetes. *Diabetes.* 1998;47:1748.

Connolly J, et al. Primary closure of infected diabetic foot wounds. A report of closed instillation in 30 cases. *J Am Podiatr Med Assoc.* 2000;90:175.

Daly M, et al. Acute effects of insulin sensitivity and diurnal metabolic profiles of a high-sucrose compared with a high-starch diet. *Am J Clin Nutri.* 1998;67:1186.

Delahanty L. Clinical significance of medical nutrition therapy in achieving diabetes outcomes and the importance of the process. *J Am Diet Assoc.* 1998;98:28.

Diabetes Care and Education Dietetic Practice Group. Scope of Practice for Qualified Dietetics Professionals in Diabetes Care and Education. *JAMA.* 2000;100:1205.

Franz M. Nutritional care in diabetes and reactive hypoglycemia. In: Mahan K, Escott-Stump S, eds. *Krause's food, nutrition, and diet therapy.* 10th ed. Philadelphia: WB Saunders, 2000.

Frost G, et al. Insulin sensitivity in women at risk of coronary heart disease and the effect of a low glycemic diet. *Metabolism.* 1998; 47:1245.

Gerich J. Is insulin resistance the principal cause of type 2 diabetes? *Diabetes Obes Metab.* 1999;1:257.

Giacca A, et al. Glucose production, utilization and cycling in response to moderate exercise in obese subjects with type 2 diabetes and mild hyperglycemia. *Diabetes.* 1998;47:1763.

Guisti J, Saul N. Nutrition evaluation and assessment of patient care: quarterly outcome analysis for diabetes mellitus. *J Am Diet Assoc.* 1997;97:31S.

Gutierrez M, et al. Utility of a short-term 25% carbohydrate diet on improving glycemic control in type 2 diabetes mellitus. *J Am Col Nutri.* 1998;17:595.

Heaps J. Cost effectiveness of medical nutrition therapy provided by dietitians for persons with diabetes mellitus. *J Am Diet Assoc.* 1997;97:101S.

Kulkarni K, et al. Nutrition practice guidelines for type 1 diabetes mellitus positively affect dietitian practices and patient outcomes. *J Am Diet Assoc.* 1998;98:62.

Lakka H, et al. Hyperinsulinemia and the risk of cardiovascular death and acute coronary and cerebrovascular events in men: the Kuopio Ischaemic Heart Disease Risk Factor Study. *Arch Int Med.* 2000;160:1160.

Lipkin E. New strategies for the treatment of type 2 diabetes. *J Am Diet Assoc.* 1999;99:329.

Lorenz R, et al. Diabetes training for dietitians: needs assessment, program description, and effects on knowledge and problem solving. *J Am Diet Assoc.* 2000;100:225.

Louheranta A, et al. A high stearic-acid diet does not impair glucose tolerance and insulin sensitivity in healthy women. *Metab: Clin and Experimental.* 1998;47:529.

Meigs J, et al. Hyperinsulinemia, hyperglycemia, and impaired homeostasis: the Framingham Offspring Study. *JAMA.* 2000;283:221.

Meigs J, Stafford R. Cardiovascular disease prevention practices by U.S. physicians for patients with diabetes. *J Gen Int Med.* 2000;15:220.

Ogilvy-Stuart A, et al. Hypoglycemia and resistance to ketoacidosis in a subject without functional insulin receptors. *J Clin Endocrinol Metab.* 2001;86:3319.

Ozata M, et al. Improved glycemic control increases fasting plasma acylation-stimulating protein and decreases leptin concentrations in type II diabetic subjects. *J Clin Endocrinol Metab.* 2001;86: 3659.

Pennison E, Egerman R. Perinatal outcomes in gestational diabetes: a comparison of criteria for diagnosis. *Am J Obstet Gynecol.* 2001; 184:1118.

Tuominen J, et al. Bone mineral density in patients with type 1 and type 2 diabetes. *Diab Care.* 1999;22:1196.

Yang W, et al. Weight reduction increases plasma levels of an adipose-derived anti-inflammatory protein, adiponectin. *J Clin Endocrinol Metab.* 2001;86:3815.

Young C, et al. Gestational diabetes screening in subsequent pregnancies of previously healthy patients. *Am J Obstet Gynecol.* 2000; 182:1024.

Zinman B, et al. Effectiveness of human ultralente versus NPH insulin in providing basal insulin requirement for an insulin lispro multiple daily injection regimen. *Diabetes Care.* 1999;22:603

SECTION 10

Weight Management, Undernutrition, and Malnutrition

CHIEF ASSESSMENT FACTORS

- HEIGHT
- WEIGHT HISTORY, PRESENT WEIGHT, USUAL BODY WEIGHT
- REFERENCE OR HEALTHY BODY WEIGHT
- BODY MASS INDEX (BMI)
- GOAL WEIGHT
- PERCENTAGE OF GOAL BODY WEIGHT; RECENT CHANGES (SUCH AS 5% CHANGE IN USUAL WEIGHT IN 1 MONTH OR 10% CHANGE IN USUAL BODY WEIGHT IN 3–6 MONTHS)
- TRICEPS SKINFOLD MEASUREMENTS (TSF)
- ARM MUSCLE CIRCUMFERENCE (AMC) MEASUREMENTS
- FRAME SIZE—SMALL, MEDIUM, LARGE
- WAIST CIRCUMFERENCE
- LABORATORY VALUES—GLUCOSE, BLOOD UREA NITROGEN (BUN), ALBUMIN/PREALBUMIN, HEMOGLOBIN AND HEMATOCRIT (H&H), CHOLESTEROL (CHOL), TRIGLYCERIDES (TRIG), TOTAL LYMPHOCYTE COUNTS
- SLEEP APNEA, ALTERED LUNG FUNCTION
- ANOREXIA, NAUSEA, VOMITING, DIARRHEA—FREQUENCY, LENGTH OF TIME
- HYPERTENSION
- ACTIVITY LEVELS
- HISTORY OF EATING DISORDERS (ANOREXIA NERVOSA, BULIMIA, BINGE EATING), CANCER, SMOKING, USE OF ALCOHOL, OTHER CONDITIONS OR DISEASE STATES

TYPES OF MALNUTRITION

Undernutrition may be primary—from insufficient intake or secondary—from impaired utilization. Among elderly patients, failure to thrive is known as "the dwindles" and may come from the "11 D's:" disease, drinking alcohol, drugs, deficits (sensory), desertion/isolation, dementia, delirium, dysphagia, depression, destitution, and despair. If a person has too low a BMI (see Tables 10–1 to 10–3), there is an increased risk of malnutrition or starvation. A woman with a low BMI may also have difficulty becoming pregnant.

Overnutrition is caused from excessive calorie intake and/or inadequate activity (Table 10–4). BMI over 30 is the initial calculated measure used to determine obesity. If a person has too high a BMI, he or she is at increased risk for high blood pressure, high blood cholesterol, diabetes, orthopedic problems, gallstones, gout, osteoarthritis, sleep apnea, and some cancers like breast, colon, and gall bladder. A woman may have problems with her menstrual cycle and may have difficulty becoming pregnant if she is obese. Epidemiological evidence clearly shows that being overweight contributes to menstrual disorders, infertility, miscarriage, poor pregnancy outcome, impaired fetal well-being, and diabetes mellitus (Norman and Clark, 1998). Changes in sensitivity to insulin may occur. Pregnant women who are obese have a higher waist circumference at 16 weeks' gestation and are more at risk for pregnancy-induced hypertension and preeclampsia (Sattar et al., 2001).

Calculation of Fat Grams

Easy way to calculate number of grams of fat needed = desired body weight divided by 2

Examples: 130 lb/2 = 65 g 170 lb/2 = 85 g

Conversion factors for common measurements are listed in Table 10–5.

TABLE 10–1 Important Weight Calculations and Body Mass Index Guidelines

The old Metropolitan Life Insurance height–weight charts are no longer used because BMI more often correctly predicts risks for chronic disease or malnutrition. Calculation of percent usual body weight = (actual weight/usual weight) × 100. Calculation of percent weight change = (usual weight–actual weight/usual weight) × 100.

Calculation of lean body mass: Body composition is often measured using dual-energy X-ray absorptiometry (DEXA) or electrical impedance absorptiometry. Underestimation of body fat percentage measured by bioelectrical impedance analysis compared to dual X-ray absorptiometry has been suggested as a concern (Eisenkolbl et al., 2001).

(continued)

TABLE 10–1 Important Weight Calculations and Body Mass Index Guidelines (*Continued*)

Waist measurements: Evidence from epidemiologic studies (NHLBI, 1998) shows waist circumference to be a better marker of abdominal fat content than waist:hip ratio (WHR), and that it is the most practical anthropometric measurement for assessing a patient's abdominal fat content before and during weight loss treatment. Computed tomography and MRI are both more accurate but impractical for routine clinical use. Waist circumference correlates with intra-abdominal adipose tissue. Upper body obesity is defined as a waist circumference of greater than 40 inches for men and greater than 35 inches for women. This is the "apple shape." If more of the weight is around the hips, it is "pear shape" and metabolic risks are lower.

Calculation for BMI: Multiply weight in pounds × 703. Then multiply height in inches × height in inches. Divide the (weight × 703) by the (height × height). There are also many web sites that make it easy to calculate BMI, which may be downloaded to a hand-held device: http://www.cdc.gov/nccdphp/dnpa/bmi/calc-bmi.htm, http://www.nhlbisupport.com/bmi/, http://www.healthyweight.com.

NHLBI clinical guidelines for BMI (NHLBI, 1998): http://www.nhlbi.nih.gov/guidelines/obesity/ob_home.htm

<18.5 BMI	Underweight
18.5–24.9	Normal
25–29.9	Overweight
30–34.9	Mildly obese (Class I Obesity)
35–39.9	Moderately obese (Class II Obesity)
40+	Extremely obese (Class III Obesity)

Using these standards, 55% of American adults are overweight or obese (Strawbridge et al., 2000).

Lowest mortality (Stevens, 2000):

Ages 20–29	BMI Men 21.4; Women 19.5
Ages 30–39	BMI Men 21.6; Women 23.4
Ages 40–49	BMI Men 22.9; Women 23.2
Ages 50–59	BMI Men 25.8; Women 25.2
Ages 60–69	BMI Men 26.6; Women 27.3

BMIs for pregnant women

The amount of weight a woman should gain during her pregnancy depends on her pre-pregnant BMI. The woman wants to gain enough weight to have a healthy baby but not too much weight to avoid complications and long-term health risks. For **twins,** ideal weight gain is about 35–45 pounds (National Academy of Sciences, http://books.nap.edu/books/0309041384/html/220.html#pagetop).

Pre-pregnant BMI	Weight gain during pregnancy
Less than 19.5	28–40 lbs
19.6–26	25–35 lbs
27–29	15–25 lbs
greater than 30	about 13 pounds

(continued)

TABLE 10–1 Important Weight Calculations and Body Mass Index Guidelines (*Continued*)

BMIs for children (See also section 3, Childhood Obesity)

Growth charts are used for children to watch the pattern of their growth. Charts cannot be used to diagnose obesity or malnutrition; if a child is over the 85th percentile or lower than the 5th percentile on the charts, the child should see a doctor. The curves on the growth chart show the pattern of growth. Growth charts for infants and children have been recently revised, calculated the same as for adults but interpreted differently based on BMI. Children are not just small adults; as they grow their BMI will change. For example, it may be healthy for a 2-year-old child to have a BMI of 16.1 and for that same child to have a BMI of 15.5 at age 6 years and then a BMI of 20 at age 15 years. Growth charts can be found at http://www.cdc.gov/growthcharts/.

BMIs for adolescents

An expert consensus panel suggests that a BMI of 95% for age and gender should define obesity. BMI charts are used for their age and sex. Over the 95th percentile on this chart is "overweight;" 85th percent tile and 95th percentile are "at risk of overweight." Children under the 5th percentile should be examined to see if they are normal but small children or have a problem that prevents formal growth rate. http://www.pediatrics.org/ cgi/content/full/102/3/e29

TABLE 10–2 Body Mass Index Tables

BMIs 19–35

Body Mass Index Chart

Height (inches)	19	20	21	22	23	24	25	26	27	28	29	30	31	32	33	34	35
								Body Weight (pounds)									
58	91	96	100	105	110	115	119	124	129	134	138	143	148	153	158	162	167
59	94	99	104	109	114	119	124	128	133	138	143	148	153	158	163	168	173
60	97	102	107	112	118	123	128	133	138	143	148	153	158	163	168	174	179
61	100	106	111	116	122	127	132	137	143	148	153	158	164	169	174	180	185
62	104	109	115	120	126	131	136	142	147	153	158	164	169	175	180	186	191
63	107	113	118	124	130	135	141	146	152	158	163	169	175	180	186	191	197
64	110	116	122	128	134	140	145	151	157	163	169	174	180	186	192	197	204
65	114	120	126	132	138	144	150	156	162	168	174	180	186	192	198	204	210
66	118	124	130	136	142	148	155	161	167	173	179	186	192	198	204	210	216
67	121	127	134	140	146	153	159	166	172	178	185	191	198	204	211	217	223
68	125	131	138	144	151	158	164	171	177	184	190	197	203	210	216	223	230
69	128	135	142	149	155	162	169	176	182	189	196	203	209	216	223	230	236
70	132	139	146	153	160	167	174	181	188	195	202	209	216	222	229	236	243
71	136	143	150	157	165	172	179	186	193	200	208	215	222	229	236	243	250
72	140	147	154	162	169	177	184	191	199	206	213	221	228	235	242	250	258
73	144	151	159	166	174	182	189	197	204	212	219	227	235	242	250	257	265
74	148	155	163	171	179	186	194	202	210	218	225	233	241	249	256	264	272
75	152	160	168	176	184	192	200	208	216	224	232	240	248	256	264	272	279
76	156	164	172	180	189	197	205	213	221	230	238	246	254	263	271	279	287

To use this table, find the appropriate height in the left-hand column. Move across to a given weight. The number at the top of the column is the BMI at that height and weight. Pounds have been rounded off. http://www.nhlbi.nih.gov/guidelines/obesity/bmi_tbl.htm

TABLE 10–3 Body Mass Index Tables

BMIs 36–54

Body Mass Index Table

	36	37	38	39	40	41	42	43	44	45	46	47	48	49	50	51	52	53	54
Height (inches)								**Body Weight (pounds)**											
58	172	177	181	186	191	196	201	205	210	215	220	224	229	234	239	244	248	253	258
59	178	183	188	193	198	203	208	212	217	222	227	232	237	242	247	252	257	262	267
60	184	189	194	199	204	209	215	220	225	230	235	240	245	250	255	261	266	271	276
61	190	195	201	206	211	217	222	227	232	238	243	248	254	259	264	269	275	280	285
62	196	202	207	213	218	224	229	235	240	246	251	256	262	267	273	278	284	289	295
63	203	208	214	220	225	231	237	242	248	254	259	265	270	278	282	287	293	299	304
64	209	215	221	227	232	238	244	250	256	262	267	273	279	285	291	296	302	308	314
65	216	222	228	234	240	246	252	258	264	270	276	282	288	294	300	306	312	318	324
66	223	229	235	241	247	253	260	266	272	278	284	291	297	303	309	315	322	328	334
67	230	236	242	249	255	261	268	274	280	287	293	299	306	312	319	325	331	338	344
68	236	243	249	256	262	269	276	282	289	295	302	308	315	322	328	335	341	348	354
69	243	250	257	263	270	277	284	291	297	304	311	318	324	331	338	345	351	358	365
70	250	257	264	271	278	285	292	299	306	313	320	327	334	341	348	355	362	369	376
71	257	265	272	279	286	293	301	308	315	322	329	338	343	351	358	365	372	379	386
72	265	272	279	287	294	302	309	316	324	331	338	346	353	361	368	375	383	390	397
73	272	280	288	295	302	310	318	325	333	340	348	355	363	371	378	386	393	401	408
74	280	287	295	303	311	319	326	334	342	350	358	365	373	381	389	396	404	412	420
75	287	295	303	311	319	327	335	343	351	359	367	375	383	391	399	407	415	423	431
76	295	304	312	320	328	336	344	353	361	369	377	385	394	402	410	418	426	435	443

To use this table, find the appropriate height in the left-hand column. Move across to a given weight. The number at the top of the column is the BMI at that height and weight. Pounds have been rounded off. http://www.nhlbi.nih.gov/guidelines/obesity/bmi_tbl.htm

TABLE 10–4 Calculation of Kilocalorie Needs for Adults (Short Methods):

	Level of Activity or Illness		
Goal:	**Low**	**Moderate**	**High**
Lose weight	15 kcal/kg	20 kcal/kg	25 kcal/kg
Maintain weight	20 kcal/kg	25 kcal/kg	30 kcal/kg
Gain weight	25 kcal/kg	30 kcal/kg	35 kcal/kg

Calorie need based on size for adults

There is a simple equation that can be used that may give a calorie level for size and activity level. To calculate the number of calories an adult needs to select the appropriate number and multiply it times the person's current weight.

	Calories needed for each pound of body weight
Men, active women	15
Most women, sedentary men and adults over 55 years	13
Sedentary women, obese adults	10
Pregnant women 1st trimester	13–15
2nd and 3rd trimester	16–17
Lactating women	15–17

Calorie need based on size for children

There is a general decline in the calories needed per pound, as a child gets older.
Calculate the calorie needs using the information in the table.

Age	**Calories needed for each pound of body weight**
0–12 mos	55
1–10 yrs	45–36
11–15 yrs–young women	17
11–15 yrs–young men	30
16–20 yrs–young women	15
16–20 yrs–young men	18

*Note that these figures may not be accurate for children who are obese

TABLE 10–5 Conversion Factors

1 foot = 30.48 cm
1 inch = 2.54 cm
1 cm = 0.39 inches
1 m = 39.37 inches
1 fluid oz = 29.57 mL
1 oz = 28 g
1 pound = 0.453 kg
1 kg = 2.2 pounds

OBESITY

NUTRITIONAL ACUITY RANKING: LEVEL 2

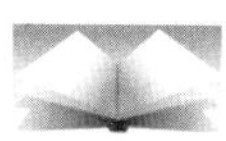

DEFINITIONS AND BACKGROUND

Obesity is the most common form of disturbed nutrition in the United States; undernutrition of specific nutrients is common. BMI standards are used to determine weight evaluations. BMI correlates well with body fat and is, therefore, a good predictor of chronic disease and mortality, except in highly trained athletes. Overweight is defined as BMI of 25–29; obesity is defined as BMI over 30. The prevalence of overweight (BMI over 25) and obesity (BMI over 40) doubled for all sex and race groups from 1985–1995 (Lewis et al., 2000). About 60% of American adults are overweight accordingly; 25% are obese.

According to Bray and Ryan (2000), the syndromes of obesity can be classified in several ways: The first is an anatomic classification based on the size, number, and distribution of fat cells and fat tissue. The second is an etiologic classification based on identification of specific diseases and settings that produce obesity (including hypothalamic injury and endocrine disease such as Cushing's disease and the polycystic ovary syndrome). The most common causes, however, are stopping smoking, over-consumption of high-fat foods, a decrease in the level of activity, and aging. Understanding the background for an individual provides a framework in which to design preventive or therapeutic strategies (Table 10–6).

Obesity is probably genetically predisposed; National Institute of Health (NIH) estimates that environment contributes 40–60%. Among children older than age 3, obesity is a strong predictor of adult obesity; parental obesity more than doubles the risk of adult obesity among both obese and nonobese children under 10 (Whitaker et al., 1997). Parents and the media have a strong impact on weight concerns and dieting among children and adolescents (Field et al., 2001). Apoprotein E is being studied for its role in obesity as well as in dyslipidemias (Srinivasan et al., 2001).

BMI and other cardiovascular risk factors without abdominal obesity measurement are sufficient to predict who needs weight loss (Kiernan and Winkleby, 2000) (Table 10–7). True height loss during aging must be taken into account when indexes based on height (such as BMI) are used; the rate of decrease in height is greater in women than in men. Height loss begins at age 30 and accelerates with increasing age; this degree of height loss would account for the "artifactual" increase in BMI that occurs for both men and women with aging (Sorkin et al., 1999).

Waist circumference is a predictor of mortality and chronic disease; it is a prognostic indicator along with BMI (Folsom et al., 2000). Use of DEXA is an accurate measurement method (Kamel et al., 1999). Hydrostatic weighing without head submersion in morbidly obese persons provides an accurate, acceptable, and convenient alternative method. Bioelectrical impedance analysis (BIA) can also be used but has been found to under-predict percentage body fat compared with hydrostatic weighing (Heath et al., 1998).

Percentage body fat and BMI are different among different ethnic groups; BMI cut-off points should, therefore, be population-specific. African Americans and Polynesians have BMIs a few points higher than those of whites; Chinese, Ethiopians, Indonesians, and Thais tend to have BMIs that are lower than whites (Deurenberg et al., 1998). Black women have lower metabolic rates than white women, and black men tend to have lower levels of fat oxidation than white men; these differences may contribute to greater obesity (Weyer et al., 1999). Among black women, BMI is inversely associated with self-image and satisfaction with body size; these perceptions may help motivate black women to lose weight (Riley et al., 1998). Among native Hawaiians, prevalence of overweight is 30% higher than among the general U.S. population in spite of similar diets and physical activity; therefore, genetics seem to play a larger role (Grandinetti et al., 1999). Ethnic disparity has no current consensus and is an emerging area of study.

Overweight and obesity increase risks of chronic diseases, secondary symptoms, and impaired quality of life. Obesity is positively related to depression in many individuals (Roberts et al., 2000). The prevalence of 2 or more health conditions increases with increasing BMI in all racial and ethnic groups (Must et al., 1999). Initial BMI and longer duration of overweight or obesity are positively related to the development of type 2 diabetes (Wannamethee et al., 1999). Concerns that dieting induces eating disorders have not been substantiated (National Task Force, 2000).

All health problems are more common in obese women than in men, except for the risk of cardiac heart disease (CHD) (Lean et al., 1999). Excess weight and even modest weight gain substantially increase risk of hypertension (HPN) in adult women; weight loss reduces the risk (Huang et al., 1998). Women who smoke and have a BMI over 30 (or under 20) have delayed conception (Bolumar et al., 2000).

Morbid obesity (over 40 BMI) is a strong predictor for premature death and moderate obesity (BMI between 25 and 32) is not associated with excess mortality whereas systolic blood pressure (BP), glucose intolerance, diabetes mellitus (DM), and smoking are related (Bender et al., 1998). In spite of surgical risks in the morbidly obese, weight loss provides greater overall benefits. Among patients with morbid obesity, quality of life is better after surgically induced weight loss than before, even if this effect decreases with time (Van Gemert et al., 1998).

A large percentage of Americans have lost 10% of their maximum weight and have maintained this loss for over 1 year, contrary to the belief that few people maintain their weight loss (McGuire et al., 1999). Low resting metabolic rate (RMR) in formerly obese persons may be genetic or acquired (Weyer et al., 2000) and may contribute to weight regain (Astrup et al., 1999). Visceral adipose tissue (VAT) distribution is an important determinant of RMR in men and postmenopausal women (Armellini et al., 2000).

Very-low-energy diets (VLED) combined with behavior therapy (BT) results in better maintenance of weight loss after 5 years than BT alone (Pekkarinen and Mustajoki, 1997). Several case reports and small studies of patients receiving starvation diets have reported hypotension, ventricular arrhythmias, and sudden cardiac death (Ahmed et al., 2001). Orthostatic hypotension may complicate very-low-calorie protein diets because of sodium depletion and depressed sympathetic nervous system activity. Bariatric surgery is associated with disproportionately high mortality rates in both the perioperative and postoperative periods (Ahmed et al., 2001).

Night-eating syndrome (NES) consists of morning anorexia, evening hyperphagia, and insomnia. Night eaters awaken more often during the night than others and have a lower nocturnal rise in plasma melatonin and leptin levels, with significantly higher circadian levels of plasma cortisol than controls (Birketvedt et al., 1999). Men tend to be more affected by NES (Aronoff et al., 2001). Shift work (alternating work schedules including night shift) appears to be positively related to BMI in men and women; it is unknown whether this is related to dietary habits or metabolic effects (Van Amelsvoort et al., 1999).

Obesity markedly influences serum insulin, leptin, growth hormone (GH) secretion, and free fatty acid (FFA) levels. In obese adolescent girls there is a blunted relative diurnal excursion in leptin levels; a nocturnal rise in leptin is paralleled by a nocturnal rise in GH and FFA levels (Heptulla et al., 2001) (see Table 10–8). Additional studies are needed.

Thermic effect of food (TEF) contributes to satiety. Overfeeding is a potent stimulus of thermogenesis and amplifies small individual variations associated with normal overfeeding (Dulloo et al., 1999). High protein meals also result in the greatest sensation of fullness (Crovetti et al., 1998).

It has been shown that a combination of diet and physical activity is the best treatment in weight management because physical activity influences energy balance, effects resting metabolic rate, and improves body composition, along with other benefits (Rippe et al., 1998). Self-esteem, body image, self-efficacy, locus of control, motivation, stress management, problem solving and decision making, and assertiveness are all important as well as the stage of change and environmental influences (Senekal et al., 1999).

About 5% of medical costs can be attributed to obesity, including health, life, disability insurance, and paid sick leave costs (Thompson et al., 1998). Sustained modest weight loss by obese adults would result in substantial health and economic benefits. A sustained weight loss of 10% would reduce the expected lifetime duration of HPN, hyperlipoproteinemia (HLP), and type 2 DM by 1.2–2.9, 0.3–0.8, and .5–1.7 years, respectively; reduction in lifetime costs for these 5 diseases would be $2,200–5,300 per patient (Oster et al., 1999). The American Dietetic Association recommends eight medical nutrition therapy visits for adult weight management (http://www.knowledgelinc.com/ada/mntguides/).

TABLE 10–6 Role of the Dietitian in Weight Management

The position of the American Dietetic Association on weight management calls for a multifaceted approach to working with clients. Healthful diet, moderate physical activity, reduced focus on weight, improved self-esteem, a more positive body image, and a functional support system are needed. White women seem to be especially vulnerable to body dissatisfaction in the U.S.; body image is closely related to self-esteem, especially in women. Preoccupation with thinness contributes to unhappiness and also interferes with development of rational eating and exercise behav iors. "Body size acceptance" is used to describe the goal of

(continued)

TABLE 10–6 Role of the Dietitian in Weight Management (*Continued*)

helping clients to challenge and replace the normative discontent that has become common (Parham, 1999). A major step forward has been to consider obesity as a chronic and debilitating disease that is associated with increased morbidity and mortality as in other diseases. Dietitians can be effective case managers in helping to monitor patient risks (St Jeor, 1997). Assessment of the individual's readiness to change stage will be most important in the initial visit (Snetselaar, 2000).

Increased intake of food away from home, especially fast food, probably contributes to the increasing prevalence of obesity (Binkley et al., 2000). Health care providers rarely advise patients to lose weight; those they do advise are already obese (Sciamanna et al., 2000). With the number of obesity cases rising, physicians cannot be the only care providers of these patients. A nonphysician primary obesity care provider can provide much of the care for obese patients with the physician acting as a support (Frank, 1998).

Pressure to be thin has resulted in a new set of problems that are impairing the psychological and social well-being of people who are overweight and of those who are not. It is important to help overweight and obese people be healthy regardless of weight change (Ikeda et al., 1999).

Weight management professionals have developed programs that aim to replace dieting with conventional eating habits in response to concern about the unreliability and harmful effects of dieting, i.e., the " Non-Diet" approach, which improves eating behavior, psychological well-being, and weight stability (Higgins and Gray, 1999).

Flexible and creative ways of staying in touch with participants are essential for maintaining weight loss. Problem-solving skills are needed that may require training outside the field of dietetics (Mattfeldt-Beman et al., 1999). Adults who are advised to lose weight are significantly more likely to lose weight than those who do not receive advice to lose weight (Galuska et al., 1999).

The **Mayo Clinic Healthy Weight Pyramid** is a useful tool; it suggests unlimited use of fruits and vegetables; 4–8 servings grains; 3–7 servings lean meat, fish, beans, and low fat dairy; 3–5 servings nuts, canola or olive oil, or avocados; and up to 75 calories from candy and other processed sweets.

Dietitians should play a role in achieving the goals of the Healthy Weight 2010 objectives: http://www.obesity.org/Healthy-Weight_2010. htm.:

1 Improve quality of life by reducing diseases and disability associated with obesity.
2 Increase quantity of life by reducing premature death associated with obesity.
3 Reduce disparities and social stigma related to obesity.
4 Promote healthy behaviors for weight control and weight management. Prevent weight gain that may lead to or exacerbate obesity and its comorbidities.
5 Educate public about health risks associated with obesity and its comorbidities.
6 Increase access to appropriate medical evaluation and treatment of obesity.

(continued)

TABLE 10–6 Role of the Dietitian in Weight Management (*Continued*)

7 Improve health communication dealing with weight control between health professionals, managed care organizations and patients, and providers of weight control-related services and consumers.
8 Form partnerships with organizations, businesses, and governmental health agencies (local, state, federal) to improve data collection and increase research funding with regard to obesity.

TABLE 10–7 Overweight/Obese Cutoff Points

Height in Inches	*Overweight (BMI of 25)*	*Obese (BMI of 30)*
	(pounds)	**(pounds)**
58	119	143
59	124	148
60	128	153
61	132	158
62	136	164
63	141	169
64	145	174
65	150	180
66	155	186
67	159	191
68	164	197
69	169	203
70	174	207
71	179	215
72	184	221
73	189	227
74	194	233
75	200	240
76	205	246

Derived from: National Institutes of Health (See Tables 10–2 and 10–3.)

TABLE 10–8 Role of Leptin

The hormone leptin, produced by adipocytes (fat cells), was discovered in mice; subsequently the human Ob gene was mapped to chromosome 7 (http://www.ncbi.nlm.nih.gov/disease/Obesity.html). Leptin is thought to act as a lipostat; as the amount of fat stored in adipocytes rises, leptin is released into the blood and signals to the brain that the body has enough to eat. Most overweight people have high levels of leptin in their bloodstream, indicating that other molecules also effect feelings of satiety and contribute to the regulation of body weight.

Leptin is produced within white adipose tissue, brown fat, the placenta, and fetal heart, bone, and cartilage. The hormone has multiple functions: inhibiting food intake, stimulating and maintaining energy expenditure, signaling to the reproductive sys-

(continued)

TABLE 10–8 Role of Leptin (*Continued*)

tem, and influencing metabolism (insulin secretion, lipolysis, and glucose transport). Mean plasma leptin levels are 3 times higher in obese twins than in lean twins and in women than in men (Ronnemaa et al., 1997). Leptin is involved in a variety of physiologic processes, not just energy balance. Leptin appears to be involved in physiologic regulation of hunger during negative energy balance (Keim et al., 1998). The complexity of the leptin system may reduce its potential as a target for antiobesity therapy (Trayhurn et al., 1999).

OBJECTIVES

- Determine the category of obesity—Hyperplastic–hypertrophic obesity results from increased fat cell number and lipid content of fat cells, most often in patients whose obesity began in their early years. Juvenile obesity is hyperplastic (increase in cell number). It is now believed that increases in cell number can occur throughout a lifetime.
- Decrease patient's calorie intake to induce a weight loss of ½–1 lb weekly. Ensure loss of fat, not lean body mass (LBM). Create an energy deficit of 500 kcals per day from usual intake.
- Provide a nutritionally balanced, individualized diet pattern. It is more important to balance energy expenditure with intake than to eat a very low-fat diet, which may be counterproductive (Allred, 1995). Diet histories show a trend toward underreporting of foods high in carbohydrates (CHO) and fat; this may have important implications when interpreting apparent declines in dietary fat (Heitmann et al., 2000).
- Maintain a normal or slightly higher protein intake to maintain nitrogen balance, especially with calorie-restricted diets. A diet high in protein and CHO induces a greater thermic response than a diet high in fat (Westerterp et al., 1999).
- Alleviate associated risk factors such as elevated lipids, blood pressure, uric acid, and glucose levels. Risk of HPN is positively related to central-type obesity and weight cycling (Guagnano et al., 2000).
- For patients who are morbidly obese, surgery may be indicated. Patients who undergo gastroplasty require regular follow-up, nutrition advice on diet quality and symptom management, and vitamin–mineral supplements for more than a year after surgery. Low protein intakes have adverse consequences in the long-term; iron, calcium, and zinc tend to be low (Cooper et al., 1999).
- Weigh weekly on the same scale with the same clothing on a monthly basis. BMI changes actually may be more important than weight itself.
- Avoid or correct disordered eating (abnormal eating/cheating, compulsive eating, addictive or manipulative habits, eating disorders). Emphasize healthy eating, not body fat percentages.
- Use water-dense foods. Intake of foods high in water content reduces subsequent energy intake more effectively than does intake of water with food (Rolls et al., 1999). The DASH diet also works well for this purpose.
- Prevent or improve symptoms of the Metabolic Syndrome (Syndrome X) if present. See section 9.

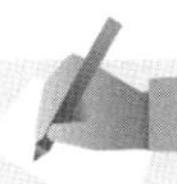

DIETARY AND NUTRITIONAL RECOMMENDATIONS

- Have the patient set his/her own goal: a weight loss of ½–1 lb per week. Each pound of body fat contains approximately 3,500 kcal.
- Schedule six to eight small meals at frequent intervals to prevent cheating and overeating. A snack eaten during satiety does not prolong the interval before individuals voluntarily eat their next meal (Marmonier et al., 1999). Breakfast is a crucial meal to prevent overeating later by some individuals.
- Diet should provide adequate fluid intake to excrete metabolic wastes. Beverages with meals increase the sensation of fullness. Rule of thumb is to use 1 ml water per 1 kcal, or 30 cc/kg of body weight.
- Decrease overall salt intake, if fluid retention is a concern.
- Intake of protein should follow recommended dietary allowances (RDAs) appropriate to the patient's age or slightly higher to maintain satiety while fat is being decreased.
- With elevated triglycerides, decrease concentrated sweets and sugars, fats, and alcohol. The latest NHLBI guidelines recommend use of 35% kilocalories from fat, with more from monounsaturated sources and not saturated fats.
- Increase fiber content; it takes longer to chew, is low in kilocalories, and increases satiety. High fiber cereal at breakfast seems to curb appetite at lunch slightly. Encourage 25–30 g per day.
- Teach patient to splurge by plan, not by impulse. Intake of a wide variety of sweets, snacks, condiments, entrees and CHO, and intake of a low variety of vegetables are positively related with energy intake and body fatness (McCrory et al., 1999).
- For a modified fast, a physician may prescribe Optifast, which gives 420 kcal, 70 g of egg-white and milk protein, essential fatty acids (EFAs), a small percentage of CHO, and standard vitamins and minerals. Medifast is another example.
- Very low calorie diets (VLCDs) may cause reduced resting energy expenditure (REE) by 20%; moderation is better.
- Decrease alcohol intake, with 7 kcal/g. Excesses may contribute to many cases of obesity (Suter et al., 1992).
- Use lots of raw fruits and vegetables, which contain a high water content compared with other choices.
- Extra vitamin D may be needed in obese persons; this may be due to its deposition in body fat compartments (Wortsman et al., 2000).
- The American Dietetic Association supports a "total diet approach" where the overall food pattern is more important than one food or meal. If food is consumed in moderation with appropriate portion size and regular activity, a more positive approach to food makes the client feel less anxious and guilty (American Dietetic Association, 2002).

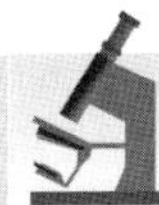

PROFILE

Clinical/History		Lab Work
Height	Percentage of body fat	Uric acid
Weight	BP	T3, T4
BMI	Skinfold thickness	Glucose (gluc)
Desirable BMI	Waist circumference	Albumin (alb), prealbumin
Weight changes	Sleep apnea?	Chol
Percentage of excess weight		Triglycerides (Trig)
		Hypoxemia

Common Drugs Used and Potential Side Effects

- Appetite suppressants may cause excitability, gastrointestinal (GI) distress, and other problems. This is especially true of drugs containing amphetamine. If an anorexiant has been prescribed, avoid using excesses of caffeine in the diet; this is not necessary if using a lipase inhibitor. Ionamin (Fastin) is a stimulant-like amphetamine; dry mouth can occur. Phentermine (Adipex-P) remains on the market; it is also an amphetamine derivative.
- Sibutramine (Meridia) increases energy expenditure (EE) and satiety, which may contribute to weight-reducing properties. It acts via the central nervous system (CNS) as serotonergic and noradrenergic reuptake inhibitor. About 25% of increased heart rate can be attributed to increased thermogenesis; plasma epinephrine, plasma glucose, and BP are all significantly elevated (Hansen et al., 1998).
- Orlistat (Xenical) decreases pancreatic lipase and decreases fat absorption. Soft stools and anal leakage may occur, especially if a diet high in fat (over 90 g) is consumed. Orlistat helps minimize weight regain after weight loss (Hill et al., 1999) and appears to be well tolerated. High-density lipoprotein (HDL) levels are much higher, overall total cholesterol (TC) levels drop, Vitamin E and beta-carotene levels are significantly higher in Orlistat users (Finer et al., 2000). Fat-soluble vitamins may be required during chronic therapy, because absorption may be decreased. Patients on Xenical should have a BMI over 27 with risk factors, over 30 without risk factors; the drug is not for everyone. Be sure to teach the patient about fat intake, or its side effects may cause failure of the plan.
- Dexedrine causes elevated glucose levels, dry mouth, unpleasant taste, dizziness, diarrhea, anorexia, extreme weight losses, GI disturbances, and drowsiness. It can cause growth disturbances in children.

- Olestra, a food fat substitute, decreases serum carotenoid and other fat-soluble vitamin absorption. Health effects reported are those found commonly in the general population and analyses of the data find no biological reason to conclude that serious or meaningful health effects are the result of olestra consumption (Allgood et al., 2001). Overall, there have been positive impacts on dietary fat intakes and serum cholesterol levels among consumers who use olestra-containing foods (Patterson et al., 2000).
- Prozac may cause headaches, dry mouth, nausea, diarrhea, and hyperglycemia. Other antidepressants have specific side effects that should be addressed. Prozac is often used for patients with bulimia nervosa.
- Fenfluramine HCl (Pendimin) and Redux (dexfenfluramine HCl) were taken off the market because of side effects, the most dangerous of which is pulmonary HPN and valvular problems (Weissman, 2001).
- Psychotropic medications may cause weight gain. Selective serotonin reuptake inhibitors, selective serotonin reuptake inhibitors (SSRIs) (Prozac, Zoloft, Paxil, Luvox, Celexa) cause weight loss at first, then weight gain later; Paxil causes the most weight change. Tricyclic antidepressants (TCAs) can cause much weight gain from slowed metabolism and increased CHO cravings; these include Elavil, Asendin, Aventyl, Pamelor, Adaptin, Sinequan, Tofranil, Norpramin, Anafranil, and Vivactil. Monoamine oxidase inhibitors (MAOI) have categories that cause more weight gain (i.e., nonselective reversibles, or Marplan, Nardil, Parnate). MAOI selective reversible drugs (RIMAs) manerix or Humoryl are not as weight enhancing. Mood stabilizers made with lithium can cause weight gain, as can the antipsychotics Haldol, Mellaril, Moban, Clozaril, Zyprexa, Serlect, Risperdal, Seroquel, and Zeldox.
- Anticonvulsants (Depakote, Tegretol, Lamictal, Neurontin, Topamax) can increase appetite and insulin levels. Insulin, prednisone, oral contraceptive (such as Depo-Provera) and other drugs have weight gain as a potential side effect. Monitor closely.
- Ursodeoxycholic acid administered during VLCD seems to have a protective role against developing gallstones (Festi et al., 2000).

Herbs, Botanicals and Supplements

- Herbs and botanical supplements should not be used without discussing with physician.
- Ephedra and Ma Huang contain ephedrine and derivative alkaloids and work as anorexiants. Do not take with digoxin, hypoglycemic agents, antihypertensives, oxytocin, theophylline, caffeine, and dexamethasone steroids to prevent antagonistic and dangerous combinations that affect heart rate and BP. The Food and Drug Administration (FDA) warns not to take more than 8 mg three times daily; some forms have been removed from the market.
- Chitosan is a major ingredient in many over-the-counter (OTC) products that claim to reduce excess body weight by reducing fat absorption. Weight and serum levels of cholesterol, TG, vitamins A, D, and E, and beta-carotene were not significantly different between two groups studied (Pittler et al., 1999).
- Stanols (Take Control) and sterols (Benacol) do not affect weight but are often used by overweight individuals. They are safely used as directed to lower elevated cholesterol levels.
- Hydroxycitric acid and garcinia are no more effective than placebo for treatment of obesity (Morelli and Zoorob, 2000). Garcinia has cytotoxic effects and has been demonstrated to have a toxic effect in animals.
- Chromium picolinate has been reported to improve glucose and lipid metabolism. Results of one study indicate that its use during a 4-week diet-and-exercise weight-loss program accelerated the rate of body fat loss and helped to maintain fat-free mass (lean tissue), thereby producing favorable changes in body composition (Hoeger et al., 1998).
- Phenylpropanolamine (PPA) produces dose-related, life-threatening cardiovascular and central nervous toxicity from adrenergic overstimulation. Because of these effects and the risk of hemorrhagic stroke, FDA requested that manufacturers stop using PPA in OTC cold medicines and prescription diet aids (Mersfelder, 2001).

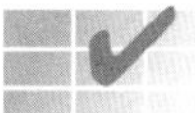

PATIENT EDUCATION

- ✓ A multidimensional program is best: formulation of reasonable goals, prevention of unnecessary weight loss or gain, weight loss when necessary, prevention of relapse, acceptance of an overweight/obese physique when necessary (Senekal et al., 1999). Individualize according to psychosocial, behavioral, and biological factors.
- ✓ Instruct patient how to maintain a proper diet; use of menus, recipes; portion control; eating at parties; low-calorie snacking; food preparation methods; and tips on restaurant dining. Frequency of restaurant food consumption positively correlates to body fatness (McCrory et al., 1999).
- ✓ Behavior therapy may be helpful in self-monitoring (food diaries, weights, activity). Teach stimulus control of cues, family intervention, and slowing down of eating. Be wary of eating in groups, at parties, and during breaks.
- ✓ Identify the mind–body connection. Teach patient about physical hunger–satisfaction rating scale (from 1–10) to identify true hunger from emotional "hunger." Emotional hunger results from anxiety, guilt, depression, loneliness, boredom, reward, and excess celebration. Steps to normalize eating include awareness training, changing thoughts and beliefs about food, handling issues of deprivation and guilt, and refocusing on areas other than food and weight. More information is available from http://www.med.unc.edu/nutr/nim. The scale is ranked as shown in Figure 10–1.

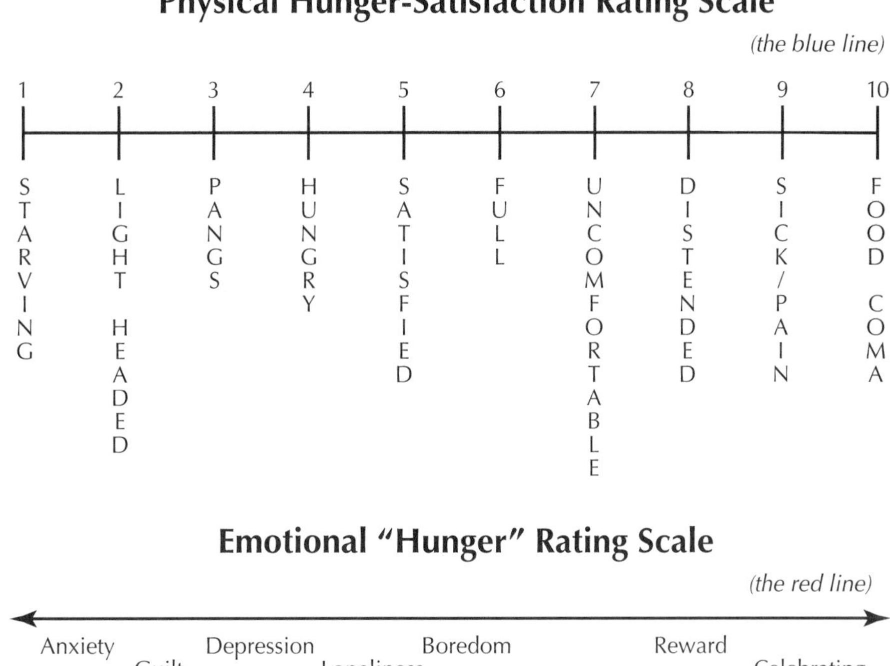

Figure 10–1 Hunger Rating Scale. (Courtesy of Claudia S. Plaisted, MS, RD, LDN, http://www.med.unc.edu/nutr/nim).

- ✔ To delay automatic eating, drink a glass of water instead of eating and wait 20 minutes; if the sensation still persists, it is probably hunger.
- ✔ One pound requires many extra capillary blood vessels for the additional circulation.
- ✔ Physical activity is an integral part of weight loss maintenance. Encourage moderate levels of physical activity for 30–45 minutes, 3–5 days a week. All adults should set a long-term goal to accumulate at least 30 minutes or more of moderate-intensity physical activity each day of the week (http://www.nhlbi.nih.gov/guidelines/obesity/sum_rec.htm). There is no such thing as cellulite; an active lifestyle can help to achieve a more fit body.
- ✔ Strategies aimed at reducing weight in childhood are important but only affect adult health if weight loss is maintained during adulthood (Gunnell et al., 1998).
- ✔ Make meals last 20 minutes or longer.
- ✔ Eat slowly; chew well. Sugarless gums can help.
- ✔ Avoid bizarre, fad dieting, skipping meals, and emphasis on any one dietary component.
- ✔ Soup before a meal and fructose-sweetened beverages can retard appetite.
- ✔ Noncalorie sweeteners are useful tools in weight management. However, low-sugar drinks do not necessarily facilitate a reduced energy intake (Holt et al., 2000).
- ✔ Although continuous exercise is hard to maintain, intense intervals of exercise can be easily endured and may be an important adjunct to lifestyle modifications for control of body weight (Hunter et al., 1998). Guidelines that suggest moderate-intensity exercise 30 minutes daily are better accepted by obese subjects than the old guideline of 20–60 minutes 3 times weekly (Weyer et al., 1998). Resistance training increases muscle mass. Aerobic exercise should be directed at 70% of maximal oxygen consumption. See Table 10–9.
- ✔ Be careful! Do not provide too low a calorie level (hypophagia); sudden death syndrome may occur.
- ✔ Caloric intake less than 1,200 kcal for women and 1,500 kcal for men requires an additional multivitamin supplement.
- ✔ Premenstrual weight gain may include 2–5 lb of fluid. Women should not assume that the menstrual cycle accounts for weight gains.
- ✔ Beware of a cultural emphasis on thinness, which may lead to unhealthy weight loss measures (Katzmarzyk and Davis, 2001). Enhancement of self-esteem is an important element (McArthur and Howard, 2001).
- ✔ Individuals vary in their ability to adjust intakes (Rolls et al., 1994). Nutritional counseling should be highly individualized as a result. Tables 10–10 and 10–11 describe cases for sleep apnea, Pickwickian syndrome, and smokers.
- ✔ Recipe modifications are useful for replacing fat in recipes (e.g., use applesauce or pear puree for muffins or sponge cake; prune or black bean puree in brownies or spice cake or chocolate cake; white bean puree in cookies).
- ✔ Table 10–12 provides a handy portion adjustment guide using everyday objects; Table 10–13 provides a chart with fad diets and how they compare.

TABLE 10–9 Physical Activity Equivalents

Warm Weather	Calories/Hr.	Cold Weather
Jogging 6 mph	450	Jumping rope
Hiking on steep hills	400	Indoor rappelling
Aerobics (low impact)	400	Snow shoveling, light
Rowing	400	Rowing machine
Swimming	400	Skiing cross-country
Tennis, singles	390	Racquetball
Cycling 10 mph	300	Stationary bike 10 mph
Golf with walking	300	Splitting logs
Gardening	280	Window cleaning
Mowing lawn	275	Mopping floors
Tennis, doubles	235	Indoor Basketball
Badminton	250	Indoor Volleyball
Walking 3 mph	250	Mall walking

TABLE 10–10 Weight Management for Sleep Apnea and Pickwickian Syndrome

Obstructive sleep apnea (OSA) is characterized by short duration (less than a minute) of repetitive episodes of impaired breathing during sleep. It occurs in 3% of adults in the U.S., 70% of whom are obese, which contributes to pharyngeal obstruction. Cardiovascular morbidity or even mortality may be increased (Loube et al., 1997). Continuous positive airway pressure (CPAP) is a primary treatment used at night to keep the pharynx from collapsing. Morbid obesity can also be associated with excessive daytime sleepiness even in the absence of sleep apnea (Resta et al., 2001).

A patient with Pickwickian syndrome (obesity-hypoventilation) is obese and hypersomnolent with cor pulmonale, polycythemia, nocturnal enuresis, and personality changes. Even mild obesity can affect lung function, especially in men. Weight loss can decrease symptoms and is a desired intervention.

TABLE 10–12 Portion Adjustments Using Everyday Objects (Source: Oregon State University Extension–used with permission)

Bread, Cereal, Rice, Pasta:
1 cup potatoes, rice, or pasta = 1 tennis ball or 1 ice cream scoop or a fist
One pancake = 1 compact disc (CD)
½ cup cooked rice = a cupcake wrapper full
One piece cornbread = bar of soap
One slice bread = audiocassette tape

Vegetables
1 cup green salad = 1 baseball or a fist
One baked potato = a fist
¾ cup tomato juice = small Styrofoam cup
½ cup broccoli = 1 scoop ice cream or one light bulb
½ cup serving = 6 asparagus spears, 7–8 baby carrots, or one ear of corn on the cob

Fruit
½ cup grapes (15) = a light bulb
½ cup fresh fruit = 7 cotton balls
One medium size fruit = a tennis ball or a fist
1 cup cut-up fruit = a fist
¼ cup raisins = large egg

Milk, Yogurt, Cheese
1–½ oz cheese = 9 volt battery, or 3 dominos
1 oz cheese = pair of dice, or your thumb
1 cup ice cream = large scoop the size of a baseball

Meat, Poultry, Fish, Dry Beans, Eggs, Nuts
2 Tbsp peanut butter = ping pong ball
1 tsp peanut butter = fingertip
1 Tbsp peanut butter = thumb tip
3 oz cooked meat, poultry, fish = your palm; a deck of cards; a cassette tape
3 oz grilled or baked fish = a checkbook
3 oz cooked chicken = chicken leg, thigh, or breast

Fats, Oils
1 tsp butter or margarine = size of a stamp, the thickness of your finger or thumb tip
2 Tbsp salad dressing = ping pong ball

TABLE 10–11 Weight Control and Smoking Cessation

Smoking cessation can lead to weight gain because of increased caloric consumption and changes in activity levels. Smoking increases the basal metabolic rate, so when it ceases the rate also decreases, making weight loss more difficult. High frequency of weight gain among adults who quit smoking demonstrates the need for interventions that address weight control (O'Hara et al., 1998). Moderate-to-heavy smokers who attempt to quit may need to reduce intake by 100–200 kcal daily just to maintain weight. Fruit often helps relieve the craving for sweets.

In general, smokers tend to consume more calories, fat, and ethanol/ethyl alcohol (ETOH) (McPhillips et al., 1994). Past smokers are more likely to be obese than current smokers, but smoking cessation lengthens life by several years and is worth it. Smoking cessation lowers cardiovascular and cancer risks more than compensating for possible weight gain.

Among both boys and girls, contemplation of and experimentation with smoking is related to weight concerns, as is daily exercise among boys and monthly purging or daily dieting among girls (Tomeo et al., 1999). Women who quit smoking typically gain 6–12 lbs in the first year after quitting; they fear weight gain more than men; smoking education information is available from the Office on Women's Health at www.4woman.gov.

TABLE 10–13 Fad Diets: How They Compare

Eating Plan	*Premise*	*Author's Background*	*Dietary Recommendations*	*Caloric Guidelines*	*Low/Missing Nutrients*	*Negative Health Implications*	*Scientific Evidence*
Food Guide Pyramid (FGP)	One component of a healthy lifestyle that includes nutrition and physical activity. The FGP includes all food groups; grains, fruits, veggies, dairy, meat/protein, and fats/sweets.	USDA and Health and Human Service dietitians developed the FGP, and a panel of health experts reviewed the plan.	50–60% Carbohydrate (CHO) 20–30% Fat 10–20% Protein	1,600–2,800 depending upon whether individual is male or female and activity level.	None, if the Pyramid is followed.	None, if the Pyramid is followed.	Scientific studies have proven that the most effective weight-loss program balances a healthful eating plan with regular exercise. To maintain weight loss, lose no more than 1–2 pounds a week.
Sugar Busters!	Recommends no sugar in diet. Authors say sugar is toxic to the body, causing it to release insulin and store excess sugar as body fat.	Authors are a corporate CEO and three medical doctors.	No firm guidelines. Advises against CHOs, especially simple/refined CHOs (which would eliminate some grains, fruits, and vegetables). Focuses more on protein and fat.	800–1,200	Carbohydrates Vitamins Minerals Fiber	Long-term effects may include increase risk for heart disease, kidney, and liver damage; short-term effects may include fatigue, weakness, and irritability.	Testimonial claims support it. Evidence is based on opinions, not proven scientific facts.
The Zone	Claims CHOs make you fat. It says most of our bodies over produce insulin when we eat CHOs. Does promote exercise.	Author Barry Sears has a Ph.D. in biochemistry and no formal training in nutrition.	40% Carbohydrate 30% Protein 30% Fat	800–1,200	Carbohydrates Vitamins Minerals Fiber	Takes pleasure out of eating by regarding food as a medicine prescription. Also, may experience fatigue, weakness, and irritability.	It has not been proven scientifically and is supported by testimonials and poorly conducted studies.
Diet Revolution	A throwback to the 70s high-protein, low-CHO diets. Says CHOs make you fat. Claims diet works fast and keeps you satisfied.	Dr. Atkins is a medical doctor and has no formal training in nutrition.	As much meat and fat as you want.	800	Carbohydrates Vitamins Minerals Fiber	May increase risk for heart disease and puts added work on the kidneys. May also experience fatigue, weakness, and irritability due to caloric restriction.	It has not been proven scientifically and is supported by testimonials.

(continued)

TABLE 10–13 Fad Diets: How They Compare

Eating Plan	*Premise*	*Author's Background*	*Dietary Recommendations*	*Caloric Guidelines*	*Low/Missing Nutrients*	*Negative Health Implications*	*Scientific Evidence*
Protein Power	A high-protein, low-CHO diet, the book claims the body has no need for CHOs, therefore, they should be avoided.	Authors Michael and Mary Eades are medical doctors with no formal training in nutrition.	30–50% Fat 30–45% Protein 15–35% Carbohydrate	No guidelines are provided, but they warn against eating less than 850–1,000 calories per day.	Carbohydrates Vitamins Minerals Fiber	May add stress to kidneys and increase risk for heart disease. May also experience fatigue, weakness, and irritability.	Claims success through testi monials and book sales.
Dr. Bob Arnot's Revolutionary Weight Control Program	Claims foods are drugs. Some foods make you feel good and others make you feel bad. Refined CHOs are the equivalent of "crack" and a big factor of weight gain.	Author Bob Arnot is a medical doctor but admits he is not a weight-loss expert.	55–65% Carbohydrate 20–25% Protein 15–20% Fat	No guidelines are provided.	Some forms of carbohydrates Vitamins Minerals	This book may take a psychological toll on its followers. Labeling food "good" or "bad" may make some feel like a bad person when they eat a "bad" food.	Arnot's theory lacks supporting scientific studies. His proof comes "from my producers at work, scientific colleagues, 100,000 readers of *Turning Back the Clock,* my wife, children, and friends."
Eat For Your Blood Type	Claims that people absorb nutrients and "react" to foods differently depending on blood type, which is based on our prehistoric ancestors.	Peter D'Adamo is a Naturopathic Physician.	Type O=Eat mostly meats Type A=Eat mostly fruits, vegetables, and grains Type B=Eat oats and rice flours, bananas, and other prescribed foods Type AB=Eat foods like tofu, sardines, oats, and rice	1,200 or less	Depending on blood type, whole food groups are eliminated. Vitamins Minerals	By eliminating entire food groups, some essential nutrients are deficient or absent.	No scientific evidence using blood type as an eating guide to lose weight. No data showing that prehistoric people with any particular blood type ate this way.

Source: Wheat Food Council and Washington State Dairy Council, #DC64, 1999. May be reproduced for educational purposes.

For More Information

- American Dietetic Association
  Weight Management protocol
  www.eatright.org
- CDC National Center for Chronic Disease Prevention and Health Promotion
  Report of the Surgeon General on Physical Fitness
  http://www.cdc.gov/nccdphp/sgr/summ.htm
- DASH Diet in Weight Management
  http://www.nhlbi.nih.gov/hbp/prevent/h_weight/h_weight.htm
- Gastric Surgery for Severe Obesity
  http://www.niddk.nih.gov/health/nutrit/pubs/gastsurg.htm
- Genome Studies of Obesity
  http://www.ncbi.nlm.nih.gov/disease/Obesity.html
- National Association to Advance Fat Acceptance (NAAFA)
  http://www.naafa.org/
- National Institutes of Health
  http://www.nhlbi.nih.gov/
- NHLBI Cholesterol and Metabolic Syndrome Guidelines
  http://www.nhlbi.nih.gov/guidelines/cholesterol/index.htm
- NHLBI Obesity Education Initiative
  NHLBI Health Information Network
  P.O. Box 30105
  Bethesda, Maryland 20824-0105
  (301) 592-8573
  Fax (301) 592-8563
  http://www.nhlbi.nih.gov
- President's Council on Physical Fitness
  http://www.surgeongeneral.gov/ophs/pcpfs.htm
- Shape Up America
  http://www.shapeup.org/
- Surgeon General
  http://www.surgeongeneral.gov/topics/obesity/
- Weight Control Information Network (WIN)
  1 Win Way
  Bethesda, MD 20892-3665
  1-877-946-4627
  Fax: (202) 828-1028
  http://www.niddk.nih.gov/health/nutrit/win.htm
- Weight Watchers International
  http://www.weightwatchers.com/
- Xenical—Roche Laboratories
  Xenicare Personal Program for use of Xenical
  1-800-936-4227

UNDERWEIGHT AND/OR GENERAL DEBILITY

NUTRITIONAL ACUITY RANKING: LEVEL 2

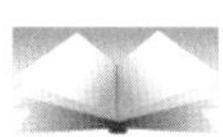

DEFINITIONS AND BACKGROUND

Being underweight is defined as having BMI below 18.5; about 8–9% of the population is underweight. Weight gain may be difficult for healthy individuals because of genetic tendency toward leanness, excessive activity, or inadequate eating patterns. Low BMI is a significant predictor of mortality, among young as well as old hospitalized patients (Landi et al., 2000). There are serious health risks associated with low weight and efforts to maintain an unrealistically lean body mass (Strawbridge et al., 2000). Self-esteem building should be a component in any nutrition education program aimed at preventing unhealthy dieting behaviors; it is important to identify individuals who are attempting weight loss despite being of normal or low body weight (Pesa, 1999).

Body fat is 80% of total fuel storage; body storage of glycogen is approximately 1,100 calories; body storage of protein equals 40,000 kcal of muscle tissue (loss of 30–50% is incompatible with survival). The Ancel Keys studies (1950) demonstrated that starvation results in food preoccupation, unusual eating habits, increased use of caffeine and tea, binge eating, depression, anxiety, social withdrawal, poor judgment, apathy, egocentrism, edema, sleep disturbances, hypothermia, GI disturbances, and lowered basal metabolism. Death in starvation is often from decreased respiratory muscle function and terminal pneumonia.

In elderly individuals, progressive debility leads to failure to thrive. Debility refers to unplanned and excessive weight loss, in which lean body mass has been lost. Patients with cardiac cachexia or chronic obstructive pulmonary disease (COPD) are often considered to be debilitated, if they have lost weight fairly rapidly; they generally seem to be quite emaciated. Chronic pancreatic insufficiency of unknown cause and intestinal bacterial overgrowth are more common than realized in the elderly and must be considered in any older patient with unexplained weight loss or failure to thrive (Holt, 2001). In the elderly, micronutrient deficiency is a common result and should be addressed.

The extent of hyperphagia after a period of starvation is largely determined by autoregulatory feedback mechanisms from fat and lean tissues (Dulloo et al., 1997). Blunted responsiveness to neuropeptide Y (NPY), a feeding stimulant, occurs concurrently with age-related anorexia and hypophagia (Pu et al., 2000). Older men are especially vulnerable to hypophagia after a period of weight loss (Roberts et al., 1994). The American Dietetic Association recommends three medical nutrition therapy visits for adults who have had unintentional weight loss (http://www.knowledgelinc.com/ada/mntguides/).

OBJECTIVES

- Increase body weight gradually.
- Encourage weight gain of approximately 1 lb weekly.
- In the case of recent debility, provide diet as tolerated to improve nutritional status. Progress slowly—it may take several days to stimulate the patient's appetite. If confusion exists, dehydration may be a factor.

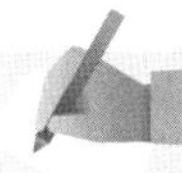

DIETARY AND NUTRITIONAL RECOMMENDATIONS

- Calculate patient's goal weight: (see Table 10–1) calculate patient's basal energy requirements and add kilocalories according to activity or stress factors. If patient's height and age are not available, it may be reasonable to use a simplified method such as, women: 100 lb for the first 5 feet plus 5 lb for each inch, plus or minus 10%, men: 106 lb for the first 5 feet plus 6 lb for each inch, plus or minus 10%.
- Calculate patient's metabolic rate. Each pound of fat requires 3,500 kcal; therefore, diet should be increased by 500 kcal daily to promote a weight gain of 1 lb per week.
- Use a high-protein/high-calorie diet with frequent feedings. Tube feed if needed. (See Decision Tree, section 17.)
- Diet should provide adequate amounts of zinc (Zn) to stimulate appetite, plus a general vitamin–mineral supplement, if needed.
- Plan meals and snacks according to appetite and preferences; encourage a snack about every 2–3 hours.

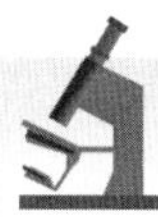

PROFILE

Clinical/History

Height
Weight
Usual weight
Recent weight changes
BMI
Desirable BMI
TSF, Mid-arm circumference (MAC), Mid-arm muscle circumference (MAMC)
BP
Intake and Output (I & O)

Lab Work

Hemoglobin and Hematocrit (H&H)
Trig
Alb, prealbumin
Chol
BUN, Creatinine (creat)
K+, Na+
Nitrogen (N) balance
Alkaline phosphatase (alk phos)
Ca++, Mg++
Total lymphocyte count (TLC)

Common Drugs Used and Potential Side Effects

- Appetite may be stimulated through use of medications such as Reglan, but not everyone responds positively with an increased appetite. Dry mouth and nausea may result.
- Antidepressants may be warranted when a qualified professional has documented depression. Monitor for dry mouth and other side effects specific to ordered medication.

Herbs, Botanicals and Supplements

- Herbs and botanical supplements should not be used without discussing with physician.

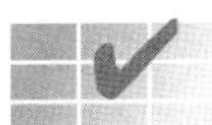

PATIENT EDUCATION

- ✓ Help patient make meals in a simple manner, using attractive foods.
- ✓ Identify spices, seasonings, and other flavor enhancements to stimulate the senses.
- ✓ Some identification of high-energy foods (sweets) may be useful in refeeding programs in which patient refuses to eat or take supplements. Adding or "hiding" kilocalories and protein in food also may be feasible, e.g., use of dry milk powder in soups or mashed potatoes.
- ✓ Promote lean body mass development through strength training—see Table 10–14.
- ✓ Offer tips on weight gain such as eating a small snack every 2–3 hours. A high-calorie bedtime snack is often beneficial.

TABLE 10–14 National Institute on Aging–Strength Training Tips

1. Start with a weight you can lift without too much effort (5 times).
2. When that is easy, rest a few minutes, and do it again (2 sets).
3. Increase to 3 sets.
4. Lift weight 10 times in each set.
5. Lift weight 15 times in each set.
6. Slowly increase weight and sets.

Source: Exercise: A Guide from the National Institute on Aging, 1-800-222-2225.

For More Information:

- American Dietetic Association
  Unintentional Weight Loss Prevention protocol
  http://www.eatright.org

PROTEIN–CALORIE MALNUTRITION (KWASHIORKOR, MARASMUS, MIXED, PCM)

NUTRITIONAL ACUITY RANKING: LEVEL 4

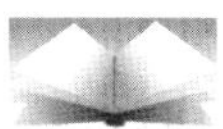

DEFINITIONS AND BACKGROUND

Of patients admitted to hospitals, 35–55% are malnourished on admission; 25–30% more become malnourished during stay. Approximately 50% of hospitalized patients are malnourished to some degree. In one study, 1.3–17.4% of hospitalized children were found to have severe or mild PCM (Hendricks et al., 1995). Malnutrition decreases cardiac output, BP, O2 consumption, TLC, T cells, and glomerular filtration rate (GFR) and increases infection rate, fatty infiltration, energy, emphysema and pneumonia, anemia, GI tract atrophy, bacterial overgrowth, and hepatic mass losses (Tables 10–15 and 10–16). Tissue catabolism usually begins with lowered albumin and plasma proteins, red blood cells (RBCs), and leukocytes, then later wasting of organs, skeletal muscle, bone, skin, and subcutaneous tissue. The CNS is the last tissue to be catabolized. Total starvation is fatal in 8–12 weeks.

Nutritional assessment, then intervention, saves approximately $2.40 for every $1 spent on a nutrition support team (Gallagher-Allred et al., 1996). It is important to use the designated International Classification of Diagnoses, 9th edition (ICD.9) codes in the medical record so that proper reimbursement for PCM is possible. As reported in more than 150 clinical studies, malnutrition is a health problem of huge magnitude, potentially affecting more than half of hospitalized patients in the United States (Bickford et al., 1999).

Albumin shifts intravascularly in marasmus and extravascularly in kwashiorkor. PCM risks: severe = albumin below 2.5 or prealbumin below 10; moderate = albumin 2.5–3.2 or prealbumin 10–17; mild-to-no risk = albumin 3.2 or prealbumin over 17.

In **kwashiorkor (ICD.9 code 260),** patient appears well nourished or even overnourished but has had recent stress with protein intake insufficient to maintain visceral stores. Albumin is usually lower than 3.0 gm/dL, and transferrin levels are depressed. TSF and weight for height are often normal. Depressed cellular immunity also exists. TLC, BUN, and creatinine are low. Pitting edema leads to the description of a "wet" PCM, and an enlarged fatty liver may occur. This takes place over a few weeks to months.

In **marasmus (ICD.9 code 261),** patient seems to be chronically starved. Decreased anthropometric values (MAMC, TSF, etc.) are produced by chronically inadequate diets and a moderate catabolic illness. Patient may have normal albumin and transferrin levels. Even muscle mass may be within normal limits. This is a "dry," dehydrated PCM in most cases. Absence of subcutaneous fat is common; TSF and weight for height are low. This occurs over months or years from low calorie intake.

In **mixed marasmic-kwashiorkor (ICD.9 code 262),** patient is severely depleted of somatic and visceral protein stores and consequently is less able to withstand added metabolic stress and catabolic illness. Anthropometric measures, muscle mass, and serum values are generally low. This may occur over a few weeks. Patient appears cachectic or may have edema (with a more normal appearance).

In **moderate PCM (ICD.9 code 263.0),** patient's weight is 75–84% of ideal or healthy body weight. Lymphocytopenia, energy, and anemia exist. Edema, generally, is not present. In **mild PCM (ICD.9 code 263.1)** usual body weight may be 85–95% of normal, TSF about 40–50 percentile, and serum albumin 2.8–3.5 g/dL. PCM is common in GI patients, especially inflammatory bowel disease (IBD), ventilator, radiation or chemotherapy, burn and surgical patients, and patients with renal failure.

Other PCM (ICD.9 code 263.8), other severe PCM (ICD.9 code 262), and **unspecified PCM (ICD.9 code 263.9)** are also codes for classifying various stages of PCM. **Slow fetal growth and fetal malformation (ICD.9 code 764)** and **low birthweight due to short gestation (ICD.9 code 765)** are used in the neonatal population.

OBJECTIVES

- Prevent weight loss, weakness, apathy, infections, and poor wound healing (see Table 10–15). For kwashiorkor: correct protein deficiency, edema, and fatty liver. For marasmus: provide energy immediately. Correct complications, which can include dehydration, electrolyte imbalances, infections, and vitamin–mineral deficiencies (see Table 10–16).
- Prevent complications (sepsis, overfeeding with hyperosmolar-nonketotic coma or hyperglycemia, congestive heart failure [CHF]).
- Avoid hazards of refeeding (hypophosphatemia, low Mg++, low K+). Fluid administration must be monitored carefully. Parenteral feeding is more of a problem than oral or enteral methods. Risk profiles include patients with anorexia nervosa, alcoholism, morbid obesity with rapid weight loss, prolonged fasting, or chronic malnutrition and underfeeding (Solomon and Kirby, 1990).

TABLE 10–15 Complicating Effects of Chronic Malnutrition (Protein-Calorie Deprivation) on Body Systems

Digestive Tract—Frequent, chronic, or even fatal diarrhea; bacterial translocation in gut; low HCl production in stomach; progressive weight loss; GI tract shrinks
Nervous System—Irritability, weakness and apathy even if intellect remains intact
Muscular System—Decreased activity; delayed physical rehabilitation; decreased muscle size and strength; delayed hospital discharge and ability to perform work
Skin and Skeleton—Pale, thin, dry inelastic skin; pressure ulcers; decreased subcutaneous fat; loss of bone density
Immune System—Depressed cell-mediated immunity; increased infection, particularly gram-negative sepsis; impaired wound healing; more wound infections or disruption; impaired ability to fight infections; delayed response to cancer chemotherapy or radiation therapy
Pulmonary System—Depressed ventilatory response to hypoxia; decreased lung capacity; slow breathing; pneumonia and eventually respiratory failure
Cardiac and Hematological System—Anemia; altered clotting time; decreased heart size; decreased amount of blood pumped; slow heart rate; decreased BP; heart failure; decreased number of blood cells
Renal System—Fluid, electrolyte and acid-base malfunctioning; increased frequency of urinary tract infections; elevated BUN from muscle and tissue breakdown; decreased GFR
Endocrine System—Decreased body temperature (hypothermia); fluid accumulation in skin from lower subcutaneous fat and decreased albumin; vitamin–mineral deficiencies
Reproductive System—Decreased size of ovaries or testes; decreased libido; cessation of menstruation
Quality of Life—Increased and prolonged use of hospitals, critical care units, expensive drugs, and excessive requirements of hospital support

TABLE 10–16 Selected Biochemical Changes Observed in Severe PCM

Body Composition	**Marasmus**	**Edematous PCM**
Total body water	High	High
Extracellular water	High	Higher
Total body potassium	Low	Lower
Total body protein	Low	Low
Serum or Plasma		
Transport proteins (transferrin, ceruloplasmin, retinol-, cortisol- and thyroxine-binding proteins, beta-lipoproteins)	Normal or low	Low
Branched-chain amino acids	Normal or low	Low
Tyrosine:phenylalanine ratio	Normal or low	Low
Enzymes (in general), such as amylase, alkaline phosphatase	Normal	Low
Transaminase	Normal or high	High
Liver		
Fatty infiltration	Absent	Severe
Glycogen	Normal or low	Normal or low
Urea cycle and other enzymes such as xanthine oxidase, glycolic acid oxidase, cholinesterase	Low	Lower
Amino acid synthesizing enzymes	High	Not as high

Data from: Torun B, Viteri F. Protein-energy malnutrition. In: Warren K, Mahmood A, eds. *Tropical and geographical medicine*. 2nd ed. New York: McGraw-Hill, 1990.

TABLE 10–17 Characteristics That Indicate Poor Prognosis in Patients with PCM

Age less than 6 months
Deficit in weight for height greater than 30%, or in weight for age greater than 40%
Signs of circulatory collapse: cold hands and feet, weak radial pulse, diminished consciousness
Stupor, coma, or other alterations in awareness
Infectious, particularly bronchopneumonia or measles
Petechiae or hemorrhagic tendencies (purpura is usually associated with septicemia or a viral infection)
Dehydration and electrolyte disturbances, particularly hypokalemia and severe acidosis
Persistent tachycardia, signs of heart failure or respiratory difficulty
Total serum proteins below 30 g/L
Severe anemia with clinical signs of hypoxia
Clinical jaundice or elevated serum bilirubin level
Extensive exudative or exfoliative cutaneous lesions or deep decubitus ulcerations
Hypoglycemia
Hypothermia

Source: Shils M, et al. *Modern nutrition in health and disease.* 9th ed. Baltimore: Williams & Wilkins, 1998.

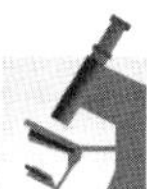

PROFILE

Clinical/History	Lab Work	
Height or arm length/knee length	Alb, prealbumin	TLC, white blood cell count (WBC) (decreased)
Weight	Chol, Trig (decreased)	Na+, K+, Cl−
BMI (see Table 10–1)	Serum Fe	Total iron-binding capacity (TIBC) (<250 mg/dL)
Recent weight; weight changes	Alk phos (decreased)	Serum B12
Usual weight	Transferrin	Serum folacin
Desirable BMI	Gluc (increased or decreased)	Ca++, Mg++
I & O	H&H	Serum Cu (decreased)
BP	Urine acetone	Oxygen saturation levels
Edema	T3, T4	
Muscle wasting	Mg++	
TSF	BUN (decreased)	
MAMC, MAC	Creatinine	

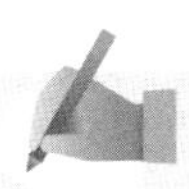

DIETARY AND NUTRITIONAL RECOMMENDATIONS

- **PCM:** Sufficient calories and protein, gradually increasing to meet needs. Vitamin–mineral supplementation is needed to treat all of these conditions.
- **Kwashiorkor:** Begin initial treatment with small amounts of skim milk, perhaps lactose-treated. After 1 week, gradually add a mixed diet. Start treatment with 2.5–3 g protein/kg body weight, 0.8–1.0 × BEE at first. Diet should provide adequate CHO and caloric intake to spare protein and correct weight loss. Use tube feeding (TF) or total parenteral nutrition (TPN), if appropriate (see section 17). Add thiamin if needed.
- **Marasmus:** Start treatment with intravenous or oral glucose. Gradually add lactose-treated skim milk to diet, adding solids later. Provide high biologic value (HBV) proteins and calories adequate to use N effectively. Avoid overfeeding (use 25–30 kcal/kg), progressing gradually to 35–40 kcal/kg. Add a vitamin–mineral supplement, if necessary, including thiamin. TF, if needed--start with continuous versus intermittent or bolus feedings.
- **Important Protein Measurements:** Somatic (muscle mass, renal function), visceral (albumin, transferrin), general (N balance)

Herbs, Botanicals and Supplements

- Herbs and botanical supplements should not be used without discussing with physician.

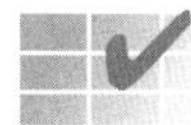

PATIENT EDUCATION

- ✓ Emphasize importance of gradual refeeding.
- ✓ Unless nutritional therapy is aggressive, infection is a major risk. Surgery becomes life threatening, and sepsis is more likely.
- ✓ PCM can increase fistula formation, reduce recovery and wound healing after surgery, and lead to pneumonia or poor drug tolerance.
- ✓ Allow patients to participate in feeding decisions. Set goals and help plan together with family.
- ✓ Discuss complicating effects of protein–calorie deprivation.

For More Information:

- American Dietetic Association
  Unintentional Weight Loss Prevention protocol
  http://www.eatright.org
- Web-search for ICD.9 Codes
  http://clinweb2.kumc.edu/Codes/icd9desc.asp

REFEEDING SYNDROME

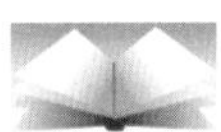

DEFINITIONS AND BACKGROUND

Refeeding syndrome is mostly hypophosphatemia, which follows aggressive refeeding after a period of starvation. The metabolic adaptation of semistarvation (in conditions such as anorexia nervosa) is impaired during refeeding with an increase in the thermic effect of food and a high risk of refeeding syndrome (Melchior, 1998).

Abnormal metabolism results, with a shift from body fat to CHO as substrate. Insulin is secreted excessively, and glucagon decreases with reduced gluconeogenesis, glycogenolysis, and fatty acid mobilization. Glucose is taken up rapidly into the cells, and phosphorus is driven inside the cells. Severe hypophosphatemia may occur more quickly with parenteral nutrition (PN) than with enteral or oral feeding. Adenosine triphosphatase (ATP) levels decrease as a result, with major effects on the cardiac, pulmonary, CNS, hematologic, and muscular systems. Signs of hypophosphatemia include anorexia, bone pain, dizziness, muscle weakness, respiratory failure, and myocardial dysfunction.

Other problems encountered in refeeding syndrome include sodium derangements, possibly leading to CHF; potassium shifts into cells with resulting hypokalemia and arrhythmias; magnesium shifts intracellularly with tetany and seizures. Thiamin deficiency also has been noted with refeeding, because it is a cofactor in CHO metabolism.

OBJECTIVES

- ▲ Gradually correct starvation without overloading the system with nutrients of any type. Use less than full levels of calorie and fluid needs.
- ▲ Advance calories and volume with careful monitoring of cardiac and respiratory side effects.
- ▲ Monitor for neurologic, hematologic, and metabolic complications such as hypokalemia, hypophosphatemia, hyperglycemia, and sodium retention.
- ▲ Correct vitamin and mineral deficiencies, especially with symptoms.

DIETARY AND NUTRITIONAL RECOMMENDATIONS

- Estimate previous calorie intake during starvation and begin with that amount of calories or with 20 kcal/kg.
- Protein should be calculated at 1.2–1.5 g/kg as tolerated to protect and restore some lean body mass.
- Restrict CHO intake at first to 150–200 g/day to prevent sudden insulin production.
- Fat calories should make up the difference.
- Gradually increase calories after 3–5 days as tolerated, to reach goal kilocalories by 10–14 days.
- Maintain fluid balance; adjust when edema exists (e.g., fluid restriction according to I & O, tachycardia, peripheral edema).
- Adjust for sodium and potassium intakes dependent on laboratory values until normal.
- Supplement with thiamin and other vitamins and minerals as needed. Excesses are not required.

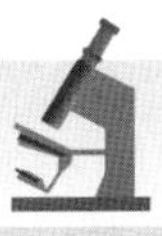

PROFILE

Clinical/History

Height
Weight
BMI
Desirable BMI
Percentage of weight
History of weight changes
I & O
Edema
Tachycardia
Temperature

Lab Work

Gluc (serum, urinary)
Urinary acetone
Alb, prealbumin
Chol, Trig
H&H, Serum Fe
K+
Na+
Mg+
BUN
Alk Phos; Serum phosphorus
Creatinine
Partial pressure of carbon dioxide (pCO_2), partial pressure of oxygen (pO_2)

Common Drugs Used and Potential Side Effects

- Replacement of potassium may be needed, if serum levels are depleted. Monitor specific medications used and their side effects, e.g., GI distress.
- Insulin is often used to correct high hyperglycemia levels. Watch for signs of hypoglycemia, if food intake is unusually low.

Herbs, Botanicals and Supplements

- Herbs and botanical supplements should not be used without discussing with physician.

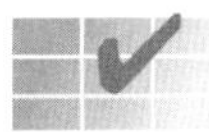

PATIENT EDUCATION

- ✓ Discuss ways in which future periods of starvation can be avoided.
- ✓ Offer guidelines according to discharge intervention plan for use at home or elsewhere. Physician may suggest long-term medication use or therapies.

REFERENCES

Cited References

Ahmed W, et al. Cardiovascular complications of weight reduction diets. *Am J Med Sci.* 2001;321:280.

Allgood G, et al. Postmarketing surveillance of new food ingredients: results from the program with the fat replacer olestra. *Rgul Toxicol Pharmacol.* 2001;33:224.

American Dietetic Association. Position of the American Dietetic Association: total diet approach to communicating food and nutrition information. *J Am Diet Assoc.* 2002;102:100.

Armellini F, et al. Postabsorptive resting metabolic rate and thermic effect of food in relation to body composition and adipose tissue distribution. *Metabolism: Clin & Experimental.* 2000;49:6.

Aronoff N, et al. Gender and body mass index as related to night eating syndrome in obese patients. *J Am Diet Assoc.* 2001;101:102.

Astrup A, et al. Meta-analysis of resting metabolic rate in formerly obese subjects. *Am J Clin Nutri.* 1999;69:1117.

Barlow S, Dietz W. Obesity evaluation and treatment: expert committee recommendations. The Maternal and Child Health Bureau, Health Resources and Services Administration, and the Department of Health and Human Services. *Pediatr.* 1998;102:E29.

Bender R, et al. Assessment of excess mortality in obesity. *Am J Epid.* 1998;147:42.

Binkley, et al. The relation between dietary change and rising U.S. obesity. *Int J of Obesity and Related Metabolic Disorders.* 2000;24:1032.

Birketvedt G, et al. Behavioral and neuroendocrine characteristics of the night-eating syndrome. *J Am Med Assoc.* 1999;282:657.

Bolumar F, et al. Body mass index and delayed conception: a European multicenter study on infertility and subfecundity. *Am J Epid.* 2000;151:1072.

Bray G, Ryan D. Clinical evaluation of the overweight patient. *Endocrine.* 2000;13:167.

Cooper P, et al. Nutritional consequences of modified vertical gastroplasty in obese subjects. *Int J Obesity and Related Metabolic Disorders.* 1999;23:382.

Crovetti R, et al. The influence of thermic effect of food on satiety. *Euro J Clin Nutri.* 1998;52:482.

Deurenberg P, et al. Body mass index and percent body fat: a meta analysis among different ethnic groups. *Int J Obesity and Related Metabolic Disorders.* 1998;22:1164.

DiBuono M, et al. Weight loss due to energy restriction suppresses cholesterol biosynthesis in overweight, mildly hypercholesterolemic men. *J Nutri.* 1999;129:1545.

Dulloo A, et al. Low protein overfeeding: a tool to unmask susceptibility to obesity in humans. *Int J Obesity and Related Metabolic Disorders.* 1999;23:1118.

Dulloo A, et al. Poststarvation hyperphagia and body fat overshooting in humans: a role for feedback signals from lean and fat tissues. *Am J Clin Nutri.* 1997;65:717.

Eisenkolbl J, et al. Underestimation of percentage fat mass measured by bioelectrical impedance analysis compared to dual energy X-ray absorptiometry method in obese children. *Eur J Clin Nutri.* 2001;55:423.

Festi D, et al. Review: low caloric intake and gall bladder motor function. *Aliment Pharmacol Ther.* 2000;14:51S.

Field A, et al. Peer, parent, and media influences on the development of weight concerns and frequent dieting among preadolescent and adolescent girls and boys. *Pediatr.* 2001;107:54.

Finer N, et al. One-year treatment of obesity: a randomized, double-blind, placebo controlled, multicenter study of orlistat, a gastrointestinal lipase. *Int J Obesity & Related Metab Disorders.* 2000;24:306.

Folsom A, et al. Associations of general and abdominal obesity with multiple health outcomes in older women: the Iowa Women's Health Study. *Arch Int Med.* 2000;160:2117.

Frank A. A multidisciplinary approach to obesity management: the physicians' role and team care alternatives. *J Am Diet Assoc.* 1998;98:10S.

Franz M. Managing obesity in patients with comorbidities. *J Am Diet Assoc.* 1998;98:10S.

French S, et al. Is dieting good for you? Prevalence, duration, and associated weight and behavior changes for specific weight loss strategies over 4 years in U.S. adults. *Int J Obesity and Related Metabolic Disorders.* 1999;23:320.

Gallagher-Allred C, et al. Malnutrition and clinical outcomes: the case for medical nutrition therapy. *J Am Diet Assoc.* 1996;361:366.

Galuska D, et al. Are health care professionals advising obese patients to lose weight? *J Am Med Assoc.* 1999;282:1576.

Grandinetti A, et al. Prevalence of overweight and central adiposity is associated with percentage of indigenous ancestry among native Hawaiians. *Int J Obesity and Related Metabolic Disorders.* 1999;23:733.

Guagnano M, et al. Risk factors for hypertension in obese women: the role of weight cycling. *Euro J Clin Nutri.* 2000;54:356.

Gunnell D, et al. Childhood obesity and adult cardiovascular mortality: a 57-year follow-up study based on the Boyd Orr cohort. *Am J Clin Nutri.* 1998;67:1111.

Hakala P, et al. Environmental factors in the development of obesity in identical twins. *Int J Obesity and Related Metabolic Disorders.* 1999;23:746.

Hansen D, et al. Thermogenic effects of sibutramine in humans. *Am J Clin Nutri.* 1998;68:1180.

Heptulla R, et al. Temporal patterns of circulating leptin levels in lean and obese adolescents: relationships to insulin, growth hormone, and free fatty acids rhythmicity. *J Clin Endocrinol Metab.* 2001;86:90.

Heath E, et al. Bioelectric impedance and hydrostatic weighing with and without head submersion in persons who are morbidly obese. *J Am Diet Assoc.* 1998;98:8.

Heitmann B, et al. Do we eat less fat, or just report so? *Int J Obesity & Related Metab Disorders.* 2000;24:435.

Higgins L, Gray W. What do antidieting programs achieve? *Australian J Nutr and Dietetics.* 1999;56:128.

Hill J, et al. Orlistat, a lipase inhibitor, for weight maintenance after conventional dieting. *Am J Clin Nutri.* 1999;69:1108.

Hoeger W, et al. Four-week supplementation with a natural dietary compound produces favorable changes in body composition. *Adv Ther.* 1998;15:305.

Holt P. Diarrhea and malabsorption in the elderly. *Gastroenterol Clin North Am*. 2001;30:427.

Holt S, et al. The effects of sugar-free vs sugar-rich beverages on feelings of fullness and subsequent food intake. *Int J Food Sci Nutri*. 2000;51:59.

Huang Z, et al. Body weight, weight change, and risk for hypertension in women. *Ann Int Med*. 1998;128:81.

Hunter G, et al. A role for high intensity exercise on energy balance and weight control. *Int J Obesity and Related Metabolic Disorders*. 1998;22:489.

Ikeda J, et al. A commentary on the new obesity guidelines from NIH. *J Am Diet Assoc*. 1999;99:918.

Kamel E, et al. Measurement of abdominal fat by magnetic resonance imaging, dual-energy X-ray absorptiometry and anthropometry in nonobese men and women. *Int J Obesity and Related Metabolic Disorders*. 1999;23:686.

Keim N, et al. Relation between circulating leptin concentrations and appetite during a prolonged moderate energy deficit in women. *Am J Clin Nutri*. 1998;68:794.

Keys A, et al. *The biology of human starvation*. Vol. 1. Minneapolis: University of Minnesota Press, 1950.

Kiernan M, Winkleby M. Identifying patients for weight loss treatment: an empirical evaluation of the NHLBI Obesity Education Initiative Expert Panel Treatment recommendations. *Arch Int Med*. 2000;160:2169.

Landi F, et al. Body mass index and mortality among hospitalized patients. *Arch Int Med*. 2000;160:2641.

Lean M, et al. Impairment of health and quality of life using new U.S. federal guidelines for the identification of obesity. *Arch Int Med*. 1999;159:837.

Lewis C, et al. Weight gain continues in the 1990s: 10 year trends in weight and overweight from the CARDIA Study. *Am J Epid*. 2000; 151:1172.

Loube D, et al. Continuous positive airway pressure treatment results in weight loss in obese and overweight patients and obstructive sleep apnea. *J Am Diet Assoc*. 1997;97:896.

Marmonier C, et al. Metabolic and behavioral consequences of a snack consumed in satiety state. *Am J Clin Nutri*. 1999;70:854.

Mattfeldt-Beman M, et al. Participants' evaluation of a weight-loss program. *J Am Diet Assoc*. 1999;99:66.

McArthur L, Howard A. Dietetics majors' weight reduction beliefs, behaviors, and information sources. *J Am Col Health*. 2001;49:175.

McCrory M, et al. Dietary variety within food groups: Association with energy intake and body fatness in men and women. *Am J Clin Nutri*. 1999;69:440.

McCrory M, et al. Overeating in America: association between restaurant food consumption and body fatness in healthy adult men and women ages 19–80. *Obesity Research*. 1999;7:564.

McGuire M, et al. The prevalence of weight loss maintenance among American adults. *Int J Obesity and Related Metabolic Disorders*. 1999;23:1314.

McPhillips J, et al. Dietary differences in smokers and nonsmokers from two southeastern New England communities. *J Am Diet Assoc*. 1994;94:287.

Melchior J. From malnutrition to refeeding during anorexia nervosa. *Curr Opin Clin Nutr Metab Care*. 1998;1:481.

Mersfelder T. Phenylpropanolamine and stroke: the study, the FDA ruling, the implications. *Cleve Clin J Med*. 2001;68:208.

Morelli V, Zoorob R. Alternative therapies: part 1. Depression, diabetes, obesity. *Am Fam Phys*. 2000;62:1051.

Must A, et al. The disease burden associated with overweight and obesity. *J Am Med Assoc*. 1999;282:1523.

National Heart, Lung, and Blood Institute Expert Panel on the identification, evaluation, and treatment of overweight and obesity in adults. Executive summary of the clinical guidelines on the identification, evaluation, and treatment of overweight and obesity in adults. *J Am Diet Assoc*. 1998;98:10.

NHLBI Clinical Guidelines on the Identification, Evaluation and Treatment of Overweight and Obesity in Adults-the Evidence Report. *Obesity Research*. 1998;53 Suppl.

National Task Force on the Prevention and Treatment of Obesity. *Arch Int Med*. 2000;160:2581.

Nieman D, et al. Influence of obesity on immune function. *J Am Diet Assoc*. 1999;99:294.

Norman R, Clark A. Obesity and reproductive disorders: a review. *Reprod Fertil Dev*. 1998;10:55.

Olson J, et al. Evidence for a major gene influence on abdominal fat distribution: the Minnesota breast cancer family study. *Genet Epidemiol*. 2001;220:458.

Oster G, et al. Lifetime health and economic benefits of weight loss among obese persons. *Am J Public Health*. 1999;89:1536.

Parham E. Promoting body size acceptance in weight management counseling. *J Am Diet Assoc*. 1999;99:920.

Patterson R. Changes in diet, weight, and serum lipid levels associated with Olestra consumption. *Arch Intern Med*. 2000;160:2600.

Pekkarinen T, Mustajoki P. Comparison of behavior therapy with and without very-low-energy diet in the treatment of morbid obesity. *Arch Int Med*. 1997;157:1581.

Pesa J. Psychosocial factors associated with dieting behaviors among female adolescents. *J Sch Health*. 1999;69:196.

Pittler M, et al. Randomized double-blind trial of chitosan for body weight reduction. *Euro J Clin Nutri*. 1999;53:379.

Pu S, et al. Neuropeptide Y counteracts the anorectic and weight reducing effects of ciliary neurotropic factor. *J Neuroendocrinol*. 2000;12:827.

Resta O, et al. Sleep-related breathing disorders, loud snoring and excessive daytime sleepiness in obese subjects. *Int J Obes Relat Metab Disord*. 2001;25:669.

Riley N, et al. Relation of self-image to body size and weight loss attempts in black women: The CARDIA Study. *Am J Epid*. 1998; 148:1062.

Rippe J, et al. The role of physical activity in the prevention and management of obesity. *J Am Diet Assoc*. 1998;98:10S.

Roberts R, et al. Are the obese at greater risk for depression? *Am J Epid*. 2000;152:163.

Roberts S, et al. Control of food intake in older men. *JAMA*. 1994; 272:1601.

Rolls B, et al. Satiety after preloads with different amounts of fat and carbohydrate: implications for obesity. *Am J Clin Nutri*. 1994;60: 476.

Rolls B, et al. Water incorporated into a food but not served with a food decreases energy intake in lean women. *Am J Clin Nutri*. 1999;70:448.

Ronnemaa T, et al. Relation between plasma leptin levels and measures if body fat in identical twins discordant for obesity. *Ann Int Med*. 1997;126:26.

Sattar N, et al. Antenatal waist circumference and hypertension risk. *Obstet Gynecol*. 2001;97:268.

Sciamanna C, et al. Who reports receiving advice to lose weight? *Arch Int Med*. 2000;160:2334.

Senekal M, et al. A multidimensional weight-management program for women. *J Am Diet Assoc.* 1999;99:1257.

Snetselaar L. Counseling for change. In: Mahan K, Escott-Stump S, eds. *Krause's food, nutrition, and diet therapy.* 10th ed. Philadelphia: WB Saunders, 2000.

Solomon S, Kirby D. The refeeding syndrome: a review. *J Parenter Enteral Nutri.* 1990;14:90.

Sorkin J, et al Longitudinal change in height of men and women: implications for interpretation of the body mass index. The Baltimore Longitudinal Study of Aging. *Am J Epid.* 1999;150:969.

Srinivasan S, et al. Apolipoprotein E polymorphism modulates the association between obesity and dyslipidemias during young adulthood: the Bogalusa Heart Study. *Metabolism.* 2001;50:696.

St Jeor S. New trends in weight management. *J Am Diet Assoc.* 1997; 97:1096.

Strain G. Response to promoting size acceptance in weight management counseling. *J Am Diet Assoc.* 1999;99:926.

Strawbridge W, et al. New NHBI clinical guidelines for obesity and overweight: Will they promote health? *Am J Pub Health.* 2000;90: 340.

Stevens J. Impact of age on associations between weight and mortality. *Nutr Rev.* 2000;58:129.

Suter P, et al. The effect of ethanol on fat storage in healthy subjects. *N Engl J Med.* 1992;326:983.

Thompson D, et al. Estimated economic costs of obesity to U.S. business. *Am J Health Promotion.* 1998;13:120.

Tomeo C, et al. Weight concerns, weight control behaviors, and smoking initiation. *Pediatrics.* 1999;104:918.

Trayhurn P, et al. Leptin: fundamental aspects. *Int J Obesity and Related Metabolic Disorders.* 1999;23:22.

Van Amelsvoort L, et al. Duration of shift work related to body mass index and waist to hip ratio. *Int J Obesity and Related Metabolic Disorders.* 1999;23:948.

Van Gemert W, et al. Quality of life assessment of morbidly obese patients: effect of weight-reducing surgery. *Am J Clin Nutri.* 1998; 67:197.

Wannamethee S, et al. Weight change and duration of overweight and obesity in the incidence of type 2 diabetes. *Diab Care.* 1999; 22:1266.

Weissman N. Appetite suppressants and valvular heart disease. *Am J Med Sci.* 2001;321:285.

Westerterp K, et al. Diet induced thermogenesis measured over 24h in a respiration chamber. *Int J Obesity and Related Metabolic Disorders.* 1999;23:287.

Weyer C, et al. Energy metabolism after 2 years of energy restriction: the Biosphere experiment. *Am J Clin Nutri.* 2000;72:946.

Weyer C, et al. Energy metabolism in African Americans: potential risk factors for obesity. *Am J Clin Nutri.* 1999;70:13.

Weyer C, et al. Implications of the traditional and the new ACSM physical activity recommendations on weight reduction in dietary treated obese subjects. *Int J Obesity and Related Metabolic Disorders.* 1998;22:1071.

Whitaker R, et al. Predicting obesity in young adulthood from childhood and parental obesity. *N Engl J Med.* 1997;337:337.

Wortsman J, et al. Decreased bioavailability of vitamin D in obesity. *Am J Clin Nutri.* 2000;72:690.

Suggested Readings

American Dietetic Association. Position of the ADA: fat replacers. *J Am Diet Assoc.* 1998;98:463.

Appleby P, et al. Low body mass index in nonmeat eaters: the possible roles of animal fat, dietary fiber and alcohol. *Int J Obesity and Related Metabol Disorders.* 1998;22:454.

Arcaro G, et al. Body fat distribution predicts the degree of endothelial dysfunction in uncomplicated obesity. *Int J Obesity and Related Metabolic Disorders.* 1999;23:936.

Aronne L. Modern medical management of obesity: the role of pharmaceutical intervention. *J Am Diet Assoc.* 1998;98:10S.

Bano G, et al. Reduced bone mineral density after surgical treatment for obesity. *Int J Obesity and Related Metabolic Disorders.* 1999; 23:361.

Bathalon G, et al. Psychological measures of eating behavior and the accuracy of 3 common dietary assessment methods in healthy postmenopausal women. *Am J Clin Nutri.* 2000;71:739.

Benedetti G, et al. Body composition and energy expenditure after weight loss following bariatric surgery. *J Am Col Nutri.* 2000;19: 270.

Brondel L, et al. Postprandial thermogenesis and alimentary sensory stimulation in human subjects. *Int J Obesity and Related Metabolic Disorders.* 1999;23:34.

Calle E, et al. Body mass index and mortality in a prospective cohort of U.S. adults. *N Eng J Med.* 1999;341:1097.

Carey I, et al. The effect of adiposity and weight change on forced expiratory volume decline in a longitudinal study of adults. *Int J Obesity and Related Metabolic Disorders.* 1999;23:979.

Clark M, Ogden J. The impact of pregnancy on eating behavior and aspects of weight concern. *Int J Obesity and Related Metabolic Disorders.* 1999;23:34.

Evans E, et al. Body composition changes with diet and exercise in obese women: a comparison of estimates from other clinical methods and a 4-component model. *Am J Clin Nutri.* 1999;70:5.

Fanghanel G, et al. A clinical trial of the use of sibutramine for the treatment of patients suffering essential obesity. *Int J Obesity and Related Metabolic Disorders.* 2000;24:144.

Ferguson M, et al. Fat distribution and hemostatic measures in obese children. *Am J Clin Nutri.* 1998;67:1136.

Field A, et al. Weight cycling, weight gain, and risk of hypertension in women. *Am J Epid.* 1999;150:573.

Fine J, et al. A prospective study of weight change and health-related quality of life in women. *JAMA.* 1999;282:2136.

Fontaine K, et al. Body mass index, smoking, and mortality among older American women. *J Women's Health.* 1998;7:1257.

Forbes G. Longitudinal changes in adult fat-free mass: influence of body weight. *Am J Clin Nutri.* 1999;70:1025.

Foreyt J, et al. The role of the behavioral counselor in obesity treatment. *J Am Diet Assoc.* 1998;98:10S.

Foster G, et al. Changes in resting energy expenditure after weight loss in obese African American and white women. *Am J Clin Nutri.* 1999;69:13.

Golay A, et al. Similar weight loss with low-energy food combining or balanced diets. *Int J Obesity & Related Metab Disorders.* 2000; 24:492.

Glueck C, et al. Metformin reduces weight, centripetal obesity, insulin, leptin, and low-density lipoprotein cholesterol in nondiabetic, morbidly obese subjects with body mass index greater than 30. *Metabolism.* 2001;50:856.

Hebebrand J, et al. Epidemic obesity: Are genetic factors involved via increased rates of assortative mating? *Int J Obesity & Related Metab Disorders.* 2000;24:345.

Heitmann B, et al. Mortality associated with body fat, fat-free mass and body mass index among 60-year old Swedish men—a 22-

year follow-up. The study of men born in 1913. *Int J of Obesity and Related Metabolic Disorders*. 2000;24:33.

Johansson L, et al. Under- and overreporting of energy intake related to weight status and lifestyle in a nationwide sample. *Am J Clin Nutri*. 1998;68:266.

Karason K, et al. Weight loss and progression of early atherosclerosis in the carotid artery: A 4-year controlled study of obese subjects. *Int J Obesity and Related Metabolic Disorders*. 1999;23:948.

Katzmarzyk P, Davis C. Thinness and body shape of Playboy centerfolds from 1978 to 1998. *Int J Obesity Relat Metab Disord*. 2001;25:590.

Kennedy E, et al. Popular diets: correlation to health, nutrition, and obesity. *J Am Diet Assoc*. 2001;101:411.

Kortelainen M, Sarkioja T. Visceral fat and coronary pathology in male adolescents. *Int J Obesity Relat Metab Disord*. 2001;25:228.

Laquatra L. Weight management. In: Mahan K, Escott-Stump S, eds. *Krause's food, nutrition, and diet therapy*. 10th ed. Philadelphia: WB Saunders, 2000.

Ludwig D, et al. Dietary fiber, weight gain, and cardiovascular disease factors in young adults. *J Am Med Assoc*. 1999;282:1539.

MacIntosh C, et al. Effects of age on concentrations of plasma cholecystokinin, glucagon-like peptide 1, and peptide YY and their relation to appetite and pyloric motility. *Am J Clin Nutri*. 1999;69:999.

Mokdad A, et al. The spread of the obesity epidemic in the United States, 1991–1998. *J Am Med Assoc*. 1999;282:1519.

Nawitz H, et al. Weight loss counseling by health care providers. *Am J Pub Health*. 1999;89:764.

Nonas C. A model for chronic care of obesity through dietary treatment. *J Am Diet Assoc*. 1998;98:10S.

Okosun I, et al. Impact of birth weight on ethnic variations in subcutaneous and central adiposity in American children aged 5–11 years. A study from the National Health and Nutrition Examination Survey. *Int J Obesity & Related Metab Disorders*. 2000;24:479.

Ravelli A, et al. Obesity at age 50 in men and women exposed to famine prenatally. *Am J Clin Nutri*. 1999;70:811.

Reeves R, et al. Nutrient intake of obese female binge eaters. *J Am Diet Assoc*. 2001;101:209.

Rogers P. Eating habits and appetite control: a psychobiological perspective. *Proc Nutr Soc*. 1999;58:59.

Rolls B, et al. Energy density but not fat content of foods affected energy intake in lean and obese women. *Am J Clin Nutri*. 1999;69:863.

Rosmond R, Bjorntorp P. Psychosocial and socio-economic factors in women and their relationship to obesity and regional body fat distribution. *Int J Obesity and Related Metabolic Disorders*. 1999;23:138.

Ross R, Janssen I. Physical activity, total and regional obesity: dose-response considerations. *Med. Sci. Sports Exerc*. 2001;33:521S.

Savendahl L, Underwood L. Fasting increases serum total cholesterol, LDL cholesterol, and apolipoprotein B in healthy, nonobese humans. *J Nutri*. 1999;129:2005.

Serdula M, et al. Prevalence of attempting weight loss and strategies for controlling weight. *J Am Med Assoc*. 1999;282:1353.

Shick S, et al. Persons successful at long-term weight loss and maintenance continue to consume a low-energy, low-fat diet. *J Am Diet Assoc*. 1998;98:408.

Skov A, et al. Randomized trial on protein vs carbohydrate in ad libitum fat reduced diet for the treatment of obesity. *Int J Obesity and Related Metabolic Disorders*. 1999;23:528.

Speechly D, et al. Acute appetite reduction associated with an increased frequency of eating in obese males. *Int J Obesity and Related Metabolic Disorders*. 1999;23:1151.

Stein T, et al. Plasma leptin influences gestational weight gain and postpartum weight retention. *Am J Clin Nutri*. 1998;68:1236.

Sturm R, Wells K. Does obesity contribute as much to morbidity as poverty or smoking? *Public Health*. 2001;115:229.

Sullivan D, Walls R. Protein-energy undernutrition and the risk of mortality within six years of hospital discharge. *J Am Col Nutri*. 1998;17:571.

Tomoyasu N, et al. Missreporting of total energy intake in older men and women. *J Am Geriatric Society*. 1999;47:710.

Wadden T, Vogt R, Foster G, Andersen D. Exercise and the maintenance of weight loss: 1-year follow-up of a controlled clinical trial. *J Consult Clin Psychol*. 1998;66:429.

Yanovski J, et al. A prospective study of holiday weight gain. *N Engl J Med*. 2000;342:861.

Zorrilla G. Hunger and satiety: deceptively simple words for the complex mechanisms that tell us when to eat and when to stop. *J Am Diet Assoc*. 1998;98:10

SECTION 11

MUSCULOSKELETAL, ARTHRITIC, AND COLLAGEN DISORDERS

CHIEF ASSESSMENT FACTORS

- ACTUAL HEIGHT MEASUREMENTS, ANNUALLY
- HEIGHT LOSS
- PAIN IN MUSCLES, JOINTS, BONES
- EDEMA
- EXTREMITY WEAKNESS
- MOVEMENT PROBLEMS, STIFFNESS
- WEIGHT LOSS, ANOREXIA, DEPRESSION
- INSOMNIA
- EASY FATIGUE
- UNSTEADY GAIT AND PROPENSITY TO FALL
- CONTRACTURES
- INFLAMMATION (JOINTS, ETC.)
- ARTHRITIS—WARNING SIGNS: EARLY MORNING STIFFNESS, SWELLING IN ONE OR MORE JOINTS, OBVIOUS REDNESS AND WARMTH IN A JOINT, UNEXPLAINED WEIGHT LOSS, FEVER, OR WEAKNESS COMBINED WITH JOINT PAIN, SYMPTOMS SUCH AS THESE THAT LAST MORE THAN 2 WEEKS.
- USE OF BONE-WASTING MEDICATIONS
- BONE DENSITY ASSESSMENT

OVERVIEW

The National Arthritis Data Workgroup reviewed data from available surveys and found that an estimated 15% (40 million) of Americans had some form of arthritis in 1995; by the year 2020, an estimated 18.2% (59.4 million) will be affected (Lawrence et al., 1998). Rheumatic disorders include rheumatoid arthritis, juvenile rheumatoid arthritis, spondylarthropathies, systemic lupus erythematosus, scleroderma, polymyalgia rheumatica, giant cell arteritis, gout, and fibromyalgia.

For example, polymyalgia rheumatica (PMR) causes aching, severe muscle stiffness and pain. Symptoms start suddenly and may affect several areas in the neck, shoulders, upper arms, lower back, hips, and/or thighs. It usually goes away with treatment but may reoccur. Symptoms include mild joint stiffness and swelling, depression, night sweats, fatigue, mild fever, and anorexia. PMR is not associated with any other disease. Some people also have inflammation of large blood vessels that become narrow and blocked (giant cell arteritis) with symptoms of double vision, severe headaches, and vision loss. The cause of PMR is not known but may be related to aging. Diagnosis is difficult. Treatment includes exercise, medications: glucocorticoids, NSAIDs, and rest. There are no specific dietary treatments recommended.

Controlled scientific studies of many patients can prove that a particular treatment is beneficial and that an apparent improvement is incidental. Some studies have been done in alternative therapies, particularly diet in the treatment of arthritis, but none has shown any real benefit in the long term (http://rheumb.bham.ac.uk/alt.html). Some patients do seem to benefit from complementary therapies, either because the treatment truly works or because of psychologic (placebo) effects. The important consideration is that treatment should do no harm. Specific diets and use of herbal or botanical products should only be undertaken with medical consultation.

For More Information

- American Academy of Orthopaedic Surgeons
  http://www.aaos.org/
- American Academy of Physical Medicine & Rehabilitation
  1-800-825-6582
  http://www.aapmr.org
- American Autoimmune-Related Diseases Association (AARDA)
  22100 Gratiot Ave.
  E. Detroit, MI 48021
  810-776-3900
  http://www.aarda.org/
- American College of Rheumatology
  http://www.rheumatology.org/
- American Osteopathic Association
  1-800-621-1773
  http://www.aoa-net.org
- American Pain Foundation
  http://www.painfoundation.org/
- American Society for Bone and Mineral Research
  http://www.asbmr.org/
- Arthritis Foundation
  http://www.arthritis.org/
- Disability Resources
  http://www.halftheplanet.org/
- Drug List
  http://www.rxlist.com/alternative.htm
- National Association of Orthopaedic Nurses
  http://www.naon.inurse.com/
- National Institute of Arthritis and Musculoskeletal and Skin Disorders
  Building 31, Room 4C05
  31 Center Drive, MSC 2350
  Bethesda, MD 20892-2350
  301-496-8190
  www.nih.gov/niams
- National Institutes of Health
  http://www.osteo.org/links.html
- National Osteoporosis Foundation
  http://www.nof.org/
  Powerful Bones Campaign for Girls – http://www.nof.org/powerfulbones/index.htm
- Quack Watch for Unproven Remedies
  http://www.quackwatch.com/
- Rheumatic Diseases Internet Journal
  http://www.rheuma21st.com/

ANKYLOSING SPONDYLITIS (SPINAL ARTHRITIS)

NUTRITIONAL ACUITY RANKING: LEVEL 1

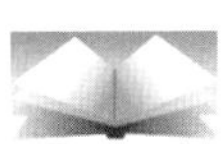

DEFINITIONS AND BACKGROUND

Among the 100 different rheumatic diseases, which affect the joints and muscles, is a group of five diseases called spondylarthropathies. These include: ankylosing spondylitis, reactive arthritis/Reiter's Syndrome, psoriatic arthritis/spondylitis, spondylitis of inflammatory bowel disease, and undifferentiated spondyloarthropathy

Spondylitis is inflammation of the joints linking the vertebrae (a fused spine is not uncommon). In ankylosing spondylitis (AS), inflammation of connective tissue recedes but leaves hardened and damaged joints that fuse together the bones of the spinal column; etiology is unknown. The sacroiliac joints generally are affected first. The condition is most common in men aged 16–35 years and may run in families. Genetic marker HLA-B27 is detected from blood work. Spondylitis affects about 300,000 Americans. It is more common in Caucasians than in African Americans.

Symptoms and signs include chronic lower back pain, early morning stiffness in the lower back where lower spine is joined to pelvis, vague chest pains, tender heels, weight loss, anemia, anorexia, slight fever and chest pain, and recurring iritis or reddened eyes. Valvular heart disease may also occur. Pain may occasionally start in the knees and shoulders. Surgery to replace a joint may relieve pain. Exercise to strengthen muscles that tend to cause pain on stooping or bending may be useful and may also relieve lower back pain; good posture will reduce some types of pain.

OBJECTIVES

- ▲ Reduce pain and inflammation.
- ▲ Improve appetite and intake.
- ▲ Control weight loss.
- ▲ Correct anorexia, nausea, and febrile state.
- ▲ Improve ability to participate in physical activity.

DIETARY AND NUTRITIONAL RECOMMENDATIONS

- A normal diet is useful, with weight loss/calorie control, if needed, to normalize weight.
- Food preferences can be offered to stimulate appetite.
- It is prudent to increase dietary intake of foods rich in antioxidants such as vitamins E and C, selenium, fish oils, and rich sources of omega-3 fatty acids.

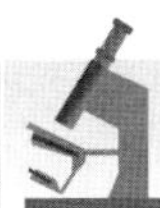

PROFILE

Clinical/History	Lab Work	
Height	Ca++	Blood urea nitrogen (BUN), Creatine (Creat)
Weight	Erythrocyte sedimentation rate (ESR) (high)	Phosphorus (P)
Body mass index (BMI)	HLA-B27 gene test (found in 90%)	Hemoglobin and hematocrit (H&H)
Weight changes	Alkaline phosphatase (alk phos)	Aspartate aminotransaminase (AST), Alanine aminotransferase (ALT)
Anorexia	Albumin (alb), prealbumin	
Temperature	X-rays	
Lower back pain		
Pain in knees or shoulders		
Iritis		

Common Drugs Used and Potential Side Effects

- Anti-inflammatory drugs such as COX2 inhibitors, indomethacin (Indocin), or phenylbutazone may be used. Many side effects can result such as hyperglycemia, hyperkalemia, or anemia. Nausea, dizziness, and headache can also result.
- Fenoprofen (Nalfon) can cause constipation, nausea, and vomiting.
- Etanercept, an anti-tumor necrosis factor (TNF) therapy, which has been used to treat rheumatoid arthritis, may cause significant improvement in pain and mobility, according to research. Etanercept works by blocking a naturally occurring protein (tumor necrosis factor-alpha) that, when present in elevated levels, is believed to be one of the causes of inflammation and bone destruction in AS.

Herbs, Botanicals and Supplements

- Herbs and botanical supplements should not be used without discussing with physician.
- Ginger, corn, pineapple, pigweed, and vegetarianism have been recommended; there are no clinical trials that prove efficacy.

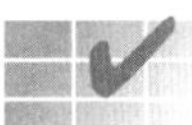

PATIENT EDUCATION

- ✔ Exercise is crucial, especially swimming, to relieve back pain.
- ✔ Patient should practice deep breathing exercises for pain relief. Stretching and strengthening exercises also are important.
- ✔ Patient should be sleeping on a hard bed, supine.
- ✔ Discuss role of calories in weight control.

For More Information

- Ankylosing spondylitis International Federation
  http://www.asif.rheumanet.org/index.htm
- National Ankylosing Spondylitis Society (NASS) – United Kingdom
  http://www.nass.co.uk/
- Spondylitis Association of America
  P. O. Box 5872
  Sherman Oaks, CA 91413
  1-800-777-8189 (Info. Line)
  818-981-1616 (Los Angeles)
  http://www.spondylitis.org
- Spondylitis Exercises
  http://www.spondylitis.org/html/exercise_what.htm
- Spondylitis Library
  http://spondylibrary.com/

EXTENDED IMMOBILIZATION

NUTRITIONAL ACUITY RANKING: LEVEL 2

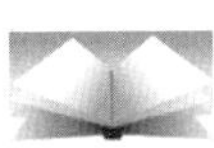

DEFINITIONS AND BACKGROUND

Immobilization, for various reasons, may be nutritionally depleting. Patients with orthopedic injuries may lose 15–20 lb from stress, immobilization, trauma, and bed rest. Immobilization hypercalcemia involves nausea, vomiting, abdominal cramps, constipation, headache, and lethargy. Nitrogen and calcium losses often are extensive. Unloading of weight bearing bones as induced by microgravity or immobilization has significant impacts on the calcium and bone metabolism; it is the most likely cause for space osteoporosis (Heer et al., 1999).

OBJECTIVES

- Correct negative nitrogen balance from increased losses (perhaps up to 2–3 g of nitrogen per day). Prevent pressure ulcers and infections.
- Prevent deossification and osteoporosis of bones. Prevent hypercalcemia from low serum levels of albumin, which normally binds calcium.
- Prevent kidney and bladder stones.
- Provide adequate fluid intake to aid excretion of nutrients.
- Prevent constipation, impactions, and obstruction.
- Prevent anemias that result from inadequate nitrogen balance.
- Prevent venous thrombosis.

DIETARY AND NUTRITIONAL RECOMMENDATIONS

- Diet should provide adequate intake of high biologic value (HBV) proteins to correct nitrogen balance. An intake of 1.2 g protein/kg body weight is recommended. Provide adequate carbohydrates (CHOs), plus 1–2% total kilocalories as essential fatty acids (EFAs).
- Increased intake of phosphorus during the first few weeks may be useful.
- Encourage adequate intake of calcium. A high-protein diet raises the body's calcium requirements.
- Diet should provide a high fluid intake.
- Intake of vitamin C and zinc should be adequate to protect against skin breakdown. Various organs and the skeleton are zinc deficient in immobilized patients (Higashi et al., 1993).
- Diet should provide adequate amounts of fiber to prevent constipation. Avoid overuse of fiber with impaction.
- Reduce intake of excessive amounts of fats and sugars, because immobilized persons may have CHO and lipid abnormalities (Baumann and Spungen, 1994).

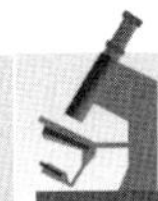

PROFILE

Clinical/History

Height or arm length/knee length
Weight
BMI
Weight changes
Triceps skinfold (TSF), midarm muscle circumference (MAMC), midarm circumference (MAC)

Lab Work

Dual-energy x-ray absorbtiometry (DEXA)
P
H&H
Alb
Prealbumin, Retinol-binding protein (RBP)
Ca++ (increased); parathormone (PTH)
Urinary Ca++
Nitrogen (N) balance
Red blood cell count (RBCs)
BUN, Creat

Common Drugs Used and Potential Side Effects

- Medications may be used to treat underlying conditions; they may have side effects that contribute to nutrient losses.

Herbs, Botanicals and Supplements

- Herbs and botanical supplements should not be used without discussing with physician.

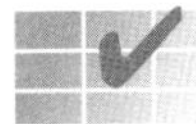

PATIENT EDUCATION

- Explain to patient that early ambulation is the best treatment possible.
- Explain that calcium and nutrient intakes will have to be monitored for patients who will be tube fed or on a liquid diet for extended periods of time.
- Explain need for adequate fiber and fluid intake to prevent constipation, urinary tract infections, etc.

FIBROMYALGIA

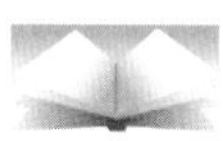

DEFINITIONS AND BACKGROUND

Myofascial pain syndromes are a group of disorders characterized by achy pain and stiffness in soft tissues, including muscles, tendons, and ligaments. The pain and stiffness of fibromyalgia may be widespread throughout the body or localized, especially along the spine. Persistent symptoms may be disruptive but are not life threatening. Symptoms include sleep disturbance, depression, fatigue, headaches, diarrhea and/or constipation, numbness in the hands and feet, weakness, memory changes, and dizziness. In the United States, the fibromyalgia estimate is 2–4% of adults.

Plant foods are rich natural sources of antioxidants in addition to other nutrients. Use of an uncooked vegan diet in this population shows highly increased serum levels of beta and alpha carotenes, lycopene, lutein, and vitamins C and E (Hanninen et al., 2000). Diet is also especially rich in fiber, quercetin, myristin, and kaempherol. The shift of fibromyalgic subjects to this living food (LF) diet results in a decrease of joint stiffness and pain as well as an improvement of self-reported quality of life (Hanninen et al., 2000).

OBJECTIVES

- Relieve pain.
- Correct any infections; prevent injury.
- Lose weight, if obese.
- Correct underlying problems such as hypertension.
- Lifestyle changes, including stress reduction, relaxation techniques, and exercise, can be useful.

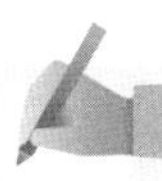

DIETARY AND NUTRITIONAL RECOMMENDATIONS

- An uncooked vegan diet may be beneficial (Hanninen et al., 2000). The LF diet includes berries, fruits, vegetables and roots, nuts, germinated seeds, and sprouts. The Food Guide Pyramid is also a useful tool.
- A weight loss plan may be needed.

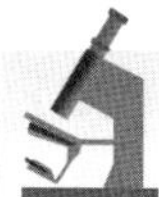

PROFILE

Clinical/History	Lab Work	
Height	Triglycerides (Trig)	BUN
Weight	Cholesterol (chol)	Creat
BMI	ESR (Sed Rate)	Na+
Tender areas, back pain	Alb, prealbumin	K+
Headache		Glucose (gluc)
		Alk Phos

Common Drugs Used and Potential Side Effects

- Analgesics may be used. Monitor for vitamin C depletion and other side effects.
- Antidepressants may be useful in some cases. Medications that decrease pain and improve sleep may be prescribed.

Herbs, Botanicals and Supplements

- Herbs and botanical supplements should not be used without discussing with physician.

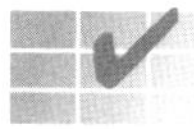

PATIENT EDUCATION

- Discuss weight management goals such as weight loss for obesity.
- Daily exercise will be important for strengthening weak muscles.
- Address any problems with sleep disturbances, which are common.

For More Information:

- American Fibromyalgia Syndrome Association, Inc.
  http://www.afsafund.org/
- Fibromyalgia Network
  http://www.fmnetnews.com/
- National Fibromyalgia Partnership, Inc
  http://www.fmpartnership.org/FMPartnership.htm

GOUT

NUTRITIONAL ACUITY RANKING: LEVEL 1

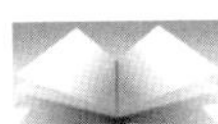

DEFINITIONS AND BACKGROUND

Gout is a disorder that has sudden and recurring attacks of painful arthritis, caused by abnormal metabolism of purines, with inflamed joints (usually the big toe, ankle, knees, and feet). Uric acid is the end product of purine nucleotide metabolism in humans. In gout, hyperuricemia results, with deposition of monosodium urate crystals in various tissues.

Obesity leads to and exacerbates many serious disorders, including gout and osteoarthritis; weight loss is generally associated with a decrease in risk factors and the alleviation of clinical symptoms (Pi-Sunyer, 1996). Risk factors for gout besides obesity include high alcohol intake, high levels of uric acid (may be genetic), some hypertensive drugs, and high intake of purines. The disease may be triggered by injury, starvation, intake of large amounts of alcohol or protein-rich foods, emotional stress, or illnesses such as diabetes, sickle cell anemia, or chronic renal disease.

The disease tends to affect men, especially between the ages of 30 and 50 and is sometimes hereditary. More than 1 million people in the United States are afflicted with gout, an estimated 840 out of every 100,000 people (http://www.rheumatology.org/patients/factsheet/gout.html). Almost 20% of individuals with gout will also develop kidney stones.

Severe pain usually occurs, more so at night. The joint swells and skin turns warm, red, purplish, and shiny. Acute gout most commonly affects the first metatarsal joint of the foot, but other joints may also be involved. Tophi, hard lumps of urate crystals, can be deposited under the skin around the joints; these may be permanent. Patients with asymptomatic hyperuricemia do not require treatment, but efforts should be made to lower their urate levels by encouraging them to make changes in diet or lifestyle (Harris, 1999). Common phases of gout are listed in Table 11–1.

TABLE 11–1 Phases of Gout (Harris et al., 1999)

1. Asymptomatic hyperuricemia
2. Acute gouty arthritis
3. Intercritical gout
4. Chronic tophaceous gout

OBJECTIVES

- Instruct patient to lose weight if obese and to do so gradually to prevent increased purine release.
- Increase excretion of urates where desirable.
- Force fluid intake to prevent uric acid kidney stones.
- Correct any existing hyperlipidemia.
- Prevent complications such as renal disease, hypertension, and stroke.
- Encourage lifestyle changes, if needed (e.g., reduction in weight, alcohol intake, etc.)

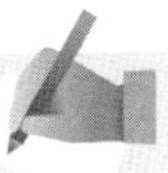

DIETARY AND NUTRITIONAL RECOMMENDATIONS

- A high-carbohydrate diet increases excretion of urates, as does a low-fat intake; increase CHO ingestion and decrease fat ingestion. Balance this within a weight loss plan if needed.
- If patient's condition is acute, avoid excessive intake of purines (Emmerson, 1996) by limiting ingestion of anchovies, smoked meat, sardines, liver, kidney, brain, heart, caviar, herring, and gravies.
- Diet should exclude alcoholic beverages.
- Ensure a high fluid intake.
- Cut down on large amounts of simple CHOs and total fat if triglycerides are elevated.

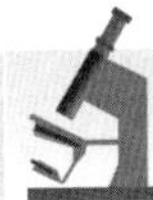

PROFILE

Clinical/History	Lab Work	
Height	Uric acid (increased)	Chol
Weight	Na+, K+	Alb, prealbumin
BMI	Trig (increased)	BUN (increased)
Urate crystals in urine	Birefringent crystals in the synovial fluid	Creat
Use of alcoholic beverages		Gluc
		AST, ALT

Common Drugs Used and Potential Side Effects

- Treatment includes NSAIDs, colchicine, corticosteroids, and analgesics. NSAIDs are favored unless risk of side effects (gastrointestinal [GI] distress or bleeding) is too high (Emmerson, 1996).
- Colchicine and analgesics may cause vomiting. Avoid using them with uricosuric drugs. Take with adequate fluids. Monitor for sufficient intake of vitamin C.
- Uricosuric drugs: Probenecid (Benemid) and sulfinpyrazone (Anturane) block renal absorption of urates. Adequate intake of fluid is needed. Anorexia, nausea, vomiting, and sore gums may result.
- Allopurinol (Zyloprim) blocks uric acid formation. Adequate intake of fluid is needed. Mild GI upset, taste changes, or diarrhea can occur; take after meals.
- Indocin or adrenocorticotropic hormone (ACTH) (corticotropin). Used to reduce fever and inflammation, Indocin or ACTH may require restricted sodium intake. Beware of elevated glucose levels.

Herbs, Botanicals and Supplements

- Herbs and botanical supplements should not be used without discussing with physician.
- Celery, avocado, turmeric, cat's claw, chiso, and devil's claw have been recommended; there are no clinical trials that prove efficacy.

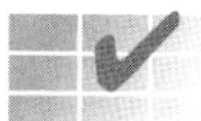

PATIENT EDUCATION

- ✓ Advise patient that alcohol may precipitate a gouty attack.
- ✓ Have patient avoid fasting.
- ✓ For some individuals, stress may precipitate an acute attack. Encourage relaxation and pleasant activities.
- ✓ It is thought that the inflammatory response may be suppressed by an increase in omega-3 fatty acids, as found in fatty fish (mackerel, herring, and salmon). Use of these types of fish instead of meat entrees several times a week may be beneficial.

For More Information

- American College of Rheumatology
  http://www.rheumatology.org/patients/factsheet/gout.html

MUSCULAR DYSTROPHY

NUTRITIONAL ACUITY RANKING: LEVEL 2

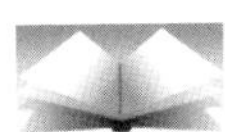

DEFINITIONS AND BACKGROUND

Actually a group of 9 disorders, muscular dystrophy (MD) involves a hereditary condition with progressive degenerative changes in the muscle fibers, leading to weakness and atrophy. Several of the disorders are described below.

In the Duchenne type (DMD) of MD, the facial muscles are involved, and the patient cannot suck, close lips, bite, chew, or swallow. Aggressive forms appear gradually in males aged 1–15 years, with frequent falls and difficulty in climbing. Some patients may also have heart failure. Generalized weakness and muscle wasting affects limb and trunk muscles first; calves are often enlarged. It is an X-linked recessive disorder; females are carriers. Survival is rare after the late twenties. Becker muscular dystrophy (BMD) is very similar to Duchenne, but patients live longer.

Emery-Dreyfus muscular dystrophy (EDMD) has onset in childhood to the early teens. Weakness and wasting of shoulder, upper arm and shin muscles, and joint deformities are common. Disease usually progresses slowly. Frequent cardiac complications are common

Limb-Girdle muscular dystrophy (LGMD) has an onset in late childhood to middle age. Weakness and wasting affects shoulder and pelvic girdles first. Progression is slow, with cardiopulmonary complications often occurring in later stages of the disease. It is inherited as an autosomal recessive, autosomal dominant trait.

Fascioscapulohumeral muscular dystrophy (FSHMD) begins in childhood to early adulthood, with facial muscle weakness and weakness and wasting of the shoulders and upper arms. It progresses slowly with some periods of rapid deterioration and may span many decades. Inheritance is autosomal dominant.

Myotonic dystrophy has onset anywhere from birth to middle age. Generalized weakness and muscle wasting affect the face, feet, hands, and neck first. Delayed relaxation of muscles after contraction. Congenital myotonic form is more severe. Progression is slow, sometimes spanning 50–60 years. Inheritance is autosomal dominant.

Oculopharyngeal muscular dystrophy (OPMD) has onset in early adulthood to middle age. It first affects muscles of eyelid and throat and slowly progresses with swallowing problems common as disease progresses. Inheritance is autosomal dominant.

Distal muscular dystrophy first shows signs between ages 40–60, with weakness and muscle wasting of the hands, forearms, and lower legs. It progresses slowly. It is passed on as an autosomal dominant trait.

Muscular biopsy is required for the definitive diagnosis of specific congenital muscular dystrophy. Extremely elevated serum creatine kinase (CK) levels may indicate muscle disease; muscle biopsy sometimes confirms diagnoses of muscular dystrophy in patients with unexplained elevations of AST, ALT, and lactic acid dehydrogenase (LDH) (Korones et al., 2001). Myoblast transfer therapy is under investigation as a possible treatment. Vitamin E, selenium, and calcium have been studied for their roles in the onset of these disorders.

The prognosis of MD varies according to type and progression. Some cases may be mild and very slowly progressive, with normal lifespan, while other cases may have more marked progression of muscle weakness, functional disability, and loss of ambulation. Life expectancy may depend on the degree of progression and late respiratory deficit; in DMD, death usually occurs in the late teens to early 20s (http://www.ninds.nih.gov/health_and_medical/disorders/md.htm).

OBJECTIVES

- Encourage patient to lead an active life; exercise programs can help prevent contractures.
- Prevent obesity, which may result from inactivity. Obesity complicates therapy.
- Avoid constipation, because fecal impaction is frequent.
- Encourage activities other than eating to prevent dependency on food as a source of pleasure.
- Adapt to feeding difficulties.
- Malnutrition is a serious threat to patients with muscular disease, especially if there is also respiratory muscle weakness. Monitor nutritional status on a regular basis.

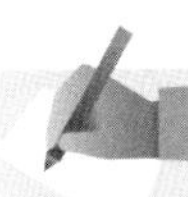

DIETARY AND NUTRITIONAL RECOMMENDATIONS

- Work with the Food Pyramid as a basic guide. Use a low-calorie diet if necessary to control or lessen obesity. Check patient's BMI and adjust accordingly.
- Use foods that are easy to chew and swallow for DMD. Use pureed or blenderized foods when needed. Tube feed only if necessary.
- Provide adequate fiber (prune juice, bran, etc.), if constipation becomes a problem. Beware of excesses as well.

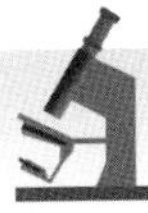

PROFILE

Clinical/History	Lab Work	
Height	BUN, N balance	Creatine kinase (CK) (increased)
Weight	H&H	PO4
BMI	CK levels (often increased)	Alb, prealbumin
Ability to swallow	LDH (increased)	Gluc
Ability to chew	Creat (often decreased)	AST
Hand-to-mouth coordination		ALT

Common Drugs Used and Potential Side Effects

- The myotonia (delayed relaxation of a muscle after a strong contraction) may be treated with medications such as phenytoin or quinine.

Herbs, Botanicals and Supplements

- Herbs and botanical supplements should not be used without discussing with physician.

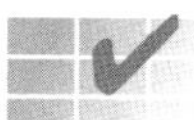

PATIENT EDUCATION

- ✓ Provide low-calorie snacks for patients who are obese.
- ✓ Help patient modify food textures to meet needs.
- ✓ Discuss problems related to inactivity or weight gain.

For More Information

- Facioscapulohumeral Dystrophy (FSHD) Society
  3 Westwood Road
  Lexington, MA 02420
  http://www.fshsociety.org
- Muscular Dystrophy Association
  National Headquarters
  3300 E. Sunrise Dr.
  Tucson, AZ 85718
  1-800-572-1717
  http://www.mdausa.org/
- Muscular Dystrophy Association of Canada
  http://www.mdac.ca/
- Muscular Dystrophy Family Foundation
  http://www.mdff.org/
- National Institute of Neurological Disorders and Stroke
  National Institutes of Health
  Bethesda, MD 20892
  http://www.ninds.nih.gov/health_and_medical/disorders/md.htm
- Parent Project for Muscular Dystrophy Research
  1012 North University Blvd.
  Middletown, OH 45042
  ParentProject@aol.com
  http://www.parentprojectmd.org
  Tel: 413-424-0696, 1-800-714-KIDS (5437)

OSTEOARTHRITIS AND DEGENERATIVE JOINT DISEASE

NUTRITIONAL ACUITY RANKING: LEVEL 1–2

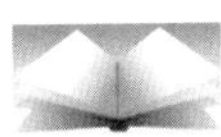

DEFINITIONS AND BACKGROUND

Osteoarthritis (OA) may be primary (more common in elderly individuals) or may follow an injury or disease involving the articular surfaces of synovial joints; it is technically "Osteoarthrosis." Symptoms and signs include pain, swelling, and synovial joint stiffness. A fracture increases the risk for degenerative joint disease (DJD) later in life, especially if across an articular surface.

An estimated 43 million Americans report having arthritis, and of those, an estimated 7.8 million report that the arthritis limits their daily activities, according to the Centers for Disease Control (CDC). While most of the increase can be attributed to an aging population, a larger proportion of Americans are overweight, causing strain on joints over the years (MMWR, 5/4/01).

OA of the knee occurs in more than 3 million people in the United States; women older than 45 years of age are especially affected (Gershoff, 1996). Vitamins A, C, D, and E may be related to the processes that impede or give rise to OA, because they have major roles in modulating oxidative stress, participating in immune responses, and contributing to cell differentiation (Sowers and Lachance, 1999). Low intake serum levels of vitamin D may be associated with increased risk of progression of OA (McAlindon et al., 1996). Interestingly, vitamin D is shunted to fat cells rather than to circulation in obese patients; their needs may be higher than one would expect.

Spondylosis is OA of the spine (see entry at the beginning of this section). Infective arthritis is septic, from bacterial invasion from nearby joints, from chickenpox, rubella, or mumps. In seronegative arthritis, blood tests for rheumatoid arthritis are negative; autoimmune disorders, Crohn's disease, and psoriasis may be associated. These are usually not related to DJD.

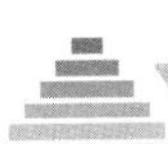

OBJECTIVES

- If patient is obese, lessen pressure on weight-bearing joints.
- Encourage patient (especially if elderly) to consume adequate amounts of protein and calcium. Fat and carbohydrate intake should be limited if these prevail in the diet.
- Evaluate for any food allergies to rule out symptoms unrelated to arthritis.
- Joint replacement may be necessary; prepare accordingly.
- Fish oils and certain plant seed oils may impact immune and inflammatory responses, with their roles as precursors of eicosanoids. Less pain may be experienced (Eriksen et al., 1996).
- Maintain integrity of cartilage in affected joints.

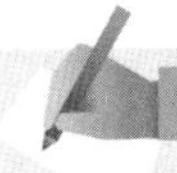

DIETARY AND NUTRITIONAL RECOMMENDATIONS

- Use a calorie-controlled diet if obesity is present.
- Dry skim milk can be used as a lower-calorie, less expensive source of calcium than fluid whole milk.
- Suggest an increased use of fish and fish oils (e.g., cod liver oil) in diet to increase availability of omega-3 fatty acids (Eriksen et al., 1996). Ensure adequate intake of zinc plus antioxidants vitamins C and E (Fairburn et al., 1992).
- Use of folic acid and vitamin B12 may supplement the use of NSAIDs and gradually lower their necessity (Flynn, 1994).
- Milk, fatty fish such as salmon, eggs, some fortified cereals, and multivitamin supplements may be used under supervision to provide vitamin D. Vitamin D, taken in doses up to twice the recommended dietary allowance (RDA) under a doctor's care, has been speculated to protect against disease advancement (Gershoff, 1996).
- Consume sources of beta-carotene, and six fruits and vegetables daily

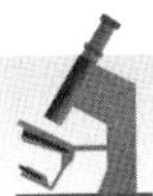

PROFILE

Clinical/History

Height
Weight
BMI

Lab Work

Antinuclear bodies (to rule out other conditions)
Antistreptolysin titer (ASO), lupus erythematosus (LE) prep (to rule out other conditions)
Anti-rheumatoid factor
BUN, Creat
X-rays; DEXA
Sedimentation rate
C-reactive protein
Gluc
Alk phos
Uric acid
K+, Na+
Serum folate
Serum vitamin B12

Common Drugs Used and Potential Side Effects

A useful on-line drug information guide is available at http://www.arthritis.org/conditions/DrugGuide/drug index.asp

- Aspirin can be taken with meals to reduce gastric distress. Prolonged use can cause GI bleeding; intake of folate should be increased.
- Steroids may cause sodium retention, calcium, nitrogen, and potassium depletion, truncal obesity, and hyperglycemia. Generally, they are not to be used with OA.
- NSAIDs may increase risks of acquiring hypertension (Gurwitz et al., 1994). Indomethacin (Indocin) and sulindac (Clinoril) may cause nausea, renal failure, or diarrhea. Lodine (etodolac) may cause renal failure or ab-

dominal pain. Naprosyn can cause abdominal pain, nausea, or heartburn. Tolectin causes abdominal pain, nausea and vomiting (N & V), and GI upsets. Ibuprofen (Advil/Motrin) may cause nausea and vomiting. Trilisate (choline magnesium trisalicylate) may cause constipation, diarrhea, and N & V. Take NSAIDs with food; anorexia, flatulence, and GI distress may result otherwise. Add extra folic acid and vitamin B12 to diet.

- Cytotec (misoprostol) reduces stomach acid if NSAIDs are used. Abdominal cramps may occur.
- Vioxx (rofecoxib) and Celebrex (celecoxib) have fewer GI side effects than NSAIDs; ulcers are not a consequence. Both decrease prostaglandin production. Some other side effects are being evaluated, such as hypertension in Vioxx users. There may be increased risk for myocardial infarction or stroke, because they block COX-2 but not COX-1, which facilitates blood clotting. Some recommendations may include taking one baby aspirin daily.
- After 3 years of studying glucosamine sulphate in a knee OA trial, researchers from the University of Liege in Belgium found that the supplement reduced cartilage damage and decreased pain associated with OA in the group of patients taking the supplement (*Lancet*, 1/27/01). These trials suggest that oral glucosamine sulfate and chondroitin may help relieve symptoms of OA (McAlindon et al., 2000). X-rays have shown that cartilage thickness is somewhat protected over several years. Sulfate may be a key factor (Hoffer et al., 2001).

Herbs, Botanicals and Supplements (see Table 11–2 also)

- Herbs and botanical supplements should not be used without discussing with physician.
- S-adenosylmethionine (SAMe) is being studied for its role in rebuilding eroded joint cartilage; it is also useful for mild depression. Enteric coating is needed.
- Glucosamine or chondroitin sulfate has some positive results; an National Institutes of Health (NIH) study has been undertaken. Glucosamine can increase blood glucose levels and aggravate shellfish allergy, because it is made from these shells. Chondroitin may alter blood-clotting activity in a manner similar to that of aspirin.
- Ginger, red pepper, celery seed, pineapple, stinging nettle, and turmeric have been recommended; there are no clinical trials that prove efficacy.
- A study suggests that taking vitamin E gamma tocopherol may worsen arthritis; the authors of the study recommend that people who take vitamin E should take alpha tocopherol. (NYTimes, Science Times, 11/23/99). A double-blind study in Australia found no relief of symptomatic pain (Brand et al., 2001).
- A supplement guide is available from http://www.arthritis.org/conditions/SupplementGuide/default.asp.

TABLE 11–2 Side effects of Common Herbs Used for Arthritis (Excerpted from *The Arthritis Foundation's Guide to Alternative Therapies at* http://www.arthritis.org/conditions/alttherapies/nature.asp.)

Bromelain	May increase effects of blood-thinning drugs and tetracycline antibiotics.
Echinacea	Might counteract immune-suppressant drugs such as glucocorticoids taken for lupus and rheumatoid arthritis. Might increase side effects of methotrexate.
Evening Primrose oil	Can counteract the effects of anticonvulsant drugs.
Fish oil	May increase effects of blood-thinning drugs and herbs.
Folic acid	Interferes with methotrexate; ask your doctor how to take it.
Gamma linoleic acid (GLA)	May increase effects of blood-thinning drugs and herbs.
Garlic	Can increase effects of blood-thinning drugs and herbs.
Ginger	Can increase NSAID side effects and effects of blood-thinning drugs and herbs.
Ginkgo	May increase effects of blood-thinning drugs and herbs.
Ginseng	May increase effects of blood-thinning drugs, estrogens, and glucocorticoids; shouldn't be used by those with diabetes; may interact with monoamine oxidase (MAO) inhibitors.
Kava	Can increase effects of alcohol, sedatives, and tranquilizers.
Magnesium	May interact with blood pressure medications.
St. John's Wort	May enhance effects of narcotics, alcohol, and antidepressants; increase risk of sunburn; interfere with iron absorption.
Valerian	Can increase the effects of sedatives and tranquilizers.
Zinc	Can interfere with glucocorticoids and other immunosuppressive drugs.

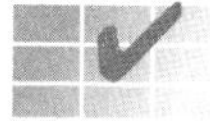

PATIENT EDUCATION

✓ Encourage patient to avoid fad diets for "arthritis cure."
✓ Ensure patient's diet is balanced and includes all nutrients.
✓ Degenerative joint disease is seldom a serious problem and has no life-threatening risks.
✓ "Rest frequently and sleep on a firm bed" is wise advice.
✓ Do not allow muscles around the joints to become weak through disuse. Exercise and stretching should be suggested for daily application to maintain flexibility. Long-term weight training and aerobic walking programs significantly improve balance in older adults with OA of the knee in particular.
✓ Cartilage or stem cell transplants are being tested for pain relief.
✓ Acupuncture may be useful to relieve pain.

For More Information

- American Juvenile Arthritis Foundation http://www.arthritis.org/Answers/about_AJAO.asp
- Arthritis Resource Center at Healingwell http://www.healingwell.com/arthritis
- Johns Hopkins Arthritis Center http://www.hopkins-arthritis.som.jhmi.edu/

OSTEOMYELITIS, ACUTE

NUTRITIONAL ACUITY RANKING: LEVEL 2

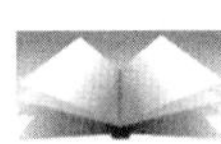

DEFINITIONS AND BACKGROUND

The acute form of osteomyelitis may be caused by localized infection of the long bones or injury to bone and surrounding soft tissue. *Staphylococcus aureus* is implicated in most patients with acute hematogenous osteomyelitis; *Staphylococcus epidermidis, S. aureus, Pseudomonas aeruginosa, Serratia marcescens,* and *Escherichia coli* are commonly isolated in patients with chronic osteomyelitis (Carek et al., 2001).

When a bone is infected, the bone marrow swells and compresses against the rigid outer wall of bone and blood vessels may be compressed or die; abscesses may form. Symptoms and signs include sudden, acute pain (often in the joint nearest the site of infection), fever, chills, tachycardia, diaphoresis, nausea and vomiting, dehydration, electrolyte imbalance, contractures in affected extremities, and pressure ulcers. If not treated properly, condition may become chronic. Treatment generally involves evaluation, staging, determination of etiology, antimicrobial therapy, and debridement or stabilization of bone (Carek, 2001).

OBJECTIVES

- ▲ Decrease febrile state.
- ▲ Correct nausea and vomiting.
- ▲ Characterize and treat the infection. Prevent further infection, dehydration, and other complications.
- ▲ Promote recovery and healing.

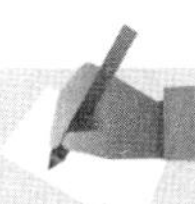

DIETARY AND NUTRITIONAL RECOMMENDATIONS

- Encourage adequate fluid intake.
- Maintain a normal-to-high-calorie and protein intake, with adequate amounts of vitamins and minerals included (e.g., zinc, vitamin A, and vitamin C).

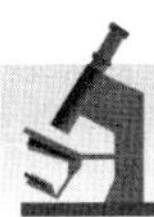

PROFILE

Clinical/History	Lab Work	
Height	ESR (increased)	White blood cell count (WBC) (increased)
Weight	Alb, prealbumin	Gluc
BMI	BUN, Creat	Bone densitometry
Intake and output (I & O)	AST, ALT	
Temperature	K+	
Blood pressure (BP)	Na+	
	Ca++	

Common Drugs Used and Potential Side Effects

- Antibiotics are needed to correct infections that are present. Monitor for specific side effects and timing of meals. For optimal results, antibiotic therapy must be started early, with antimicrobial agents administered parenterally for at least 4–6 weeks (Carek, 2001).
- Analgesics may be used for pain. GI distress is a common side effect. Extra vitamin C may be needed.

Herbs, Botanicals and Supplements

- Herbs and botanical supplements should not be used without discussing with physician.

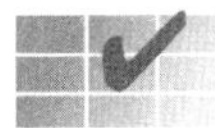

PATIENT EDUCATION

- ✓ Discuss role of nutrition in wound healing, immunity, and other conditions related to this disorder.
- ✓ Discuss signs that may indicate reversal of status or recovery.

OSTEOMALACIA

NUTRITIONAL ACUITY RANKING: LEVEL 2

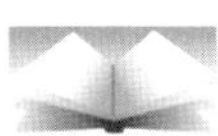

DEFINITIONS AND BACKGROUND

Deossification of the bone (osteomalacia or adult rickets) results from deficiency of vitamin D, calcium, or phosphorus. Osteomalacia may occur in conjunction with bone loss and hip fractures, but more commonly from vitamin D deficiency that occurs with Crohn's disease, colon resection, chronic renal failure, cystic fibrosis, or celiac disease. Anticonvulsant-induced osteomalacia may also occur.

For adults, the 5 ug (200 IU) vitamin D RDA may prevent osteomalacia in the absence of sunlight, but more is needed to help prevent osteoporosis and secondary hyperparathyroidism (Vieth, 1999). Severe vitamin D deficiency leads to secondary hyperparathyroidism, increased bone turnover and loss, and osteomalacia; deficiency is common in elderly people, especially the institutionalized (Lips et al., 2001). Bones become softened and deformed. Other symptoms include muscular weakness, listlessness, aching, and bowing of bones.

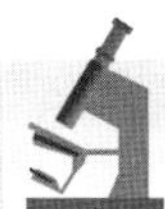

PROFILE

Clinical/History		
Height	Serum Mg++	Bone densitometry; DEXA
Weight	Serum Ca++ (decreased)	X-ray ("washed out" bones) —not useful for measuring bone mineral density
BMI	Urinary Ca++	Bone biopsy (rarely)
Bone pain	Alk phos (increased)	
Lab Work	Alb, prealbumin	
Serum P (decreased)	BUN	
	Creat	

Common Drugs Used and Potential Side Effects

- Treatment with calcium salts should be monitored frequently to prevent hypercalcemia; use with plenty of liquids. Avoid taking with iron supplements or bulk-forming laxatives. High calcium diets may reduce zinc absorption and balance and may, therefore, increase zinc requirements (Wood and Zheng, 1997).
- TPN solutions may need to exclude vitamin D, which may be one cause of osteomalacia.
- Anticonvulsant therapy may deplete vitamin D and calcium.
- Tranquilizers, sedatives, muscle relaxants, and oral diabetic agents may also deplete vitamin D.
- Phosphate binders with aluminum may precipitate the disorder. Calcium carbonate may be an effective substitute; do not take with whole grains, bran, high oxalate foods, or iron tablets.
- Drugs that inhibit calcium absorption include neomycin, thyroid hormone, triamterene, heparin, steroids, or cholestyramine. Furosemide (Lasix) may cause hypercalciuria.
- Ergocalciferol is a vitamin D analog that is used with calcium for complete healing in approximately 6 months. Diet should be corrected, and the drug can be discontinued for patients with normal GI function.

OBJECTIVES

- Provide correct amount of calcium, phosphorus, or vitamin D.
- Prevent or reverse, if possible, bone density loss resulting from calcium loss in the bone matrix.
- Monitor long-term use of total parenteral nutrition (TPN); check contents of calcium and vitamin D and adjust accordingly.

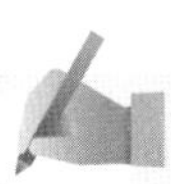

DIETARY AND NUTRITIONAL RECOMMENDATIONS

- Encourage use of milk, especially vitamin D-fortified milk. Diet should be high in calcium; adults will need 1,200–1,500 mg.
- If patient is lactose-intolerant, try Lact-Aid or other forms of lactose-free milk.
- Alkaline-producing dietary components (K+, Mg++, and fruits and vegetables) may contribute to maintenance of bone mineral density (BMD) (Tucker et al., 1999). Include diet high in fruits and vegetables.

Herbs, Botanicals and Supplements

- Herbs and botanical supplements should not be used without discussing with physician.

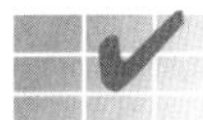

PATIENT EDUCATION

✔ Explain which foods are good sources of calcium, phosphorus, and vitamin D. Encourage patient to spend time in the sun for skin synthesis of vitamin D; avoid sunburn. Total-body sun exposure easily provides the equivalent of 250 ug (10,000 international units [IU]) vitamin D daily, suggesting that this is a physiologic limit (Vieth, 1999).

✔ Explain that fortified margarine and milk are dietary sources of vitamin D.

✔ Vegetarians who avoid dairy products may be at risk for calcium and vitamin D depletion; discuss alternative sources from diet or from necessary supplementation.

OSTEOPOROSIS

NUTRITIONAL ACUITY RANKING: LEVEL 2

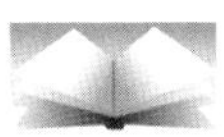

DEFINITIONS AND BACKGROUND

Adequate provision of nutrients composing the bone matrix and regulating bone metabolism should be provided from birth to achieve maximal bone mass, dependent upon individual genetic background and to prevent osteoporosis later in life (Branca and Vatuena, 2001). Minerals and trace elements other than calcium are involved in skeletal growth, some are matrix constituents (magnesium and fluoride) and others are components of enzymatic systems involved in matrix turnover (zinc, copper, and manganese). Vitamin D plays a role in calcium metabolism; Vitamins C and K are cofactors of key enzymes for skeletal metabolism (Branca and Vatuena, 2001).

Osteoporosis is a progressive decrease in the density of bones, which makes them porous, brittle, and more likely to fracture. Bone mineral density is often more than 2.5 standard deviations below the mean of healthy young white adult women (Writing Group, 1996). At first there are no symptoms, but eventually fractures can occur that are very painful and loss of height may result. Of women older than 50 years of age, 10% have some form of osteoporosis; lactase deficiency is a common finding.

About 28 million Americans have this disease (http://www.osteo.org/osteo.html); 80% are women. Osteoporosis is responsible for more than 1.5 million fractures annually, including 300,000 hip fractures, approximately 700,000 vertebral fractures, 250,000 wrist fractures, and more than 300,000 fractures at other sites (http://www.osteo.org/osteo.html). Women with low bone density and multiple risk factors are especially prone to hip fractures. Men are also prone to this disease, often secondary to chronic renal failure or from use of medications such as corticosteroids, anticonvulsants, or barbiturates. Currently, a major study about osteoporosis in men is underway in the United States (Amin and Felson, 2001). See Table 11–3.

Excessive use of alcohol or cigarette smoking may aggravate the condition. Postmenopausal women who have a history of diabetes are also at higher risk (Nicodemus et al., 2001). Elderly women with high BMD have an increased risk of breast cancer, especially advanced cancer, compared with women with low BMD, suggesting an association between two of the most prevalent conditions affecting an older woman's health (Zmuda et al., 2001).

Type I osteoporosis is accelerated phase osteoporosis, occurring in women 5–20 years after menopause, with pain in the vertebrae, rounding of shoulders, height loss, and proneness to fractures (especially of the spine, hip, and wrist). Bone mineral density decreases rapidly in women within 5 years of menopause as a result of hypoestrogenemia (Speroff et al., 1996). Type I responds best to estrogen replacement.

Type II is slow phase osteoporosis. Of individuals older than 85 years of age, 4% sustain a serious fracture related to osteoporosis each year. Symptoms and signs range from asymptomatic conditions to severe backache. Type II may respond to calcium increases.

The best protection against osteoporosis is acquisition of a high peak bone mass (reaching genetic potential) by 30 years of age and reducing bone losses later in life. Physical activity has different effects on bone, depending on its intensity, frequency, duration, and the age at which it is started, with greater anabolic effects in adolescence and as a result of weight-bearing exercise (Branca and Vatuena, 2001). Adequate intakes of calcium appear necessary for exercise to have its bone-stimulating action. Milk intake during adolescence is associated with BMD of the total body, spine, and radius; current calcium intakes may be associated with bone marrow content of the spine (Teegarden et al., 1999).

Women may lose bone during lactation because of calcium lost in breast milk. Calcium supplementation does not prevent bone loss during lactation and only slightly enhances the gain in bone density after weaning (Kalkwarf et al., 1997). Epidemiologic studies have not shown a relationship between numbers of births or lactations with later bone mineral density; other factors play a role. There is currently no consensus on the effect of dietary protein intake on the skeleton, but there is some suggestion that low calcium intakes adversely influence the effect of dietary protein on fracture risk. Increasing protein intake may have a favorable effect on change in BMD in elderly subjects supplemented with calcium citrate, malate, and vitamin D (Dawson-Hughes and Harris, 2002.)

Alkaline-producing dietary components ($K+$, $Mg+$, and fruits and vegetables) may contribute to maintenance of BMD (Tucker et al., 1999). Low intakes of magnesium and potas-

TABLE 11–3 Osteoporosis Risk Factors

<u>Factors that cannot be changed:</u>
Female gender
Family history of osteoporosis
Slender frame; low BMT and low muscle mass
Caucasians, especially women of Northern European extraction; and Asian women
Advancing age

<u>Factors that might be altered:</u>
Premature menopause, amenorrhea, low estrogen in women and low testosterone in men
Excessive use of alcohol
Smoking—Low levels of vitamin D and PTH are noted among smokers (Brot et al., 1999)
Lifetime diet low in calcium and vitamin D (poor diet, excess fiber)
Sedentary lifestyle or extended bed rest
Low vitamin D intake or sunlight exposure
Hypogonadism, as from low estrogen levels or anorexia nervosa
Use of certain medications such as glucocorticoids or some anticonvulsants
Depression, past or current
Hypertension—Associated with abnormal calcium metabolism and, in older white women, bone loss at femoral neck (Cappucino et al., 1999)

sium and high intakes of alcohol are significantly related to total bone mass (New et al., 2000). High intake of retinol may be associated with osteoporosis; in one study, for every 1-mg increase in daily intake of retinol, risk for hip fracture increased 68% (Melhus et al., 1998). Caffeine does not appear to influence bone loss in healthy postmenopausal women (Lloyd et al., 1997) or in teenage girls (Lloyd et al., 1998).

Recent studies suggest that over 300 mg/day of caffeine can negatively impact the vitamin D receptor gene (VDR). The STOP-IT study (Site Testing Osteoporosis Prevention and Intervention Trial) found that greater amounts of caffeine affected BMD (Rapuri et al., 2001). Therefore, both genetic and lifestyle factors play a role in BMD and risk for osteoporosis.

In healthy people, total body weight often influences BMD (Edelstein and Barrett-Connor, 1993). In older women, moderate drinking (1–3 glasses of wine daily) is associated with increased trochanteric BMD; higher intakes may be associated with lower BMD (Ganry et al., 2000). Vitamin D receptors may also influence bone density; this is somewhat controversial. Another factor to consider is past or current depression, which has been associated with decreases in BMD (Michelson et al., 1996; Robbins et al., 2001).

Currently, bone remodeling is being studied for its role, along with estrogen replacement, cytokines, parathyroid hormones, and the hormones osteocalcin and osteonectin. The Postmenopausal Estrogen/Progestin Interventions (PEPI) Trial studied 875 healthy women between the ages of 45 and 64 over a 3-year period. This multicenter, randomized, double-blinded study found that postmenopausal women assigned to the estrogen therapy group increased BMD rather than lost it at the spine and hip; their conclusion was that estrogen replacement therapy increases BMD at clinically important sites (Writing Group, 1996).

In men and women 65 and older, dietary supplementation with 500 mg calcium and 700 IU vitamin D moderately reduces bone loss measured in the femoral neck, spine, and total body and reduces the incidence of nonvertebral fractures (Dawson-Hughes et al., 1997).

A new procedure, percutaneous vertebroplasty, inserts a special cement to fill bone crevices. It holds promise and reduces pain but is still under study.

OBJECTIVES

- Preserve height; support independece, and improve functional status (Nutrition Screening Initiative, 2002.
- Lessen the risk of spontaneous fractures by supporting dietary adequacy and reducing excessive exercise while encouraging adequate activity levels.
- Decrease precipitating factors: anticonvulsants, corticosteroids, lactase deficiency, low milk intake, general low intake of calcium or calcium malabsorption, and sedentary lifestyle. Maintain reasonable weight for height.
- Provide adequate time for improvement, which takes 6–9 months.
- Ultimately, decrease morbidity and mortality by retarding future bone loss through medical nutrition therapy (Packard and Heaney, 1997).
- Intake of animal proteins is inversely related to risk of hip fracture in postmenopausal women (Munger et al., 1999). Assure adequate intakes.
- Intake of fruit and vegetables appears to be positively associated with bone health; magnesium and potassium are significantly related to total bone mass (New et al., 2000).
- Avoid excesses of caffeine (over 300 mg), and alcohol (limit to 1 drink daily for women, 2 for men.)
- Soft drinks should not replace daily use of milk products.

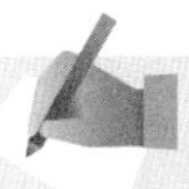

DIETARY AND NUTRITIONAL RECOMMENDATIONS

- Diet should be adequate in calcium, at least 1,000–1,200 mg daily before menopause, 1.5 g daily over age 65 or after menopause (unless on estrogen replacement). To fulfill the requirement, 1 quart of milk daily can be recommended. Calcium supplements can be used if dairy products are not tolerated; calcium absorption averages approximately 30–40% from most sources. Space the supplements throughout the day; over 500 mg at one time is not absorbed as well.
- If fluid milk is not consumed, dry skim milk powder can be added to many foods. Cheese is also a good source of calcium, especially aged cheese. Live-culture yogurt is beneficial.
- In early stages of treatment, try maintaining the Ca:P ratio from dietary sources; a 1:1 ratio is recommended. Phosphorus reduces urinary calcium excretion, but excessive amounts increase PTH and lower serum Ca++.
- Isoflavones may also prove to be beneficial, as in 2–3 servings of soy foods daily (Messina, 1994). Recent research is ongoing in this area.
- If patient is obese, use a calorie-controlled diet that provides adequate vitamins, minerals, and calcium.
- Check that the water is fluoridated in the area.
- Consume at least the RDA of vitamin D; this means 10–20 μg or 200–400 IU daily. Fortified milk, cod liver oil, egg yolks, and fatty fish are good dietary sources. One cup milk =100 IU vitamin D; would need 4–6 cups to get sufficient amounts from diet. Do not exceed 2,000 IU daily.
- Adequate manganese (as from meat and poultry) may be beneficial to improve absorption of calcium. Vitamins C and K, potassium, and magnesium also should be consumed to meet at least the RDA levels.
- Beware excesses of fiber (especially wheat bran), because it increases calcium excretion (Avenell, 1994). Phytates and oxalates also tend to aggravate losses of calcium.
- Sodium also must be controlled; decrease excesses of sodium while increasing potassium and magnesium. Decreasing sodium intake by 50% may be as effective as increasing calcium by more than 800 mg daily (Devine et al., 1995).
- Manage protein intake and maintain at RDA levels. Dairy foods contain a good Ca:protein ratio and should be included in the dietary plan when possible (Dawson-Hughes and Harris, 2002.).
- Intake of caffeine in coffee does not seem to be a problem if calcium (such as milk) is consumed in adequate amounts, i.e., two or more cups daily (Barrett-Connor et al., 1994; Harris and Dawson-Hughes, 1994).
- Include alkaline-producing dietary components (K+, Mg++, and fruits and vegetables) that contribute to maintenance of BMD (Tucker et al., 1999).

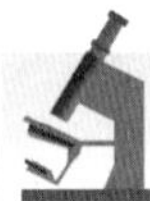

PROFILE

Clinical/History	Lab Work	
Height Weight BMI Back pain BP	Ca++, serum Urinary Ca++ Alk phos Mg++ Alb, prealbumin PTH (useful in	some patients) Serum P (may be decreased with hyperparathyroidism) Bone densitometry; DEXA

Common Drugs Used and Potential Side Effects

- Adequate calcium and vitamin D intake are crucial to develop optimal peak bone mass and to preserve bone mass throughout life. Supplementation of these two components in bioavailable forms may be necessary in individuals who do not achieve recommended intake from dietary sources (National Institutes of Health, 2000).
- Calcium, with or without estrogen replacement, retards bone loss (Aloia, 1994) and reduces bone turnover in postmenopausal women, especially in those with low intakes of dietary calcium (Fardellone et al., 1998). Elemental calcium varies in supplements—see Table 11.4. Calcium carbonate (Tums, Roxane, Os-Cal, Calciday, Oyst-Cal, Oystercal, Caltrate, Gencalc) contains 40%, calcium chloride contains 36%, calcium acetate (Phos-Ex, PhosLo) contains 25%, calcium citrate (Citracal) contains 21%, calcium lactate contains 13%, and calcium gluconate contains 9%. Tricalcium phosphate provides 39% calcium. Note that rates of absorption also vary. Calcium maleate is better absorbed than even calcium carbonate (Dawson-Hughes et al., 1990; Lloyd et al., 1993). Bone meal or Dolomite may include contaminants and should be avoided (even with a 33% calcium content).

  Calcium carbonate (Tums, Titralac, Fosfree, Calcet + Vitamin D) temporarily decreases gastric acidity, which is needed for calcium absorption. Dietary calcium is better absorbed; need 1,000–1,500 mg/day. Excesses of calcium supplements can cause hypercalcemia; monitor intakes carefully. Beware of excess vitamin D, which can cause vitamin D calcinosis. Avoid taking with iron supplements. Use extra water. Reduce high intakes of protein, phosphorus, sodium, and caffeine. High-calcium diets may reduce net zinc absorption and balance and may increase zinc requirements (Wood and Zheng, 1997).
- Hormone or estrogen replacement therapy (ERT) has some merit as well as controversy. In the CHART study (Speroff, 1996), daily treatment with estrogen (estradiol) was well tolerated and protected the endometrium from hyperplasia. Estrogen tends to increase the risk of cancer of the endometrium if not opposed with progesterone. Ensure adequate calcium intake while using estrogen; this enhances the positive effect of estrogen on bone mass at all skeletal sites and may enhance the positive effect of calcitonin on bone mass in the spine (Nieves et al., 1998). Selective estrogen receptor modulators (SERMs) are useful in mimicking estrogen while having fewer side effects such as breakthrough bleeding.
- Intermittent etidronate therapy prevents the loss of vertebral and trochanteric bone in corticosteroid-treated patients (Adachi et al., 1997). Metallic taste, nausea, diarrhea, and decreased potassium and magnesium may be problems.
- According to the National Osteoporosis Foundation: the FDA approves estrogen, calcitonin, alendronate, raloxifene, and risedronate for the treatment of postmenopausal osteoporosis. Estrogen, alendronate, risedronate, and raloxifene are approved for the prevention of the disease. Alendronate is approved for the treatment of osteoporosis in men. Alendronate and risedronate are approved for use by men and women with glucocorticoid-induced osteoporosis. Zoledronic acid is under study.

  Fosamax (alendronate) was the first nonhormonal drug approved; it reverses bone loss while decreasing bone resorption. It is taken with plain water only, first thing in the morning. Patients with severe renal disease or those who are pregnant or breastfeeding should not take it. Nausea, heartburn, irritation or pain of the

TABLE 11–4 Common Calcium Supplements

Product	*Source of calcium and mg of elemental calcium/tablet*	*Number of tablets/day to provide about 900–1,000 mg calcium*
Caltrate 600 ®	Carbonate (600 mg)	1.5
Caltrate 600 + Vitamin D ®	Carbonate (600 m g)	1.5
Os-Cal 500 ®	Carbonate from oyster shell (500 mg)	2
Os-Cal 500 + Vitamin D ®	Carbonate from oyster shell (500 mg)	2
Posture ® (600 mg)	Phosphate (600 mg)	1.5
Posture-Vitamin D ®	Phosphate (600 mg)	1.5
Citracal ®	Citrate (200 mg)	5
Citracal ® + Vitamin D	Citrate (315 mg)	3
Citracal Liquitab ®	Citrate (500 mg)	2
Tums ® 500 mg	Carbonate from limestone (500 mg)	2
Tums E-X ® 300 mg	Carbonate from limestone (300 mg)	3.5
Tums Ultra ®	Carbonate from limestone (400 mg)	2.5
Calcet ® + Vitamin D	Carbonate, lactate, gluconate (300 mg)	3.5
Fosfree ®	Carbonate, gluconate, lactate (175 mg)	6

Source: Shils M, et al. eds. *Modern nutrition in health and disease*. Baltimore, MD: Lippincott Williams & Wilkins, 1999.

esophagus, vomiting, dysphagia, sensation of fullness, and constipation or diarrhea may occur. It seems to be effective even if taken once weekly with resulting increases in bone density.

Actonel (risedronate) can cause dysphagia, esophageal ulcer, and stomach ulcer. Take on an empty stomach 30 minutes before meals. Take additional vitamin D and calcium. Headache, GI distress, diarrhea, nausea, constipation, and rash may occur, although rarely.

Evista (raloxifene) protects against thin, weak bones and fractures. It lowers total cholesterol by 7% and low-density lipoproteins (LDL) by 11%. It may trigger menopausal symptoms, including hot flashes, but is less likely to have an estrogen-like increase in cancer risk.

Calcitonin (Miacalcin) makes calcium more available to bones. It is given as an injection or nasal spray. Injectable calcitonin may cause allergic reactions and flushing of the face and hands, urinary frequency, nausea, and skin rash. Bone loss is reduced and bone mass increases, although not in the hip. A modest increase in bone mass occurs.

- Calcitriol (1,25-dihydroxyvitamin D) is the active form of vitamin D hormone, which increases GI absorption of calcium from the gut, kidney reabsorption of calcium, stimulates bone resorption, decreases PTH production, and stimulates skeletal osteoblasts/clasts. It is more commonly used in renal osteodystrophy. Ergocalciferol is a vitamin D analog that is used with calcium supplements; monitor for side effects such as hypercalcemia.
- Use of oral contraceptives for more than 6 years increases bone density (Kritz-Silverstein and Barrett-Connor, 1993). Folic acid depletion may occur.
- Sodium fluoride can cause changes in bone quality and may actually increase fractures, unless used with calcium citrate (Pak, 1995). The slow-release form may increase bone formation and decrease the risk of fractures. In patients with mild-to-moderate osteoporosis, long-term supplements with fluoride plus calcium result in lower rates of vertebral fracture than supplementation with calcium alone. Intake of fluoride in drinking water at 1 ppm does not appear to be associated with increased risk of hip fracture (Hillier et al., 2000).
- Anabolic therapy is being studied; bone formation is directly stimulated by fluoride, growth hormone (GH), insulin-like growth factor I, the statins, and PTH (Rosen and Bilezikian, 2001).
- Teriparatide (Forteo), should get clearance by the FDA to combat osteoporosis. Forteo actually builds new bone. It's the first drug to mimic human parathyroid hormone, which triggers the formation of new bone.
- Anti-seizure drugs (phenytoin, barbiturates) and glucocorticoids may lead to lost bone density. Monitor chronic use carefully.

Herbs, Botanicals and Supplements

- Herbs and botanical supplements should not be used without discussing with physician. Cabbage, pigweed, dandelion, avocado, and parsley have been recommended, but there is no proof of efficacy.
- There is not enough evidence to support use of soy.

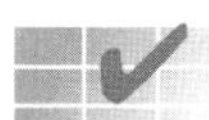

PATIENT EDUCATION

- ✓ Prevention is the best medicine. Encourage patient to stand upright, rather than sit or recline, as often as feasible.
- ✓ Regular exercise, especially resistance and high-impact activities, contributes to development of high peak bone mass and may reduce the risk of falls in older individuals (National Institutes of Health, 2000). Aerobic strengthening exercises and lifting weights may be beneficial. Change a sedentary lifestyle. Walking or running is beneficial. However, excessive weight-bearing exercise can cause amenorrhea in women when a low-calorie diet is consumed.
- ✓ Explain that efficiency of calcium absorption declines with age. Adequate calcium and vitamin D are important throughout life. The overall benefit of healthful eating must be overemphasized; it may also be cost effective to consider public health initiatives such as calcium and vitamin D supplementation in the elderly (Prince, 1997).
- ✓ Describe use of milk and other alternate calcium sources in diet. Broccoli, kale, other greens, and soybeans are useful.
- ✓ Decrease use of alcohol (Felson, 1995; Greendale, 1995) and smoking.
- ✓ Caffeine poses a smaller risk and generally presents no problems; BMD is not affected by caffeine if at least one glass of milk is consumed daily (Bennett-Connor et al., 1994).
- ✓ Encourage adequate exposure to sunlight (10–30 minutes daily), but be wary of sunburn and overexposure with its risks of skin cancer. (Nutritional Screening Initiative, 2002.)
- ✓ Beware of vegetarian diets that are low in absorbable manganese, a factor in bone reformation/maintenance.
- ✓ Remind all teenagers that osteoporosis actually begins with acquisition of an adequate skeleton by 20 years of age and that calcium intake is crucial during the teens and twenties. Osteoporosis is "kid stuff" in that maintenance of weight-bearing activity is important during the growing years. Consumption of carbonated beverages instead of milk is a big concern.
- ✓ Some mineral waters are excellent sources of calcium; bioavailability is good (Couzy et al., 1995).
- ✓ Those persons with previous fractures should be monitored carefully for osteoporosis (NIH Consensus Development Panel, 2001).
- ✓ Avoid long-term use of high doses of retinol from fortified foods or supplements (Feskanich et al., 2002).

For More Information

- ✦ National Osteoporosis Foundation
  1232 22nd St., NW
  Washington, DC 20037-1292
  202-223-2226
  http://www.nof.org/
- ✦ National Institutes of Health Osteoporosis and Related Bones Diseases
  National Resource Center
  http://www.osteo.org/about.html
- ✦ National Bone Health Campaign
  http://www.nof.org/powerfulbones/index.htm
- ✦ Osteoporosis Society of Canada
  http://www.osteoporosis.ca/index.shtml

PAGET'S DISEASE (OSTEITIS DEFORMANS)

NUTRITIONAL ACUITY RANKING: LEVEL 2

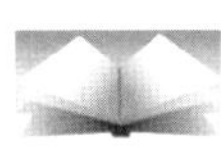

DEFINITIONS AND BACKGROUND

Paget's disease is a chronic disorder of the skeleton, where areas on bone grow abnormally, enlarging and becoming soft. It is of unknown etiology, with excessive bone destruction and repairing. Of all persons older than 50 years of age, 3% have an isolated lesion; the actual clinical disease is much less common.

Paget's disease of bone is the second most common bone disease in the world. The disease tends to run in families. Approximately 3 million Americans have the disease, and it rarely occurs before age 40. The disease was higher in frequency in people who were in the older decades of life with the highest prevalence of 2% in the 65- to 74-year-old people; there is a slight male predominance in the 45- to 74-year age group (Altman et al., 2000).

Symptoms and signs include deep "bone pain," joint pain, back pain, skull enlargement, hearing loss or headaches, thickening of long bones, bowing of limbs, curvature of the spine, heart failure (especially in severe form), spontaneous fractures, anemia, or bone sarcoma. Prognosis is good in mild cases.

OBJECTIVES

- Prevent complications, especially related to the nervous system (e.g., blindness, fractures, vertebral collapse, and deafness).
- Prevent side effects of drug therapy.
- Promote full recovery when possible.
- Differentiate from other conditions with bone lesions.

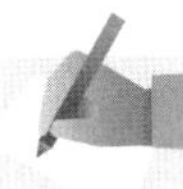

DIETARY AND NUTRITIONAL RECOMMENDATIONS

- Adequate protein is important, with adequate calories to spare protein.
- Adequate levels of calcium and vitamins C and D may be needed.
- To correct anemia, monitor serum levels of iron and vitamin B12 to determine need for an altered diet.

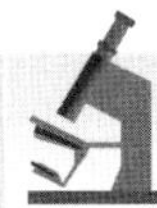

PROFILE

Clinical/History

Height
Weight
BMI

Lab Work

Ca++
Alb, prealbumin
PTH (abnormal)
Uric acid (UA) (often elevated)
Transferrin
Serum Phosphorus
Alk phos (increased)
Urinary Ca++ (altered)
H&H
Serum B12
Radiolabeled bisphosphonate
X-rays (denser, expanded bones)
Bone scans

Common Drugs Used and Potential Side Effects

- Drugs that inhibit bone resorption—bisphosphonates (etidronate, pamidronate, clodronate, or alendronate)—may be used to slow the progression. Risedronate is a new bisphosphonate and thus can be used in various bone conditions involving increased levels of bone resorption such as Paget's disease of bone. Bisphosphonates are pyrophosphate analogs that bind to bone at active sites of remodeling (Theriault and Hortobagyi, 2001).
- Thyrocalcitonin or synthetic calcitonin may be used to decrease passage of calcium from bones to bloodstream. It is often parenteral as salmon Calcimar. Monitor for nausea or vomiting. Newer methods of administration include a nasal spray.
- Aspirin is often used to relieve bone pain; monitor GI effects. Vitamin C may be depleted.
- Vitamin D may be used (e.g., 50,000 IU three times weekly). Monitor for side effects of toxicity.
- Estrogen or testosterone may be given if osteoporosis coexists. Increases in endometrial cancer have been noted with high doses of estrogens when progesterone is not also used.
- Actonel (risedronate sodium) can cause dysphagia, esophageal ulcer, and stomach ulcer. Take on an empty stomach 30 minutes before meals. Take additional vitamin D and calcium. Headache, diarrhea, nausea, constipation, and rash may occur, although they are rare.

Herbs, Botanicals and Supplements

- Herbs and botanical supplements should not be used without discussing with physician.

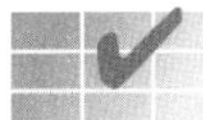

PATIENT EDUCATION

- ✔ Discuss appropriate dietary alterations for patient's condition, individualized for the current condition and status. Include good food sources of calcium, B-complex vitamins, iron, protein, and vitamin D. Monitor carefully, if supplements are used, in addition to dietary guidance.
- ✔ Discuss side effects for the specific drugs ordered.

For More Information

- ✦ National Association for the Relief of Paget's Disease
  http://www.paget.org.uk/
- ✦ National Institutes of Health Osteoporosis and Related Bones Diseases
  http://www.osteo.org/pdisbone.html
- ✦ The Paget Foundation for Paget's Disease of Bone and related Disorders
  120 Wall Street, Suite 1602
  New York, NY 10005
  1-800-23-PAGET
  Fax: (212) 509-8492
  http://www.paget.org/

POLYARTERITIS NODOSA

NUTRITIONAL ACUITY RANKING: LEVEL 2

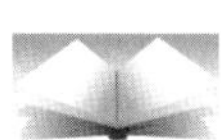

DEFINITIONS AND BACKGROUND

In polyarteritis nodosa (PAN), segments of medium arteries become inflamed in several organs, causing damage (often in brain, heart, liver, GI tract, and renal tissues). The condition is rare and fatal if not treated. It is 2–3 times more common in men and usually develops in men aged 40–50. Viral or bacterial infections such as hepatitis B seem to trigger it, but the specific cause is not known. Small-to-medium-sized arteries are involved by inflammatory necrosis. Aneurysms with inflammatory destruction also occur.

Symptoms and signs include chest pains (heart), shortness of breath (lungs), abdominal pain (liver and intestines), weakness and numbness (nerves), edema, and hematuria (kidneys). Fatigue, aches and pains, persistent fever, anorexia, kidney damage, weight loss, and tachycardia may result. Some skin changes may occur, including rash, nodules, or Raynaud syndrome.

Renal involvement eventually develops in most and is accompanied by hypertension in half of patients. PAN also commonly involves the gut (abdominal angina, hemorrhage, perforation), heart (myocarditis, myocardial infarction), or eye (scleritis); rupture of renal or mesenteric microaneurysms can simulate an acute abdomen (http://vasculitis.med.jhu.edu/pan2.htm).

OBJECTIVES

- Treat as soon as possible to decrease heart and renal damage.
- Improve appetite and intake.
- Prevent weight loss.
- Increase calorie intake to counteract fever.
- Reduce edema and anorexia.

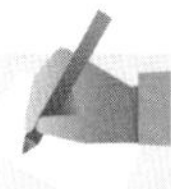

DIETARY AND NUTRITIONAL RECOMMENDATIONS

- Adequate-to-high-calorie intake may be beneficial in case of weight loss.
- A normal-to-high-protein intake generally is required.
- Fluid or sodium intake may be limited with excessive edema or with use of steroids.

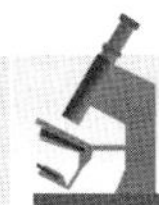

PROFILE

Clinical/History		
Height	Temperature	Alb, prealbumin
Weight	BP	BUN, Creat
BMI	**Lab Work**	Na+
Hematuria	Hepatitis B antigen	Transferrin
I & O	K+	H&H
Edema		Serum Ca++

Common Drugs Used and Potential Side Effects

- Steroids such as prednisone may be used. Side effects of long-term use include negative nitrogen and potassium balances; decreased calcium and zinc levels; CHO intolerance; and excessive sodium retention. Weight gain is also common; a calorie-controlled diet may be useful.
- Pain relievers may be needed; monitor individually for side effects such as GI distress.
- Immunosuppressive drugs such as cyclophosphamide may be used; long-term effects can reduce the ability to fight infections.

Herbs, Botanicals and Supplements

- Herbs and botanical supplements should not be used without discussing with physician.

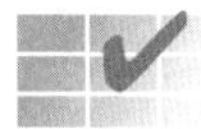

PATIENT EDUCATION

- ✓ Discuss alternate dietary guidelines as appropriate for medications and side effects of the disease.
- ✓ Discuss sources of nutrients as appropriate for the ordered diet.

For More Information

- Johns Hopkins Vasculitis Center http://vasculitis.med.jhu.edu/pan.htm

RHEUMATOID ARTHRITIS

NUTRITIONAL ACUITY RANKING: LEVELS 1–2

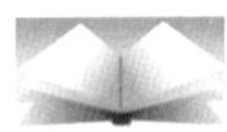

DEFINITIONS AND BACKGROUND

A chronic polyarthritis mainly affecting the smaller peripheral joints, rheumatoid arthritis (RA), is accompanied by general ill health. Crippling deformities can occur. Arthritis and other rheumatic conditions are common conditions associated with ambulatory medical care (Hootman et al., 2000). To diagnose RA, symptoms must have been present for at least 6 weeks and four of seven criteria of the American Rheumatism Association (ARA) must be met: morning stiffness in and around joints, lasting more than 1 hour; arthritis of 3 or more joint areas involved simultaneously; arthritis of at least 1 area in a wrist, metacarpophalangeal (MCP) or proximal interphalangeal (PIP) joint; symmetric arthritis involving the same joint areas; rheumatoid nodules; positive serum rheumatoid factor; radiographic changes typical of RA on hand and wrist radiographs, including erosions, or unequivocal bony decalcification in or adjacent to the involved joints; should not have evidence of other disease such as PAN or lupus (http://www.nih.gov/niams/healthinfo/info.htm).

Cause of RA is likely to be either infectious (mycoplasma or chlamydia) or autoimmunity (increased cytokine production, etc.). Inflammation of synovial tissues is the dominant manifestation; hand involvement occurs in 85% of cases and knees or ankles/feet in 80%. Of all cases, 75% are in women. Most patients are between ages 20–40; it affects 2 million Americans. Respiratory and aerobic exercises may be needed to improve respiratory muscle strength and endurance and aerobic capacity in these patients. Leg muscle strength is an important and independent determinant of walking ability.

Increased cytokine production causes decreased body cell mass (Roubenoff, 1994), especially TNF-a (Firestein and Zvaifler, 1997). Recent studies have investigated inadequate antioxidant use over time as a potential factor. Treatment with TNF-R:Fc results in improvement in the inflammatory symptoms of RA (Moreland et al., 1997).

Omega-3 polyunsaturated fatty acids (PUFA) have been widely documented to reduce inflammation in diseases such as rheumatoid arthritis by down regulation of T-cell proliferation (Arrington et al., 2001). Intakes of cooked vegetables and olive oil are independently associated with risk of RA; mechanisms underlying these associations are uncertain (Linos et al., 1999).

Tumor necrosis factor-alpha has been shown to be a central mediator of inflammatory and joint destructive processes in rheumatoid arthritis (Kast, 2001). Supplementation with gamma-linolenic acid reduces generation of mediators of inflammation and attenuates symptoms, but it also causes potentially harmful increases in serum arachidonic acid unless eicosapentanoic acid (EPA) is also used (Barham et al., 2000). Recent double-blind studies have shown some benefit of borage oil in treatment of RA; the gamma linolenic acid component of borage oil increases prostaglandin E levels that increase cAMP levels that in turn suppress tumor necrosis factor-alpha synthesis.

Chronic anemia is common in this population; serum ferritin may be lower in the presence of RA. Plasma transferrin receptor level is a reliable index for assessing iron status in populations with RA (Lammi-Keefe et al., 1996). Patients benefit from dietary supplements of nutrients when intake does not reach RDAs.

Juvenile RA (Still's disease) (JCA) can occur in children or adults. Salicylates, gold salts, or glucocorticoids may be used. Hands and feet are affected most commonly. Children suffering from JCA have reduced serum levels of beta-carotene, retinol, and zinc compared with healthy children (Helgeland, 2000).

Sjögren's syndrome is a variant form of RA, with insufficient production of lacrimal and salivary secretions. Artificial tears, artificial saliva, and glucocorticoids may be needed. Sjögren's syndrome is an autoimmune disorder, striking 2–4 million Americans and many more worldwide (http://www.sjogrens.org/).

Felty syndrome is a triad of RA, granulocytopenia, and splenomegaly. Infections, leg ulcers, burning eyes, and anemia also can complicate the condition. Sometimes, splenectomy is indicated. Drug therapy may be helpful to others. Felty syndrome affects about 1% of patients with RA.

Rheumatoid vasculitis can be life threatening and usually occurs in patients with severe deforming arthritis and a high titer of rheumatoid factor. Vasculitic lesions include rheumatoid nodules, small nail fold infarcts, and purpura. Fatigue, weight loss, fever, organ ischemia, CNS infarctions, myocardial infarction (MI), and peripheral neuropathy can occur. D-penicillamine and prednisone generally are used to treat it.

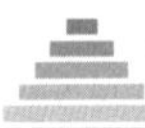

OBJECTIVES

- Maintain satisfactory nutritional status; malnutrition is common in this condition. Monitor weight changes.
- Suggest ways of simplifying meal preparation.
- Restrict sodium intake, if needed.
- Modify patient's diet if hyperlipidemia is present.
- Avoid or correct constipation.
- Consume antioxidant sources (vitamin E and selenium) and vitamin D-rich foods in higher than usual amounts (Fairburn et al., 1996; Gershoff, 1996).
- A vegetarian diet may also have significant benefits (Agren et al., 2001). It is not a cure.
- Promote growth in children with RA; stunting can occur from use of glucocorticoids.

DIETARY AND NUTRITIONAL RECOMMENDATIONS

- Use a high-protein/high-calorie diet if patient is malnourished. Include fatty fish such as salmon, fish oils, and vitamin D to lessen inflammation when possible (Eriksen et al., 1996; McAlindon et al., 1996).
- An uncooked vegan diet may be useful (Hanninen et al.,

2000). This LF diet includes berries, fruits, vegetables and roots, nuts, germinated seeds, and sprouts. Adequate fluid, fiber, vitamins, and minerals are important. Beta-carotene, selenium, and vitamins C and E may be beneficial; choose nutrient-dense foods wisely.

- Restrict saturated fats and sodium if other problems such as hypercholesterolemia or hypertension are also present or if steroids are used.
- Provide nonirritating meals, if the drugs being used cause gastric irritation.
- Ensure diet provides adequate intake of protein, calcium, magnesium, B-complex vitamins, potassium and zinc (Woolf and Manore, 1999).
- With dysphagia, tube feed or use soft/thick, pureed foods as needed.
- Increase folic acid if methotrexate is used; either use diet or folic acid supplements (Morgan et al., 1994).

PROFILE

Clinical/History

- Height
- Weight
- BMI
- Temperature

Lab Work

- RBC
- C-reactive protein (CRP)
- LE prep
- Creat (may be decreased)
- ESR–increases with inflammation
- Antinuclear Antibodies (ANA)
- Rheumatoid Factor (RF)
- Antistreptococcal antibody titer
- Immunoglobulins (may be elevated in Sjögren's)
- Ceruloplasmin (may be increased)
- H&H
- Serum B12
- Ferritin
- Transferrin
- Serum folate, RBC folate
- Serum copper
- Total protein
- Alb, prealbumin
- Gluc
- BUN

Common Drugs Used and Potential Side Effects

- Salicylate/aspirin. Prolonged use can cause GI bleeding. Intake of vitamin C and folate should be increased.
- Phenylbutazone (Butazolidin) can cause peptic ulceration. This is rarely used now.
- Indomethacin (Indocin) also can cause GI ulceration, renal failure, and hyperkalemia.
- Gold salt (Ridaura) was sometimes used in the past. Abdominal pain, nausea, vomiting, and diarrhea may result.
- Fenoprofen (Nalfon), ibuprofen (Motrin), and naproxen (Naprosyn) can cause headaches, nausea, abdominal pain, bloating, or anorexia.
- Methotrexate can cause anemia, nausea, vomiting, and stomatitis. Extra folic acid should be provided (Morgan et al., 1994).
- Flurbiprofen (Ansaid) or piroxicam (Feldene) may cause GI bleeding, nausea, and diarrhea.
- Tenidap reduces interleukin production. No specific nutritional side effects have been noted, but there are other side effects (Moreland, 1997).
- Minocycline, doxycycline, and other antibiotics are being piloted for use.
- Hydroxychloroquine sulfate (Plaquenil) may cause anorexia, nausea, abdominal cramps, and diarrhea.
- Prescription medications, Salagen (pilocarpine hydrochloride), and Evoxac (cevimeline) are available to treat dry mouth associated with Sjögren's; they simulate the salivary glands. Depending on severity of symptoms, other medications include NSAIDs, steroids, and immunosuppressive drugs.
- Cyclosporine is sometimes used with severe RA; monitor for GI side effects.

Herbs, Botanicals and Supplements

- Herbs and botanical supplements should not be used without discussing with physician.
- Younger female patients tend to use alternative treatments for RA more than males; perception of negative impact of the disease on several aspects of life seems to play a large part (Jacobs et al., 2001). Psychosocial intervention may be beneficial.
- With use of methotrexate (Rheumatrex), avoid Echinacea for potential damage to the liver.
- St. John's wort and Echinacea should not be used with cyclosporine.
- MSM (methylsulfonylmethane) has been promoted for use in RA and other types of arthritis. Evidence is minimal and side effects may include nausea, diarrhea, and headaches.
- With use of borage oil, concomitant NSAID use may undermine borage oil effects, and borage oil would be contraindicated in pregnancy given the teratogenic and labor-inducing effects of prostaglandin E agonists (Kast, 2001).

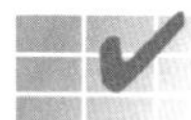

PATIENT EDUCATION

- ✓ Instruct patient about simplified planning and preparation tips.
- ✓ No nutrients can replace blood transfusions if needed for anemia.
- ✓ Discourage quackery and substitute sound health practices. The "Dong" diet is useless, for example. A collagen solution made from chicken cartilage was tried in 1992 at Beth Israel Hospital in Boston, but no confirming studies have followed.
- ✓ CHO tolerance must reflect individual needs; sometimes, CHO intolerance occurs because of chronic inflammation and use of steroids.
- ✓ Inflammatory responses may be reduced by inclusion of omega-3 fatty acids for their roles as precursors of eicos-

anoids. Herring, salmon, tuna, and mackerel are good dietary sources.

- ✔ Strengthening exercises may help improve patient's ability to walk and may decrease joint pain and fatigue.
- ✔ Check BMD; there is a high incidence of osteoporosis in this population.
- ✔ Encourage nutrient-dense foods. If intake is poor, a vitamin–mineral supplement may be needed (woolf and Manore, 1999).

For More Information

- ✦ Arthritis Foundation
  1-800-283-7800
  http://www.arthritis.org
- ✦ American Autoimmune Related Diseases Association
  1-800-598-4668
  http://www.aarda.org
- ✦ National Institute of Dental and Craniofacial Research
  National Institutes of Health
  Gene Therapy and Therapeutics Branch
  Bethesda, MD 20892
  http://www.nidr.nih.gov/
- ✦ National Sjögren's Syndrome Association
  1-800-395-6772
- ✦ Sjögren's Syndrome Foundation
  1-800-475-6473
  http://www.sjogrens.org/

RUPTURE OF INTERVERTEBRAL DISK

NUTRITIONAL ACUITY RANKING: LEVEL 1

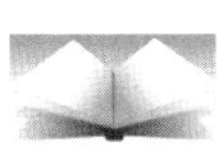

DEFINITIONS AND BACKGROUND

Other names for a slipped or ruptured disk include cervical radiculopathy, herniated intervertebral disk, lumbar radiculopathy, prolapsed intervertebral disk, and radiculopathy. In this condition, slipping or prolapse of a cervical or lumbar disk occurs, with neck/shoulder pain or low back pain accordingly. Degenerating changes in the disks begin around 30 years of age. Percutaneous automated diskectomy (PAD) surgery can be performed in some cases; this surgery breaks up the disc and removes fragments. A laminectomy surgically removes the lamina of a vertebra.

With lumbar radiculopathy, ambulation may be painful and limping can occur. Muscular weakness, severe back pain that radiates to buttocks or legs and feet, pain that worsens with coughing or laughing, tingling or numbness in legs or feet, and muscle contractions or spasms may also result. With cervical radiculopathy, neck pain in back and sides is deep; pain may radiate to shoulders, upper arm, or forearm and worsens with coughing or laughing; spasm of neck muscles and pain worsening at night may occur.

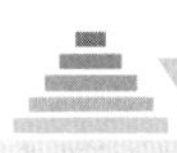

OBJECTIVES

- ▲ Maintain adequate rest and activity levels, as assigned by physician.
- ▲ Prevent weight gain from decreased activity.
- ▲ Encourage adequate hydration.
- ▲ Prevent constipation and straining.
- ▲ Assist with feeding, if patient is in traction.
- ▲ Relieve pain and promote healing.

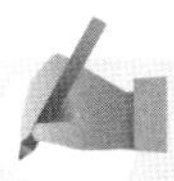

DIETARY AND NUTRITIONAL RECOMMENDATIONS

- A regular diet generally is sufficient. For some, a more strict calorie-controlled diet may be beneficial to promote weight loss.
- Increased fluid and fiber intake can be helpful to reduce constipation. Fresh fruits and vegetables, bran, and other foods may be needed.

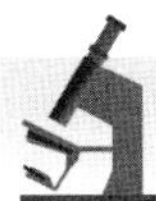

PROFILE

Clinical/History	Lab Work	
Height	H&H	MRI or CT scan
Weight	Na+, K+	Myelography
BMI	Alb, prealbumin	Diskography
I & O	BUN, Creat	Spinal or neck x-rays
BP	Ca++	Nerve conduction velocity test
Constipation	Alk phos	
Edema	Gluc	

Common Drugs Used and Potential Side Effects

- Anti-inflammatory drugs may be used. Nausea, GI distress, and anorexia may result. Follow directions regarding when to take (e.g., before or after meals).
- Analgesics may be helpful to relieve pain. Chronic use of aspirin may cause GI bleeding.
- Muscle relaxants may be ordered. GI distress or nausea can occur.

Herbs, Botanicals and Supplements

- Herbs and botanical supplements should not be used without discussing with physician.

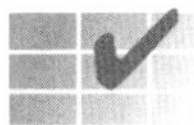

PATIENT EDUCATION

- ✔ Instruct patient regarding effective methods of relieving constipation.
- ✔ Discuss role of nutrition and exercise in health maintenance.
- ✔ After surgery, the role of nutrition in wound healing should be discussed.

SCLERODERMA

NUTRITIONAL ACUITY RANKING: LEVEL 3

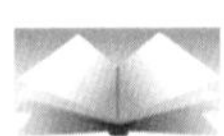

DEFINITIONS AND BACKGROUND

In scleroderma (systemic sclerosis or PSS), pathological deposition of fibrous connective tissue in the skin and visceral organs occurs. The GI tract is affected, and Raynaud's syndrome (ischemia of fingers) is common. Symptoms and signs include thickening and swelling of the ends of the fingers, dysphagia, heartburn, fibrosis of salivary and lacrimal glands, abdominal pains, flatulence, weight loss, nausea and vomiting, diarrhea, and constipation.

As the disease progresses, large areas of the skin may be affected or only the fingers (sclerodactyly). Skin on the face tightens and causes a masklike appearance. Spider veins (telangiectasia) occur on the fingers, chest, face, lips, or tongue. Calcium deposits can occur on the fingers or other bony areas; sores or contractures may result from the scarring. Scarring of the esophagus may be especially detrimental, causing blockage or even cancer. Lungs can be affected, leading to shortness of breath with exercise. Multiple organ system dysfunction may occur in the cardiac and renal systems. Renal failure, pulmonary hypertension, and interstitial lung disease are major causes of morbidity and mortality in systemic sclerosis (Bar et al., 2001). There is no known cure, and the disease can be fatal.

The CREST syndrome, or limited cutaneous sclerosis, is less severe and causes less internal organ damage. Calcium deposits, Raynaud's phenomenon, esophageal dysfunction, skin damage on fingers, and telangiectasia form the acronym for CREST. Pulmonary hypertension, heart failure, or respiratory failure may result.

OBJECTIVES

- ▲ Prevent or correct protein–calorie malnutrition (PCM) and nutrient deficiencies.
- ▲ Correct xerostomia from Sjögren's syndrome (decreased saliva with dysphagia and difficulty in chewing as a result).
- ▲ Monitor dysphagia with esophageal involvement; alter mode of feeding as needed.
- ▲ Counteract vitamin B12 and fat maldigestion and absorption, which may be common.
- ▲ Monitor hypomotility of the GI tract, with altered fiber intake as appropriate. Pseudo-obstruction and gastroparesis may occur. For many patients, nutritional support and relief of symptoms remain the primary management goal of pseudo-obstruction (Quigley, 1999).

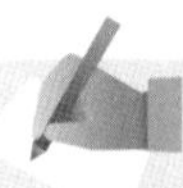

DIETARY AND NUTRITIONAL RECOMMENDATIONS

- A soft diet with moistened foods and extra fluids may be useful. Add fiber if constipation is a problem (e.g., adding crushed bran to hot cereal).
- Tube feed if patient is dysphagic. Use TPN if GI tract is too affected by the disease, with intractable diarrhea and severe malabsorption.
- Reduce lactose if intolerance occurs.
- Small, frequent feedings may be needed.
- Reduce fiber in case of obstruction; low residue or tube feeding may be needed.
- Give fat- and water-soluble vitamins in supplemental form, if needed; extra calcium may be needed if lactose is not tolerated orally.
- Calories (30–40 kcal/kg) and adequate to high protein.
- With hypertension and multiple organ system dysfunction, reduced sodium may be needed when there is fluid overload.

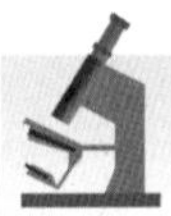

PROFILE

Clinical/History	Lab Work	
Height	Antibodies to centromeres (distinguishes mild-to-severe forms)	time (PT)
Weight	Serum folate	Alb, prealbumin
BMI	H&H	BUN, Creat
Temperature	Serum B12	Na+, K+
Skinfold measurements	Gluc	Ca++
BP	Prothrombin	Alk phos
I & O		Fecal fat test, hydrogen breath test for malabsorption

Common Drugs Used and Potential Side Effects

- Bethanechol (Urecholine) may be given to augment lower esophageal sphincter (LES) pressure. Diarrhea may occur.
- Antacids or histamine-blocking agents may be used to reduce gastric hyperacidity. Monitor for side effects specific to selected medication, including depletion of any nutrients.
- Antibiotics (such as tetracycline) may be necessary to decrease intestinal bacteria overgrowth. Read directions and take at proper timing with meals to prevent GI distress.
- Anti-inflammatory agents often are used such as steroids with their multiple effects. Monitor for nitrogen and calcium losses, altered electrolyte levels, and elevated glucose levels. Correct diet accordingly.
- Antihypertensives usually are needed; monitor blood pressure results. Potassium supplements may or may not be required; determine need according to medication selected. Angiotensin-converting enzyme (ACE) inhibitors are commonly used.
- Trental (pentoxifylline) is used for Raynaud's syndrome to improve circulation. Anorexia or GI distress may result.

Herbs, Botanicals and Supplements

- Herbs and botanical supplements should not be used without discussing with physician.
- For Raynaud's disease: evening primrose, gingko, mustard, garlic, borage, and red pepper have been suggested, but there are no clinical trials, which prove effectiveness.

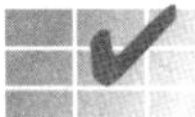

PATIENT EDUCATION

- ✓ Artificial saliva (Xero-Lube) or lemon glycerine may be useful.
- ✓ If eating orally, adequate chewing time will be required.
- ✓ For heartburn, keep head elevated after meals; decrease or limit intake of chocolate, caffeine, fatty foods, alcohol, citrus, and tomatoes.
- ✓ Physical therapy and exercise may help maintain muscle strength but cannot totally prevent joints from locking into stiffened positions.

For More Information

- Scleroderma Foundation
  89 Newbury St., Suite 201
  Danvers, MA 01923
  978-750-4499
  1-800-722-HOPE
  http://www.scleroderma.org/

SYSTEMIC LUPUS ERYTHEMATOSUS

NUTRITIONAL ACUITY RANKING: LEVEL 3

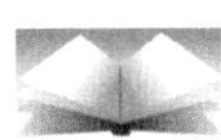

DEFINITIONS AND BACKGROUND

Systemic lupus erythematosus (SLE), or lupus, is an autoimmune disorder that involves areas of inflammation of the joints, tendons, other connective tissues, and skin. There may also be pyrexia, malaise, butterfly rash on cheeks, hepatosplenomegaly, weight loss, diarrhea, pleurisy, pericarditis, and renal damage. Women in their late teens to thirties are most affected.

Some environmental factors that may trigger the disease are: infections, antibiotics (especially those in the sulfa and penicillin groups), ultraviolet light, extreme stress, and certain drugs. There may also be a genetic tendency; close family members have a 10 times greater frequency than the general population.

More people have lupus than AIDS, cerebral palsy, multiple sclerosis, sickle-cell anemia, and cystic fibrosis combined; between 1,400,000 and 2,000,000 people reported to have been diagnosed with lupus. For most people, lupus is a mild disease affecting only a few organs. For others, it may cause serious and even life-threatening problems. Thousands of Americans die each year from lupus-related complications. There are three types of lupus: discoid, systemic, and drug-induced. Cure is not yet possible.

OBJECTIVES

- ▲ Counteract steroid therapy.
- ▲ Replenish potassium reserves.
- ▲ Reduce fever and replace nutrient losses and weight loss.
- ▲ Control disease manifestations.
- ▲ Manage cardiac effects. Pericarditis is the most common problem. Shortness of breath and chest pain can occur.
- ▲ Lupus nephritis or glomerulonephritis is the medical term for the kidney disease, which occurs in SLE; about a third of patients with lupus will develop nephritis, which requires medical evaluation and nutritional management.

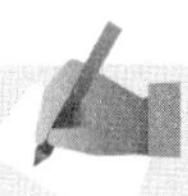

DIETARY AND NUTRITIONAL RECOMMENDATIONS

- It may be useful to use a high-potassium diet unless potassium replacements are provided.
- If needed, mildly restrict sodium intake.
- Diet should be high in protein and kilocalories to compensate for nitrogen losses during fever. If renal damage is excessive, diet can be adjusted.
- Alter diet, if needed, to lower blood pressure levels.

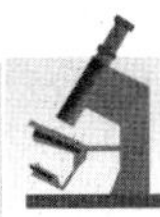

PROFILE

Clinical/History

Height
Weight
BMI
BP
I & O
Temperature

Lab Work

Alb, prealbumin
Transferrin
LE prep
Sedimentation rate
Complement test (C3, C4, CH50, CH100) to measure complementary proteins circulating in the blood
K+
Na+
H&H (decreased)
Transferrin
Serum ferritin
Antinuclear bodies (increased)
Serum Copper (increased)
Total Protein (decreased)
WBC (decreased)
Gluc (increased)
Specific gravity, urine (decreased)
Chol (increased)
BUN, Creat

Common Drugs Used and Potential Side Effects

- NSAIDs or acetaminophen currently are useful. If sodium retention occurs, alter diet as necessary.
- Steroid therapy may cause sodium retention, hyperglycemia, potassium and calcium depletion, and negative nitrogen balance. Side effects include weight gain, a round face, acne, easy bruising, fractures or osteoporosis, hypertension, cataracts, hyperglycemia or onset of diabetes, increased risk of infection, and stomach ulcers.
- Sunscreens are needed to protect against the sun's harmful rays. There generally are no systemic side effects.
- Antimalarials such as chloroquine (Aralen) or hydroxychloroquine (Plaquenil) may be used. They are most often prescribed for skin and joint symptoms of lupus. Side effects are rare and consist of occasional diarrhea or rashes. Chloroquine can affect the eyes. Plaquenil may cause anorexia, nausea, abdominal cramps, or diarrhea.
- Cytotoxic drugs such as azathioprine (Imuran) and cyclophosphamide (Cytoxan) tend to suppress the immune system. There are often GI side effects.

Herbs, Botanicals and Supplements

- Herbs and botanical supplements should not be used without discussing with physician.

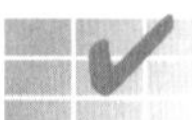

PATIENT EDUCATION

- ✔ Ensure patient has an adequate intake of fluids during febrile periods.
- ✔ Explain which foods are sources of sodium and potassium in the diet.
- ✔ Adequate rest is needed during flare-ups.
- ✔ Sunblock should be used outdoors.
- ✔ Discuss how to manage diet if elevated blood glucose persists.

For More Information

- Lupus Foundation of America
  1300 Piccard Dr., Suite 200
  Rockville, MD 20850-4303
  301-670-9292
  1-800-558-0121
  http://www.lupus.org/

REFERENCES

BONE HEALTH & OSTEOPOROSIS- Cited References

Adachi J, et al. Intermittent etidronate therapy to prevent corticosteroid-induced osteoporosis. *N Engl J Med.* 1997;337:382.

Aloia J, et al. Calcium supplementation with and without hormone replacement therapy to prevent postmenopausal bone loss. *Ann Intern Med.* 1994;120:97.

Amin S, Felson D. Osteoporosis in men. *Rheum Dis Clin North Am.* 2001;27:19.

Avenell A, et al. Bone loss associated with high fibre weight reduction diet in postmenopausal women. *Eur J Clin Nutri.* 1994;48:561.

Barrett-Connor E, Chang J, Edelstein S. Coffee-associated osteoporosis offset by daily milk consumption: the Rancho Bernardo study. *JAMA.* 1994;271:280.

Brand C, et al. Vitamin E is ineffective for symptomatic relief of knee osteoarthritis: a 6-month double-blind, randomized, placebo-controlled study. *Ann Rheum Dis.* 2001;60:946.

Brot C, et al. The influence of smoking on vitamin D status and calcium metabolism. *Euro J Clin Nutri.* 1999;53:920.

Cappucino F, et al. High blood pressure and bone-mineral loss in elderly white women: a prospective study. *Lancet.* 1999;354:971.

Carek P, et al. Diagnosis and management of osteomyelitis. *Am Fam Physician.* 2001;63:2413.

Cheng Y, et al. Relation of nutrition to bone lead and blood lead levels in middle-aged to elderly men: The Normative Aging Study. *Am J Epid.* 1998;147:1162.

Couzy F, et al. Calcium bioavailability from a calcium- and sulfate-rich mineral water, compared with milk, in young adult women. *Am J Clin Nutri.* 1995;62:1239.

Dawson-Hughes B, et al. A controlled trial of the effect of calcium supplementation on bone density in postmenopausal women. *N Engl J Med.* 1990;323:878.

Dawson-Hughes B, Harris SS. Calcium intake influences the association of protein intake with rates of bone loss in elderly men and women. *Am J Clin Nutr* 2002;75:773.

Dawson-Hughes B, et al. Effect of calcium and vitamin D supplementation on bone density in men and women aged 65 of age or older. *N Engl J Med.* 1997;337:670.

Devine A, et al. A longitudinal study of the effect of sodium and calcium intakes on regional bone density in postmenopausal women. *Am J Clin Nutri.* 1995;62:740.

Edelstein S, Barrett-Connor E. Relation between body size and bone mineral density in elderly men and women. *Am J Epidemiol.* 1993; 138:160.

Fardellone P, et al. Biochemical effects of calcium supplementation in postmenopausal women: influence of dietary calcium intake. *Am J Clin Nutri.* 1998;67:1273.

Felson D, et al. Alcohol intake and bone mineral density in elderly men and women: the Framingham study. *Am J Epidemiol.* 1995; 142:485.

Feskanich D, et al. Vitamin A intake and hip fractures among postmenopausal women. *JAMA* 2002;287:47.

Ganry O, et al. Effect of alcohol intake on bone mineral density in elderly women: the EPIDOS study. *Am J Epid.* 2000;151:773.

Greendale G, et al. Lifestyle factors and bone mineral density: the postmenopausal estrogen/progestins intervention study. *J Women's Health.* 1995;4:231.

Gurwitz J, et al. Initiation of antihypertensive treatment during nonsteroidal anti-inflammatory drug therapy. *JAMA.* 1994;272:781.

Hanninen, et al. Antioxidants in vegan diet and rheumatic disorders. *Toxicology.* 2000;155:45.

Harris S, Dawson-Hughes B. Caffeine and bone loss in healthy postmenopausal women. *Am J Clin Nutri.* 1994;60:573.

Heany R, et al. Dietary changes favorably affect bone remodeling in older adults. *J Am Diet Assoc.* 1999;99:1228.

Heer M, et al. Calcium metabolism in microgravity. *Eur J Med Res.* 1999;4:357.

Higashi A, et al. Zinc kinetics in patients with bone demineralization due to physical immobilization. *J Am Col Nutri.* 1993;12:61.

Hillier S, et al. Fluoride in drinking water and risk of hip fracture in the U.K. *Lancet.* 2000;355:265.

Hoffer L, et al. Sulfate could mediate the therapeutic effect of glucosamine sulfate. *Metabolism.* 2001;50:767.

Kalkwarf H, et al. The effect of calcium supplementation on bone density during lactation and after weaning. *N Engl J Med.* 1997; 337:523.

Kraemer W, et al. Bone mineral density in elite junior Olympic weight lifters. *Med Sci Sports Exerc.* 1993;25:1103.

Kritz-Silverstein D, Barrett-Connor E. Bone mineral density in postmenopausal women as determined by prior oral contraceptive use. *Am J Public Health.* 1993;83:100.

Lawrence R, et al. Estimates of the prevalence of arthritis and selected musculoskeletal disorders in the United States. *Arthritis Rheum.* 1998;41:778.

Lips P, et al. A global study of vitamin D status and parathyroid function in postmenopausal women with osteoporosis: baseline data from the multiple outcomes of raloxifene evaluation clinical trial. *J Clin Endocrinol Metab.* 2001;86:1212.

Lloyd T, et al. Calcium supplementation and bone mineral density in adolescent girls. *JAMA.* 1993;270:841.

Lloyd T, et al. Dietary caffeine intake and bone status of postmenopausal women. *Am J Clin Nutri.* 1997;65:1826.

Lloyd T, et al. Dietary caffeine intake is not correlated with adolescent bone gain. *J Am Col Nutri.* 1998;17:454.

Marczynski W, et al. Fractures of thoracic and lumbar spine; treatment and follow-up. *Ann Transplant.* 1999;4:46.

Melhus H, et al. Excessive dietary intake of vitamin A is associated with reduced bone mineral density and increased risk for hip fracture. *Ann Int Med.* 1998;129:770.

Messina M. *Osteoporosis—not just deficiency disease. The soy connection 2:2.* Chesterfield, MO: United Soybean Board, 1994.

Michelson D, et al. Bone mineral density in women with depression. *N Engl J Med.* 1996;335:1176.

Munger R, et al. Prospective study of dietary protein intake and risk of hip fracture in postmenopausal women. *Am J Clin Nutri.* 1999; 69:147.

National Institutes of Health. Osteoporosis prevention, diagnosis, and therapy. *NIH Consens Statement.* 2000;17:1.

New S, et al. Dietary influences on bone mass and bone metabolism:

further evidence of a positive link between fruit and vegetable consumption and bone health? *Am J Clin Nutri*. 2000;71:142.

Nicodemus K, et al. Type 1 and type 2 diabetes and incident hip fractures in postmenopausal women. *Diabetes Care*. 2001;24:1192.

Nieves J, et al. Calcium potentiates the effect of estrogen and calcitonin on bone mass: review and analysis. *Am J Clin Nutri*. 1998; 67:18.

NIH Consensus Development Panel on Osteoporosis Prevention, Diagnosis, and Therapy. Osteoporosis prevention, diagnosis, and therapy. *JAMA*. 2001;285:785.

Nutrition Screening Inditiative. A physician's guide to nutrition in chronic disease management for older adults. http://www.aafp.org/nsi/physiciansguide.pdf

Packard P, Heaney R. Medical nutrition therapy for patients with osteoporosis. *J Am Diet Assoc*. 1997;97:414.

Pak C, et al. Treatment of postmenopausal osteoporosis with slow-release sodium fluoride: final report of a randomized controlled trial. *Ann Intern Med*. 1995;123:401.

Prince R. Diet and the prevention of osteoporotic fractures (Editorial). *N Engl J Med*. 1997;337:701.

Robbins J, et al. The association of bone mineral density and depression in an older population. *J Am Geriatr Soc*. 2001;49:732.

Rosen C, Bilezikian J. Clinical review 123: anabolic therapy for osteoporosis. *J Clin Endocrinol Metab*. 2001;86:957.

Sowers M, Lachance L. Vitamins and arthritis. The roles of vitamins A, C, D, and E. *Rheum Dis Clin North Am*. 1999;25:315.

Speroff L, et al. The comparative effect on bone density, endometrium, and lipids of continuous hormones as replacement therapy (CHART study). *JAMA*. 1996;276:1397.

Teegarden D, et al. Previous milk consumption is associated with greater bone density in young women. *Am J Clin Nutri*. 1999;69: 1014.

Tucker K, et al. Potassium, magnesium, and fruit and vegetable intakes are associated with greater bone mineral density in elderly men and women. *Am J Clin Nutri*. 1999;69:727.

Wood R, Zheng J. High dietary calcium intakes reduce zinc absorption and balance in humans. *Am J Clin Nutri*. 1997;65:1803.

Writing Group for the PEPI Trial. Effects of hormone therapy on bone mineral density: results from the postmenopausal estrogen-progestin interventions (PEPI) trial. *JAMA*. 1996;276:1389.

Zmuda J, et al. Bone mass and breast cancer risk in older women: differences by stage at diagnosis. *J Natl Cancer Inst*. 2001;93:930.

BONE HEALTH AND OSTEOPOROSIS—Suggested Readings

Anderson J. Bone health. In: Mahan K, Escott-Stump S, eds. *Krause's food, nutrition, and diet therapy*. 10th ed. Philadelphia: WB Saunders, 2000.

Kinyamu H, Gallagher J, et al. Dietary calcium and vitamin D intake in elderly women: effect on serum parathyroid hormone and vitamin D metabolites. *Am J Clin Nutri*. 1998;67:342.

Laskey M, et al. Bone changes after 3 months of lactation: influence of calcium intake, breast-milk output, and vitamin D-receptor genotype. *Am J Clin Nutri*. 1998;67:685.

Musgrave D, et al. Back problems among postmenopausal women taking estrogen replacement therapy: the study of osteoporotic fractures. *Spine*. 2001;26:1606.

New S, et al. Nutritional influences on bone mineral density: a cross-sectional study in premenopausal women. *Am J Clin Nutri*. 1997; 65:1831.

Peterson B, et al. The effects of an educational intervention on calcium intake and bone mineral content in young women with low calcium intake. *Am J Health Promotion*. 2000;14:149.

Reddy M, Cook J. Effect of calcium intake on nonheme iron absorption from a complete diet. *Am J Clin Nutri*. 1997;65:1820.

Ritchie L, et al. A longitudinal study of calcium homeostasis during human pregnancy and lactation and after resumption of menses. *Am J Clin Nutri*. 1998;67:693.

Sambrook P, Eisman J. Osteoporosis prevention and treatment. *Med J Aust*. 2000;172:226.

Ullom-Minnich P. Prevention of osteoporosis and fractures. *Am Fam Physician*. 1999;60:194.

Vieth R. Vitamin D supplementation, 25-hydroxyvitamin D concentrations, and safety. *Am J Clin Nutri*. 1999;69:842.

Wolf R, et al. Update on the epidemiology of osteoporosis. *Curr Rheumatol Rep*. 2000;2:74.

OTHER MUSCULOSKELETAL DISEASES—Cited References

Agren J, et al. Divergent changes in serum sterols during a strict uncooked vegan diet in patients with rheumatoid arthritis. *Br J Nutri*. 2001;85:137.

Altman R, et al. Prevalence of pelvic Paget's disease of bone in the United States. *J Bone Miner Res*. 2000;15:461.

Arrington J, et al. Docosahexaenoic acid suppresses function of the CD28 costimulatory membrane receptor in primary murine and Jurkat T cells. *J Nutri*. 2001;131:1147.

Bar J, et al. Pulmonary-renal syndrome in systemic sclerosis. *Semin Arthritis Rheum*. 2001;30:403.

Barham J, et al. Addition of eicosapentaenoic acid to gamma-linolenic acid-supplemented diets prevents serum arachidonic acid accumulation in humans. *J Nutri*. 2000;130:1925.

Bauman W, Spungen A. Disorders of carbohydrate and lipid metabolism in veterans with paraplegia or quadriplegia: a model of premature aging. *Metab Clin Exp*. 1994;43:749.

Branca F, Vatuena S. Calcium, physical activity and bone health—building bones for a stronger future. *Public Health Nutri*. 2001;4: 117.

Emmerson B. The management of gout. *N Engl J Med*. 1996;334:445.

Eriksen W, et al. Does dietary supplementation of cod liver oil mitigate musculoskeletal pain? *Eur J Clin Nutri*. 1996;50:689.

Fairburn K, et al. Alpha-tocopherol, lipids and lipoproteins in knee-joint synovial fluid and serum from patients with inflammatory joint disease. *Clin Sci*. 1992;83:657.

Firestein G, Zvaifler N. Anticytokine therapy in rheumatoid arthritis (editorial). *N Engl J Med*. 1997;337:195.

Flynn M, et al. The effect of folate and cobalamin on osteoarthritic hands. *J Am Col Nutri*. 1994;13:351.

Gershoff S. Vitamin D keeps a form of arthritis in check. *Tufts University Diet and Nutrition Letter*. 1996;14:1.

Harris M, et al. Gout and hyperuricemia. *Am Fam Physician*. 1999; 59:925.

Helgeland M, et al. Dietary intake and serum concentrations of antioxidants in children with juvenile arthritis. *Clin Exp Rheumatol*. 2000;18:637.

Hootman J, et al. Characteristics of chronic arthritis and other rheumatic condition-related ambulatory care visits, United States, 1997. *Ann Epidemiol*. 2000;10:454.

Jacobs J, et al. Why do patients with rheumatoid arthritis use alternative treatments? *Clin Rheumatol*. 2001;20:192.

Kast R. Borage oil reduction of rheumatoid arthritis activity may be mediated by increased cAMP that suppresses tumor necrosis factor-alpha. *Int Immunopharmacol.* 2001;1:2197.

Korones D, et al. "Liver function tests" are not always tests of liver function. *Am J Hematol.* 2001;66:46.

Lammi-Keefe C, et al. Day-to-day variation in iron status indexes is similar for most measures in elderly women with and without rheumatoid arthritis. *J Am Diet Assoc.* 1996;96:247.

Linos A, et al. Dietary factors in relation to rheumatoid arthritis: a role for olive oil and cooked vegetables? *Am J Clin Nutri.* 1999; 70:1077.

McAlindon T, et al. Glucosamine and chondroitin for treatment of osteoarthritis: a systematic quality assessment and meta-analysis. *J Am Med Assoc.* 2000;283:1469.

McAlindon T, et al. Relation of dietary intake and serum levels of vitamin D to progression of osteoarthritis of the knee among participants in the Framingham study. *Ann Intern Med.* 1996;125:353.

Moreland L, et al. Treatment of rheumatoid arthritis with a recombinant human tumor necrosis factor receptor (p75)-Fc protein. *N Engl J Med.* 1997;337:141.

Morgan S, et al. Supplementation with folic acid during methotrexate therapy for rheumatoid arthritis: a double-blind, placebo-controlled trial. *Ann Intern Med.* 1994;121:833.

Quigley E. Chronic intestinal pseudo-obstruction. *Treat Options Gastroenterol.* 1999;2:239.

Pi-Sunyer F. A review of long-term studies evaluating the efficacy of weight loss in ameliorating disorders associated with obesity. *Clin Ther.* 1996;18:1006.

Rapuri P, et al. Caffeine intake increases the rate of bone loss in elderly women and interacts with vitamin D receptor genotypes. *Am J Clin Nutri.* 2001;74:694.

Roubenoff R, et al. Rheumatoid cachexia: cytokine-driven hypermetabolism accompanying reduced body cell mass in chronic inflammation. *J Clin Invest.* 1994;93:2379.

Theriault R, Hortobagyi G. The evolving role of bisphosphonates. *Semin Oncol.* 2001;28:284.

Vollertsen R, Conn D. Vasculitis associated with rheumatoid arthritis. *Rheum Dis Clin North Am.* 1990;16:445.

Woolf K, Manore M. Nutrition, exercise, and rheumatoid arthritis. *Top Clin Nutr.* 1999; 14:30.

OTHER MUSCULOSKELETAL DISEASES—Suggested Readings

Evers A, et al. Cognitive, behavioral, and physiological reactivity to pain as a predictor of long-term pain in rheumatoid arthritis patients. *Pain.* 2001;93:139.

Franzese T. Nutritional care in rheumatic disease. In: Mahan K, Escott-Stump S, eds. *Krause's food, nutrition, and diet therapy.* 10th ed. Philadelphia: WB Saunders, 2000.

Kanik K, Wilder R. Hormonal alterations in rheumatoid arthritis, including the effects of pregnancy. *Rheum Dis Clin North Am.* 2000;26:805.

Lawrence R, et al. Estimates of the prevalence of arthritis and selected musculoskeletal disorders in the United States. *Arthritis Rheum.* 1998;41:778.

Weaver C. Calcium requirements of physically active people. *Am J Clin Nutri.* 2000;72:579S.

Zollinger P, et al. Effect of vitamin C on frequency of reflex sympathetic dystrophy in wrist fractures: a randomized trial. *Lancet.* 1999; 354:2025.

SECTION 12

Hematology: Anemias and Blood Disorders

CHIEF ASSESSMENT FACTORS

- CONCURRENT ILLNESS/DISEASES (CEREBROVASCULAR DISEASE MYOCARDIAL INFARCTION, ASTHMA, HEMORRHAGE, CANCERS, RENAL DISEASE)
- PAST DIAGNOSIS OF BLOOD DISORDER
- BLEEDING TENDENCIES
- BLOOD TRANSFUSION
- BLOOD TYPE
- BRUISING
- EXPOSURE TO RADIATION
- LYMPHADENOPATHY
- SURGERY, ESPECIALLY GASTRIC, HEPATIC, OR RENAL
- INFECTIONS, SEPSIS
- FAMILY HISTORY (LEUKEMIAS, CANCER, ANEMIAS, IMMUNE DISORDERS, ALLERGIES)
- ALCOHOL AND NICOTINE USE
- DIETARY HABITS (HEME VERSUS NONHEME IRON, ETC.)
- OCCUPATION
- DECREASED PROTEIN INTAKE
- MEDICATIONS (PRESCRIPTIONS, OVER-THE-COUNTER)
- USE OF HERBAL OR BOTANICAL MEDICATIONS
- ANOREXIA, FATIGUE
- BEEFY, RED TONGUE; OTHER SIGNS OF DEFICIENCIES
- EXPOSURE TO LEAD PAINT, OTHER TOXINS

GENERAL INFORMATION ABOUT ANEMIAS

Anemias are a set of hematological disorders with a reduced number of red blood cells, amount of hemoglobin, or number of volume-packed red cells (hematocrit); the main consequences include hypoxia and decreased oxygen-carrying capacity. Common causes include excessive bleeding, decreased red blood cell production, or increased red blood cell destruction. The erythrocyte life span is 120 days. Erythropoeitin is a hormone that stimulates red blood cell production.

Anemias can be encountered in generalized or specific nutritional deficiencies (Table 12–1). According to Dr. Victor Herbert, "Nutritional anemias are caused by lack and are corrected by provision." Anemia should not be accepted as an inevitable consequence of aging; chronic disease and iron deficiency (Table 12–2) are the most common causes (Smith, 2000). Vitamin B12 deficiency, folate deficiency, chronic gastrointestinal bleeding, and myelodysplastic syndrome are among other causes of anemia in the elderly. Anemias are more common in the hospitalized elderly than among those who live independently.

Unabsorbed dietary iron may increase free radical production in the colon to a level that could cause mucosal cell damage or increased production of carcinogens; low carbohydrate (CHO) intake is associated with free radical generation (Lund et al., 1999). Studies about the role of iron in health have now expanded beyond knowledge about anemias and deficiency syndromes.

Tables 12–3 and 12–4 provide descriptions of various types of anemia, including those not covered in this text.

TABLE 12–1 Nutritional Factors in Blood Formation

Iron
Vitamin C
Vitamin E
Protein
Vitamin B12
Folic acid
Vitamin B6
Copper and Riboflavin in minute amounts

Table 12–3 Definitions

Microcytic anemias—Usually caused by or resulting in iron deficiency; red blood cells are small in size.
Macrocytic anemias—Folic acid or vitamin B12 insufficiency; red blood cells are larger than usual.
Megaloblastic anemias—Anemias in which there are large, nucleated abnormal red blood cells, irregular in shape, as in pernicious anemia. It may also result from use of certain immunosuppressive or antitumor drugs.
Normocytic anemias—From inhibition of marrow by infection or chronic disease; red blood cells are of usual size.
Normochromia—Blood with a normal color and level of hemoglobin.
Hyperchromia—Blood that is excessively pigmented.
Hypochromia—Blood condition in which there is a low level of hemoglobin.

Table 12–2 Significance of Iron Stores in Various Anemias

Type of Anemia	*Ferritin*	*Total Iron-Binding Capacity (TIBC)*	*Marrow Iron*	*Treatment*
Iron deficiency	Low	High	Absent	Iron supplements; treat sources of blood loss.
Renal Disease	Normal	Normal or Low	Normal	Give erythropoeitin. Iron supplementation may also be needed.
Anemia of Chronic Disease	Normal or High	Normal or Low	Normal or Increased	Treat underlying disease.
Thalassemia minor	Normal	Normal	Normal	None specifically.
Megaloblastic anemias	Normal to High	Usually normal	Normal or Low	Treat cause of megaloblastic anemia; shift in hemoglobin to reticuloendothelial stores can occur.

Based on data from Abramson and Abramson, 1999.

Table 12–4 Anemias Not Covered in This Text

Acquired Autoimmune Hemolytic Anemia: A rare autoimmune disorder characterized by the premature destruction of red blood cells. Normally, red blood cells have a life span of 120 days before the spleen removes them, but in this condition, red blood cells are destroyed prematurely. Bone marrow production of new cells can no longer compensate. This anemia occurs in individuals who previously had a normal red blood cell system.

Anemia of Chronic Disease (ACD): Condition of impaired iron utilization where functional iron (hemoglobin) is low, but tissue iron (such as in storage) is normal or high. ACD is seen in a wide range of chronic autoimmune, cancerous or leukemic, inflammatory, and infectious disease conditions. In rheumatoid arthritis there is frequently co-existence of ACD and iron deficiency anemia resulting from gastrointestinal (GI) bleeding due to drug therapy. ACD is known as hypoferremia of inflammatory disease and anemia of inflammation and is often diagnosed as mild iron deficiency anemia. The difference is that low hemoglobin, low TIBC, and low transferrin with elevated ferritin are identified. Supplementation with iron for those with ACD can be harmful and even result in death. A genetically engineered form of erythropoietin, or epoetin, may be helpful in certain patients with severe ACD and eliminate the need for transfusions, but it is very expensive. Levels of erythropoietin are reduced in ACD; the genetically engineered form can correct anemia caused by cancer in about 50–60% of patients and may improve survival in HIV patients with anemia (WebMD, 7/21/01).

Anemia of Prematurity: Vitamin E supplementation given to preterm infants does not reduce the severity of the anemia of prematurity (Fishman et al., 2000).

Anemia of Renal Disease (Abramson and Abramson, 1999): This anemia occurs in both acute and chronic renal failure. It is often normochromic, normocytic, and sometimes microcytic. The buildup of uremic toxins and decreased erythropoietin production adversely affect erythropoiesis. The accumulation of toxic metabolites, which are normally excreted by the kidneys, shortens the life span of circulating red blood cells. There is an inverse relationship between blood urea nitrogen (BUN) levels and red blood cell life span, but there is also diminished renal production of erythropoietin that results in decreased red blood cell production.

Anemia in Persistent Nephrotic Syndrome: Anemia is common before the deterioration of kidney function. Nephrotic patients have erythropoietin (EPO) deficiency with a blunted response to anemia; EPO therapy is recommended for this group of patients (Feinstein et al., 2001).

Blackfan-Diamond Anemia: A rare blood disorder of unknown cause characterized by deficiency of red blood cells at birth (congenital hypoplastic anemia) and other symptoms including slow growth, abnormal weakness and fatigue, pallor, characteristic facial abnormalities, protruding shoulder blades (scapulae), webbing or abnormal shortening of the neck due to fusion of certain bones in the spine (cervical vertebrae), hand deformities, congenital heart defects, and/or other abnormalities. The physical findings vary greatly from case to case. Blackfan-Diamond anemia may be inherited as either an autosomal dominant or recessive genetic trait.

Familial Hemolytic Jaundice (Spherolytic Anemia): A hereditary anemia in which red blood cells are shaped like spheres rather than their normal, donut-like shape. Jaundice and anemia occur from destruction of the abnormal cells by the spleen. Surgical removal of the spleen usually is indicated. There is no permanent cure.

Fanconi's Anemia: A cancer-prone genetic disease, Fanconi's anemia is characterized by delayed bone marrow failure with a progression to aplastic anemia that requires bone marrow transplantation. It is a rare disorder that may be apparent at birth or during childhood, characterized by deficiency of all bone marrow elements including red blood cells, white blood cells, and platelets (pancytopenia). Fanconi's anemia may also be associated with cardiac, kidney, or skeletal abnormalities as well as patchy, brown discolorations (pigmentation changes) of the skin. There are several different subtypes of Fanconi's anemia, each of which is thought to result from abnormal mutations of different genes. More information is available from: Fanconi's Anemia Research, 66 Club Road, Suite 390, Eugene, OR 97401; (503) 687–4658.

Hereditary Nonspherocytic Hemolytic Anemia: A group of rare genetic blood disorders characterized by defective red blood cells (erythrocytes) that are not abnormally "sphere-shaped" (spherocytes). Membranes of red blood cells, abnormal metabolism of a chemical contained in hemoglobin (porphyrin), and deficiencies in certain enzymes such as glucose-6-phosphate dehydrogenase (G6PD) or pyruvate kinase are thought to be the cause of these disorders.

For More Information

- NIH/National Heart, Lung and Blood Institute Information Center
  P.O. Box 30105
  Bethesda, MD 20824--0105
  (301) 592–8573
- National Organization for Rare Disorders
  P.O. Box 8923, New Fairfield, CT 06812-8923
  (203) 746–6518
  www.rarediseases.org

APLASTIC ANEMIA

NUTRITIONAL ACUITY RANKING: LEVEL 2

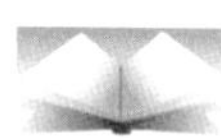

DEFINITIONS AND BACKGROUND

Aplastic anemia is a rare bone marrow disorder with normocytic, normochromic anemia in which normal marrow is replaced with fat. Symptoms and signs include increasing fatigue and weakness, slow thought processes, headache, dizziness, irritability, wax-like pallor, petechiae, ecchymosis, hemorrhagic diathesis (gums, nose, GI tract, urinary tract, vagina), tachycardia, tachypnea, dyspnea, increasing or persistent infections, and hemosiderosis with resulting cirrhosis, diabetes, heart failure, and bronzing of skin. In about 50% of cases, the exact cause is not known; in other cases, certain toxic agents (e.g., inorganic arsenic) or drugs (e.g., phenylbutazone, choramphenicol, etc.) may be the cause.

OBJECTIVES

- Prevent infections or sepsis.
- Reduce bleeding tendencies and hemorrhages.
- Prepare for splenectomy or bone marrow transplantation.
- Reduce febrile status.
- Prevent further complications and decline in cardiovascular and hepatic functions.
- Ensure adequate periods of rest.

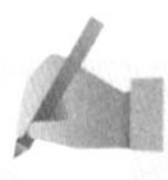

DIETARY AND NUTRITIONAL RECOMMENDATIONS

- Replenish nutrient stores.
- Provide a balanced diet with six small feedings.
- Provide extra fluid unless contraindicated (e.g., 3 L daily).
- If patient has mouth lesions, avoid excesses in hot or cold foods, spicy or acidic foods, or foods with rough textures.
- If steroids are used, limiting sodium intake may be beneficial.

Common Drugs Used and Potential Side Effects

- Corticosteroids may be used. Watch side effects of chronic use such as elevated serum sodium levels, decreased potassium and calcium levels, and negative nitrogen balance. Hyperglycemia may occur; alter diet accordingly.
- Aspirin should be avoided, because it may aggravate blood losses.
- Antibiotics may be required when infections are present. Monitor for GI distress and other side effects.
- Other drugs that may aggravate the condition include chloramphenicol, phenylbutazone, sulfa drugs, and ibuprofen. These each have specific GI side effects that should be monitored (see index for more information).

Herbs, Botanicals and Supplements

- Herbs and botanical supplements should not be used without discussing with physician.

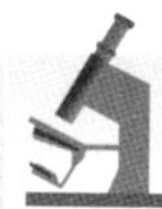

PROFILE

Clinical/History

Height
Weight
Body mass index (BMI)
Blood pressure (BP)
Fatigue and weakness
Headache, irritability
Wax-like pallor
Petechiae, ecchymosis
Hemorrhagic diathesis (gums, nose, GI tract, urinary tract, vagina)
Tachycardia, tachypnea, dyspnea
Persistent infections
Bronzing of skin.

Lab Work

Red blood cell count (RBC) (decreased)
Pro Time(PT)
Serum Fe
Glucose (gluc)
Granulocytes (decreased)
TIBC
Transferrin
Hemoglobin and hematocrit (H&H)
Platelets (decreased)
White blood cell count (WBC) (less than 1,500)
Albumin (alb), prealbumin
Alanine aminotransferase (ALT), aspartate aminotransaminase (AST), bilirubin

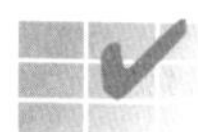

PATIENT EDUCATION

- Discuss needs of the patient that are specific for signs and symptoms and for side effects of any medications.
- Discuss simplified, but nutritious, meal planning.
- If patient has diabetes, heart failure, or cirrhosis, counsel specifically to those issues for dietary management.

For More Information

- Aplastic Anemia and MDS International Foundation, Inc.
http://www.aplastic.org/

COPPER DEFICIENCY ANEMIA

NUTRITIONAL ACUITY RANKING: LEVEL 2

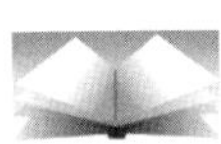

DEFINITIONS AND BACKGROUND

Copper is needed in minute amounts for the formation of hemoglobin. People with poor diets who have a high intake of milk may become deficient in copper. The copper-deficient anemias actually may be related to iron and protein deficiencies or zinc excess. One study found this anemia in a person who swallows pennies (Hassan et al., 2000). Gastrectomy may also cause a potential deficiency of copper.

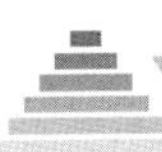

OBJECTIVES

- Correct anemia.
- Instruct patient regarding good sources of protein, iron, and copper to prevent recurrences.
- Monitor use of zinc in supplements, diet, and enteral or parenteral sources to avoid overdosing and related copper depletion.

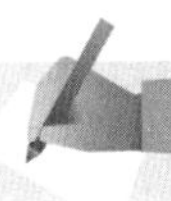

DIETARY AND NUTRITIONAL RECOMMENDATIONS

- Good sources of copper include oysters, liver, nuts, dried legumes, and raisins.
- Protein should be at least 1 g/kg; iron intake adequate for age and sex.
- Monitor use of multivitamin and mineral supplements to avoid large doses of zinc. In vitro, ascorbic acid can act as a pro-oxidant in the presence of transition metals such as iron or copper; large doses of vitamin C are not recommended (Gerster, 1999).

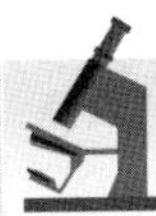

PROFILE

Clinical/History	Lab Work	
Height	Complete blood count (CBC)	Transferrin
Weight	Alb, prealbumin	H&H , Serum Fe
BMI	Serum copper (low)	Retinol-binding protein (RBP)
Pallor	Ceruloplasmin	Hypochromic anemia
		Serum Zinc (Zn)

Herbs, Botanicals and Supplements

- Herbs and botanical supplements should not be used without discussing with physician.

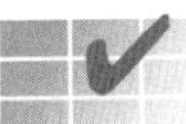

PATIENT EDUCATION

- Indicate which foods are good sources of copper, iron, and protein.
- Have patient avoid fad diets. Monitor vegetarian (nonheme iron) diets carefully.
- Zinc in large doses may deplete copper levels; discuss use of mineral supplements.

FOLIC ACID DEFICIENCY ANEMIA

NUTRITIONAL ACUITY RANKING: LEVEL 2

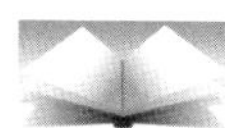

DEFINITIONS AND BACKGROUND

Folic acid is needed for the synthesis of DNA and maturation of red blood cells. Folic acid deficiency anemia generally is caused by inadequate diet, intestinal malabsorption, alcoholism, or pregnancy. It is a hyperchromic, macrocytic, megaloblastic anemia with signs and symptoms of weight loss, anorexia, malnutrition, smooth and sore red tongue, diarrhea, easy fatigue, lethargy, poor wound healing, and coldness of extremities. Because similar hematologic changes occur with B12 deficiency, it is important to check the Schilling test and serum levels of B12 along with folate tests. Folate is best measured by red blood cell folate, because serum levels are misleading.

Conditions that increase folate requirements include burns, hepatitis, infection, inflammatory diseases, cancers, pregnancy and lactation, surgery, and hemolytic anemias. Malabsorptive states also affect folate status (i.e., celiac disease, blind-loop syndrome, congenital or acquired megacolon, Crohn's disease). Folate is also lost easily with alcoholism or during dialysis. In cardiac disease, homocysteine levels may be elevated in the presence of folic acid deficiency (Boushey, 1995).

OBJECTIVES

- Increase folic acid in diet to alleviate anemia.
- Improve diet to provide nutrients needed to make red blood cells: folate and other B-complex vitamins, iron, protein, etc.
- Instruct patient to correct faulty diet habits, if they are causing the anemia.
- Check for malabsorption syndromes (celiac disease, blind-loop syndrome, congenital or acquired megacolon, Crohn's disease) and correct these as far as possible through use of medications and other treatments. Monitor folate status regularly.

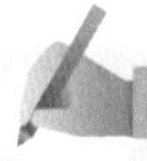

DIETARY AND NUTRITIONAL RECOMMENDATIONS

- Provide a diet that is high in folic acid, protein, copper, iron, and vitamins C and B12.
- Ingestion of one fresh fruit or vegetable would provide sufficient folic acid, but other sources include fish, legumes (dried beans and peas), whole grains, leafy dark green vegetables, broccoli, citrus fruits and juices such as grapefruit, berries, and meats. The U.S. Food and Drug Administration (FDA) ordered all food manufacturers to fortify grains with folic acid starting January 1, 1998. These fortified foods include most enriched breads, flours, corn meal, rice, noodles, macaroni, and other grain products.
- Diets that provide bland, liquid, or soft foods may be needed for patient's with a sore mouth; 6–8 small meals may be helpful.

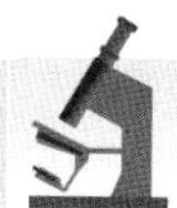

PROFILE

Clinical/History

Height
Weight
BMI
Weight loss
Anorexia, malnutrition
Smooth and sore red tongue
Diarrhea
Fatigue, lethargy
Poor wound healing
Coldness of extremities
History (Hx) of alcohol abuse?

Lab Work

Serum folate (less than 3 ng/mL)
RBC folate (more reliable than serum)
Serum homocysteine (elevated)
Low RBC
H&H
CBC (macrocytic cells)
Transferrin
Serum B12
Serum Fe (increased)
Mean cell volume (MCV)
Leukopenia, WBC
Forminoglutamic acid (FIGLU)
Schilling test

Common Drugs Used and Potential Side Effects

- Supplements of folic acid (Folvite) are better than diet alone to alleviate the anemia. Folate deficiency is treated with 1 mg of folic acid daily (Smith, 2000). Leucovorin is an active reduced form. The only major side effect is that high levels of folate may mask a B12 deficiency.
- Folic acid antagonists (cancer treatments) affect body's use of folic acid. Methotrexate, for example, is especially depleting; it is common to administer leucovorin at the same time as a "folinic acid rescue."
- Other medications that may cause folate deficiency include pentamidine isethionate (antiprotozoal), pyrimethamine (antimalarial), triamterene (diuretic), and trimethoprim (antibiotic).
- Drugs that cause folate malabsorption include oral contraceptives, cimetidine (Tagamet, an H2 antagonist), which is now sold over the counter, sulfasalazine (Azulfidine) for Crohn's disease, and isoniazid (INH, for tuberculosis). Anticonvulsants (primidone, phenytoin, phenobarbitol) also interfere with the body's use of folic acid. It is common to hold meals or a tube feeding for 1 hour before and after administration of phenytoin/dilantin.

- Multivitamin preparations do not always contain folic acid, because folacin masks a vitamin B12 deficiency. Check labels. Vitamin B12 helps folate travel into cells via transport form (5-methyl tetrahydrofolate).

Herbs, Botanicals and Supplements

- Herbs and botanical supplements should not be used without discussing with physician.

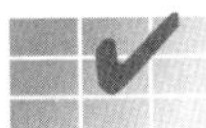

PATIENT EDUCATION

- ✓ Vitamin C promotes absorption of folic acid from foods.
- ✓ Pregnant women should receive appropriate counseling; 30% may have a folate deficiency. Daily needs increase by approximately 200 μg over the adult requirements of 400 μg. Folate protects against neural tube defects in the first trimester.
- ✓ Large intakes of folate (1+ mg/day, etc.) can cure the anemia but may mask a correlated vitamin B12 anemia; monitor carefully.
- ✓ Attractive meals may help appetite.
- ✓ Fad and restrictive diets should be avoided.
- ✓ Alcoholic beverages interfere with folate metabolism and absorption.
- ✓ Food folates are oxidized easily and destroyed by lengthy cooking (Hine, 1996). Advise patients accordingly.

HEMOLYTIC ANEMIA FROM VITAMIN E DEFICIENCY

NUTRITIONAL ACUITY RANKING: LEVEL 2

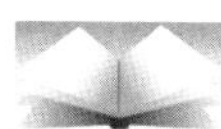

DEFINITIONS AND BACKGROUND

In hemolytic anemia caused by a vitamin E deficiency, red blood cells have an abnormal membrane, which results in hemolysis. Red blood cells are destroyed faster than they can be produced in bone marrow. This condition often occurs in infants who receive polyunsaturated fatty acids (PUFAs) without adequate vitamin E. Children with cystic fibrosis should be screened for vitamin E deficiency; this population may be susceptible to vitamin E-deficient hemolytic anemia (Wilfond et al., 1994).

Symptoms and signs include edema, anemia and paleness of skin, intolerance for physical activity, and puffy eyelids. In severe cases in infancy, encephalomalacia can result.

Other types of hemolytic anemias include aplastic anemia, hemoglobin-SC disease, hemolytic anemia due to G6PD deficiency, hereditary elliptocytosis, hereditary spherocytosis, idiopathic autoimmune hemolytic anemia, nonimmune hemolytic anemia caused by chemical agents, secondary immune hemolytic anemia, and sickle thalassemia. The incidence of all types of hemolytic anemias occurs in 4/100,000 persons in the U.S. Most are not affected specifically by vitamin E. Symptoms in these types of anemia include pallor, shortness of breath, rapid heart rate, jaundice, dark urine, splenomegaly, nosebleeds, chills, fatigue, bleeding gums, heart murmur, weakness, confusion, or dizziness.

G6PD deficiency is seen in about 10% of African-American males in the U.S. and is also common in persons from the Mediterranean area or Asia. The severity differs among different populations. In the most common form in the African-American population, the deficiency is mild and the hemolysis affects primarily older red blood cells. In Caucasians, G6PD deficiency tends to be more serious, as even young red blood cells are affected.

OBJECTIVES

- ▲ Correct vitamin E deficit.
- ▲ Prevent further complications.
- ▲ Correct anemia.

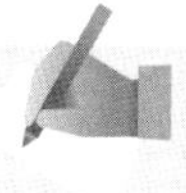

DIETARY AND NUTRITIONAL RECOMMENDATIONS

- Decrease excessive PUFA intake, which depletes vitamin E.
- Provide diet as usual for age and sex.
- Avoid excesses of iron.
- Ensure adequate intake of zinc, which may become deficient.

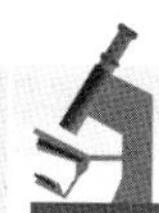

PROFILE

Clinical/History

Height
Weight
BMI
Growth percentile
BP
Heart rate (rapid?)
Shortness of breath
Dizziness
Edema
Pallor
Nosebleeds
Dark urine?
Puffy eyelids

Lab Work

RBC (low)
Hemoglobin (low)
Reticulocyte count (increased)
Serum a-tocopherol levels
Hemoglobin in urine
Hemosiderin in urine
TIBC
Bilirubin (elevated)
Transferrin
Gluc
AST (increased)
Blood test for G6PD

Common Drugs Used and Potential Side Effects

- Water-soluble vitamin E (a-tocopherol) is likely to be given daily. Avoid taking with an iron supplement, which could interfere with utilization.
- Persons with G6PD deficiency need to avoid exposing themselves to certain medicines such as aspirin (acetylsalicylic acid), certain antibiotics used to treat infections, fava beans, and moth balls.

Herbs, Botanicals and Supplements

- Herbs and botanical supplements should not be used without discussing with physician.

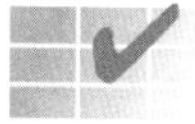

PATIENT EDUCATION

- ✓ Discuss, in layman's terms, the role of vitamin E in lipid oxidation and utilization. Discuss sources of PUFAs and why excesses should be controlled.
- ✓ Discuss sources of vitamin E in the diet. Natural sources are more bioavailable than synthetic sources.
- ✓ Discuss exercise tolerance and ability to eat sufficient amounts of food, as related to fatigue.

IRON DEFICIENCY ANEMIA

NUTRITIONAL ACUITY RANKING: LEVEL 2

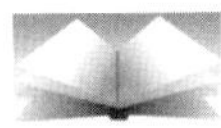

DEFINITIONS AND BACKGROUND

The nutrient most commonly deficient in the world is iron, affecting approximately 40% of the world's population (up from 30% in 1980). Iron deficiency anemia (IDA) results from inadequate intake, impaired erythropoiesis or absorption of iron, blood loss, or demands from closely repeated pregnancies. When caused by an inadequate diet, it may take years to produce symptoms when there are adequate iron stores. In the elderly, chronic blood loss is the most common cause of IDA.

Iron is the basic nutritional component of heme, a protein. Hemoglobin is the iron-containing protein in red blood cells that carries oxygen to all body cells. Hematocrit is the measure of red blood cells in a given volume of blood, packed by centrifuge. Transferrin is the carrier protein that picks up iron from the intestines (ferric state). Serum ferritin is the most useful test to differentiate IDA from anemia of chronic disease (Smith, 2000).

See Table 12–5 for content of iron in various body sources. Absorption of iron occurs in the ferrous form; storage is in the liver, spleen, and bone marrow. In one study, the only dietary factors found to be useful in estimating nonheme iron absorption from a meal were animal tissue, phytate, and vitamin C (Reddy et al., 2000).

Serious systemic consequences of IDA include impaired cognitive function, blue sclerae, koilonychia, impaired exercise tolerance, and functional changes of the bowel (Bruner et al., 1996). Other symptoms and signs include weakness, fatigue, vertigo, headache, irritability, heartburn, dysphagia, flatulence, vague abdominal pains, anorexia, glossitis, stomatitis, pale skin, ankle edema, tingling extremities, and palpitations.

TABLE 12–5 Iron Distribution in the Body

Forms	*Men (mg iron/kg BW)*	*Women (mg iron/kg BW)*
Storage–Ferritin	9	4
Storage–Hemosiderin	4	1
Transport Protein–Transferrin	Less than 1	Less than 1
Functional Hemoglobin	31	31
Functional Myoglobin	4	4
Enzymes	2	2
TOTAL	50	42

Based on data from: Insel, et al. *Nutrition*. Sudbury, MA: Jones & Bartlett Publishers, 2001.

Approximately 90% of the body's store of iron is reused. Diet replaces iron lost through sweat, feces, and urine. The duodenum (upper small intestine) is where iron is best absorbed. Damage or surgery here can greatly inhibit total iron absorption, thus leading to greater risk of deficiency.

Iron deficiency is still relatively common in toddlers, adolescent girls, and women of childbearing age (Looker et al., 1997). Severe IDA occurs in a substantial number of young infants, more commonly in Southeast Asians and less so among African Americans (Kwiatkowski et al., 1999). Ingestion of cow's milk causes occult intestinal blood loss in young infants. Infants aged 7.5 months lose less blood than younger infants; the loss declines by age 12 months (Ziegler et al., 1999). The hemoglobin (Hb) content of reticulocytes (young RBCs) is a good indicator of iron deficiency and IDA in children (Brugnara et al., 1999).

Risk of iron deficiency may be underestimated in some high-risk populations, even those served by Women, Infants, and Children's Supplemental Feeding Program (WIC). Low iron levels are more prevalent among African American children and are related to age of the child, perception of feeding difficulty by the mother, and concurrent medical illness in the child (Gupta et al., 1999). Efforts to prevent mild and moderate mental retardation should include adequate nutrition during early childhood (Hurtado et al., 1999).

While iron deficiency is the major cause of nutritional anemia, changes in vitamins A, B12, C and E, folic acid and riboflavin status have also been linked to its development and control (Fishman et al., 2000). Vitamin A can improve hematologic indicators and enhance the efficacy of iron supplementation; when vitamin A deficiency is endemic, a single dose of vitamin A is often sufficient to correct iron deficiency in children (Gupta, 1999). Riboflavin enhances the hematologic response to iron, and its deficiency may account for a significant proportion of anemia in many populations (Fishman et al., 2000).

Menstruation increases iron losses by 30 mg per month; thus, women tend to become iron deficient more easily than men. Low hemoglobin levels before surgery or significant blood losses increase complications among patients with cardiovascular disease (Carson et al., 1996). Patients with acute inflammation often present altered iron status indices that resemble those observed in anemia of chronic disease; iron levels, TIBC, and serum ferritin then lose their diagnostic value (Chiari et al., 1995). When there is not enough hemoglobin, free erythrocyte protoporphyrin (FEP) accumulates and is a reasonable test for this condition (Herbert and Subak-Share, 1995).

Pica is seen in approximately 50% of patients with iron deficiency. Pica generally is a consequence, rather than a cause, of iron deficiency; it is relieved by iron supplementation (Moore and Sears, 1994). Exposure to lead also has a significant affect on hemoglobin and hematocrit levels (Hu et al., 1994). Lead poisoning reduces hemoglobin production, causes iron deficiency, and elevates FEP as the precursor.

In gastritis, cure of *H. pylori* infection is associated with reversal of dependence on iron supplements and recovery from IDA (Annibale et al., 1999).

OBJECTIVES

- Alleviate anemia and associated anorexia. Correct causation.
- Provide adequate oral iron to replace losses or deficits, especially heme sources of protein (e.g., liver, beef, oysters, lamb, pork, ham, tuna, shrimp, other fish, chicken).
- Provide an acid medium to favor better absorption. Enhancers include gastric juice and ascorbic acid. Food sources of vitamin C should be included daily.
- Monitor and correct geophagia (clay-eating), amylophagia (starch-eating), ice-eating, and other forms of pica.
- Avoid or correct constipation.
- Screen for dilutional sports anemia in athletes; it may just be an adaptation to aerobic conditioning (Taunikar and Sabio, 1992).
- Reduce iron inhibitors: excessive fiber (as in whole grains), phytic acid (as in spinach, bran, legumes, and soy products), tannins in tea, and polyphenols in coffee or red wine.

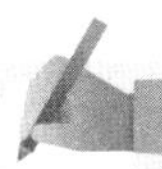

DIETARY AND NUTRITIONAL RECOMMENDATIONS

- If IDA is related to inadequate iron in diet, usually adding three portions of lean red meat (heme iron sources) per week, along with all other essential vitamins and minerals will correct anemia. The average mixed diet contains approximately 6 mg of iron per 1,000 kcal. Iron absorption increases as stores become depleted. Sources of iron include liver, eggs, kidney, beef, dried fruits, enriched whole-grain cereals, molasses, and oysters. Heme iron is found readily in beef, pork, and lamb; consume with fruit or fruit juice.
- Use liberal amounts of high biologic value (HBV) proteins that are needed for production of red blood cells and hemoglobin. Foods with HBV proteins include meat, cheese, and eggs.
- Increase intake of vitamin C (oranges, grapefruit, tomatoes, broccoli, cabbage, baked potatoes, strawberries, cantaloupe, green pepper), especially when patient is taking an iron pill to increase acid medium.
- Detect pica and discuss with patient. Pica substance may displace other important foods, leading to nutrient malnutrition. The ingested substance may also be toxic.
- Heme iron is absorbed well, regardless of other foods in the diet, whereas nonheme iron absorption is greatly affected by other foods. Absorption of nonheme iron is best in the presence of foods rich in vitamin C or with heme-containing sources.
- Approximately one-half of the iron in human milk is absorbed; only about 4% of the iron in iron-fortified infant formula is absorbed.
- Tea, coffee, wheat brans, and soy products tend to inhibit absorption of nonheme iron. Monitor use carefully; avoid excesses.

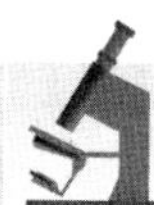

PROFILE

Clinical/History

Height
Weight
BMI
Pallor
Brittle, spoon-shaped fingernails (koilonychias)
Stool exam for occult blood
Impaired cognitive function
Blue sclerae
Impaired exercise tolerance
Weakness, fatigue
Vertigo
Headache, irritability
Heartburn
Dysphagia
Flatulence, vague abdominal pains
Anorexia
Diarrhea
Glossitis, stomatitis
Ankle edema
Tingling extremities
Palpitations

Lab Work

H. pylori test
Serum iron (low)
H&H (hemoglobin [Hgb]) more sensitive)
Mean cell hemoglobin (MCH), Mean cell hematocrit (MCHC) (decreased)
CBC
Transferrin (increased)
*Transferrin iron saturation percentage= Serum Fe/TIBC × 100 (normal = 35 + 15%)
*FEP—NL = 30 mg
*Ferritin (decreased stores in liver, spleen, bone marrow; levels are below 20 g/L)
MCV (lower than 80)
RBC (small, microcytic, hypochromic)
WBC/differential (increased)
TIBC (increased over 350 mcg/dL)
Serum Cu
Cholesterol (chol)
Reticulocyte count

*Best tests for IDA.

Common Drugs Used and Potential Side Effects

- If anemia is caused by increased demand for iron such as a growth spurt (toddlers, adolescents) or pregnancy, oral supplementation may be necessary. Short-term supplementation with moderate doses (30–60 mg daily) of oral iron, combined with increased consumption of heme-rich sources of iron may be sufficient to address iron demands. Multivitamin supplementation may raise hemoglobin concentration, but few studies have isolated the effect of multivitamins from iron on hematological status; the public health impact of vitamin supplementation in controlling or correcting anemia is not totally clear (Fishman et al., 2000). Further research is needed to understand the roles of individual and combined vitamin deficiencies on anemia.
- Ferrous salts (Feosol, Fer-In-Sol, Mol-Iron) are better used for iron therapy than other forms; a few studies have shown that prolonged-release ferrous sulfate (Slow Fe) improved iron absorption with fewer side ef-

fects than standard ferrous sulfate pills. Other forms include ferrous fumarate (Femiron, Feostat, Fumerin, Hemocyte, Ircon) or ferrous gluconate (Fergon, Ferralet, Simron). Regardless of source, large doses of supplemental oral iron have not proven to be beneficial. It takes 4–30 days to note improvements after iron therapy, especially in hemoglobin levels. Iron stores are replaced after 1–3 months of treatment. Treat only when indicated; many individuals receive oral iron without justification. Increased supplementation in normal individuals can cause additional, unnecessary iron to go into storage as reflected by ferritin elevation.

- Iron tablets (Feostat, Fergon, Feosol) may cause gastric irritation and constipation.
- When hemoglobin levels are seriously low, the heart is particularly vulnerable. Whole blood transfusion or IV iron may be needed to stabilize hemoglobin levels. Parenteral or IV iron can be administered by injection or infusion. This therapy is reserved for cases of trauma where blood loss is life-threatening and not used for insufficiency due to inadequate dietary iron intake. Imferon can be given intramuscularly, if oral iron is not tolerated; pain and skin discoloration may result.
- Enteric-coated or sustained-release remedies are more expensive and often carry the iron past maximal absorption site in the upper intestine.
- Aspirin or corticosteroids can increase GI bleeding or cause peptic ulceration. Vitamin C and nutrient levels may be decreased.
- Some medications, including antacids, can reduce iron absorption. Iron tablets may also reduce the effectiveness of other drugs, including the antibiotics tetracycline, penicillamine, and ciprofloxacin and the anti-Parkinson's drugs methyldopa, levodopa, and carbidopa. Wait 2 hours between doses of these drugs and iron supplements.

Herbs, Botanicals and Supplements

- Herbs and botanical supplements should not be used without discussing with physician.

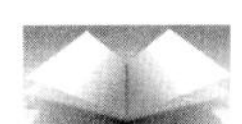

PATIENT EDUCATION

- ✓ Hemoglobin is made from protein, iron, and copper. Red blood cells are made from vitamin B12, folacin, and amino acids.
- ✓ Explain nonfood pica—clay, starch, plaster, paint chips—and the relationship to nutrition. In food pica in which singular foods are eaten instead of balanced meals, the foods chosen are often crunchy or brittle. Excessive consumption of Lifesavers candies, lettuce, ice, celery, snack chips, and chocolate has been noted; after iron supplementation, cravings often become a revulsion.
- ✓ Explain which foods are good sources of iron, protein, vitamin C, and related nutrients.
- ✓ Changes in stool color (green or tarry and black) are common with supplements.
- ✓ Beware of excessive phytates, phosphates, oxalates, fiber, alkalis, antacids, tannins, and calcium phosphates. Discuss food sources.
- ✓ To avoid side effects of supplements, take them with meals or milk. "Food iron" has fewer side effects.
- ✓ The average American diet contains 10–20 mg of iron daily, roughly 10% of which is absorbed.
- ✓ Overdosing (200 mg of iron or more daily) with supplements does no good. The body can only synthesize 5–10 mg of hemoglobin per day. The process cannot be expedited.
- ✓ Local or systemic infections interfere with iron absorption and transport.
- ✓ Three months of moderate-intensity endurance exercise (walking, running, or cycling) does not negatively affect selected measures of iron status in previously untrained women with normal iron stores (Bourique et al., 1997).

For More Information

- ✦ Iron Disorders Institute
  http://www.irondisorders.org/disorders/ida/

PERNICIOUS ANEMIA AND B_{12} DEFICIENCY ANEMIA

NUTRITIONAL ACUITY RANKING: LEVEL 2

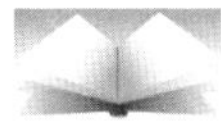

DEFINITIONS AND BACKGROUND

Pernicious anemia is a rare blood disorder characterized by inability of the body to properly utilize vitamin B12 (a cobalamin), which is essential for development of red blood cells. Pernicious anemia is thought to be an autoimmune disorder, and certain people may have a genetic predisposition. The three forms of pernicious anemia include congenital pernicious anemia, juvenile pernicious anemia, and adult onset pernicious anemia. The forms are based on the age at onset and the precise nature of the defect causing impaired B12 utilization (e.g., absence of intrinsic factor). Defective RBC production occurs, caused by a lack of intrinsic factor of the stomach. If there is no intrinsic factor, extrinsic factor (vitamin B12) is not absorbed. Thyroid disease, gastric surgery, anorexia nervosa or bulimia nervosa, diabetes mellitus, myxedema, family history of pernicious anemia, and Northern European ancestry seem to be risk factors.

With poor intake of extrinsic factor (vitamin B12) a megaloblastic anemia occurs and is corrected by use of oral cyanocobalamin once weekly for a month. **Vitamin B12 deficiency** may take 5–6 years to appear. It occurs mostly in vegetarians and among the elderly. Reduced intestinal absorption is more commonly the cause of B12 deficiency than is lack of adequate nutritional intake, e.g., persons with celiac disease may have a B12 deficiency (Dahele and Ghosh, 2001). Low serum levels cannot identify all cases of B12 deficiency; serum methylmalonic acid level may be useful for diagnosis of B12 deficiency (Smith, 2000). Homocysteine levels are also useful as part of the profile.

Studies have shown that *Helicobacter pylori* infection is a cause of B12 deficiency via diminished production of intrinsic factor by atrophied gastric glands and subsequent failure to absorb the vitamin (Kaptan et al., 2000). Atrophic gastritis with hyochlorhydria may also be a predisposing factor for poor B12 absorption. Low levels of cobalamin in older persons cannot be explained on the basis of either the aging process or on atrophic gastritis alone; hidden blood loss should also be evaluated (van Asselt et al., 1996).

There may be almost 800,000 older adults in the United States who have undiagnosed and untreated B12 deficiency; it may be masked by high folate intakes (Carmel, 1996). Megaloblastic anemia (MA) due to vitamin B12 deficiency is a reversible form of ineffective hematopoiesis; myelodysplastic syndrome (MDS) is an acquired, irreversible disorder of ineffective hematopoiesis, characterized by stem cell dysfunction as a consequence of DNA damage. MA and MDS can occur simultaneously (Drabick et al., 2001).

Symptoms of either type of anemia may include fatigue, flatulence, nausea and vomiting, diarrhea, upset stomach, constipation, anorexia, weight loss, pale waxy skin, tachycardia, cardiomegaly, achlorhydria, and glossitis. Recurring episodes of anemia (megaloblastic) and an abnormal lemon-yellow coloration of the skin (jaundice) are also common.

The Schilling test is performed to detect vitamin B12 absorption; B12 levels are measured in the urine after the ingestion of radioactive B12. With normal absorption, the ileum absorbs more B12 than the body needs and excretes excess into the urine. With impaired absorption, however, little or no B12 is excreted into the urine.

OBJECTIVES

- Alleviate anemia and causation when possible.
- Provide foods that won't hurt a sore mouth. Glossitis (beefy, red tongue) decreases desire to eat.
- Correct patient's anorexia.

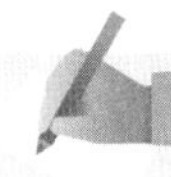

DIETARY AND NUTRITIONAL RECOMMENDATIONS

The following suggestions are supportive measures for the required B12 injections in pernicious anemia:

- Diet should make liberal use of HBV proteins.
- If patient has a sore mouth, use a soft or liquid diet, especially with bland foods.
- Supplement diet with iron, vitamin C and other B-vitamins (folic acid), and copper.
- Good sources of vitamin B12 include liver, other meats, fish, poultry, eggs, and fortified products such as soy milk. The daily average intake is 2–30 mg.

Common Drugs Used and Potential Side Effects

- Vitamin B12 deficiency is effectively treated with oral vitamin B12 supplementation (Smith, 2000). Crystamine or Rubramin PC is cyanocobalamin in drug form for vitamin B12 deficiency.
- For pernicious anemia, vitamin B12 injections must be given daily until remission, after which 6–8 injections yearly will suffice. The usual dose is 100 μg per dose; avoid megadoses. Injections can be painful; intranasal applications are quickly absorbed and have no side effects (Slot et al., 1997).
- Trinsicon contains vitamin B12, ferrous fumarate, vitamin C, folacin, and intrinsic factor. It is less effective when taken with dairy products.

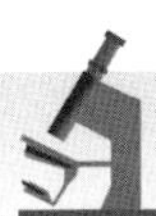

PROFILE

Clinical/History		
Height	Yellow or waxy skin	Schilling test (decreased)
Weight	BP	Transferrin
BMI	Postural hypotension	Gastrin (increased)
Weight loss?	**Lab Work**	Serum B12
Fatigue	RBC	MCV, MCHC, MCH (increased)
Flatulence, nausea, and vomiting	Macrocytic/nucleated cells	TIBC
Diarrhea	Lactic acid dehydrogenase (LDH) (may be increased)	Urinary methylmalonic acid for B12 status
Constipation	CBC	Serum folate
Anorexia		Serum homocysteine
Tachycardia, cardiomegaly		
Achlorhydria		
Glossitis		
Beefy, red tongue		

Herbs, Botanicals and Supplements

- Herbs and botanical supplements should not be used without discussing with physician.

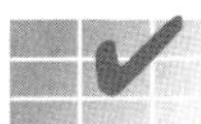

PATIENT EDUCATION

- ✔ Beware of vegetarian diets because vitamin B12 is found only in animal foods. Avoid fad diets as well.
- ✔ Pernicious anemia develops after total gastrectomy unless vitamin B12 is administered. The problem can occur in patients with only partial gastrectomy or in patients who have had gastrojejunostomies.
- ✔ Avoidance of fatigue is essential.
- ✔ Megaloblastic B12 anemia may be common in elderly individuals; careful food choices are essential.
- ✔ For pernicious anemia, lifelong B12 injections are necessary.

PROTEIN DEFICIENCY ANEMIA

NUTRITIONAL ACUITY RANKING: LEVEL 2

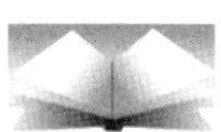

DEFINITIONS AND BACKGROUND

Protein is required for production of hemoglobin and red blood cells. When intake is deficient, the body frees protein from red blood cells for other uses. Protein deficiency anemia usually occurs in combination with other deficiencies. It may occur in patients with nephrosis.

OBJECTIVES

- Gradually reintroduce patient to a high-protein diet if patient has had deficient protein intake for a long time.
- Correct concurrent deficiencies of other nutrients.
- Supply adequate amounts of calories and CHOs so amino acids can be used for erythropoiesis.

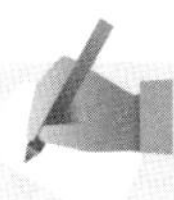

DIETARY AND NUTRITIONAL RECOMMENDATIONS

- Use a normal, well-balanced diet with emphasis on HBV proteins.
- Ensure diet supplies adequate amounts of iron, B12, and folic acid to support red blood cell formation. Pyridoxine also should be adequate.
- Ensure diet includes 1.5–3 g protein/kg body weight (approximately 100–150 g for adults).
- Ensure diet is high in CHOs and calories to spare protein for other functions.

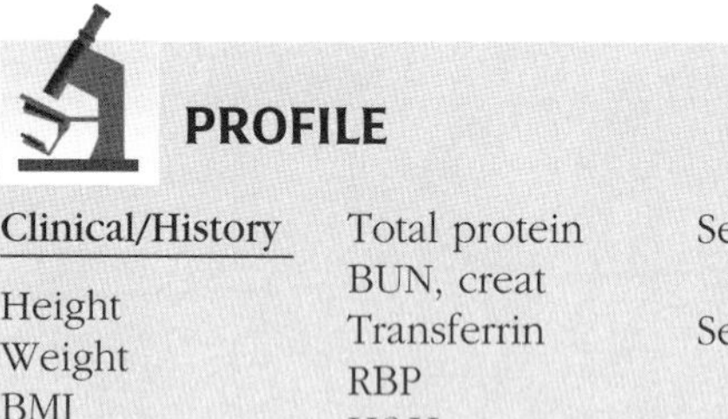

PROFILE

Clinical/History

Height
Weight
BMI

Lab Work

Alb, prealbumin
Total protein
BUN, creat
Transferrin
RBP
H&H
CBC, WBC
Serum Fe
Serum B12
Serum folacin
Serum pyridoxine
Serum copper

Common Drugs Used and Potential Side Effects

- A multiple vitamin-mineral supplement may be useful to replenish depleted nutrient stores.
- Trinsicon contains vitamin B12, ferrous fumarate, vitamin C, folacin, and intrinsic factor. It is less effective when taken with dairy products.

Herbs, Botanicals and Supplements

- Herbs and botanical supplements should not be used without discussing with physician.

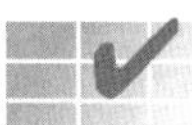

PATIENT EDUCATION

- Protein deficiency leads to nutritional edema, which may mask signs of poor nutrition.
- When food budgets are limited and when indicated, discuss foods that are low-cost sources of protein (e.g., textured vegetable protein, peanut butter). Two tablespoons of peanut butter contain 8 g of protein and 0.6 mg of iron. Teach patients how to combine appropriate foods to obtain complete proteins.
- Explain that less expensive cuts of meat contain as much protein as expensive ones. Some cuts may require longer cooking times or lower temperatures to avoid becoming tough.

PARASITIC INFESTATION ANEMIA

NUTRITIONAL ACUITY RANKING: LEVEL 2

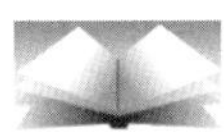

DEFINITIONS AND BACKGROUND

Infestation of the GI tract by parasitic worms that feed on blood (hookworm) or on nutrients (tapeworm) may occur. Anemia can result as a side effect of blood loss or deficiencies in iron, vitamin B12, or folic acid. Symptoms include anemia, fatigue, abdominal discomfort, nausea, vomiting, fever, and irritability (see also the Ascariasis and Trichinosis entries in Section 15).

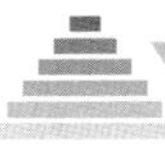

OBJECTIVES

- Correct anemia from blood losses; eliminate parasitic infestation.
- Prevent GI tract perforation or obstruction, when likely to exist.
- Improve nutritional status and appetite.

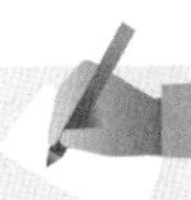

DIETARY AND NUTRITIONAL RECOMMENDATIONS

- A diet high in protein, B-complex vitamins, and iron may be appropriate.
- Provide adequate calories to meet individual's needs for anabolism, if needed.
- Heme iron sources and vitamin C should be included in foods chosen.
- Iron inhibitors should be excluded from diet as far as possible until recovery is complete.

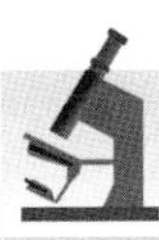

PROFILE

Clinical/History

Height
Weight
BMI
Fatigue
Abdominal discomfort
Nausea, vomiting
Fever
Irritability

Lab Work

Serum B12
Anemia
TIBC
Alb
Serum Fe
Serum folic acid
H&H
Transferrin
Gluc

Common Drugs Used and Potential Side Effects

- If needed, oral or parenteral iron may be given to correct anemia more rapidly. Beware of excessive use of oral supplements because of their potential side effects with iron overloading; monitor all sources (including iron-enriched foods).

Herbs, Botanicals and Supplements

- Herbs and botanical supplements should not be used without discussing with physician.

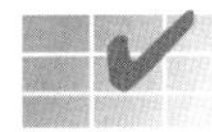

PATIENT EDUCATION

- Discuss ways to prevent further parasitic infestations, as with small children playing in soil.
- Discuss ways to prepare foods high in necessary nutrients and methods to increase bioavailability (e.g., combining orange juice at breakfast with an iron-fortified cereal, etc.).

SICKLE CELL ANEMIA

NUTRITIONAL ACUITY RANKING: LEVEL 2

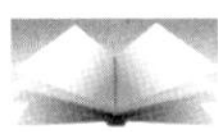

DEFINITIONS AND BACKGROUND

Sickle cell anemia is a hereditary hemolytic anemia. Cells are crescent-shaped and become rigid; they lodge themselves in the capillaries of the peripheral blood system outside the heart. Capillaries become clogged, preventing normal flow of oxygen to tissues. Sickle cell disease has several forms including sickle cell anemia, sickle cell hemoglobin C disease, and sickle cell thalassemia disease.

It is usually detected within the first year of life. The largest population in the world with sickle cell anemia is in Africa. While this condition most commonly affects blacks of African descent, it is also found in people of Middle Eastern, East Indian, and Mediterranean origin. About 100,000 Americans have sickle cell disease, approximately 1 in every 400–500 African Americans. The origins of sickle cell anemia probably occurred thousands of years ago, and the trait probably helped people resist malaria.

Chronic anemia, pallor, and jaundice result. These sickled cells do not last as long as normal blood cells. Bone marrow functions at six times the normal rate. Because there are fewer cells, the blood is thinner or anemic. When red cells are destroyed, bilirubin is released into the blood and turns the whites of the eyes to a shade of yellow.

Inadequate dietary intakes of folate are common, while vitamin B12 intakes are usually adequate (Kennedy et al., 2001). Low RBC folate levels may occur. Serum homocysteine (tHcy) levels may be elevated in this population; greater intakes than normal of folate may be needed to normalize serum tHcy levels, even if transfusions are used (Lowenthal et al., 2000). Additional research is needed to explore the effects of improved folate status, the need for folate supplementation, and the relationship of folate, vitamin B12, and homocysteine levels and the risk for vascular damage and stroke in children with sickle cell disease (Kennedy et al., 2001).

Caution is needed about iron overloading, especially after transfusions. Iron deficiency, through reduction of MCHC, actually may be beneficial for longer RBC survival and oxygen affinity.

Infants and children who have sickle cell anemia are at risk for nutritional deficiencies during acute illnesses, when inadequate intake of energy and macronutrients may occur (Malinauskas et al., 2000). Frequent episodes of acute illness are common, where fever and pain occur. Health professionals must be aware of the risks of nutritional inadequacy with loss of body mass (Malinauskas et al., 2000).

"Acute chest syndrome" can be triggered by infections and fat clots in the lungs; it is the leading cause of death in this disorder. At one time, most patients died by age 20. Bone marrow transplantation may be one consideration for patients with severe disease, in which a perfect match must be available from a sibling (Walters et al., 1996). These days, aggressive antibiotic therapy and transfusions can save lives.

After 1–2 years of conventional transfusions, variable tissue iron concentrations and tissue damage are observed in patients with sickle cell disease and in some patients, iron chelation therapy may not be appropriate after 1 year of transfusions while clearly indicated in others by this time to prevent tissue injury (Olivieri, 2001).

OBJECTIVES

- Supplement treatment with missing nutrients. Correct any malnutrition.
- Reduce oxygen debt. Improve patient's ability to participate in the activities of daily life.
- Reduce painful cramps, liver dysfunction, cholelithiasis, jaundice, and hepatitis.
- Lessen likelihood of pressure ulcers, infections, and renal failure.
- Promote normal growth and development, which could be stunted in children.
- Resting energy expenditure (REE) in patients with sickle cell anemia is best determined by indirect or direct measurement of energy expenditure. Metabolic rate is altered and special formulas may be needed (Kopp-Hoolihan et al., 1999).

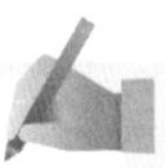

DIETARY AND NUTRITIONAL RECOMMENDATIONS

- Use vitamin B6 and folic acid supplements and adequate diet.
- Diet should include HBV proteins and adequate vitamin B12.
- Diet should provide adequate intake of vitamin C, zinc, riboflavin, vitamin E, vitamin A, and calories. Avoid excesses of vitamin C and iron, including from tube feedings or total parenteral nutrition (TPN) or multivitamin-mineral supplements.
- Nightly tube feeding can help to improve nutritional status.

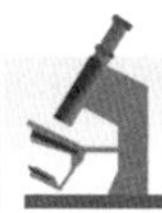

PROFILE

Clinical/History

Height
Weight
BMI
Chronic anemia, pallor
Jaundice

Lab Work

Serum Fe (increased from hemolysis)
Alb (normal)
RBP (decreased)
H&H
tHcy-may be elevated
Percentage of transferrin saturation
Serum B_{12}
Urinary zinc
N balance
Chol, Triglycerides (trig) (decreased)
MCV, Serum ferritin
TLC
pO2, pCO2
Serum folacin
Uric acid (increased)
Homocysteine

Common Drugs Used and Potential Side Effects

- Antibiotics may be used aggressively. Monitor for all side effects and GI distress.

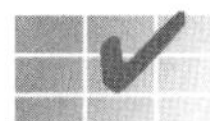

PATIENT EDUCATION

- ✔ Indicate which foods are good sources of folic acid, HBV proteins, vitamin C, zinc, riboflavin, and vitamins A, E, and B6.
- ✔ Discuss ways for easy meal preparation, because fatigue tends to be a problem.

For More Information

- Sickle Cell Information Center
  PO Box 109
  Grady Memorial Hospital
  80 Butler St.
  Atlanta, GA 30335
  http://www.emory.edu/PEDS/SICKLE/
- Sickle Cell Society
  http://www.sicklecellsociety.org/
- Sickle Cell Disease Association of America
  Hartford Regional Center
  Gengras Ambulatory Center
  114 Woodland St., Suite 2101
  Hartford, Conneticut 06105-1299
  860-527-0119
  860-714-5540
  http://www.sicklecellct.org/
- National Hotline—Sickle Cell Disease Association of America
  8:30–5 M-F Pacific Time
  1–800-421–8453
  310-216-6363

SIDEROBLASTIC/SIDEROTIC ANEMIA

NUTRITIONAL ACUITY RANKING: LEVEL 2

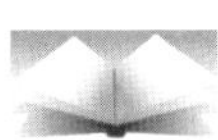

DEFINITIONS AND BACKGROUND

Sideroblastic anemias are a group of blood disorders characterized by an impaired ability of the bone marrow to produce normal red blood cells. The iron inside red blood cells is inadequately used to make hemoglobin, despite adequate or increased amounts of iron. Abnormal red blood cells called sideroblasts are found in the blood of people with these types of anemia.

This anemia is a microcytic, hypochromic anemia similar to that caused by iron deficiency, except that serum iron is normal or elevated. In some cases, a vitamin B6 deficiency impairs hemoglobin synthesis. The disorder also may have non-nutritional causes such as cancer, isoniazid (INH) use (nonsupplemented), collagen disorders, and chronic alcoholism. Signs and symptoms are the same as those found in iron deficiency anemia.

OBJECTIVES

- Correct problems and symptoms.
- Identify causes and solutions.
- Correct any suppression of bone marrow, iron-loading, etc.

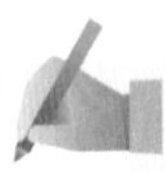

DIETARY AND NUTRITIONAL RECOMMENDATIONS

- A diet high in vitamin B6 may be beneficial (drugs are often used).
- Protein and CHO intake should be adequate, calories as well.
- Folic acid also may be needed.
- Alcohol intake should be severely limited.
- Balanced meals and snacks, as necessary, may be appropriate.

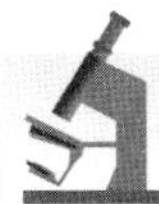

PROFILE

Clinical/History	Lab Work	
Height	Transferrin saturation (often elevated)	Serum folic acid
Weight	RBC	WBC
BMI		Serum Fe
		B6 levels
		Serum Cu

Common Drugs Used and Potential Side Effects

- Vitamin B6 may be ordered; age-dependent doses are specified.
- Chloramphenicol may cause drug-induced bone marrow suppression, resulting in sideroblastic anemia.
- INH and cycloserine can cause abnormal vitamin B6 metabolism. Monitor for GI side effects.

Herbs, Botanicals and Supplements

- Herbs and botanical supplements should not be used without discussing with physician.

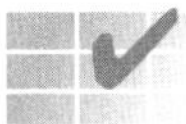

PATIENT EDUCATION

- Discuss adequate sources of all needed nutrients such as vitamin B6—especially if deficiency was causative.
- Discuss attractive menu planning and balancing of meals, because appetite and intake may be poor chronically. Discuss snacks and frequency.

HEMOCHROMATOSIS (IRON OVERLOADING)

NUTRITIONAL ACUITY RANKING: LEVEL 2

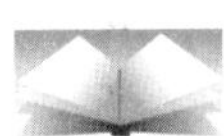

DEFINITIONS AND BACKGROUND

Hemochromatosis is a condition in which iron stores are deposited in excess, often from excess intake or liver/pancreatic diseases, renal dialysis, or frequent and long-term transfusions. Hereditary hemochromatosis (HH) is a genetic disorder of iron storage characterized by excessive intestinal absorption of dietary iron.

Healthy people may accumulate up to 1 g of iron, but people with this condition accumulate 15–30 g. Increased iron absorption leads to excessive accumulation of iron deposits within cells of the liver, heart, pituitary gland, pancreas, and other organs, gradually causing tissue damage and impaired functioning of affected organs. HH is considered one of the most common genetic disorders in Caucasians, affecting 1 in 250 people. The disorder is recessive, requiring the gene from two carrier parents. It is more common in Hispanics or people of Mediterranean and Irish or northeastern European descent and is 10 times more common in males.

Symptoms and signs include bronzing of the skin, profound fatigue, joint pain or arthritis, loss of body hair, loss of libido, lack of menstruation or early menopause, abdominal pain, chronic intermittent diarrhea, irregular heartbeat, cardiomegaly with congestive failure, cirrhosis or hepatomegaly, enlarged spleen, diabetes mellitus, hypothyroidism, and depression. Iron overload from hemochromatosis is not associated with an increased prevalence of coronary artery disease (Miller and Hutchins, 1994). Because hemochromatosis has so many possible symptoms, it often goes undiagnosed. However, early detection is important and may prevent organ failure that can occur if it is left untreated.

OBJECTIVES

- Remove excess iron from body (usually with phlebotomies of 500 mL weekly), performed by physician using chelation therapy. This may take a few months or years, then therapy several times annually for rest of life.
- If excess iron intake is a problem, discontinue use in supplements and fortified foods. Read labels carefully.
- Teach principles of nutrition and menu planning to incorporate adequate intake of other nutrients that may be depleted with excessive phlebotomies (e.g., folate and other B-complex vitamins, protein).

DIETARY AND NUTRITIONAL RECOMMENDATIONS

- Provide a normal diet, unless renal or hepatic function is altered. Do not consume foods rich in iron and vitamin C in large amounts; read cereal labels and avoid those with 100% of the recommended dietary allowance (RDA) for these two nutrients.
- Ensure adequate protein intake and provide calories to meet needs and activity.
- Check food labels for iron fortification; discuss alternatives.
- Avoid alcohol because of potential damage to a vulnerable liver.

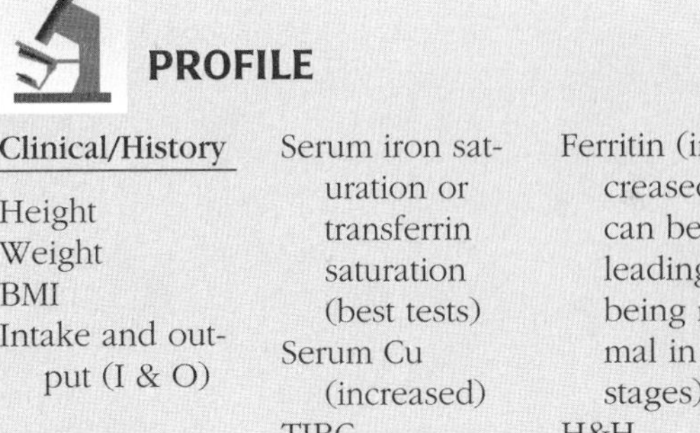

PROFILE

Clinical/History

Height
Weight
BMI
Intake and output (I & O)

Lab Work

Transferrin (increased)
Serum iron saturation or transferrin saturation (best tests)
Serum Cu (increased)
TIBC
Alb
Serum Fe
Ferritin (increased—can be misleading by being normal in early stages)
H&H
Gluc

Common Drugs Used and Potential Side Effects

- Avoid use of multivitamin supplements that contain iron and vitamin C, because these can increase iron absorption.

Herbs, Botanicals and Supplements

- Herbs and botanical supplements should not be used without discussing with physician.

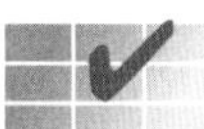

PATIENT EDUCATION

- Discuss nutrient sources as appropriate for the individual.
- Highlight iron fortification and review food labeling issues.
- Genetic testing of other family members is recommended for those with inherited type.

For More Information

- Hemochromatosis Foundation
  PO Box 8569
  Albany, NY 12208-0569
  518-489-0972
  http://www.hemochromatosis.org/
- Iron Overload Diseases Association, Inc.
  Hemochromatosis Diagnosis, Treatment, and Maintenance
  433 Westwind Dr.
  North Palm Beach, FL 33408-5123
  561-840-8512
  http://www.ironoverload.org/
- Iron Disorders Institute
  864-241-0111
  http://www.irondisorders.org

HEMORRHAGE, ACUTE OR CHRONIC

NUTRITIONAL ACUITY RANKING: LEVEL 2

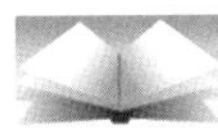

DEFINITIONS AND BACKGROUND

Hemorrhage is the excessive discharge of blood from a ruptured vessel. The bleeding (bright red and in spurts from an artery; dark red and in a steady flow from a vein) can be external, internal, or into skin or other tissue. When massive, a hemorrhage can cause such symptoms as rapid, shallow breathing; cold, clammy skin; thirst; visual disturbances; and extreme weakness. Loss of more than 20% of blood volume causes hypotension and tachycardia; loss of more than 1 quart of blood may lead to shock. Peptic ulcer, hemophilia, or stroke may be causes.

To stop a hemorrhage, blood must clot properly. Blood clots when its fibrinogen is converted to fibrin by action of thrombin. Table 12–6 shows blood clotting and how nutritional factors play a role.

Table 12–6 Blood Clotting

Clotting factors involving nutrition include:
I. Fibrinogen
II. Prothrombin
III. Thromboplastin
IV. Calcium

OBJECTIVES

- ▲ Medical management is designed to control bleeding, take care of the underlying cause of the bleeding, and replace lost blood. Transfusions may be given.
- ▲ Less severe hemorrhages may require iron, vitamin B12, and folic acid to help replace red blood cells.
- ▲ Support erythropoiesis.
- ▲ Control intestinal effects from GI bleeding, which can cause a protein overload.
- ▲ Prevent hypovolemic shock (low cardiac output, decreased blood pressure, and decreased urinary output).

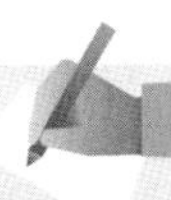

DIETARY AND NUTRITIONAL RECOMMENDATIONS

- Ensure diet is rich in proteins, iron, folic acid, vitamin B12, and copper.
- Check need for vitamin K in the diet. If medications to replace vitamin K are used, diet should provide a balance without excess.
- Monitor content of enteral feedings and multivitamin supplements carefully to ensure that all RDAs are met without excesses.

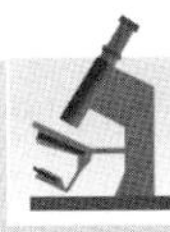

PROFILE

Clinical/History	Lab Work	
Height	Transferrin	Serum Fe
Weight	RBC	Serum B12
BMI	Alb	Serum folate
Pulse	BUN	PT
Temperature	CBC	TIBC (increased)
BP	H&H	Creatinine
		Occult blood

Herbs, Botanicals and Supplements

- Herbs and botanical supplements should not be used without discussing with physician.

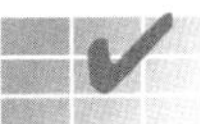

PATIENT EDUCATION

- ✓ Blood donors should be alerted to the need to replace daily iron intake by 0.7 mg for a year. Every pint is equivalent to 250 mg of iron lost.
- ✓ Discuss adequate dietary replacement for lost nutrients.

POLYCYTHEMIA VERA (OSLER'S DISEASE)

NUTRITIONAL ACUITY RANKING: LEVEL 1–2

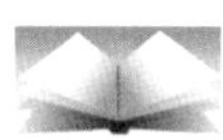

DEFINITIONS AND BACKGROUND

Polycythemia vera is a chronic, progressive disease in which increased blood volume and increased erythrocyte levels occur. Signs and symptoms may include belching, fullness, thirst, flatulence, constipation, headache, vertigo, lassitude, tinnitus, blurred vision, diplopia, dyspnea on exertion, chest pain, paresthesias, pruritus, dusky reddish skin on face and hands, thrombosis, gout, hemorrhagic tendency, hypertension, enlarged spleen, seizures, confusion, slurred speech, peptic ulcer, or congestive heart failure (CHF).

The average age at diagnosis is 50–60 years. Incidence is highest among those of Jewish ancestry, occurring in 1/100,000 of the population. Its cause is unknown, and the disease is considered a hematologic malignancy. The disease develops slowly and may progress to acute myelogenous leukemia. Increased viscosity of the blood and the number of platelets can result in a high potential for clot formation, which can cause stroke, hemorrhage, or myocardial infarction. With treatment, individuals with this condition may live 15–20 years.

OBJECTIVES

- Prepare patient for phlebotomy by ensuring adequate nutrient stores.
- Prepare, as needed, for chemotherapy or radiation therapy, which may be provided.
- Correct or control condition.
- Manage any side effects such as CHF, peptic ulcer disease, gastric bleeding, gout, leukemia, and seizures.

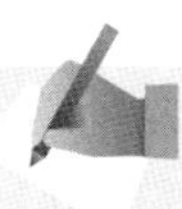

DIETARY AND NUTRITIONAL RECOMMENDATIONS

- A diet of preferred foods and balanced meals should be offered.
- Extra fluids will be helpful, e.g., 3–4 L daily (unless contraindicated, as with CHF).
- Changes in dietary texture or content may be needed if radiation or chemotherapy alter nutrient or dietary needs.

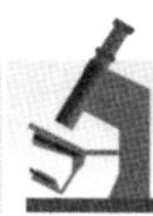

PROFILE

Clinical/History

- Height
- Weight
- BMI
- BP
- I & O

Lab Work

- Hgb (elevated)
- Hct (elevated above 54% for men and 49% for women)
- Platelets (elevated)
- Leukocytes (elevated)
- Erythropoeitin (low)
- TIBC
- Erythrocyte sedimentation rate (ESR)
- Leukocyte alkaline phosphatase
- Serum ferritin
- Gluc
- RBC (7–12 million)
- Alb, prealbumin
- Chol, Trig
- BUN, Creat
- Uric acid (elevated)
- Serum B12 (often elevated)
- Bone marrow biopsy

Common Drugs Used and Potential Side Effects

- Chemotherapeutic agents (busulfan, chlorambucil, cyclophosphamide) may be used. Nausea and vomiting are common side effects.
- Antihistamines can help reduce itching sensation.
- Myelosuppressive agents may be prescribed.
- Interferon-alpha or anagrelide may be used in younger patients.
- Low-dose aspirin is sometimes used in patients with thrombotic or ischemic conditions.
- Other medications may be necessary based on complications (CHF, etc.)

Herbs, Botanicals and Supplements

- Herbs and botanical supplements should not be used without discussing with physician.

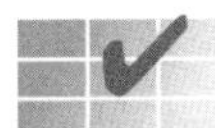

PATIENT EDUCATION

- ✔ Discuss need to maintain a healthy lifestyle and to eat adequate protein and calories because of the frequent phlebotomies (where completed).
- ✔ Discuss ways to prepare meals that are nutritious yet simple to prepare.

For More Information

- ✦ Myeloproliferative Disorders
  MPD RESEARCH CENTER, Inc.
  115 East 72nd Street, New York, NY 10021
  http://www.acor.org/diseases/hematology/MPD/

THALASSEMIA (COOLEY'S ANEMIA)

NUTRITIONAL ACUITY RANKING: LEVEL 2

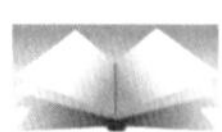

DEFINITIONS AND BACKGROUND

Thalassemia (Cooley's anemia) is a hereditary disease with an increased rate of destruction of red blood cells. Frequency of thalassemia is dependent on ethnic origins of the patient population; it is most common in persons with Mediterranean ancestry. β-Thalassemia is well recognized in persons of Greek and Italian descent, whereas alpha-thalassemic syndromes have an increased frequency in African, American Indian, and Asian populations. Collectively, the thalassemias are among the most common inherited disorders (Jandl, 1987).

The red blood cells are fragile and contain abnormal hemoglobin. Signs and symptoms include anemia, bone abnormalities, jaundice, enlarged spleen, and leg ulcers. The most common form, β-thalassemia, may allow a normal lifespan; some other forms may be fatal. In alpha-thalassemia one or more of the genes is actually missing. In beta-thalassemia, both globin genes are present but fail to produce hemoglobin. When a beta globin gene fails, beta-thalassemia results; when the alpha globin fails, alpha-thalassemia results.

In thalassemia major, symptoms can begin as early as 3 months of age. In the first year or two of life and in the absence of transfusion, a child can demonstrate severe anemia and expansion of the facial and other bones. These children may be pale or jaundiced, have a poor appetite, fail to grow normally, and have an enlarged spleen, liver, or heart. The incidence of gallstones is unusually common in this population (Premawardhena et al., 2001).

Because treatment involves frequent blood transfusion (approximately once every month) iron overload occurs (Olivieri, 1999). Excess iron accumulates leading to liver, heart, and pituitary damage and failure of these organs. If splenomegaly occurs, a splenectomy may be needed.

OBJECTIVES

- Offer temporary relief with blood transfusions.
- Improve hematologic status with oxygen availability.
- Correct failure to thrive and GI problems, which complicate the condition in infants.
- Reduce or correct infections.
- Promote healing of any ulcerations.
- Prevent or correct side effects of iron overloading from frequent transfusions.

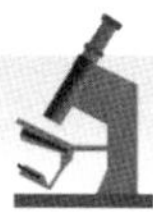

PROFILE

Clinical/History	Lab Work	
Height	Alk phos	percentage (increased)
Weight	Gluc	Serum Fe (increased)
BMI	RBC	Serum ferritin (increased)
Jaundice	CBC	TIBC (decreased)
I& O	H&H	Alb
Leg ulcers	Transferrin (decreased)	
Bone abnormalities	Transferrin iron saturation	
Enlarged spleen		

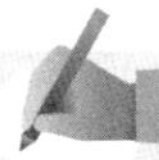

DIETARY AND NUTRITIONAL RECOMMENDATIONS

- A diet high in quality protein, calories, B-complex vitamins (especially folic acid), and zinc will be beneficial.
- Provide adequate fluid intake.
- With iron overload, avoid use of multivitamin-mineral supplements that contain iron and vitamin C in large amounts.

Herbs, Botanicals and Supplements

- Herbs and botanical supplements should not be used without discussing with physician.

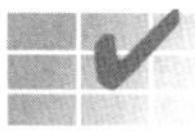

PATIENT EDUCATION

- ✔ Discuss ways to improve nutritional intake, when deficient.
- ✔ Discuss importance of diet in the maintenance of hematological health.

For More Information

- Cooley's Anemia Foundation
  1–800-522–7222
  www.thalassemia.org

THROMBOCYTOPENIC PURPURA

NUTRITIONAL ACUITY RANKING: LEVEL 1–2

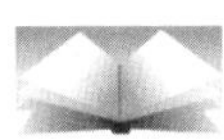

DEFINITIONS AND BACKGROUND

There are many different reasons for the development of decreased marrow production or platelet destruction that causes thrombocytopenic purpura. These can sometimes be determined by examination of bone marrow. Other forms of thrombocytopenia may be associated with hereditary factors.

Idiopathic thrombocytopenic purpura (ITP) is caused by platelet destruction by antibodies, causing bleeding disorders. Thrombotic thrombocytopenic purpura (TTP) is a platelet disorder manifested by vascular lesions. Essential thrombocytopenia is a rare blood disease affecting the clotting factor (platelets) of the blood, characterized by an abnormally low platelet count and a shorter than normal (10 days) platelet survival time.

Headache, slurred speech, numbness and weakness of extremities, increased temperature, and bleeding (as in ITP) occur. Tendency to bleed excessively into the skin or mucous membranes (e.g., in the nose), especially during menstruation, may also occur. In this illness, only after splenectomy is a complete remission obtained, defined as a normal platelet count, mean platelet life, and platelet production (Louwes et al., 2001).

OBJECTIVES

▲ Avoid infections, especially upper respiratory infections and flu to prevent coughing, which increases intracranial pressure.
▲ Rest adequately.
▲ Prepare patient for splenectomy, if indicated. Ensure adequate nutrient stores.
▲ Reduce bleeding tendency and complicating results.

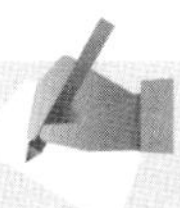

DIETARY AND NUTRITIONAL RECOMMENDATIONS

- Maintain diet of preference or as ordered. Use small, frequent feedings if patient has nausea or vomiting.
- Adequate folic acid will be needed.
- Increase fluids (e.g., 3 L daily) unless contraindicated.
- After splenectomy, patient will need adequate protein, calories, zinc, and vitamins A and C for wound healing.
- Vitamin K in the diet may need to be monitored.

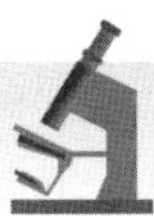

PROFILE

Clinical/History	Lab Work	
Height	Alb, prealbumin	Casts in urine
Weight	RBP	Proteinuria
BMI	N balance	H&H (decreased)
Bleeding	PT	Ca++
BP		K+, Na+

Common Drugs Used and Potential Side Effects

- Corticosteroids such as prednisone may be used to control bleeding. Side effects are numerous and may affect nutritional status—e.g., decreased serum Ca++, K1, and nitrogen; increased serum Na+; glucose intolerance.

Herbs, Botanicals and Supplements

- Herbs and botanical supplements should not be used without discussing with physician.

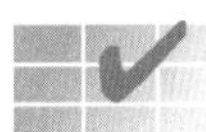

PATIENT EDUCATION

✔ Discuss altering nutrients as needed, dependent on medications ordered and their use over time, surgery, if required, and ability to eat adequately.

For More Information

- The ITP Society of the Children's Blood Foundation
  New York NY
  http://www.ultranet.com/˜7Eitpsoc/
- Platelet Disorder Support Foundation
  http://www.itppeople.com/

REFERENCES

Cited References

Abramson S, Abramson N. 'Common' uncommon anemias. *Am Fam Physician*. 1999;59:851.

Annibale B, et al. Reversal of iron deficiency anemia after Helicobacter pylori eradication in patients with asymptomatic gastritis. *Ann Int Med*. 1999;131:668.

Bourique S, et al. Twelve weeks of endurance exercise training does not affect iron status measures in women. *J Am Diet Assoc*. 1997; 97:1116.

Boushey C, et al. A quantitative assessment of plasma homocysteine as a risk factor for vascular disease: probable benefits of increasing folic acid intakes. *J Am Med Assoc*. 1995;274:1049.

Brugnara C, et al. Reticulocyte hemoglobin content to diagnose iron deficiency in children. *J Am Med Assoc*. 1999;281:2225.

Bruner A, et al. Randomized study of cognitive effect of iron supplementation in nonanemic iron-deficient adolescent girls. *Lancet*. 1996;348:892.

Carmel R. Prevalence of undiagnosed pernicious anemia in the elderly. *Arch Intern Med*. 1996;156:1097.

Carson J, et al. Effect of anemia and cardiovascular disease on surgical mortality and morbidity. *Lancet*. 1996;348:1055.

Chiari M, et al. Influence of acute inflammation on iron and nutritional status indexes in older inpatients. *J Am Geriatr Soc*. 1995; 43:767.

Dahele A, Ghosh S. Vitamin B12 deficiency in untreated celiac disease. *Am J Gastroenterol*. 2001;96:745.

Drabick J, et al. Concurrent pernicious anemia and myelodysplastic syndrome. *Ann Hematol*. 2001;80:243.

Feinstein S, et al. Erythropoietin deficiency causes anemia in nephrotic children with normal kidney function. *Am J Kidney Dis*. 2001;37:736.

Fishman S, et al. The role of vitamins in the prevention and control of anemia. *Public Health Nutri*. 2000;3:125.

Gerster H. High-dose vitamin C: a risk for persons with high iron stores? *Int J Vitam Nutr Res*. 1999;69:67.

Gupta S, et al. Childhood iron deficiency anemia, maternal nutritional knowledge and maternal feeding practices in a high-risk population. *Preventive Med*. 1999;29:152.

Hassan H, et al. Zinc-induced copper deficiency in a coin swallower. *Am J Gastroenterol*. 2000;95:2975.

Herbert V, Subak-Sharpe G. *Total nutrition: the only guide you'll ever need*. New York: St. Martin's Press, 1995; 521–522.

Hine J. What practitioners should know about folic acid. *J Am Diet Assoc*. 1996;96:451.

Hu H, et al. The relationship between bone lead and hemoglobin. *JAMA*. 1994;272:1512.

Hurtado E, et al. Early childhood anemia and mild or moderate mental retardation. *Am J Clin Nutri*. 1999;69:115.

Insel P, Turner R, Ross D. *Nutrition*. Sudbury, MA: Jones & Bartlett Publishers, 2001.

Jandl J. *Blood: textbook of hematology*. Boston: Little, Brown, 1987; 207.

Kaptan K, et al. *Helicobacter pylori* - is it a novel causative agent in vitamin B12 deficiency? *Arch Int Med*. 2000;160:1349.

Kennedy T, et al. Red blood cell folate and serum vitamin B12 status in children with sickle cell disease. *J Pediatr Hematol Oncol*. 2001;23:165.

Kopp-Hoolihan L, et al. Elevated resting energy expenditure in adolescents and sickle cell anemia. *J Am Diet Assoc*. 1999;99:195.

Kwiatkowski J, et al. Severe iron deficiency anemia in young children. *J Pediatr*. 1999;135:514.

Looker A, et al. Prevalence of iron deficiency in the United States. *J Am Med Assoc*. 1997;277:973.

Louwes H, et al. Effects of prednisone and splenectomy in patients with idiopathic thrombocytopenic purpura: only splenectomy induces a complete remission. *Ann Hematol*. 2001;80:728.

Lowenthal E, et al. Homocysteine elevation in sickle cell disease. *J Am Col Nutri*. 2000;19:608.

Lund E, et al. Oral ferrous sulfate supplements increase the free radical generating capacity of feces from healthy volunteers. *Am J Clin Nutri*. 1999;69:250.

Malinauskas B, et al. Impact of acute illness on nutritional status of infants and young children with sickle cell disease. *J Am Diet Assoc*. 2000;100:330.

Miller M, Hutchins G. Hemochromatosis, multiorgan hemosiderosis, and coronary artery disease. *JAMA*. 1994;272:231.

Moore D, Sears D. Pica, iron deficiency and the medical history. *Am J Med*. 1994;97:390.

Olivieri N. Progression of iron overload in sickle cell disease. *Semin Hematol*. 2001;38:57.

Olivieri N. The b-Thalassemias. *N En J Med*. 1999;341:99.

Premawardhena A, et al. Genetic determinants of jaundice and gallstones in hemoglobin E beta-thalassaemia. *Lancet*. 2001;357:1945.

Reddy M, et al. Estimation of nonheme iron bioavailability from meal composition. *Am J Clin Nutri*. 2000;71:937.

Slot W, et al. Normalization of plasma vitamin B12 concentration by intranasal hydroxocobalamin in vitamin B12 deficient patients. *Gastro*. 1997;113:430.

Smith D. Anemia in the elderly. *Am Fam Physician*. 2000;62:1565.

Taunikar R, Sabio H. Anemia in the adolescent athlete. *Am J Dis Child*. 1992;146:1201.

van Asselt D, et al. Free and protein-bound cobalamin absorption in healthy middle-aged and older subjects. *J Am Geriatr Soc*. 1996;44:949.

Walters M, et al. Bone marrow transplantation for sickle cell disease. *N Engl J Med*. 1996;335:369.

Wilfond B, et al. Severe hemolytic anemia associated with vitamin E deficiency in infants with cystic fibrosis. Implications for neonatal screening. *Clin Pediatr*. 1994;33:2.

Ziegler E, et al. Cow's milk and intestinal blood loss in late infancy. *J Pediatr*. 1999;135:720.

Suggested Readings

Allen L, et al. Lack of hemoglobin response to iron supplementation in anemic Mexican preschoolers with multiple micronutrient deficiencies. *Am J Clin Nutri*. 2000;71:1485.

Hunt J, Roughead Z. Adaptation of iron absorption in men con-

SECTION 13

Cancer

CHIEF ASSESSMENT FACTORS

American Cancer Society's Seven Warning Signs of Cancer:

- CHANGE IN BOWEL/BLADDER HABITS
- SORE THAT DOES NOT HEAL
- UNUSUAL BLEEDING OR DISCHARGE
- THICKENING OR LUMP IN BREAST OR ELSEWHERE
- INDIGESTION OR DYSPHAGIA
- OBVIOUS CHANGE IN WART OR MOLE
- NAGGING COUGH OR HOARSENESS

Other Concerns:

- WEIGHT CHANGES—UNINTENDED WEIGHT LOSS OR BMI LESS THAN 22
- CHANGES IN FOOD INTAKE, ANOREXIA OR NAUSEA
- PAIN
- ALTERED LABORATORY RESULTS (INCLUDING ALBUMIN BELOW 3.5 G/DL OR UNINTENDED DECLINE IN CHOLESTEROL BELOW 150 MG/DL
- SIDE EFFECTS OF MEDICATIONS, COMPLEMENTARY AND ALTERNATIVE MEDICINE, OR OTHER THERAPIES
- CHANGES IN USUAL FUNCTIONAL CAPACITY OR ENERGY LEVELS
- MUSCLE WASTING
- EDEMA OR ASCITES
- ANOREXIA OR NAUSEA
- DIARRHEA
- MOUTH SORES
- VOMITING
- PROBLEMS WITH NAUSEATING ODORS
- DYSPHAGIA, MUCOSITIS OR ESOPHAGITIS
- DRY MOUTH
- DEPRESSION
- HISTORY OF TOBACCO USE, EXCESSIVE ALCOHOL USE, ENVIRONMENTAL RISK EXPOSURE

GENERAL INFORMATION ABOUT CANCER, CANCER PREVENTION, AND RISK REDUCTION

There are 100+ variations of cancer; it is the number two killer in the United States, causing 25% of all deaths.

Natural carcinogens include ultraviolet (UV) radiation, dyes, environmental chemicals, (smoke, mines), viruses, nitrosamines, aflatoxins, and safrole. Eventually, one out of every three Americans will develop some form of cancer. Today, 40% of patients survive at least 5 years after diagnosis.

Nutritive and nonnutritive dietary constituents can promote or hinder development of chronic diseases such as cancer, obesity, inflammatory diseases, diabetes and cardiac heart disease (CHD). One-third of cancers are now linked to diet, developing over a long period of time. There is growing evidence that excess body weight increases the risk of cancer at several sites, including kidney, endometrium, colon, prostate, gallbladder, and breast in postmenopausal women (Bergstrom et al., 2001).

Currently, the Human Genome Project has identified 30,000 genes; they are 99.9% identical in all races and ethnic groups. Research has unveiled some of the molecular and cellular events that are involved in cancer specifically (Kim et al., 1999). Tumor cells may derive energy from metabolism of glucose to lactate in the Cori cycle rather than from complete oxidation to carbon dioxide and water in the Krebs cycle (Tisdale, 1993). DNA methylation is important in the control of gene expression; certain genes could be possible targets for chemotherapy (Momparler and Bovenzi, 2000).

Evidence from recent diet and nutrition studies showed that fruit and vegetable intake is critically important in risk reduction (Van Duyn and Pivonka, 2000). Antioxidants protect against free radical damage (American Institute for Cancer Research, 1994). Chromosomal damage is directly related to cancer and cell mutation; B-carotene is believed to protect against x-rays (Umegaki et al., 1994). Not eating enough antioxidant foods is the equivalent of irradiating oneself (Voelker, 1995).

There are more than 60 flavonoids that possess a wide range of properties, including anti-inflammatory and antitumor activity, inhibition of blood clots, and strong antioxidant activity (Craig, 1997). Currents and raisins contain high levels of isoflavones, genistein, and daidzein and should be included in the diet as protective (Liggins et al., 2000). High tomato consumption and blood lycopene levels are most protective against cancers of the prostate, lung, and stomach and are also protective against cancers of the pancreas, colon, rectum, esophagus, oral cavity, breast, and cervix (Giovannucci, Tomatoes. . . , 1999). Improving resistance of lymphocytes to oxidative stress is one goal (Porrini and Riso, 2000). Caution to the reader is suggested in that these are often small studies and generalizing these results to the entire population may not be entirely accurate; the results may not hold up in large, randomized trials. Overall, antioxidant and phytochemical effects can be obtained from eating a wide variety of fruits and vegetables.

Intake of B-carotene supplements is not as effective as dietary sources (Lee, 1999). Vegetarians seem to have lower cancer rates. For example, lower levels of deoxycholic acid, a cancer-promoting bile acid, in the feces may protect against colon cancer among vegetarians (van Faasen et al., 1993). People who eat the most fruits and vegetables have approximately one-half the rates of other members of their population; the "5-A-Day" message should be encouraged and expanded to state that "5 is the minimum."

Patients with cancer, especially those with weight loss, have higher rates of lipid oxidation and use more exogenous lipids than patients without cancer. An increase in fat intake may help prevent further losses or even increase body weight (BW) in these patients (Korber et al., 1999). High dietary intakes or serum levels of polyunsaturated fatty acids (PUFAs) do not seem to be associated with increased risk of fatal cancers (Simon et al., 1998).

Drinking green tea may help prevent cancer (Imai, 1997). A single dose of black or green tea induces a significant rise in plasma antioxidant activity (Leenan et al., 2000). Additionally, a complete anticancer grocery list would include dark green, yellow, and orange fruits or vegetables, red grapes, cruciferous vegetables, orange juice, tomatoes, olive and canola oils, garlic, legumes, and whole grains.

Use of complementary and alternative medicine (CAM) therapy has increased in the cancer population. Some products are harmless, but some may lead to serious problems. A study was designed to evaluate use of CAM therapies and found that vitamins were most commonly used (81%); herbal remedies were used by 54%, and relaxation techniques by 32.5% (Bernstein and Grasso, 2001). Multivitamins, herbal remedies, including green tea, Echinacea, and shark cartilage, and vitamins C and E as single supplements were most common. Advice may be needed to prevent the reduced effectiveness of chemotherapy or radiation therapy from antioxidant or herbal therapies (Bernstein and Grasso, 2001).

Although slightly more than half of U.S. adults understand that there is a relationship between diet and cancer risk, few are aware of specific nutrients and foods that influence risk (Harnack et al., 1998). Suggested nutrients that are protective or preventive for cancer are listed in Table 13–1; some of the latest guidelines about phytochemicals in cancer prevention are listed in Table 13–2. Table 13–3 provides a list of risk factors in different types of cancer.

TABLE 13–1 Protective/Preventive Nutritional Factors in Cancer

Recommendations–Protective Nutrients

Adequate vitamin A, especially in B-carotene and lycopenes (beware of excesses–they may act as pro-oxidants in some cases)
200–800 International Units (IU) vitamin E (Natural sources, d-alpha-tocopherol = need 22 IU daily for basic needs; synthetic sources, dl-alpha-tocopherol is less available = need 33 IU for basic needs)
Omega-3 fatty acids
Phytochemicals
Vitamin D3
250–500 mg vitamin C
50–200 mg selenium
Vitamin B6
Folate, thiamine, niacin, and riboflavin
Fiber from fruits, vegetables, and whole grains

Other preventive suggestions: (Note–80–90% of cancers are environmental/preventable)

1. Stop smoking.
2. Increase use of all phytochemicals, fruits and vegetables (5–10 per day), fiber, low fat milk, soy products, and fish.
3. Decrease use of alcoholic beverages.
4. Control weight; avoid obesity. Exercise daily for 30 minutes at a minimum.
5. Decrease fat (saturated or unsaturated) intake. Follow the 25/25 rule–25% kcal from fat and 25 g of fiber daily.
6. Reduce frying, grilling, and use of smoked and salt-cured foods.

TABLE 13–2 Phytochemicals

*Phytochemicals are ingredients that occur naturally in fruits, vegetables, and grains. They have not been shown to be essential nutrients and their functions in the body are under investigation. Some phytochemicals function as antioxidants to squelch free radicals. Currently, the emphasis remains on food sources, not supplements or pills.

Phytochemical Family	*Food Sources*
Allyl sulfides (allium, as S-allyl-cysteine or SAC; diallyl sulfide; allyl methyl trisulfide) *Role: decreases tumor cell growth; inhibits kinase activity; arterial vasodilator*	Onions, garlic (especially oil), leeks, chives, scallions, and red pepper
Carotenoids (a, b, lutein) and lycopenes *Role: increases activity of killer cells slightly; photoprotective agent*	Carrots, broccoli, spinach, and other green leafy vegetables, winter squash, papaya, mango, cantaloupe, tomatoes, and watermelon
Coumarins *Role: anticoagulant effect; inhibits proteolysis & lipoxygenase; anti-inflammatory agent*	Leafy green vegetables and citrus fruits
Dithiolthiones (containing sulfur) *Role: antimutagenic; chemoprotective for epithelial cells*	Cruciferous vegetables (broccoli, cauliflower, cabbage, kale, Brussels sprouts, collard greens, mustard, and turnip greens)
D-limonene, Terpenes *Role: decreases bacterial and fungal growth; decreases cancer cell growth*	Citrus fruit oils (orange, grapefruit, lemon), cherries, and citrus fruit peel
Epigallocatechin gallate (EGCG) *Role: decreases growth of hydroquinone oxidase; decreases COX-2 gene expression and cancer cell growth; decreases nitric oxide toxicity*	Green and black tea
Flavonoids (quercetin, kaempferol, myricetin) *Role: Fights free radicals*	Citrus fruits, apples, whole grains, and potato skins
Folate *Role: decreases cancer cell multiplication; efficient DNA synthesis and repair; regulates cellular S-adenosylmethionine levels and gene expression*	Leafy greens and orange juice
Herbs not commonly eaten Astragalus *Role: increases macrophages* Echinacea *Role: increases immune cells (interferon, killer cells, interleukin 2)* Ginseng *Role: increases lymphocytes*	Not available from foods at this time

(continued)

TABLE 13–2 Phytochemicals (*Continued*)

Herbs, spices, seasonings *Roles:* *1. Preserves alpha-tocopherol; decreases liver inflammation* *2. Protects plasmid DNA from degradation by radiation* *3. Decreases ATPase* *4. Lowers lipid peroxidation; maintains antioxidant effect* *5. Contains flavonoids, which decrease ascorbate-dependent free radical oxidation; decreases inflammation, tumorigenesis, and malarial impact*	1. Turmeric/cumin, rosemary, thyme, sage, and oregano 2. Chili powder, black pepper, and turmeric 3. Cinnamon, caraway, cumin, coriander, and turmeric 4. Ginger 5. Licorice (glycyrrhiza)
Indole-3-carbinol *Role: Modulates and down-regulates effects of estrogen and testosterone on tumor formation and growth; inhibits cell adhesion*	Cruciferous vegetables (broccoli, cauliflower, cabbage, kale, Brussels sprouts, collard greens, mustard, or turnip greens)
Isoflavones (genistein, daidzein, biochanin A) *Role: Phytoestrogens, which attach to estrogen receptors and block real estrogens; they also lower cholesterol levels and decrease cancer activity.*	Soybeans (tofu, soy milk); legumes; raisins, and currants
Isothiocyanates (sulphorophane, etc.) *Role: Increases period of cancer latency; effective agents against fungi such as Aspergillus*	Cruciferous vegetables (broccoli, cauliflower, cabbage, kale, Brussels sprouts, collard greens, mustard, or turnip greens)
Lignans *Role: phytoestrogens, which attach to estrogen receptors and block real estrogen; they also lower cholesterol levels and decrease cancer activity.*	Flaxseed, whole grains, berries, and vegetables
Monounsaturated fats *Role: decreases tumorigenesis*	Canola and olive oils
Oligosaccharides *Role: Increase short chain fatty acid formation; decrease cholesterol and lowers insulin levels*	Whole grains
Phenolic acids (polyphenols)—these are also flavonoids *Role: superoxide anion radical (SOR)-scavenging activity; interaction of the tumor promoter benzoyl peroxide (BPO) with murine peritoneal macrophages; protects against oxidation of LDL*	
Ellagic acid, ferulic acid	Tomatoes, citrus fruits, carrots, whole grains, and nuts; grapes and wine
Gallic acid	Green and black grape juices
Chlorogenic acid	Cherry juice
Tannic acid, caffeic acid *Role: inhibit proliferation of cancer cells*	Green and black tea and coffee
Phytates *Role: can decrease oxidative damage to cells*	Whole grains
Protease Inhibitors *Role: Inhibit action of protein-splitting enzymes; may prevent cancer cell formation or may decrease tumor size*	Whole grains
Resveratrol *Role: Decreases platelet activity*	Red grapes, wine, and grape juice
Saponins *Role: Decrease heart disease and cancer risks*	Beans and legumes, soybeans
Selenium and Glutathione *Role: Increase immune cell functioning; DNA methylation; regulation of cytokine production*	Brazil nuts, lean meats, and seafood; potatoes (glutathione)
Vitamin B6 *Role: Increases lymphocyte numbers*	Legumes, whole grains, chicken, pork, and bananas
Vitamin C *Role: Minimizes damage to neutrophils*	Citrus fruits, peppers, broccoli, tomatoes, and strawberries
Vitamin E *Role: increases antibody production + B and T cell functioning*	Wheat germ, mayonnaise, creamy salad dressings, pistachios, almonds, peanuts, and walnuts
Zinc *Role: increases neutrophil function and killer cell numbers; decreases cytokines; increases T and B cell numbers*	Wheat germ, lean beef, seafood, and black eyed peas

Derived from: Environmental Nutrition newsletters (January–February 2001); Steinmetz and Potter, 1996; American Institute for Cancer Research, 1994; Dwyer et al., 1994.

TABLE 13–3 Cancers and Potential Dietary Risk Factors

Cancers of the GI Tract:

Salivary Cancer (CA)–Tumors in the salivary glands are rare. Intake of over 200 mg vitamin C per day is associated with lower risk of salivary gland cancer compared with intake of under 100 mg/day; fiber intake from beans is associated with less risk; cholesterol intake is associated with higher risk (Horn-Ross, 1997).

Oral CA–Smoking cigarettes, cigars, or pipes; use of smokeless tobacco; alcohol; low use of fruits and vegetables (B-carotene and vitamin E) and lycopene (Giovannucci, Tomatoes. . . , 1999); low use of whole grains (Levi et al., 2000).

Less clear roles: low use of milk, allium compounds, green or black tea, and fish.

Esophageal CA–Smoking cigarettes; use of smokeless tobacco; alcohol; low use of green leafy vegetables and citrus fruits (vitamin C and beta carotene) and lycopene (Giovannucci, Tomatoes. . . , 1999); low use of whole grains (Levi et al., 2000).

Less clear roles: use of pickled vegetables, excessively high temperature beverages or soups; low use of green or black tea and fish.

Laryngeal CA–High use of alcohol; smoking; low use of dark green and orange vegetables and B–carotene (Zheng, 1992); low use of whole grains (Levi et al., 2000). Salted fish seems to be a risk for nasopharyngeal cancer.

Less clear roles: low use of green or black tea.

Stomach CA–Smoking; low carotenoids (Zheng et al., Retinol . . . , 1995); low intake of vitamins C and E; low use of indoles (cruciferous vegetables). Lycopene may be protective (Giovannucci, Tomatoes . . . , 1999). Intake of fish is associated with reduced risk (Fernandez et al., 1999). Onions are protective; leeks and garlic supplements are not (Dorant et al., 1996). Fruits are also protective. Refrigeration of food decreases possible risks.

Less clear roles: alcohol; salted, grilled, smoked, cured or pickled foods; exposure to nitrosamines or amino acid pyrosalates in broiled meat and fish; low use of fish and whole grains. Nonherbal tea drinking also may be protective in postmenopausal women (Zheng et al., 1996). Increased use of starches may be related to risks.

Liver CA–Alcohol abuse; low intake of vegetables (carotenoids).

Less clear roles: exposure to high levels of aflatoxins.

Gallbladder or Biliary CA–Obesity; untreated chronic gallstones.

Less clear roles: low vegetable and high sugar intakes (Moerman et al., 1995).

Pancreatic CA–Smoking; low intake of citrus fruit, beans or legumes (phytoestrogens), and fiber. Lycopene may be protective (Giovannucci, Tomatoes . . . , 1999). Obesity, inactivity, and insulin resistance are also implicated.

Less clear roles: low fiber intake; high intakes of meat and dietary cholesterol.

Colorectal CA–Low use of vegetables (folate, carotenoids, cruciferous vegetables [indoles]); high calories and saturated fats; obesity, sedentary lifestyle and lack of exercise. Long-term use of multivitamin supplements may reduce risk of colon cancer, may be due to folic acid content (Giovannucci et al., Multivitamin use. . . , 1998). Lycopene (Giovannucci, Tomatoes. . . , 1999); fish (Fernandez et al., 1999); and calcium may be protective. Exposure to chlorination by-products in drinking water may increase risk of colon cancer (Doyle et al., 1997). Olive oil may decrease risk (J Epid 10/00).

Less clear roles: High intake of alcohol, eggs, and meats; low use of vitamins C or D and bran; allium (garlic) intake (Steinmetz et al., 1994). Nonherbal tea drinking also may be protective in postmenopausal women (Zheng et al., 1996). Grilling, broiling, total fat and high saturated fats, and high sugar may increase risks as well.

Reproductive System Cancers:

Breast CA–Lycopene may be protective (Giovannucci, Tomatoes . . . , 1999). Dietary intake of vegetables is protective among premenopausal women. Vitamin C, alpha-tocopherol, folate, a- and beta-carotene, zeaxanthin, and dietary fiber from fruits and vegetables are most protective (Freudenheim et al., 1996). High intakes of beef and pork are related to breast cancer (Djuric et al., 1998). Breastfeeding 2+ years reduces risk by half (Zheng, 2001). Obesity and rapid early growth; low exercise; alcohol use greater than 1 serving daily.

Less clear: low omega-3 or monounsaturated fatty acids (Hunter, 1993); low use of soy or lutein.

CA of the Cervix–Smoking; low fruit and vegetable intakes (vitamins C, E, B-carotene, and folate). Lycopene may also be protective (Giovannucci, Tomatoes . . . , 1999). Low folate is implicated with human papilloma virus.

Less clear roles: low intakes of nonfat milk products.

Endometrial CA–Obesity. Low intake of fruits, vegetables, especially tomatoes for lycopene; low fiber intake.

Less clear roles: high intake of saturated fat from meat (Shu et al., 1993; Zheng et al., Dietary . . . , 1995); low intake of carotene (Barbone, 1993).

Ovarian CA–Nulliparity and use of talcum powder are factors. Oral contraceptive use, early pregnancy, and menopause tend to be protective. High vegetable intake, especially green leafy vegetables, is protective (Kushi et al., 1999). Studies suggest Vitamin E, lutein, beta-carotene may protect.

Less clear roles: Women with ovarian cancer tend to drink more milk and use more dairy products; lactose ingestion and lactase persistence may play a role–galactose may be an oocyte toxin (Meloni et al., 1999).

Prostate CA–Obesity, lack of exercise; high total and saturated fat intake; high dairy product intake; high intake of red meats (Ross and Henderson, 1994). Vegetables and lycopene may be protective (Giovannucci, Tomatoes . . . , 1999). Grape seed extract, soy genistein, lutein, and green tea are also being studied for their protective aspects.

Less clear roles: high linoleic acid; low intake of isoflavones, vitamin E, nuts, selenium, and essential fatty acids.

(continued)

TABLE 13–3 Cancers and Potential Dietary Risk Factors (*Continued*)

Other Cancers:
Brain CA—Protective—use of fresh vegetables (specifically Chinese cabbage and onion), fruit, fresh fish, and poultry (Hu, LaVecchia et al., 1999). Less clear roles: Interaction between the effects of N-nitroso compounds and protein or cholesterol intakes (Kaplan et al., 1997); chlorinated water among those with high intakes of tap water and for lifetime exposure to trihalomethanes (Cantor et al., 1999).
Lung CA—Smoking. Low use of fruits, vegetables, vitamins E and C, quercetin and other flavonoids, selenium, and carotenoids (Michaud et al., 2002). Lycopene may be protective (Giovannucci, Tomatoes . . . , 1999). Exposure to frying oils at high temperatures. Higher body mass index (BMI) (Rauscher et al., 2000); low physical activity. Less clear roles: high use of alcohol, animal fats, red meat, and saturated fats.
Non-Hodgkin's Lymphoma—High meat intake and a high intake of fat from animal sources are associated with an increased risk of non-Hodgkin lymphoma in older women (Chiu et al., 1996).
Thyroid CA—Low fruit and vegetable intake; high iodine exposure.
Skin CA and actinic keratoses—Possibly high fat diets, which depress the immune system (Black, 1998). *Melanoma*—Possibly from low vitamin B6, carotenoids, and soy proteins (isoflavones). Less clear roles: low use of green or black tea. Diet restricted in tyrosine and phenylalanine may be useful.
Kidney CA—Smoking; obesity (Chow et al., 2000). Less clear roles: low intake of vegetables; high intake of meats and dairy products.
Bladder and Urinary Tract CA—Nonherbal tea drinking may be protective in postmenopausal women (Zheng et al., 1996). Fruits, retinol, vitamin C, multivitamin use (Bruemmer et al., 1996), and vegetables may be protective. Smoking seems to be related to bladder cancer. Less clear roles: high use of fried foods and coffee.

For More Information

- AMC Cancer Research Center and Foundation
  1600 Pierce St.
  Denver, CO 80214
  1–800-321–1557
  http://www.amc.org/
- American Cancer Society
  http://www.cancer.org/
- American College of Surgeons
  633 N. St Clair St.
  Chicago, IL 60611-3211
  312-202-5000
  http://www.aoa.dhhs.gov/aoa/dir/28.html
- American Dietetic Association
  http://eatright.org/
- American Institute for Cancer Research (AICR)
  http://www.aicr.org/
- Cancer Information and Counseling Line
  1–800-525–3777
  http://www.amc.org/cicl.htm
- National Cancer Institute
  1–800-4-CANCER
  http://www.nci.nih.gov/
- Oncology Nursing Society
  http://www.ons.org/

CANCER, GENERAL GUIDE

NUTRITIONAL ACUITY RANKING: LEVEL 3

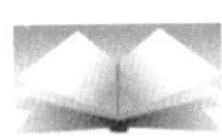

DEFINITIONS AND BACKGROUND

Total parenteral nutrition (TPN) should not be used to prolong life for patients at the end stages of disease but may be appropriate for patients with responsive cancers when enteral and oral feedings are poorly tolerated. In critical illness, calculation of energy requirements of obese teens with chronic diseases such as cancer is complicated by growth and disease state; use of indirect calorimetry may be more helpful (Ringwald-Smith et al., 1999).

Table 13–4 provides some basic cancer definitions. Table 13–5 defines the types of nutritional care offered in cancer care. Table 13–6 describes the nutritional implications of cancer treatments. Table 13–7 offers suggestions for coping with side effects of treatments and other common problems of cancer. Table 13–8 lists several chemotherapy drug combinations. Fatigue is probably the most common experience of patients with cancer (Kalman and Villani, 1997). Otherwise, each cancer tends of have its own set of side effects.

Table 13–4 Cancer Definitions

Adenocarcinoma. Cancer that starts in the glands.
Adenoma. Benign growth that may or may not transform to cancer.
Basal Cell Carcinoma. Most common form of skin cancer, affecting 800,000 Americans each year. In fact, it is the most common of all cancers. Chronic exposure to sunlight is the cause of almost all basal cell carcinomas, which occur most frequently on exposed parts, e.g., face, ears, neck, scalp, shoulders, and back.
Blood-Related cancers: Leukemia and myeloma are cancers that originate in the bone marrow; lymphoma originates in lymphatic tissues. Leukemia, lymphoma, and myeloma are considered to be related, because they involve the uncontrolled growth of cells with similar functions and origins; they result from an acquired (not inherited) genetic injury to the DNA of a single cell, which becomes abnormal (malignant) and multiplies continuously. The accumulation of malignant cells interferes with the body's production of healthy blood cells and makes the body unable to protect itself against infections.
Cancer. Abnormal, uncontrolled growth of cells in a lump or mass that also destroys normal tissue. Oncogenes in a tumor cell may be identifying markers.
Carcinoma. A form of cancer involving epithelial tissue and coverings of internal and external surfaces. Lungs, colon, breast, stomach, uterus, skin, and tongue cancers are included in this group, which comprise 80–90% of all cancers.
Epithelioma. Carcinoma consisting of many epithelial cells.
Metastasis. A transfer of disease from one organ to another that is not directly connected to it; especially the spread of carcinoma.

(continued)

Table 13–4 Cancer Definitions (*Continued*)

Oat cell carcinoma. A rapidly spreading, highly fatal cancer of the bronchus.
Oncology. Scientific study of tumors.
Sarcoma. Cancer arising from bone or connective tissue, which sometimes spreads into blood or lymphatic tissues.
Small Cell Carcinoma. A carcinoma that most commonly arises in the lung but can occur as a cancer in other body sites including the prostate, cervix, and head and neck; almost always responsive to chemotherapy and radiation therapy.

TABLE 13–5 Categories of Nutritional Care in Cancer

A. Preventive care
B. Maintenance care in therapy
C. Recovery and posttreatment
D. Palliative care in terminal patients

OBJECTIVES

- Overcome side effects of treatment. Diminish toxicity of treatment. Coordinate total care plan with doctor, nurse, patient, family, etc.
- Correct cachexia from weakness, anorexia, redistribution of host nutrients, and nutritional depletion. Control cancer and complications such as anemia or multiple organ dysfunction.
- Prevent or minimize weight loss from increased basal metabolic rate (usual increase is 15%). Some patients are hypometabolic; others hypermetabolic by 10–30% above normal rates. Greatest losses occur from protein stores and body fat. Early nutritional status is a good prognostic indicator.
- Prevent further depletion of humoral and cellular immunity from malnutrition.
- Prevent infection or sepsis, further morbidity, or death from starvation or infections.
- Provide appropriate micronutrients.
- Control gastrointestinal (GI) symptoms, which are more common with weight loss greater than 10%.
- For some, synthetic retinoids are being used to prevent recurrence after surgery. Further studies are warranted.
- Improve quality of life through resolution of treatment-related side effects.

TABLE 13–6 Nutritional Implications of Cancer Treatments

Surgery	
Oropharynx	Difficulty with chewing and swallowing, dysgeusia, xerostomia, odynophagia
Esophagus	Heartburn, loss of normal swallowing, decreased motility, obstruction
Stomach	Dumping syndrome, delayed emptying, anemia, malabsorption
Pancreas	Exocrine or endocrine insufficiency (i.e., insulin)
Small intestines	Lactose intolerance, bile acid depletion, steatorrhea, fat malabsorption, B12 deficiency and anemia, short-gut syndrome
Colon	Loss of electrolytes and water, diarrhea, constipation, gas, bloating
Chemotherapy	
Alkylating agents	Nausea, vomiting
Antibiotics	Anorexia, diarrhea, nausea and vomiting, stomatitis
Antimetabolites	Diarrhea, nausea, vomiting, stomatitis
Corticosteroids	Sodium and fluid retention, weight gain
Sex hormones	Anorexia, nausea, vomiting, sodium and fluid retention
Vinca alkaloids	Nausea and vomiting
Radiation	
Head–neck	Anorexia, dysgeusia, weight loss, odynophagia, dysphagia, difficulty chewing, xerostomia
Thorax	Nausea, esophagitis, vomiting
Abdominal, intestinal	Early: lactose intolerance, diarrhea, distention, abdominal pain, nausea and vomiting
	Late: intestinal stenosis, edema, fluid and electrolyte loss, weight loss, enteritis

Updated from: *A guide to nutritional care*. Evansville, IN: Mead Johnson Nutritional Division, 1980.

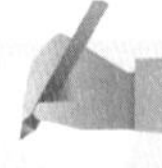

DIETARY AND NUTRITIONAL RECOMMENDATIONS

- In general, intake of protein should be high (1–1.5 g/kg body weight to maintain; 1.5–2 g/kg body weight to replete losses). Intake of calories should be high (25–35 kcal/kg body weight to maintain; 35–50 kcal/kg body weight to replete body stores). Add calories if the patient is febrile or septic. Fat should be 30–50% nonprotein calories (NPCs).
- Schedule larger meals earlier in the day. If needed, schedule five to six small meals daily, tube feeding, or intravenous feeding. If the gut works, use it.
- Use TPN if enteral nutrition is contraindicated. Parenteral nutrition (PN) is not likely to benefit advanced cancer that is unresponsive to treatment (Bloch, 1994). Caution use of TPN therapy with chemotherapy because of the risks from sepsis.
- Provide adequate, but not excessive, micronutrient supplementation (Blot, 1993; Bass and Cox, 1995), vitamin B6, pantothenic acid, folic acid, vitamins A, E, and C. Use more foods high in B-carotene; include lots of fruits and vegetables in appropriate forms. Do not use excesses of iron, but correct anemias when possible; use recommended dietary allowance (RDA) levels as a guide.
- Nutritional treatment for specific cancers: see specific entries. Alter dietary therapy as needed; each person's needs vary before and after treatments and various therapies.
- Review each case individually and honor patient's wishes regarding more aggressive intervention.
- Increased need for leucine, methionine, and branched chain amino acids have been suggested; data are not conclusive.
- After surgery or abdominal radiation, glutamine may be useful to protect from enteropathy, to lower morbidity, augment tumor cell kill, and boost natural killer cell (NK) activity.
- Control simple sugars with carbohydrate (CHO) intolerance, as with corticosteroid therapy.
- Use adequate fluid for hydration.

Common Drugs Used and Potential Side Effects

- Methotrexate. Folate preparations can alter drug response. Folate, lactose, vitamin B12, and fat are less well absorbed. Mouth sores are common.
- Other antineoplastic agents: side effects include nausea, anorexia, stomatitis, diarrhea, taste alterations, some vomiting, sloughing of colonic mucosa. Hyperuricemia, nausea, and vomiting are common with alkylating agents.
- Immunotherapy (interleukin-2 and interferon are used). Lymphokine is administered to decrease tumor growth. Side effects include nausea, vomiting, abdominal pain, fatigue, and anorexia. In addition, low levels of folate and vitamins A and B6 may result.
- Antibiotics and steroids also alter nutritional status. Monitor their use carefully.
- Antiemetics (granisetron or ondansetron) may also be used to relieve nausea and vomiting after chemotherapy. Headache may result.
- Reglan and Compazine may be useful for cases of anorexia/cachexia syndrome. Nausea, diarrhea, increased gastric emptying, or drowsiness can result. Zofran (odansetan), Kytril (granisetron), and Anzemet (dolasetron), if administered at the same time over 24–48 hours, can prevent nausea and vomiting in chemotherapy, but abdominal pain and constipation may occur.
- Monoclonal antibodies (MAbs) attack only abnormal elements of cells have begun to emerge; drug design for "kinder and gentler" cancer therapies. These drugs target only abnormal cells and correct the abnormal enzyme that causes cancerous cells to grow out of control. Campath-1H, Rituxan, and Bexxar are sample

TABLE 13–7 Side Effects of Treatment and Common Problems of Cancer

1. Fatigue is probably the most common experience of patients with cancer (Kalman and Villani, 1997). For fatigue, meals may be prepared in quantity when the patient is less tired. To prevent further fatigue, foods that require less chewing may be used. Provide frequent rest periods, especially before meals.

2. Loss of teeth makes the patient's mouth more sensitive to cold, heat, and sweets. Try serving foods at room temperature.

3. Xerostomia, dry mouth from surgical removal of salivary glands, atrophy of mucous membranes, or from permanent damage from radiation to salivary glands may cause difficulty in eating and swallowing. Use salivary substitutes, lip balm, sugarless gum and candies, gravies, and sauces. Increase fluids and use softened, moist foods (custard, stews, soups). Sip beverages with each bite of food. Cut food into small pieces. Ice chips and popsicles also can help. Pureed or baby foods often are useful. Avoid salty foods. Tart foods and beverages such as lemonade may help to stimulate saliva production. Sucking on popsicles, lemon drops, hard candy can also help. Sip on water or other fluids frequently throughout the day. Synthetic saliva products such as Optimoist or MouthKote may help. Use caution with tart foods if oral lesions are present. Radiation therapy patients benefit from a thorough dental examination before treatment. Use of fluoride trays, rinses, and other measures may be helpful.

4. For poor dentition and caries, avoid sweets and use sodium fluoride three times daily. Mouth care should be provided several times daily. Persons receiving irradiation to the head and neck area may benefit from use of fluoride trays and stannous fluoride.

5. Thick saliva can produce more caries. Use less bread, milk, gelatin, and oily foods. Blenderize foods such as fruits and vegetables. Encourage intake of plenty of fluids to decrease viscosity of oral secretions. Encourage good oral intake and regular oral rinses.

6. Sore mouth and throat (stomatitis, mucositis, or esophagitis) result from local bleeding, mucosal irritation, and lesions. Pain and inflammation are common. Modify the texture and consistency of foods as needed. Use a diet with fewer spices and seasonings such as nutmeg, chili powder, or cloves. Have patient rinse mouth with water and sodium bicarbonate. Avoid acidic juices, salty foods or soups, dry toast, and coarse or grainy breads or cereals. Grind meats. Use the "mechanical soft diet" as needed. Offer fluids frequently and by straw—cold or tepid. Popsicles and cold liquid foods may help. Smaller meals are useful. Cut foods into smaller pieces; grind or puree if needed. Mix food with sauces or gravies to make it easier to swallow. Swish mouth with lidocaine before meals; some changes in taste or enjoyment of foods may result. Avoid smoking and use of alcohol.

7. Mouth blindness (dysgeusia) is defined as disinterest and aversion to foods. Emphasize the aroma and colors of foods. Provide a variety of foods and use garnishes. Acidic foods (e.g., lemonade) may help stimulate patient's ability to taste foods. Use highly flavored foods and sauces. Try milk shakes that are coffee or mint flavored. Fresh vegetables, special breads, highly flavored snacks, olives, and pickles may be well received by the patient. Add sauces to meats. Foods that are served warm or hot have more flavor and aroma.

8. Anorexia may be caused by coping with the diagnosis and treatment-related side effects, medications, GI distress, altered sensory experiences, or tumors. The condition leads to cachexia. Cachexia is the clinical consequence of a chronic, systemic inflammatory response; depletion of skeletal muscle and redistribution of the body's protein are major changes that occur (Kotler, 2000). Anorexia cachexia syndrome (ACS) is caused by numerous factors; altered glucose metabolism may be one of them. Use small, frequent feedings and supplements. Teach ways to increase calories and protein. Fortify foods when possible. Relieve symptoms before meals whenever possible. Anabolic and anticatabolic agents such as Megace and Oxandrine may be able to mitigate cachexia (Kotler, 2000).

9. Weight loss can be treated by adding fats to foods, dry milk to mashed potatoes and shakes, and extra sugar to coffee and cereals. Use small, frequent feedings and the patient's favorite foods. Use 40–50 kcal/kg for repletion. Add cream sauces, extra meat or cheeses in casseroles, and gravies. Encourage patients to be as physically active as possible, especially using long muscles to promote lean body mass.

10. To treat diarrhea, alter fiber in diet. Beware of lactose intolerance secondary to disease process, drug therapy, or abdominal or pelvic radiation therapy. Decrease fatty foods. Increase fluids that contain sodium and potassium; a clear liquid diet for 24 hours may be helpful. Use cool or room temperature foods instead of very hot or very cold foods. Evaluate all medications carefully. Avoid dairy products if they increase indigestion or diarrhea. Consume small amounts of fluid and food throughout the day.

11. Constipation requires fiber and fluids (8 cups) to be added to the diet. Milk also may be beneficial, if tolerated. Fresh or dried fruits, all vegetables, and bran may help. A hot drink may help. Get adequate exercise. Use of over-the-counter bulking agents may be useful in some cases. Avoid gas-forming foods and beverages in excess.

12. Aversion to foods and specific tastes. For some patients, a lower threshold for urea causes aversion to meat; these patients may say that the meat "smells rotten." Substitute milk, cottage cheese, eggs, peanut butter, legumes, poultry, fish, and cheese. In addition, patient may have a decreased ability to taste salt and sugar. Add other seasonings, sauces, and more salt or sugar as desired by the patient; however, do not allow sweet foods to replace nourishing foods. Some people are "super tasters" and have a lot of taste buds, with extra sensitivity to sweet and sour foods; some are normal; some are nontasters, with dull sensitivity to foods. Ensure adequate zinc intake. Foods served at cool or cold temperatures often have a less offensive taste and aroma.

(continued)

TABLE 13–7 Side Effects of Treatment and Common Problems of Cancer (*Continued*)

13. Preference for cold foods. Cold foods may be better accepted than hot foods. Use cold, clear fluids, carbonated beverages, ices, gelatin, watermelons, grapes and peeled cucumbers, cold meat platters, ice cream, and salted nuts. Serve supplements over ice, between meals. Shakes, puddings, and custards are other alternatives.

14. Nausea can be treated by slow, deep breathing, ice chips, or sips of carbonated beverages. Try a dry diet also (liquids between meals). Try relaxation measures. Antivert or other medications may be helpful. Eat small meals; rest afterward. Keep crackers or salty potato chips handy. Eat toast, yogurt, sherbet, popsicles, pretzels, angel food cake, canned fruit, baked chicken, and hot cereal such as oatmeal, clear liquids, or broth. Cut down on greasy, spicy, fried or fatty foods. Some people prefer tart lemonade to sweetened beverages. Foods with strong odors and excessive sweetness may not be tolerated. Sit upright for meals and snacks. Avoid tight clothing. If breakfast is the best meal, it can also be the largest of the day. Encourage patients to use anti-emetics as directed by physician; under-usage may contribute to nausea. As directed, use of other agents may be more effective in nausea management.

15. If meals are interrupted by treatment, encourage a good breakfast and snacks to make up for interrupted meals. Keep kitchen well stocked. Meals-on-demand may be a useful way to serve meals to this population.

16. To treat pain, give pain medications with the first few bites of a meal or have patient eat when pain is lowest. Encourage trying foods again after time lapse. Try biofeedback or muscle relaxation.

17. Loneliness may affect eating habits. Social eating may improve food intake. Visitors should be encouraged to bring gifts of food, as appropriate.

18. In the case of malabsorption, elemental diets can only be used if patient has an intact duodenum and jejunum. TPN can be used only in some cases, considering risks of infection. Elemental diets are often prescribed by mouth with poor patient compliance; work with patient on ways to improve compliance. Use of tart beverages with mixed product can be useful (e.g., lemonade).

19. For difficulty in swallowing (dysphagia), use moist foods. Add gravies and sauces to foods. Some patients tolerate semisolid foods better than liquids. Patient should sip fluids throughout meal. To prevent aspiration, patient should try placing liquid under tongue. Some patients may also find that tilting their heads will be useful. Thickeners are available for liquids, if thin beverages are not tolerated well (as with choking, coughing with each swallow). Use of a straw may be beneficial. Spoons are easier to control than forks in the mouth. Avoid very hot or very cold foods. Pureed foods may be better tolerated than regular foods.

20. For anemias, a balanced diet with 50% high biologic value proteins, B-complex vitamins, iron (using caution), and vitamin C may be helpful. Use of heme sources of iron, if possible, will increase iron bioavailability.

21. Early satiety can be a problem. Rather than stressing plain water, encourage use of a calorie-containing beverage. Take liquids between meals. Avoid fatty, greasy foods, because they are more slowly digested and absorbed. Use small meals and frequent snacks, "nibbling."

22. During periods of vomiting, use sips of clear liquids every 10–15 minutes after vomiting episodes cease; keep head elevated. "Flat" carbonated beverages are useful. Call doctor if abdominal pains persist. Antiemetics may be needed.

23. Insulin resistance is common from tumor itself (Yoshikawa et al., 1994). Control of CHO intake may be indicated when this occurs. Various medications also may be used to treat, such as oral agents.

24. Fluid retention may require elevating the legs at rest, staying physically active (walking, etc.), and reducing salt intake overall. The doctor will prescribe diuretics, if indicated.

25. After curative surgery, direct efforts at restoring nutritional health to pre-illness status. Promote healing and management of all side effects.

26. Radiotherapy (usually given daily for 2–8 weeks) can cause nausea or vomiting if administered to the brain or abdominal/pelvic fields. A light meal is encouraged before treatment. Diarrhea may occur in radiation enteritis; glutamine may be useful in supplements or in tube feeding (TF)/TPN.

27. With all types of chemotherapy (given daily, weekly, monthly for 1–2 months, or even years), prompt attention to side effect management and appropriate use of supportive care (medications, nutrition, etc. will be needed). Increase fluid intake for adequate hydration. After chemotherapy, cardiac, kidney, or pulmonary toxicity may occur. Some chemotherapy agents may cause infertility in both men and women. Nausea and vomiting can now be well controlled; drugs include Zofran (odansetan), Kytril (granisetron), and Anzemet (dolasetron), if administered at the same time. Hemopoietic agents (Neupogen, Procrit, GSCF, GM-SCF) may be needed if red blood cell production is too low; transfusions are used as a last resort. Avoid risk of infection and cuts during chemotherapy. Monitor for nosebleeds, bruising, black or bloody stools, or reddish urine.

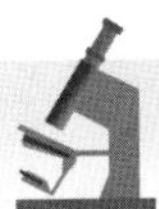

PROFILE

Clinical/History

Height
Weight
BMI
Weight changes
Temperature
Nausea or vomiting
Diarrhea
Taste changes
Food aversion
Ascites
Dysphagia
Sore mouth
Chewing problems
Choking
Intake and output (I & O)
Tumor stage
Tumor grade (growth rate)
Constipation
Edema

Lab Work

Triglycerides (Trig)
Cholesterol (Chol) (often low)
Nitrogen (N) balance, Retinol-binding protein (RBP)
Alkaline phosphatase (alk phos), PO4
Magnesium (Mg++)
White blood cell count (WBC)
Erythrocyte sedimentation rate (ESR)
Type of cells
Ceruloplasmin (increased)
Calcium (Ca++)
Hemoglobin and hematocrit (H&H)
Sodium (Na+), K+
Partial pressure of carbon dioxide (pCO2), partial pressure of oxygen (pO2)
Serum Fe, ferritin
Aspartate amino-transaminase (AST), alanine amino-transferase (ALT)
Lactate (increased five times), from lactic acid
Glucose (gluc) (often increased)
MRI or CT scan
Albumin (alb) (level of 2 g/dL may allow sepsis)
Chloride (Cl−)
Blood urea nitrogen (BUN) (often decreased)
Creatinine
Mean cell volume (MCV)
Platelets
Urinary acetone
Ca++ (increased with bone resorption)
Uric acid
S-phase fraction (SPF) = percentage of cells that are in the synthesis stage of division
Monoclonal bodies (anti-body-seeking CA cells)
Transferrin, total iron-binding capacity (TIBC)
Transferrin saturation (often increased)
Total lymphocyte count (TLC) (not reliable here)

drugs in this category. The anti-epidermal-growth-factor-receptor (EGFR), cetuximab, specifically binds to the EGFR with high affinity, blocking growth-factor binding, receptor activation, and subsequent signal-transduction events leading to cell proliferation (Baselga, 2001).

- Aspirin and other pain relievers may prevent some types of cancer, including colon cancer. Use of herbal NSAIDs may eventually be recommended along with these medications to enhance effectiveness.

Herbs, Botanicals and Supplements

- **State clearly to patient whether "guidance" or "promotion" is being offered; herbs and botanical supplements should not be used without discussing with physician.**
- The Natural Product Cancer Chemopreventive Agents study through the National Cancer Institute has found about 200 active chemical ingredients in over 15,000 products. These chemicals are being studied for their roles in cancer prevention and treatment.
- Popular products used by cancer patients include (Spaulding-Albright, 1997): astragalus (stimulates interferon), cat's claw (contains alkaloids), Essiac (contains Indian rhubarb, sheepshead sorrel, slippery elm, burdock root plus watercress, red clover, blessed thistle, and kelp), Hoxsey Herbal treatment (contains arsenic and cascara, which can be toxic), kombucha tea, pycnogenol (contains bioflavonoids), shitake mushrooms (contains polysaccharide lentinan, which stimulates T cell and NK cell production). Milk thistle (contains flavolignans, 80% Silymarin) and perhaps has a role in decreasing skin or prostate cancer; it is being studied but is known to have some hepatic side effects.
- **Herbs with documented toxic side effects** include aconite (bushi), arnica (wolfbane, mountain tobacco), belladonna (deadly nightshade), blue cohosh (squaw root), borage, broom (broom tops, Irish broom), calamus (sweet root/flag), chaparral (creosote bush), coltsfoot, comfrey, convallaria (lily of the valley), ephedra (ma huang), germander, jimson weed, jin bu huan, laetrile, licorice (glycyrrhiza glabra), liferoot (golden senecio, ragwort), lobelia (Indian or wild tobacco), mandrake, mistletoe (iscador), Pau d'Arco (Taebuia), pennyroyal, periwinkle, poke root, sassafras, wormwood (madder, mug, and Ming wort, artemisia), and yohimbe (Spaulding-Albright, 1997).
- St. John's wort has not been proven effective against acute depression, but more studies are underway for its effect on reducing alcohol consumption in alcohol-dependent individuals, etc. It accelerates the effects of coumadin and tamoxifen and must be used cautiously.
- Green tea contains polyphenols and may be encouraged.
- Garlic seems to have reduced gastric cancer in China and Italy; its sulfur compounds tend to be chemoprotective. Supplements are not as effective as the real garlic for allicin and s-allylcysteine activity.
- Herbals NSAIDs have been proposed as useful—grapes and cherries, onions, citrus, garlic, willow bark, turmeric, and other herbs are being studied for their effect. Gingko biloba has antioxidant and anti-inflammatory effects; the role in cancer is not known.
- Indian mulberry (noni juice) is being studied for its antitumor activity.
- Skullcap (Scutellaria) is being studied for skin cancer. It should not be taken orally.
- Soy isoflavones have a role in prostate, breast, and bone cancers. Exact dosage and effects on specific genes are

Table 13–8 Chemotherapy Drug Combinations (http://www.bmtsupport.ie/resources.html)

ACOB—Doxorubicin, cyclophosphamide, vincristine, bleomycin
ABVD—Doxorubicin, vinblastine, bleomycin, DTIC
ARA-C—Cytarabine ATRA—all-trans retinoic acid or Vesanoid
BACOP—Bleomycin, doxorubicin, cyclophosphamide, vincristine, prednisone
BEAM—Busulfan, etoposide, ara-c, melphalan
BLEO—Bleomycin 2CdA – 2-chlorodeoxyadenosine (Generic name = cladribine)
C-MOPP—Cyclophosphamide, Oncovin, procarbazine, prednisone
CCNU—(1–2-chloroethyl)-3-cyclohexyl-1-nitrosourea)
CHOD—Cyclophosphamide, doxorubicin, vincristine, dexamethasone
CHOP—Cyclophosphamide, Adriamycin, vincristine, prednisone
COP—Cyclophosphamide, vincristine, prednisone
COPP—CCNU, – vincristine, procarbazine, prednisone, CyA – cyclosporin A DCF – 2-deoxycoformycin (pentostatin)
DTIC—Dacarbazine, 5-(3,3-dimethyl-1-triazino)imidazole-4-carboxamide
EPOCH—Etopside, prednisone, vincristine, cyclophosphamide (Cytoxan), Adriamycin
FAC—fluorouracil, Adriamycin, cyclophosphamide
Flu—Fludarabine (Fludara) IFN – Interferon (comes in alpha 2a, alpha 2b, human leukocyte, and beta)
HOP-BLEO—Cyclophosphamide, doxorubicin, vincristine, prednisone and bleomycin
IL—Interleukin mBACOD methotrexate, bleomycin, doxorubicin, cyclophosphamide, vincristine, dexamethasone
MF—Cyclophosphamide, methotrexate, fluorouracil
MOPP—Nitrogen mustard, vincristine, procarbazine, prednisone
MTX—or M methotrexate proMACE – prednisone, methotrexate with leucovorin rescue, doxorubicin, cyclophosphamide, etoposide (VP-16)

not currently known; the best advice is to encourage typical dietary use and not to change drastically at this time. Soy may not be indicated in estrogen-dependent breast cancer.

- Shark cartilage is being studied in clinical trials for lung cancer.
- Chinese medicine PC-SPES (which contains chrysanthemum, licorice, ginseng, saw palmetto, and other herbal products) seems to have some anti-estrogenic effects and is being studied in clinical trials, as well, for prostate cancer as adjuvant therapy.

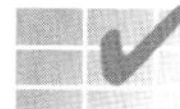

PATIENT EDUCATION

- ✓ The patient's improved nutritional status may allow neoplastic cells to become more susceptible to medical treatment. This may make patients more suitable for treatments for which they were denied previously. An improved nutritional status also reduces side effects, promotes better rehabilitation, and improves quality of life while perhaps increasing survival rates. Malnutrition can potentiate toxicity of antineoplastic agents.
- ✓ Malnutrition does not have to be accepted in the case of the cancer patient. Aggressive therapy = aggressive nutrition. Start "where the patient is."
- ✓ Instruct patient to use unscientific treatments with caution; including Laetrile and megavitamins. Discuss these issues with compassion and understanding of patient's perspective. Alternative therapies should be reviewed in light of potential harm versus possible benefits.
- ✓ In a small trial, daily intake of *Bifidobacterium lactis* enhanced natural immune function of older adults (Arunachalam et al., 2000). Regular use of yogurt and other naturally functional foods may be useful.
- ✓ Patients want faith in doctor's expertise, hope to provide coping and strength, and charity to fellow patients. Patient desires must be respected.
- ✓ For cancer survivors, less is known about optimal nutritional actions. Because there are different phases of cancer survivorship, from active treatment to advanced disease, existing evidence must be reviewed from which informed decisions can be made regarding dietary choices. Popular complementary and alternative methods related to dietary intervention are often used and should be carefully addressed with patients (Brown et al., 2001).
- ✓ For terminal, palliative care, emotional support, and comfort may be the best treatment. Hydration is the priority rather than meeting RDAs or calorie requirements. Food and fluid use beyond specific patient requests may play a minimal role in providing comfort to terminally ill patients (McCann et al., 1994). Counselor should be aware of the stages of death and dying to identify where patient is: (a) denial, (b) anger, (c) bargaining, (d) depression and loss, or (e) acceptance. Patient must be included in all decisions.

For More Information

- American Dietetic Association
  Cancer, Medical, and Radiation Oncology protocols
  www.eatright.org
- Antioxidants and Chemo-radiotherapy
  http://nccam.nih.gov

- Cancer Related Links
  http://www.uchsc.edu/uh/marrow/www/related.htm
- CANSearch: Guide to Cancer Resources on the Internet
  http://www.cansearch.org/canserch/canserch.htm
- Cancer Resources
  http://www.cancerresources.com
- Chemotherapy Buddies
  http://jonir.home.texas.net
- OncoLink: University of Pennsylvania Medical Center and the University of Pennsylvania Cancer Center
  http://oncolink.upenn.edu/
- Steve Dunn's Cancer Information Page
  http://www.cancerguide.org/
- Texas Cancer Data Center
  http://www.txcancer.org/

ACUTE LEUKEMIA

NUTRITIONAL ACUITY RANKING: LEVEL 3 (MAY OFTEN BE 4)

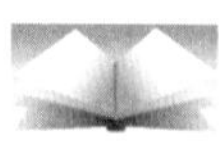

DEFINITIONS AND BACKGROUND

Leukemia involves uncontrolled proliferation of leukocytes and their precursors in blood-forming organs, with infiltration into other organs. Blood has a grayish-white appearance. Primary treatment of leukemias currently involves chemotherapy to kill attacking abnormal blood cells. Bone marrow transplantation may be feasible in some cases; see that entry. Acute leukemia is a rapidly progressing disease that results in accumulation of immature, functionless cells in the marrow and blood (http://www.leukemia-lymphoma.org). Marrow often can no longer produce enough normal red and white blood cells and platelets; anemia, frequent infections, easy bleeding, and bruising develop. Table 13–9 lists various types of leukemias.

Symptoms and signs of leukemias include easy fatigue, malaise, irritability, fever, pallor, petechiae, ecchymosis, purpura, hemorrhage, palpitations, shortness of breath, slight weight loss, bone or joint pain, cough, sternal tenderness, splenomegaly, hepatomegaly, anemia, hemorrhages such as nosebleeds, headache, nausea and vomiting, graft-versus-host disease (GVHD), and mouth ulcers.

Persons with Down's syndrome and other genetic disorders tend to have more cases of leukemia. Exposure to radiation or certain chemicals also have been implicated. Use of vitamin K at birth to prevent hemorrhage has been ruled out as a cause (Klebanoff et al., 1993). Children with acute lymphocytic leukemia (ALL) may develop transient glucose intolerance (Turner et al., 1983).

Table 13–9 Various Forms of Leukemia

1. Acute lymphocytic (lymphoblastic) leukemia, also called ALL, primarily affects bone marrow and lymph nodes. This condition mainly affects children and represents approximately 50% of all childhood leukemias. African Americans are half as likely as whites to develop ALL and have a slightly lower risk for acute myelogenous leukemia (AML). Five-year survival rate is 58%; figure is altered for children or for individuals over age 75.

2. Acute myelogenous (nonlymphocytic) leukemia (AML) consists of proliferation of myeloblasts, which are immature polynuclear leukocytes. AML is more common in adults but also accounts for just under half of cases of childhood leukemia. Average age of a patient with AML is 65-years-old. AML is slightly more common among men than women. Smoking is a known cause of AML. Chronic exposure to benzene, usually in the workplace, has been established as a cause of AML; federal and state regulations have led to a reduction in such exposures (http://www. leukemia-lymphoma.org). Extraordinary doses of irradiation can also increase the incidence of AML. Five-year survival rate is 14%; figure changes for children and persons over age 75.

3. Chronic lymphocytic leukemia (CLL) affects adults and is almost twice as common as chronic myelogenous leukemia (CML). See disease description.

4. Chronic myelogenous leukemia (CML) affects mostly adults and is very rare in children. It is half as common as CLL. See disease description.

OBJECTIVES

- Prevent hemorrhage and infections.
- Promote recovery and stabilization before bone marrow transplantation, if performed.
- Prevent constipation; correct anorexia and nausea or vomiting.
- Prevent complications and further morbidity.
- Prevent weight loss; correct as needed.
- Prevent veno-occlusive disease (VOD).

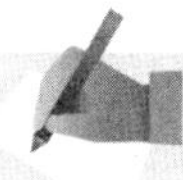

DIETARY AND NUTRITIONAL RECOMMENDATIONS

- Attractive meals should be served at proper temperatures; avoid extremes.
- Small meals may be better tolerated to avoid overwhelming patient.
- In some cases, cold or iced foods may be preferred.
- A high-protein/high-calorie/high vitamin–mineral intake should be offered; use TF or TPN if necessary.
- Extra fluids will be important during febrile states.
- Vitamin A may be beneficial; do not provide excesses.

TABLE 13–1 Protective/Preventive Nutritional Factors in Cancer

Recommendations–Protective Nutrients

Adequate vitamin A, especially in B-carotene and lycopenes (beware of excesses–they may act as pro-oxidants in some cases)
200–800 International Units (IU) vitamin E (Natural sources, d-alpha-tocopherol = need 22 IU daily for basic needs; synthetic sources, dl-alpha-tocopherol is less available = need 33 IU for basic needs)
Omega-3 fatty acids
Phytochemicals
Vitamin D3
250–500 mg vitamin C
50–200 mg selenium
Vitamin B6
Folate, thiamine, niacin, and riboflavin
Fiber from fruits, vegetables, and whole grains

Other preventive suggestions: (Note–80–90% of cancers are environmental/preventable)

1. Stop smoking.
2. Increase use of all phytochemicals, fruits and vegetables (5–10 per day), fiber, low fat milk, soy products, and fish.
3. Decrease use of alcoholic beverages.
4. Control weight; avoid obesity. Exercise daily for 30 minutes at a minimum.
5. Decrease fat (saturated or unsaturated) intake. Follow the 25/25 rule–25% kcal from fat and 25 g of fiber daily.
6. Reduce frying, grilling, and use of smoked and salt-cured foods.

TABLE 13–2 Phytochemicals

*Phytochemicals are ingredients that occur naturally in fruits, vegetables, and grains. They have not been shown to be essential nutrients and their functions in the body are under investigation. Some phytochemicals function as antioxidants to squelch free radicals. Currently, the emphasis remains on food sources, not supplements or pills.

Phytochemical Family	*Food Sources*
Allyl sulfides (allium, as S-allyl-cysteine or SAC; diallyl sulfide; allyl methyl trisulfide) *Role: decreases tumor cell growth; inhibits kinase activity; arterial vasodilator*	Onions, garlic (especially oil), leeks, chives, scallions, and red pepper
Carotenoids (a, b, lutein) and lycopenes *Role: increases activity of killer cells slightly; photoprotective agent*	Carrots, broccoli, spinach, and other green leafy vegetables, winter squash, papaya, mango, cantaloupe, tomatoes, and watermelon
Coumarins *Role: anticoagulant effect; inhibits proteolysis & lipoxygenase; anti-inflammatory agent*	Leafy green vegetables and citrus fruits
Dithiolthiones (containing sulfur) *Role: antimutagenic; chemoprotective for epithelial cells*	Cruciferous vegetables (broccoli, cauliflower, cabbage, kale, Brussels sprouts, collard greens, mustard, and turnip greens)
D-limonene, Terpenes *Role: decreases bacterial and fungal growth; decreases cancer cell growth*	Citrus fruit oils (orange, grapefruit, lemon), cherries, and citrus fruit peel
Epigallocatechin gallate (EGCG) *Role: decreases growth of hydroquinone oxidase; decreases COX-2 gene expression and cancer cell growth; decreases nitric oxide toxicity*	Green and black tea
Flavonoids (quercetin, kaempferol, myricetin) *Role: Fights free radicals*	Citrus fruits, apples, whole grains, and potato skins
Folate *Role: decreases cancer cell multiplication; efficient DNA synthesis and repair; regulates cellular S-adenosylmethionine levels and gene expression*	Leafy greens and orange juice
Herbs not commonly eaten Astragalus *Role: increases macrophages* Echinacea *Role: increases immune cells (interferon, killer cells, interleukin 2)* Ginseng *Role: increases lymphocytes*	Not available from foods at this time

(continued)

TABLE 13–2 Phytochemicals (*Continued*)

Phytochemical / Role	Sources
Herbs, spices, seasonings *Roles:* 1. *Preserves alpha-tocopherol; decreases liver inflammation* 2. *Protects plasmid DNA from degradation by radiation* 3. *Decreases ATPase* 4. *Lowers lipid peroxidation; maintains antioxidant effect* 5. *Contains flavonoids, which decrease ascorbate-dependent free radical oxidation; decreases inflammation, tumorigenesis, and malarial impact*	1. Turmeric/cumin, rosemary, thyme, sage, and oregano 2. Chili powder, black pepper, and turmeric 3. Cinnamon, caraway, cumin, coriander, and turmeric 4. Ginger 5. Licorice (glycyrrhiza)
Indole-3-carbinol *Role: Modulates and down-regulates effects of estrogen and testosterone on tumor formation and growth; inhibits cell adhesion*	Cruciferous vegetables (broccoli, cauliflower, cabbage, kale, Brussels sprouts, collard greens, mustard, or turnip greens)
Isoflavones (genistein, daidzein, biochanin A) *Role: Phytoestrogens, which attach to estrogen receptors and block real estrogens; they also lower cholesterol levels and decrease cancer activity.*	Soybeans (tofu, soy milk); legumes; raisins, and currants
Isothiocyanates (sulphorophane, etc.) *Role: Increases period of cancer latency; effective agents against fungi such as Aspergillus*	Cruciferous vegetables (broccoli, cauliflower, cabbage, kale, Brussels sprouts, collard greens, mustard, or turnip greens)
Lignans *Role: phytoestrogens, which attach to estrogen receptors and block real estrogen; they also lower cholesterol levels and decrease cancer activity.*	Flaxseed, whole grains, berries, and vegetables
Monounsaturated fats *Role: decreases tumorigenesis*	Canola and olive oils
Oligosaccharides *Role: Increase short chain fatty acid formation; decrease cholesterol and lowers insulin levels*	Whole grains
Phenolic acids (polyphenols)—these are also flavonoids *Role: superoxide anion radical (SOR)-scavenging activity; interaction of the tumor promoter benzoyl peroxide (BPO) with murine peritoneal macrophages; protects against oxidation of LDL* Ellagic acid, ferulic acid Gallic acid Chlorogenic acid Tannic acid, caffeic acid *Role: inhibit proliferation of cancer cells*	 Tomatoes, citrus fruits, carrots, whole grains, and nuts; grapes and wine Green and black grape juices Cherry juice Green and black tea and coffee
Phytates *Role: can decrease oxidative damage to cells*	Whole grains
Protease Inhibitors *Role: Inhibit action of protein-splitting enzymes; may prevent cancer cell formation or may decrease tumor size*	Whole grains
Resveratrol *Role: Decreases platelet activity*	Red grapes, wine, and grape juice
Saponins *Role: Decrease heart disease and cancer risks*	Beans and legumes, soybeans
Selenium and Glutathione *Role: Increase immune cell functioning; DNA methylation; regulation of cytokine production*	Brazil nuts, lean meats, and seafood; potatoes (glutathione)
Vitamin B6 *Role: Increases lymphocyte numbers*	Legumes, whole grains, chicken, pork, and bananas
Vitamin C *Role: Minimizes damage to neutrophils*	Citrus fruits, peppers, broccoli, tomatoes, and strawberries
Vitamin E *Role: increases antibody production + B and T cell functioning*	Wheat germ, mayonnaise, creamy salad dressings, pistachios, almonds, peanuts, and walnuts
Zinc *Role: increases neutrophil function and killer cell numbers; decreases cytokines; increases T and B cell numbers*	Wheat germ, lean beef, seafood, and black eyed peas

Derived from: Environmental Nutrition newsletters (January–February 2001); Steinmetz and Potter, 1996; American Institute for Cancer Research, 1994; Dwyer et al., 1994.

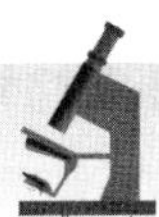

PROFILE

Clinical/History		
Height	Bone or joint pain	H&H, Serum Fe
Weight	Cough, sternal tenderness	Platelets
BMI	Splenomegaly, hepatomegaly	Lactic acid dehydrogenase (LDH) (elevated)
Weight changes (slight weight loss?)	Hemorrhages such as nosebleeds	Zinc (decreased)
Temperature (fever over 101°)	Headache	TLC (reliability varies)
Frequent infections	Nausea and vomiting	Uric acid (increased)
Malaise, irritability	Mouth ulcers	Transferrin
Pallor		Ferritin (increased)
Hemorrhage	**Lab Work**	Cytochemistry
Petechiae, ecchymosis, purpura	WBC (increased)	Flow cytometry
Palpitations, shortness of breath	Alb, prealbumin	Immunocytochemistry
	N balance	Cytogenetics
	Serum copper (increased)	Molecular genetic studies
	Gluc	

Common Drugs Used and Potential Side Effects

Chemotherapy treatments are given in the following phases (http://www3.cancer.org/cancerinfo): **Induction:** In general, the purpose of the first phase is to destroy as many cancer cells as quickly as possible and bring about a remission. **Consolidation:** The goal of this phase is to get rid of leukemia cells from where they can "hide." **Maintenance**: After the number of leukemia cells has been reduced by the first two phases of treatment, lower doses of chemotherapy drugs are given over a period of about 2 years. **Central nervous system treatment**: Because ALL often spreads to the coverings of the brain and spinal cord, patients often receive chemotherapy in the spinal fluid or radiation therapy of the head as a method of prevention. The toxicity of bone marrow transplant (BMT) treatment or peripheral blood stem cell transplant (PBSCT) may lead to bloody diarrhea, fever, and other symptoms of GVHD. Dietitians must understand and manage differences according to type of transplant, side effects, etc.

- Chemotherapy often used—methotrexate, 5-azacitidine, cytarabine, thioguanine, and daunorubicin may cause stomatitis, nausea, or vomiting. Coadministration of these agents with glucose may help. Adequate fluid intake is important.
- If L-asparaginase (Elspar) is used, hepatitis or pancreatitis may result; watch carefully. This drug is often used with ALL.
- Pegaspargase (Oncaspar) can cause nausea, vomiting, anorexia, and glucose changes.
- Gleevec is a signal transduction inhibitor, which interferes with an abnormal enzyme that sends signals to the nucleus of a cancer cell. Nausea and vomiting are potential side effects.
- Antifungals, antivirals, or antibiotic drugs may be used. Side effects vary by specific medication used.
- In some cases, interferon may be used.
- Prednisone may be used, with side effects related to steroids with chronic use. Alter diet and intake accordingly: calorie control, sodium control, etc.

Herbs, Botanicals and Supplements

- Herbs and botanical supplements should not be used without discussing with physician.

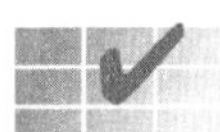

PATIENT EDUCATION

- ✓ A well-balanced diet is essential; discuss ways to improve or increase intake. (See the general cancer entry regarding side effects of disease or therapy.)
- ✓ Adequate fluid intake is important. *Tumor lysis syndrome* is a side effect caused by rapid breakdown of leukemia cells. When these cells die, they release substances into the bloodstream that can affect kidneys, heart, and nervous system. Giving patient extra fluids or certain drugs that help rid the body of these toxins can prevent this problem.
- ✓ Offer guidelines to transition from TPN or PN to enteral nutrition and oral intake.
- ✓ Discuss guidance for GVHD (acute versus chronic symptoms). Nutrition support team must recognize that short- and long-term outcomes are affected by transplant type, preparative regimens, diagnosis, disease stage, age, and nutritional status (Lenssen et al., 2001).

For More Information

- ✦ The Leukemia-Lymphoma Society
  1311 Mamaroneck Ave., White Plains, NY 10605
  http://www.leukemia-lymphoma.org

CHRONIC LEUKEMIA

NUTRITIONAL ACUITY RANKING: LEVEL 3

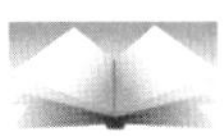

DEFINITIONS AND BACKGROUND

Chronic lymphocytic leukemia (CLL) involves a crowding out of normal leukocytes in lymph glands, interfering with body's ability to produce other blood cells. CLL is more common in people older than 50 years of age and in males. Chronic granulocytic leukemia has similar overproduction of white blood cells in the bone marrow, often believed to be developed through an abnormal acquired chromosome (Philadelphia, Ph1), perhaps as a result of ionizing radiation.

Symptoms and signs of chronic forms of leukemia include anemia, increased infections, bleeding, enlarged lymph nodes (in lymphatic form), night sweats, fever, weight loss, and anorexia. Five-year survival rates for CLL are 71%, and CML is 32%; figures differ for children and people over 75. Primary treatment of leukemias at this time involves chemotherapy to kill attacking abnormal blood cells. Bone marrow transplantation may be feasible in some cases; see appropriate entry.

OBJECTIVES

- Prevent hemorrhage, infections, further complications, and morbidity.
- Promote recovery and stabilization before bone marrow transplantation, if required.
- Prevent or correct constipation, nausea, vomiting, and anorexia.
- Alter diet according to medications and therapies such as chemotherapy.
- Maintain weight that is appropriate for height. Correct weight loss if necessary.

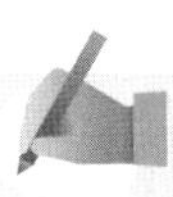

DIETARY AND NUTRITIONAL RECOMMENDATIONS

- Serve attractive meals at temperatures that are tolerated. In some cases, cold foods are preferred.
- Small, frequent meals generally are more desired than large meals.
- TF or use TPN, if appropriate or necessary, but avoid sepsis and fluid overload.
- Extra fluids will be important to reduce a febrile state. If on interferon, increased fluids can significantly decrease treatment-related nausea.

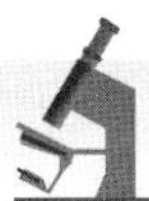

PROFILE

Clinical/History

Height
Weight
BMI
Weight changes (weight loss?)
Blood pressure (BP)
Increased infections
Bleeding
Enlarged lymph nodes (in lymphatic form)
Night sweats
Fever?
Anorexia

Lab Work

WBC
Pro Time (PT)
Transferrin
Serum ferritin (increased)
TLC (varied results)
N balance
Uric acid (increased)
Platelets
H&H
Alb

Common Drugs Used and Potential Side Effects

- Chemotherapeutic agents may be used, with varying side effects. Chlorambucil (Leukeran) and busulfan are common; nausea, severe fatigue, flu-like symptoms, low-grade temperature, vomiting, glossitis, and cheilosis may occur. Avoid hot, spicy, or acidic foods, if not tolerated.
- Antifungals, antivirals, or antibiotic drugs may be used. Side effects vary with specific medication used.
- Pegaspargase (Oncaspar) can cause nausea, vomiting, anorexia, and glucose changes.

Herbs, Botanicals and Supplements

- Herbs and botanical supplements should not be used without discussing with physician.

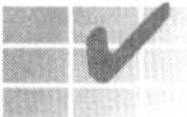

PATIENT EDUCATION

- Discuss alternative ways to make meals more attractive and appealing.
- Discuss importance of adequate fluid intake.
- For other side effects of the disease and therapies, see general cancer entry.

For More Information

- The Leukemia-Lymphoma Society
  1311 Mamaroneck Ave., White Plains, NY 10605
  http://www.leukemia-lymphoma.org

BONE MARROW TRANSPLANTATION

NUTRITIONAL ACUITY RANKING: LEVEL 4

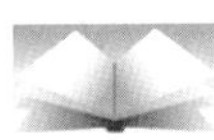

DEFINITIONS AND BACKGROUND

Bone marrow transplantation involves replacement of medically destroyed bone marrow with histocompatible donor bone marrow to establish a graft and reinstate production of normal cellular blood components. Autologous BMT (AMBT) is one's own bone marrow; allogeneic BMT comes from a matched donor. There are also syngeneic, SBMT, (from a genetically identical person such as a twin), and nonmyeloablative (treatments that do not totally eradicate stem cell lines) transplants as well. MUD is a transplant using a matched unrelated donor.

Transplantation often is necessary in leukemia, aplastic anemia, advanced breast cancer, or in multiple myeloma. BMT is being studied for use with other diseases. Interestingly, transfer of type 1 diabetes often occurs after bone marrow transplantation, supporting the belief that diabetes is immunologic in nature (Lampeter et al., 1993).

Peripheral blood stem cell transplant (PBSCT) differs from BMT in that under the influence of an administered artificial growth factor called granulocyte colony stimulating factor (G-CSF), stem cells are stimulated to grow and leave bone marrow as they increase in number to such a degree that there is not enough room for all of them within the bone marrow (http://www.bmtsupport.ie/stem_cell.html). They may be used instead of bone marrow for autografts (where patients are given high doses of chemotherapy, with their own bone marrow infused afterwards) in CML, AML, CLL, ALL, and lymphomas. PBSCT may be used during intensive chemotherapy where neutropenia may have otherwise prohibited its use.

Health professionals caring for patients undergoing peripheral blood stem cell transplantation need to understand the basics of the procedure to manage their patients (Lebel-Medieros et al., 1998). Hospitalized transplant patients resume oral intake sooner than an ambulatory group, but no differences exist in time spent on TPN or days it takes to resume good protein intake (Stern, 2000).

Side effects from stem cell transplantation can be divided into early and long-term effects. Early side effects are basically the same as those of any other type of high-dose chemotherapy, caused by damage to bone marrow and other rapidly reproducing tissues of the body. Long-term side effects could include radiation damage to the lungs with shortness of breath, GVHD, damage to the ovaries causing infertility and loss of menstrual periods, damage to the thyroid gland that causes problems with metabolism, cataracts (damage to the lens of the eye), bone damage with possible need to have part of the bone and joint replaced, and growth changes in children.

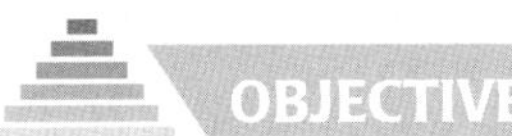

OBJECTIVES

Pretransplant:

- Provide adequate nutrient stores (glucose, calories, vitamins, and minerals as well as protein).
- Assure adequate hydration.

Posttransplant:

- Individualize needs; promote engraftment of marrow. Rejection occurs less often in well-nourished patients.
- Prevent infection, which is common. Prevent oral infections, mucositis, gastroenteritis, and pneumocystosis.
- Reduce nausea, vomiting, and diarrhea, when present.
- Improve weight status; promote anabolism.
- Correct anorexia, stomatitis, xerostomia, and depression—all of which reduce total intake. Early satiety is also common.
- Avoid or prevent GVHD with rash, erythroderma, hair loss, jaundice, abdominal pain, emaciation, pneumonitis, infections, and gastrointestinal (GI) tract problems.
- Prevent or correct hepatic veno-occlusive disease (VOD) from high doses of chemotherapy in preparation for the BMT. Rapid weight gain, elevated bilirubin, right upper quadrant (RUQ) pain, ascites, jaundice, and hepatomegaly can occur.
- Replenish nutrient stores and promote wound healing. Prevent surgical complications, including postoperative bleeding, severe pancreatitis, edema, ascites, diarrhea, or ulcers.
- Promote positive nitrogen balance when possible.
- Correct hyperglycemia from metabolic stress, insulin resistance, and medication side effects.
- Monitor closely for renal insufficiency and necessary changes for diet.
- Prevent or prepare for long-term complications such as hyperphagia and obesity, insulin resistance and diabetes, hyperlipidemia, hypertension, and osteoporosis.

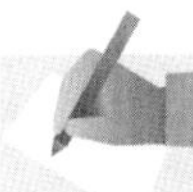

DIETARY AND NUTRITIONAL RECOMMENDATIONS

- TPN may be needed to prepare patient before transplant and to initiate recovery posttransplant. PN supports long-term survival but not short-term survival; TF has fewer complications (Klein and Koretz, 1994). Glutamine should be an additive for both TPN and TF products (McBurney et al., 1994).

- In some cases, use of a "low bacteria" (neutropenic) diet may be useful for several months before and after transplantation. Protective isolation may be needed, and products may require special preparation (as with a laminar flow hood). Keep foods at a temperature that is safe to prevent food infection. Microwave hot foods immediately before service. Ensure careful handwashing.
- Provide 35–40 kcal/kg, or calculate basal energy expenditure (BEE) × 1.3 to maintain weight or BEE × 1.5 for infection, GVHD, and neutropenia.
- Protein intake should be 1.5–2 g/kg of weight; fat intake should be 1–2.5 g/kg.
- Sterile water may be used to keep hydration at an adequate level to prevent renal problems.
- If needed, patient may need a low-lactose/low-fiber/low-fat/bland diet. Progress, as tolerated, to a normal diet over time.
- As patient recovers and no longer requires a protective setting, use of live-culture pasteurized yogurt may be beneficial to increase bowel flora. Lactobacillus acidophilus therapy also can be helpful.

PROFILE

Clinical/History

- Height
- Weight
- BMI
- Weight changes
- Temperature
- Ascites, jaundice
- I & O

Lab Work

- H&H
- Bilirubin
- Gluc
- Mg++
- Ca++
- Complete blood count (CBC)
- ANC (absolute neutrophil count) to evaluate engrafting (desired = 500)
- Na+, K+
- Alb, prealbumin
- RBP
- Serum phosphorus (low from cyclosporin A)
- Uric acid
- Chol, Trig
- TLC (varied reliability)
- Ferritin
- Transferrin
- BUN, Creat

Common Drugs Used and Potential Side Effects

- Total body irradiation (TBI) may be performed in some cases. Side effects vary for each individual, but anorexia, diarrhea, and mucositis or esophagitis are common.
- Chemotherapy drugs may be used, such as busulfan (to destroy marrow stem cells) or cyclophosphamide (Cytoxan), which can cause nausea, vomiting, diarrhea, and anorexia. Methotrexate, fludarabine, carmustine, and cyclophosphamide may cause anorexia, mucositis, and esophagitis; some also cause diarrhea.
- Antibiotics such as amphotericin may be used to fight infections. Nausea, stomach pain, or vomiting may occur.
- Clotrimazole (Mycelex) may be used for bowel preparation. Nausea or vomiting can result.
- Cyclosporine (CSA) as Sandimmune or Prednisone may be given to prevent GVHD for 1 to several months postoperatively. Numerous side effects can result (e.g., nausea and vomiting, skin rashes, hemorrhagic cystitis, altered potassium metabolism).
- Analgesics, antihistamines, and antidepressants may be used; monitor for specific side effects.
- Acyclovir may be given prophylactically to resolve oral ulcers (Woo et al., 1993). Headaches, GI distress, or diarrhea may occur.
- Gleevec interferes with an abnormal enzyme that sends signals to the nucleus of a cancer cell. Nausea and vomiting are potential side effects.
- Neutropenia secondary to immune suppression may be managed with Neupogen and a low-bacteria diet.

Herbs, Botanicals and Supplements

- Herbs and botanical supplements should not be used without discussing with physician.
- St. John's wort and Echinacea should not be taken with cyclosporine, because they alter drug functioning.

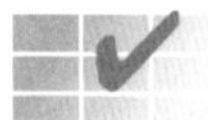

PATIENT EDUCATION

- ✓ Discuss needed protection against environmental infections (safe food handling and preparation, keeping foods below 40° or above 140°, use of sterile water, etc.).
- ✓ The "low-bacteria" (also called neutropenic) diet used in some cases may include careful use of raw fruits and vegetables, milk, and shellfish—all of which may be contaminated easily with bacteria. Results from this diet are not conclusive but often are recommended by BMT units.
- ✓ Small, frequent meals of bland, cold consistency may be well tolerated.
- ✓ Discuss any necessary nutritional support methods and procedures to be used at home or in discharge planning. Transition from TPN and PN to enteral nutrition or oral diet will be helpful.

For More Information

- Bone Marrow Support Group
  http://www.bmtsupport.ie/stem_cell.html

LYMPHOMAS AND TUMORS

BRAIN TUMOR

NUTRITIONAL ACUITY RANKING: LEVEL 3

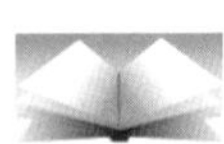

DEFINITIONS AND BACKGROUND

A neoplasm arising from intracranial cells, a brain tumor may be benign if it is unlikely to spread or malignant if it is likely to spread. In children, brain tumors are most common in girls aged 5–9 years. Constituting 50% of brain tumors, a glioma is a tumor of neurological origin. A neuroma, a tumor composed of nerve cells, may occur along any nerve and is not necessarily associated with a brain tumor. A glioblastoma multiforme is a CNS neoplasm, especially related to the cerebrum. Meningiomas affect the meninges.

Dietary factors may play an important role in development of brain tumors (gliomas and meningiomas). In a case-controlled study in China (Hu, LaVecchia et al., 1999), consumption of fresh vegetables (specifically Chinese cabbage and onion), fruit, fresh fish, and poultry was inversely related to the risk of developing brain cancer. A protective effect was also seen for vitamin E intake, calcium and, although insignificantly, beta-carotene and vitamin C. Risk of brain cancer increased with consumption of salted vegetables and salted fish.

Data have suggested an interaction between the effects of N-nitroso compounds and protein or cholesterol intakes (Kaplan et al., 1997). Antioxidants are also being studied at this time.

Iowa residents with brain cancer and healthy controls completed a mail survey about lifetime residential history, sources of drinking water, beverage intake, and other potential sources of risk for brain cancer. Association of chlorinated water was stronger among those who had above-median intakes of tap water; similar findings were found for estimates of mean lifetime exposure to trihalomethanes (Cantor et al., 1999). More research is needed.

Symptoms and signs include headache, vertigo, altered consciousness or convulsions, inability to follow commands, mental or personality changes, unequal pupil response, hemianopsia, blurred or decreased vision, ptosis, tinnitus, altered gait, dysphagia, vomiting with or without nausea, aphasia, elevated blood pressure, and loss of sense of smell.

OBJECTIVES

- Provide adequate calories without excess.
- Avoid constipation and straining.
- Prevent upper respiratory infections with coughing, which can increase intracranial pressure.
- Counteract side effects of therapy—radiation, surgery, etc.
- Correct hypoalbuminemia.
- Monitor carefully for elevated blood glucose levels, which may occur secondary to corticosteroids that are used to control brain edema.

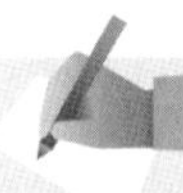

DIETARY AND NUTRITIONAL RECOMMENDATIONS

- Maintain diet, as ordered, with extra fluid, unless contraindicated.
- Provide adequate fiber in diet.
- Alter texture and liquids, if necessary, for dysphagia. If necessary, TF or offer TPN.
- Limit sodium to 4–6 g daily to correct cerebral edema.

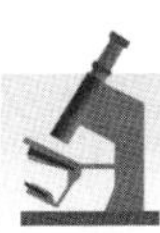

PROFILE

Clinical/History

- Height
- Weight
- BMI
- Weight changes
- Aphasia
- BP (elevated?)
- Cerebral edema, headaches
- Vertigo
- Altered consciousness or convulsions
- Inability to follow commands
- Mental or personality changes
- Unequal pupil response
- Hemianopsia, blurred or decreased vision
- Tinnitus
- Altered gait
- Dysphagia
- Vomiting with or without nausea
- Loss of sense of smell.
- Temperature

Lab Work

- Gluc (elevated)
- Cerebrospinal fluid (CSF)—elevated protein
- Alb, prealbumin, RBP
- TLC, WBC (altered)
- WBC in CSF (Normal [NL] or increased)
- Transferrin
- ALT (elevated)
- CT scan
- Skull x-ray
- Electroencephalogram (EEG)

Common Drugs Used and Potential Side Effects

- Steroid therapy may be used. Decrease sodium and increase potassium if appropriate. Negative nitrogen balance or hyperglycemia may result over time. Maintain near normal blood glucose levels if possible.
- Anticonvulsants are often used. Side effects may include a decrease in serum folacin levels and other nutrients; monitor individually.
- Analgesics generally are used to relieve pain. Vitamin C depletion is common.
- Use of procarbazine (an antineoplastic) may warrant restriction of tyramine-containing foods secondary to its monoamine oxidase (MAO)-inhibitor–like action.

Herbs, Botanicals and Supplements

- Herbs and botanical supplements should not be used without discussing with physician.

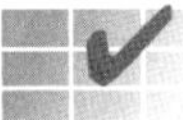

PATIENT EDUCATION

- ✓ The importance of regular and attractive meals should be stressed to help appetite if fair or poor. Keep in mind that sense of smell may have declined recently.
- ✓ Discuss importance of a balanced diet with good sources of protein at meals.

For More Information

- Clinical Trials and Noteworthy Treatments for Brain Tumors: Musella Foundation
  1100 Peninsula Blvd
  Hewlett, NY 11557
  516-295-4740
  http://www.virtualtrials.com/musella.cfm
- Brain Cancer
  http://cancernet.nci.nih.gov/wyntk_pubs/brain.htm
- National Brain Tumor Foundation
  1–800-934-CURE
  www.braintumor.org
- Onco-Link—Brain Cancer
  http://cancer.med.upenn.edu/disease/brain/

BREAST CANCER

NUTRITIONAL ACUITY RANKING: LEVEL 2–3

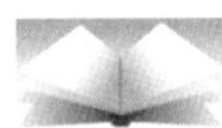

DEFINITIONS AND BACKGROUND

Breast cancer (mammary carcinoma) is the second most common site of CA in women, affecting one in nine women at some point in their lives. Studies have now identified genetic predictors such as the HER-2 gene. BRCA-1 is a gene located on chromosome 17 which, if mutated, may predict high risk. Onset of breast cancer is more common after age 30 but is not limited to one specific decade of life. Breast cancer in men is uncommon and generally is preceded by gynecomastia.

Fertility and ovarian function probably play a role in onset of breast cancer; estrogen exposure seems to be the critical factor. Fetal and childhood nutrition may have a greater impact on risk for breast cancer than diets during adulthood. Exposure to diets that produce high levels of estrogen seem to be most important in utero and after menopause. High estrogen levels during reproductive years seem to be protective.

Incidence of breast cancer is higher in women who have a family or personal history of breast cancer or a history of breast tissue dysplasia. Early menarche (before 12 years of age) yields a four times higher risk; obesity, nulliparity, or late age for first pregnancy and late age at menopause yield higher than average risks (Hankin, 1993). Lactation is not always found to be protective. Prolonged breastfeeding appears to be associated with only a marginal decrease in risk of breast cancer (Lipworth et al., 2000). However, a large cohort study in Iceland found that ever lactating was associated with a decreased risk of breast cancer, and longer duration was more protective (Tryggvadottir et al., 2001).

Protective effect of obesity against premenopausal breast cancer applies mainly to teenaged girls. Obesity and Western dietary patterns may independently provoke hyperinsulinemic insulin resistance at puberty. In teen girls this has been related to abnormal ovarian steroidogenesis and anovulation, which may decrease mammary carcinogenesis. If obesity continues after adolescence, higher plasma levels of insulin-like growth factor 1 (IGF-1) associated with hyperinsulinemia can interact with estrogen receptors in mammary epithelium and lead to increased proliferative activity (Stoll, 1998).

The heaviest and tallest women in their 40s and 50s have two times the risk of developing breast cancer. Higher bone mineral density predicts risk of breast cancer in older women (Cauley et al., 1996). Physical activity during leisure time and at work is associated with reduced risk of breast cancer (Thune et al., 1997).

Weight gain and use of estrogen replacement therapy (ERT) appear to be positively associated with breast cancer risk in postmenopausal women (Jernstrom, 1999). Avoiding weight gain after menopause may contribute importantly to prevention of breast cancer (Huang et al., 1997; Trentham-Dietz et al., 1997). Weight gain in the years preceding onset is critical; increased fat cell adiposity increases estrogen availability.

Weight gain is a common observation among women after diagnosis of breast cancer (Demark-Wahnefried et al., 1997). Gains in weight range up to 50 pounds and are influenced by menopausal status, nodal status, and type/duration and intensity of treatment. Weight gain appears to be greater among premenopausal women, among those who are node positive, and among those receiving higher-dose, multiagent, and longer-duration regimens. Weight gain during therapy may increase risk of recurrence and decrease survival. African-American ethnicity, time, adjuvant chemotherapy, current energy intake, and postmenopausal status are important factors; lower physical activity and higher energy intake are most influential (Rock et al., 1999). Changes in rates of metabolism, physical activity, and dietary intake are all plausible mechanisms and call for more research.

Among women with radiologically dense tissue in over 50% of the breast area, consumption of a low-fat, high-CHO diet for 2 years reduces area of density but not percentage of dense tissue; in addition, weight loss and becoming postmenopausal allow reductions in area of dense breast tissue (Boyd et al., 1997). Fat intake during adulthood does not seem to be associated with overall risk for breast cancer, except in women with no history of benign breast disease where intake of unsaturated fat (oleic, especially) appears to be a risk (Velie et al., 2000).

Risk of breast cancer is increased with intake of well-done meats, probably because of heterocyclic amines formed during high temperature cooking (Zheng et al., 1998). In addition, high alcohol intakes tend to increase risks in postmenopausal women (van den Brandt et al., 1995). Saturated fat intake has not been proven to be a definitive risk. In the Nurses Health Study, no association was found between type and amount of fat intake and risk of breast cancer (Holmes et al., 1999).

Tumors are frequently found in the upper/outer quadrant of the breast (45%) and nipple area (25%), with 30% identified in other breast areas. In early stages, a single nontender, firm, or hard mass with poorly defined margins may exist. Later, skin or nipple retraction, axillary lymphadenopathy, breast enlargement, redness, mild edema, and pain may occur. In late stages, ulceration, moderate edema, and metastases to bone, liver, or brain are common. Staging of breast cancer is described in Table 13–10.

TABLE 13–10 Staging of Breast Cancer

Stage 0	In situ
Stage I	Rarely metastasizing/noninvasive (less than 1 inch in diameter)
Stage II	Rarely metastasizing/invasive (1–2 inches in diameter)
Stage III	Moderately metastasizing/invasive (2 inches or larger)
Stage IV	Highly metastasizing/invasive

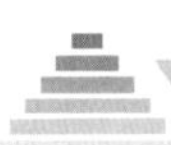

OBJECTIVES

- Control side effects of therapy and treatments (local or extensive mastectomy, chemotherapy, external beam radiation therapy, brachytherapy).
- Promote good nutritional status to reduce future incidents and recurrence. Risks for deficiency of vitamins B12, folacin, thiamin, iron, and riboflavin are common (Ames et al., 1993).
- Encourage regular breast self-examinations.
- Maintain or attain appropriate weight for height. Patient should lose weight before treatment, if obese, but be careful not to lose lean body mass (LBM).
- Increase likelihood of survival and wellness.
- For mastectomy patients, promote wound healing and prevent infection.
- Monitor genetic responsiveness to 6-n-propylthiouracil (PROP) and preferences for fruits and vegetables. Generally, lower acceptance of cruciferous and selected green and raw vegetables occurs in women who report disliking such foods; they tend to be medium or super tasters of PROP (Drewnowski, 2000). PROP-sensitive tasters may seek to reduce bitterness by adding fat, sugar, or salt to their vegetables.

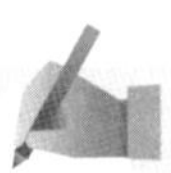

DIETARY AND NUTRITIONAL RECOMMENDATIONS

- A diet with control of excessive calories and fat may be helpful. Some theories suggest that obesity may promote original tumor growth, and calories seem to play greatest role. A 20% fat intake, with decrease in saturated fatty acids (SFAs) to 7%, has been suggested.
- At least 5–9 fruits and vegetables and 6 grain foods daily should be encouraged for access to important nutrients and phytochemicals. A serving is: 1 piece of fresh fruit, 6 oz (¾ cup) 100% fruit juice, ½ cup cooked vegetables or canned fruit, 1 cup leafy vegetables or salad, 1 handful (¼ cup) dried fruit, ½ cup dried peas or beans.
- Alcoholic beverages should be discouraged strongly, because there is some possible etiological role.
- Dietary sources of vitamins and minerals that meet Dietary Reference Intake (DRI) and RDA levels are usually adequate, but a general supplement also may be safely recommended. Demographic and personal characteristics, time passed since diagnosis, and stage of cancer at diagnosis are predictive of dietary supplement use by women at risk for breast cancer recurrence; supplement use is common in 80% of women with a history of breast cancer (Newman, 1998).
- Intake of soy seems to be protective for most women unless they are estrogen-sensitive. An intake of soy daily does not seem to be a risk factor for cancer promotion; more studies are underway.

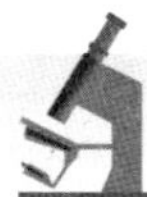

PROFILE

Clinical/History

Height
Weight
BMI
Weight changes
Anorexia, nausea
Breast self-examination–masses?
Calcifications
Biopsy
Skin or nipple retraction
Axillary lymphadenopathy
Breast enlargement
Redness, mild edema, pain
Ulceration, moderate edema
I & O
Temperature

Lab Work

Serum estrogen
Estrogen receptors (positive or negative)
Carcinoembryonic antigen (CEA)
Prolactin
TLC (varies)
Ca++
H&H
ESR to evaluate metastasis
Gluc
Alk phos
CBC
Chol, Trig
Alb, prealbumin
Mammography

Common Drugs Used and Potential Side Effects

- For patients who are estrogen receptor positive, hormonal therapy may be a breast cancer promoter; oral contraceptive use should be monitored or discontinued. Estrogen replacement (to prevent osteoporosis) increases risk levels by 2.5% annually but reduces risks for stroke, hip fracture, and CHD. Antiestrogen therapy with tamoxifen (Noraldex) is common. Tamoxifen may be prescribed to treat estrogen-dependent breast cancer or to be used preventively for women at high risk. Nausea, vomiting, and hot flashes are common side effects.
- For patients who are estrogen receptor negative, hormonal therapy actually may be recommended (e.g., progesterone and androgen therapy). Megestrol acetate (a hormonal antineoplastic drug, a synthetic derivative of progesterone) can reverse anorexia and weight loss in some women. Appetite improvement often is noted.
- Chemotherapy also may be used. Taste alterations are common for beef, chicken, and coffee. Cytoxan (cyclophosphamide) requires extra fluid intake. Doxorubicin, 5-fluorouracil, and methotrexate are also commonly used; many GI side effects are noted.
- Arimidex can cause anorexia, weight changes, nausea, vomiting, dry mouth, constipation, and diarrhea.
- Hormone replacement therapy (HRT) may lower chances of return of cancer; larger studies are needed (O'Meara et al., 2001).

Herbs, Botanicals and Supplements

- Herbs and botanical supplements should not be used without discussing with physician.
- Dehydroepiandrosterone (DHEA, taken to delay aging) may stimulate late promotion of breast cancer in postmenopausal women and should be avoided. Human mammary cancer cells are depressed by DHEA in presence of high estrogen levels but stimulated by DHEA in presence of low estrogen levels (Stoll, 1999).
- With use of methotrexate (Rheumatrex), avoid Echinacea for potential damage to liver.

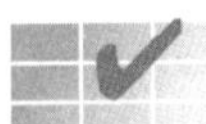

PATIENT EDUCATION

- ✓ For prevention and to reduce risk of recurrence, breast cancer detection projects are available throughout the United States. Check with local chapter of the National Cancer Institute (NCI) and the American Cancer Society (ACS). Early detection of new tumors is crucial as lower stage tumors are much easier to control.
- ✓ Discuss ways to make meals more appetizing, especially if appetite is poor.
- ✓ Counsel patient regarding a prudent diet to prevent weight gain or to lose weight if needed.
- ✓ Swimming and brisk walking tend to reduce risk levels (Hankin, 1993). Exercise seems to be an important preventive factor.
- ✓ Daughters of women with breast cancer should have a first mammogram before 40 years of age as a baseline and annually every 1–2 years thereafter. Lumps and changes should be reported immediately to a physician.
- ✓ Reduction or elimination of alcoholic beverage intake should be considered.
- ✓ For treatment and recovery, maintain healthy weight for height, increase fruit and vegetable intake, limit use of alcoholic beverages, decrease overall fat and increase overall fiber intakes, and promptly identify and manage treatment-related side effects.

For More Information

- American Cancer Society
  Reach to Recovery Program
  1–800-227–2345
- Breast Cancer Risk Assessment Tool (BCRAT)
  http://bcra.nci.nih.gov/hrc
- Cornell University Program on Breast Cancer and Environmental Risk Factors in New York State
  http://www.cfe.cornell.edu/bcerf/
- National Alliance of Breast Cancer Organizations
  http://www.nabco.org/
- National Breast Cancer Coalition
  http://www.natlbcc.org/
- Onco-Link
  http://cancer.med.upenn.edu/disease/breast/general/
- Y-Me
  1–800-221–2141
  http://www.y-me.org/

CHORIOCARCINOMA

NUTRITIONAL ACUITY RANKING: LEVEL 3

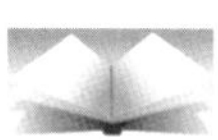

DEFINITIONS AND BACKGROUND

Choriocarcinoma involves a highly malignant neoplasm from the chorionic epithelium; it may develop after a hydatidiform mole, a miscarriage, or a full-term delivery. Rarely, it may occur in males (testes). Symptoms and signs include profuse or intermittent vaginal bleeding, discharge between menses, cough, hemoptysis, headache, nausea and vomiting, hypertension, tachypnea, vaginal or vulvar lesion, anemia, sepsis, weight loss, and cachexia. Alternative names include chorioblastoma, trophoblastic tumor, chorioepithelioma, invasive/malignant mole, gestational trophoblastic disease, and gestational trophoblastic neoplasia

After an initial diagnosis, a careful history and examination are done to rule out metastasis (spread to other organs). Chemotherapy is treatment of choice today; a hysterectomy is rarely indicated. Over 90% of women with malignant but nonmetastatic disease are able to maintain reproductive capacity.

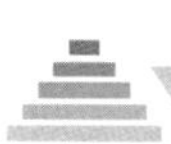

OBJECTIVES

- ▲ Maintain appropriate weight for height. Correct weight loss and cachexia.
- ▲ Correct side effects of chemotherapy if used.
- ▲ Treat and correct all other side effects of therapy and disease state.
- ▲ Prepare patient for surgery, if necessary.

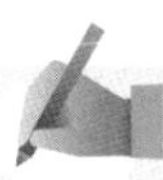

DIETARY AND NUTRITIONAL RECOMMENDATIONS

- Modify diet to patient preferences.
- Increase liquids as needed.
- Provide adequate protein, B-complex vitamins, iron, calories, and other nutrients for wound healing, as appropriate. Use RDA and DRI levels as a guide.
- Alter texture of diet if patient is fatigued at mealtimes or if stomatitis occurs after chemotherapy.

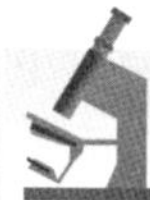

PROFILE

Clinical/History

- Height
- Weight
- BMI
- Weight loss?
- Nausea, vomiting
- Temperature
- I & O
- BP; Hypertension?
- Vaginal bleeding
- Discharge between menses
- Cough, hemoptysis
- Headache
- Nausea and vomiting
- Tachypnea
- Vaginal or vulvar lesion
- Sepsis?
- Cachexia?

Lab Work

- Human chorionic gonadotropin (HCG) titer
- Alb, prealbumin
- Transferrin
- Gluc
- H&H
- Serum Fe
- Ca++, Mg++
- TLC (varies)
- Na+, K+
- ALT (increased)

Common Drugs Used and Potential Side Effects

- Methotrexate may be used; nausea and vomiting are common side effects. Administer with glucose to reduce toxicity.
- Vincristine or dactinomycin may also be used. Constipation or dysphagia can occur with vincristine. Dry mouth or stomatitis/esophagitis may occur with dactinomycin.

Herbs, Botanicals and Supplements

- Herbs and botanical supplements should not be used without discussing with physician.

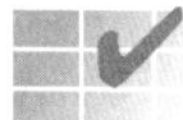

PATIENT EDUCATION

- ✔ Nausea or vomiting may require small, frequent feedings and control of fluid intake at mealtimes.
- ✔ See general cancer entry for more suggestions specific to individual patient's side effects from therapy.

For More Information

- ✦ Onco-Link—Choriocarcinoma
http://cancer.med.upenn.edu/specialty/gyn_onc/gestat/

COLORECTAL CANCER (INTESTINAL CARCINOMAS)

NUTRITIONAL ACUITY RANKING: LEVEL 3–4

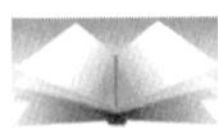

DEFINITIONS AND BACKGROUND

Between 50,000 and 60,000 deaths occur annually from colorectal cancer; approximately 7,000 of these are from rectal CA. Colorectal cancer currently is the second most common type of CA. Family history of colorectal cancer is a risk factor. High risk for intestinal cancer also exists among patients with ulcerative colitis and Crohn's disease after 8 years' duration. Incidence of colorectal cancer rises significantly after age 50 and doubles with each successive decade. Fecal occult blood test and flexible sigmoidoscopy are methods of choice.

In cancer of the small intestine, malignancy generally is found in the lower duodenum and lower ileum, with a high rate of mortality and few early symptoms; it presents in approximately 5% of cases. In the large intestine, slow-growing malignancies are usually found in the cecum, lower ascending, and sigmoid colon; prognosis is optimistic but few early symptoms are found. Rectal CA is more common in men than in women and often occurs after middle age, with bleeding, pain, and irregular bowel habits.

The adenomatous polyp is the precursor of most, if not all, colorectal cancers. The average 10–12 years that it takes for a polyp to undergo malignant degeneration provides a window of opportunity to identify and remove benign polyps before they become invasive cancers (Cohen, 1996). The Polyp Prevention Trial identified that low-fat, high dietary fiber diets do not always protect against colorectal cancer or adenomas (Fuchs et al., 1999; Schatzkin et al., 2000). Another study identified that a high-fiber wheat bran supplement does not protect against polyps recurrence either (Alberts et al., 2000). Overall, the American Gastroenterology Association (2000) still supports the use of whole grains, fruits, and vegetables to achieve an intake of 30–35 g per day.

Taking 1,200 mg as calcium carbonate daily is associated with moderate but significant reduction in risk of recurrent colorectal adenomas (Baron et al., 1999). Dietary calcium, vitamin D, and lactose may play a role in protection against colorectal cancer (Ma et al., 2001).

Evidence from epidemiologic studies suggests that folate status is inversely related to risk of certain cancers—especially colorectal cancer (Choi and Mason, 2000). Folate's role in formation of S-adenosylmethionine, the universal methyl donor, and in the formation of purine and thymidine for synthesis of DNA and RNA has been postulated.

Studies suggest that intake of vitamin C may reduce the recurrence of polyps (Cahill, 1993). Other studies have suggested that intake of fruits and vegetables is more crucial, perhaps from phytochemical or resistant starch content (Greenberg et al., 1994; Phillips et al., 1995). Increased dietary intake of foods high in lutein (spinach, broccoli, lettuce, tomatoes, oranges, orange juice, carrots, celery, and greens) may help prevent colon cancer. Beta-carotene, alpha-carotene, lycopene, zeaxanthins are not specifically related to risk of colon cancer (Slattery et al., 2000). Persons with higher intakes of these and vitamin C have lower relative risks overall for colon cancer (Zhang et al., Dietary carotenoids, 1999).

High alcohol use is also a risk (Giovannucci et al., Alcohol. . ., 1995). Excessive iron intake should be avoided because of the tendency to increase adenoma formation (Nelson et al., 1994).

Excess body weight is a risk factor for colon cancer in both men and women (Ford et al., 1999). Abdominal obesity and its metabolic effects of increased blood glucose and insulin levels are positively associated with risk of colorectal cancer (Schoen et al., 1999). Physical inactivity and obesity may increase risk of colon cancer via an increase in synthesis of prostaglandin E2 (PGE2) in the rectal mucosa (Martinez et al., 1999).

Intakes of red and white meat appear to be important risk factors for colon cancer. High BMI, high intake of red meat, and low legume intake seem to triple the level of risk (Singh et al., 1998). Intake of heterocyclic amines (formed in meat and fish during cooking) within the usual dietary range is unlikely to cause cancer of colon, rectum, bladder, or kidney; however, very high intakes (over 1,900 mg) may increase risk of cancer (Augustsson, 1999). Both heterocyclic aromatic amines (HAAs) and polycyclic aromatic hydrocarbons (PAHs) are mutagens in well-cooked meats that are counterbalanced by lower fat content when consumed in moderate amounts (Muscat and Wynder, 1994).

Symptoms and signs of intestinal cancers include: weakness, weight loss, anorexia, anemia, dehydration, electrolyte imbalance, intestinal obstruction, bowel abscess, fistula, and metastases to other organs (lungs, kidneys, and bone). For GI cancers, symptoms include nausea and vomiting, anorexia, upper abdominal pain, weight loss, and anemia. In colorectal cancers, symptoms include altered bowel habits, rectal bleeding, abdominal cramping, pain, and distention. The right side of the colon (ascending) absorbs fluids and salts; cancer spreads upward here; obstruction is rare. The left side of the colon (the descending colon) stores feces; cancer here tends to encircle the bowel and cause obstructions. If surgery is required, maintaining the ileocecal valve is crucial.

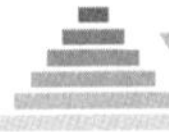

OBJECTIVES

- ▲ Decrease residue, especially with obstruction, until fiber is better tolerated. Whole-grain breads (especially rye) seem to be effective in lowering fecal bile acids (Korpela et al., 1992).
- ▲ Prevent further weight loss; correct anemia and dehydration.

- Counteract side effects of therapies; resection is common (see short gut syndrome entry in Section 7). Chemotherapy or radiation is also used in some cases.
- Provide nutrients in a tolerable form—oral, parenteral, or enteral.
- Provide sufficient calcium, vitamin D, and dairy products; low levels have been found to be correlated with colon cancer (Bostick et al., 1993). Calcium may block tumor-producing effects of dietary fats by binding free fatty acids in the lumen.
- Prevent or ameliorate starvation diarrhea.

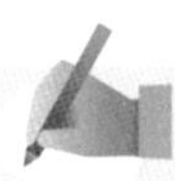

DIETARY AND NUTRITIONAL RECOMMENDATIONS

- TPN or TF may be needed for an extended period of time. Include glutamine in either type of solution.
- Administer parenteral fluids with adequate electrolytes, vitamins C and K, and selenium (if used over a long time). Vitamin D, calcium, iron, and fat intakes also should be monitored for adequacy. Zinc may also be low (Song et al., 1993).
- With ileal resection—vitamin B12 deficiency can occur; bile salts may be lost in diarrhea; hyperoxaluria and renal oxalate stones can be a problem. With massive bowel resection, malabsorption, malnutrition, metabolic acidosis, and gastric hypersecretion may result.
- Ileostomy and colostomy—salt and sodium/water balance are problems. Ostomy diets may be needed (see ileostomy and colostomy entries in Section 7).
- Increase calories; ensure adequate protein.
- As needed, decrease residue; eventually increase (as tolerated) wheat bran, cereal, and vegetable fibers (insoluble), including rye bread.
- Increased intakes of calcium and folate would be prudent.
- Monitor carefully for possible lactose intolerance. Decrease intake of lactose or use lactase enzyme products when indicated.

Common Drugs Used and Potential Side Effects

- Steroid therapy may be administered. Sodium retention, hyperglycemia, nitrogen, and calcium losses may occur.
- Chemotherapy may be used; monitor side effects accordingly, because these agents may further impact bowel function.
- Fluorouracil plus levamisole, methotrexate, mitomycin, lomustine, vincristine, and similar agents are used commonly. Diarrhea, nausea, vomiting, low WBC, and mouth sores can occur.
- Regular low doses of aspirin may help prevent colon cancer by reducing prostaglandin production.

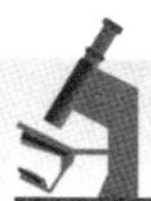

PROFILE

Clinical/History

Height
Weight (loss?)
BMI
Rectal bleeding, pain
Irregular bowel habits
Weakness
Anorexia
Dehydration, electrolyte imbalances
Intestinal obstruction, bowel abscess
Fistula

Lab Work

Colon lavage cytology
H&H (decreased)
Serum Fe
Transferrin
Na+
K+ (often decreased)
Chol, Trig
TLC (varies)
WBC, ESR (increased)
Alb, prealbumin
RBP
Mg++
Ca++
Serum zinc
Proctoscopy, colonoscopy
Melena (stool test)
Digital rectal examination

Herbs, Botanicals and Supplements

- Herbs and botanical supplements should not be used without discussing with physician.
- Long-term use of multivitamin supplements may reduce risk of colon cancer; this effect may be due to folic acid content (Giovannucci et al., Multivitamin use. . . , 1998).
- With use of methotrexate (Rheumatrex), avoid Echinacea for potential damage to the liver.
- Low-dose fish oil supplementation may be useful to normalize cell proliferation (Anti et al., 1994).

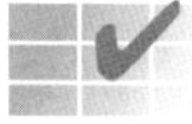

PATIENT EDUCATION

- Discuss appropriate dietary regimen for specific problems generated by therapy.
- Encourage family participation in all levels of care.
- Discuss how to prevent further tumors or polyps. Increasing intake of vitamin D and calcium in dairy products, vitamin C, and B-carotene in fruits or vegetables, rye, and whole grain breads and cereals should be used as tolerated.
- Encourage physical activity when feasible.
- Family members (offspring and other first degree relatives) should have a digital examination annually at 40 years of age, stool tests for blood after 50 years of age, and sigmoidoscopy or colonoscopy after age 50 every 3–5 years. An annual fecal occult blood test (FOBT) can also be useful. Yet less than 50% of the eligible population has undergone any type of screening.
- Encourage consumption of milk for its useful calcium, vitamin D, and lactose content. If necessary, use lactase enzymes if intolerance exists; monitor also for verified milk allergy and avoid milk in those cases.

For More Information

- American Society of Colon and Rectal Surgeons
  85 W. Algonquin Rd., Suite 550
  Arlington Heights, IL 60005
  http://www.fascrs.org/brochures/colorectal-cancer.html
- Colorectal Cancer Network
  http://www.colorectal-cancer.net/
- Colorectal Cancer Prevention and Control Initiatives
  http://www.cdc.gov/cancer/colorctl/colorect.htm
- Colorectal Cancer Screening
  http://www.gastro.org/public/cc_screening.html#Diagnosed
- Johns Hopkins Hereditary Colorectal Cancer
  http://www.hopkins-coloncancer.org/subspecialties/heredicolor_cancer/overview.htm
- Medline Information–Colorectal Cancer
  http://www.nlm.nih.gov/medlineplus/colorectalcancer.html
- National Colorectal Research Alliance
  http://www.nccra.org/
- National Colorectal Cancer Action Campaign
  http://www.cdc.gov/cancer/screenforlife/

ESOPHAGEAL CANCER

NUTRITIONAL ACUITY RANKING: LEVEL 3 (MAY OFTEN BE 4)

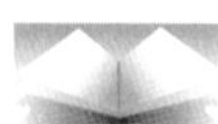

DEFINITIONS AND BACKGROUND

Esophageal cancer develops in the middle or lower third of the esophagus. It is one of the more common types of head and neck cancer, primarily adenocarcinoma or squamous cell cases with surgical resection (Brennan et al., 1995). Formerly, it was almost always fatal because the condition often was advanced before symptoms appeared. This condition is more common in persons older than 50 years of age, especially males, and generally is found only in 5–7/100,000 persons.

Barrett's esophagus (BE) is a premalignant condition associated with esophageal adenocarcinoma. Cyclooxygenase-z (COX-2) is an inducible enzyme that is overexpressed in BE as in colon cancer.

In patients with head and neck cancer, zinc status is a better indicator of tumor size and stage of disease than overall nutritional status (Doerr et al., 1997). Increasing tumor size and overall stage of disease is positively correlated with Zn deficiency, but not with alcohol intake or smoking status.

Causes may include low intake of fruit and vegetables or obesity (Brown et al., 1995) or low vitamin C intake (Goodwin and Brodwick, 1995). Among Hong Kong Chinese, in whom a high incidence occurs, alcohol excesses, tobacco use, ingestion of pickled vegetables, infrequent use of citrus fruits and green leafy vegetables, and consuming drinks and soups at very high temperatures seem to be the greatest risk factors (Cheng et al., 1992). Moldy corn and popcorn may also pose a risk when contaminated with fungal moniliform (Norred and Voss, 1994). Low use of whole grains and high use of refined grains may be a risk factor as well (Levi et al., 2000).

Symptoms and signs include dysphagia, painful swallowing, substernal pain, feeling of fullness, weight loss, malaise, malnutrition, dehydration, anemia, regurgitation after eating, electrolyte imbalance, hiccups, foul breath, aspiration, increased salivation, hoarseness and coughing, and hepatomegaly. Approximately one-third of patients are mild to moderately malnourished at the time of diagnosis.

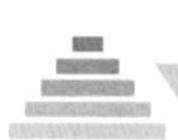

OBJECTIVES

- ▲ Prevent sepsis, further weight loss, malnutrition, cachexia, and aspiration.
- ▲ Hydrate adequately; encourage fluids between meals and limit fluid intake at meals to improve intake of other foods.
- ▲ Feed adequately if resection is needed; some fat malabsorption, reflux, dumping syndrome, increased mediastinal pressure, and increased food transit time may be side effects.
- ▲ Omit alcoholic beverages, especially if ethanol/ethyl alcohol (ETOH) abuse has occurred by history.
- ▲ Promote positive nitrogen balance and prevent loss of LBM.
- ▲ Prepare for treatments (usually surgery but sometimes radiation or chemotherapy as well).
- ▲ Correct anemia.
- ▲ Compensate for progressive dysphagia.
- ▲ Improve quality of life (QOL).

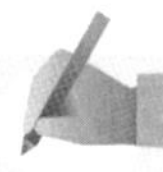

DIETARY AND NUTRITIONAL RECOMMENDATIONS

- Patient often is nil per os (NPO, nothing by mouth), with parenteral (PPN or TPN) or gastrostomy feedings. While less common, jejunostomy is useful for correcting lost weight (Pearlstone et al., 1995). In this patient population, initiation of oral feeding 48 hours after total laryngectomy is a safe clinical practice (Medina and Khafif, 2001).
- If swallowing is possible, provide a diet high in calories and protein with bland or pureed foods as required. Adjust individually to meet patient's needs.
- Increase fluid intake as tolerated, with up to 3.5 L daily unless contraindicated.
- Medium-chain triglycerides (MCTs) may be beneficial if fat malabsorption exists, especially with steatorrhea.
- Increase intake of vitamins A and C, zinc, and other nutrients that may be low. Use more fruits and vegetables (Li et al., 1993).
- If esophagectomy has been performed, gastric stasis can occur. Fat maldigestion has been a common complaint; a lower fat diet may be better tolerated.
- Calorie requirements may equal 35–40 kcals/kg; 1.5–2 g protein/kg.
- Limit simple sugars and carbonated beverage intake if there is dumping syndrome.
- In advanced cases, palliative care may be needed.

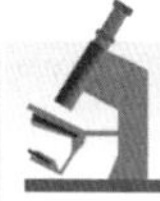

PROFILE

Clinical/History

- Height
- Weight (loss?)
- BMI
- Weight changes
- BP
- I & O; Dehydration?
- Temperature
- Dysphagia, painful swallowing
- Substernal pain
- Feeling of fullness
- Malaise
- Malnutrition
- Anemia
- Regurgitation after eating
- Hiccups, foul breath
- Aspiration
- Increased salivation
- Hoarseness and coughing
- Hepatomegaly

Lab Work

- Alb, prealbumin
- Transferrin
- H&H
- ALT (increased)
- Gluc
- T3, T4
- Thyroid-stimulating hormone (TSH)
- Barium swallow
- Endoscopy

Common Drugs Used and Potential Side Effects

- Cisplatin can cause nausea, vomiting, altered taste, changes in renal function, and diarrhea.
- Bleomycin and methotrexate can also aggravate nausea, vomiting, anorexia, or stomatitis.
- Aspirin is now believed to reduce esophageal cancer risk by 90% by reducing prostaglandin production. Further studies are needed in larger population groups.

Herbs, Botanicals and Supplements

- Herbs and botanical supplements should not be used without discussing with physician.
- With use of methotrexate (Rheumatrex), avoid Echinacea for potential damage to the liver.
- With cyclosporine, avoid use with Echinacea and St. John's wort because of counterproductive effects on the drug.

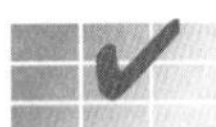

PATIENT EDUCATION

- ✓ If patient can eat orally, encourage him or her to chew slowly.
- ✓ If jejunostomy feeding is required after esophagastric surgery, teach patient/family/caretaker how to prepare feedings and how to produce the item in a clean environment.
- ✓ Encourage help from speech therapy services.
- ✓ Hypothyroid status can cause dysphagia; counsel accordingly.

For More Information

- CancerLinks USA
  http://www.cancerlinksusa.com/esophagus/wynk/
- Cancer Net–Esophageal Cancer
  http://cancernet.nci.nih.gov/cancer_types/Esophageal cancer.shtml
- Medline–Esophageal Cancer
  http://www.nlm.nih.gov/medlineplus/esophageal-cancer.html
- Onco-Link–Esophageal Cancer
  http://www.nlm.nih.gov/medlineplus/esophageal-cancer.html
- Oncology Channel
  http://www.oncologychannel.com/esophagealcancer/
- OnTumor.com
  http://www.ontumor.com/esophageal.htm

GASTRIC CARCINOMA

NUTRITIONAL ACUITY RANKING: LEVEL 3–4

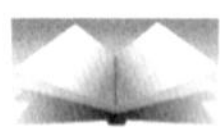

DEFINITIONS AND BACKGROUND

Gastric carcinoma most commonly occurs in the pyloric segment and along the lesser curvature. Often, no early definitive signs are evident. Symptoms and signs include a feeling of fullness, indigestion, dysphagia, anorexia, weight loss, anemia, pallor, vertigo, nausea and vomiting, malnutrition, melena, occult blood, and dehydration.

During chronic inflammation associated with GI malignancies, demand for amino acids outstrips dietary supply and skeletal muscle protein may be mobilized to meet this demand; inefficient body nitrogen economy occurs (Preston, 1998).

Gastric cancer often follows long-term pernicious anemia, Menetrier's disease, or chronic gastritis. It is generally found in males aged 50–70 years, often among smokers. Vitamin C seems to be protective against gastric cancer (Goodwin and Brodwick, 1995). Green tea does not necessarily protect against it. It is believed that *H. pylori* infection may play some role in up to 40–60% of all stomach cancers (http://www.canadianhp.com/english/gastric_cancer.html).

In patients with GI cancer who receive chemotherapy before surgery, administration of PN during chemotherapy improves short-term nutritional status without significantly increasing the number of tumor cells and prevents postoperative complications (Jin et al., 1999). In a rare form of previously incurable stomach cancer known as gastrointestinal stromal tumor (GIST), newly approved Gleevec may shrink tumors by more than half with minimal side effects, leading to an extended remission.

OBJECTIVES

- Prevent or reverse weight loss and further malnutrition.
- Encourage fluids.
- Counteract side effects of chemotherapy, radiation, or gastrectomy. If gastrectomy is performed, dumping syndrome or hypochlorhydria may result.
- Correct protein-losing enteropathy.
- Improve QOL.

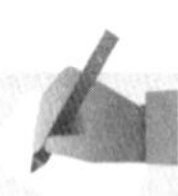

DIETARY AND NUTRITIONAL RECOMMENDATIONS

- Parenteral therapy or TPN may be used, especially before surgery. After removal of parts of the stomach, patients are often volume-sensitive and need small meals and snacks with fluids between meals.
- If oral intake is allowed, try light meals that are nutrient-dense and well balanced. A high-protein/high-calorie diet will be needed.
- Generally, 2–3 L of fluid is required throughout the day, unless contraindicated for other reasons.
- Postgastrectomy, beware of dumping syndrome (see postgastrectomy entry in Section 7). Small, frequent feedings may be better tolerated; concentrated CHO, alcohol, and use of carbonated beverages may need to be limited.
- Jejunostomy at resection may be indicated.
- Be sure that dietary intake (or supplementation) includes selenium and other key nutrients for wound healing and correction of anemia. Take minerals with food because they are often not tolerated on an empty stomach.
- As possible, increase intake of fruits and vegetables (Li et al., 1993).

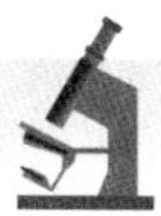

PROFILE

Clinical/History

Height
Weight (loss?)
BMI
I & O, dehydration?
BP
Feelings of fullness, indigestion
Dysphagia, anorexia
Anemia, pallor
Vertigo
Nausea or vomiting
Temperature
Anorexia

Lab Work

Alb, prealbumin
Na+, K+
TLC (varies)
Gluc
H&H
Transferrin
ALT (increased)
Melena, occult blood
Barium swallow
Endoscopy

Common Drugs Used and Potential Side Effects

- Cytotoxic drugs such as mitomycin C may cause fever, nausea, vomiting, anorexia, and stomatitis can result.
- With 5-fluorouracil (5-FU), anorexia and nausea are common. Sore mouth, taste changes, and vomiting also may result.
- For some cases, added thiamine is needed with 5-FU treatment.
- Antibiotic therapy to eradicate *H. pylori* bacteria may be needed, if present.

Herbs, Botanicals and Supplements

- Herbs and botanical supplements should not be used without discussing with physician.

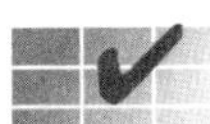

PATIENT EDUCATION

- ✔ Encourage patient to chew slowly and well, when and if oral intake is possible.
- ✔ Feeding tubes may be useful in home setting (e.g., jejunostomy).

For More Information

- ✦ Canadian Helicobacter Pylori Website
  http://www.canadianhp.com/english/gastric_cancer.html
- ✦ Onco-Link—Gastric Cancer
  http://cancer.med.upenn.edu/disease/gastric/
- ✦ National Cancer Institute–Gastric Cancer
  http://www.graylab.ac.uk/cancernet/304880.html

HEAD & NECK CANCERS

NUTRITIONAL ACUITY RANKING: LEVEL 3

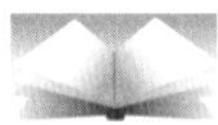

DEFINITIONS AND BACKGROUND

Head and neck cancers account for 40,000 new cases in the U.S. each year, with the highest overall incidence rate in black males. Mortality rate of 12,000 U.S. deaths annually. Etiology is linked to tobacco use for all tumor sites, as every form of tobacco is known to result in dysplastic and carcinogenic injuries. Alcohol is thought to play a synergistic role with tobacco.

Oral cavity may have gingival swelling, pain, bleeding, and loosening teeth. Oral cancer is more prevalent in persons with chronically unclean mouths or in persons with poorly fitted dentures. A goal includes elimination of irritation and infections. The disorder is rare in persons younger than 40 years of age. Risk of metastasis is great.

In cancers of the nose and paranasal sinuses, unilateral obstruction and epistaxis are common symptoms. In the nasopharynx, signs include pain, otologic changes, and nasal obstruction. In the oropharynx, there may be a dull ache, dysphagia, referred otalgia, and trismus. In the laryngeal area, symptoms include voice changes, dysphagia, odynophagia, and dyspnea. In cancer of the salivary gland, unilateral symptoms and impaired jaw mobility can occur.

Low vitamin C intake may be related to head and neck cancers (Goodwin and Brodwick, 1995); it is not known whether vitamin C should be available in combination with other antioxidants. Low use of whole grains and high use of refined grains may be a risk factor as well in oral cancer (Levi et al., 2000).

Rarely do mouth ulcers from stress or trauma indicate any major sign of a health problem. A physician should see ulcers that fail to heal after 10 days or those that recur. Leukoplakia, thickened white patches, should be biopsied if they exist for a prolonged time.

Radiation therapy is the main treatment modality for these head and neck cancers. Side effects often include odynophagia, dysphagia, mucositis, esophagitis, xerostomia (with occasional osteoradionecrosis), dental caries, weight loss, taste changes, and decreased appetite. Prognosis for cure worsens as depth of tumor invasion increases. Nutritional status and overexpression or mutation of the p53 gene may also play a role (http://cancer.med.upenn.edu/md2b/headneck.html).

OBJECTIVES

- Abstain from smoking, alcohol, and irritants to the mouth such as chewing tobacco and snuff.
- Prevent abscesses and infection; provide good mouth care.
- Monitor dysphagia and difficulty with chewing.
- Correct for side effects (mucositis, xerostomia, fibrosis, dental caries, weight loss, etc.) of treatment.
- Prevent weight loss and malnutrition.

DIETARY AND NUTRITIONAL RECOMMENDATIONS

- Decrease use of condiments if they are irritating (e.g., black pepper, chili powder) and dilute acidic fruits or juices, such as orange, grapefruit, and tomato.
- Tolerance will vary for hot and cold foods and drinks. Monitor and alter intake accordingly.
- TPN or gastrostomy feeding may be needed at least temporarily or for an extended period of time.
- A dysphagia diet (thick pureed foods, decrease in thin liquids) may be needed if swallowing is difficult.
- For other side effects, see Table 13–7.

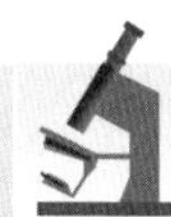

PROFILE

Clinical/History

Height
Weight (loss?)
BMI
Weight changes
Gingival swelling, pain, bleeding
Odynophagia
Mucositis, esophagitis
Xerostomia
Dental caries
Taste changes, decreased appetite
Loosening teeth
Palpable mass
Gingival hyperplasia
Nonhealing ulcerative oral lesions
Glottic tumors
Dysphagia
BP

Lab Work

Alb, prealbumin
RBP
Transferrin
Na+, K+
Ca++, Mg++
H&H
TLC (varies)
Gluc
Chol
ALT (may be increased)
Nasopharyngoscopy
Direct laryngoscopy, esophagoscopy
Cranial nerve defects
Biopsy

Common Drugs Used and Potential Side Effects

- Steroids may be used to reduce inflammation; sodium retention, potassium depletion, and negative nitrogen balance can result. Hyperglycemia also can occur.
- Chemotherapy medications may be used. Monitor according to medication used.

Herbs, Botanicals and Supplements

- Herbs and botanical supplements should not be used without discussing with physician.

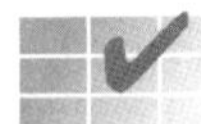

PATIENT EDUCATION

- ✓ Relaxation therapy or biofeedback can be beneficial.
- ✓ Discuss a diet rationale that is appropriate for patient's condition.

For More Information

- American Oral Cancer Clinic
  http://www.tonguecancer.com/
- Oral Cancer Awareness Initiative
  http://www.oral-cancer.org/
- NIH Cancer Information
  http://www.nidr.nih.gov/Spectrum/NIDCR3/3menu.htm

HEPATIC CARCINOMA

NUTRITIONAL ACUITY RANKING: LEVEL 3–4

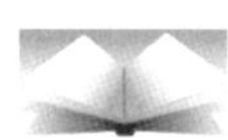

DEFINITIONS AND BACKGROUND

Malignant hepatic tumors commonly are due to metastatic lesions from other organs. Primary tumors are common with alcohol abuse, aflatoxin ingestion, or chronic hepatitis B or C (Levin and Amos, 1995). Cirrhosis may be a necessary intermediate for the development of hepatocellular carcinoma among alcoholics (Kuper et al., 2001).

Symptoms and signs of hepatic cancer include slow onset, anorexia, weakness, progressive weight loss, nausea and/or vomiting, increased flatulence, steatorrhea, diarrhea, abdominal fullness, low-grade fever, dehydration, anemia, malnutrition, abnormal liver function tests (LFTs) , decreased albumin levels, portal hypertension, dyspnea, jaundice, ascites, and hepatic coma. Untreated liver cancer may rapidly lead to death in 5–6 months.

According to McGlynn et al. (2001), primary liver cancer (PLC) has been common in many areas of the developing world, but uncommon in most of the developed world. There are some PLC increases in incidence in developed countries, whereas developing countries have experienced declines. The increased seroprevalence of hepatitis-C (HCV) in the developed world and the elimination of hepatitis-B (HBV)-cofactors in the developing world are likely to have contributed to the patterns. Progress may be seen in the developing world once the HBV-vaccinated segment of the population reaches adulthood.

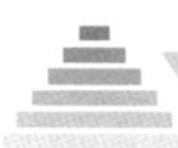

OBJECTIVES

- ▲ Reduce fluid retention, ascites.
- ▲ Correct serum protein levels and production.
- ▲ Prevent further nausea and vomiting, weight loss, anorexia, and malnutrition.
- ▲ Counteract side effects of therapy (e.g., surgery, chemotherapy, radiation).
- ▲ Improve overall nutritional and hematologic status.
- ▲ Improve prognosis as long as possible.
- ▲ Improve QOL.

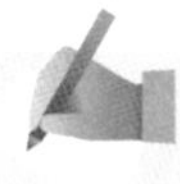

DIETARY AND NUTRITIONAL RECOMMENDATIONS

- Patient may be NPO with parenteral/TPN as needed.
- Progress, if and when tolerated, to high-calorie/high-protein diet with an increased CHO intake. If hepatic coma occurs, decreased protein with supplemented amino acids will be needed. (See hepatic encephalopathy/coma entry in Section 8.)
- Reduce sodium if ascites and edema are significant. Monitor need for extra protein if albumin is also low.
- Monitor serum levels of other values to determine other restrictions or needed alterations.
- Supplemental vitamins A, D, K, and B-complex may be beneficial. Be careful of toxic levels because of poor hepatic clearance.
- With surgery, monitor nutrients needed for adequate wound healing and recovery.
- Encourage regular meals and snacks. Manage decreased appetite.

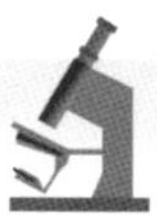

PROFILE

Clinical/History

Height
Weight
BMI
Progressive weight loss
GI bleeding
I & O, dehydration
Anorexia, weakness
Nausea and/or vomiting
Increased flatulence
Steatorrhea, diarrhea
Abdominal fullness
Low-grade fever
Anemia, malnutrition
Portal hypertension
Dyspnea
Jaundice, ascites, or hepatic coma
Melena
Hepatomegaly
Therapy—surgery, etc.
Temperature (fever?)

Lab Work

PT (prolonged)
H&H
Transferrin
AST, ALT (abnormal)
Sedimentation rate (increased)
Na+
Ammonia
Alb (decreased), prealbumin
RBP
Gluc (decreased)
Alk phos
K+
TLC (varies)

Common Drugs Used and Potential Side Effects

- Antiemetics may be used for vomiting.
- Diuretics are used commonly; monitor side effects carefully.

Herbs, Botanicals and Supplements

- Herbs and botanical supplements should not be used without discussing with physician.

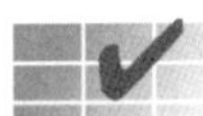

PATIENT EDUCATION

- ✔ Teach patient about signs of deficiency of vitamins K and C such as bleeding gums.
- ✔ Discuss signs of hepatic coma that require dietary alterations.

For More Information

- ✦ Onco-Link–Liver Cancer
  http://cancer.med.upenn.edu/disease/liver/

LUNG CANCER (BRONCHIAL CARCINOMA)

NUTRITIONAL ACUITY RANKING: LEVEL 3 (MAY OFTEN BE 4)

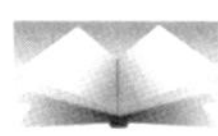

DEFINITIONS AND BACKGROUND

There are several kinds of lung cancer, but only bronchial cancer is common. This cancer is the most common type of cancer in the Western world, among males and females. Squamous cell cancer is common and oat cell carcinoma is less common. Small cell lung carcinomas tend to respond to specific chemotherapy protocols. For most cases, radiation and chemotherapy are needed because the cancer is discovered too late for surgical intervention or is not clinically indicated. Oat cell CA is a rapidly spreading, highly fatal lung CA; aggressive chemotherapy is needed.

In 85% of cases, smoking causes lung cancer. Heavy smokers are 25 times more susceptible to lung cancer. Cigarette smoking cannot fully explain high lung cancer rates in Taiwanese women, despite a low prevalence of smoking. Lung cancer was positively related to the number of meals cooked per day using Chinese quick-frying methods and not using fans to ventilate cooking oils (Ko et al., 2000). Other causes include exposure to industrial chemicals, radon, or passive smoke.

Dietary factors play a protective role. There seems to be a clear relationship between lung cancer risk and saturated fatty acid consumption in nonsmoking women; regular intake of beans and peas may be protective (Alavanja et al., 1993). Foods rich in flavonoids may protect against certain types of lung cancer, possibly by inhibiting P450 enzymes, which decrease bioactivation of carcinogens (Le Marchand et al., 2000). Onions and apples appear to be the most protective for their quercetin; white grapefruit provides naringin. Dietary onions are quite protective against squamous cell lung cancer.

Risk of cancer in the respiratory tract seems positively related to intake of refined grains and negatively related to intake of whole grains (Levi et al., 2000). Previous reports of lower plasma levels of vitamin E and carotenoids in smokers vs. nonsmokers may have been caused by differences in dietary habits between the two groups; smoking is associated with lower levels of vitamin C, which can be replaced by supplementation (Lykkesfeldt et al., 2000).

In men, high intakes of beer and spirits (average 3+ drinks daily) are associated with increased risk of lung cancer (Prescott et al., 1999). Wine intake may protect against lung cancer possibly because it contains antioxidants.

Signs and symptoms of lung cancer include persistent cough, bloody sputum, chest pain, recurring pneumonia, weight loss, or bronchitis. Cancer cells of the lung often spread to the brain, bone, liver, and skin.

OBJECTIVES

- Patient must be encouraged to stop smoking.
- Prepare patient for therapy—surgery, radiation, and chemotherapy.
- Meet calorie needs (with basal metabolic rate [BMR] elevated by approximately 30%).
- Counteract side effects such as cachexia, infections, atelectasis, and SIADH.
- Prevent or correct other side effects such as weight loss and anorexia.
- Maximize pulmonary health.
- Improve QOL.

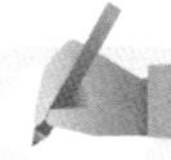

DIETARY AND NUTRITIONAL RECOMMENDATIONS

- Increase calories and protein, CHO, and fluids.
- Alter diet as appropriate for side effects (see general cancer entry).
- Small, frequent meals may be beneficial.
- Adequate vitamin/mineral provision will be needed. Vitamins A and C are especially important. Include fruits and vegetables, dried beans and peas, and other phytochemical sources. Apples are a good source of quercetin.
- Encourage decreased alcohol intake if common in patient's history.

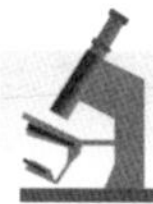

PROFILE

Clinical/History

Height
Weight (loss?)
BMI
Persistent cough
Bloody sputum
Chest pain
Recurring pneumonia or bronchitis
I & O

Lab Work

Alb, prealbumin
Na+
Gluc
Ca++
Mg++
TLC (varies)
pCO2, pO2
K+
ALT (increased)
Bronchoscopy
Biopsy
MRI, CT scan
Sputum cytology
Chest x-ray
Thoracentesis

Common Drugs Used and Potential Side Effects

- Cytotoxic drugs are often used. Vincristine can cause severe constipation; with methotrexate, nausea and vomiting are common; doxorubicin (Adriamycin) causes stomatitis, anorexia, hair loss, and diarrhea. Coadministration of methotrexate with intravenous glucose may alleviate some of the toxic GI effects.
- Cyclophosphamide (Cytoxan) and other combinations of therapy may be used. Anorexia, stomatitis, nausea, or vomiting may occur.
- With immunotherapy, Bacillus Calmette-Guerin (BCG) vaccine often is tried as therapy.
- New experimental agents include molecular-targeted therapies. AstraZeneca and OSI Pharmaceutical companies are testing these drugs.

Herbs, Botanicals and Supplements

- Herbs and botanical supplements should not be used without discussing with physician.

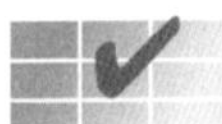

PATIENT EDUCATION

- ✔ Discuss alternate methods of eating if meals are not consumed as usual.
- ✔ Discuss side effects of drugs being used.
- ✔ Smokers who quit will allow their lung tissues to repair much of the damage. Those who cannot quit should use a brand of cigarettes with lower nicotine and low tar. Chewing tobacco and snuff is also carcinogenic.
- ✔ Avoid smoking prior to meals or with meals as smoking may decrease appetite.

For More Information

- Alliance for Lung Cancer
  http://www.alcase.org/
- Cancer Net–Lung Cancer
  http://cancernet.nci.nih.gov/wyntk_pubs/lung.htm
- Focus on Lung Cancer
  http://www.lungcancer.org/
- Lung Cancer Information Library
  http://www.meds.com/lung/lunginfo.html
- Lung Cancer OnLine
  http://www.lungcanceronline.org/
- Onco Link–Lung Cancer
  http://cancer.med.upenn.edu/disease/lung1/

HODGKIN'S DISEASE

NUTRITIONAL ACUITY RANKING: LEVEL 3

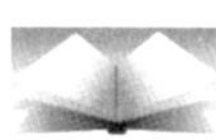

DEFINITIONS AND BACKGROUND

A malignant tumor of lymphoid tissue, Hodgkin's disease usually presents with enlarged lymph nodes that are firm and rubbery, pruritus, generalized and severe, jaundice, night sweats, fatigue and malaise, weight loss, slight fever, alcohol-induced pain, cough, dyspnea, and chest pain. Patients who have HIV infection are more prone to Hodgkin's disease.

Patients who present with weight loss initially have a worse prognosis than those without weight loss. It is most common between ages 15 and 34 and again over age 60. Treatment involves radiation and chemotherapy. Stage 1 is limited to one body part; stage 2 involves two or more areas on the same side of the diaphragm; stage 3 involves lymph nodes above and below the diaphragm; stage 4 involves lymph nodes and other areas such as lungs, marrow, and liver. The five-year survival rate for Hodgkin's is 83%; it is one of the more curable forms of cancer.

OBJECTIVES

- ▲ Prevent infections such as candidiasis.
- ▲ Counteract side effects of chemotherapy, radiation, and other treatments.
- ▲ Prevent or correct weight loss, fever, and malaise.

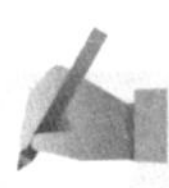

DIETARY AND NUTRITIONAL RECOMMENDATIONS

- A diet as tolerated is acceptable. Bland foods may be better accepted for a while.
- Increase protein, kilocalories, and fluids.
- Six small feedings are generally better tolerated than three large meals.
- Alter diet according to symptoms.
- In hyperglycemia, manage intake of carbohydrates and overall energy.

Common Drugs Used and Potential Side Effects

- Chemotherapy is often given in combination. MOPP = mechlorethamine (nitrogen mustard), vincristine (Oncovin), procarbazine, and prednisone; this may cause nausea, vomiting, diarrhea, weakness, constipation, and mouth sores. ChlVPP 5 chlorambucil, vinblastine, procarbazine, and prednisone may cause similar side effects.
- Corticosteroids can aggravate electrolyte status and will decrease calcium, potassium, and nitrogen balance over time. Hyperglycemia also may occur; monitor blood glucose levels.

Herbs, Botanicals and Supplements

- Herbs and botanical supplements should not be used without discussing with physician.

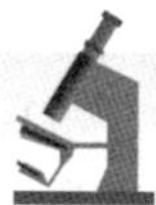

PROFILE

Clinical/History

Height
Weight (loss?)
BMI
Enlarged lymph nodes that are firm and rubbery
Pruritus, severe
Jaundice
Night sweats
Fatigue and malaise
Slight fever, temperature
Alcohol-induced pain
Cough, dyspnea, and chest pain
Diarrhea
I & O

Lab Work

Ceruloplasmin (increased)
Reed-Sternberg cells (more than one nucleus)
ESR (Sedimentation rate)
TLC (varies)
Uric acid (increased)
TP (increased)
Gluc
Serum Cu (increased)
H&H
Bilirubin (increased)
Alk phos (often increased)
Ferritin (increased)
ALT (increased)
Serum lipids—chol, trig
Lymphangiogram
X-ray or CT scan
Bone marrow biopsy (bx)

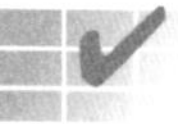

PATIENT EDUCATION

- ✓ Discuss methods of improving appetite by use of attractive meals.
- ✓ Encourage rest periods before and after meals to reduce fatigue.

For More Information

- Lymphoma Information Network
  http://www.lymphomainfo.net/hodgkins/
- Onco Link
  http://cancer.med.upenn.edu/disease/hodgkins/

LYMPHOMAS, NONHODGKIN'S

NUTRITIONAL ACUITY RANKING: LEVEL 3

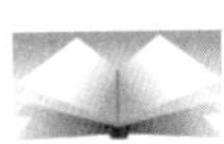

DEFINITIONS AND BACKGROUND

Non-Hodgkin's lymphomas are malignant tumors of lymphoid tissue other than Hodgkin's disease. They generally result from invasion of the lymph nodes and other tissues by lymphocytes. The bacterium, *H. pylori,* is associated with the development of lymphoma in the stomach wall. Patients with HIV have a much higher risk of developing lymphoma (www.leukemia-lymphoma.org). Burkitt's lymphoma in Africa is associated with prior infection with the Epstein-Barr virus; it may also play a role in the development of some lymphomas. Burkitt's lymphoma is most common in children, young adult males, or patients with AIDS; it originates from a B-lymphocyte and requires chemotherapy for treatment. T-cell lymphoma of the intestine is a form of extranodal, non-Hodgkin's lymphoma with an enteropathy that involves the GI tract and has no specific treatment available at this time.

Non-Hodgkin's lymphoma is relatively common among individuals whose immune system is suppressed, and some types of dietary fat and protein have been associated with decreased immune responses. Rural lifestyle, farming, and exposure to certain chemicals in herbicides and pesticides have been suspected to have an increased risk of lymphoma. Dietary intake of beef, pork, or lamb as a main dish may also be related to the disease; intake of trans fatty acids and broiling or barbecuing meats may promote the disease (Zhang et al., Dietary fats. . . , 1999).

Symptoms and signs are similar to those of Hodgkin's disease and those of enlarged tonsils and adenoids. Difficulty breathing, swelling of face, thickened or dark, itchy skin areas, increased incidence of bacterial infections, night sweats, weight loss, fever, anemia, and pleural effusion can occur. It is possible, as well, to develop chylous ascites or chyloperitoneum. By time of diagnosis, it is often widely spread. Radiation is a common treatment for early stages. A cure is less likely for those over age 60. Five-year survival rate for non-Hodgkin's lymphoma is 52%.

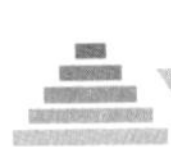

OBJECTIVES

- Correct dysphagia, nausea and vomiting, and anorexia.
- Prevent infections, candidiasis, etc.
- Prevent or counteract weight loss.
- Control protein-losing enteropathy, chylous ascites, and other side effects.
- Modify diet according to side effects of therapy (radiation, chemotherapy).

DIETARY AND NUTRITIONAL RECOMMENDATIONS

- A normal diet is allowed, as tolerated. Bland foods may be preferred, at least temporarily.
- Six small feedings are often better tolerated.
- Increase protein and calories as appropriate to maintain or gain weight.
- MCT and decreased long-chain triglycerides (LCT) may be appropriate for chylous ascites.
- Attend to side effects by altering diet as needed.

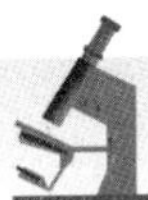

PROFILE

Clinical/History

Height
Weight, weight loss
BMI
Enlarged tonsils and adenoids.
Difficulty breathing
Swelling of face
Thickened or dark, itchy skin areas
Bacterial infections
Night sweats
Fever, temperature
I & O

Lab Work

Abnormal lymphocytes
Bilirubin (increased)
Ceruloplasmin (increased)
Na+, K+
Gluc
Ca++ (increased)
Positive antiglobulin test (Coombs' test)
Chol, Trig
Serum copper (increased)
Alb, prealbumin
LDH (increased)
Uric acid (increased)
Gamma globulin (increased)
RBP
ALT (increased)
Pleural effusion
CT scan
Gallium scan
Lymphangiogram

Common Drugs Used and Potential Side Effects

- Chemotherapy is often given in combination. CHOP= Cyclophosphamide, doxorubicin, vincristine (Oncovin), and prednisone may cause nausea, vomiting, anorexia, diarrhea, and other GI side effects.
- Single agents may also be used. Methotrexate causes GI pain, mouth ulcers, and nausea; it also depletes folic acid levels.

Herbs, Botanicals and Supplements

- Herbs and botanical supplements should not be used without discussing with physician.

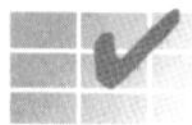

PATIENT EDUCATION

- ✔ Discuss any specific side effects of chemotherapy or radiation.
- ✔ Highlight methods for making meals more attractive.
- ✔ Discuss fiber as an alternative to stool softeners, when appropriate.

For More Information

- Cancer Links
  http://www.ontumor.com/lymphoma/
- Onco-Link–Non-Hodgkin's Lymphoma
  http://cancer.med.upenn.edu/disease/nonhodgkins/

MELANOMA AND SKIN CANCERS

NUTRITIONAL ACUITY RANKING: NOT RANKED

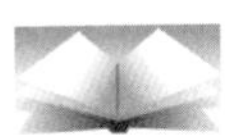

DEFINITIONS AND BACKGROUND

Skin cancers are increasing. Omega-3 fatty acids may be especially useful as protective agents for the skin (Liu et al., 2001). Low intake of total fat and high intake of specific vitamins have been hypothesized to reduce risk of basal cell carcinoma of the skin, but more long-term studies are needed (van Dam et al., 2001). Basal cell tumors start as small, shiny, firm nodules that enlarge slowly; they may bleed and scab then heal and then repeat the cycle. Basal cell tumors should be removed to avoid destruction to other tissues.

Squamous cell carcinoma originates in the middle layer of epidermis and may develop on sun-damaged skin, or even in the mouth lining or tongue. This type begins as a reddened area with a scaly, crusted surface that does not heal. It may have the appearance of a wart and eventually becomes an open sore. Removal is important before spreading can occur.

Melanoma originates in the melanocytes and tends to spread rapidly. Biopsy is essential. It is the most common cancer for women 25–29 and the second most common cancer for women 30–34 and is increasing faster than any other cancer. An American's lifetime risk of developing melanoma is about one in 75. Potentially disfiguring surgery is not always necessary to remove a melanoma, the deadliest kind of skin cancer. Stages are found in Table 13–11.

TABLE 13–11 Stages of Melanoma

Stage I Definition: Cancer is found in the outer layer of the skin (epidermis) and/or the upper part of the inner layer of skin (dermis), but it has not spread to nearby lymph nodes. The tumor is less than 1.5 mm (1/16 of an inch) thick.

Stage II Definition: The tumor is 1.5–4 mm (less than 1/6 of an inch) thick. It has spread to the lower part of the inner layer of skin (dermis) but not into the tissue below the skin or into nearby lymph nodes.

Stage III Definition: Any of the following mean that the tumor is stage III—the tumor is more than 4 mm (approximately 1/6 of an inch) thick; tumor has spread to the body tissue below the skin; additional tumor growths within one inch of the original tumor (satellite tumors); tumor has spread to nearby lymph nodes or there are additional tumor growths (satellite tumors) between the original tumor and the lymph nodes in the area.

Stage IV Melanoma treatment may be one of the following: Surgery to remove lymph nodes that contain cancer or tumors that have spread (metastasized) to other areas of the body; radiation therapy to relieve symptoms; systemic chemotherapy and/or biological therapy; biologic agents injected directly into the tumors that have spread.

OBJECTIVES

- Maintain appropriate weight for height.
- General healthy Dietary Guidelines should be followed.
- Prevent or correct nutritional deficiencies, and improve patient tolerance of treatment.
- Minimize potential treatment side effects.
- Optimize immune function to increase effectiveness of therapy
- Enhance QOL.

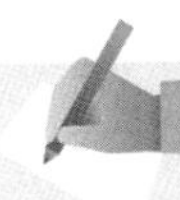

DIETARY AND NUTRITIONAL RECOMMENDATIONS

- Eat a variety of foods
- Choose a diet moderate in fat while controlled in saturated fat and cholesterol. Include good sources of omega-3 fatty acids regularly (i.e., salmon, tuna, mackerel, herring, sardines).
- Choose a diet with plenty of vegetables, fruits, and grain products.
- Use sugars only in moderation
- Use salt and sodium only in moderation
- Use alcoholic beverages in moderation only.
- If anemic, a diet that meets at least RDA and DRI requirements for blood-forming nutrients will be needed.
- Include more fiber-rich foods in diet.
- Reduce use of salt-cured, smoked, and nitrate-preserved foods.

Common Drugs Used and Potential Side Effects

- Interferon alfa 2b (Intron-A) is used in adult patients who have surgically treated melanoma considered at high risk of recurring, according to results of a definitive study at the University of Pittsburgh that evaluated the use of this agent.
- Immunomodulating agent, histamine dihydrochloride (Maxamine), when used in combination with interleukin-2 (IL-2), improves survival for stage IV malignant melanoma patients compared with those treated with the same doses of IL-2 alone. These studies have been done at the University of Pittsburgh National Cancer Institute.

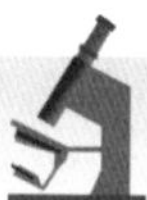

PROFILE

Clinical/History		Lab Work
Height	Itching, bleeding of mole	Alb
Weight	Nausea and vomiting	H&H
BMI	Anorexia	Serum ferritin
Changes in skin or mole		Transferrin

Herbs, Botanicals and Supplements

- Herbs and botanical supplements should not be used without discussing with physician.

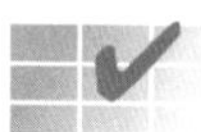

PATIENT EDUCATION

- ✔ Discuss rationale for spacing meals throughout day to avoid fatigue.
- ✔ Offer recipes and meal plans that provide nutrients required to improve status and immunological competence.
- ✔ Patients undergoing treatment should be allowed flexibility in their food selections, while focusing on high-calorie, high-protein choices whenever possible.
- ✔ Offer recipes and menu options for individual planning.
- ✔ Patient must use sunscreen or avoid the sun in most cases.
- ✔ Biofeedback and stress management techniques may be useful.

For More Information

- Melanoma Research Foundation
  23704–5 El Toro Rd., #206
  Lake Forest, CA 92630
  http://www.melanoma.org/

MYELOMA, MULTIPLE

NUTRITIONAL ACUITY RANKING: LEVEL 3

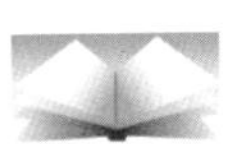

DEFINITIONS AND BACKGROUND

Multiple myeloma is a malignant plasma cell cancer of the hematopoietic system in which plasma cells proliferate, invade bone marrow, and produce abnormal immunoglobulin. The condition is rare, affecting 4 in 100,000 persons. Males are affected more often than females, and the disorder usually strikes after 50 years of age. It represents only 1% of all cancers.

Multiple myeloma affects several areas of bone marrow. Symptoms and signs include bone pain, weight loss, infections, pathologic fractures, shortened stature, paraplegia, fatigue, weakness, apathy, sudden confusion, renal disorders, bleeding tendency (especially gums), nausea and vomiting, anorexia, URIs, and urinary tract infections (UTIs).

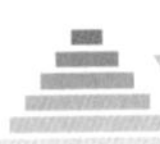

OBJECTIVES

- Avoid fasting. Space meals and snacks adequately.
- Counteract episodes of fatigue and weakness.
- Manage pain effectively.
- Counteract side effects of antineoplastic therapy, steroid therapy, and radiotherapy.
- Avoid infections and febrile states.
- Prevent spontaneous fractures, as far as possible.
- Correct anorexia, nausea and vomiting, and weight loss.

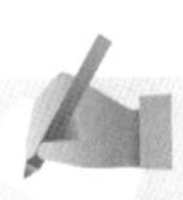

DIETARY AND NUTRITIONAL RECOMMENDATIONS

- Provide diet as usual, with six small feedings rather than large meals.
- A higher protein intake may be useful to counteract losses.
- Provide adequate calories to meet needs of weight control, preventing unnecessary losses.
- Avoid dehydration by including adequate fluid intake (e.g., 3 L daily). This is important.
- Ensure sufficient intake of vitamins, minerals, and phytochemicals, especially from fruits and vegetables.

Common Drugs Used and Potential Side Effects

- Melphalan (Alkeran) or nitrosoureas are used commonly. Monitor side effects such as anorexia, anemia, nausea, vomiting, and stomatitis.
- Prednisone, if used chronically, can increase nitrogen losses and potassium and magnesium depletion and can cause hyperglycemia and sodium retention.
- Pamidronate may be used. Ensure adequate fluid intake but not excess. Avoid use with calcium and vitamin D supplements. Extra phosphorus may be needed.

Nausea, vomiting, GI bleeding or distress, and constipation can occur.

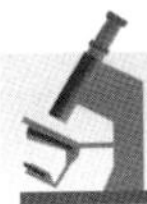

PROFILE

Clinical/History

Height
Weight, weight loss
BMI
Bone pain infections
Fractures, shortened stature
Paraplegia
Fatigue, weakness, apathy
Sudden confusion
Renal disorders
Bleeding tendency (especially gums)
Frequent infections, urinary or respiratory
Skeletal survey
I & O
BP
Nausea and vomiting
Anorexia
History (hx) bleeding

Lab Work

Ca++ (increased)
Total protein
Parathormone (PTH) (increased)
TLC (varies)
Hypercalciuria
Alb (often increased)
Transferrin
H&H
Proteinuria (Bence Jones proteins)
Sedimentation rate (increased)
Uric acid (increased)
RBP
ALT (increased)

Herbs, Botanicals and Supplements

- Herbs and botanical supplements should not be used without discussing with physician.

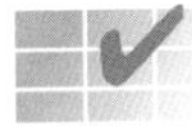

PATIENT EDUCATION

- Discuss rationale for spacing meals throughout day to avoid fatigue.
- Offer recipes and meal plans that provide nutrients required to improve status and immunologic competence.

For More Information

- Cleveland Clinic–Multiple Myeloma Programs
  http://www.clevelandclinic.org/myeloma/
- International Myeloma Foundation
  http://www.myeloma.org/
- Mayo Clinic Myeloma Amyloidosis
  http://www.mayo.edu/mmgrg/rst/mmpage.htm
- Multiple Myeloma Education Network
  http://www.healthtalk.com/mmen/
- Multiple Myeloma Foundation
  http://www.multiplemyeloma.org/

OSTEOSARCOMA

NUTRITIONAL ACUITY RANKING: LEVEL 3

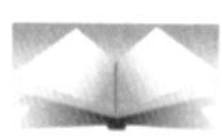

DEFINITIONS AND BACKGROUND

Osteosarcoma involves rapidly growing malignant bone tumor(s) of unknown origin, occurring most often in the long bones of young people (generally males between 10 and 25 years of age). Symptoms and signs include pain over one affected extremity, weight loss, limited use of the extremity, fatigue, warmth in a local area, fever, and cough. This type of cancer often spreads to the lung.

OBJECTIVES

- Prevent dehydration; correct fever (often 103–104°).
- Relieve pain; prolong life.
- Counteract effects of surgery (perhaps amputation), radiation therapy.
- Meet needs related to growth and elevated metabolic rate.

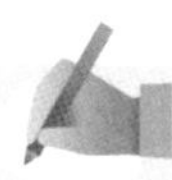

DIETARY AND NUTRITIONAL RECOMMENDATIONS

- A balanced diet (high in calories and protein) will be needed.
- Extra fluids (e.g., 3 L) are used, unless contraindicated.
- Supplement with foods or nutrients that are low in patient's intake.
- Small, frequent feedings may be better tolerated than large meals.
- A diet rich in zinc, vitamins A and C, and other key nutrients will help with wound healing after surgery.

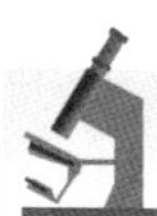

PROFILE

Clinical/History

Height
Weight, weight loss?
BMI
Pain and limited use of affected extremity
Fatigue
Warmth in a local area
Fever, temperature
Cough
I & O

Lab Work

Ca++ (increased)
H&H
Alk phos (increased)
Gluc
Na+, K+
Alb, RBP
TLC (varies)
ALT (increased)

Common Drugs Used and Potential Side Effects

- Hormone therapy may be given, usually with temporary results.
- Doxorubicin may be used with side effects effecting intake. Dry mouth, anemia, stomatitis, nausea, esophagitis, or vomiting may occur.

Herbs, Botanicals and Supplements

- Herbs and botanical supplements should not be used without discussing with physician.

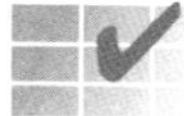

PATIENT EDUCATION

- Discuss ways to make meals more attractive and appetizing.
- Discuss with patient and family how to adjust diet for therapies given (see general cancer entry).

For More Information

- American Cancer Society's Osteosarcoma Resource Center http://www3.cancer.org/cancerinfo/load_cont.asp?ct=52
- Onco Link–Osteosarcoma http://cancer.med.upenn.edu/disease/osteosarc/
- Pediatric Osteosarcoma http://kidshealth.org/parent/medical/cancer/cancer osteosarcoma.html

PANCREATIC CARCINOMA

NUTRITIONAL ACUITY RANKING: LEVEL 3–4

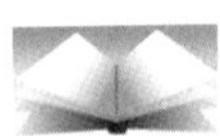

DEFINITIONS AND BACKGROUND

Pancreatic cancer is the fifth most common cause of death from cancer, primarily occurring between 65 and 79 years of age. Malignancy in the pancreas has a high mortality rate from lack of early symptoms, symptoms that mimic other conditions, and rapid metastasis to other organs. About 50–70% have cancer in the head of the pancreas, and 50% have cancer in the body and tail. There is a two times higher risk for pancreatic cancer in smokers than in nonsmokers; a history of alcohol abuse is also common. No elevation of risk has been found between coffee consumption and pancreatic cancer (Partanen et al., 1995). Abnormal glucose metabolism may play a role in etiology of pancreatic cancer, and in men only; high BMI and serum uric acid level have been related to death from this type of cancer (Gapstur et al., 2000). Obesity and insulin resistance may play a role; exercise such as walking 4 hours or more weekly may be protective.

Good folate and pyridoxine status helps reduce risk of pancreatic cancer associated with smoking cigarettes, possibly because an adequate supply of this methyl cofactor helps maintain the stability of DNA and chromosomes (Stolzenberg-Solomon et al., 1999). In patients with pancreatic cancer, the acute-phase protein response seems to be associated with weight loss and shorter survival; this may be stabilized by use of fish oil supplements (Barber et al., 1999).

Symptoms and signs include midepigastric pain, signs of biliary obstruction, rapid weight loss, anorexia, pancreatic insufficiency, hyperglycemia, steatorrhea, nausea and vomiting, fatigue, ascites, thrombophlebitis, and hepatomegaly. A fistula or diarrhea may also occur; jaundice occurs in approximately 50% of cases. Prostate stem-cell antigen (PSCA) is highly overexpressed in approximately 60% of primary pancreatic cancers (http://www.path.jhu.edu/pancreas).

Whipple's procedure (pancreas to duodenectomy) involves many operations; the entire duodenum is usually removed and the pancreas, gallbladder, and spleen may also be removed.

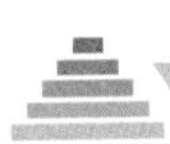

OBJECTIVES

- Reduce nausea and vomiting; control future episodes.
- Prevent or correct weight loss.
- Restore LBM.
- Control side effects of therapy and the disease such as diabetes.
- Counteract therapies—surgery, chemotherapy, and/or radiation.
- Provide foods or supplements that include all necessary nutrients to prolong life and health.
- Augment nutritional status; correct anemia.

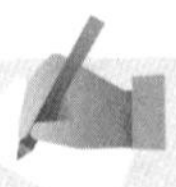

DIETARY AND NUTRITIONAL RECOMMENDATIONS

- TPN may be beneficial for short or long term, altering nutrients according to serum values. The decision must include a generally poor prognosis, weighing risks and benefits. For Whipple's procedure, TPN or TF may be required.
- Small, frequent meals may be better tolerated when and if patient can eat orally.
- Increased calories and protein should be provided to restore weight, unless patient is hyperglycemic or has extensive liver impairment.
- Eventually, a CHO-controlled diet may be needed to manage diabetes if appropriate, considering progress.
- MCT and fat-soluble vitamins (water-miscible form) may be added to the diet. Essential fatty acids (EFAs) should also be included.
- Selenium may be needed for some patients, especially with TPN solutions.
- As tolerated, increase fiber and decrease fat; increase vegetables (Carter et al., 1993).
- Use of pancreatic enzymes may be needed if steatorrhea is present.

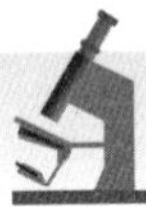

PROFILE

Clinical/History

Height
Weight
BMI
Rapid weight loss
Midepigastric pain
Signs of biliary obstruction
Anorexia
Pancreatic insufficiency
Steatorrhea
Nausea and vomiting
Fatigue
Ascites
Thrombophlebitis
Hepatomegaly
Temperature
BP

Lab Work

Alk phos (increased)
PT (increased)
Gluc (increased)
Serum lipase (increased)
Secretin
PSCA levels
Transferrin
Serum insulin
TLC (varies)
Bilirubin (increased)
Cholecystokinin
Alb
Chol, Trig
Serum amylase (increased)
H&H
ALT, AST (increased)
X-rays, CT scan

Common Drugs Used and Potential Side Effects

- Pancreatic enzymes (pancrelipase and pancreatin) are given only if serum levels of nutrients are inadequate. NOTE: All enzymes are digested when taken as an oral supplement. Enteric coating aids in maintaining integrity of enzymes until they reach small intestine.
- Insulin may be needed if patient is hyperglycemic. In islet cell tumors, hypoglycemia may occur instead. Monitor with meal timing.
- Vitamin B12 supplements may be required with total pancreatectomy, especially with steatorrhea.
- Antiemetics, antibiotics, antacids, diuretics, and analgesics may be needed. Monitor side effects according to medications prescribed. Streptozocin and other antibiotics can cause or aggravate nausea.
- Bile salts also may be needed, especially with extensive diarrhea and steatorrhea.

Herbs, Botanicals and Supplements

- Herbs and botanical supplements should not be used without discussing with physician.

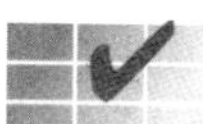

PATIENT EDUCATION

- ✔ Discuss specific dietary recommendations appropriate for patient's condition and therapies.
- ✔ With pancreatectomy, a diabetic diet may be absolutely essential. Discuss rationale with patient.
- ✔ Explain how diet affects malabsorption in regard to fat, protein, vitamins, and minerals.

For More Information

- Cancer Net—Pancreatic Cancer
  http://cancernet.nci.nih.gov/wyntk_pubs/pancreas.htm
- Johns Hopkins—Pancreatic Cancer Home Page
  http://www.path.jhu.edu/pancreas
- Lustgarten Foundation for Pancreatic Cancer Research
  http://www.lustgartenfoundation.org/
- Medline—Pancreatic Cancer
  http://www.nlm.nih.gov/medlineplus/pancreaticcancer.html
- National Pancreas Foundation
  http://www.pancreasfoundation.org/
- Pancreatic Cancer Action Network
  http://www.pancan.org/
- Onco Link—Pancreatic Cancer
  http://cancer.med.upenn.edu/disease/pancreas/

PROSTATE CANCER

NUTRITIONAL ACUITY RANKING: LEVEL 2

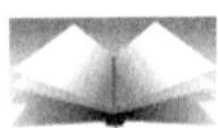

DEFINITIONS AND BACKGROUND

Prostate cancer is the second leading cause of cancer deaths in men. Incidence increases with age, mostly after 65 years of age. Prevalence is higher in northwestern Europe and the United States; incidence among African Americans is the highest in the world. Abdominal obesity in men may increase frequency and severity of urinary obstruction and incidence of prostatectomy (Giovannucci et al., 1994). Male smokers may have reduced incidence of and mortality from prostate cancer (Heinonen et al., 1998).

Risk of prostate cancer is inversely related to intake of grains, nuts, cereals, and soy products; protective effect of soy is 4 times greater than for any other factor (Silverman et al., 1998). Dietary red meat, total fat, and SFA intake may be significant in etiology (Giovannucci et al., 1993). BMI, hip circumference, and waist:hip ratios are not correlated, but large waist circumference is associated with benign prostatic hypertrophy (BPH).

Phytochemicals such as lycopene are also protective (Giovannucci et al., Intake . . ., 1995). High intake of vegetables, especially cruciferous types, is associated with lower risk of prostate cancer; lutein and zeaxthanin are important, but fruit intake does not make any difference. Alpha-tocopherol seems to be protective (Klein et al., 2001); selenium may also be protective and a special study is underway (Zhong and Oberley, 2001).

Signs and symptoms of prostate cancer include urinary dribbling, frequency, pain, or burning. Persistent pain in the pelvis, lower back, or upper thighs also may occur. Surgical intervention is most common; hormonal therapy is second.

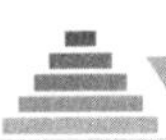

OBJECTIVES

- Prepare patient for therapy (surgery, radiation, medications, or chemotherapy). Hormone therapy and chemotherapy are used less commonly.
- Prevent side effects such as nausea, vomiting, and diarrhea.
- Prevent or correct weight loss.
- Maintain weight that is appropriate for height. If patient is obese, a weight control plan may be needed.
- Prepare for treatments such as brachytherapy (internal radiation therapy, in which small radioactive pellets are inserted or implanted into prostate gland).

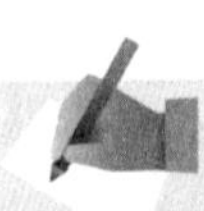

DIETARY AND NUTRITIONAL RECOMMENDATIONS

- Provide adequate calories and protein; avoid excesses.
- If surgery has been performed, a multiple vitamin–mineral supplement may be indicated to promote wound healing.
- Monitor need for lowering sodium if corticosteroids are prescribed.
- Increase use of fruits and vegetables, especially green and yellow–orange. Tomatoes, pizza sauce, strawberries, and similar products are important for their lycopene content.
- Increase isoflavinoids from beans, soybeans, lentils, tofu, tempeh, soy nuts, soymilk, and dried fruit.
- Low-fat and high-fiber diets may be indicated (Carter et al., 1993). Increased use of omega-3 fatty acids has been shown in some preliminary studies to be useful; include salmon, sardines, tuna, mackerel, and herring in diet.

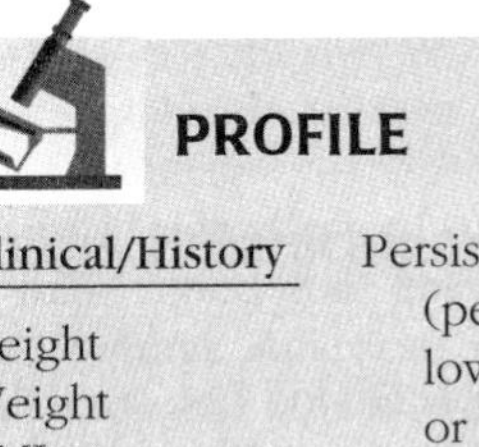

PROFILE

Clinical/History		Lab Work
Height Weight BMI Weight changes Urinary dribbling, frequency, pain, burning	Persistent pain (pelvis, lower back, or upper thighs) BP Rectal examination I & O	Alb, prealbumin TLC BUN, Creat Transferrin H&H Na+, K+ Ca++, Mg++

Common Drugs Used and Potential Side Effects

- Hormonal therapy may be used. Weight gain is often experienced.
- Proscar is not an effective treatment for prostatic cancer. Proscar may be useful to shrink an enlarged prostate gland.
- Chemotherapy drugs have varying side effects; monitor closely.
- Radiation therapy may cause temporary changes in bowel habits (such as increased frequency, increased flatulence, bowel cramping) and urinary frequency. Various medications may aggravate the same effects.

Herbs, Botanicals and Supplements

- Herbs and botanical supplements should not be used without discussing with physician.
- Saw palmetto has some proven efficacy. Avoid taking with estrogens, testosterone, anabolic steroids, oral contraceptives, or finasteride because herb and drug function in similar ways and additive effects are possible.
- Pygeum, nettle, and isoflavones in soy and red clover are being studied at this time for their efficacy in BPH.

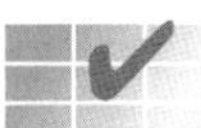

PATIENT EDUCATION

- ✔ Discuss lifestyle and dietary changes that are recommended (i.e., lowering intake of red meats, saturated fats, increasing fruits and vegetables, especially tomato products, increasing fiber).
- ✔ Discuss side effects of any specific therapy offered.
- ✔ Discuss long-term plans for recovery.
- ✔ Discuss menu plans for sufficient intakes of all indicated nutrients.

For More Information

- Association for the Cure of Prostate Cancer
  http://www.capcure.org/
- Onco Link—Prostate Cancer
  http://cancer.med.upenn.edu/disease/prostate/
- Prostate Cancer Info Link
  http://www.comed.com/Prostate/
- Prostate Cancer Research Institute
  http://www.prostate-cancer.org/
- Prostate Cancer Support Group
  http://www.ustoo.com/
- Urologic Oncology Program
  http://www.cancer.med.umich.edu/prostcan/prostcan.html

RADIATION COLITIS AND ENTERITIS

NUTRITIONAL ACUITY RANKING: LEVEL 3

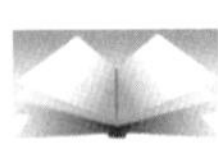

DEFINITIONS AND BACKGROUND

Radiotherapy may involve high-energy radiation from x-rays, cobalt-60, radium, etc. Brachytherapy provides internal, continuous local delivery of radiation to site of malignancy (concealed). Teletherapy provides external radiation to a localized area; 7,000 rads usually causes damage, especially to small intestine (radiation enteritis).

Serious injury to the intestinal epithelium and arterioles of the small or large intestines results in cell death, fibrosis, and obstruction after radiation therapy. Radiation to the ileum is especially devastating. If radiation must be given chronically, resection may be needed. The ability of the intestines to become hyperplastic and to increase absorptive capacity is thus prevented. Of patients who are given abdominal or pelvic radiotherapy, 5–40% will develop radiation enteritis or colitis. Of these persons, many will require home TPN or chronic PN because of the effects on the intestinal tract.

About 50–80% of patients, who have radiation to the pelvis, end up with radiation enteritis; onset can occur up to years later. Symptoms and signs of radiation enteritis or colitis include nausea, vomiting, mucoid diarrhea, abdominal pain, and bleeding (later—colic, decrease in stool caliber, and progressive obstipation with stricture and fibrosis).

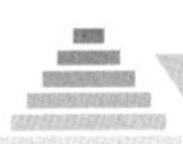

OBJECTIVES

- ▲ Correct malnutrition and malabsorption from diarrhea, bacterial overgrowth, protein exudative losses, CHO loss from decreased enzymes, and steatorrhea from ileal damage.
- ▲ Prevent or correct intestinal ischemia.
- ▲ Prepare patient for surgery, if needed, to relieve obstruction.
- ▲ Meet hypermetabolic needs from infection and complications.
- ▲ Prevent gallstones, renal stones, and other effects after radiation.
- ▲ Replace folic acid and vitamin B12 if ileal damage has occurred.
- ▲ Ensure adequate electrolyte and fluid intake.
- ▲ Boost natural killer (NK) cell activity.

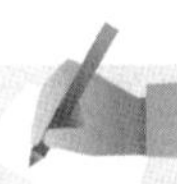

DIETARY AND NUTRITIONAL RECOMMENDATIONS

- An elemental diet may be best tolerated, especially if obstruction or constipation has occurred. If taken orally, these products should be sipped slowly to avoid dumping effect. Encourage patient to consider them medications.
- Low residue, low fat, and low lactose diets have been suggested (Sekhon, 2000). An individualized approach is needed in every case to avoid excessive restrictions. TPN also may be appropriate for the patient, before or after surgery.
- If oral intake is possible, six to eight small feedings may be better tolerated. A low-residue, low-fat, and gluten-free diet may be necessary.
- Gradually add foods back to diet as tolerance increases.
- Fluid and electrolyte balance and intake should be maintained carefully.
- Glutamine and short-chain fatty acids are likely to be used to protect gut and decrease morbidity; 0.5–1.0 g/kg daily may be useful. Investigations are ongoing.

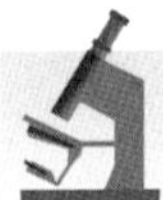

PROFILE

Clinical/History

Height
Weight
BMI
Weight changes
Nausea, vomiting
Mucoid diarrhea
Abdominal pain
Bleeding or decrease in stool caliber
Constipation with stricture and fibrosis
I & O

Lab Work

Alb, RBP
Transferrin
Hydrogen (H) breath test
Gluc
Ca++, Mg++
Fecal fat test
H&H, Serum Fe
Na+, K+
Schilling test
ALT
Intestinal biopsy

Common Drugs Used and Potential Side Effects

- Sedatives may be used as needed.
- Antispasmodics may be used if intestinal colic persists.
- Corticosteroids may cause or aggravate sodium or potassium depletion, negative nitrogen balance, hyperglycemia, and other problems.
- Sulfasalazine has side effects that should be monitored carefully (such as anorexia, nausea, diarrhea, GI distress). Extra folate is needed.
- Preliminary data suggest that use of amifostine may reduce radiation damage in prostate cancer treatment. Further study is needed.

Herbs, Botanicals and Supplements

- Herbs and botanical supplements should not be used without discussing with physician.

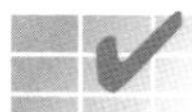

PATIENT EDUCATION

- ✔ Home TPN may be needed for short- or long-term use.
- ✔ Discuss ways to make meals appetizing and palatable and how to decrease nausea (see general cancer entry).

For More Information

- American Dietetic Association
  Radiation Oncology protocol
  www.eatright.org

URINARY TRACT CANCERS: RENAL, BLADDER, AND WILMS' TUMOR (EMBRYOMA OF THE KIDNEY)

NUTRITIONAL ACUITY RANKING: LEVEL 3

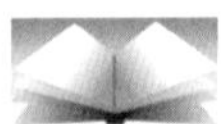

DEFINITIONS AND BACKGROUND

Urinary tract cancer, especially of the bladder, affects more than 50,000 Americans each year. Men are more prone to this type of cancer than are women. Renal cell cancer accounts for about 2% of cancers worldwide; it is increasing in incidence in North America and northern Europe but not in other areas of the world (McLaughlin and Lipworth, 2000). In the United States, the highest rates are now seen among blacks. Blood in the urine and increased frequency of urination are the most common symptoms. Smoking is the most common risk factor; exposure to dyes, rubber, and leather products at work may also pose a risk. Obesity is another factor (Chow et al., 2000).

Surgery is usually required for removal of urinary tract tumors; prognosis with early intervention is good. Survival has improved. See Table 13–12 for tumor staging.

Intake of fruit, retinol, vitamin C, or daily multivitamin supplements tends to be protective, whereas intake of fried foods increases risk (Bruemmer et al., 1996). Drinking nonherbal tea also may prove to be a protective factor (Zheng et al., 1996). Fluid intake is inversely related to risk of bladder cancer in men; daily intake of over 6 cups vs. less than 1 cup of water is associated with less bladder cancer (Michaud et al., 1999).

Wilms' tumor, also called nephroblastoma or embryoma of the kidney, is a highly malignant tumor occurring almost exclusively in young children (younger than 6 years of age); 62% are aged 1–4 years. Metastasis to lungs, liver, and brain can occur. Symptoms and signs include weight loss, anorexia, enlarged kidney, hypertension, fever, anemia, and abdominal pain. A cure may be possible, if metastasis has not occurred before nephrectomy.

OBJECTIVES

- ▲ Prepare patient for surgery (e.g., nephrectomy) and for postsurgical wound healing.
- ▲ Control side effects of radiotherapy and chemotherapy.
- ▲ Promote normal growth and development, as far as possible, in children with Wilms' tumor.
- ▲ Control hypertension; correct anemia. These conditions are common with any of the renal tumors.

TABLE 13–12 Renal Tumor Staging

Stage I	Limited to kidneys (can be excised)
Stage II	Extension into perirenal tissue occurs; excision still may be possible
Stage III	Tumor is not completely resectable
Stage IV	Metastasis occurs
Stage V	Bilateral renal involvement occurs

DIETARY AND NUTRITIONAL RECOMMENDATIONS

- ● Provide adequate calories and protein according to age. If needed, include a safety measure for weight loss that has occurred. In obese adults, weight loss regimens are not recommended until several months after surgery.
- ▲ Ensure adequate intake of foods high in HBV proteins, iron, and B-complex vitamins to help prevent worsening of anemia.
- ▲ Restrict excessive sodium with hypertension. Monitor calcium and magnesium levels as well; supplement if necessary.
- ▲ Monitor protein tolerance; increase as tolerated.
- ▲ Ensure adequate fluid intake, especially water, unless restriction is needed for some other medical reason.

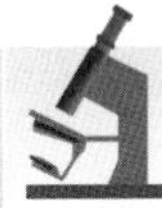

PROFILE

Clinical/History

- Height
- Weight
- Weight changes
- BMI
- Growth percentile in child
- Hematuria
- BP (increased)
- Anorexia
- Enlarged kidney?
- Fever, temperature
- Anemia
- Abdominal pain
- I & O
- Smoking history

Lab Work

- Ca++
- Alb, prealbumin
- Creat
- Mg++
- Gluc
- TLC (varies)
- BUN
- H&H, Serum Fe
- Serum ferritin
- Transferrin
- Liver function tests
- ALT
- Abdominal CT scan
- X-ray

Common Drugs Used and Potential Side Effects

- Dactinomycin or vincristine may cause dry mouth, dysphagia, stomatitis, esophagitis, diarrhea, nausea, and other side effects. Monitor accordingly.
- Doxorubicin also may be used for renal tumors. Dry mouth, nausea, vomiting, esophagitis, or stomatitis may occur.
- For bladder cancer, chemotherapy often involves 5-fluorouracil, cisplatin, cyclophosphamide, methotrexate, or vinblastine. Many GI side effects are common, including nausea, anorexia, diarrhea, or vomiting.

Herbs, Botanicals and Supplements

- Herbs and botanical supplements should not be used without discussing with physician.

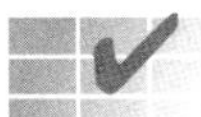

PATIENT EDUCATION

- ✔ Discuss side effects patient is experiencing in light of therapies used (e.g., radiation therapy, chemotherapy, and surgery).
- ✔ Discuss normal growth and/or desirable weight for patient.
- ✔ Highlight meals that are attractive so patient eats as well as possible.
- ✔ Discuss how to correct anemia through appropriate medications and dietary measures.

For More Information

- Cancer Links–USA
  http://www.ontumor.com/kidney.htm
- Kidney Cancer Association
  http://www.nkca.org/selfcare.html
- Med-Line—Kidney Cancer
  http://www.nlm.nih.gov/medlineplus/kidneycancer.html
- National Kidney Cancer Association
  http://www.nkca.org/
- National Cancer Institute Kidney Cancer Web
  http://web.ncifcrf.gov/research/kidney/
- Pediatric Onco Link—Wilms Tumor
  http://cancer.med.upenn.edu/disease/ped_wilms/
- Renal Cell Cancer
  http://www.graylab.ac.uk/cancernet/201070.html

REFFERENCES

Cited References

Alberts D, et al. Lack of effect of a high-fiber cereal supplement on the recurrence of colorectal adenomas. *N Engl J Med.* 2000;342: 1156.

Alavanja M, et al. Saturated fat intake and lung cancer risk among nonsmoking women in Missouri. *J Natl Cancer Inst.* 1993;85: 1906.

Alpha-Tocopherol, Beta-Carotene Cancer Prevention Study Group. The effect of vitamin E and beta-carotene on the incidence of lung cancer and other cancers in male smokers. *N Engl J Med.* 1994;330:1029.

American Gastroenterology Association. Medical position statement: impact of dietary fiber on colon cancer occurrence. Clin Pract and Practice Economics Committee. *Gastroenterol.* 2000;118:1233.

American Institute for Cancer Research. *Taking a closer look at antioxidants.* Pamphlet #E47-TLA/E62. Washington, DC: American Institute for Cancer Research, 1994.

Ames H, et al. Taste perception and breast cancer: evidence of a role for diet. *J Am Diet Assoc.* 1993;93:541.

Anti M, et al. Effects of different doses of fish oil on rectal cell proliferation in patients with sporadic colonic adenomas. *Gastroenterology.* 1994;107:1709.

Arunachalam K, et al. Enhancement of natural immune function by dietary consumption of *Bifidobacterium lactis* (HN109). *Euro J Clin Nutri.* 2000;54:263.

Augustsson K, et al. Dietary heterocyclic amines and cancer of the colon, rectum, bladder and kidney—A population-based study. *Lancet.* 1999;353:703.

Barber M, et al. Fish oil-enriched nutritional supplement attenuates progression of the acute-phase response in weight-losing patients with advanced pancreatic cancer. *J Nutri.* 1999;129:1120.

Barbone F, et al. Diet and endometrial cancer: a case-control study. *Am J Epidemiol.* 1993;137:393.

Baron J, et al. Calcium supplements for the prevention of colorectal adenomas. *N Engl J Med.* 1999;340:101.

Baselga J. The EGFR as a target for anticancer therapy-focus on cetuximab. *Eur J Cancer.* 2001;37:16S.

Bass F, Cox R. The need for dietary counseling of cancer patients as indicated by nutrient and supplement intake. *J Am Diet Assoc.* 1995;95:1319.

Bergstrom A, et al. Overweight as an avoidable cause of cancer in Europe. *Int J Cancer.* 2001;91:421.

Bernstein B, Grasso T. Prevalence of complementary and alternative medicine use in cancer patients. *Oncology.* 2001;15:1267.

Black H. Influence of dietary factors on actinically-induced skin cancer. *Mutat Res.* 1998;422:185.

Bloch A. Feeding the cancer patient: where have we come from, where are we going? *Nutr Clin Pract.* 1994;9:87.

Blot W, et al. Nutrition intervention trials in Linxian, China: supplementation with specific vitamin/mineral combinations, cancer incidence, and disease-specific mortality in the general population. *J Natl Cancer Inst.* 1993;85:1483.

Boyd N, et al. Effects at two years of a low-fat, high carbohydrate diet on radiologic features of the breast: results from a randomized trial. *J Natl Cancer Inst.* 1997;89:488.

Brennan J, et al. Molecular assessment of histopathological staging in squamous-cell carcinoma of the head and neck. *N Engl J Med.* 1995;332:429.

Brown J, et al. Nutrition during and after cancer treatment: a guide for informed choices by cancer survivors. *Cancer J Clin.* 2001;51: 153.

Brown L, et al. Adenocarcinoma of the esophagus: role of obesity and diet. *J Natl Cancer Inst.* 1995;87:104.

Bruemmer B, et al. Nutrient intake in relation to bladder cancer among middle-aged men and women. *Am J Epidemiol.* 1996;144: 485.

Cantor K, et al. Drinking water source and chlorination byproducts in Iowa. III. Risk of brain cancer. *Am J Epid.* 1999;150:552.

Carter J, et al. Hypothesis: dietary management may improve survival from nutritionally linked cancers based on analysis of representative cases. *J Am Col Nutri.* 1993;12:209.

Cauley J, et al. Bone mineral density and risk of breast cancer in older women: the study of osteoporotic fractures. *JAMA.* 1996; 276:1404.

Cheng K, et al. Pickled vegetables in the etiology of esophageal cancer in Hong Kong Chinese. *Lancet.* 1992;33:1314.

Chiu B, et al. Diet and risk of non-Hodgkin lymphoma in older women. *J Am Med Assoc.* 1996;275:1315.

Choi S, Mason J. Folate and carcinogenesis: an integrated scheme. *J Nutri.* 2000;130:129.

Chow W, et al. Obesity, hypertension, and the risk of kidney cancer in men. *N Engl J Med.* 2000;343:1305.

Cohen J, et al. Fruit and vegetable intake and prostate cancer risk. *J Natl Cancer Inst.* 2000;92:61.

Cohen L. Colorectal cancer: a primary care approach to screening. *Geriatrics.* 1996;51:45.

Craig W. Phytochemicals: guardians of our health. *J Am Diet Assoc.* 1997;97:S199.

Demark-Wahnefried W, et al. Weight gain in women diagnosed with breast cancer. *J Am Diet Assoc.* 1997;97:519.

Djuric Z, et al. Oxidative DNA damage levels in blood from women at high risk for breast cancer are associated with dietary intakes of meats, vegetables, and fruits. *J Am Diet Assoc.* 1998;98:524.

Doerr T, et al. Zinc deficiency in head and neck cancer patients. *J Am Col Nutri.* 1997;16:418.

Dorant E, et al. Consumption of onions and a reduced risk of stomach carcinoma. *Gastroenterology.* 1996;110:12.

Doyle T, et al. The association of drinking water source and chlorination by-products with cancer incidence among postmenopausal women in Iowa: a prospective cohort study. *Am J Pub Health.* 1997;87:1168.

Drewnowski A, et al. Genetic taste markers and preferences for vegetables and fruit of female breast cancer patients. *J Am Diet Assoc.* 2000;100:191.

Dwyer J, et al. Tofu and soy drinks contain phytoestrogens. *J Am Diet Assoc.* 1994;94:739.

Fernandez E, et al. Fish consumption and cancer risk. *Am J Clin Nutri.* 1999;70:85.

Ford E, et al. Body mass index and colon cancer in a national sample of adult U.S. men and women. *Am J Epid.* 1999;150:390.

Freudenheim J, et al. Premenopausal breast cancer risk and intake of vegetables, fruits, and related nutrients. *J Natl Cancer Inst*. 1996;88:340.

Fuchs C, et al. Dietary fiber and the risk of colorectal cancer and adenoma in women. *N Engl J Med*. 1999;340:169.

Gapstur S, et al. Abnormal glucose metabolism and pancreatic cancer mortality. *JAMA*. 2000;283:2552.

Giovannucci E, et al. A prospective study of dietary fat and risk of prostate cancer. *J Natl Cancer Inst*. 1993;85:1571.

Giovannucci E, et al. Alcohol, low-methionine/low-folate diets and risk of colon cancer in men. *J Natl Cancer Inst*. 1995;87:265.

Giovannucci E, et al. Intake of carotenoids and retinol in relation to risk of prostate cancer. *J Natl Cancer Inst*. 1995;87:1767.

Giovannucci E, et al. Multivitamin use, folate and colon cancer in women in the Nurses's Health Study. *Ann Int Med*. 1998;129:517.

Giovannucci E, et al. Obesity and benign prostatic hyperplasia. *Am J Epidemiol*. 1994;140:989.

Giovannucci E. Tomatoes, tomato-based products, lycopene and cancer: Review of the epidemiologic literature. *J Natl Cancer Inst*. 1999;91:317.

Goodwin J, Brodwick M. Diet, aging and cancer. *Clin Geriatr Med*. 1995;11:577.

Hankin J. Role of nutrition in women's health: diet and breast cancer. *J Am Diet Assoc*. 1993;93:994.

Harnack L, et al. Cancer prevention-related nutrition knowledge, beliefs, and attitudes of U.S. adults: 1992 NHIS Cancer Epidemiology Supplement. *J Nutr Ed*. 1998;30:131.

Heinonen O, et al. Prostate cancer and supplementation with a-tocopherol and B-carotene: incidence and mortality in a controlled trial. *J Cancer Institute*. 1998;90:440.

Holmes M, et al. Association of dietary intake of fat and fatty acids with risk of breast cancer. *J Am Med Assoc*. 1999;281:914.

Horn-Ross P. Diet and the risk of salivary gland cancer. *Am J Epid*. 1997;146:171.

Hu J, La Vecchia C, et al. Diet and brain cancer in adults: a case-control study in northeast China. *Int J Cancer*. 1999;81:20.

Huang Z, et al. Dual effects of weight and weight gain on breast cancer risk. *J Am Med Assoc*. 1997;278:1407.

Imai K, et al. Cancer-preventive effects of drinking green tea among a Japanese population. *Preventive Med*. 1997;26:769.

Jernstrom H, et al. Obesity, weight change, fasting insulin, pro-insulin, C-peptide and insulin-like growth factor-1 levels in women with and without breast cancer. *J Women's Health and Gender-Based Medicine*. 1999;8:1265.

Jin D, et al. Effects of parenteral nutrition support and chemotherapy on the phasic concentration of tumor cells in gastrointestinal cancer. *J Parenter Enteral Nutrition*. 1999;23:237.

Kalman D, Villani L. Nutritional aspects of cancer-related fatigue. *J Am Diet Assoc*. 1997;97:650.

Kaplan S, et al. Nutritional factors in the etiology of brain tumors: potential role of nitrosamines, fat, and cholesterol. *Am J Epid*. 1997;146:832.

Kim S, et al. National Institutes of Health workshop: role of nutrient regulation of signal transduction in metabolic diseases. *Am J Clin Nutri*. 1999;70:544.

Klein E, et al. SELECT: the next prostate cancer prevention trial. Selenum and Vitamin E Cancer Prevention Trial. *J Urol*. 2001;166:1311.

Klein S, Koretz R. Nutrition support in patients with cancer: what do the data really show? *Nutr Clin Pract*. 1994;9:87.

Klebanoff M, et al. The risk of childhood cancer after neonatal exposure to vitamin K. *N Engl J Med*. 1993;329:905.

Ko Y, et al. Chinese food cooking and lung cancer in women nonsmokers. *Am J Epid*. 2000;151:140.

Korber J, et al. Increased lipid utilization in weight losing and weight stable cancer patients with normal body weight. *Euro J Clin Nutri*. 1999;53:740.

Kotler D. Cachexia. *Ann Int Med*. 2000;133:622.

Kuper H, et al. The risk of liver and bile duct cancer in patients with chronic viral hepatitis, alcoholism, or cirrhosis. *Hepatology*. 2001;34:714.

Kushi L, et al. Prospective study of diet and ovarian cancer. *Am J Epid*. 1999;149:21.

Lampeter E, et al. Transfer of insulin-dependent diabetes between HLA-identical siblings by bone-marrow transplantation. *Lancet*. 1993;341:1243.

Lebel-Medieros N, et al. Rationale, process, and nutritional implications of peripheral blood stem cell transplantation. *J Am Diet Assoc*. 1998;98:9.

Lee I. B-carotene supplementation and incidence of cancer and cardiovascular disease: The Women's Health Study. *J Inst Nutri*. 1999;91:2102.

Leenan R, et al. A single dose of tea with or without milk increases plasma antioxidant activity in humans. *Euro J Clin Nutri*. 2000;54:87.

Le Marchand L, et al. Intake of flavonoids and lung cancer. *J Natl Cancer Inst*. 2000;92:154.

Lenssen P, et al. Nutrient support in hematopoietic cell transplantation. *J Parenter Enteral Nutri*. 2001;25:219.

Levi F, et al. Refined and whole grain cereals and the risk of oral, esophageal, and laryngeal cancer. *Euro J Clin Nutri*. 2000;54:487.

Levin B, Amos C. Therapy of unresectable hepatocellular carcinoma. *N Engl J Med*. 1995;332:1294.

Liggins J, et al. Daidzein and genistein content of fruits and nuts. *J Nutr Biochem*. 2000;11:326.

Lipworth L, et al. History of breastfeeding in relation to breast cancer risk: a review of the epidemiological literature. *J Natl Cancer Inst*. 2000;92:302.

Liu G, et al. Omega-3 but not omega-6 fatty acids inhibit AP-1 activity and cell transformation in JB6 cells. *Proc Natl Acad Sci*. 2001;298:7510.

Lykkesfeldt J, et al. Ascorbate is depleted by smoking and replanted by moderate supplementation: a study in male smokers and nonsmokers with matched dietary antioxidant intakes. *Am J Clin Nutri*. 2000;71:530.

Ma J, et al. Milk intake, circulating levels of insulin-like growth factor-I, and risk of colorectal cancer in men. *J Natl Cancer Inst*. 2001;93:1330.

Martinez M, et al. Physical activity, body mass index, and prostaglandin E2 levels in rectal mucosa. *J National Cancer Inst*. 1999;91:950.

McBurney M, et al. A cost-evaluation of glutamine-supplemented parenteral nutrition in adult bone marrow transplantation. *J Am Diet Assoc*. 1994;94:1263.

McCann R, et al. Comfort care for terminally ill patients: the appropriate use of nutrition and hydration. *JAMA*. 1994;272:1263.

McGlynn K, et al. International trends and patterns of primary liver cancer. *Int J Cancer*. 2001;94:290.

McLaughlin J, Lipworth L. Epidemiologic aspects of renal cell cancer. *Semin Oncol*. 2000;27:115.

Medina J, Khafif A. Early oral feeding following total laryngectomy. *Laryngoscope*. 2001;111:368.

Meloni G, et al. Lactose absorption in patients with ovarian cancer. *Am J Epid*. 1999;150:183.

Michaud D, et al. Fluid intake and the risk of bladder cancer in men. *N Engl J Med.* 1999;340:1390.

Michaud D, et al. Intake of specific carotenoids and risk of lung cancer in two prospective U.S. cohorts. *Am J Clin Nutri.* 2000;72:990.

Moerman C, et al. Consumption of foods and micronutrients and the risk of cancer of the biliary tract. *Prev Med.* 1995;24:591.

Momparler R, Bovenzi V. DNA methylation and cancer. *J Cell Physiol.* 2000;183:145.

Muscat J, Wynder E. The consumption of well-done red meat and the risk of colorectal cancer. *Am J Public Health.* 1994;84:856.

Nelson R, et al. Body iron stores and risk of colonic neoplasia. *J Natl Cancer Inst.* 1994;86:455.

Newman V, et al. Dietary supplement use by women at risk for breast cancer recurrence. *J Am Diet Assoc.* 1998;98:285.

Norred W, Voss K. Toxicity and role of fumonisins in animal diseases and human esophageal cancer. *J Food Protect.* 1994;57:522.

O'Meara E, et al. Hormone replacement therapy after a diagnosis of breast cancer in relation to recurrence and mortality. *J Natl Cancer Inst.* 2001;93:754.

Partanen T, et al. Coffee consumption not associated with risk of pancreas cancer in Finland. *Prev Med.* 1995;24:213.

Pearlstone D, et al. Effect of enteral and parenteral nutrition on amino acid levels in cancer patients. *J Parenter Enteral Nutri.* 1995; 19:204.

Porrini M, Riso P. Lymphocyte lycopene concentration and DNA protection from oxidative damage is increased in women after short period of tomato consumption. *J Nutri.* 2000;130:189.

Prescott E, et al. Alcohol intake and the risk of lung cancer: influence of type of alcoholic beverage. *Am J Epid.* 1999;149:463.

Preston T, et al. Fibrinogen synthesis is elevated in fasting cancer patients with an acute phase response. *J Nutri.* 1998;128:1355.

Rauscher G, et al. Relation between body mass index and lung cancer risk in men and women never and former smokers. *Am J Epid.* 2000;152:506.

Ringwald-Smith K, et al. Comparison of energy estimation equations with measured energy expenditure in obese adolescent patients with cancer. *J Am Diet Assoc.* 1999;99:844.

Risch H, et al. Dietary fat intake and risk of epithelial ovarian cancer. *J Natl Cancer Inst.* 1994;86:1409.

Rock C, et al. Factors associated with weight gain in women after diagnosis of breast cancer. *J Am Diet Assoc.* 1999;99:1212.

Ross R, Henderson B. Do diet and androgens alter prostate cancer risk via a common etiologic pathway? *J Natl Cancer Inst.* 1994; 86:252.

Schatzkin A, et al. Lack of effect of a low-fat, high fiber diet on the recurrence of colorectal adenomas. *N Engl J Med.* 2000;342:1149.

Schoen R, et al. Increased blood glucose and insulin, body size and incident colorectal cancer. *J National Cancer Inst.* 1999;91:1147.

Sekhon S. Chronic radiation enteritis: Women's food tolerances after radiation treatment for gynecologic cancer. *J Am Diet Assoc.* 2000;100:941.

Shu X, et al. A population-based case-control study of dietary factors and endometrial cancer in Shanghai, People's Republic of China. *Am J Epidemiol.* 1993;137:155.

Silverman D, et al. Dietary and nutritional factors and pancreatic cancer: a case-controlled study based on direct interviews. *J Natl Cancer Inst.* 1998;90:1710.

Simon J, et al. Serum fatty acids and the risk of fatal cancer. *Am J Epid.* 1998;148:854.

Singh P, et al. Dietary risk factors for colon cancer in a low-risk population. *Am J Epid.* 1998;148:761.

Slattery M, et al. Carotenoids and colon cancer. *Am J Clin Nutri.* 2000; 71:575.

Steinmetz K, et al. Vegetables, fruit, and colon cancer in the Iowa Women's Health Study. *Am J Epidemiol.* 1994;139:1.

Steinmetz K, Potter J. Vegetables, fruit, and cancer prevention: a review. *J Am Diet Assoc.* 1996;96:1027.

Stern J. Impact of a randomized, controlled trial of liberal vs conservative hospital discharge criteria on energy, protein, and fluid intake in patients who received marrow transplants. *J Am Dietetic Assoc.* 2000;100:1015.

Stoll B. Dietary supplements of dehydroepiandrosterone in relation to breast cancer risk. *Euro J Clin Nutri.* 1999;53:771.

Stoll B. Teenage obesity in relation to breast cancer risk (a review). *Int J Obesity and Related Metabolic Disorders.* 1998;22:1035.

Stolzenberg-Solomon R, et al. Pancreatic cancer risk and nutrition-related methyl-group availability indicators in male smokers. *J Natl Cancer Inst.* 1999;91:535.

Thune I, et al. Physical activity and the risk of breast cancer. *N Engl J Med.* 1997;336:1269.

Tisdale M. Cancer cachexia. *Anticancer Drugs.* 1993;4:115.

Trentham-Dietz A, et al. Body size and risk of breast cancer. *Am J Epid.* 1997;145:1011.

Tryggvadottir L, et al. Breastfeeding and reduced risk of breast cancer in an Icelandic cohort study. *Am J Epid.* 2001;154:37.

Turner G, et al. Relative hyperglucagonemia in L-asparaginase-and prednisone-induced glucose intolerance in management of acute lymphocytic leukemia. *Clin Pediatr.* 1983;22:363.

Umegaki S, et al. Beta-carotene prevents x-ray induction of micronuclei in human lymphocytes. *Am J Clin Nutri.* 1994;59:409.

van Dam R, et al. Diet and basal cell carcinoma of the skin in a prospective cohort of men. *Am J Clin Nutri.* 2000;71:135.

van Faasen A, et al. Bile acids and pH values in total feces and in fecal water from habitually omnivorous and vegetarian subjects. *Am J Clin Nutri.* 1993;58:917.

van den Brandt P, et al. Alcohol and breast cancer: results from the Netherlands Cohort Study. *Am J Epidemiol.* 1995;141:907.

Van Duyn M, Pivonka E. Overview of the health benefits of fruit and vegetable consumption for the dietetics professional: selected literature. *J Am Diet Assoc.* 2000;100:1511.

Velie E, et al. Dietary fat, fat subtypes, and breast cancer in postmenopausal women: a prospective cohort study. *J Natl Cancer Inst.* 2000;92:833.

Voelker R. Ames agrees with mom's advice: eat your fruits and vegetables. *JAMA.* 1995;273:1077.

Woo S, et al. A longitudinal study of oral ulcerative mucositis in bone marrow transplant recipients. *Cancer.* 1993;72:1612.

Yoshikawa T, et al. Effects of tumor removal and body weight loss on insulin resistance in patients with cancer. *Surgery.* 1994;116: 62.

Zhang S, et al. Dietary carotenoids and vitamins A, C, and E. *J Natl Cancer Inst.* 1999;91:547.

Zhang S, et al. Dietary fat and protein in relation to risk of non-Hodgkin's lymphoma among women. *J Natl Cancer Inst.* 1999;91: 175.

Zheng T, et al. Lactation and breast cancer risk: a case-control study in Connecticut. *Br J Cancer.* 2001;84:1472.

Zheng W, et al. Diet and other risk factors for laryngeal cancer in Shanghai, China. *Am J Epidemiol.* 1992;136:178.

Zheng W, et al. Dietary intake of energy and animal foods and endometrial cancer incidence: the Iowa women's health study. *Am J Epidemiol.* 1995;142:388.

Zheng W, et al. Retinol, antioxidant vitamins, and cancers of the upper digestive tract in a prospective cohort study of postmenopausal women. *Am J Epidemiol.* 1995;142:955.

Zheng W, et al. Tea consumption and cancer incidence in a prospective cohort study of postmenopausal women. *Am J Epidemiol.* 1996;144:175.

Zheng W, et al. Well-done meat intake and the risk of breast cancer. *J Natl Cancer Inst.* 1998;90:1724.

Zhong W, Oberley T. Redox-mediated effects of selenium on apoptosis and cell cycle in the LNCaP human prostate cancer cell line. *Cancer Res.* 2001;61:7071.

Suggested Readings

American Institute for Cancer Research. *Food, nutrition, and the prevention of cancer: a global perspective.* Washington, DC: AICR, 1997.

Coghlin-Dickson T. Clinical Pathway nutrition management for outpatient bone marrow transplantation. *J Am Diet Assoc.* 1997;97:61.

de Kleijn K, et al. Intake of dietary phytoestrogens is low in postmenopausal women in the United States: the Framingham Study. *J Nutri.* 2001;131:1826.

Drewnowski A, et al. Both food preferences and food frequency scores predict fat intakes of women with breast cancer. *J Am Diet Assoc.* 2000;100:1325.

Eriksson K, et al. Nutrition and acute leukemia in adults: relation between nutritional status and infectious complications during remission induction. *Cancer.* 1998;82:1071.

Frankmann C. Nutritional care in cancer and neoplastic disease. In: Mahan K, Escott-Stump S, eds. *Krause's food, nutrition, and diet therapy.* 10th ed. Philadelphia: WB Saunders, 2000.

Goodman G, et al. Predictors of serum selenium in cigarette smokers and the lack of association with lung and prostate cancer risk. *Cancer Epidemiol Biomarkers Prev.* 2001;10:1069.

Hasler C, et al. How to evaluate the safety, efficacy, and quality of functional foods and their ingredients. *J Am Diet Assoc.* 2001;101:733.

Hebert J, et al. Change in women's diet and body mass following extensive intervention for early-stage breast cancer. *J Am Diet Assoc.* 2001;101:421.

Hoque A, et al. Molecular epidemiologic studies within the Selenium and Vitamin E Cancer Prevention Trial (SELECT). *Cancer Causes Control.* 2001;12:627.

Jansen M, et al. Cohort analysis of fruit and vegetable consumption and lung cancer mortality in European men. *Int J Cancer.* 2001;92:913.

Kappel A, et al. Serum carotenoids as biomarkers of fruit and vegetable consumption in the New York Women's Health Study. *Public Health Nutri.* 2001;4:829.

Köhlmeier M, et al. Introducing cancer nutrition to medical students: effectiveness of computer-based instruction. *Am J Clin Nutri.* 2000;71:873.

McCarty M. Mortality from Western cancers rose dramatically among African-Americans during the 20th century: are dietary animal products to blame? *Med Hypotheses.* 2001;57:169.

Minami Y, et al. Determinants of infant feeding method in relation to risk factors for breast cancer. *Prev Med.* 2000;30:363.

Rivadeneira D, et al. Nutritional support of the cancer patient. *Cancer J Clin.* 1998;48:69.

Spaulding-Albright N. A review of some herbal and related products commonly used in cancer patients. *J Am Diet Assoc.* 1997;97:S208.

Yong L, et al. Prospective study of relative weight and risk of breast cancer: The Breast Cancer Detection Demonstration Project Follow-Up Study. *Am J Epid.* 1996;143:985.

SECTION 14

Surgical Disorders

CHIEF ASSESSMENT FACTORS

Presurgical Status:

- HISTORY OF ILLNESS—ACUTE OR CHRONIC (DIABETES, CEREBROVASCULAR DISEASE, CORONARY HEART DISEASE, ETC.)
- RECENT WEIGHT CHANGES, ESPECIALLY UNINTENTIONAL LOSS
- SERUM ALBUMIN, TRANSFERRIN, RETINOL BINDING PROTEIN (RBP)
- HYDRATION STATUS
- ELECTROLYTE STATUS
- BLOOD PRESSURE, ABNORMAL
- ANEMIA
- NAUSEA, VOMITING
- SURGICAL PROCEDURE (GASTROINTESTINAL [GI] VERSUS NON-GI INVOLVEMENT)
- OBESITY
- INFECTIONS
- RESPIRATORY FUNCTION (e.g., OXYGEN SATURATION LEVELS)
- RECENT STARVATION STATUS

Postsurgical Status:

- BREATHING RATE, PNEUMONIA
- ELECTROLYTE BALANCE
- PAIN, SLEEP DISTURBANCE
- NAUSEA, VOMITING, CONSTIPATION
- IMPAIRED SKIN INTEGRITY, DEHISCENCE OF WOUND
- URINARY TRACT INFECTION, SEPSIS
- ATELECTASIS
- PARALYTIC ILEUS, ABDOMINAL DISTENTION
- RESPIRATORY FUNCTION (e.g., OXYGEN SATURATION LEVELS)
- FEVER

TABLE 14–1 Emergency Versus Major Surgery

Elective Surgery—Minimal increases in nitrogen loss and 10–15% increase in calorie needs; Major Surgery—Greater intensity and duration will increase catabolic effects. Preoperative nutrition may be needed for up to 1 month, if possible (Cerra, 1984).

TABLE 14–2 Extent of Body Reserves of Nutrients

Nutrient	*Time Required to Deplete Reserves in Well-Nourished Individuals*
Amino acids	Several hours
Carbohydrate	13 hours
Sodium	2–3 days
Water	4 days
Zinc	5 days
Fat	20–40 days
Thiamin	30–60 days
Vitamin C	60–120 days
Niacin	60–180 days
Riboflavin	60–180 days
Vitamin A	90–365 days
Iron	125 days (women); 750 days (men)
Iodine	1,000 days
Calcium	2,500 days

From: Guthrie H. *Introductory nutrition*. 7th ed. St Louis: Times Mirror/ Mosby College Publishers, 1989.

GENERAL SURGERY

NUTRITIONAL ACUITY RANKING: LEVEL 2

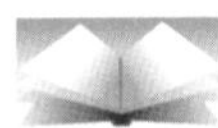

DEFINITIONS AND BACKGROUND

Nutritional risk of surgery (Table 14–1) may be related to the extent of surgery, prior nutritional state of patient, and effect of surgery on patient's ability to digest and absorb nutrients. After surgery or injury, plasma cortisol generally increases rapidly with an acceleration in the breakdown of fat to fatty acids and glycerol. The metabolic response to surgical or accidental injury is characterized by the breakdown of skeletal muscle protein and the transfer of amino acids to visceral organs and the wound, where the substrate serves to enhance host defenses and support vital organ function and wound repair (Wilmore, 2001).

Increased excretion of nitrogen and sodium retention occur but is reversed in approximately 5–7 days (or as late as 12–14 days in elderly individuals); this may be prolonged after severe burns. Increased excretion of potassium occurs but begins to reverse itself 1–2 days after surgery. An increased excretion of calcium is seen after skeletal trauma or during immobilization. Major surgery or stress to soft tissue is followed by increased calcium excretion in children and adults and decreased calcium excretion in elderly individuals. Vitamin C may be destroyed by extensive inflammation in postoperative condition. Table 14–2 indicates extent of body reserves of nutrients, which are an advantage when considering specific intervention and patient population (Heyland et al., 2001).

Malnutrition is prevalent among surgical patients and is associated with higher surgical complication rates and mortality. Some causes of poor nutritional status are related to the underlying disease, socio-economic factors, age, and length of hospitalization. While medical teams often overlook malnutrition, and screening of these patients is not routine, it is important to identify patients at risk for malnutrition to prevent related complications (Correia et al., 2001).

In a population of patients preparing for GI or hernia surgery, nutritional status was assessed by using Subjective Global Assessment; malnutrition was present in 55% of patients, with 19% severely malnourished (Correia et al., 2001). The presence of cancer, infection, age over 60 years, upper GI disease, and longer length of hospital stay all negatively influenced nutritional status.

Nutritional status plays an important role in determining outcome after many types of operations. For example, impaired nutrition is an important predictor of death or the need for reventilation after operations for lung cancer (Jagoe et al., 2001). High-risk patients with head and neck cancer (e.g., heavy alcohol users) need a feeding gastrostomy at the time of their initial surgical therapy (Schweinfurth et al., 2001).

A fever causes increased nutritional needs; for every 1° increase, there is an increased caloric need of 7–8%. With wounds, burns, and hemorrhage, there is an increased protein need. Major wounds and burns can cause a loss of 50 g protein or more per day. With hemorrhage or major blood loss, or even when much blood is drawn for laboratory tests, loss of iron and plasma protein may be great; loss of 1 L of blood is equivalent to 500 mg of iron and 50 g of plasma protein. Fluids should also be increased.

Patient risk factors predictive of postoperative morbidity include serum albumin level, anesthesia classification, complexity of operation, and 17 other preoperative risk variables (Daly et al., 1997). See Table 14–3.

Remember that D5W has only 170 kcal/L. After surgery, patients fed a regular diet have less morbidity when compared with those fed a clear liquid diet (Martindale, 1998).

Postoperative enteral nutrition (EN) with supplemental arginine, ribonucleic acid, and omega-3 fatty acids, instead of standard tube feeding (TF), significantly improves surgical outcomes through decreases in infection, wound complications, and hospital lengths of stay (Daly et al., 1992). Patients who receive this enteral immunonutrition before and after major upper GI surgery have a significantly lower incidence of infections and lower treatment costs (Senkal et al., 1999). Patients who have surgery for cancer have fewer infections and significantly shorter lengths of stays (cut by 1–2 days) when they receive EN supplemented with immunonutrients (Braga et al., 1999).

Glutamine (GLN) accounts for approximately one third of the translocated nitrogen. GLN supplementation has important effects in catabolic surgical patients, but the exact mechanisms to explain these events remain unknown, and more research is required to explain the apparent benefits of dietary GLN (Wilmore, 2001). Immunonutrition may decrease infectious complication rates, but it is not associated with overall mortality.

Slow wound healing and dehiscence are more common among persons older than age 60. A complete, balanced therapeutic diet is recommended. Protein beyond 1.5 g/kg may dehydrate the patient (Thomas, 1996). Correcting a nutritional deficit may not affect the underlying illness. Table 14–4 describes postsurgical stages and their impact on nutritional status.

TABLE 14–3 Role of Albumin in Surgical Outcomes

Serum albumin concentration predicts surgical outcomes better than many other patient characteristics (Gibbs et al., 1999). About 54,215 subjects were studied in the National VA Surgical Risk Study for whom preoperative serum albumins were available. Patients were monitored for 30 days after surgery. Albumin over 4.6 had mortality of 1% and morbidity 10%; albumin less than 2.1—mortality 29% and morbidity 65%. Serum albumin level before surgery was a stronger predictor of mortality and morbidity than age, gender, smoking history (hx), alcohol use, emergency vs. elective surgery, presence of comorbidity with all major organ systems, and 14 preoperative lab values. Presurgery serum albumin is an especially strong predictor of certain types of morbidity, particularly sepsis, renal failure, and major infections.

Plasma albumin half-life is markedly shorter in hypoalbuminemic patients receiving total parenteral nutrition (TPN) (Spiess et al., 1996). The fall in serum albumin associated with acute illness—sepsis, trauma, burns, or surgery—is probably explained by increased catabolism and decreased synthesis.

OBJECTIVES

Preoperative:

- ▲ Maintain reserves. Proper nourishment should be emphasized to prepare for surgical stress, wound healing, hemorrhage, and potential dehydration. Some authors suggest glucose/potassium intravenous loading in nondiabetic, nonrespiratory patients for preoperative preparation.
- ▲ Monitor patients who are grossly overweight. Fatty tissues are not resistant to infections; they are hard to suture. Dehiscence may occur. Controlled weight loss should be instituted before surgery whenever possible.

Postoperative

- ▲ Maintain or replete nutrient stores.
- ▲ Correct electrolyte and fluid imbalances (water, sodium, potassium).
- ▲ Prevent extended time for wound healing. Wound has priority for first 5–10 days; tensile strength peaks at 40–50 days.
- ▲ Restore lost protein and iron from hemorrhage/bleeding.
- ▲ Replace important nutrients (vitamin C, 100–200% recommended dietary allowance (RDA); vitamin K, zinc, vitamin A). Arginine triggers anabolic hormones (insulin, growth hormone) and secretin and has been shown to speed wound healing; it is as a potent secretagogue and vasodilator (Kirk et al., 1993). Select an immune-enhanced tube-feeding product for this purpose (Daly, 1992).
- ▲ Minimize weight loss, which is not obligatory. Prevent or correct protein–calorie malnutrition (PCM).
- ▲ Attend to special needs such as fever, trauma, pregnancy, infancy, or childhood.
- ▲ Prevent infection, which can occur in more than 10% of surgical cases.

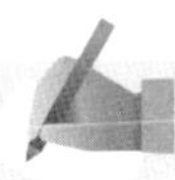

DIETARY AND NUTRITIONAL RECOMMENDATIONS

Preoperative:

- Use a high-protein/high-calorie diet. TF or TPN if needed.
- If patient is obese, use a low-calorie diet that includes carbohydrates (CHOs) adequate for glycogen stores.
- Ensure that intakes of zinc, vitamins C, and K are adequate.
- Gradually restrict diet to clear liquids and then NPO, nothing by mouth.

Postoperative:

- Immediately after surgery, use intravenous glucose and electrolytes as needed. As treatment progresses, diet may be changed as tolerated.

TABLE 14–4 Postsurgical Phases

3–7 days: Marked catabolic response
2–5 weeks: Turning point and anabolic phase at which spontaneous improvement begins
6 weeks or longer: Fat gain phase, in which vigorous nutritional support could promote excessive fat stores

- Because tolerances vary after surgery, a postoperative diet allows a combination of liquid and solid items (Travis and Barr, 1997).
- If oral feeding is not possible, use enteral nutrition whenever possible. Initiate TF within 12–18 hours for less sepsis and fewer complications; gut can generally tolerate early feedings (Moore et al., 1991; Zaloga 1992; Erickson and Perrault, 1993). Intrajejunal feedings may offer maximal gains for patients with GI distress.
- When necessary, because of prolonged GI compromise or conditions such as short bowel syndrome, use TPN. Short-term TPN also tends to reverse undesirable T-cell lymphokine and immunologic responses in malnourished surgical patients (Welsh et al., 1996).
- Patient's increased appetite requires a high calorie intake, high biologic value (HBV) proteins, and increased fluid, zinc, and vitamins C and A; 40–45 kcal/kg and 1.5 g protein/kg are needed.
- Increase branched-chain amino acids (BCAAs) for stress greater than usual.
- Alter care plans by degree of net catabolism (losses of 5–15 g of nitrogen daily may be common). Alter calories accordingly.
- With infection, use precautions against excesses of zinc and iron, because they are bacterial nutrients. It may be beneficial to omit zinc and iron from TPN solutions for a few days in cases where sepsis is a risk.
- Delayed wound healing and dehiscence are three times more common after 60 years of age (Thomas, 1996). A complete, balanced diet is best recommended, using caution not to exceed protein over 1.5 g/kg because of risk of dehydration. Excess vitamin and mineral supplementation provides no improvement in healing rate.
- Arginine sources include shrimp, lean ground beef, pumpkin seeds, garbanzo beans, cottage cheese, peanuts, and soymilk; use where possible.

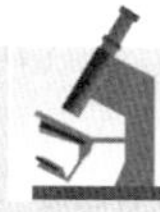

PROFILE

Clinical/History

Height
Weight
Body mass index (BMI)
Weight changes
Intake and output (I & O)
Nausea, vomiting
Constipation
Anorexia
Urinary tract infection (UTI)
Skin integrity

Lab Work

Albumin (alb), prealbumin
Blood urea nitrogen (BUN), Creatine (creat)
Potassium (K+)
N balance
Transferrin
Sodium (Na+)
Glucose (gluc)
Pro Time (PT) or INR
Hemoglobin and hematocrit (H&H), Serum Fe
RBP
Phosphorus (P)
Total lymphocyte count (TLC)
Calcium (Ca++)
Magnesium (Mg++)
Vitamin B12

Common Drugs and Anesthesia Used and Potential Side Effects

- Anesthesia delays peristalsis; nausea is common. Patient may eat ice chips or sip carbonated beverages until nausea subsides.
- Nitrous oxide anesthesia may cause neurologic damage in patients with a vitamin B12 deficiency (Flippo and Holder, 1993).
- Pain medications should be taken sufficiently in advance of meals to allow a pleasant, pain-free mealtime.
- Treatment with warfarin (Coumadin), a blood thinner used to prevent emboli, requires that patient reduce excessive intake of vitamin K foods (cabbage, kale, and spinach) to control levels. The vegetarian should be watched in particular. Heparin has no dietary consequences.
- Metoclopramide (Reglan) may help with postoperative ileus. Dry mouth or nausea can result after prolonged use.

Herbs, Botanicals and Supplements

- Herbs and botanical supplements should not be used without discussing with physician.
- Three physicians recently described the interactions between herbs, anesthesia, and surgery and suggested ways to reduce associated risks. For surgical patients, herbs can affect sedation, pain control, bleeding, heart function, metabolism, immunity, and recovery, and studies suggest that as many as one-third of presurgical patients take herbal medications, but that many of those patients fail to disclose herbal use during preoperative assessment, even when prompted (Ang-Lee, Moss, Yuan, 2001). Table 14–5 describes these potential interactions.

TABLE 14–5 Effects of Herbal Medications and Recommendations for Discontinued Use Before Surgery

Herb (other names)	*Relevant effects*	*Perioperative concerns*	*Recommendations*
Echinacea	Boosts immunity	Allergic reactions, impairs immune suppressive drugs, can cause immune suppression when taken long-term, could impair wound healing.	Discontinue as far in advance as possible, especially for transplant patients or those with liver dysfunction.
Ephedra (ma huang)	Increases heart rate, increases blood pressure	Risk of heart attack, arrhythmias, stroke, interaction with other drugs, and kidney stones.	Discontinue at least 24 hours before surgery.
Garlic (ajo)	Prevents clotting	Risk of bleeding, especially when combined with other drugs that inhibit clotting.	Discontinue at least 7 days before surgery.
Ginko (duck foot, maidenhair, silver apricot)	Prevents clotting	Risk of bleeding, especially when combined with other drugs that inhibit clotting.	Discontinue at least 36 hours before surgery.
Ginseng	Lowers blood glucose, inhibits clotting	Lowers blood-sugar levels. Increases risk of bleeding. Interferes with warfarin (an anti-clotting drug).	Discontinue at least 7 days before surgery.
Kava (kawa, awa, intoxicating pepper)	Sedates, decreases anxiety	May increase sedative effects of anesthesia. Risk of addiction; tolerance and withdrawal unknown.	Discontinue at least 24 hours before surgery.
St John's wort (amber, goat weed, Hypericum, Klamath weed)	Inhibits re-uptake of neurotransmitters (similar to Prozac)	Alters metabolisms of other drugs such as cyclosporin (for transplant patients), warfarin, steroids, protease inhibitors (vs HIV). May interfere with many other drugs.	Discontinue at least 5 days before surgery.
Valerian	Sedates	Could increase effects of sedatives. Long-term use could increase amount of anesthesia needed. Withdrawal symptoms resemble Valium addiction.	If possible, taper dose weeks before surgery. If not, continue use until surgery. Treat withdrawal symptoms with benzodiazepines.

Source: Ang-Lee M, Moss J, Yuan C. Herbal medicines and perioperative care. *JAMA*. 2001;286:208. Reprinted with permission.

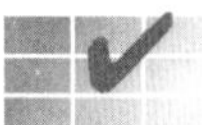

PATIENT EDUCATION

- ✔ Immobilization of patient can produce unwanted side effects. Have patient drink plenty of fluids and ambulate as soon as possible.
- ✔ Patients tend to lose 0.5 lb daily early in postoperative period. Weight gain during this time suggests fluid excess.
- ✔ Eat and drink slowly to prevent gas formation from swallowed air.
- ✔ Discuss the role of surgery as planned trauma, allowing adequate time for return to homeostasis.
- ✔ Discuss wound healing priority, tensile strength, role of nutrients (zinc, vitamin C, vitamin A, and amino acids). Substrate failure can decrease anabolism, delaying scar tissue formation.
- ✔ Zinc deficiency impairs wound healing. Supplementation in people who are not deficient does not accelerate wound-healing rates. Avoid excesses that can interfere with immune system function and copper absorption and may cause GI distress.
- ✔ During rehabilitative, anabolic stage (3 months–1 year postoperatively), calories should be adequate but not excessive.

For More Information

- ✦ U.S. Surgical
  http://www.ussurg.com/health-care/index.html
- ✦ American Academy of Physical Medicine and Rehabilitation
  One IBM Plaza, Suite 2500
  Chicago, IL 60611-3604
  312-464-9700
  http://www.aapmr.org/

HYPONATREMIA

NUTRITIONAL ACUITY RANKING: LEVEL 2

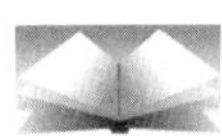

DEFINITIONS AND BACKGROUND

Low serum sodium concentration (hyponatremia) can occur as a result of loss of sodium in excess of osmotically obligated water (primary salt depletion), a dehydration in which sodium loss is greater than water loss. In this case, contracted extracellular fluid volume is evident, and a hypertonic or isotonic saline solution is given (perhaps along with salty broths). Heavy exercise may also induce a rare form of hyponatremia (Montain et al., 2001).

Retention of water in excess of sodium also can cause hyponatremia (with water intoxication, dilutional hyponatremia, syndrome of inappropriate antidiuretic hormone [SIADH], etc.). In dilutional hyponatremia, impaired water excretion occurs (as in congestive heart failure [CHF], cirrhosis, or nephrotic syndrome); sodium is abnormally retained, and a low-sodium diet with diuretics may be indicated. With water intoxication, fluid will be restricted. SIADH occurs in such conditions as oat cell cancer (CA), pulmonary diseases, cerebrovascular accident (CVA), brain tumor, thiazides, sulfonylureas, and myxedema; see SIADH entry.

Signs and symptoms of hyponatremia include lethargy, anorexia, nausea, vomiting, cramping, muscular twitching, confusion, fingerprinting over the breastbone, seizures, and coma.

OBJECTIVES

- Correct hyponatremic state.
- Prevent future episodes, as far as possible.
- Avoid giving large water flushes with isotonic tube feeding.

DIETARY AND NUTRITIONAL RECOMMENDATIONS

- Provide appropriate dietary alterations, as indicated above by causation.
- Monitor effects on serum sodium levels; prevent further problems.
- Replace sodium only under doctor's supervision. Hypertonic saline solutions are dangerous.

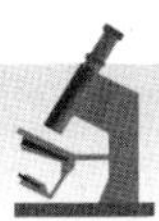

PROFILE

Clinical/History	Lab Work	
Height Weight BMI I & O Underlying problems	Serum Na+ (less than 135 mEq/L) Urinary Na+ Osm (less than 285 mOsm/Kg) K+	BUN, Creat Chloride (Cl-) Partial pressure of carbon dioxide (pCO2), partial pressure of oxygen (pO2)

Common Drugs Used and Potential Side Effects

- In appropriate cases, a 3% or 5% NaCl solution may be given.
- V2 vasopressin antagonists may become therapeutic agents in hyponatremic disorders (Palm et al., 2001).
- D5W used in excess can cause hyponatremia in water intoxication. Furosemide (Lasix) and vigorous diuretic therapy may also cause hyponatremia.
- Other drugs that interfere with renal water excretion include vincristine, oxytocin, and some tranquilizers.

Herbs, Botanicals and Supplements

- Herbs and botanical supplements should not be used without discussing with physician.
- Table 14–5 lists specific herbs and botanicals that should be discontinued before surgery.

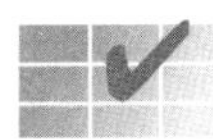

PATIENT EDUCATION

- ✓ Inform patient about good sources of necessary electrolytes.
- ✓ Advise against self-medication with unusual diets or supplements—discuss need to adhere carefully to medical suggestions.

HYPERNATREMIA

NUTRITIONAL ACUITY RANKING: LEVEL 2

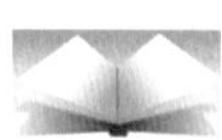

DEFINITIONS AND BACKGROUND

Hypernatremia usually occurs in water deprivation or in persons who cannot obtain sufficient water to replace losses (after head trauma, carbon monoxide poisoning, diabetes insipidus, etc.). Some people may have damage to the thirst center while undergoing surgery for aneurysms. Sodium intoxication may result from excess intake of NaCl or sodium bicarbonate. Steroids also can cause hypernatremia. High-protein tube feedings without adequate water flushes, excessive diaphoresis, diabetes insipidus, or watery diarrhea may be other causes. In infants, severe prolonged hypernatremia can impair intellectual and physical development (Birnbaumer, 2001).

Signs and symptoms of hypernatremia include thirst, dry and sticky mucous membranes, fever, dry and swollen tongue, disorientation, and seizures.

OBJECTIVES

- Correct dehydration.
- Monitor thirst, the first sign of water loss.
- Flushing, fever, loss of sweating, dry tongue, and mucous membranes may result from hypernatremia. Tachycardia, hallucinations, or coma can result, if condition is not corrected.

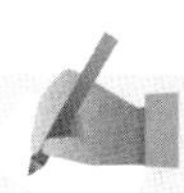

DIETARY AND NUTRITIONAL RECOMMENDATIONS

- Determine patient's fluid needs (generally 30 mL/kg or 1 mL/kcal given in TF or TPN). Elderly individuals may need more or less according to their renal or cardiovascular status.
- Hyperosmolar nonketotic hyperglycemia (HNKH) or diabetes insipidus also can cause water loss; replace water appropriately—orally or parenterally.
- Monitor use of all tube feedings carefully; high-protein formulas can cause simple dehydration.
- Patients with dysphagia may have difficulty obtaining enough fluid if they cannot tolerate thin liquids. Monitor closely.

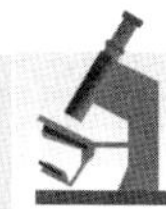

PROFILE

Clinical/History	Lab Work	
Height	Serum Na+ (more than 135 mEq/L)	Urinary-specific gravity (more than 1.015)
Weight	Urinary Na+	BUN, Creat
BMI	K+	pCO2, pO2
Temperature	Osm (more than 295 mOsm/kg)	
I & O		
Thirst		
Underlying conditions		
Skin turgor		

Common Drugs Used and Potential Side Effects

- High doses of steroids can cause hypernatremia; monitor carefully.
- Monitor solutions, which contain NaCl and other sodium additives, closely. Over-the-counter (OTC) analgesics that contain sodium should not be used without physician's awareness.

Herbs, Botanicals and Supplements

- Herbs and botanical supplements should not be used without discussing with physician.
- Table 14–5 lists specific herbs and botanicals that should be discontinued before surgery.

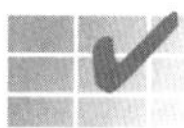

PATIENT EDUCATION

- ✔ Discuss appropriate fluid intake for age and underlying condition(s).
- ✔ Discuss sources of fluid as alternatives to beverages alone (i.e., plain gelatin, sherbets, fruit ices, ice chips, thin soups).
- ✔ Monitor fluid losses and gains, behavior changes, and fever.
- ✔ Offer fluids at regular intervals to increase intake.

HYPOKALEMIA

NUTRITIONAL ACUITY RANKING: LEVEL 2

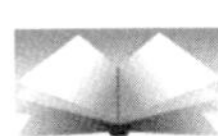

DEFINITIONS AND BACKGROUND

Hypokalemia results from inadequate intake, excessive GI losses from diarrhea, gastric suction, vomiting, or fistulas, and urinary losses of adrenal or renal origin. Diuretic therapy is a common cause. Chronic use of aspirin and penicillin, refeeding syndrome after starvation (Crook et al., 2001), alcoholism, and anorexia nervosa are also potential causes.

Symptoms and signs include severe muscle weakness, EKG changes and arrhythmias, lethargy, hypotension, shallow breathing, fatigue, anorexia, constipation, confusion, and impaired CHO tolerance. Chloride depletion usually accompanies hypokalemia; alkalosis also is common.

OBJECTIVES

- ▲ Replace potassium (generally with KCl, except in renal tubular acidosis).
- ▲ Prevent future episodes of hypokalemia, wherever possible.

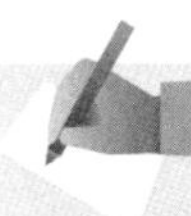

DIETARY AND NUTRITIONAL RECOMMENDATIONS

- A potassium-rich diet includes bananas, oranges, grapefruit, potatoes, and most other fruits and vegetables. In addition, most salt substitutes contain potassium (read labels). Avoid overuse.
- Monitor sodium intake to prevent under- and overdoses.
- Discuss fiber sources if constipation is a problem.
- Fluid intake should be adequate.

Common Drugs Used and Potential Side Effects

- Diuretics can cause potassium wastage (e.g., furosemide [Lasix]).
- When used, penicillin and aspirin can cause or aggravate potassium depletion.
- Steroids in combination with diuretics can especially deplete potassium levels.
- Kaochlor, Kay-Ciel, K-Lor, K-Lyte, K-Tab, Klotrix, Micro-K, K-Dur, Klor-Con, Ten-K, and Slow-K are all sources of potassium. Be aware that an overdose of potassium may cause blood in the stools or even cardiac arrest. There have been reports of GI bleeding unless taken with meals. Diarrhea, nausea, or vomiting also may occur; take with meals. Some products are slow-release.

Herbs, Botanicals and Supplements

- Herbs and botanical supplements should not be used without discussing with physician.
- See Table 14–5, which lists the specific herbs and botanicals that should be discontinued before surgery.

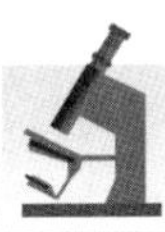

PROFILE

Clinical/History	Lab Work	
Height	K+ (less than 3.5 mEq/L)	Na+
Weight	EKG	BUN
BMI	Osm	Cl−
Constipation		Creat
I & O		Gluc

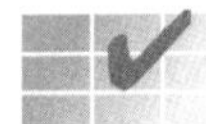

PATIENT EDUCATION

- ✔ Discuss dietary sources of potassium (oranges, grapefruit, baked potatoes, bananas, lima beans).
- ✔ Discuss importance of following medical advice carefully and of reading labels of all supplements to avoid overdoses of K+ on the opposite extreme.
- ✔ Notify physician when necessary.

HYPERKALEMIA

NUTRITIONAL ACUITY RANKING: LEVEL 2

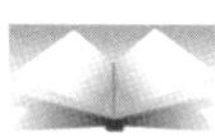

DEFINITIONS AND BACKGROUND

Because the distal nephron has such a large capacity for secreting potassium, even in advanced renal failure, hyperkalemia occurs only when an additional problem exists (e.g., oliguria, tissue catabolism, K+ supplementation, use of penicillin G, severe acidosis, excessive spironolactone or triamterene therapy, deficiency of endogenous steroids, end-stage renal disease [ESRD], crush injury, or adrenal insufficiency). Symptoms and signs of hyperkalemia include weakness, anxiety, altered EKGs (with more than 7 mEq/L, a fatal arrhythmia can occur), flaccid muscle paralysis, or even respiratory arrest, if severe.

OBJECTIVES

- ▲ Treat immediately to prevent arrhythmias, bradycardia, heart block, and respiratory arrest.
- ▲ Prevent constipation and fecal impaction.
- ▲ If all else fails, dialysis may be needed.

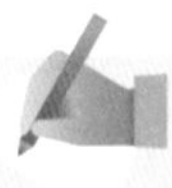

DIETARY AND NUTRITIONAL RECOMMENDATIONS

- Intravenous feedings are likely to be used (glucose, insulin, bicarbonate) to shift K+ intracellularly; Na+ and Ca++ may also be needed as physical antagonists to K+. Infusions will be given until excess K+ is permanently removed. Monitor closely.
- When patient can eat orally, a controlled K+ intake will be needed to avoid further exacerbation. Avoid dried fruits, bananas, orange juice, baked potatoes, dried beans, milk, milk-based products, cocoa, coffee, and whole grain breads in excess of planned amounts.

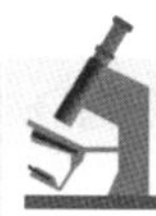

PROFILE

Clinical/History	Temperature	BUN, Creat
Height	**Lab Work**	Serum K+ (more than 5.5 mEq/L)
Weight	EKG	Ca++, Mg++
BMI	Na+	Gluc
I & O	Cl−	

Common Drugs Used and Potential Side Effects

- Sodium polystyrene sulfonate (Kayexalate) may also be needed (given with sorbitol to prevent constipation). Take separately from calcium or antacids. Anorexia or potassium depletion will occur.
- Discuss use of potassium-sparing diuretics, which can cause problems. Aldactone (spironolactone) may cause nausea or vomiting.

Herbs, Botanicals and Supplements

- Herbs and botanical supplements should not be used without discussing with physician.
- See Table 14–5, which lists specific herbs and botanicals that should be discontinued before surgery.

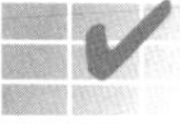

PATIENT EDUCATION

- ✔ Discuss potassium sources from diet and how medications affect serum levels.
- ✔ Use salt substitutes sparingly, if at all.
- ✔ Notify physician of any problems.

HYPOCALCEMIA

NUTRITIONAL ACUITY RANKING: LEVEL 2

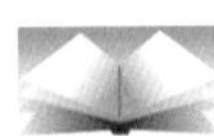

DEFINITIONS AND BACKGROUND

Vitamin D deficiency caused by nutritional deficiency or malabsorption, renal insufficiency, hepatic dysfunction, hypoparathyroidism, hyperphosphatemia, acute pancreatitis, or calcitonin-producing tumors of the thyroid will cause hypocalcemia. In addition, malnutrition or hypoalbuminemia may aggravate hypocalcemia because calcium is transported bound to serum albumin. Symptoms and signs of hypocalcemia include tetany, seizures, and cardiac arrest. In the long term, bone demineralization with bone pain and compression fractures may result.

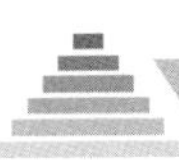

OBJECTIVES

- ▲ Correct symptomatic condition (usually calcium gluconate intravenously).
- ▲ Be careful when correcting coexisting acidosis with sodium bicarbonate.
- ▲ Provide adequate vitamin D3 supplementation, as needed.

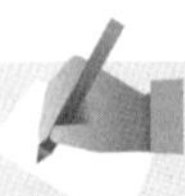

DIETARY AND NUTRITIONAL RECOMMENDATIONS

- Once able to eat, offer calcium-rich foods. Discuss with patient.
- Beware of excesses of caffeine, oxalates, fiber, and aluminum-containing antacids.
- Increase consumption of vitamin D and lactose-containing foods, if tolerated.

Common Drugs Used and Potential Side Effects

- Corticosteroids, furosemide, isoniazid (INH), and tetracycline can reduce calcium availability.

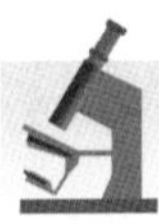

PROFILE

Clinical/History	Lab Work	
Height	Mg++	Ca++
Weight	Phosphorous	Alb
BMI	T3, T4	Na+, K+
I & O	Alkaline phosphatase (Alk phos)	Osm
		Urinary Ca++

- Calcium carbonate (as in Tums) provides 40% elemental calcium. Drink extra water. Avoid use of iron supplements at the same time.
- Aluminum in antacids can reduce calcium bioavailability.
- Citrated blood transfusions may cause hypocalcemia.

Herbs, Botanicals and Supplements

- Herbs and botanical supplements should not be used without discussing with physician.
- See Table 14–5, which lists the specific herbs and botanicals that should be discontinued before surgery.

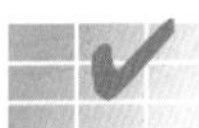

PATIENT EDUCATION

- ✓ Beware of bone meal and dolomite because of their toxic metal content.
- ✓ Calcium is found in milk, cheese, leafy greens, and yogurt. Dry milk can be added to foods.
- ✓ Oxalates in chocolate seem to have no adverse effect on calcium bioavailability in chocolate milk.
- ✓ Spinach should be limited because of its effect on calcium bioavailability.

HYPERCALCEMIA

NUTRITIONAL ACUITY RANKING: LEVEL 2

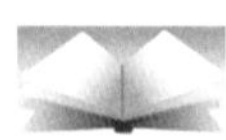

DEFINITIONS AND BACKGROUND

Hypercalcemia can be caused by increased parathormone activity, increased vitamin D activity (as in tuberculosis [TB] or sarcoidosis), enhanced bone resorption from bone tumors, multiple myeloma, immobilization, milk-alkali syndrome, adrenal insufficiency, breast cancer, or head/neck cancer. Malignant disease produces hypercalcemia via bone destruction or metastasis with resulting release of calcium into the bloodstream.

Symptoms and signs of hypercalcemia include drowsiness, lethargy, stupor, muscle weakness, decreased reflexes, nausea and vomiting, anorexia, constipation, ileus, polyuria, renal stones, azotemia, nocturia, hypertension, bradycardia, pruritus, and eye abnormalities. Short-term therapy generally is undertaken in the intensive care unit (ICU).

OBJECTIVES

- Correct underlying condition with rehydration (usually with normal saline) and hemodilution.
- Intravenous organic phosphate can help remove excess calcium. Neutra-Phos or Phospho-Soda may be used. Steroids are an alternative.
- Prevent recurrence.
- Correct nausea, vomiting, constipation, and other side effects of elevated calcium.

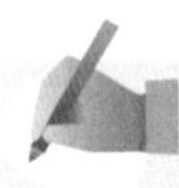

DIETARY AND NUTRITIONAL RECOMMENDATIONS

- Be careful not to provide excesses of milk, vitamins D or A, calcium supplements or antacids, and lactose until condition has been normalized.
- Caffeine, oxalates, fiber, and phytates will decrease calcium absorption and help promote greater excretion.
- Monitor potassium and magnesium losses with treatment; these are common. Correct diet accordingly.

Common Drugs Used and Potential Side Effects

- Furosemide and ethacrynic acid can help increase calcium excretion. Impaired renal function may contraindicate use. Monitor serum potassium levels.
- Prednisone can be used to decrease vitamin-D-mediated calcium absorption. Monitor effect on serum glucose, sodium, etc. Nausea, metallic taste, diarrhea, and vomiting may result.
- Didronel (intravenous) can decrease calcium levels. Nausea and vomiting may result.
- Antacids with aluminum can also be used to increase excretion. Be aware of high calcium levels in Tums, an OTC drug.
- Lithium and thiazides may increase serum calcium levels; monitor carefully.

Herbs, Botanicals and Supplements

- Herbs and botanical supplements should not be used without discussing with physician.
- See Table 14–5, which lists specific herbs and botanicals that should be discontinued before surgery.

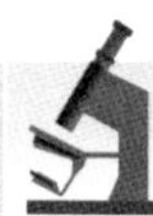

PROFILE

Clinical/History	Lab Work	
Height	Alk phos	Ca++
Weight	Mg++	Na+, K+
BMI	Serum P	BUN
I & O	Osm	Alb
		Urinary Ca++

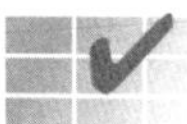

PATIENT EDUCATION

- ✔ Discuss calcium content of supplements, TF, and antacids—highlight need for physician to be aware of all products taken.
- ✔ Discuss how to avoid future problems from diet and medications.

HYPOMAGNESEMIA

NUTRITIONAL ACUITY RANKING: LEVEL 2

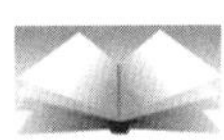

DEFINITIONS AND BACKGROUND

Hypomagnesemia is usually seen with diarrhea, protein–calorie malnutrition (PCM), malabsorption, or alcoholism. Of patients in tertiary care units, 10% may have this condition. Rarely, hypomagnesemia is seen with hyperparathyroidism, diabetic ketoacidosis or hypercalcemia, excessive diuretic therapy, renal tubular disease, or acute pancreatitis. Hypomagnesemia may contribute to development of foot ulcers in patients with diabetes (Rodriguez-Moran and Guerrero-Romero, 2001).

Symptoms and signs include anxiety, hyperirritability, confusion, hallucinations, seizures, tremor, hyperreflexia, tetany, tachycardia, hypertension, arrhythmias, vasomotor changes, profuse sweating, muscle weakness, grimaces of facial muscles, and refractory hypocalcemia.

OBJECTIVES

- ▲ Correct low serum magnesium levels.
- ▲ Prevent sudden death.
- ▲ Correct symptoms and side effects of condition.

DIETARY AND NUTRITIONAL RECOMMENDATIONS

- No specific foods are exceptionally excellent sources; chocolate, nuts, fruits and green vegetables, beans or potatoes, wheat, and corn are considered good sources. Meats, seafood, and dairy products are fair to poor.
- Discuss long-term measures to prevent further episodes. Long-term use of magnesium-free TPN can be one aggravating source of problem. Monitor intake from all sources—oral, TF, or TPN.

Common Drugs Used and Potential Side Effects

- Many medications can cause hypomagnesemia—furosemide, ethacrynic acid, thiazides, some antibiotics, cisplatin, and cyclosporine.

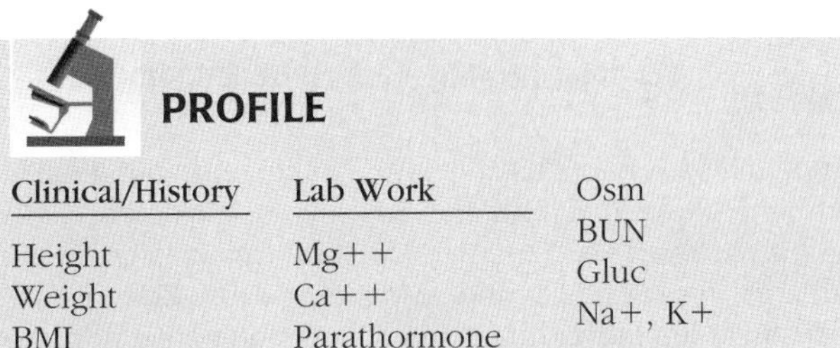

PROFILE

Clinical/History	Lab Work	
Height	Mg++	Osm
Weight	Ca++	BUN
BMI	Parathormone (PTH)	Gluc
Blood pressure (BP)		Na+, K+

- Normal renal function is needed for use of MgSO4. Diarrhea can occur.
- Milk of magnesia (MOM) can be used for liquid form of magnesium hydroxide. Nausea, cramps, or diarrhea may result.

Herbs, Botanicals and Supplements

- Herbs and botanical supplements should not be used without discussing with physician.
- See Table 14–5, which lists specific herbs and botanicals that should be discontinued before surgery.

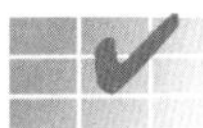

PATIENT EDUCATION

- ✔ Discuss food and drug sources of magnesium and their appropriate inclusion in overall care plan.
- ✔ Discuss role of magnesium in the body and as related to underlying disorder.

HYPERMAGNESEMIA

NUTRITIONAL ACUITY RANKING: LEVEL 2

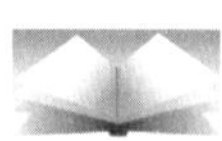

DEFINITIONS AND BACKGROUND

Hypermagnesemia is usually found in patients with renal failure who are treated with antacids such as Maalox or Gelusil or with cathartics such as MOM. Symptoms and signs include lethargy, hyporeflexia, and respiratory depression. Fatal effects include bradycardia, myocardial infarction, and respiratory failure (Schelling, 2000).

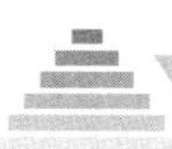

OBJECTIVES

- Reduce or eliminate sources of exogenous magnesium.
- Treat respiratory depression with calcium, gluceptate, or other medications.
- Prevent further morbidity and side effects.

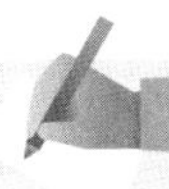

DIETARY AND NUTRITIONAL RECOMMENDATIONS

- No specific dietary alterations are required, except omission of magnesium-rich sources until condition is corrected.
- Monitor intake of all magnesium (as with TPN solutions).

Common Drugs Used and Potential Side Effects

- Calcium-containing medications may be given to help with excretion of excessive magnesium.
- TPN solutions should be monitored carefully for all electrolytes.
- Use caution with multivitamin–mineral therapies that require megadoses (McGuire et al., 2000).

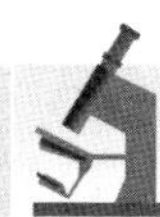

PROFILE

Clinical/History		
Height	BP	Ca++
Weight	I & O	Na+, K+
BMI		Gluc
	Lab Work	Osm
	Mg++	

Herbs, Botanicals and Supplements

- Herbs and botanical supplements should not be used without discussing with physician.
- See Table 14–5, which lists specific herbs and botanicals that should be discontinued before surgery.

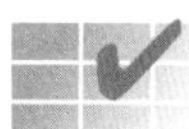

PATIENT EDUCATION

- Discuss effects of magnesium on the body, sources from diet, and as OTC medications and supplements.
- Discuss prevention of toxic levels of magnesium.

PHOSPHATE IMBALANCES

NUTRITIONAL ACUITY RANKING: LEVEL 2

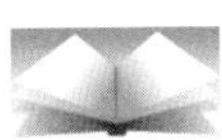

DEFINITIONS AND BACKGROUND

Phosphorus is a major component of bone and is one of the most abundant constituents of all metabolic processes and tissues; 85% is found in the skeleton. Only about 12% is bound to proteins, so a typical laboratory assessment is of elemental P, with some additional values for HPO4 and NaHPO4 as well.

Hypophosphatemia: ingestion of CHO acutely depresses serum phosphorus levels, probably resulting from cellular uptake and phosphate formation. Lowered plasma phosphorus can occur from alkalosis, hyperparathyroidism, hypovitaminosis D, malabsorption syndrome, starvation or cachexia, chronic alcoholism, renal tubular defects, acid-base disturbances, diabetic ketoacidosis, and genetic hypophosphatemia. Hypophosphatemia also can occur as a result of unmonitored TPN. Rapid delivery of intravenous glucose, such as with TPN, may accentuate phosphorus depletion syndrome and can lead to convulsions, muscle weakness, and hemolytic anemia.

In hypophosphatemia, anorexia, weakness, bone pain, dizziness, and waddling gait may be observed. In severe cases, elevated creatine phosphokinase (CPK) levels are seen, with rhabdomyolysis superimposed on myopathy. CHF can result if phosphorus is not administered. Additionally, low serum phosphorus levels will result in lowered 2,3-diphosphoglyceric acid (2,3-DPG), which facilitates oxyhemoglobin dissociation (leading to tissue hypoxia and low pO2).

Hyperphosphatemia can result from renal insufficiency, hypoparathyroidism, or hypervitaminosis D. In hyperphosphatemia, calcium phosphate may be deposited in abnormal sites. In addition, abnormal renal phosphorus clearance occurs. Phosphorus levels tend to be higher in children and to rise in women after menopause.

OBJECTIVES

- ▲ Normalize serum phosphorus levels.
- ▲ Prevent further abnormalities and complications.
- ▲ Control phosphorus delivery to all tissues.

DIETARY AND NUTRITIONAL RECOMMENDATIONS

- ● Appropriate levels of phosphorus should be provided according to age and serum status.
- ▲ Monitor glucose intake, especially from parenteral nutrition (PN) or TPN. Check all tube feedings for phosphorus content as well.
- ▲ During treatment, keep a normal Ca:P ratio.

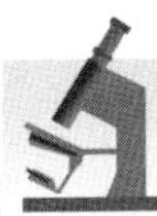

PROFILE

Clinical/History	Lab Work	
Height	Alk phos	CPK
Weight	Serum P or phosphate	BUN, Creat
BMI	Gluc	Serum Ca++
I & O		Alb
		H&H, Serum Fe
		pO2, pCO2

- ▲ Monitor dietary intake of milk, meat, and other foods high in phosphorus. Observe serum levels regularly, especially in renal patients.

Common Drugs Used and Potential Side Effects

- Antacids containing aluminum will prevent phosphorus absorption in intestinal lumen. They are used to correct hyperphosphatemia, as in renal disease, but can aggravate or cause hypophosphatemia in other conditions.
- Diuretics may affect phosphorus to a varying degree, depending on chemical content. Monitor accordingly.
- Potassium acid phosphate (K-Phos Original), an acidifier, can be used to correct hypophosphatemia. It may cause nausea, vomiting, or diarrhea.

Herbs, Botanicals and Supplements

- Herbs and botanical supplements should not be used without discussing with physician.
- See Table 14–5, which lists the specific herbs and botanicals that should be discontinued before surgery.

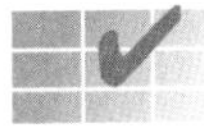

PATIENT EDUCATION

- ✔ Appropriate measures should be provided to patient according to his or her condition. For example, a low-phosphorus diet with high calcium and adequate vitamin D will be needed for patients with renal osteodystrophy. For conditions causing hypophosphatemia (such as Reye's syndrome and other infectious illnesses), adequate dietary phosphorus would be warranted. Balance is required.
- ✔ Patient may be advised that approximately 50–60% of dietary phosphorus is absorbed from dietary intakes (more in depleted persons).

AMPUTATION

NUTRITIONAL ACUITY RANKING: LEVEL 2

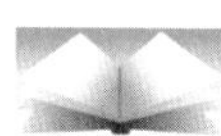

DEFINITIONS AND BACKGROUND

Amputations may result from trauma, peripheral vascular disease (PVD), congenital deformity, chronic infections, gangrene, or tumors such as osteosarcoma. In diabetes mellitus, poor nutritional control plays a part in increased risk for amputation.

"A-K" denotes above the knee; "B-K" denotes below the knee amputation. In amputation, the percentage of total body weight lost depends on body part lost: foot, 1.8%; below the knee, 6%; above the knee, 13%; entire lower extremity, 18.5%; hand, 1%; below elbow, 3%; entire upper extremity, 6.5%. BMI tables are not altered for amputees and are not always useful (Tzamaloukas et al., 1994). Figure 14–1 indicates how body proportions are commonly calculated (i.e., what percentage has been removed by the amputation).

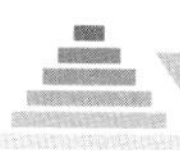

OBJECTIVES

Immediately Postoperative:

- Provide adequate protein and calories for healing.
- Provide adequate intake of vitamins and minerals (zinc, vitamins C, K, and A, etc.). Low albumin levels, serum carotene, zinc, and vitamin C are commonly found.

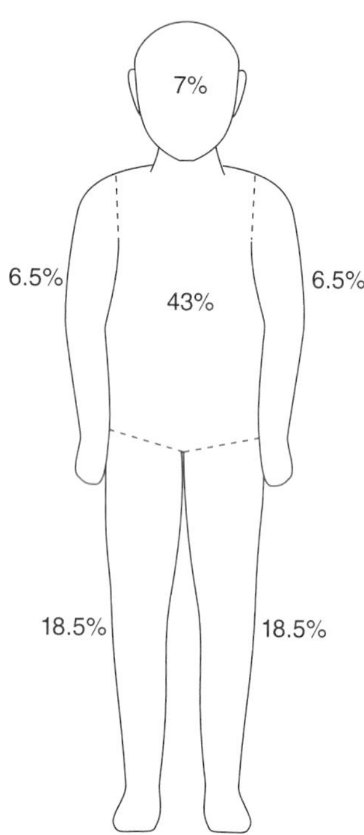

FIGURE 14–1 Weight proportions of body segments in percentage of total body weight (from cadavers of young adult men).
(Data from Brunnstrom S. *Clinical kinesiology*. Philadelphia: FA Davis, 1972.)

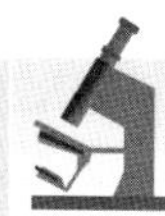

PROFILE

Clinical/History	Lab Work	
Preoperative/postoperative height	Alb	K+, Na+
Preoperative weight, present weight		pCO2, pO2
Preoperative/postoperative BMI		H&H
Percentage of body weight (BW) of amputated area		Gluc
I & O		PT
BP		Transferrin, RBP
Arteriography		Skin perfusion pressure

Long Term:

- Patients with an A-K amputation who walk (with/without prosthesis) use 25% more energy than a normal person who walks at the same speed. These patients may have difficulty maintaining weight. Otherwise, immobilized patients may tend to gain weight and will need control measures.
- Other types of amputations will alter care plans accordingly.

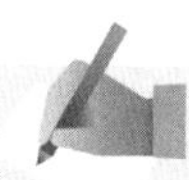

DIETARY AND NUTRITIONAL RECOMMENDATIONS

Immediately Postoperative:

- Use a high-protein/high-calorie diet.
- Supplement diet with vitamins and minerals, especially zinc, vitamins A, C, and K, and arginine. TF, if necessary, with an immune-enhanced product.

Long Term:

- Provide a low-calorie diet, if needed.
- For patients who lose weight, a high-calorie diet should be used to compensate for increased energy use.

Common Drugs Used and Potential Side Effects

- Anesthesia delays peristalsis; nausea is common. Patient may eat ice chips or sip carbonated beverages until nausea subsides.
- Nitrous oxide anesthesia may cause neurologic damage in patients with a vitamin B12 deficiency (Flippo and Holder, 1993). Monitor for verified deficiency levels.
- Pain medications should be taken sufficiently in advance of meals to allow a pleasant, pain-free mealtime.

Herbs, Botanicals and Supplements

- Herbs and botanical supplements should not be used without discussing with physician.
- See Table 14–5, which lists the specific herbs and botanicals that should be discontinued before surgery.

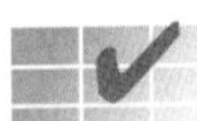

PATIENT EDUCATION

- ✔ Describe role of nutrition in wound healing.
- ✔ Describe role of activity in synthesis of protein tissues.
- ✔ Indicate how to control or increase calories in diet for energy use.
- ✔ For hand or arm amputations, consider adaptive feeding equipment. Occupational therapist (OT) specialists can help. Discuss meal preparation.

For More Information

- American Amputee Foundation
  P.O. Box 250218
  Little Rock, AR 72225
  501-666-2523
- Amputee Coalition of America
  http://www.amputee-coalition.org/
- Amputee Resource Foundation of America
  6480 Wayzata Blvd.
  Golden Valley, MN 55426
  http://www.amputeeresource.org/
- Dietitians in Physical Medicine and Rehabilitation
  c/o The American Dietetic Association
  216 West Jackson Boulevard
  Chicago, IL 60606-6995
  1–800-877–1600

APPENDECTOMY

NUTRITIONAL ACUITY RANKING: LEVEL 1

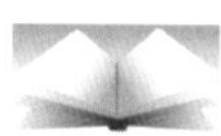

DEFINITIONS AND BACKGROUND

Appendectomy generally is an uncomplicated procedure with minimal recovery time. It is believed that a low-fiber diet contributes to appendicitis, which precedes surgery.

OBJECTIVES

- ▲ Reduce any febrile condition that exists.
- ▲ Lower risks of infection, sepsis, peritonitis, or abscess formation.
- ▲ Replace nutrient losses.

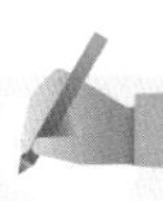

DIETARY AND NUTRITIONAL RECOMMENDATIONS

- Use a high-protein/high-calorie diet. Ensure diet provides adequate amounts of zinc, vitamins C, K, and A.
- Use soft diet to lessen fiber content.
- When patient is able to eat fiber, include foods high in fiber, as tolerated.

Common Drugs Used and Potential Side Effects

- Avoid use of excessive laxatives, which may deplete electrolytes. When able to progress, use a higher fiber intake and plenty of liquids.
- Antibiotics may be needed; monitor specific side effects for selected medication.
- Pain medications should be taken sufficiently in advance of meals to allow pleasant, pain-free mealtime.

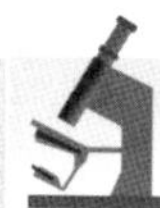

PROFILE

Clinical/History	Lab Work	
Height	Gluc	White blood cell count (WBC)
Weight	K+, Na+	Erythrocyte sedimentation rate (ESR) (increased in appendicitis)
BMI	H&H	
I & O	Alb, prealbumin	
BP	PT	
Temperature	Gluc	
	Ultrasonography	
	Abdominal x-rays	

Herbs, Botanicals and Supplements

- Herbs and botanical supplements should not be used without discussing with physician.
- See Table 14–5, which lists the specific herbs and botanicals that should be discontinued before surgery.

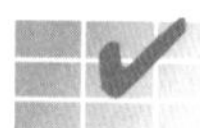

PATIENT EDUCATION

- ✓ Indicate which foods are sources of protein and calories in the diet.
- ✓ Evaluate presurgical intake. A history of poor fiber intake may be evident. Low intake of green vegetables and tomatoes may have altered the bacterial environment of the intestinal tract.

BOWEL SURGERY

NUTRITIONAL ACUITY RANKING: LEVEL 3

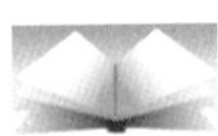

DEFINITIONS AND BACKGROUND

Most people with short bowel syndrome (SBS) experience spontaneous small bowel adaptation over time, when they can be weaned from PN. There are some individuals who cannot be weaned and are potential candidates for techniques to promote intestinal adaptation and intestinal lengthening (Vernon and Georgeson, 2001).

Perioperative use of a special supplemented formula modulates cytokine production and enhances cell-mediated immunity and synthesis of proteins with short half-lives (Giannotti et al., 1999). In patients who undergo elective open colon resection, early postoperative feeding is safe and effective and results in a shorter hospital stay than traditional feeding; however, more men than women do not tolerate early feeding (DiFronzo et al., 1999).

Patients who have had an ileostomy lose a considerable amount of fluid that contains sodium and potassium. Fat and vitamin B12 absorption are reduced. Table 14–6 describes absorptive capacity of the small bowel after resection.

Check for electrolytes from ileostomy drainage. Prune juice should be avoided because of its laxative effects. Moderately low-fiber foods may be added gradually. Avoid foods high in roughage: nuts, cabbage, prunes, celery, corn, pineapple, beans, onions, etc. Use large amounts of fluids. (See appropriate entry and short-gut syndrome in Section 7.) Patients who have had a colostomy may follow the same pattern after oral feedings have been resumed.

Patients who have had a hemorrhoidectomy usually tolerate a low-residue diet to delay defecation and allow healing at operative site. After patient is healed, it is important to have patient return to a high-fiber diet to prevent constipation. (See appropriate entry in Section 7.)

Residual small bowel length remains an important predictor of duration of PN use in infants with SBS but other factors such as use of breast milk plays a role in intestinal adaptation. In addition, prompt restoration of intestinal continuity is associated with lowered risk of cholestatic liver disease; early enteral feeding after surgery is associated both with reduced duration of PN and less cholestasis (Andorsky et al., 2001).

Small bowel transplantation has become the treatment of choice for patients with chronic intestinal failure, whose illness cannot be maintained on home PN (HPN). Rejection and sepsis rates are higher for patients who have had small bowel transplantation than for those who have received other organs; bacterial translocation from the gut is the main problem (Ghanekar and Grant, 2001). See Section 7 also.

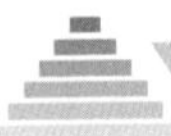

OBJECTIVES

Preoperative:

- ▲ Relieve distress.
- ▲ Replenish depleted reserves.
- ▲ Use special immune-enhanced formulas to prepare system for surgery.

TABLE 14–6 Absorptive Role of Small Intestine

The small intestine has a large adaptive capacity, with resection of small segments generally not causing nutritional problems. If the terminal ileum is removed, vitamin B12 and bile salts will not be reabsorbed.

Diarrhea can be massive if the ileocecal valve is removed with the terminal ileum, with great electrolyte losses and hypovolemia. Cholestyramine may be needed to bind bile salts. Fat malabsorption with steatorrhea and inadequate vitamins A, D, E, and K absorption may also occur. Medium-chain triglycerides (MCT) and water-miscible supplements may be necessary. Hyperoxaluria and renal stones may occur. Calcium supplements, altered polyunsaturated fatty acids (PUFA) intake, and aluminum hydroxide binders may be needed.

Postoperative:

- ▲ Reduce bowel residue while healing occurs. Early enteral feeding is generally recommended, although both enteral and PN have good results after bowel surgery (Pacelli et al., 2001).
- ▲ Slowly progress back to a normal diet. Diarrhea may be induced by a dairy-based (full liquid) diet after bowel surgery; progress from clear liquids to soft–solid diet and avoid dairy products as needed (Stike et al., 2001).
- ▲ Modify diet, as needed, for part of bowel that was affected.
- ▲ Prevent complications. Patients on HPN because of SBS are at high risk of developing systemic osteoporosis but not for deterioration of teeth or periodontal structures (von Wowern et al., 1996).
- ▲ Successful small bowel transplant recipients can resume unrestricted oral diets (Ghanekar and Grant, 2001).

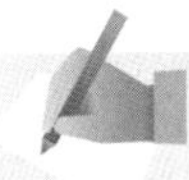

DIETARY AND NUTRITIONAL RECOMMENDATIONS

Preoperative:

- Regress from soft diet to full liquids and then clear liquids. If needed, use an elemental diet, jejunostomy, or other enteral/parenteral mode.

Postoperative:

- Use an elemental diet or TPN as needed. For some patients, enteral nutrition may be primary therapy (Booth et al., 1994). Growth hormone, glutamine, short-chain fatty acids, and fermentable fiber sources may be useful (Byrne et al., 1992; Ziegler et al., 1994).
- Slowly progress from a low-residue to a normal diet.
- Good sources of sodium include milk and broth/bouillon.
- Good sources of potassium include juices, milk, and cocoa.
- For patients who received a jejunoileal bypass, long-term follow-up is necessary to prevent or correct nutritional deficits (see Table 14–7).

Table 14–7 Jejunoileal Bypass Surgery

Previously used to treat morbid obesity, jejunoileal bypass surgery causes food to bypass 90% of the small intestine. Jejunoileal bypass surgery appears to result in decreased energy intake by reducing patients' desire to eat and preference for foods high in CHO and fat. In the case of a jejunoileostomy, food bypasses 90% of the small intestine. Prolonged gastric emptying and altered gut hormones may have the impact; overall, higher levels of neurotensin are found after bypass (Naslund et al., 1997). Long-term side effects include cholelithiasis, liver or renal disease (Hocking et al., 1998), oxalate renal stones, root caries from decreased salivation (Greenway and Greenway, 2000), nonalcoholic steatohepatitis (Diehl, 1999), reduced bone mineral density and osteoporosis (Bano et al., 1999), and arthritic syndromes (Boman et al., 1998). Long-term follow-up of patients is recommended.

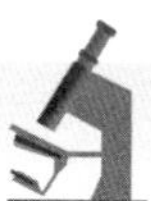

PROFILE

Clinical/History		
Height	I & O	H&H
Weight	Stoma drainage	Gluc
BMI	**Lab Work**	Electrolytes
BP	Alb, prealbumin	Na+, K+
Temperature		PT or INR
		BUN, Creat

Common Drugs Used and Potential Side Effects

- Anesthesia delays peristalsis; nausea is common. If permitted, patient may eat ice chips or sip carbonated beverages until nausea subsides.
- Nitrous oxide anesthesia may cause neurologic damage in patients with a vitamin B12 deficiency (Flippo and Holder, 1993). Monitor for verified deficiency levels.
- Pain medications should be taken sufficiently in advance of meals to allow a pleasant, pain-free mealtime.

Herbs, Botanicals and Supplements

- Herbs and botanical supplements should not be used without discussing with physician.
- See Table 14–5, which lists the specific herbs and botanicals that should be discontinued before surgery.

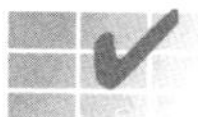

PATIENT EDUCATION

- ✓ Suggest patient eat slowly and chew foods well.
- ✓ Excessive intake of roughage should be avoided.
- ✓ Control fluids carefully to include adequate amounts.
- ✓ Long-term nutritional support may be needed.

GASTRIC RESTRICTIVE SURGERY: BYPASS, STAPLING, OR GASTROPLASTY

NUTRITIONAL ACUITY RANKING: LEVEL 3

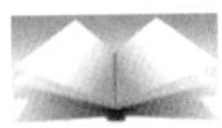

DEFINITIONS AND BACKGROUND

Gastric reduction (gastroplasty) is a bariatric surgical procedure used to bypass a portion of the stomach as a method of weight loss in the morbidly obese patient. Over 10 million Americans are severely obese. Most patients lose more than 60% of their excess weight after surgery. Delayed stomach emptying increases satiety, reducing overall intake.

Candidates should be 100 lb or more over ideal weight range, have a BMI higher than 40 kg/m2, or a BMI over 35 kg/m2, if there are serious medical comorbidities (Albrecht and Pories, 1999). Patients with diabetes mellitus do well with this surgery and often need no further medication. Gastric reduction and bypass have been found to be safe and to maintain loss of 35 lb or more over 5 years, reducing complications of morbid obesity (Reinhold, 1994).

The adjustable silicone gastric banding (ASGB), vertical gastric banding (VBG), and gastric bypass (GB) have produced the most reliable results (Albnrecht and Pories, 1999). Each has advantages and disadvantages, with GB producing greater sustained weight loss in the long-term, with a slightly higher risk of metabolic complications. However, bypass can cause deficiencies in vitamin B12 and iron. Both procedures reduce capacity to 40–60 mL. Stretching the pouch postoperatively can defeat the purpose of the procedure.

Weight loss from these operations can relieve and bring diseases such as diabetes and hypertension into full long-term remission (Albrecht and Pories, 1999). The most widely performed procedure, Roux-en-Y gastric bypass, achieves permanent (over 14 years) and significant weight loss (more than 50% of excess body weight) in more than 90% of patients (Mun et al., 2001).

According to Pories and Albrecht (2001), the Greenville version of the gastric bypass induces long-term remission of type II diabetes mellitus in morbidly obese patients, returning those with impaired glucose tolerance to euglycemia, usually in a matter of days. These authors suggest that the reason is not the loss of weight (i.e., reduction in fat mass) but the result of the exclusion of food and alteration in incretin signals from the antrum, duodenum, and proximal jejunum to the islet cells of the pancreas.

Patients who receive enteral immunonutrition (formula supplemented with arginine, ribonucleic acid, and n-3 fatty acids) before and after major upper GI surgery have a significantly lower incidence of infections and lower treatment costs than those who receive a control formula (Senkal et al., 1999).

Use of a multidisciplinary clinical pathway, preprinted orders, discharge home instruction sheet, and daily guidelines for patients has been shown to decrease length of stay, average total charges, and percentage of wound infections (Rouse et al., 1998).

Currently, surgical therapy is the most effective modality in terms of extent and duration of weight reduction in selected patients with acceptable operative risks.

OBJECTIVES

Preoperative:

- Provide adequate glycogen stores and vitamins C and K for surgical procedure. Consider enteral immunonutrition.
- Patients with diabetes should be under fairly good glucose control or at least stable.

Postoperative:

- Promote wound healing and restoration of depleted glycogen in the liver.
- Prevent side effects during weight loss.
- Prevent complications (alkaline reflux gastritis, esophagitis, perforation, gastric dilation, stomal obstruction, peptic ulcer, staple line disruption, and excessive vomiting).
- At 4–6 weeks postoperatively, patients often report that foods taste sweeter and will modify intakes accordingly. Some have aversions to meat (Burge et al., 1995).
- Prevent neurologic, hematologic, and cardiovascular side effects of vitamin B12 deficiency (Summer et al., 1996).

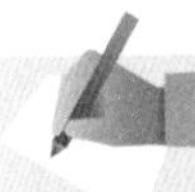

DIETARY AND NUTRITIONAL RECOMMENDATIONS

Preoperative:

- Use a balanced diet with adequate calories, protein, vitamins, and minerals. Enteral immunonutrition may be useful.
- Diet should regress from liquids to nil per os (NPO, nothing by mouth).

Postoperative:

- During a period of several days, progress to full liquids. Enteral feeding with a high-calorie product may be useful.
- Until weight loss is achieved, semisolid foods should be added in small amounts. Initial gastric capacity is 30–60 mL; progression is up to 120–150 mL.
- Some patients have problems with vomiting if they eat too rapidly, chew improperly, drink fluids right after eating, lie down after eating, or overeat. Recommend eating slowly and consuming liquids separately from meals (30 minutes before or after).
- Dehydration or dumping syndrome also can occur.
- Avoid high-fat, high-CHO foods.
- Monitor for vitamin B12 deficiency; correct through diet or supplemental sources as needed.

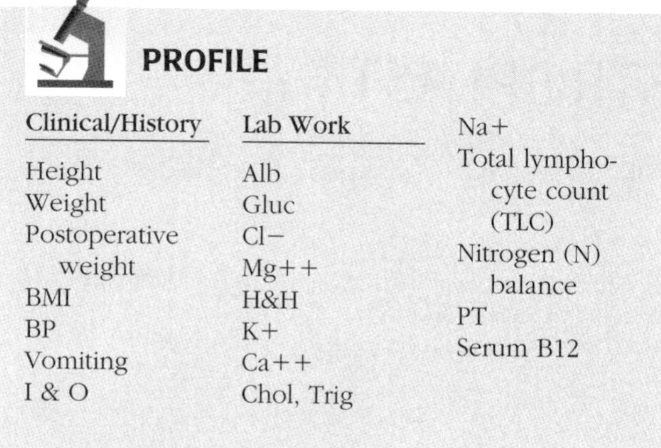

PROFILE

Clinical/History	Lab Work	
Height	Alb	Na+
Weight	Gluc	Total lymphocyte count (TLC)
Postoperative weight	Cl−	Nitrogen (N) balance
BMI	Mg++	PT
BP	H&H	Serum B12
Vomiting	K+	
I & O	Ca++	
	Chol, Trig	

Common Drugs Used and Potential Side Effects

- Anesthesia delays peristalsis; nausea is common. If permitted, patient may eat ice chips or sip carbonated beverages until nausea subsides.
- Nitrous oxide anesthesia may cause neurologic damage in patients with a vitamin B12 deficiency (Flippo and Holder, 1993). Monitor for verified deficiency levels.
- Pain medications should be taken sufficiently in advance of meals to allow a pleasant, pain-free mealtime.

Herbs, Botanicals and Supplements

- Herbs and botanical supplements should not be used without discussing with physician.
- See Table 14–5, which lists the specific herbs and botanicals that should be discontinued before surgery.

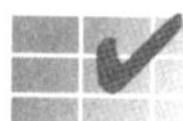

PATIENT EDUCATION

- ✔ Indicate appropriate quantities and qualities of foods that will be consumed. Overeating may stretch stoma.
- ✔ Help patient progress to normalized diet with 120–150 mL per meal. Increase awareness of eating/satiety process.
- ✔ Have patient eat and sip liquids slowly to prevent vomiting. Meat and bread/toast should be taken in small bites.
- ✔ A multivitamin–mineral preparation generally is needed. Vitamin B12, folacin, iron, potassium, and vitamin A are especially at risk.
- ✔ Discuss methods of blenderizing foods.
- ✔ Discuss high-protein supplemental beverages.
- ✔ Fasting can cause hypoglycemia; discuss this detail.
- ✔ Surgery may empower clients to take control of their lives

For More Information

- American Society for Bariatric Surgery
  140 N.W. 75th Dr., Suite C
  Gainesville, FL 32607
  352-331-4900
  http://www.asbs.org/

CESAREAN DELIVERY (C-SECTION)

NUTRITIONAL ACUITY RANKING: LEVEL 1

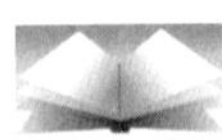

DEFINITIONS AND BACKGROUND

A cesarean delivery (C-section) is performed for numerous reasons, including maternal diabetes or edema-proteinuria-hypertensive (EPH)-gestosis. Delivery of a fetus through a uterine incision could have such complications as hemorrhage, infection, fever, drainage, cystitis, or pneumonia after the operation.

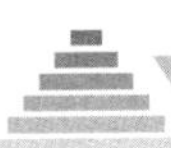

OBJECTIVES

- ▲ Replenish stores of nutrients from blood and fluid losses.
- ▲ Reduce fever; prevent or correct infections.
- ▲ Promote wound healing.
- ▲ Correct any anemia as a result of pregnancy (PG) or hemorrhage.
- ▲ Encourage mother to breastfeed.

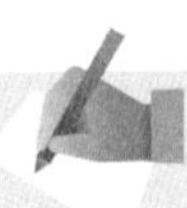

DIETARY AND NUTRITIONAL RECOMMENDATIONS

- ● NPO with intravenous or clear liquids will be given until nausea subsides.
- ▲ Progress to usual diet, with increased fiber to soften stools.
- ▲ Increase fluids to 2–3 L, unless contraindicated.
- ▲ High-calorie/high-protein intake will be essential to promote adequate wound healing. An iron supplement or vitamins C, A, and zinc in a multiple vitamin–mineral capsule may be beneficial.

Common Drugs Used and Potential Side Effects

- Anesthesia delays peristalsis; nausea is common. If permitted, patient may eat ice chips or sip carbonated beverages until nausea subsides.
- Nitrous oxide anesthesia may cause neurologic damage in patients with a vitamin B12 deficiency (Flippo and Holder, 1993). Monitor for verified deficiency levels.

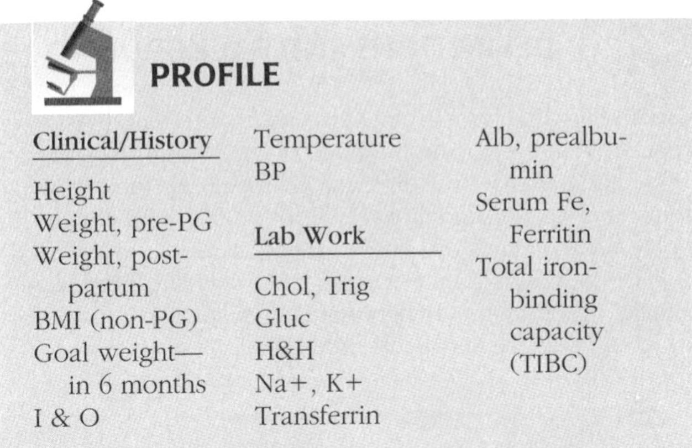

PROFILE

Clinical/History	Temperature	Alb, prealbumin
Height	BP	Serum Fe, Ferritin
Weight, pre-PG	**Lab Work**	Total iron-binding capacity (TIBC)
Weight, postpartum	Chol, Trig	
BMI (non-PG)	Gluc	
Goal weight—in 6 months	H&H	
I & O	Na+, K+	
	Transferrin	

- Pain medications should be taken sufficiently in advance of meals to allow a pleasant, pain-free mealtime.
- A prenatal supplement can be used for several months postpartum, or an iron supplement may be given. Ferrous salts are more beneficial and bioavailable than ferric salts. Iron supplements may cause or aggravate constipation. Use any of them as directed by physician.

Herbs, Botanicals and Supplements

- Herbs and botanical supplements should not be used without discussing with physician.
- See Table 14–5, which lists the specific herbs and botanicals that should be discontinued before surgery.

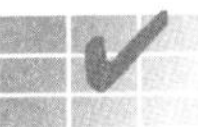

PATIENT EDUCATION

- ✔ Discuss importance of nutrition for wound healing, recovery of blood losses, lactation, etc.
- ✔ Stress that mother should not diet excessively for at least 6 weeks (longer if breastfeeding) to allow healing.

CRANIOTOMY

NUTRITIONAL ACUITY RANKING: LEVEL 2

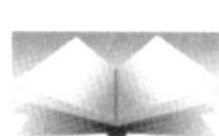

DEFINITIONS AND BACKGROUND

Craniotomy involves an operative procedure that consists of removing and replacing the bone of the skull to provide access to intracranial structures, usually for a brain tumor. Symptoms and signs to monitor during or after the procedure involve altered states of consciousness, nausea and vomiting, seizures, paralysis of face or extremities, drainage from the site, shock, aspiration, hyperthermia, dysphagia, thrombophlebitis, diabetes insipidus, or SIADH.

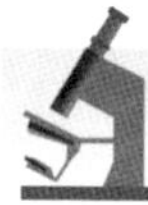

PROFILE

Clinical/History	I & O	Lab Work
Height	Nausea, vomiting	H&H
Weight	Gag reflex	Alb
BMI	Electroencephalogram (EEG)	WBC, ESR
CT scan		Na+, K+
BP		TLC
Consciousness		CSF

OBJECTIVES

- Prevent aspiration.
- Limit fluids if necessary.
- Prevent or correct dysphagia, constipation, UTI, nausea and vomiting, and diabetes insipidus.
- Normalize electrolyte levels.

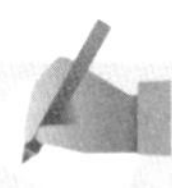

DIETARY AND NUTRITIONAL RECOMMENDATIONS

- NPO is needed until nausea and vomiting subside.
- Progress from liquids to soft diet as ordered; patient should be fed while lying on his/her side or with his/her head elevated 30° to prevent aspiration. Check swallowing reflex.
- Spoon-feed as needed.
- Adequate fiber may be beneficial.
- If necessary, TF (such as gastrostomy) may be helpful.
- If steroids are used, reduce sodium intake to 4–6 g daily (or less).

Common Drugs Used and Potential Side Effects

- Steroids may be used, with numerous consequences (such as sodium retention, nitrogen depletion, potassium or calcium losses, hyperglycemia). Alter diet as needed.
- Anticonvulsants may be used (phenytoin [Dilantin], etc.). Monitor specific drugs accordingly. Folic acid depletion is common.
- Analgesics may be used as pain relief. Take them sufficiently in advance of meals for adequate pain relief.

Herbs, Botanicals and Supplements

- Herbs and botanical supplements should not be used without discussing with physician.
- See Table 14–5, which lists the specific herbs and botanicals that should be discontinued before surgery.

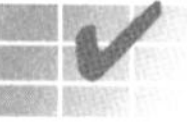

PATIENT EDUCATION

- Discuss importance of diet in correcting any malnutrition or anemia. As needed, teach family about a diet for dysphagia (e.g., thick, pureed foods with reduced thin liquids).
- When and if patient can eat, teach him or her to chew slowly and thoroughly.
- Promote eventual self-feeding.
- Discuss anxiety related to pain, poor vision, headaches, and seizures. Some patients may be aphasic.

HYSTERECTOMY, ABDOMINAL

NUTRITIONAL ACUITY RANKING: LEVEL 1

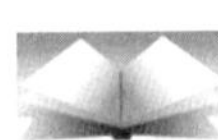

DEFINITIONS AND BACKGROUND

An abdominal hysterectomy is the surgical removal of the uterus through an abdominal incision. An abdominal approach is used if the uterus is enlarged or if an oophorectomy (ovary removal) and salpingectomy (removal of the fallopian tubes) are performed at the same time. In extensive surgery, 5–10 pints of blood may be lost. Laser surgery for some women may prevent need for a more extensive surgery.

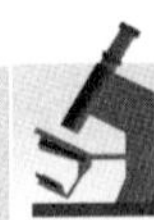

PROFILE

Clinical/History	Lab Work	
Height	Alb, prealbumin	K+, Na+
Weight		H&H
BMI		Serum Fe, ferritin
BP		Gluc
I & O		PT or INR
Blood losses		
Temperature		

OBJECTIVES

- Promote wound healing and rapid recovery.
- Replete nutrient reserves and glycogen stores.
- Replace protein, iron, and vitamin K from heavy blood losses (when they occur).
- Prevent complications such as UTIs, incisional infections, fever, nausea, and vomiting.

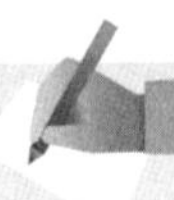

DIETARY AND NUTRITIONAL RECOMMENDATIONS

- Use a high-protein/high-calorie diet.
- Increase fluid intake.
- Ensure adequate fiber is provided for alleviation of constipation.
- Supplement diet with iron, zinc, and vitamins K, C, and A.

Common Drugs Used and Potential Side Effects

- Anesthesia delays peristalsis; nausea is common. If permitted, patient may eat ice chips or sip carbonated beverages until nausea subsides.
- Nitrous oxide anesthesia may cause neurologic damage in patients with a vitamin B12 deficiency (Flippo and Holder, 1993). Monitor for verified deficiency levels.
- Pain medications should be taken sufficiently in advance of meals to allow a pleasant, pain-free mealtime.

Herbs, Botanicals and Supplements

- Herbs and botanical supplements should not be used without discussing with physician.
- See Table 14–5, which lists the specific herbs and botanicals that should be discontinued before surgery.

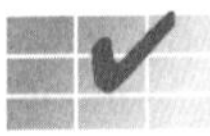

PATIENT EDUCATION

- ✓ Explain that resumption of normal activity may be slow but exercise improves nutrient repletion and tissue repair.
- ✓ Emphasize importance of nutrition for wound healing.

PELVIC EXENTERATION

NUTRITIONAL ACUITY RANKING: LEVEL 1

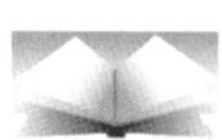

DEFINITIONS AND BACKGROUND

Pelvic exenteration surgery involves removal of all reproductive organs and adjacent tissues in the female patient (i.e., radical hysterectomy, pelvic node dissection, cystectomy and formation of an ileal conduit, vaginectomy, and rectal resection with colostomy). The procedure is a major operation. Reasons for this surgery generally involve cancer.

Fanning and Andrews (2001) reported evidence-based medicine with the following conclusions: postoperative colonic stasis occurs after major abdominal surgery and persists for approximately 3 days; early feeding after major gynecologic surgery results in emesis but does not increase incidence of aspiration pneumonia, dehiscence, or intestinal leaks and decreases hospital stay; slow advancement of postoperative diet after major gynecologic surgery is probably unnecessary; after major abdominal gynecologic surgery, there appear to be minimal medical benefits (decreased infection rate) of early postoperative feeding; after radical hysterectomy, postoperative bowel stimulation decreases length of hospital stay.

OBJECTIVES

- Preoperatively, a low-residue or elemental diet may be needed, regressing to clear liquids, NPO. Vitamin K may be needed 24–48 hours before the procedure.
- Postoperatively, promote wound healing and recovery.
- Prevent hemorrhage, infection, urinary or GI problems, shock, fever, and sepsis.
- Correct anemia or other problems.
- Provide colostomy-teaching if needed.

DIETARY AND NUTRITIONAL RECOMMENDATIONS

- Parenteral fluids with electrolytes may be needed (3–4 L daily unless contraindicated). TPN or TF may also be appropriate (see Fanning and Andrews' findings above).
- Progress, as tolerated, to a high-protein/high-calorie intake with snacks (eggnog, custard, etc.).
- If nausea is an extensive problem, using fluids between, instead of with, meals may help.
- Adequate iron, zinc, and vitamins A and C will help with wound healing process.
- For colostomy, see appropriate information in Section 7.

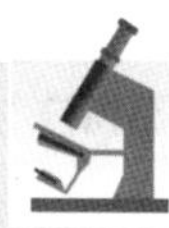

PROFILE

Clinical/History		
Height	BP	H&H
Weight	Colostomy	Serum Fe
BMI	**Lab Work**	Alb, prealbumin
Temperature, fever	PT	Gluc
I & O	Transferrin	Serum Zn
	TLC, WBC	

Common Drugs Used and Potential Side Effects

- Anesthesia delays peristalsis; nausea is common. If permitted, patient may eat ice chips or sip carbonated beverages until nausea subsides.
- Nitrous oxide anesthesia may cause neurologic damage in patients with a vitamin B12 deficiency (Flippo and Holder, 1993). Monitor for verified deficiency levels.
- Pain medications should be taken sufficiently in advance of meals to allow a pleasant, pain-free mealtime.
- Antibiotics help correct bacterial infections. Monitor side effects relevant to specific medication.
- Iron in ferrous form may be used. Monitor for constipation.
- Other drugs may be used to correct UTIs and other complications. Monitor accordingly for side effects.

Herbs, Botanicals and Supplements

- Herbs and botanical supplements should not be used without discussing with physician.
- See Table 14–5, which lists the specific herbs and botanicals that should be discontinued before surgery.

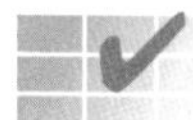

PATIENT EDUCATION

- Nutrients needed for wound healing must be discussed with patient and family.
- The need to take rest with mealtimes and not to become fatigued should be addressed.
- Recovery may take 6 months or longer.
- Colostomy teaching should be performed as necessary.

OPEN HEART SURGERY (CORONARY ARTERY BYPASS OR VALVE REPLACEMENT)

NUTRITIONAL ACUITY RANKING: LEVEL 3

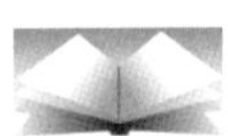

DEFINITIONS AND BACKGROUND

Open heart procedures require use of a cardiopulmonary machine for extracorporeal circulation. In coronary artery bypass graft (CABG) surgery, narrowed or blocked arteries are bypassed. The vein usually comes from the leg. Blood can then flow directly into the heart muscle. CABG usually takes 4–5 hours. Valve replacement is not as extensive; it involves replacing the damaged valve with a mechanical prosthesis (St. Jude valve) or biologic tissue valve.

In patients with cardiac disease and hypoalbuminemia, postoperative morbidity and mortality are related to severity of the underlying cardiac disease rather than malnutrition cachexia (Rady et al., 1997). All types of hypoalbuminemia, except malnutrition cachexia, are positively associated with postoperative organ dysfunction—cardiac, pulmonary, renal, hepatic and neurologic, GI bleeding, nosocomial infections, duration of mechanical ventilation, length of stay (LOS) in the cardiac ICU, and death while in hospital.

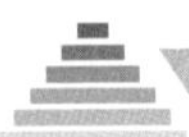

OBJECTIVES

Preoperative:

- Monitor serum levels of electrolytes, albumin, and glucose.
- Provide a normal diet as ordered by physician (diet may be sodium-restricted, calorie-controlled, etc.).
- Provide ample amounts of glycogen for stores. Use PN support, as needed, for malnourished cardiac patients (see congestive heart failure and cardiac cachexia entries in Section 6).

Postoperative:

- Promote wound healing.
- Restore normal fluid and electrolyte balance.
- Promote weight control.
- Wean from ventilator support when possible.
- Prevent hyperosmolar nonketotic hyperglycemia (HNKH) coma, sepsis, atelectasis, renal failure, cardiac tamponade, or wound dehiscence.
- Maintain comfort and educate regarding follow-up.
- Long-term, avoid excessive weight gain, which can further aggravate heart condition.

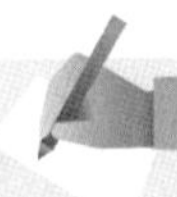

DIETARY AND NUTRITIONAL RECOMMENDATIONS

- Control fluid intake by measuring previous day's output plus 500 mL for insensible losses.
- Control sodium and potassium intake by monitoring serum levels, controlling edema, and measuring blood pressure. Modify diet as needed.
- As treatment progresses, control intake of cholesterol in diet (check serum levels and discuss history with patient). Modify sodium intake as needed. At home, 2–4 g of sodium is reasonable.
- Provide adequate protein and calories for wound healing; provide adequate zinc and vitamins A, C, and K as well.
- The National Cholesterol Education Program guidelines for diet may be used.
- TF or use TPN if severely malnourished. Replete slowly and keep head of bed elevated 30° to prevent worsening of CHF. Low-sodium TF products would be needed; high-calorie, low-density volumes may be useful.

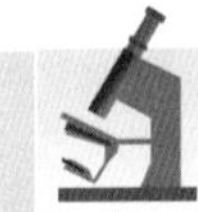

PROFILE

Clinical/History

Height
Weight
BMI
BP
I & O
Heart failure?
Edema

Lab Work

Chol
Lactic acid dehydrogenase (LDH) (increased)
Prothrombin time (PTT), PT
Na+
Alb, prealbumin
H&H
Trig
CPK
K+
Ca++
Gluc
RBP
Transferrin
Serum insulin
Acetone
EKG, chest x-rays
Radionucleotide imaging screening
Coronary angiography

Common Drugs Used and Potential Side Effects

- Anesthesia delays peristalsis; nausea is common. If permitted, patient may eat ice chips or sip carbonated beverages until nausea subsides.
- Nitrous oxide anesthesia may cause neurologic damage in patients with a vitamin B12 deficiency (Flippo and Holder, 1993). Monitor for verified deficiency levels.
- Pain medications should be taken sufficiently in advance of meals to allow a pleasant, pain-free mealtime.
- Diuretics and digoxin may deplete potassium. Monitor carefully. Anorexia, nausea, and diarrhea may occur. Hypoalbuminemia may cause digoxin toxicity.
- Beta-blockers, ace inhibitors, and other cardiac drugs may have been used for some time. Monitor for side effects. Some require use of low-sodium, low-calorie diets for most effectiveness.
- Insulin may be needed with hyperglycemia.

Herbs, Botanicals and Supplements

- Herbs and botanical supplements should not be used without discussing with physician.
- See Table 14–5, which lists the specific herbs and botanicals that should be discontinued before surgery.

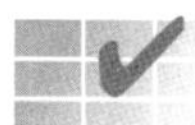

PATIENT EDUCATION

- ✔ Teach appropriate measures for changes in daily diet to prevent further problems while wound is healing.
- ✔ Discuss need to alter lifestyle (diet, exercise, and stress) to prevent additional problems. Many patients continue to have atherogenic activity after heart surgery.
- ✔ Restriction of excesses of simple sugars and alcohol may be needed for patients with diabetes or hypertriglyceridemia.

PANCREATIC SURGERY

NUTRITIONAL ACUITY RANKING: LEVEL 3

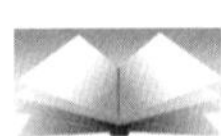

DEFINITIONS AND BACKGROUND

Surgery of the pancreas may include total pancreatectomy with/without islet cell autotransplant for chronic pancreatitis and cancer; subtotal for islet cell tumor and CA; or pancreatoduodenectomy (Whipple's operation) for carcinoma. The standard Whipple's procedure results in dumping syndrome, diarrhea, dyspepsia, ulceration at gastroenterostomy site, and postoperative weight loss of 10–40 kg (Kozuschek et al., 1994). A new pylorus-preserving method is more protective of the upper intestine.

Chronic pancreatitis in childhood is a rare but potentially debilitating disorder. Distal pancreatectomy and pancreaticojejunostomy are effective treatments for this difficult group of patients, with long-term pain relief and reduced need for re-hospitalization (Weber and Keller, 2001).

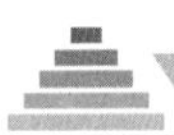

OBJECTIVES

- Monitor any history of ETOH abuse (with resulting malnutrition and malabsorption problems).
- Encourage nourishing, well-balanced meals, if ordered and tolerated.
- Monitor medications and replacement enzymes or hormones, if ordered.
- Reduce an elevated temperature.

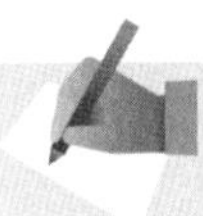

DIETARY AND NUTRITIONAL RECOMMENDATIONS

- NPO will be needed preoperatively, with PN or TPN to prepare patient for a major operation.
- Postoperatively, TPN or oral intake may progress as tolerated. Clear liquid to soft diet is a general order.
- A calorie-controlled diabetic diet may be needed.
- Small, frequent feedings may be helpful.
- Force fluids unless contraindicated.
- Alter fat source if malabsorption or steatorrhea occurs.

Common Drugs Used and Potential Side Effects

- Anesthesia delays peristalsis; nausea is common. If permitted, patient may eat ice chips or sip carbonated beverages until nausea subsides.
- Nitrous oxide anesthesia may cause neurologic damage in patients with a vitamin B12 deficiency (Flippo and Holder, 1993). Monitor for verified deficiency levels.
- Pain medications should be taken sufficiently in advance of meals to allow a pleasant, pain-free mealtime.
- Antibiotics may be used for bacterial infections. Monitor for GI distress or other side effects.
- Insulin may be needed for patients with hyperglycemia. Time meals and snacks accordingly.
- Vitamin K can help with clotting. There are generally no side effects with this injection.
- Pancreatic enzymes and bile salts may be needed. If too much is used, diarrhea or loose stools may result.

Herbs, Botanicals and Supplements

- Herbs and botanical supplements should not be used without discussing with physician.
- See Table 14–5, which lists specific herbs and botanicals that should be discontinued before surgery.

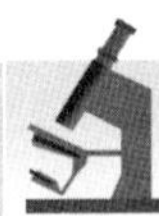

PROFILE

Clinical/History	Lab Work	
Height	PT or INR	Chol (may be increased)
Weight	Acetone	Alb, prealbumin
BMI	Na+, K+	Lipase
Temperature, fever	Cl−	Glucosuria
I & O	Hemoglobin A1c test (HbA1c)	H&H, Serum Fe
	Serum insulin	Gluc
		Amylase

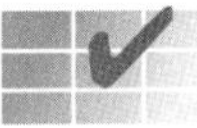

PATIENT EDUCATION

- ✓ Resources are available to help with diabetes, if patient becomes a new diabetic.
- ✓ The need for balanced meals will be essential for wound healing and recovery.
- ✓ If patient has any history of ETOH abuse, discuss how alcohol affects the pancreas.

PARATHYROIDECTOMY

NUTRITIONAL ACUITY RANKING: LEVEL 1

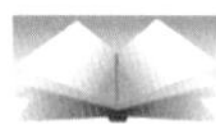

DEFINITIONS AND BACKGROUND

Surgical removal of the parathyroid glands may cause hypoparathyroidism (with tingling, tetany, hoarseness, and seizures).

OBJECTIVES

- Prepare patient preoperatively for surgery.
- Force fluids unless contraindicated.
- Alter calcium, vitamin D, and phosphorus intake if needed.

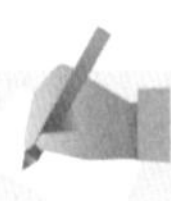

DIETARY AND NUTRITIONAL RECOMMENDATIONS

- Immediately after surgery, intravenous feeding or TF may be needed. TPN may not be recommended because of potential for sepsis in the neck area.
- Approximately, 3–4 L of fluid may be needed.
- A high-calcium/low-phosphorus diet may be necessary. Monitor carefully.

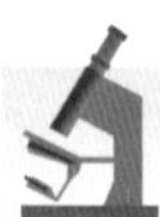

PROFILE

Clinical/History	Lab Work	
Height	Ca++	Na+, K+
Weight	Alk phos	H&H
BMI	TLC	Serum P
BP	PT or INR	Alb, prealbumin
I & O	Gluc	BUN, Creat
Temperature	Mg++	

Common Drugs Used and Potential Side Effects

- Anesthesia delays peristalsis; nausea is common. If permitted, patient may eat ice chips or sip carbonated beverages until nausea subsides.
- Nitrous oxide anesthesia may cause neurologic damage in patients with a vitamin B12 deficiency (Flippo and Holder, 1993). Monitor for verified deficiency levels.
- Pain medications should be taken sufficiently in advance of meals to allow a pleasant, pain-free mealtime.
- Vitamin D, calcium chemotherapy, and a low-phosphorus diet with aluminum hydroxide (Amphojel) may be ordered for symptoms of hypoparathyroidism. Constipation is one side effect of Amphojel.

Herbs, Botanicals and Supplements

- Herbs and botanical supplements should not be used without discussing with physician.
- See Table 14–5, which lists specific herbs and botanicals that should be discotinued before surgery.

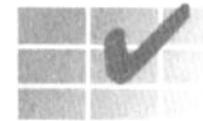

PATIENT EDUCATION

- ✓ Counsel patient regarding follow-up measures according to prescribed dietary regimen or medication side effects.
- ✓ Extra fluids are necessary.

SPINAL SURGERY

NUTRITIONAL ACUITY RANKING: LEVEL 2

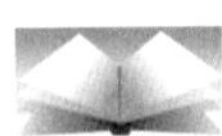

DEFINITIONS AND BACKGROUND

Spinal surgery generally is performed to relieve pressure on spinal nerves or cord due to herniated discs, trauma, displaced fractures, osteoporosis, or incomplete vertebral dislocation from rheumatoid arthritis (RA). A laminectomy, diskectomy, or spinal fusion may be performed.

OBJECTIVES

- ▲ Preoperatively, nutrients may be needed for adequate stores (e.g., glucose, protein, vitamins A, C, and K, and zinc).
- ▲ Correct nausea and vomiting, if these complications have been a problem.
- ▲ Avoid weight gain.
- ▲ Prevent calculi, UTIs, and pressure ulcers.

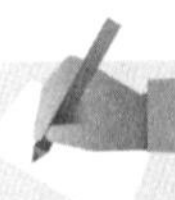

DIETARY AND NUTRITIONAL RECOMMENDATIONS

- Parenteral fluids may be given as ordered.
- A balanced diet, when patient is ready, with control of total calories to prevent excessive weight gain, may be used.
- If patient has been malnourished, a gradual increase in calories may be beneficial.
- Adequate hydration with 3 L of fluid will be necessary unless contraindicated. Monitor to prevent overhydration.
- Increasing fiber intake may be helpful if constipation is a problem. Prune juice, crushed bran, and other items may be used if chewing is a problem for patient. Otherwise, extra fruits and raw vegetables may be used.

Common Drugs Used and Potential Side Effects

- Anesthesia delays peristalsis; nausea is common. If permitted, patient may eat ice chips or sip carbonated beverages until nausea subsides.
- Nitrous oxide anesthesia may cause neurologic damage in patients with a vitamin B12 deficiency (Flippo and Holder, 1993). Monitor for verified deficiency levels.
- Pain medications should be taken sufficiently in advance of meals to allow a pleasant, pain-free mealtime.
- Antibiotics may be used with bacterial infections. Monitor for GI distress and other side effects.
- Anti-inflammatory drugs may have been used before surgery; monitor for consequential side effects.

Herbs, Botanicals and Supplements

- Herbs and botanical supplements should not be used without discussing with physician.
- See Table 14–5, which lists specific herbs and botanicals, which should be discontinued before surgery.

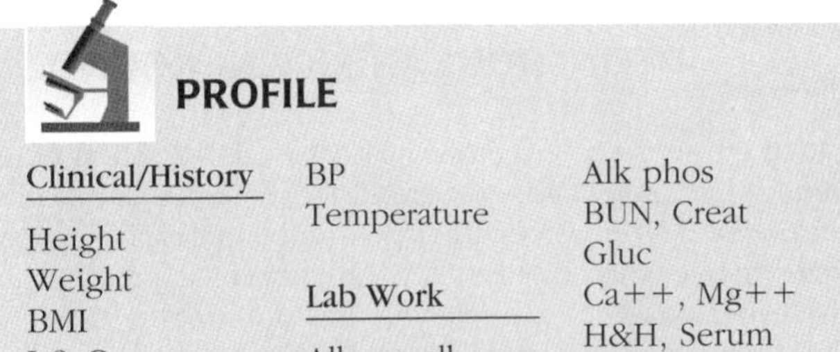

PROFILE

Clinical/History

Height
Weight
BMI
I & O
BP
Temperature

Lab Work

Alb, prealbumin
Na+, K+, Cl-
Alk phos
BUN, Creat
Gluc
Ca++, Mg++
H&H, Serum Fe
CSF

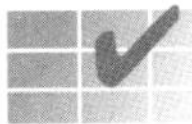

PATIENT EDUCATION

- ✔ Discuss importance of hydration in prevention of UTIs and other problems such as renal stones.
- ✔ Discuss how fiber can prevent or correct constipation.

TOTAL HIP ARTHROPLASTY

NUTRITIONAL ACUITY RANKING: LEVEL 2

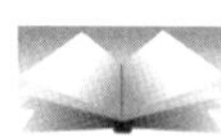

DEFINITIONS AND BACKGROUND

A total hip replacement (arthroplasty) is the formation of an artificial hip joint. Prostheses are either cemented in place or uncemented. The procedure is performed in cases of severe degenerative joint disease, RA, or congenital deformities. Those persons with a prior wrist fracture may be twice as likely to break a hip later in life.

Nutritional status before arthroplasty is a good predictor of surgical outcomes after surgery; albumin levels over 3.4 are predictors of a better outcome (Lavernia et al., 1999).

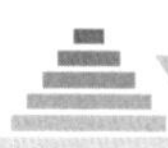

OBJECTIVES

- ▲ Replenish stores pre- and postoperatively.
- ▲ Prevent side effects of immobilization (renal calculi, pressure ulcers, and UTIs).
- ▲ Promote adequate wound healing.
- ▲ Regain maximum mobility.

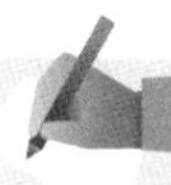

DIETARY AND NUTRITIONAL RECOMMENDATIONS

- Use a high-protein/high-calorie diet.
- Supplement diet with zinc and vitamins A, C, and K. Check patient's iron stores to determine whether replenishing is needed after blood loss.
- If weight loss is needed, provide a balanced, low-calorie diet after wound healing is completed.
- Diet should provide adequate amounts of calcium and phosphorus—calculi should be prevented and bone tissue adaptation to the new joint should be promoted.

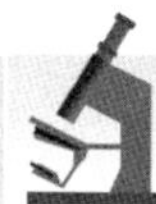

PROFILE

Clinical/History	Lab Work	
Height	PT	BUN, Creat
Weight	Alb, prealbumin	Alk phos
BMI	Ca++	Phosphorus
I & O	Gluc	Transferrin
BP	H&H	K+
		RBP

Common Drugs Used and Potential Side Effects

- Anesthesia delays peristalsis; nausea is common. If permitted, patient may eat ice chips or sip carbonated beverages until nausea subsides.
- Nitrous oxide anesthesia may cause neurologic damage in patients with a vitamin B12 deficiency (Flippo and Holder, 1993). Monitor for verified deficiency levels.
- Pain medications should be taken sufficiently in advance of meals to allow a pleasant, pain-free mealtime.

Herbs, Botanicals and Supplements

- Herbs and botanical supplements should not be used without discussing with physician.
- See Table 14–5, which lists specific herbs and botanicals that should be discontinued before surgery.

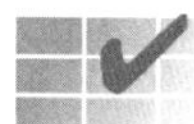

PATIENT EDUCATION

- ✔ Ambulation, when possible, will promote healing and increase strength.
- ✔ Have patient eat small, frequent meals if nausea is a problem.

TONSILLECTOMY AND ADENOIDECTOMY

NUTRITIONAL ACUITY RANKING: LEVEL 1

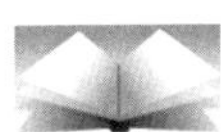

DEFINITIONS AND BACKGROUND

Removal of tonsils and adenoids (tonsillectomy and adenoidectomy) is less common than a few decades ago. This tissue is considered to be part of the protective immune system, and removal is now a last resort, especially for children with chronic ear, throat, and sinus infections.

OBJECTIVES

- Supply adequate nourishment for glycogen stores preoperatively.
- Postoperatively provide cold liquids that will not produce discomfort and progress to nonirritating foods.
- Prevent or correct vomiting and nausea.

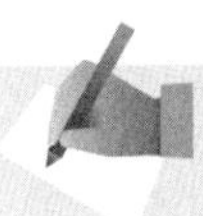

DIETARY AND NUTRITIONAL RECOMMENDATIONS

- Postoperatively, give cold liquids (sherbet, ginger ale, nectars, and gelatin). Avoid milk products only if patient cannot tolerate them.
- On second or third day, use soft, smooth foods (pudding, strained cereals, soft-cooked eggs).
- Progress to regular diet as tolerated. A soft diet may be preferred for a few more days.
- Use supplements of vitamin C if patient cannot tolerate juices. Evaluate zinc intake and encourage dietary sources when possible.
- Use adequate fluid intake (e.g., 3 L for adults and 2 L for children).

Common Drugs Used and Potential Side Effects

- Anesthesia delays peristalsis; nausea is common. If permitted, patient may eat ice chips or sip carbonated beverages until nausea subsides.
- Pain medications should be taken sufficiently in advance of meals to allow a pleasant, pain-free mealtime.

Herbs, Botanicals and Supplements

- Herbs and botanical supplements should not be used without discussing with physician.
- See Table 14–5, which lists specific herbs and botanicals that should be discontinued before surgery.

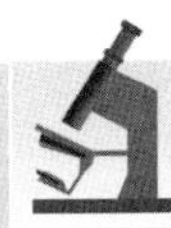

PROFILE

Clinical/History		
Height	I & O	K+, Na+
Weight	BP	H&H
BMI	**Lab Work**	Alb, prealbumin
	Gluc	

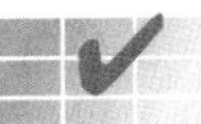

PATIENT EDUCATION

- ✓ Help patient select nonirritating foods for use at home. Avoidance of hot, spicy foods, raw vegetables, toast and crackers, citrus juices, and other related foods until full recovery will be recommended.
- ✓ Straws should not be used, temporarily.
- ✓ Taking large swallows of water causes less pain than small swallows.
- ✓ Patient should remain on cool liquids until pain subsides.
- ✓ Some doctors recommend avoidance of red gelatin to distinguish from hemorrhage.

REFERENCES

Cited References

Albrecht R, Pories W. Surgical intervention for the severely obese. *Baillieres Best Pract Res Clin Endocrinol Metab.* 1999;13:149.

Andorsky D, et al. Nutritional and other postoperative management of neonates with short bowel syndrome correlates with clinical outcomes. *J Pediatr.* 2001;139:27.

Bano G, et al. Reduced bone mineral density after surgical treatment for obesity. *Int J Obes Relat Metab Disord.* 1999;23:361.

Birnbaumer M. The V2 vasopressin receptor mutations and fluid homeostasis. *Cardiovasc Res.* 2001;51:409.

Boman L, et al. Do arthralgias occur after bilio-intestinal bypass for morbid obesity. *Obes Surg.* 1998;8:261.

Booth I. Enteral nutrition as primary therapy in short bowel syndrome. *Gut.* 1994;1:69S.

Braga M, et al. Perioperative immunonutrition in patients undergoing cancer surgery: results of a randomized double-blind phase 3 trial. *Arch Surg.* 1999;134:428.

Burge J, et al. Changes in patients' taste acuity after Roux-en-Y gastric bypass for clinically severe obesity. *J Am Diet Assoc.* 1995; 95:666.

Byrne T, et al. Growth hormone, glutamine, and fiber enhance adaptation of remnant bowel following massive intestinal resection. *Surg Forum.* 1992;43:151.

Cerra F. *Pocket manual of surgical nutrition.* St. Louis: CV Mosby, 1984.

Correia M, et al. Risk factors for malnutrition in patients undergoing gastroenterological and hernia surgery: an analysis of 374 patients. *Nutr Hosp.* 2001;16:59.

Crook M, et al. The importance of the refeeding syndrome. *Nutrition.* 2001;17:632.

Daly J, et al. Enteral nutrition with supplemental arginine, RNA and omega-3 fatty acids in patients after operation: immunologic, metabolic and clinical outcome. *Surgery.* 1992;112:56.

Daly J, et al. Risk adjustment of the postoperative morbidity rate for the comparative assessment of the quality of surgical care: results of the National Veterans Affairs Surgical Risk Study. *J Am Col Surg.* 1997;185:328.

Diehl A. Nonalcoholic steatohepatitis. *Semin Liver Dis.* 1999;19:221.

DiFronzo L, et al. Factors affecting early postoperative feeding following open colon resection. *Arch Surg.* 1999;134:94.

Erickson L, Perrault K. Early postoperative feeding—results of a North American survey. *J Can Diet Assoc.* 1993;54:190.

Fanning J, Andrews S. Early postoperative feeding after major gynecologic surgery: evidence-based scientific medicine. *Am J Obstet Gynecol.* 2001;185:1.

Flippo T, Holder W. Neurologic degeneration associated with nitrous oxide anesthesia in patients with vitamin B12 deficiency. *Arch Surg.* 1993;128:1391.

Ghanekar A, Grant D. Small bowel transplantation. *Curr Opin Crit Care.* 2001;7:133.

Gianotti L, et al. A prospective, randomized clinical trial on perioperative feeding with an arginine-, omega 3 fatty acid-, and RNA-enriched enteral diet: effect on host response and nutritional status. *J Parenter Enteral Nutri.* 1999;23:314.

Gibbs J, et al. Preoperative serum albumin level as a predictor of operative mortality and morbidity: results from the National VA Surgical Risk Study. *Arch Surg.* 1999;134:36.

Greenway S, Greenway F. Root surface caries: a complication of the jejunoileal bypass. *Obes Surg.* 2000;10:33.

Heyland D, et al. Should immunonutrition become routine in critically ill patients? A systematic review of the evidence. *JAMA.* 2001;286:944.

Hocking M, et al. Long-term consequences after jejunoileal bypass for morbid obesity. *Dig Dis Sci.* 1998;43:2493.

Kirk S, et al. Arginine stimulates wound healing and immune function in aged humans. *Surgery.* 1993;114:155.

Kozuschek W, et al. A comparison of long term results of the standard Whipple procedure and the pylorus preserving pancreatoduodenectomy. *J Am Col Surg.* 1994;178:443.

Lavernia C, et al. Nutritional parameters and short-term outcome in arthroplasty. *J Am Col Nutri.* 1999;18:274.

Martindale R. Clear liquid diets: tradition or intuition? *Nutr Clin Practice.* 1998;13:186.

McGuire J, et al. Fatal hypermagnesemia in a child treated with megavitamin/megamineral therapy. *Pediatrics.* 2000;105:18.

Montain S, et al. Hyponatremia associated with exercise: risk factors and pathogenesis. *Exerc Sport Sci Rev.* 2001;29:113.

Moore F, et al. Early enteral feeding, compared with parenteral, reduces postoperative septic complications: the results of a meta-analysis. *Ann Surg.* 1991;216:172.

Mun E, Blackburn G, Matthews J. Current status of medical and surgical therapy for obesity. *Gastroenterology.* 2001;120:669.

Naslund E, et al. Reduced food intake after jejunoileal bypass: a possible association with prolonged gastric emptying and altered gut hormone patterns. *Am J Clin Nutri.* 1997;66:26.

Pacelli F, et al. Enteral vs parenteral nutrition after major abdominal surgery: an even match. *Arch Surg.* 2001;136:933.

Palm C, et al. The role of V2 vasopressin antagonists in hyponatremia. *Cardiovasc Res.* 2001;51:403.

Pories W, Albrecht R. Etiology of type II diabetes mellitus: role of the foregut. *World J Surg.* 2001;25:527.

Rady M, et al. Clinical characteristics of preoperative hypoalbuminemia predict outcome of cardiovascular surgery. *J Parenter Enter Nutri.* 1997;21:81.

Reinhold R. Late results of gastric bypass surgery for morbid obesity. *J Am Col Nutri.* 1994;13:326.

Rodriguez-Moran M, Guerrero-Romero F. Low serum magnesium levels and foot ulcers in subjects with type 2 diabetes. *Arch Med Res.* 2001;32:300.

Rouse A, Tripp B, et al. Meeting the challenge of managed care through clinical pathways for bariatric surgery. *Obes Surg.* 1998; 8:530.

Schweinfurth J, et al. Preoperative risk assessment for gastrostomy tube placement in head and neck cancer patients. *Head Neck.* 2001; 23:376.

Schelling J. Fatal hypermagnesemia. *Clin Nephrol.* 2000;53:61.

Senkal M, et al. Outcome and cost-effectiveness of perioperative enteral immunonutrition in patients undergoing elective upper gastrointestinal tract surgery. *Arch Int Med.* 1999;134:1309.

Spiess A, et al. Albumin kinetics in hypoalbuminemic patients receiving total parenteral nutrition. *J Parenter Enter Nutri.* 1996;20:424.

Stike R, et al. Dairy product-induced diarrhea after bowel surgery: a performance improvement opportunity. *Nutr Clin Prac.* 2001;16:147.

Summer A, et al. Elevated methylmalonic acid and total homocysteine levels show high prevalence of vitamin B12 deficiency after gastric surgery. *Ann Intern Med.* 1996;124:469.

Thomas D. Nutritional factors affecting wound healing. *Ostomy/Wound Mgmt.* 1996;42:40.

Travis K, Barr S. Rethinking postoperative diets for short-stay orthopedic patients. *J Am Diet Assoc.* 1997;97:971.

Tzamaloukas A, et al. Body mass index in amputees. *J Parenter Enteral Nutri.* 1994;18:355.

Vernon A, Georgeson K. Surgical options for short bowel syndrome. *Semin Pediatr Surg.* 2001;10:91.

von Wowern N, et al. Bone loss and oral state in patients on home parenteral nutrition. *J Parenter Enter Nutri.* 1996;20:105.

Weber T, Keller M. Operative management of chronic pancreatitis in children. *Arch Surg.* 2001;136:550.

Welsh F, et al. Reversible impairment in monocyte major histocompatibility complex class II expression in malnourished surgical patients. *J Parenter Enteral Nutri.* 1996;20:344.

Wilmore D. The effect of glutamine supplementation in patients following elective surgery and accidental injury. *J Nutr.* 2001;131: 2543S.

Zaloga G, et al. Immediate postoperative enteral feeding decreases weight loss and improves wound healing after abdominal surgery in rats. *Crit Care Med.* 1992;20:115.

Ziegler T, et al. Effects of glutamine and IGF-1 administration on intestinal growth and the IGF-1 pathway after partial small bowel resection. *J Parenter Enteral Nutri.* 1994;18:20.

Suggested Readings

Buettiker V, et al. Somatostatin: a new therapeutic option for the treatment of chylothorax. *Intensive Care Med.* 2001;27:1083.

Burden S, et al. Validation of a nutrition-screening tool: testing the reliability and validity. *J Hum Nutr Diet.* 2001;14:269.

Cohen H, et al. High and low serum potassium associated with cardiovascular events in diuretic-treated patients. *J Hypertens.* 2001;19:1315.

DelSalvio G, et al. Preoperative nutritional status and outcome of elective total hip replacement. *Clin Orthop.* 1996;326:153.

Guesbeck N, Hickey M, et al. Substrate utilization during exercise in formerly morbidly obese women. *J Appl Physiol.* 2001;90:1007.

Heyland D, et al. Effect of postpyloric feeding on gastroesophageal regurgitation and pulmonary microaspiration: results of a randomized controlled trial. *Crit Care Med.* 2001;29:1495.

Jagoe R, et al. The influence of nutritional status on complications after operations for lung cancer. *Ann Thorac Surg.* 2001;71:936.

Klein, et al. Nutrition support in clinical practice: review of published data and recommendations for future research directions. *Am J Clin Nutri.* 1997;66:683.

Kushner R. Managing the obese patient after bariatric surgery: a case report of severe malnutrition and review of the literature. *J Parenter Enteral Nutri.* 2000;24:126.

Sax L. The institute of medicine's "dietary reference intake" for phosphorus: a critical perspective. *J Am Col Nutri.* 2001;20:271.

Waldorf H, Fewkes J. Wound healing. *Adv in Dermatol.* 1995; 10:77.

Winkler M, Manchester S. Nutritional care in metabolic stress. In: Mahan K, Escott-Stump S, eds. *Krause's food, nutrition, and diet therapy.* 10th ed. Philadelphia: WB Saunders, 2000.

SECTION 15

Hypermetabolic, Infectious, Traumatic, and Febrile Conditions

CHIEF ASSESSMENT FACTORS

- RECENT ILLNESSES, SURGERY
- PRESENCE OF CHRONIC DISEASES
- MEDICATIONS (PRESCRIPTION AND OVER-THE-COUNTER [OTC])
- ANEMIA, ANOREXIA, MALNUTRITION
- FEVER, CHILLS
- ACCIDENTS, OTHER TRAUMA
- METABOLIC RATE
- EDEMA
- INFECTIOUS PROCESSES OR SEPSIS (HEAT, PAIN, REDNESS, SWELLING, OR DRAINAGE IN ANY AREA)
- RAPID PULSE RATE
- ALTERED BREATHING
- URINARY CHANGES (FREQUENCY, URGENCY, BURNING)
- ALTERED WHITE BLOOD CELL COUNT (WBC) AND DIFFERENTIAL
- INDICATORS OF IMMUNITY SUCH AS T CELLS, OTHER LYMPHOCYTES
- CULTURE RESULTS, SPECIMENS
- FLUID STATUS
- MULTIPLE ORGAN SYSTEM FUNCTION, NG

GENERAL INFORMATION ABOUT NUTRITION AND IMMUNOCOMPETENCE

The fetal and early infant origins of adult cardiovascular and metabolic diseases have been studied, but many researchers have not reported the long-term consequences of early environments for human immune function. Importance of fetal and early infant programming of thymic function suggests that early environments may have long-term implications for immunocompetence and adult disease risk (McDade et al., 2001).

Chandra (2000) verifies nutrition and physical growth continue to be important factors that affect immunocompetence and morbidity from infections (Table 15–1). Small-for-gestational age low-birth-weight infants show prolonged impairment of cell-mediated immunity, antibody responses, and phagocyte function. Recent studies indicate the beneficial effect of moderate amounts of zinc given in the first 6 months of life. Thus, diet and nutrition in early life are crucial for protection against infectious disease throughout childhood and into adulthood.

Studies have been initiated regarding the role of nutrients on gene expression and related cytokine production in efforts to establish and maintain a balanced immune system throughout life (Fernandes, 1995). Specific vitamins, such as vitamin A and minerals such as zinc have been demonstrated to play important roles in protecting individuals from severity in illnesses such as diarrhea and human immunodeficiency virus (HIV) infection. Reactive oxygen species are usually kept in control by antioxidant systems in the body. If these systems are overwhelmed by oxidative stress, antioxidant supplementation may be used. Caution should be used, though, because there may be possible adverse effects (Oldham et al., 1998).

The role of large doses of vitamin C to reduce duration or severity of cold symptoms has been inconclusive, for example. Several clinical trials support the evidence against taking large amounts of vitamin C to treat the common cold (Audera et al., 2001).

Gut-associated lymphoid tissue (GALT) is the dominant location for initiation of mucosal immune response, which is dependent on nutritional elements, including fats, amino acids, and micronutrients (Cunningham-Rundles, 2001). A healthy gastrointestinal mucosal immune system provides barriers against systemic access for food antigens and microbes.

In surgical patients, preoperative oral intake of immunonutrition containing omega 3-fatty acids, arginine, and nucleotides at home may prevent the risks of hospitalization and may lead to immunomodulating effects, which can improve nutritional status (see section 14.) Adopting sound nutritional practices, reducing life stressors (Figure 15–1 , maintaining good hygiene and sanitation, obtaining adequate rest, and maintaining a healthy exercise routine can enhance immunocompetence and reduce risks of infection in any population.

Older adults are at risk for malnutrition, which contributes to increased risk of infection. Nutritional supplementation strategies have been proposed to reduce this risk and reverse some of the immune dysfunction associated with advanced age. Nutritional interventions have been examined in clinical trials of older adults; data support use of a daily multivitamin or trace-mineral supplement that includes elemental zinc over 20 mg/day and selenium (100 μg/day), with additional vitamin E to achieve a daily dosage of 200 mg/day (High, 2001).

Table 15–2 provides important nutritional factors to consider in patients who are critically ill. Table 15–3 provides a list of key nutrients for immunocompetence.

Table 15–1 Immunocompetence and Immunity

Almost all nutrients in the diet play a crucial role in maintaining an "optimal" immune response, such that deficient and excessive intakes can have negative consequences on immune status and susceptibility to a variety of pathogens.

Assessment of immunocompetence by available methods can identify individuals who are most in need of appropriate nutritional support and thus provide crucial prognostic information in terms of risk of disease, duration of hospitalization, and chances of survival (Puri and Chandra, 1985).

Iron and vitamin A deficiencies and protein-energy malnutrition are highly prevalent worldwide and are important to public health in terms of immunocompetence (Field et al., 2002).

Glutamine, arginine, fatty acids, vitamin E—Additional benefits for immunocompromised persons or patients who suffer from various infections (Field et al., 2002).

Zinc deficiency—Reduced numbers of lymphocytes in the peripheral immune system appear to be a significant cause of the loss in host defense capacity in humans and animals that are zinc deficient; both marrow and thymus are affected, with large losses noted among the pre-B and pre-T cells (Fraker and King, 2001).

Long-chain polyunsaturated omega-3 fatty acids, vitamin E, vitamin C, selenium, and nucleotides—Nutrients that may specifically modulate host defense to infectious pathogens (Field et al., 2002).

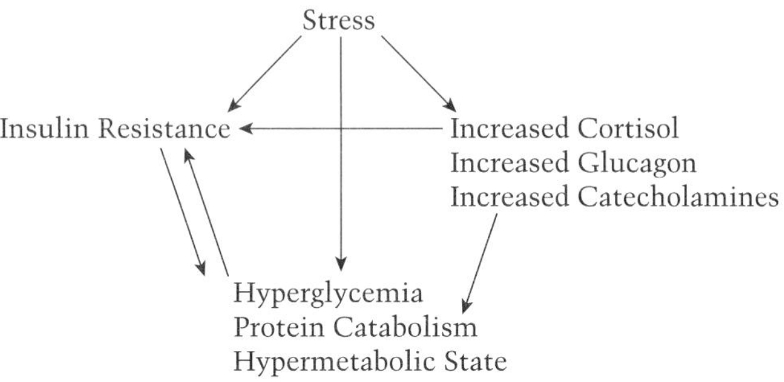

FIGURE 15–1 Hormonal response to stress. (From Matthews D. *Hormonal response to stress*. Presented at the ASPEN Conference, Miami, FL, January, 1995.)

TABLE 15–2 Factors of Importance in Critical Care

1. Estimated calorie needs in critical illness (25–30 kcal/kg actual body weight (ABW); intensive care, 20–25 kcal/kg ABW; 30% kilocalories as fat). Maintain protein at approximately 1.5 g/kg ABW. ABW is better as a calculation in obese persons than is ideal body weight (IBW) (Ireton-Jones and Turner, 1991).
2. Indirect calorimetry decreases complications from overfeeding and saves costs by reducing length of stay (LOS) (McClave and Snider, 1992). When carbon dioxide excretion levels are altered, use actual measured values (Porter and Cohen, 1996).
3. In critical illness, glutamine levels are much higher in the duodenal mucosa than in starvation (Ahlman et al., 1995). Vitamin E levels tend to be low in this population; monitor intake and supplementation accordingly (Kelly, 1994).
4. Studies suggest that arginine, dietary nucleotides (RNA), and omega-3 fatty acids promote host defense. Products such Advera (Ross) have been designed to include these nutrients at higher levels.
5. Pharmacologic doses of arginine can be used safely for up to 14 days and may have beneficial metabolic effects (Hurson et al., 1995). After 2 weeks, subjects who take arginine aspartate supplements (diet not altered) have higher insulin-like growth factors, more positive nitrogen (N) balance, decreased total serum cholesterol levels, and low-density lipoprotein (LDL) levels; high-density lipoprotein (HDL) levels are unchanged.
6. Metabolic complications can occur from overfeeding critically ill patients (Klein et al., 1998).

TABLE 15–3 Nutritional and Host Factors in Immunity

Infectious Disease Determinants
- Host immunity, including nutritional status
- Microorganismic virulence
- Environmental sanitation
- Personal hygiene

Host-Resistance Factors
- Physical barriers (skin, mucous membranes)
- Mucus and cilia on epithelial surfaces
- Phagocytes (leukocytes, macrophages)
- Complement system
- Immunoglobulins and antibodies (B cells) from bone marrow
- Cell-mediated immunity (T cells) from thymus

Immune System
- Bone marrow
- Spleen
- Lymph nodes
- Thymus
- Tonsils
- Lymphoid tissue (Peyer's patches in gut; Luster patches in bronchioles)

Groups at Greatest Risk for Infectious Illnesses
- Infants
- Elderly patients
- Malnourished and hospitalized persons

Nutrients of Immunocompetence
- Vitamin A (Bowman et al., 1990; Kramer, 1993; Field et al., 2002); B-carotene
- B-complex, especially vitamin B6 and folacin
- Vitamin C
- Vitamin E (Meydani et al., 1984; Field et al., 2002) and selenium (Levander and Buck, 1994)
- Iron and zinc (Fraker and King, 2001); beware of excesses, especially intramuscular or intravenous
- Copper (Prohaska, 1993)
- Iodine
- Magnesium (Kubena, 1993)
- Fatty acids to avoid essential fatty acid deficiency (Field et al., 2002); beware of excess poly-unsaturated fatty acids (PUFA) and obesity
- Omega-3 fatty acids (Moore et al., 1994)
- Amino acids such as arginine (Barbul, 1990) and glutamine (Burke et al., 1989; Field et al., 2002)

Excesses of Nutrients and Effect on Immunocompetence: (Puri and Chandra, 1985; Chandra and Sarchielli, 1993; and Shronts, 1993)
- Beware of excesses of iron, zinc, vitamin E, and PUFA because of their effects on immunity when taken in large doses. Parenteral iron and zinc are not appropriate in cachetic patients or in sepsis, except with careful consideration by the physician.
- Total parenteral nutrition (TPN) is contraindicated in septic patients.
- In addition, potential for nutrient–nutrient interactions is significant and not totally understood.
- Excess calcium interferes with leukocyte function by displacing magnesium ions and reducing cell adhesion (Kubena and McMurray, 1996).
- As with most nutritional guidance, variety, balance, and moderation are recommended.

AIDS AND HIV INFECTION

NUTRITIONAL ACUITY RANKING: LEVEL 4

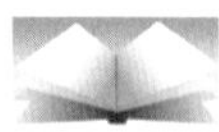

DEFINITIONS AND BACKGROUND

Acquired immune deficiency syndrome (AIDS) is a viral infection caused by human immunodeficiency virus (HIV) that has progressed to AIDS after the infected person developed an "opportunistic" infection (OI) or tumor (one that might not have developed if HIV had not been present) or a "helper" T-cell count in the blood of less than 200 cells/mm^3. Levels of CD4+ (helper) and CD8+ (nonhelper) subsets of T cells are used to evaluate immunologic competency in HIV/AIDS. Patients with marasmus, kwashiorkor, and general protein–energy malnutrition also have reduced levels of these indicators. After levels have been identified, stages of HIV infection are used to facilitate clinical evaluation and plan therapeutic interventions (CDC, 1992). Severity ranges from stages 1 to 3 according to level of depletion.

HIV is not easily transmitted but can be transmitted through exchange of bodily fluids during sexual contact, by receipt of infected blood through a blood transfusion or blood products, by sharing contaminated needles for intravenous drug abuse, or from an HIV-infected mother to neonate (children now represent 15–20% of the affected population). Persons at higher risk include homosexual or bisexual males, hemophiliacs, intravenous drug addicts, heterosexuals with multiple partners, and infants of HIV-positive mothers (especially those who are breastfed). Breastfeeding (BF) by HIV-infected mothers results in HIV transmission by approximately 14% among women with chronic HIV infection. This occurs early in BF, but increased duration increases risk (Anderson, 2000); formula feeding prevents almost half of infant infections (Nduati et al., 2000). Maternal vitamin A deficiency has been associated with increased risk of perinatal HIV transmission (Anderson, 2000).

HIV targets the immune system and makes an infected person susceptible to infection and neoplasm because of an impaired ability to mount an adequate immune response. Malnutrition and its complications further impair the body. As patients with HIV develop advanced manifestations of AIDS, mutually detrimental interactions exist among nutrition, immunity, and infection (Kruse, 1998). Though effective antiretroviral treatments are available, HIV-infected people face a lifetime of vigilant polypharmacy to control HIV and wasting (American Dietetic Association, 2000).

Nutrition has both direct effects (immune-cell triggering) and indirect effects (on DNA and protein synthesis) on progression of HIV disease. Decline in body cell mass and deficiencies in vitamins and minerals—A, B_6, B_{12}, and E, riboflavin, copper, selenium, and zinc have all been reported in asymptomatic patients with HIV disease (Kruse, 1998). High intakes of niacin, vitamins C and B12, and thiamine have been found to slow the progression from HIV infection to full-blown AIDS; while increased zinc intake has been correlated significantly with rapid progression to an AIDS-defining complication (Tang et al., 1993). Some clinicians have recommended a series of antioxidant supplements (vitamins C and E, glutathione, *N*-acetylcysteine, and B-carotene) in an effort to augment antioxidant activity in the cells, but this is still not conclusive (Fields-Gardner, 1997).

HIV infection involves multiple organs. Symptoms and signs include fever, chills, sore throat, headache, tachypnea, anxiety, fatigue, night sweats, hypoxemia, dyspnea on exertion, rales or rhonchi, cyanosis, pneumonia, diarrhea, cryptococcosis, several viral infections, ulcerating herpes simplex lesions, meningitis, anorexia, inflamed mouth or esophagus, malabsorption, weight loss, and poor nutritional status. Because of the crucial role that nutrition plays throughout the course of HIV, medical nutrition therapy should be considered an integral part of disease management at all stages.

In starvation, there generally is loss of adipose tissue with maintenance of lean body mass (LBM); in HIV/AIDS, there is loss of LBM while maintaining body fat (wasting). Wasting syndrome is defined as the involuntary loss of at least 10% of body weight and is a common AIDS-defining diagnosis reported in close to 20% of cases (Kruse, 1998). Weight loss is an independently prognostic indicator of outcome and mortality; when ABW approaches 60% of IBW, death is likely to occur, even in the absence of specific underlying diseases. Body cell mass at death is often 54% of usual levels (Flier and Underhill, 1992). A high cholesterol level is also not favorable for clinical outcome (Chlebowski et al., 1995). Weight loss, fatigue, anorexia, diarrhea, and low-grade fevers may be early, nonspecific signs of an OI. Failure to monitor body weight may result in a missed OI, which may further contribute to malnutrition and wasting. As long as an infection remains untreated, nutritional support regimens will meet with only limited success.

Fat redistribution as part of a syndrome known as peripheral lipodystrophy has been seen in patients receiving active antiretroviral therapy (Batterham et al., 1999). Etiology is unknown; women seem to be particularly prone to truncal obesity. Abnormal fatty deposits, which may be disfiguring, have been reported in the neck and dorsocervical area ("buffalo hump"). These changes may or may not be accompanied by development of hyperlipidemia and/or diabetes mellitus. Body composition measures must be accurate and ideally should be taken prior to initiation of antiretroviral therapy (Anderson, 2000). Bioelectrical impedance analysis (BIA) has been found to be useful, as are skinfold measurements. Skinfold measurements tend to overestimate fat-free mass and underestimate fat mass.

Gastrointestinal (GI) complications are common in AIDS. Weight loss is often multifactorial in etiology, but reduced oral intake is the most common factor (American Gastroenterological Association, 1996). Treatment of the underlying disease often results in weight gain. Nutritional supplements, dietary counseling, tube feeding (TF), and, if needed, parenteral nutrition (PN) may be used. Chronic diarrhea requires diagnostic testing; antimicrobial therapy may be needed.

There is substantial evidence that medical nutrition therapy for HIV/AIDS patients can reduce illness, hospital stays and related medical costs, and save lives (Young, 1997). The

American Dietetic Association recommends three medical nutrition therapy visits per year for adults with Stage 1 HIV/AIDS; 3–6 per year for adults with Stage 2 or 3 HIV/AIDS; and a minimum of five medical nutrition therapy visits for children or adolescents with HIV/AIDS (http://www.knowledgelinc.com/ada/mntguides/).

OBJECTIVES

- Improve nutrition-related immune function.
- Support prevention of OIs such as oral candidiasis by strengthening immunity.
- Enhance response to therapy through continuous counseling to manipulate diet and enhance drug levels (Fields-Gardner, 1997).
- Maintain body weight at 95–100% of usual body weight levels. LBM is especially affected. Prevent additional weight loss from fever, oral pain, infection, nausea, diarrhea, and vomiting by early nutritional intervention.
- Reduce mealtime fatigue to encourage better intake. Avoid unnecessary distractions and stresses.
- Lower temperature to normal, when febrile.
- Diagnose and treat diarrhea, malabsorption, vomiting, and HIV-induced enteropathy.
- If necessary, use TPN to prevent further weight loss and potential malnutrition (TPN will stop weight loss, but it will not prevent further immunodeficiency.).
- Keep body well hydrated. Fluids are critical to keeping body well hydrated as well as flushing the system sufficiently to prevent kidney stones and other complications.
- Support depleted levels of such nutrients as linolenic acid, selenium, and vitamin B12.
- Counteract such problems as dysphagia, mouth pain, difficulty swallowing, taste alterations (dysgeusia), and difficulty chewing.
- Alleviate nutritional effect of fatigue, anemia, anorexia, depression, and dyspnea. Efforts to optimize nutritional status are extremely important (American Dietetic Association, 2000).
- Maintain honest discussions regarding use of alternative therapies such as herbs, special diets, and megavitamin therapy, which have been shown to have no particular benefits (Luder et al., 1995).
- Maintain fat intake at prudent levels (30% total kilocalories; 7% saturated fatty acids [SFA]; cholesterol less than 300 mg). High fat and cholesterol intakes are not protective against clinical decline (Chlebowski et al., 1995).
- Alter dietary regimen if there is renal or hepatic impairment (check electrolytes, protein, etc.).

DIETARY AND NUTRITIONAL RECOMMENDATIONS

- Maintain diet as appropriate for patient's condition (e.g., high-calorie/high-protein diet with adequate nutritional supplementation). Weight gain and/or maintenance is possible in patients with HIV infection and early stages of AIDS by use of oral liquid supplements. A majority of patients with secondary infections, however, lose weight in spite of use of supplements (Stack et al., 1996).
- Use TF, especially gastrostomy, if warranted. Low-lactose/low-fat TF products may be needed (such as Impact or Advera fed continuously to reduce gastroenteritis [GE] reflux). An oral semi-elemental diet (SED) may reverse weight loss and wasting in patients with AIDS and malabsorption (Kotler et al., 1998). TPN costs four times as much as SED.
- From 2–2.5g protein/kg and 35–45 kcal/kg are needed. Fever and infection may further elevate need for these nutrients. Threonine and methionine are limiting amino acids for protein synthesis in patients with AIDS (Laurichesse et al., 1998). Calories may be needed at 1.5 times normal during bouts of infection, fever, and pneumonia.
- TPN may be necessary for weight loss exceeding 20% of usual body weight.
- Keep body well hydrated. Approximately 9–12 (8 oz) cups are recommended (Kruse, 1998).
- Increase use of omega-3 fatty acids and decrease saturated fats. There may be advantages to using a medium-chain triglyceride (MCT)-based formula in the treatment of AIDS-associated malabsorption (Craig et al., 1997).
- Small, frequent feedings (6–9 times daily) are usually better tolerated but may be difficult to achieve given complex medication regimens, which must be adhered to as well.
- In some cases, lactose or gluten is not tolerated. Reduce intake, if necessary, but avoid further anorexia when possible by offering some preferred foods and beverages. Sucrose and d-xylose may also need to be limited.
- A general multivitamin–mineral supplement should be recommended not to exceed 100% of the recommended dietary allowance (RDA). Diet and supplements should provide adequate zinc, vitamins C and B12, copper, vitamin E (Odeleye and Watson, 1992), selenium, vitamin A (Semba et al., 1993), and B-complex (see Table 15–3). Two times the RDA of all water-soluble vitamins may be useful; maintain fat-soluble vitamins at RDA levels. Vitamin K deficiency is common with antibiotic use.
- Nutrient-dense snacks may be beneficial (i.e., ice cream or pudding, if tolerated, nonacidic juices for sore mouth, ices made with tolerated juices, sandwiches made with cold meat salads, etc.). Add protein powders (dry milk powder, Pro-Mod, Pro-Mix, Casec) and glucose polymers (Polycose), if desired. Products such as Advera may be used orally as a supplement, if needed; each can has 303 kcal (Cameron, 1994). Try not to recommend particular products unless a list of several is used. Products to suggest include Advera, Ensure, Resource, Boost Plus, and Carnation Instant Breakfast.
- With bouts of diarrhea, use small meals and avoid extremes in temperatures (room temperature is best). Avoid high-fat foods; eat soft cooked chicken, turkey, fish, and lean beef. Replace electrolytes (sodium, potassium, magnesium, and chloride). If lactose intolerant, avoid milk and use a low-lactose or lactose-free diet. Avoid excesses of caffeine and alcohol. Avoid high-fiber foods including bran; substitute with high-soluble fiber foods such as oatmeal, barley, and applesauce (Fields-Gardner, 1997; Federation of American Societies for Experimental Biology, 1990).

- Children present unique nutritional needs, which are further compounded by HIV infection. See Table 15–4.

Common Drugs Used and Potential Side Effects

- Protease inhibitors (saquinavir, indinavir, ritonavir, nelfinavir): only nelfinavir has been approved for use in pediatrics (Heller, 1997). Disguising their taste is important—adding a small amount to cold foods such as ice cream, shakes, fruit ices; thick sweet foods such as honey, jellies, frozen juice; or small amounts of peanut butter, pudding, applesauce, or yogurt. Saquinavir: best absorbed after a high-energy, high-fat meal; contains some lactose; may cause diarrhea or nausea. Indinavir: best absorbed on an empty stomach or with a light, nonfat snack and increased fluids (but not skim milk, coffee, or tea), even juice if calories are needed; nausea and vomiting (N & V), change in taste, or diarrhea can occur. Ritonavir: take with a high-energy, high-fat meal; side effects include weakness, diarrhea, N & V, loss of appetite, abdominal pain, abnormal mouth sensations of burning or prickling, high chol, or TG levels. Nelfinavir (Viracept): take with food; flatulence, loose stools, or diarrhea can occur. Nevirapine (Viramune): take with food or on an empty stomach; fever, headache, hepatitis, general fatigue, mouth sores, and rash can occur. Foscarnet (Foscavir) is used for CMV retinitis (used by IV only) and may cause anorexia, N & V, abdominal pain, or diarrhea. Ganciclovir (Cytovene): may cause diarrhea, fever, neuropathy, elevated BUN and creatinine, and hypoglycemia. Lamivudine (Epivir) may cause N & V, pancreatitis, and depression. Zalcitabine (HIVID) can cause oral ulcers, N & V, and dry mouth.
- Reverse transcriptase inhibitors (ddI, ddC, d4T, 3TC) and azidothymidine/zidovudine (AZT, Retrovir) can cause severe bone marrow depletion and anemia, altered taste, constipation, nausea, indigestion, or vomiting. It works better in sequence with acyclovir. Adequate folate and vitamin B12 may prevent toxicity. Ribavirin (Virazole) may cause dyspnea and anemia.

Table 15–4 Nutrition for Children with HIV/AIDS

In HIV-infected children, malabsorption, enteric infections, malnutrition, and immune deficiency contribute significantly to shorter survival (Winter, 1996). In children with AIDS, failure to thrive (FTT) and protein–calorie malnutrition (PCM) are common; regular monitoring and interventions are needed (Gorbea-Robles et al., 1998). Early identification of children with HIV/AIDS, who are at nutritional risk, is essential; aggressive nutritional support is critical. Nocturnal, continuous feedings are useful.

Not long ago, 80% of patients with HIV/AIDS died malnourished. Today, the important role of nutrition support is well recognized. Every child with the infection should be assessed at baseline and every 4–6 months thereafter to determine risk of nutritional compromise. Severity or degree of nutritional risk in 4 sections is defined: anthropometric, biochemical, dietary intake, and medical data were graded 0–4 with 0 being low risk (Heller, 2000). Of 38 factors studied, 11 are reliable—height for age, weight for age, clinical class, somatic protein stores, mid-arm circumference, weight for height, serum albumin, immunologic status, body mass index, energy intake, and opportunistic infections.

Protein needs are 1.5–2 times the RDA for age and gender (Heller, 1997; Heller, 2000). Energy needs may vary from 50–200% of the RDA. Children with severe encephalopathy may be bed-fast and require fewer total calories. Weight loss may be due to poor energy intake, malabsorption, and OIs. A multivitamin supplement is needed to provide at least 100% of the RDA. Poor absorption may be a problem for vitamins A, C, B6, B12, folate, iron, selenium, and zinc. Calcium is needed to prevent loss of bone mass, which may persist (O'Brien et al., 2001). Herbal remedies are not recommended. Stunting and FTT have been identified in up to 94% of HIV-infected children. Skinfold measurements should be taken for comparison. The goal is simply to preserve LBM.

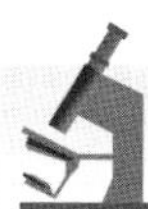

PROFILE

Clinical/History	Lab Work
Height Pre-illness weight Current weight Body mass index (BMI) Weight changes Head circumference (to 36 months of age) Herpes outbreaks Nausea, vomiting Temperature (fever, chills) Night sweats Dysphagia Chewing problems Stomatitis Blood pressure (BP) Intake and output (I & O) Diarrhea	CD4 lymphocytes (active AIDS = less than 200) Percentage of CD4 and T-lymphocyte count CD8 lymphocytes Viral load P24 antigen Total lymphocyte count (TLC) Albumin (alb), prealbumin (decreased) Retinol-binding protein (RBP) Glucose (gluc) Liver function tests Complete blood count (CBC) Hemoglobin and hematocrit (H&H) (decreased) Ferritin (increased) Platelets Creatine (creat), blood urea nitrogen (BUN) Transferrin Lactose test Schilling test Serum B12 (decreased) Serum Folate (decreased) Cholesterol (chol) Triglycerides (TG) (increased) Fecal fat test Biopsies (lymph nodes, skin lesions) DEXA scan

- Antineoplastic agents (Adriamycin, bleomycin, vincristine) or interferon—for Kaposi's sarcoma. Numerous side effects occur, including N & V, diarrhea, anorexia, stomatitis, and weight loss.
- Doxorubicin HCl administration with riboflavin to decrease toxicity. Dry mouth, esophagitis, stomatitis, nausea, or vomiting is common.
- Analgesics—Over time, aspirin may aggravate anemias. Extra vitamin C may be needed.
- Acyclovir (Zovirax) may cause headache, nausea, anorexia, sore throat, fatigue, altered taste, and diarrhea.
- Steroids—Sodium retention and potassium, calcium, and vitamin C depletion can occur; protein malnutrition can occur with extended use. Glucose intolerance also may result.
- Trimethoprim-sulfamethoxazole (Bactrim, Septra) may be used for *Pneumocystis carnii* pneumonia (PCP) for approximately 1 month. Drug may cause hepatitis, azotemia, anorexia, stomatitis, and thrombocytopenia. Monitor carefully. Folate may be needed.
- Antifungals (amphotericin-B, clotrimazole, flucytosine, ketoconazole) may cause N & V, diarrhea, weight loss, metallic taste, and GI distress.
- Pancreatic enzymes have been used with some benefit when malabsorption exists.
- Reglan, Periactin, or Megace (Megestrol acetate) may be useful to stimulate appetite and intake (Von Roenn et al., 1994). Dronabinol (marijuana derivative) takes 4–6 weeks to show effects; somnolence and impaired memory can occur.
- Oxandrolone (anabolic steroid) promotes weight gain, linear growth, and increased muscle mass. Long-term studies are needed. Psyllium (Metamucil) may be used to lower elevated total and LDL cholesterol levels. It may also help to lower blood glucose levels. Long-term studies are needed to determine any untoward side effects.
- Vitamin A supplementation improves linear growth in infants who are infected with HIV and decreases risk of stunting associated with persistent diarrhea (Villamor et al., 2002).

Herbs, Botanicals and Supplements

- Herbs and botanical supplements should not be used without discussing with physician. Licorice, St John's wort, oregano, astragalus, and burdock have been suggested but are not yet proven as efficacious.
- Echinacea is used as an antiviral agent. Do not use with warfarin or immunosuppressants.
- Garlic and St John's wort may make saquinavir or indinavir less effective.

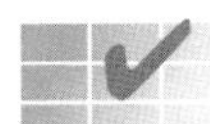

PATIENT EDUCATION

- ✔ Exceptional handwashing techniques should be used by all caregivers and by patient. Safe food-handling techniques are imperative to reduce exposure to cryptosporin, giardia, and salmonella.
- ✔ In the short term, nutrition counseling with or without oral supplementation can achieve a substantial increase in energy intake in about 50% of malnourished HIV-infected patients (Rabeneck et al., 1998). Importance of maintaining a balanced, nutritious diet should be addressed. Rest periods before and after meals are suggested.
- ✔ Diet must be altered whenever necessary; continuing contact with a nutritionist is essential regarding alternative feeding methods, the need for home-delivered meals, menu planning, and treatment of GI side effects.
- ✔ The role of nutrition in infection and immunity should be discussed. In addition, patients should be encouraged to decrease use of drugs and alcohol and cigarette smoking because of their effects on overall health status and immunocompetence.
- ✔ Patient and caregivers should report all weight loss, anorexia, and fever to doctor.
- ✔ Adequate education should address gradual and likely decline in self-care abilities, as well as alternative therapies and consequences. Resistance and strengthening exercises should be maintained to keep LBM intact. While chronic exercise and high-fat diets are often associated with immune suppression, exercise has mixed effects and a high-fat diet has no adverse effect on runners' immune systems (Venkatraman et al., 1997).
- ✔ In home care, TPN may be used. Adequate and continuing education should be offered to caregivers to prevent transmission of the disease and to reduce further likelihood of infection.
- ✔ New mothers who are HIV-positive may want to use formula instead of breastfeeding.
- ✔ Aversion to meat may be counteracted by use of cold protein foods such as cottage cheese, yogurt, skim milk, and cheeses.
- ✔ For children, consistency of caretaking is essential.

For More Information

- ✦ American Dietetic Association
  HIV/AIDS protocol for adults
  HIV/AIDS protocol for children
  www.eatright.org
- ✦ American Foundation for AIDS Research
  http://www.amfar.org/
- ✦ CDC National AIDS Hotline
  http://www.ashastd.org/nah/nah.html
- ✦ National AIDS Information Clearinghouse (NAIC)
  http://www.cdcnpin.org/
- ✦ U.S. Department of Health and Human Services
  http://www.dhhs.gov/
- ✦ HIV/AIDS Treatment Information Service
  http://www.hivatis.org

ASCARIASIS

NUTRITIONAL ACUITY RANKING: LEVEL 1

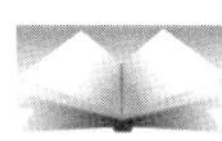

DEFINITIONS AND BACKGROUND

Intestinal roundworms (ascariasis) are the most common intestinal helminth and are usually found in warm or humid climates or when personal hygiene is inadequate. Adult worms live in the small intestine, with eggs that pass out in human feces. These eggs become infective within 2–3 weeks. When ingested by humans through fecally contaminated food or water, the eggs hatch and penetrate the intestines. Eventually, they reach the heart. Larvae mature within 2–3 months, and adult worms may live for 1 year or longer. Hemorrhage can occur in lung tissue and cause pneumonitis. Vague abdominal discomfort can occur with small intestine involvement.

OBJECTIVES

- Prevent or correct protein malnutrition.
- Prevent blockage, inflammation, volvulus, and bowel perforation.
- Differentiate symptoms from other disorders.
- Prevent further complications.

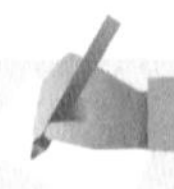

DIETARY AND NUTRITIONAL RECOMMENDATIONS

- Increase protein if patient is malnourished.
- Increase or ensure adequate calorie intake.
- Provide balanced intake of all vitamins and minerals.

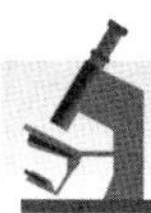

PROFILE

Clinical/History

Height
Weight
BMI

Lab Work

Alb, prealbumin
H&H, Serum Fe
Transferrin
Sodium (Na+), Potassium (K+)
Calcium (Ca++), Magnesium (Mg++)
TLC, WBC
Gluc
Total iron-binding capacity (TIBC)
Stool examination

Common Drugs Used and Potential Side Effects

- Pyrantel pamoate (Povan)—Rarely, vomiting or diarrhea may occur.

Herbs, Botanicals and Supplements

- Herbs and botanical supplements should not be used without discussing with physician.

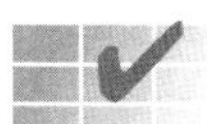

PATIENT EDUCATION

- Discuss importance of personal hygiene in maintaining a sanitary environment and in preventing reinfestation.
- Children who play outside should always wash their hands before eating meals or snacks.

BACTERIAL ENDOCARDITIS

NUTRITIONAL ACUITY RANKING: LEVEL 3

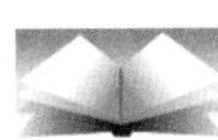

DEFINITIONS AND BACKGROUND

Bacterial endocarditis is a bacterial infection (often *Streptococcus*) of the membrane lining the heart chambers. Symptoms and signs include fever, chills, joint pain, lassitude, and malaise. Acute forms have rapid onset; the subacute form begins slowly. Anorexia and weight loss are common side effects. Most afflicted persons have had a previous heart condition such as rheumatic fever. Bacterial endocarditis accounts for 2% of all cases of organic heart disease.

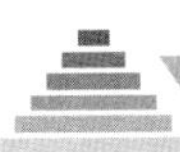

OBJECTIVES

- ▲ Restore patient's nutritional status to normal.
- ▲ Replenish electrolytes and fluids.
- ▲ Reduce edema, if present.
- ▲ Prevent heart failure, infections, flu, anemia, embolism, and nephritis.

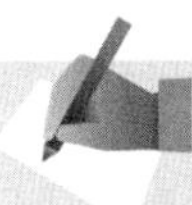

DIETARY AND NUTRITIONAL RECOMMENDATIONS

- Use a high-calorie diet. The patient's need to replenish stores of protein may require a high-protein diet.
- Ensure intake of an adequate amount of fluids, especially fruit juices.
- If patient's appetite is poor, encourage intake of favorite foods.
- Ensure adequate intake of vitamins and minerals, especially vitamins A and C.

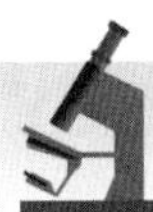

PROFILE

Clinical/History		
Height	Edema	BP
Weight	Temperature	Alb, prealbumin
BMI	I & O	RBP
Weight changes	**Lab Work**	K+, Na+
Anorexia	H&H, Serum Fe	WBC, TLC

Common Drugs Used and Potential Side Effects

- Check specific antibiotics for appropriate timing of meals and drugs. Penicillin, erythromycin, and other combinations may be used.

Herbs, Botanicals and Supplements

- Herbs and botanical supplements should not be used without discussing with physician.

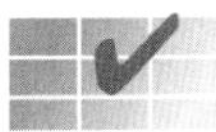

PATIENT EDUCATION

- ✔ Indicate which foods are sources of protein and calories in the diet.
- ✔ Dental care may require special attention. Abscesses should be treated immediately.

BURNS (THERMAL INJURY)

NUTRITIONAL ACUITY RANKING: LEVEL 3 (MINOR), LEVEL 4 (MAJOR BURNS)

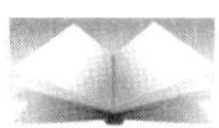

DEFINITIONS AND BACKGROUND

Electrical, thermal, chemical, or radioactive agents can cause burns. Burns are the third leading cause of accidental death in the United States; 35% of burn victims are children. Burns from microwave ovens are mostly scalds; these burns are lower in frequency than thermal burns from stoves (Powell and Tanz, 1993).

With a first-degree burn, simple redness of epidermis occurs. In a second-degree burn, redness and blistering occur. In a third-degree burn, skin and tissue destruction occurs. In a fourth-degree burn, there is extensive involvement of muscle, bone, and other tissues.

Total burn thickness seems to affect metabolic rate more than body surface area (BSA). Increased catecholamine production, body temperature, evaporative losses, and infections may occur. Local mediators (cytokines) are released from inflammatory cells, attracting more to affected area. Interleukin-1 and interleukin-6 as well as tumor necrosis factor (TNF) are involved. A 25–30% total body surface area (TBSA) burn leads to systemic edema and catabolic responses. Growth hormone (GH) may be used to decrease the catabolic effect of burns.

Loss of 1 g of nitrogen equals a 30-g loss of LBM. N balance becomes a matter of life and death in a major body burn. Survival depends on medical treatment and early, effective nutritional support (weight loss of up to 10% is acceptable; 40–50% can lead to mortality). The GI tract may become nonfunctional in a 40–50% TBSA burn; use of parenteral support may be needed.

Addition of high doses of ascorbic acid (rate of 25 mg/mL) to resuscitation fluid administered during the first 24 hours after severe burns significantly reduces resuscitation fluid volume, body weight gain, wound edema, and severity of respiratory dysfunction (Tanaka et al., 2000).

Healing takes place in three stages: establishment of the epithelial barrier, scar tissue formation (dermal replacement), and contraction (shrinkage). Severity of thermal injury and presence of systemic infection are risk factors for development of ischemic bowel disease. Systemic infection may alter integrity of the bowel, causing enteral feeding intolerance (Kowell-Vern et al., 1997).

OBJECTIVES

- Relieve pain.
- Restore fluid and electrolyte balance to prevent hypovolemic shock and to stabilize body temperature. Beware of exudate losses, which may be 20–25% of total daily nitrogen losses.
- Prevent renal insufficiency or failure from decreased plasma volume, cardiac output, and excessive pigment overload (from necrosis, toxins, and hemolysis). Correct syndrome of inappropriate antidiuretic hormone (SIADH), hypertonic dehydration, and overhydration.
- Minimize catabolism of protein tissues to avoid consequences of PCM (impaired immunity, decreased wound healing, decreased vigor and muscle strength, retarded synthesis of blood proteins and hemoglobin, increased likelihood of infection). Patients with burns have an elevated measured metabolic rate 1.2–1.3 times normal rate, increased further by percentage of burn surface.
- Promote wound healing and graft retention. Close wound surface to reduce likelihood of multiple organ system dysfunction. Grafts may be autograft (own body) or from cultured keratinocytes.
- Avoid weight losses greater than 10% of preburn weight (if that weight corresponds to patient's IBW). In children, growth must continue; maintain weight.
- Achieve positive N balance and minimize losses.
- Treat stress hyperglycemia; correct overfeeding.
- Reduce evaporative water losses, especially with occlusive wound dressings.
- Restore skin's protection to reduce infection. Sepsis is a major cause of mortality, often 2–3 weeks postinjury.
- Prevent Curling's ulcer by starting TF within a few hours after burn injury.
- Monitor obese patients carefully; they are at risk for complications from increased ventilation, more exogenous insulin requirements, and more likelihood of sepsis or bacteremia (Gottschlich et al., 1993).

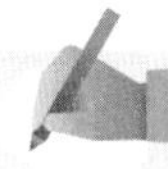

DIETARY AND NUTRITIONAL RECOMMENDATIONS

- Immediately use intravenous fluids to replace deficits; prevent gastric distention and paralytic ileus. Prevent overhydration. Add vitamin C as 25 mg/mL to promote healing.
- TF may be possible; start within a few hours for best results to decrease hypermetabolic response to injury. Use Impact, Trauma-Cal, or similar products. Intact proteins may be better used than amino acids. Increased use of branched-chain amino acids (BCAAs) has not been proven

TABLE 15-5 Common Methods for Calculating Calorie Needs in Burns

- BEE × 1.5–2
- Indirect calorimetry: more accurate for individual patients (determine or measure respiratory quotient [RQ] twice weekly)
- 35–45 kcal/kg BW for adults may be needed

conclusively to be beneficial for burn patients. Glutamine may help to preserve gut function (Ogle et al., 1994).

- Protein intake should be 1.5–3 g/kg IBW each 24 hours (infants need 3–4 g/kg IBW, young children need 1.2–2 g/kg, and older children need 1.5–2.5 g/kg). Add Pro-Mod, Pro-Pac, Casec, or other modular supplements as needed to increase protein.
- Table 15–5 provides methods commonly used to determine energy needs. Use 20–25% protein, 50% carbohydrates (CHO), and 25–30% fat (2–4% essential fatty acids [EFAs] and slight increase in omega-3 fatty acids). Low-fat TF have been shown to reduce rates of pneumonia and to speed healing (Garrel et al., 1995). CHO may be given at rate of 5 mg/kg/minute, intravenous lipids at 4 g/kg maximum in pediatrics. Add Polycose or other CHO supplements as needed.
- Gradually progress to oral diet when possible; use a high-calorie, high-protein diet with 5–6 small meals and snacks. Suitable snacks may include peanut butter cookies, brownies, cake, shakes, pasteurized eggs in milkshakes or eggnog, protein in broths, and dextrins added to coffee. (See tips for adding protein and calories to the diet in Section 5.)
- Provide adequate fluid intake: encourage intake of fruit juices (cranberry, grapefruit, prune, or orange juice) for adequate supplies of potassium. Water losses may be 10–12 times normal during first few weeks.
- Supplement diet with 5–10 times the RDA of vitamin C; zinc sulfate (two times the RDA); and 2–3 times the RDA for vitamin B-complex. Two times the RDA for vitamins A and D may be useful at first. Vitamins K and B12 should be given at least weekly. Be careful about iron and zinc excesses in patients with sepsis.
- For children, vitamins should be given at twice the RDA until recovery.
- Provide adequate copper (for collagen cross-linkage). Arginine (up to 2% of kilocalories) and carnitine also may be beneficial. Phosphorus should be added, intravenously as K+ PO4, enterally or orally as Neutra-Phos.
- Be careful to avoid excesses of linoleic acid, which can depress immunocompetence. Add fish often for omega-3 fatty acids, but there is no increased rate of healing from use in TF (Garrel et al., 1995).

Suggested Nutritional Interventions

- Obtain dietary history of patient's food preferences, allergies, and dislikes.
- Calculate percentage of body that has been burned: head and neck, 9%, each arm, 9%, anterior trunk, 18%, posterior trunk, 18%, each leg, 18%, and perineum, 1%.
- Assist in feeding patient and help determine proper feeding method to use (oral, enteral, parenteral). For children, eliminate distractions at mealtime.
- Avoid painful procedures before patient's mealtime. Do not interrupt mealtime for laboratory tests.
- Discourage consumption of empty-calorie foods or beverages. Medications can be taken with supplements, milk, or juice.
- Anticipate 2–3 months total for optimal recovery time.

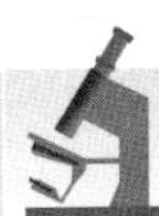

PROFILE

Clinical/History

Height
Preburn weight
Weight changes
Daily weight (beware heavy exudate, edema)
BMI
Measured energy expenditure (MEE)
Burn classification (1st, 2nd, 3rd, 4th)
Edema
I & O
Temperature
Urine acetone, sugars
Ability to chew
Ability to swallow
Hypovolemic shock (tachycardia, low BP and decreased urinary output)

Lab Work

Alb, RBP
Prealbumin (decreased)—Review 2 times weekly because of 3-day half-life
BUN, Creat
H&H
Gluc (increased)
Aspartate aminotransaminase (AST) (increased)
Na+ (decreased)
Chloride (Cl−)
K+
Urinary N (TUN)
Ca++, Mg++
N balance (amount excreted in g × 6.25 = g protein)
Note: N balance = (24 hr N intake − [24 hr UUN + 4])
Partial pressure of carbon dioxide (pCO2), partial pressure of oxygen (pO2)
Transferrin
Chol, Trig
WBC, TLC
Serum catecholamines (increased)
Ceruloplasmin
Alkaline phosphatase (alk phos) or serum PO4

Common Drugs Used and Potential Side Effects

- Silver nitrate dressings (Silvadene). Beware of nutrient leaching of sodium, copper, potassium, magnesium, calcium, and B-complex vitamins. Patient may need added salt or supplements of potassium and calcium in diet.
- Antacids are used to prevent Curling's ulcer. Cimetidine also is useful.
- Pain medications may have some effect on GI function and appetite.
- Insulin is used for stress-induced hyperglycemia.
- Interferon gamma or α-2β has been useful to decrease keloid formation. Dry mouth, stomatitis, N & V, diarrhea, or abdominal pain may result.

Herbs, Botanicals and Supplements

- Herbs and botanical supplements should not be used without discussing with physician. St John's wort, Echinacea, aloe, garlic, gotu kola, and plantain have been suggested but are not yet proven through clinical trials.

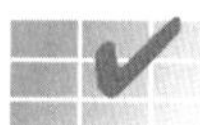

PATIENT EDUCATION

- ✔ Considering possible consequences of long-term immobilization (renal calculi, pneumonia, contractures, and pressure ulcers), have patient carefully increase activity as pain tolerance allows. Discuss importance of nutrition and physical activity.
- ✔ Review the role of fat in the diet. Fat is high in calories with low volume and is helpful in normalizing elimination. Excesses may negatively affect immunocompetence.
- ✔ Explain that adequate intake of fiber is important.
- ✔ The family's attitude toward patient's dietary intake should be firm but also patient and understanding.
- ✔ A daily kilocalorie intake record is the best way to achieve goals and assess intake.
- ✔ Discuss problems to monitor (fever, drainage, etc.).
- ✔ Offer a written care plan for home use. Table 15–6 describes the current status of use of modular products in tube feedings.

TABLE 15–6 Modular Tube Feeding for Burn Patients

In previous years, special modular tube feedings were often used in Burn Units. These included glucose powders, whole egg powder, egg white solids, corn oil and related additives. Today, Modular tube feedings are used less often because higher protein specialized enteral formulas exist. If needed, protein powders may be added either directly to the tube feeding or, if a closed-system is used, as a medication.

CANDIDIASIS

NUTRITIONAL ACUITY RANKING: LEVEL 2

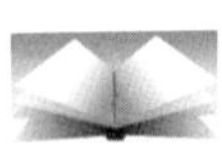

DEFINITIONS AND BACKGROUND

Candida albicans is found in mouth, feces, and vagina normally. A greater colonization occurs in debilitated persons, in whom thrush or vaginitis or cutaneous lesions are common. Persons who are susceptible include patients with hematologic malignancy, immunosuppressed patients, postoperative patients, people receiving antibiotic therapy, and people who are obese or have diabetes.

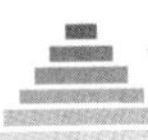

OBJECTIVES

- ▲ Prevent or treat systemic infections.
- ▲ Prevent endocarditis, emboli, splenomegaly, and other complications.
- ▲ Correct underlying conditions, where possible.

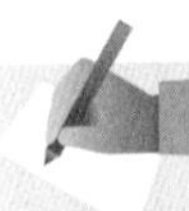

DIETARY AND NUTRITIONAL RECOMMENDATIONS

- Ensure balanced intake for all nutrients, high in quality proteins, and adequate in calories.
- Adequate fluid intake is beneficial.
- Some research suggests use of yogurt in diet; no conclusions are evident.
- Increase vitamin and mineral intake from tolerated fruits and vegetables. At least meet RDAs for vitamins A and C.

Common Drugs Used and Potential Side Effects

- Nystatin or amphotericin B may be used to correct condition. Diarrhea, nausea, and stomach pain may occur.
- Extended use of antibiotics may have caused or aggravated condition.

Herbs, Botanicals and Supplements

- Herbs and botanical supplements should not be used without discussing with physician.

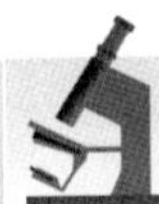

PROFILE

Clinical/History

Height
Weight
Weight changes
BMI
Lesions, symptoms
Underlying conditions

Lab Work

Gluc
Alb, prealbumin
Transferrin
TLC, WBC
H&H, Serum Fe
I & O

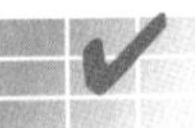

PATIENT EDUCATION

- ✔ For patients with malignant disease, a discussion about the importance of nutrition in maintaining good health status would be essential.
- ✔ Patients who are debilitated will need to understand that meals should be consumed regularly with smaller, frequent meals or snacks used, if large meals are not tolerated. Fasting and skipping meals should be avoided.

CHRONIC FATIGUE IMMUNE DYSFUNCTION SYNDROME

NUTRITIONAL ACUITY RANKING: LEVEL 2

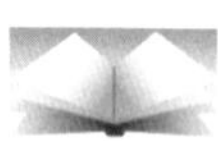

DEFINITIONS AND BACKGROUND

Chronic fatigue immune dysfunction syndrome (CFIDS), formerly called the chronic Epstein-Barr (EBV) syndrome, involves severe exhaustion and weakness, headaches, sore throat, tender lymph nodes, unrefreshing sleep, fever, muscle aches, inability to concentrate, and depression. CFIDS is a vague illness and symptoms tend to mimic depression, lupus, or even cancer. A thorough physical examination is suggested.

Etiology is unknown, but studies suggest a chronic mononucleosis caused by a herpes virus (perhaps the one known as human B-lymphotrophic virus). Research is inconclusive regarding this syndrome; some studies suggest a link to Hodgkin's disease or multiple sclerosis a few years after diagnosis. A study at Johns Hopkins has linked the condition to "neurally mediated hypotension."

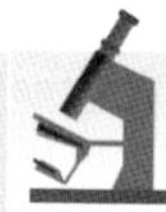

PROFILE

Clinical/History	Lab Work	
Height	Alb, prealbumin	cytomegalovirus
Weight	H&H, Serum Fe	TLC, WBC
BMI	Antibodies to measles, herpes simplex,	Gluc
Weight changes		Transferrin
Epstein-Barr viral load		Serum Fe
BP (low?)		TIBC

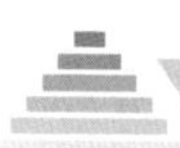

OBJECTIVES

- ▲ Improve immunologic status; prevent malnutrition.
- ▲ Prevent recurrent attacks, if possible.
- ▲ Lessen severity of symptoms.
- ▲ Prevent additional infections and stress.

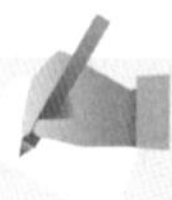

DIETARY AND NUTRITIONAL RECOMMENDATIONS

- Adequate protein should be consumed (0.8–1 gm/kg); 35 kcal/kg may be needed.
- Adequate vitamin and mineral intake should be ensured.
- Antioxidant vitamins from various foods should be included regularly in diet.
- Extra salt or fluids may be needed for hypotension.

Common Drugs Used and Potential Side Effects

- Fludrocortisone promotes sodium retention.
- Analgesics may be used for relief of muscle aches and other types of pain. Extra vitamin C may be needed.

Herbs, Botanicals and Supplements

- Zinc is often taken as an immunostimulant. Do not take with immunosuppressants, tetracycline, ciprofloxacin, levofloxacin, or ofloxacin; antagonistic effects or binding can occur.
- Herbs and botanical supplements should not be used without discussing with physician. Purslane, spinach, ginseng, and wheat grass have been suggested but are not yet proven through clinical trials.
- Do not take dandelion, fennel, or khat with ciprofloxacin or ampicillin.

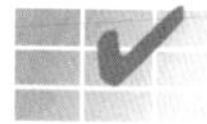

PATIENT EDUCATION

- ✓ Discuss importance of maintaining adequate nutritional intake to optimize immunologic status.
- ✓ Referral for counseling may be beneficial for some patients.
- ✓ Fad diets and special supplements should be discouraged.

For More Information

- Chronic Fatigue and Immune Dysfunction Syndrome (CFIDS)
  http://www.cfids.org/

ENCEPHALITIS AND REYE'S DISEASE

NUTRITIONAL ACUITY RANKING: LEVEL 2

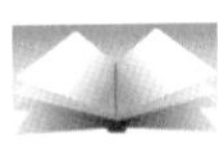

DEFINITIONS AND BACKGROUND

Encephalitis involves an inflammation of brain cells, usually by a virus such as measles, mumps, mononucleosis, or herpes simplex. It may also be caused by the tsetse fly (African sleeping sickness).

Reye's syndrome is a disease of the brain and some abdominal organs (e.g., liver), affecting mostly children and teenagers after viral illness. Etiology is unknown, but some linkage to aspirin has been suggested. Symptoms are similar to those of encephalitis, including headache, loss of energy, anorexia, irritability, restlessness, drowsiness, double vision, impaired speech and hearing, and possibly even seizures or coma.

OBJECTIVES

- Ease symptoms.
- Allow natural defense system to work.
- Assist breathing with respirator if necessary.
- Control any pernicious vomiting.

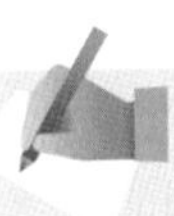

DIETARY AND NUTRITIONAL RECOMMENDATIONS

- Nasogastric (NG) TF may be needed if patient is comatose.
- When patient can eat again, a high-protein/high-calorie diet should be provided, including vitamins and minerals in adequate amounts. Vitamins A and C should be stressed from dietary sources.
- Adequate fluid intake will be important.

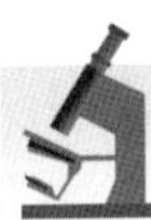

PROFILE

Clinical/History

Height
Weight
BMI
Fever, temperature
I & O
BP

Lab Work

Lactic acid dehydrogenase (LDH), creatine phosphokinase (CPK) (increased)
TLC, WBC
Ammonia (increased)
Na+, K+
Gluc (decreased)
AST, alanine aminotransferase (ALT) (increased)
BUN, uric acid (UA) (increased)
Creat
Cerebrospinal fluid
Electroencephalogram (EEG)

Common Drugs Used and Potential Side Effects

- Steroids are provided commonly. Long-term use may affect N balance or cause hyperglycemia. Sodium retention and potassium depletion can also occur. Alter diet as necessary.

Herbs, Botanicals and Supplements

- Herbs and botanical supplements should not be used without discussing with physician.

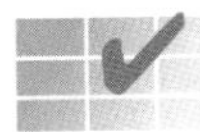

PATIENT EDUCATION

- Stress importance of consuming a balanced diet with adequate fluids.
- Help patient accept speech therapy or physical therapy, if needed.
- Discuss infection control measures in the environment, use of aspirin, etc.

FEVER

NUTRITIONAL ACUITY RANKING: LEVEL 2

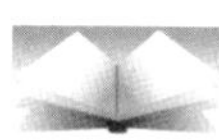

DEFINITIONS AND BACKGROUND

Fever represents disturbed thermoregulation, controlled by the hypothalamus. Fever higher than 102° (pyrexia) may be acute (with pneumonia, measles, flu, or chicken pox) or chronic (with tuberculosis, hepatitis, malaria, etc.).

Fever of unknown origin (FUO) involves illness of 3 weeks in duration with a fever higher than 100.4°; testing is needed. Results show that 40% of FUO is from infections; 20% from neoplasms, 15% from connective tissue disease, and 25% from undetermined causes.

Parenteral zinc supplementation significantly increases fever in patients with recent injury or infection, showing an exaggerated acute phase response (Braunschweig et al., 1997).

OBJECTIVES

- ▲ Meet increased nutrient needs caused by patient's hypermetabolic state, especially calorie needs. Each 1° of elevation causes 7% increase in basal metabolic rate (BMR). This equals 12% rise in basal energy expenditure (BEE) per 1°C fever above 37°C.
- ▲ Replace nitrogen losses and destroyed tissue.
- ▲ Replenish CHO; liver stores only last 24 hours.
- ▲ Normalize electrolyte status.
- ▲ Replace losses from perspiration and facilitate toxin elimination through increased urine output.
- ▲ Prevent water retention from SIADH and hypertonic dehydration.
- ▲ Treat anorexia, nausea, and vomiting when present.

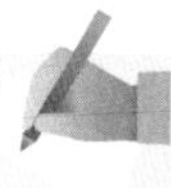

DIETARY AND NUTRITIONAL RECOMMENDATIONS

- Adults need 30–40 kcal/kg daily or an estimated 500–600 added kilocalories per 1° rise. Infants and children need additional kcals/kg as well; monitor weight changes closely.
- Adults need 1.5–2.5 g protein/kg if severe.
- Adults need adequate CHO to spare protein and restore glycogen in liver.
- Adults need 10–15 cups fluid per day. Salty broths, fruit juices, and milk can be used.
- If fever is acute, patient may need full liquids. As treatment progresses, a soft to general diet with small, frequent feedings can be used.
- With longer duration, thiamin and other nutrients should be added. Monitor need for vitamins A and C. Vitamin A supplementation may be helpful in conditions such as HIV infection and malaria in children (Villamor et al., 2002).

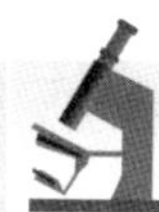

PROFILE

Clinical/History	Lab Work	
Height	N balance	Cl−
Weight	TLC, WBC	Alb, prealbumin
BMI	K+	RBP
Temperature	Carotenoids (decreased)	Specific gravity, urine (increased)
I & O	Na+	
BP		

Common Drugs Used and Potential Side Effects

- Penicillins should not be taken with acidic food or fluids such as fruit juice. Penicillin combines with serum albumins; adequate protein repletion is needed.
- Erythromycin should be taken with a full glass of water on an empty stomach. It may cause sore mouth, diarrhea, and nausea.
- Tetracycline should be taken on an empty stomach with a full glass of water. Do not give with milk or 2 hours before or after use of calcium-containing foods. Do not use for children because tetracycline can mottle teeth. Be careful with pregnant patients as well.
- Antipyretics/aspirin can cause GI distress. Take with food or milk. Avoid alcoholic beverages. Monitor use of aspirin in light of Reye's syndrome. Vitamin C depletion may occur.
- Other medications may require special instructions according to patient's problem.

Herbs, Botanicals and Supplements

- Herbs and botanical supplements should not be used without discussing with physician. Willow, elder, peppermint, meadow sweet, ginger, and red pepper have been suggested but are not yet proven through clinical trials.

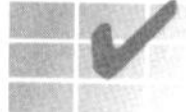

PATIENT EDUCATION

- ✔ "Feed a cold, feed a fever." Discuss how fever affects BMR.
- ✔ Stress importance of fluid intake.

FRACTURE, HIP

NUTRITIONAL ACUITY RANKING: LEVEL 2

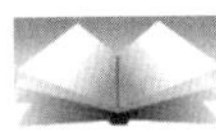

DEFINITIONS AND BACKGROUND

Broken bones result from a physical force greater than stress that cannot be withstood. "Broken hip" includes fractures of the femur head (intracapsular), femur neck (extracapsular), and greater Hesser trochanter. For some reason, those who sustain a wrist fracture are twice as likely to have hip fracture later in life.

Relative risk for hip fracture is related to many factors, such as low BMI, low milk intake, high alcohol intake, prevalent vertebral fracture, early age at menarche, and high number of children; prevention programs need to focus on reducing preventable risk factors (Fujiwara et al., 1997).

Associations between dairy product intake and hip fracture among a national sample of women aged 50 years and older have been studied; women who previously suffered hip fracture reported higher dairy use than women who had not experienced these fractures, a finding that is inconsistent with the literature (Turner et al., 1999). This behavior may reflect a change in intake of dairy products that occurs as a result of the fracture.

Pathologic fractures involve weakened bones breaking from old age, osteoporosis, and bone cancer. Incidence increases after 60 years of age, especially in women. Aggressive refeeding of malnourished patients is useful in decreasing morbidity and mortality, especially with hip fracture (Morley and Solomon, 1994).

Fatigue fractures occur from prolonged stress on normal bones. In surgical cases with open reduction with internal fixation (ORIF), adequate nutrition is necessary for wound healing and to reduce infectious processes. The most commonly broken bones are listed in Table 15–7; the hip is actually not the bone most frequently broken.

TABLE 15–7 Most Commonly Broken Bones

1. Forearm (ulna, radius)
2. Hands and feet (carpals, metacarpals, tarsals, and metatarsals)
3. Ribs
4. Fingers and thumbs (phalanges)
5. Shin bones (tibia, fibula)
6. Thigh bones (femur)
7. Skull
8. Upper arm (humerus)
9. Collarbone (clavicle)
10. Backbone (spinal bones or vertebrae)

OBJECTIVES

- Support formation of bone matrix. Complete union may take 4–8 months.
- Supply adequate nutrition for collagen formation and calcium deposition.
- Prevent side effects of long-term immobilization: renal calculi, pressure ulcers, urinary tract infections, embolus, contractures, or neurovascular dysfunction.
- Maintain optimal systemic functioning.
- Use fluoridated water supply. Hip fracture is not increased in areas where water is fluoridated (Phipps et al., 2000).

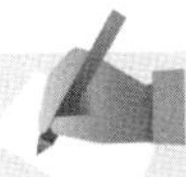

DIETARY AND NUTRITIONAL RECOMMENDATIONS

- Use a high-protein, high-calorie diet. Needs increase by 20–25%.
- Use adequate levels of calcium, phosphorus, vitamin D, and vitamin C. Encourage these nutrients to be taken in diet. Be careful of excessive vitamin D intake during immobilization.
- Ensure adequate fluid intake to excrete calcium excesses.
- Supply zinc for wound healing after surgical procedures. Watch for fever, pneumonia, and possible embolism.
- Although the main source of dietary calcium is dairy products, calcium contained in mineral water, which is as available as that of milk, could provide a valuable source of calcium.

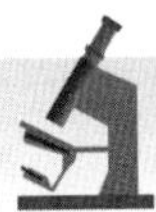

PROFILE

Clinical/History	Lab Work	
Height	Serum Ca++	Alb, prealbumin
Weight (may need chair scales)	Urinary Ca++	Gluc
BMI	BUN, Creat	WBC, TLC
I & O	H&H, Serum Fe	TIBC
BP	N balance	Alk phos (increased)

Common Drugs Used and Potential Side Effects

- Analgesics may be needed for pain. Monitor for GI distress or bleeding.
- Evaluate drugs prescribed and discuss side effects accordingly.

Herbs, Botanicals and Supplements

- Herbs and botanical supplements should not be used without discussing with physician.

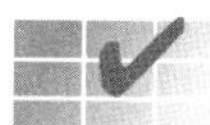

PATIENT EDUCATION

- ✔ Emphasize importance of nutrition for healing. Indicate which foods are good sources of protein in diet.
- ✔ Encourage activity and use of physical therapy after healing has progressed.
- ✔ Refer to appropriate agencies, such as Visiting Nurses Association (VNA) or Meals-on-Wheels, as needed.
- ✔ Smoking cigarettes hinders healing of bones by decreasing collagen production and oxygen availability.

FRACTURE, LONG-BONE

NUTRITIONAL ACUITY RANKING: LEVEL 2

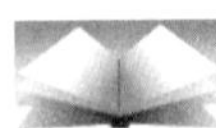

DEFINITIONS AND BACKGROUND

Along-bone fracture generally is an emergency and may be complicated by shock, wound infection, bleeding, or inadequate hydration. Traction is usually needed for internal immobilization. Simple fractures involve bones that do not protrude. A compound fracture does allow bone to protrude. With multiple fractures, BMR may increase by 20% or more for several weeks.

OBJECTIVES

- Meet calorie needs, usually increased by 20–25%.
- Provide adequate intake of all vitamins and minerals and nutrients needed to heal fracture appropriately.
- Keep nearby joints as active as possible.
- Prevent complications: pressure ulcers, renal calculi, and N & V from spinal anesthesia.

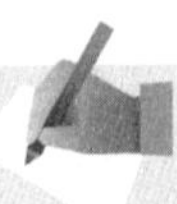

DIETARY AND NUTRITIONAL RECOMMENDATIONS

- High-protein/high-calorie intake will be needed.
- Progress from liquids to a soft diet as possible.
- Vitamin D, calcium, phosphorus, and vitamin C are especially important for bone formation.
- Zinc will help with wound healing, especially with surgery. Vitamin A is also essential.

Common Drugs Used and Potential Side Effects

- Analgesics are used for pain relief. Be careful about GI irritation or depletion of vitamin C and iron levels.
- Meperidine (Demerol) may cause vomiting, nausea, and constipation.

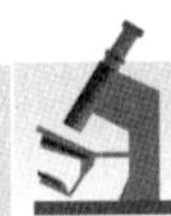

PROFILE

Clinical/History	Lab Work	
Height	Alb, prealbumin	N balance
Weight	BUN, Creat	Gluc
BMI	Pro Time (PT)	Ca++
Temperature	Phosphorus or Alk Phos (increased)	TLC
		WBC
		H&H, Serum Fe
		TIBC
		Urinary Ca++

Herbs, Botanicals and Supplements

- Herbs and botanical supplements should not be used without discussing with physician.

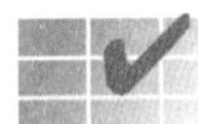

PATIENT EDUCATION

- Importance of balanced nutrition during healing should be emphasized.
- Key nutrients and their food sources should be highlighted.
- Discuss benefits of activity or physical therapy.
- Suggest smoking cessation classes for persons who smoke. Broken bones heal less quickly among smokers than nonsmokers.

HERPES SIMPLEX I AND II

NUTRITIONAL ACUITY RANKING: LEVEL 1

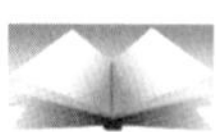

DEFINITIONS AND BACKGROUND

Herpes simplex involves a viral infection of skin or mucous membranes (herpes simplex I usually involves oral infections, herpes simplex II usually involves genital/anal infections) with vesicular eruptions of repeated frequency. Oral lesions commonly may be called "cold sores" or "fever blisters" because of their recurrence with periods of stress; they are latent in the nerve cell ganglia of the trigeminal nerve. Herpetic outbreaks are common in HIV-positive or other immunocompromised patients.

OBJECTIVES

- ▲ Reduce inflammation and duration.
- ▲ Lessen recurrences and virulence.
- ▲ Prevent spread via contact to other parts of body or to other persons.
- ▲ Reduce stress and febrile states.
- ▲ Prevent further complications such as encephalitis and aseptic meningitis.

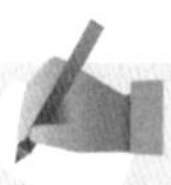

DIETARY AND NUTRITIONAL RECOMMENDATIONS

- High-quality protein and adequate calories will be essential.
- Studies have suggested that lysine may be important in lessening virulence, but research is not yet conclusive. An adequate diet contains approximately 5–8 g of lysine daily. Be aware that lysine supplementation can alter lysine:arginine ratio, which may cause elevated serum cholesterol levels.
- Increase intakes of vitamins A and C.

Common Drugs Used and Potential Side Effects

- Acyclovir (Zovirax) has been used with some success. There are some more recent antiviral agents (e.g. Valtrex) that are currently being tested as well. Nausea, vomiting, or headaches may be side effects of acyclovir.

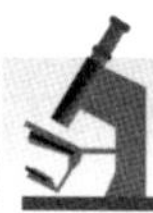

PROFILE

Clinical/History		Lab Work
Height Weight BMI Temperature Polymerase chain reaction (PCR)	test for herpes simplex virus (HSV) typing Swollen lymph nodes I & O	Alb, prealbumin Gluc H&H, Serum Fe WBC, TLC Chol, Trig CD4 and CD8 Na+, K+

- Aspirin or acetaminophen has been used for fever reduction.
- Some physicians use L-lysine monohydrochloride (1 g daily for 6 months). Monitor effects on serum cholesterol. There are no definitive results with this treatment.
- Interferon studies are being conducted in some research centers. GI distress, stomatitis, N & V, abdominal pain, or diarrhea may occur.

Herbs, Botanicals and Supplements

- Herbs and botanical supplements should not be used without discussing with physician. St John's wort, lemon balm, Echinacea, garlic, red pepper, tea, and mint have been suggested but are not yet proven through clinical trials.

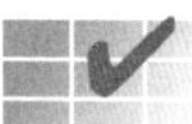

PATIENT EDUCATION

- ✔ A well-balanced diet with quality proteins should be discussed. Milk is a food that is naturally high in lysine.
- ✔ Discuss relationship of nutrition to immune status.
- ✔ Relaxation and stress reduction techniques should be highlighted.
- ✔ Immediate use of medication at signs of a breakout may be helpful to reduce severity.

HERPES ZOSTER (SHINGLES)

NUTRITIONAL ACUITY RANKING: LEVEL 1

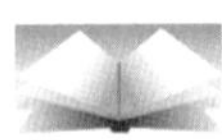

DEFINITIONS AND BACKGROUND

Herpes zoster is an acute viral infection with vesicles, usually confined to a specific nerve tract, and neuralgic pain in the area of the affected nerve. It is a reactivation of the varicella virus (chicken pox); severity correlates with age. Symptoms and signs include pain along the affected nerve tract, fever, malaise, anorexia, and enlarged lymph nodes. Bacterial infection of the lesions, poor nutritional status, and risk of dehydration may occur if rehabilitation requires a long period of time.

There is now a sensitive assay that detects simultaneous HSV-1, HSV-2, varicella-zoster virus (VZV), human cytomegalovirus (CMV), and EBV and is more comprehensive than previous assays (Markoulatos et al., 2001).

OBJECTIVES

- ▲ Prevent further systemic infection; reduce fever.
- ▲ Correct or prevent malnutrition, constipation, and encephalitis.
- ▲ Hydrate adequately.
- ▲ Prevent or correct unplanned weight loss.
- ▲ Prevent or reduce severity of postherpetic neuralgia, a very painful complication.

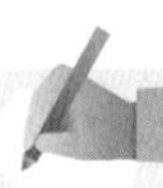

DIETARY AND NUTRITIONAL RECOMMENDATIONS

- A balanced diet with frequent, small feedings may be needed.
- Increased fiber may be useful to correct constipation.
- Facial nerves may be affected; alter diet as needed.
- Adequate vitamin E has been suggested for postherpetic neuralgia. Vitamin B12 has also been prescribed for recovery of the damaged nerve and for pain relief.
- Be sure vitamins A and C meet at least the RDA levels from dietary sources.

Common Drugs Used and Potential Side Effects

- Narcotics and analgesics may be needed to reduce pain.
- Researchers in Japan have tried injecting lidocaine and prednisone directly into spinal column for pain relief of postshingles neuralgia. A majority of patients indicated they had a positive response. Oral prednisone may be used in some cases; alter sodium intake and monitor for side effects such as glucose intolerance.
- Acyclovir is helpful if administered immediately. Newer medications may shorten duration and decrease pain; famciclovir is being studied. Monitor side effects such as GI distress, N & V, or diarrhea.
- In herpes zoster, valacyclovir is more effective than either placebo or acyclovir at facilitating cutaneous healing and healing of zoster-associated pain and postherpetic neuralgia (Baker, 2001).
- Capsaicin cream from hot peppers has proven to be useful for pain relief.
- Elavil and other antidepressants may relieve some of the neurologic overstimulation. Increased weight and appetite can result. Dry mouth and constipation are also side effects.

Herbs, Botanicals and Supplements

- Herbs and botanical supplements should not be used without discussing with physician. Lemon balm, Chinese angelica, red pepper, passionflower, and licorice have been suggested but are not yet proven through clinical trials.

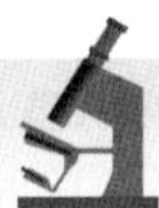

PROFILE

Clinical/History	Lab Work	
Height	Alb, prealbumin	H&H, Serum Fe
Weight	TLC, WBC	Gluc
BMI	Na+, K+	Vitamin B12
Temperature		Viral assay
I & O		

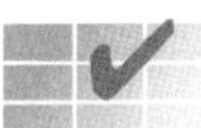

PATIENT EDUCATION

- ✔ Discuss need to increase fluid intake.
- ✔ A balanced diet will be essential in recovery. Include foods that contain vitamins E and B12.
- ✔ Infectious precautions should be discussed with patient and family. There is a link to chickenpox, and this condition may be passed to others during early stage.

INFECTION

NUTRITIONAL ACUITY RANKING: LEVEL 1–2

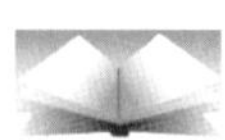

DEFINITIONS AND BACKGROUND

Infection results from successful invasion, establishment, and growth of microorganisms in a host. Responses involve general and antigen-specific immunologic defense systems. In infectious processes, vitamin A is excreted in large amounts from the urine as retinol (Stephensen et al., 1994).

Parenteral zinc supplementation significantly increased fever in patients with recent injury or infection, showing an exaggerated acute phase response (Braunschweig et al., 1997). It may be best to avoid zinc supplementation until the infection is under control.

Microbes depend on iron for growth and proliferation (Table 15–8). Iron is mostly protein-bound as transferrin.

OBJECTIVES

- ▲ Provide adequate nourishment to counteract patient's hypermetabolic state. Support body's host defense system.
- ▲ Prevent or correct dehydration, hypoglycemia, complications, and anorexia.
- ▲ Replace nutrient losses (potassium, nitrogen, magnesium, phosphorus, zinc, and sulfur).
- ▲ Correct iron-deficiency anemia, but do not overload.

TABLE 15–8 Virulence Increased by Iron

Fungi	Candida, Cryptococcus, Histoplasma, Mucor, Pneumocystis, Rhizopus
Protozoa	Entamoeba, Leishmania, Plasmodium, Toxoplasma, Trypanosoma
Acid-Fast and Gram-Positive Bacteria	Bacillus, Clostridium, Listeria, Mycobacterium, Staphylococcus, Streptococcus
Gram-Negative Bacteria	Campylobacter, Chlamydia, Escherichia, Klebsiella, Legionella, Proteus, Pseudomonas, Salmonella, Shigella, Vibrio, Yersinia

Based on data from: Robien M. Iron and microbial infection. *Support Line.* 2000;22:23.

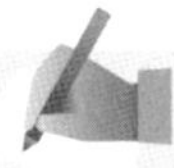

DIETARY AND NUTRITIONAL RECOMMENDATIONS

- ● Use a high-protein, high-calorie diet. Needs increase 0–20% in mild infections, 20–40% in moderate conditions, and 40–60% in sepsis.
- ▲ Increase patient's fluid intake.
- ▲ Enhance diet with vitamin A, folate, vitamin C, and B-complex food sources.
- ▲ Be careful with use of iron and zinc supplements, because these may serve as bacterial nutrients. It may be helpful to wait before providing these supplements, especially by intravenous administration, by intramuscular administration, or by TPN.

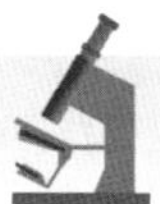

PROFILE

Clinical/History	Lab Work	
Height	Alb, prealbumin	Gluc
Weight	BUN, Creat	K+, Na+
BMI	H&H	Ceruloplasmin (decreased)
Temperature	Transferrin	Serum zinc
BP	Serum ferritin	AST (increased in acute stages)
I & O	N balance	
	TLC, WBC	

Common Drugs Used and Potential Side Effects

- Antibiotics. Administration of antibiotics with or without food is specific to the type of drug used. Avoid caffeine, sodas, and fruit juices when taking penicillins. For tetracycline, avoid milk and dairy products 2 hours before and after taking drug. With amoxicillin (Augmentin), diarrhea, nausea, and vomiting may occur.
- Griseofulvin for fungal infections should be taken with a high-fat meal. Dry mouth, nausea, and diarrhea are common effects.
- Cephalosporins (Ceclor, Cephalexin, Duricef) may cause diarrhea, N & V, and sore mouth. Hypokalemia and vitamin K deficiency may also occur.

- Gentamicin can deplete serum levels of potassium and magnesium.
- Ketoconazole (Nizoral) is used in some fungal infections and should be taken with an acidic liquid such as orange juice. Avoid taking within 2 hours of use of calcium or magnesium supplement.
- Metronidazole (Flagyl) may cause N & V, diarrhea, and anorexia. Avoid use of alcoholic beverages.

Herbs, Botanicals and Supplements

- Herbs and botanical supplements should not be used without discussing with physician.

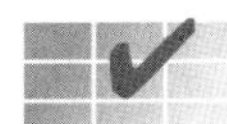

PATIENT EDUCATION

✓ Emphasize importance of eating to counteract infection and prevent new infections.

✓ Discuss role of vitamins A, C, and B6, niacin, and riboflavin in maintaining skin and mucous membrane integrity to prevent bacterial invasion and subsequent infections.

INFECTIOUS MONONUCLEOSIS

NUTRITIONAL ACUITY RANKING: LEVEL 1

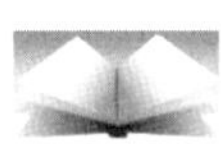

DEFINITIONS AND BACKGROUND

Infectious mononucleosis is an acute infectious disease that is believed to be caused by EB herpes virus and causes gland swellings in the neck and elsewhere (giving it its other name, "glandular fever"), with fatigue, malaise, headache, chills, and sometimes one or more other symptoms such as sore throat, fever, abdominal pain, jaundice, stiff neck, chest pain, breathing difficulty, cough, and hepatitis. Incubation is 5–15 days. It is most common between 10 and 35 years of age.

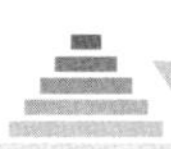

OBJECTIVES

- Restore fluid balance.
- Replenish glucose stores. Spare protein.
- Restore lost weight.
- Reduce fever. Prevent complications such as myocarditis, hepatitis, and encephalitis.

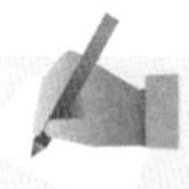

DIETARY AND NUTRITIONAL RECOMMENDATIONS

- Use a high-protein, high-calorie diet.
- Use liquids when swallowing solid foods is difficult.
- Use small, frequent feedings to improve overall nutritional quality and quantity.
- Ensure adequate intakes of vitamins A and C, especially from fruits and vegetables.

Common Drugs Used and Potential Side Effects

- Acyclovir (Zovirax) may be useful in initial infection, preventing typical persistence. Nausea, anorexia, and vomiting may occur.
- Other antibiotics may be needed for related infections.

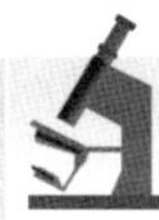

PROFILE

Clinical/History	Lab Work	
Height	H&H	CSF pressure (increased)
Weight	N balance	EBV titer
Weight changes	Alb, prealbumin	Serum agglutination test
BMI	Transferrin	UA (increased)
	WBC	AST, ALT (increased)
	TLC	Na+, K+

Herbs, Botanicals and Supplements

- Herbs and botanical supplements should not be used without discussing with physician.

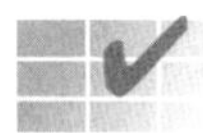

PATIENT EDUCATION

- Emphasize importance of exercise in restoring N balance.
- Instruct patient to modify food textures when swallowing is difficult.
- Discuss potential for relapse, which may be common. No specific medications are available at this time.
- Discuss frequent snacking to increase protein and calorie intakes.

INFLUENZA (FLU, RESPIRATORY)

NUTRITIONAL ACUITY RANKING: LEVEL 1

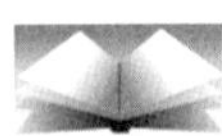

DEFINITIONS AND BACKGROUND

The influenza virus is transmitted by respiratory route, generally in the fall and winter months. Incubation is 1–4 days, with abrupt onset. Signs and symptoms include chills, fever for 3–5 days, malaise lasting 2–3 weeks, muscular aching, substernal soreness, nasal stuffiness, sore throat, some nausea, nonproductive cough, and headache.

Zinc lozenges reduce duration of symptoms of the common cold; whether this applies to influenza remains to be seen (Mossad et al., 1996). Low-dose supplementation of zinc and selenium provides significant improvement in elderly patients by increasing humoral response after vaccination and could have importance by reducing morbidity from respiratory tract infections (Girodon et al., 1999).

OBJECTIVES

- ▲ Reduce fever and relieve symptoms. Chicken soup is actually useful by providing potassium and sodium, as well as fluid; it increases mucus flow.
- ▲ Prevent complications such as Reye's syndrome, secondary bacterial infections (especially pneumonia), otitis media, and bronchitis.
- ▲ Promote bed rest, adequate hydration, and calorie intake.
- ▲ Replace fluid and electrolyte losses.

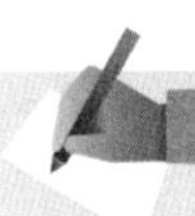

DIETARY AND NUTRITIONAL RECOMMENDATIONS

- Increase fluids (e.g., salty broths, juices).
- A high-calorie/high-protein intake should be encouraged. Small meals and snacks may be better tolerated than three large meals.
- Adequate sodium and potassium should be considered.
- Ensure adequate intakes of vitamins A and C, especially from fruits and vegetables. Citrus fruits and juices are recommended, if tolerated.

Common Drugs Used and Potential Side Effects

- Aspirin should not be used because of potential for Reye's syndrome in children. Other analgesics and pain relievers can be used. Vitamin C may be depleted.
- If bacterial infections complicate disorder, antibiotics may be needed. Monitor for proper timing of administration with food and beverages.
- Amantadine or rimantadine may be helpful, especially in type A flu. Nausea, dry mouth, and constipation may occur.
- Zinc gluconate lozenges are more useful than oral zinc because they coat the throat.
- Zinc (20 mg) and selenium (100 μg) may improve immune system response to flu vaccines.

Herbs, Botanicals and Supplements

- Herbs and botanical supplements should not be used without discussing with physician. Cardamom, horehound, mullein, ginger, mallows, and elecampane have been suggested but are not yet proven through clinical trials.

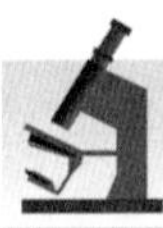

PROFILE

Clinical/History	Lab Work	
Height	H&H, Serum Fe	WBC (decreased)
Weight	Alb, prealbumin	TLC
BMI	Serum Zinc	Gluc
Weight changes		Na+, K+
I & O		Proteinuria
Temperature		

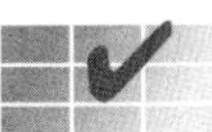

PATIENT EDUCATION

- ✔ Discuss need for rest and adequate hydration to promote rapid recovery.
- ✔ Discuss infection control, handwashing, and personal hygiene, if necessary.
- ✔ Annual vaccinations are suggested for high-risk populations, including elderly individuals or those with pulmonary diseases (asthma, COPD, etc.).
- ✔ Low humidity is often a problem, usually in cold weather.
- ✔ Psychological stress increases susceptibility.

MENINGITIS

NUTRITIONAL ACUITY RANKING: LEVEL 2

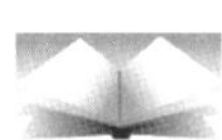

DEFINITIONS AND BACKGROUND

Infection of the meninges (meningitis) causes inflammatory reactions, usually in the pia mater or arachnoid membranes. The condition may be viral or bacterial. Bacterial forms are more likely to be fatal if left untreated. Bacterial forms include *Listeria monocytogenes, neisseria meningitides, or hemophiles influenzae, or streptococcus pneumonia.*

Meningitis can be caused by lung or ear infections or by a skull fracture. Symptoms and signs include headache, neck rigidity, fever, tachycardia, tachypnea, nausea and/or vomiting, disorientation, diplopia, altered consciousness, photophobia, petechial rash, irritability, malaise, seizure activity, and dehydration. It could lead to septic shock, respiratory failure, or death. It most commonly affects children aged 1 month–2 years of age.

OBJECTIVES

- ▲ Prevent or correct weight loss.
- ▲ Force fluids but do not overhydrate, especially if there is cerebral edema.
- ▲ Prevent or correct constipation, fever, and other symptoms.
- ▲ In the long term, control obesity, which may occur.

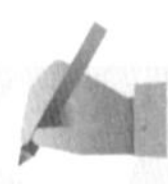

DIETARY AND NUTRITIONAL RECOMMENDATIONS

- Maintain intravenous feedings as appropriate; prevent overhydration.
- Progress diet, as possible, to high-calorie/high-protein intake.
- Unless contraindicated, provide 2–3 L of fluid.
- Adequate fiber will be beneficial to correct or prevent constipation.
- Gradually return to normal caloric intake for age.
- Ensure adequate intake of vitamins A and C from fruits, juices, and vegetables.

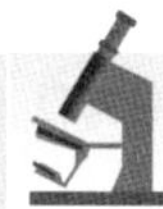

PROFILE

Clinical/History	Lab Work	
Height	Alb, RBP	H&H
Weight	Prealbumin	Na+, K+
BMI	WBC (increased)	Spinal tap; CSF (lumbar puncture)
BP	Gluc	
I & O		
Temperature		

Common Drugs Used and Potential Side Effects

- Antibiotics (penicillin, ampicillin, cephalosporin) may be used in bacterial forms or to prevent complications in viral forms. Nausea, vomiting, and diarrhea can result.
- Analgesics may be used for malaise. Vitamin C depletion may occur.
- Corticosteroids may be used; side effects may include nitrogen and calcium losses and sodium retention.

Herbs, Botanicals and Supplements

- Herbs and botanical supplements should not be used without discussing with physician.

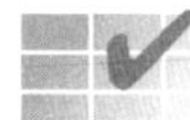

PATIENT EDUCATION

- ✔ Discuss methods to promote recovery and emphasize adequate rest.
- ✔ Discuss role of nutrition in immunologic status.
- ✔ Chronic meningitis can affect people with cancer, HIV/AIDS, and other severe disorders.

MULTIPLE ORGAN DYSFUNCTION SYNDROME

NUTRITIONAL ACUITY RANKING: LEVEL 4

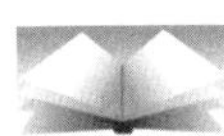

DEFINITIONS AND BACKGROUND

Multiple organ dysfunction syndrome (MODS) involves two or more systems in failure at the same time (e.g., renal, hepatic, cardiac, or respiratory). The condition always warrants hospitalization and almost always requires intensive care unit (ICU) support. Mucosal secretions rich in IgA, thick villi with tight junctions between cells, and GALT protect the gut as a barrier; many pathogens associated with MODS are endogenous to the gut (Shronts, 1996). Maintaining a healthy gut is essential for prevention and correction of MODS.

Parenteral zinc supplementation significantly increases fever in patients with recent injury or infection, showing an exaggerated acute phase response (Braunschweig et al., 1997). Avoid excesses until infections are under control.

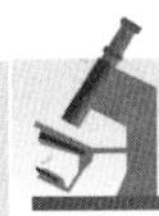

PROFILE

Clinical/History		
Height	Na+, K+	PO4
Weight	Cl−	Serum folate
BMI	Mg++, Ca++	Serum zinc
Dry weight	Phosphorus	Alanine, lactate, pyruvate (levels are higher at time of death than glucose levels, perhaps signifying accumulation or retention)
Edema, ascites	Gluc, acetone	
Temperature	ALT, AST	
I & O	Serum insulin	
	pCO2, pO2	
Lab Work	Chol, Trig	
Alb, prealbumin	Glomerular filtration rate (GFR)	
RBP	TLC, WBC	
BUN, Creat	H&H, serum Fe	
	TIBC	

OBJECTIVES

- ▲ Stabilize electrolyte and hemodynamic balances. Remove/control sources of dysfunction.
- ▲ Promote prompt and immediate responses to all changing parameters.
- ▲ Consider implications and short-term as well as long-term consequences of all actions (e.g., treatments must incorporate a consensus of opinions about which therapy precedes another).
- ▲ Promote recovery and well-being.
- ▲ Prevent further complications and sepsis.
- ▲ Promote wound healing if surgery is required.
- ▲ Provide nutritional support in appropriate mode(s); progress from parenteral to enteral or oral as rapidly as possible to preserve gut and promote immune system integrity. Support organs with appropriate substrate.
- ▲ Document all findings and recommendations immediately to allow appropriate actions to be initiated.

DIETARY AND NUTRITIONAL RECOMMENDATIONS

- Often, parenteral therapy may be required until GI dysfunction resolves. Monitoring of weight, laboratory parameters, and adequacy of nutrient intake is important.
- When patient is weaned to enteral nutrition (EN), ensure feeding is appropriate. Evaluate organ function and provide a correctly calculated feeding for patient's diagnosis and condition. (e.g., a patient with hepatic and renal failure will require a carefully chosen feeding product.) Consider using a glutamine-enriched product to preserve gut integrity and help restore normal function.
- Patients requiring ventilator support may need a higher lipid content in their feeding, even with cardiac failure.
- Progress, when possible, to oral intake. Wean gradually from both PN and EN to an appropriate oral diet, considering all disorders and parameters.
- Review current vitamin and mineral intakes; adjust according to changing needs. Antioxidants may play a role in supporting recovery. Do not use excesses of iron, zinc, PUFAs, and linoleic acid—especially parenterally—for their effects on the immune system. When possible, feed orally to acquire benefits of phytochemicals in whole foods.

Common Drugs Used and Potential Side Effects

- All medications should be reviewed for potential drug–nutrient incompatibility and stability with formulas. Try to avoid inclusion of medications with EN products because of drug–nutrient interactions, and because drugs may then be less available to patient.

- Review, as well, all vitamin and mineral supplements and enteral products to determine whether potential of hypervitaminosis and mineral toxicities exists. Discuss with physician when relevant.
- Insulin may be required because of the hyperglycemia that occurs with stress.

Herbs, Botanicals and Supplements

- Herbs and botanical supplements should not be used without discussing with physician.

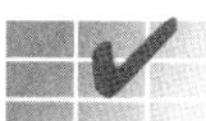

PATIENT EDUCATION

- ✔ When possible, discuss implications of organ system dysfunction in relation to nutritional support. Include a realistic assessment of potential for recovery and use of EN in the home setting, as discussed with physician.
- ✔ Family should be included in discussions about nutritional support measures that are taken.
- ✔ As appropriate, prepare patient for home nutritional needs and TPN/EN/oral intake as planned.
- ✔ Alleviate fears associated with eating or nutritional support therapies.
- ✔ Discuss any signs or problems that should require professional intervention.

PELVIC INFLAMMATORY DISEASE

NUTRITIONAL ACUITY RANKING: LEVEL 1

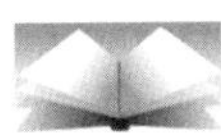

DEFINITIONS AND BACKGROUND

Pelvic inflammatory disease (PID) involves inflammation of the pelvic cavity, which may affect the fallopian tubes (salpingitis) and ovaries (oophoritis). Symptoms and signs include acute pelvic and abdominal pain, low back pain, fever, purulent vaginal discharge, N & V, UTI, diarrhea, maceration of the vulva, and leukocytosis.

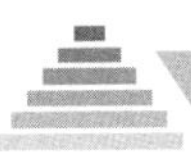

OBJECTIVES

- Promote good nutritional status to maintain weight and immunity.
- Increase hydration as tolerated.
- Lessen diarrhea, nausea, and vomiting.

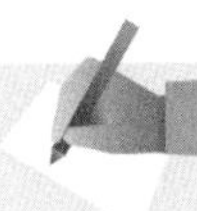

DIETARY AND NUTRITIONAL RECOMMENDATIONS

- Provide diet as tolerated with small, frequent feedings until N & V subside.
- Alter fiber and fluid, as needed, for patient's status.
- Increase calories and protein if needed to improve patient's nutritional status.
- Ensure adequate intake of all vitamins and minerals, especially vitamins A and C. Use more fruits and vegetables when possible.

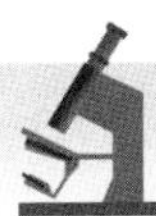

PROFILE

Clinical/History

Height
Weight
BMI
N & V
Diarrhea
Temperature
I & O

Lab Work

Alb, prealbumin
Gluc
Na+, K+
H&H, Serum Fe
TLC
WBC

Common Drugs Used and Potential Side Effects

- Antibiotics may be used. Monitor specific effects.
- Analgesics are generally used to reduce pain. Chronic use may cause GI distress and other side effects.

Herbs, Botanicals and Supplements

- Herbs and botanical supplements should not be used without discussing with physician.

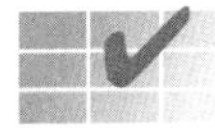

PATIENT EDUCATION

- ✓ Discuss role of nutrition in immunity.
- ✓ If N & V are extensive, discuss need for small meals and omission of fluids at mealtime. Have patient consume beverages 30 minutes before or at least 1 hour after meals.

POLIOMYELITIS

NUTRITIONAL ACUITY RANKING: LEVEL 1

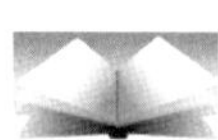

DEFINITIONS AND BACKGROUND

A highly contagious enterovirus, poliomyelitis attacks the motor neurons of the brain stem and spinal cord; it may or may not cause paralysis ("infantile paralysis"). Polio is transmitted by personal contact, by eating contaminated food, or by drinking contaminated fluids. Polio is rare in areas where the vaccine is available, but there are risks in areas where the vaccine is not administered to all members of the population. Extra immunization may be needed for persons traveling to tropical areas.

Symptoms and signs include headache, sore throat, fever, and neck and back pain. For breathing problems, a ventilator may be needed. Postpolio syndrome produces neuromuscular symptoms 25–30 years after attack; serious swallowing difficulties can ensue.

OBJECTIVES

- ▲ Beware of possible choking or aspiration in the bulbar type of paralysis—patient may be unable to swallow.
- ▲ Provide adequate nourishment.
- ▲ Prevent complications of prolonged immobilization—renal stones, pressure ulcers, and negative N balance.
- ▲ Correct electrolyte imbalance.

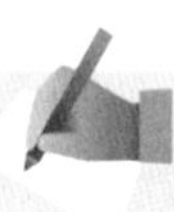

DIETARY AND NUTRITIONAL RECOMMENDATIONS

- For patient with acute paralysis, use a high-protein, high-calorie diet in liquid form. Use intravenous feeding and TF when needed.
- Use vitamin supplements 1–2 times the RDA. Extra calcium and potassium may be needed to replace losses.
- As treatment progresses, diet may be changed from a liquid to a soft, bland diet. A dysphagia diet may be useful with varying levels of thickened liquids to enhance swallowing.
- Reduce TF as oral intake increases.
- Frequent high-nutrient-density snacks are recommended.

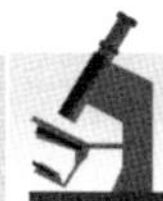

PROFILE

Clinical/History	Lab Work	
Height	H&H, Serum Fe	Na+, K+
Weight	Transferrin	Ca++
BMI	N balance	WBC, TLC
Temperature	Alb, prealbumin	Phosphorus
I & O		Ultrasound
		Video fluoroscopy

Common Drugs Used and Potential Side Effects

- Polio has no cure and antiviral drugs do not currently work.

Herbs, Botanicals and Supplements

- Herbs and botanical supplements should not be used without discussing with physician.

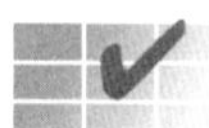

PATIENT EDUCATION

- ✓ Instruct patient regarding how to puree or blenderize foods as needed, how to add thickeners to liquids, etc.
- ✓ Discuss appropriate recipes for high-calorie/high-protein foods.

RHEUMATIC FEVER AND RHEUMATIC HEART DISEASE

NUTRITIONAL ACUITY RANKING: LEVEL 1

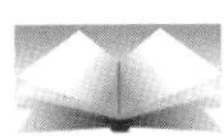

DEFINITIONS AND BACKGROUND

Rheumatic fever is an inflammatory condition affecting the connective tissues that causes joint pain, swelling, fever, rash, jerky movements (Sydenham's chorea) and facial grimacing, and carditis. It usually ensues 3 weeks after streptococcal infection. Children and adults younger than 30 years of age are more susceptible; it is rare before age 4 and after age 18. Hepatic dysfunction with clinically detectable carditis may occur, with decreased cholesterol and albumin metabolism (Panamonta et al., 1993).

Heart inflammation usually disappears but may cause permanent damage to the valves (especially the mitral valve) with a resulting heart murmur. Long-term effects are called rheumatic heart disease.

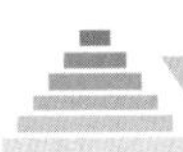

OBJECTIVES

- Cure streptococcal infection and prevent its recurrence.
- Reduce inflammation in joints and heart.
- Decrease physical activity and encourage rest while heart is inflamed.
- Recover lost weight.
- Reduce fluid retention, if present.
- Prevent complications such as bacterial endocarditis, atrial fibrillation, and heart failure.

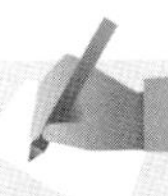

DIETARY AND NUTRITIONAL RECOMMENDATIONS

- Use a full liquid diet for acute rheumatic fever.
- As treatment progresses, gradually change diet, first to a soft diet, then to a regular diet.
- Restrict sodium intake if edema is present or if steroids are used.
- Increase intake of vitamin C, protein, and calories. Include adequate vitamin A as well.

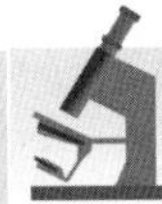

PROFILE

Clinical/History

Height
Weight
BMI
Temperature
Edema

Lab Work

Serum antibodies to streptococci
Alb, prealbumin (decreased)
RBP
WBC (increased)
Erythrocyte sedimentation rate (ESR) (increased)
TLC
Gluc
H&H, Serum Fe
TIBC
Chol (decreased)
Na+, K+
Mg++
Ca++
EKG for heart rhythm problems
Echocardiogram for heart valve problems

Common Drugs Used and Potential Side Effects

- Antibiotics are used. Monitor for specific side effects such as GI distress. Penicillin may be needed for 10 days.
- Restrict sodium if prednisone or adrenocorticotropic hormone (ACTH) is given for severe heart inflammation. Side effects include depletion of nitrogen, calcium, potassium, and hyperglycemia.
- Aspirin and non-steroidal anti-inflammatory drugs (NSAIDs) in high doses are often needed to reduce joint pain and inflammation.

Herbs, Botanicals and Supplements

- Herbs and botanical supplements should not be used without discussing with physician.

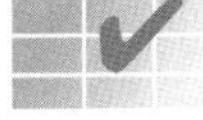

PATIENT EDUCATION

- ✔ Explain increased need for calories and protein.
- ✔ Adequate rest, exercise, and nutrition are essential.
- ✔ Discuss potential for recurrence.
- ✔ Life-long use of antibiotics before surgery and dental work is recommended to protect against bacterial invasion of cardiac tissue.

SEPSIS, SEPTICEMIA

NUTRITIONAL ACUITY RANKING: LEVEL 4

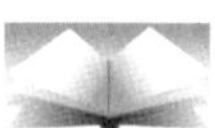

DEFINITIONS AND BACKGROUND

Sepsis involves a systemic inflammatory response (SIRS) with infection that has spread to other areas. Called septicemia when involving the bloodstream, this usually occurs from gram-negative or gram-positive bacteria (bacteremia). *Yersinia enterocolitis* can cause bacteremia, abdominal abscess, especially in states of iron overloading.

Predictors of bacteremia in elderly individuals include bladder catheter removal, fever, rigors, shock, and low TLC (Pfitzenmeyer et al., 1995). Sepsis may be a complication of vascular access devices or intravenous catheters and may be bacterial or fungal in origin. EN is associated with less sepsis than PN. Symptoms and signs of sepsis include fever, elevated WBC, pus, catabolism of LBM, and decreased glucose tolerance.

With sepsis, activated phagocytes release leukocytic endogenous mediators (LEM); hepatic uptake of amino acids occurs; increased prostaglandin synthesis occurs. Cytokines (TNF, interleukins-1 and -6) regulate hepatic protein responses, with nitrogen turnover and loss from skeletal muscle, connective tissue, and gut (Moldawer, 1996).

Metabolic responses in sepsis include increases in ACTH, aldosterone, and catecholamines (with increased gluconeogenesis, glycolysis, proteolysis, and lipolysis). Decreased T3 may reflect increased tissue levels that occur with tissue degradation and increased mobilized triglycerides.

Albumin, prealbumin, and transferrin have a transport role in the body; acute-phase proteins (C-reactive protein, α-acid glycoprotein, α-trypsin) help with host defense (Kudsk et al., 1994). These parameters go down in sepsis independent of nutritional status. Monitor all proteins in septic patients. BCAAs are useful for energy without the need to be metabolized to glucose.

Glucose turnover and amino acid catabolism are accelerated during sepsis; however, with the exception of alanine, increased amino acid catabolism is not coupled to increased glucose metabolism (Gore et al., 1995).

Parenteral zinc supplementation significantly increased fever in patients with recent injury or infection, showing an exaggerated acute phase response (Braunschweig et al., 1997).

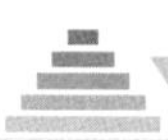

OBJECTIVES

- ▲ Treat infection or drain a local site, as possible. Support body's antimicrobial defense system. Keep environment as germ-free as possible.
- ▲ Prevent septic shock (increased cardiac output, tachycardia, low blood pressure, decreased renal output, warm flushed skin). Prevent MODS with pulmonary edema, liver failure or encephalopathy, renal failure, and other problems.
- ▲ Treat nausea, vomiting, and anorexia.
- ▲ Prevent or treat metabolic derangements during TPN, e.g., hyperglycemia, glycosuria, hyperosmolar/nonketotic coma, electrolyte abnormalities (decreased potassium, decreased phosphate, elevated chloride). If TF is used, monitor for side effects such as osmotic diarrhea.
- ▲ Prevent or correct fluid overload.
- ▲ Meet calorie needs (mild infection elevates resting energy expenditure [REE] by 15–40%; sepsis increases REE by 40–70% and doubles nitrogen losses).
- ▲ Promote tissue repair and wound healing. Protein turnover is 30–50% higher than normal (Moldawer, 1996).
- ▲ Manage blood glucose abnormalities.
- ▲ Do not overfeed.

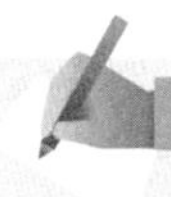

DIETARY AND NUTRITIONAL RECOMMENDATIONS

- Protein should be provided in levels of 1.5–2.0 g/kg daily (Kudsk et al., 1994). Enhanced use of BCAAs and a higher percentage of arginine, lower percentage of taurine/methionine/cysteine and lower percentage of aromatic amino acids (AAs) (phenylalanine, tyrosine, threonine).
- Provide calories at 30–35 kcal/kg (approximately 350–450 g CHO daily average, and 20% kcal as fat).
- When patient can eat, soft diet or liquids of high caloric value and nutrient density may be beneficial.
- Vitamins A and C, thiamine, vitamins D and K, and folic acid may become depleted with infection. Supplement or include in dietary intake. Urinary excretion of phosphorus, potassium, magnesium, zinc, and chromium also occur; monitor signs of malnutrition.
- Monitor fluid intake and requirements carefully. There must be adequate levels to excrete wastes properly.

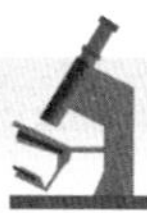

PROFILE

Clinical/History

Height
Weight
BMI
I & O
BP
Tachycardia
Temperature

Lab Work

Chol (decreased)
pO2, pCO2
WBC, TLC
Transferrin
Trig (increased)
AST (increased)
BUN, Creat
Urinary urea nitrogen (UUN)
Alb, prealbumin
RBP
Na+, K+
Cl−
Glucagon (increased)
Ca++, Mg++
H&H, serum Fe
N balance
T3 (decreased)
5-Hydroxyindole-acetic acid (5-HIAA) (increased)
Gluc (altered)
Phosphate (decreased)
Ketones
Osmolality
Glucagon: insulin ratio
Plasma lactate

Common Drugs Used and Potential Side Effects

- Antibiotics generally are used; monitor for potential side effects and GI distress.
- Steroids may be used, causing greater nitrogen depletion and hyperglycemia, sodium retention, and potassium losses. Monitor carefully.
- Insulin may be needed. Monitor for signs of hyper- and hypoglycemia.
- Iron and zinc are bacterial nutrients and should not be used automatically in TPN or PN solutions if patient is septic or at risk for sepsis.

Herbs, Botanicals and Supplements

- Herbs and botanical supplements should not be used without discussing with physician.

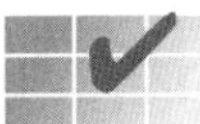

PATIENT EDUCATION

✔ Aseptic techniques will be essential.
✔ Need for a well-managed convalescence and gradual refeeding process will be needed to support patient's resistance and immunity.
✔ Reverse cycle of infection and malnutrition and reinfection with further PCM.

TOXIC SHOCK SYNDROME

NUTRITIONAL ACUITY RANKING: LEVEL 1

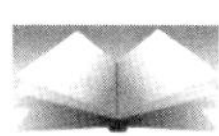

DEFINITIONS AND BACKGROUND

Toxic shock syndrome (TSS) is an acute bacterial infection caused by *Staphylococcus aureus* and most often is associated with continual use of tampons during menses. Symptoms and signs include sudden onset of high fever, severe headache, red eyes, myalgia, vomiting, watery diarrhea, red rash on palms and soles (with desquamation), decreased circulation to fingers and toes, disorientation, peripheral edema, pulmonary edema, respiratory distress syndrome, and sudden hypotension progressing to shock. Anemia, kidney, liver, and muscle damage can occur.

OBJECTIVES

- Treat patient for septic shock or respiratory distress or for other complications.
- Control diarrhea and vomiting.
- Improve well-being.
- Stabilize hydration and electrolyte balance.
- Prevent heart and lung problems and other complications.

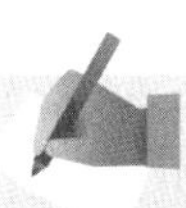

DIETARY AND NUTRITIONAL RECOMMENDATIONS

- Progress, as tolerated, from clear liquids to diet as usual. Small, frequent feedings are best tolerated.
- Increase fluids to 3 L daily, unless contraindicated.
- Ensure adequate intakes of vitamins A and C from dietary sources, including fruits, juices, and vegetables.

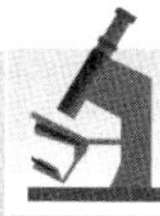

PROFILE

Clinical/History	Lab Work	
Height	WBC (increased)	Platelets (decreased)
Weight	BUN, Creat (increased)	Alb, pre-albumin
BMI	Bilirubin (increased)	CPK (increased)
Temperature	pO2, pCO2	H&H
BP	AST, ALT (increased)	Serum Fe
		Na+, K+, Cl−
		Gluc

Common Drugs Used and Potential Side Effects

- Antibiotics are required. Monitor for GI side effects. Determine how to administer specific drugs (e.g., with food, water, milk, etc.).

Herbs, Botanicals and Supplements

- Herbs and botanical supplements should not be used without discussing with physician.

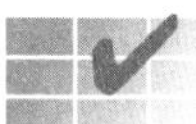

PATIENT EDUCATION

- ✓ Discuss with patient ways to decrease likelihood of reinfection such as avoiding super-absorbent tampons.
- ✓ Discuss need for adequate fluid intake and small meals, especially with vomiting or nausea.

TRAUMA

NUTRITIONAL ACUITY RANKING: LEVEL 3

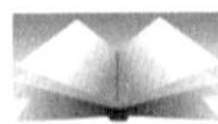

DEFINITIONS AND BACKGROUND

Trauma is caused by major injury or accidents (50% are related to traffic accidents). Trauma is related to 33% of all hospital admissions and is a leading cause of death for individuals aged 1–40 years.

Multiple traumas are complex, involving at least two injuries. Long-bone fractures, pelvis or vertebral fractures, and damage to body cavities (head, thorax, or abdomen) generally are involved. Elevated plasma catecholamines, glucocorticoids, glucagon, and glucose are noted in response to injury. The heart and brain are the organs most affected by shock.

Insulin has been shown to increase synthesis and decreased degradation of skeletal–muscle protein when amino acids are provided intravenously. The anabolic effect of insulin is not evident when nutrition is provided enterally to trauma patients; serum C-peptide and glucose levels are significantly lower after rather than before exogenous insulin is given (Clements, 1999).

Percutaneous enteroscopic gastrostomy (PEG) is a reliable form of enteral access with moderate to severe traumatic brain injury patients while intragastric feeding is well tolerated with low complication rates (Klodell et al., 2000).

Skeletal muscle is a major protein source for catabolism; BCAAs are metabolized here. Nitrogen excretion increases after injury, peaks after 7 days, and eventually stabilizes. BCAA-enriched formulas may be beneficial in trauma. The exact percentage of BCAAs is still being tested in clinical studies to identify if they make any difference in healing.

Glutamine is conditionally essential during critical stress (Gore and Jahoor, 1994). Treatment with GH has no effect on N balance in highly stressed, immobilized patients after trauma, but it does increase transferrin, albumin, and TLC levels (Behrman et al., 1995). Ascorbic acid must also be considered; plasma ascorbic acid levels tend to be 25% lower in trauma patients than in healthy persons (Schorah et al., 1996). Antioxidant defenses may be compromised in very ill individuals.

Overfeeding may be detrimental to patients with traumatic injuries, many of whom develop MODS. Patients receive the correct amount of feeding during a hospital stay less often than might be assumed (Klein and Wiles, 1997).

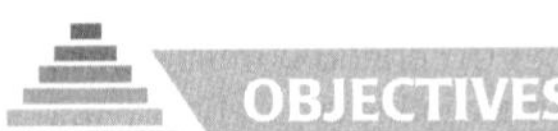

OBJECTIVES

- Assess and monitor extent of injury and resulting problems.
- Restore hemodynamic and metabolic functions, acid-base balance, and fluid balance.
- Meet elevated energy requirements (up by 20–45%). Spare proteins and LBM.
- Determine GI function; provide nutrients in most effective mode.
- Prevent complications, infection, respiratory failure, shock, and sepsis.
- For feeding, use gut first if possible. TF is a preferred route because it is safer and less expensive than parenteral route.
- Promote healing and rapid recovery.
- Treat ileus or fistula, if either occurs.
- Manage blood glucose abnormalities.
- Decrease nitrogen losses; promote N balance.
- Prevent overfeeding with respiratory distress from increased CO2 production.
- Determine and monitor fluid requirements and balance. Hydrate adequately, but do not overhydrate.
- Promote rehabilitation; correct anorexia and depression, which are common.

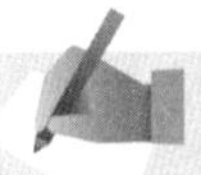

DIETARY AND NUTRITIONAL RECOMMENDATIONS

- Immediately—Intravenous feedings are given for fluid resuscitation for approximately 24 hours until stable. Life support measures and careful monitoring usually are provided.
- Days 2–5—Usually entail assessment of needs, with implementation of nutrition in most effective means (oral, enteral, or parenteral). Injury location and extent will dictate most desirable mode. Glutamine will help preserve gut integrity. Provide adequate kilocalories and nutrients until patient can eat. Begin feedings slowly and advance strength over several days; gastrostomy may be useful in head/neck trauma.
- Days 5–10—Often adaptive phase, with products like Trauma-Cal (50% BCAAs) and lipid emulsions being used when possible. Osmolarity should be monitored to be close to 300 mOsm. Predigested formula may be needed for GI injury.
- About 30–35 kcal/kg, 1.5–2 g protein/kg, and CHO given as 5 mg/kg/ minute should be calculated. The BEE often is two times normal. A diet providing 50% CHO, 15% protein, and 35% fat should be adequate.
- A slight increase in vitamin–mineral intake should be addressed, with B-complex, zinc, and vitamins A and C provided, in particular.
- In rehabilitative phase, patient can be weaned from PN to EN or oral diet and from ventilator support. Liquid to regular diets are usually tolerated at this time.

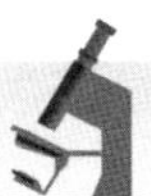

PROFILE

Clinical/History		
Height	H&H, Serum Fe	Alb, pre-albumin (fluid shifts can affect serum levels of albumin and transferrin; keep hydration status in mind when reviewing these parameters)
Weight pre-trauma	TLC	Transferrin
Weight post-trauma	WBC	RBP
Weight changes	Chol, Trig	N balance
BEE, indirect calorimetry	PO4, alk phos	
BMI	Serum hormones	
Temperature	BUN, Creat	
I & O	Gluc (increased)	
BP	Ca++, Mg++	
Lab Work	Bilirubin, AST (increased)	
Na+, K+	Serum amino acids	
Cl−	CPK (increased)	
	pCO2, pO2	

Common Drugs Used and Potential Side Effects

- Antibiotics generally are used to reduce bacterial infection. Monitor for GI distress and side effects.
- Insulin may be used for hyperglycemia. Monitor for meal and snack timing.
- Barbiturates are often used for closed head injury. They will decrease BMR.
- Analgesics, antacids, and other medications may have an effect on nutritional status. Evaluate individually.

Herbs, Botanicals and Supplements

- Herbs and botanical supplements should not be used without discussing with physician.

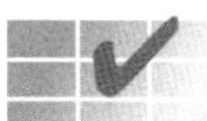

PATIENT EDUCATION

- ✓ Need for specific nutrients should be discussed.
- ✓ Rehabilitation should progress according to individual requirements and injury sites, side effects, and complications.

TRICHINOSIS

NUTRITIONAL ACUITY RANKING: LEVEL 2

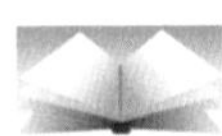

DEFINITIONS AND BACKGROUND

An acute infection caused by roundworm *Trichinella spiralis*, trichinosis is usually acquired by eating encysted larvae in raw or undercooked pork. Larvae mature and mate in the small intestine; larvae reaching striated muscle will encyst and live for years. Usual incubation is 5–15 days. The disorder has a 4% prevalence in the United States. Symptoms and signs include swelling of the upper eyelids, bleeding under the nails, skin rash, diarrhea, abdominal cramps, and malaise; later, low-grade fever, edema, sweating, dyspnea, cough, and muscle pain. In nonstriated muscle tissues such as the heart, brain, kidney, or lung, death can follow in 4–6 weeks, if untreated. Most symptoms disappear by the third month.

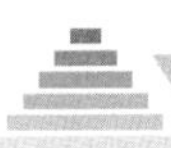

OBJECTIVES

- ▲ Correctly identify condition as rapidly as possible; treat as needed.
- ▲ Treat infections and diarrhea if severe.
- ▲ Prevent complications such as pneumonia and cardiac failure.

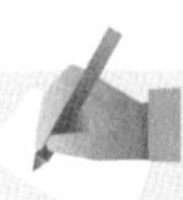

DIETARY AND NUTRITIONAL RECOMMENDATIONS

- Diet as usual can be provided. Encourage adequate intake of food sources of vitamins A and C, especially from fruits, juices, and vegetables.
- Ensure an adequate fluid intake, especially with diarrheal losses.
- Replace electrolytes with broths and juices.
- With poor appetite, offer small, frequent meals and snacks to correct any weight loss that is undesirable.

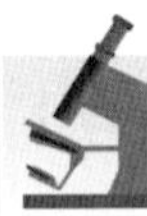

PROFILE

Clinical/History	Lab Work	
Height Weight Weight changes BMI Temperature I & O BP	Alb H&H, Serum Fe Gluc TLC, WBC Transferrin Na+, K+ Cl− Positive skin	and serologic tests for eosinophilia and leukocytosis Biopsy (bx) skeletal muscle after 4th week (for larvae or cysts)

Common Drugs Used and Potential Side Effects

- Mebendazole or thiabendazole may be used. GI distress is a common side effect.
- Aspirin or analgesics may be needed for muscular pain.
- Corticosteroids such as prednisone are often used temporarily to reduce inflammation of the heart or brain.

Herbs, Botanicals and Supplements

- Herbs and botanical supplements should not be used without discussing with physician. Chincona, elecampane, cubeb, golden seal, ipecac, and papaya have been suggested but are not yet proven through clinical trials.

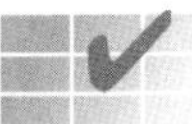

PATIENT EDUCATION

- ✔ Discuss proper handling and cooking methods for pork and other meats.
- ✔ Discuss use of thermometers, handwashing, etc.

TYPHOID FEVER

NUTRITIONAL ACUITY RANKING: LEVEL 2

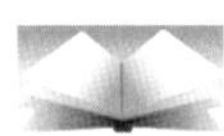

DEFINITIONS AND BACKGROUND

Typhoid fever is an infectious fever spread by contamination of food, water, or milk with *Salmonella typhi*, which can come from sewage, flies, or faulty personal hygiene. Most infections are found in people who are in contact with carriers who have persistent gallbladder or urinary tract infections. Incubation is 5–14 days. Symptoms include malaise, headache, cough, sore throat, "pea soup" diarrhea, constipation, rose spots, and splenomegaly. The problem practically has been eradicated in areas of proper sanitary practices.

OBJECTIVES

- ▲ Reduce fever and prevent irritation.
- ▲ Replace nutrient losses from diarrhea.
- ▲ Replace tissue losses.
- ▲ Prevent complications such as intestinal hemorrhage or shock.

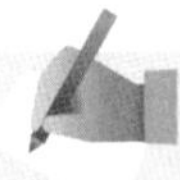

DIETARY AND NUTRITIONAL RECOMMENDATIONS

- For patients with acute fever, use a diet of high-protein, high-calorie liquids. A low-residue diet may be needed temporarily.
- As treatment progresses, gradually add soft, bland foods. Try small, frequent feedings. Gradually add pectin and other fiber.
- Include good dietary sources of vitamins A and C especially.

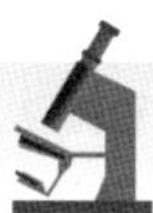

PROFILE

Clinical/History	Lab Work	
Height	Alb, prealbumin	Mg++
Weight	H&H, Serum Fe	Ca++
BMI	WBC, TLC	Stool and urine for Widal test
I & O	Gluc	
Temperature		

Common Drugs Used and Potential Side Effects

- Ampicillin should be taken 1–2 hours before or after meals. Nausea or vomiting may occur.
- Chloramphenicol may increase need for riboflavin and vitamins B6 and B12. Nausea, vomiting, or diarrhea may result.
- Achromycin (tetracycline HCl) may be used in cases of penicillin allergy. Avoid taking with milk and calcium products at mealtimes.

Herbs, Botanicals and Supplements

- Herbs and botanical supplements should not be used without discussing with physician.

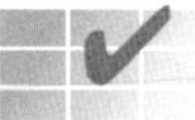

PATIENT EDUCATION

- ✔ Explain which foods are high-protein, high-calorie sources.
- ✔ Discuss control of future reinfection.

REFERENCES

Cited References

Ahlman B, et al. Intestinal amino acid content in critically ill patients. *J Parenter Enteral Nutri.* 1995;19:272.

American Dietetic Association. Position of The American Dietetic Association and Dietitians of Canada: nutrition intervention in the care of persons with human immunodeficiency virus infection. *J Am Diet Assoc.* 2000;100:708.

American Gastroenterological Association. Medical position statement: guidelines for the management of malnutrition and cachexia, chronic diarrhea, and hepatobiliary disease in patients with human immunodeficiency virus infection. *Gastroenterol.* 1996;111:1722.

Anderson J, ed. *A guide to the clinical care of women with HIV.* Rockville, MD: HIV/AIDS Bureau, U.S. Department of Health and Human Services; 2000.

Aptel I, et al. Association between calcium ingested from drinking water and femoral bone density in elderly women: evidence from the EPIDOS cohort. *J Bone Miner Res.* 1999;14:829.

Audera C, et al. Mega-dose vitamin C in treatment of the common cold: a randomized controlled trial. *Oncology.* 2001;175:359.

Baker D. Valacyclovir in the treatment of genital herpes and herpes zoster. *Expert Opin Pharmacother.* 2002;3:51.

Barbul A. Arginine and immune function. *Nutrition.* 1990;5:53.

Batterham M, et al. Measurement of body composition in people with HIV/AIDS: a comparison of bioelectrical impedance and skinfold anthropometry with dual-energy x-ray absorptiometry. *J Am Diet Assoc.* 1999;99:1109.

Behrman S, et al. The effect of growth hormone on nutritional markers in enterally fed immobilized patients. *J Parenter Enteral Nutri.* 1995;19:41.

Bowman T, et al. Vitamin A deficiency decreases natural killer cell activity and interferon production in rats. *J Nutri.* 1990;120:1264.

Braunschweig C, et al. Parenteral zinc supplementation in adult humans during the acute phase response increases the febrile response. *J Nutri.* 1997;127:70.

Burke D, et al. Glutamine supplemented total parenteral nutrition improves gut immune function. *Arch Surg.* 1989;124:1396.

Cameron A. Nutrition in HIV/AIDS. *Dietetic currents.* Vol. 21, no. 3. Columbus, OH: Ross Laboratories, 1994.

Centers for Disease Control: revised classification system for HIV infection and expanded surveillance case definition for AIDS among adolescents and adults. *MMWR.* 1992;41:1–19.

Chandra R. Food allergy and nutrition in early life: implications for later health. *Proc Nutr Soc.* 2000;59:273.

Chandra R, Sarchielli P. Nutritional status and immune response. *Clin Lab Med.* 1993;13:455.

Chlebowski R, et al. Dietary intake and counseling, weight maintenance, and the course of HIV infection. *J Am Diet Assoc.* 1995;95:428.

Clements R, et al. Insulin's anabolic effect is influenced by route of administration of nutrients. *Arch Surg.* 1999;134:274.

Craig C, et al. Decreased fat and nitrogen losses in patients with AIDS receiving medium-chain triglyceride-enriched formula vs those receiving long-chain triglyceride-containing formula. *J Am Diet Assoc.* 1997;97:605.

Cunningham-Rundles S, et al. Micronutrient and cytokine interaction in congenital pediatric HIV infection. *J Nutri.* 1996;126:2620S.

Cunningham-Rundles S. Nutrition and the mucosal immune system. *Curr Opin Gastroenterol.* 2001;17:171.

Federation of American Societies for Experimental Biology. *Nutrition and HIV infection: a review and evaluation of the extant knowledge between nutrition and HIV infection.* Bethesda, MD: Life Sciences Research Office, Federation of American Societies for Experimental Biology, 1990.

Fernandes G. Effect of calorie restriction and omega-3 fatty acids on autoimmunity and aging. *Nutr Rev.* 1995;53:S72.

Field C, et al. Nutrients and their role in host resistance to infection. *J Leukoc Biol.* 2002;71:16.

Fields-Gardner C, et al. *A clinician's guide to nutrition in HIV and AIDS.* The American Dietetic Association, 1997.

Flier J, Underhill L. Metabolic disturbances and wasting in the acquired immunodeficiency syndrome. *N Engl J Med.* 1992;327:329.

Fraker P, King L. A distinct role for apoptosis in the changes in lymphopoiesis and myelopoiesis created by deficiencies in zinc. *FASEB J.* 2001;15:2572.

Fujiwara S, et al. Risk factors for hip fracture in a Japanese cohort. *J Bone Miner Res.* 1997;12:998.

Garrel D, et al. Improved clinical status and length of care with low-fat nutrition support in burn patients. *J Parenter Enter Nutri.* 1995;19:482.

Girodon F, et al. Impact of trace elements and vitamin supplementation on immunity and infections in institutionalized elderly patients: a randomized controlled trial. *Arch Int Med.* 1999;159:748.

Gorbea-Robles M, et al. Nutrition assessment in pediatric patients infected with the human immunodeficiency virus. *Nutr Clin Practice.* 1998;13:172.

Gore D, et al. Except for alanine, muscle protein catabolism is not influenced by alterations in glucose metabolism during sepsis. *Arch Surg.* 1995;130:1171.

Gore D, Jahoor F. Glutamine kinetics in burn patients: comparison with hormonally induced stress in volunteers. *Arch Surg.* 1994;129:1318.

Gottschlich M, et al. Significance of obesity on nutritional, immunologic, hormonal, and clinical outcome parameters in burns. *J Am Diet Assoc.* 1993;93:1261.

Graham N, et al. Clinical factors associated with weight loss related to infection with human immunodeficiency virus type I in the multicenter AIDS cohort study. *Am J Epidemiol.* 1993;137:439.

Heller L, et al. Development of an instrument to assess nutritional risk factors for children infected with human immunodeficiency virus. *J Am Diet Assoc.* 2000;00:323.

Heller L. Nutrition support for children with HIV/AIDS. *J Am Diet Assoc.* 1997;97:473.

Henderson R, et al. Serum and plasma markers of nutritional status in children infected with the human immunodeficiency virus. *J Am Diet Assoc.* 1997;97:1377.

High K. Nutritional strategies to boost immunity and prevent infection in elderly individuals. *Clin Infect Dis.* 2001;33:1892.

Hurson M, et al. Metabolic effects of arginine in a healthy elderly population. *J Parenter Enter Nutri.* 1995;19:227.

Ireton-Jones C, Turner W. Actual of ideal body weight: which should be used to predict energy expenditure? *J Am Diet Assoc*. 1991; 91:193.

Kelly F. Vitamin E supplementation in the critically ill patient: too narrow a view? *Nutr Clin Pract*. 1994;9:141.

Klein C, Wiles C. Evaluation of nutrition care provided to patients with traumatic injuries at risk for multiple organ dysfunction syndrome. *J Am Diet Assoc*. 1997;97:1422.

Kleiin C, et al. Overfeeding macronutrients to critically ill adults: metabolic complications. *J Am Diet Assoc*. 1998;98:7.

Klodell C, et al. Routine intragastric feeding following traumatic brain injury is safe and well tolerated. *Am J Surg*. 2000;179:168.

Kowell-Vern A, et al. Ischemic necrotic bowel disease in thermal I jury. *Arch Surg*. 1997;132:440.

Kotler D, et al. Comparison of total parenteral nutrition and an oral, semi-elemental diet on body composition, physical function, and nutrition-related costs in patients with malabsorption due to acquired immunodeficiency syndrome. *J Parenter Enter Nutri*. 1998; 22:120.

Kramer T, et al. Lymphocyte responsiveness of children supplemented with vitamin A and zinc. *Am J Clin Nutri*. 1993;58:566.

Kruse L. Disease management: nutritional assessment and management for patients with HIV disease. *AIDS Reader*. 1998;8:121.

Kubena K. The role of magnesium in immunity. *J Nutr Immunol*. 1993; 2:107.

Kubena K, McMurray D. Nutrition and the immune system: a review of nutrient–nutrient interactions. *J Am Diet Assoc*. 1996;96:1156.

Kudsk K, et al. Visceral protein response to enteral versus parenteral nutrition and sepsis in patients with trauma. *Surgery*. 1994;116: 516.

Laurichesse H, et al. Threonine and methionine are limiting amino acids for protein synthesis in patients with AIDS. *J Nutri*. 1998; 128:1342.

Levander O, Buck R. Selenium. In: Shils M, Olson J, Shike M, eds. *Modern nutrition in health and disease*. 8th ed. Philadelphia: Lea & Febiger, 1994; 242–251.

Luder E, et al. Assessment of nutritional, clinical, and immunologic status of HIV-infected, inner-city patients with multiple risk factors. *J Am Diet Assoc*. 1995;95:655.

Macallan D, et al. Prospective analysis of patterns of weight change in stage IV human immunodeficiency virus infection. *Am J Clin Nutri*. 1993;58:417.

Markoulatos P, et al. Laboratory diagnosis of common herpesvirus infections of the central nervous system by a multiplex PCR assay. *J Clin Microbiol*. 2001;39:4426.

McClave S, Snider H. Use of indirect calorimetry in clinical nutrition. *Nutr Clin Pract*. 1992;7:207.

McDade T, et al. Prenatal undernutrition and postnatal growth are associated with adolescent thymic function. *J Nutri*. 2001;131: 1225.

Meydani S, et al. Vitamin E supplementation suppresses prostaglandin E2 synthesis and enhances the immune response in aged mice. *Mech Aging Dev*. 1984;34:191.

Moldawer L. Cytokines and the cachexia response to acute inflammation. *Support Line*. 1996;XVIII:1.

Moore F, et al. Clinical benefits of an immune-enhancing diet for early post-injury enteral feeding. *J Trauma*. 1994;37:607.

Morley J, Solomon D. Major issues in geriatrics over the last five years. *J Am Geriatr Soc*. 1994;42:218.

Mossad S, et al. Zinc gluconate lozenges for treating the common cold: a randomized, double-blind placebo-controlled study. *Ann Intern Med*. 1996;125:81.

Nduati R, et al. Effect of breastfeeding and formula feeding on transmission of HIV-1: a randomized clinical trial. *J Am Med Assoc*. 2000;283:1167.

O'Brien K, et al. Bone mineral content in girls perinatally infected with HIV. *Am J Clin Nutri*. 2001;73:821.

Odeleye O, Watson R. Potential role of vitamin E in the treatment of immunologic abnormalities during acquired immunodeficiency syndrome. *Am J Gastroenterol*. 1992;87:265.

Ogle C, et al. Effect of glutamine on phagocytosis and bacterial killing by normal and pediatric burn patient neutrophils. *J Parenter Enteral Nutri*. 1994;18:128.

Oldham K, et al. Oxidative stress in critical care: is antioxidant supplementation beneficial? *J Am Diet Assoc*. 1998;98:8.

Panamonta M, et al. Serum cholesterol levels in patients with acute rheumatic fever. *Am J Dis Child*. 1993;147:732.

Pfitzenmeyer P, et al. Predicting bacteremia in older patients. *J Am Geriatr Soc*. 1995;43:230.

Phipps K, et al. Community water fluoridation, bone mineral density, and fractures: prospective study of effects in older women. *BMJ*. 2000;321:860.

Porter C, Cohen N. Indirect calorimetry in critically ill patients: role of the clinical dietitian in interpreting results. *J Am Diet Assoc*. 1996;96:49.

Powell E, Tanz R. Comparison of childhood burns associated with use of microwave ovens and conventional stoves. *Pediatrics*. 1993; 91:344.

Prohaska J, Failla M. Copper and immunity. In: Klurfeld D, ed. *Human nutrition—a comprehensive treatise*. Vol. 8: Nutrition and immunology. New York: Plenum Press, 1993; 309–332.

Puri S, Chandra R. Nutrition and immunity. *Pediatr Clin North Am*. 1985;32:493.

Rabeneck L, et al. A randomized controlled trial evaluating nutrition counseling with or without oral supplementation in malnourished HIV-infected patients. *J Am Diet Assoc*. 1998;98:434.

Schorah C, et al. Total vitamin C, ascorbic acid, and dehydroascorbic acid concentrations in plasma of critically ill patients. *Am J Clin Nutri*. 1996;63:760.

Semba R, et al. Increased mortality associated with vitamin A deficiency during human immunodeficiency virus type I infection. *Arch Intern Med*. 1993;153:2149.

Shronts E. Basic concepts of immunology and its application to clinical nutrition. *Nutr Clin Pract*. 1993;8:177.

Shronts E. Enteral versus parenteral nutrition: a clinical review. *Support Line*. 1996;XVIII:10.

Stephensen C, et al. Vitamin A is excreted in the urine during acute infection. *Am J Clin Nutri*. 1994;60:388.

Tanaka H, et al. Reduction of resuscitation fluid volumes in severely burned patients using ascorbic acid administration: a randomized, prospective study. *Arch Surg*. 2000;135:326.

Tang A, et al. Dietary micronutrient intake and risk of progression to acquired immunodeficiency syndrome (AIDS) in human immunodeficiency virus type I (HIV-1)-infected homosexual men. *Am J Epidemiol*. 1993;138:937.

Turner L, et al. Dairy-product intake and hip fracture among older women: issues for health behavior. *Psychol Rep*. 1999;85:423.

Villamor E, et al. Vitamin A supplements ameliorate the adverse effect of HIV-1, malaria, and diarrheal infections on child growth. *Pediatrics*. 2002;109:E6.

Von Roenn J, et al. Megestrol acetate in patients with AIDS-related cachexia. *Ann Intern Med*. 1994;121:393.

Winter H. Gastrointestinal tract function and malnutrition in HIV-infected children. *J Nutri*. 1996;126:2620S.

Young J. HIV and medical nutrition therapy. *J Am Diet Assoc*. 1997;97:S161.

Suggested Readings

Chew B. Antioxidant vitamins affect food, animal immunity, and health. Conference: beyond deficiency: new views of ruminant nutrition and health. *J Nutri*. 1995;125:1804S.

Fenton M. Nutritional care in HIV infection and AIDS. In: Mahan K, Escott-Stump S, eds. *Krause's food, nutrition, and diet therapy*. 10th ed. Philadelphia: WB Saunders, 2000.

Grant J, et al. Analysis of dietary intake and selected nutrient concentrations in patients with chronic fatigue syndrome. *J Am Diet Assoc*. 1996;96:383.

Honkonen A, et al. Survey indicates need for dietitian's presence in an HIV clinic. *J Amer Diet Assoc*. 1997;97:A29.

Prelack K, et al. Urinary urea nitrogen is imprecise as a predictor of protein balance in burned children. *J Am Diet Assoc*. 1997;97:489.

Salomon S, et al. An elemental diet containing medium chain triglycerides and enzymatically hydrolyzed protein can improve gastrointestinal tolerance in people infected with HIV. *J Am Diet Assoc*. 1998;98:460.

Stack J, et al. High-energy, high-protein, oral, liquid nutrition supplementation in patients with HIV infection: effect on weight status in relation to incidence of secondary infection. *J Am Diet Assoc*. 1996;96:337.

Sun E, et al. The mechanism for the effect of selenium supplementation on immunity. *Biol Trac Elem Res*. 1995;48:231.

Suttman U, et al. Weight gain and increased concentrations of receptor proteins for tumor necrosis factor after patients with symptomatic HIV infection received fortified nutrition support. *J Am Diet Assoc*. 1996;96:565.

Tang A, et al. Low serum vitamin B12 concentrations are associated with faster human immunodeficiency virus type 1 (HIV-1) disease progression. *J Nutri*. 1997;127:345.

van Bokhorst-De van der Schuer M, et al. Differences in immune status between well-nourished and malnourished head and neck cancer patients. *Clin Nutri*. 1998;17:107.

Venkatraman J, et al. Influence of the level of dietary lipid intake and maximal exercise on the immune status in runners. *Med & Sci in Sports & Exercise*. 1997;29:333.

Winkler M, Manchester S. Nutritional care in metabolic stress. In: Mahan K, Escott-Stump S, eds. *Krause's food, nutrition, and diet therapy*. 10th ed. Philadelphia: WB Saunders, 2000.

SECTION 16

Renal Disorders

CHIEF ASSESSMENT FACTORS

- SEVEN WARNING SIGNS OF KIDNEY AND URINARY TRACT DISEASE: BURNING OR DIFFICULTY DURING URINATION, MORE FREQUENT URINATION, ESPECIALLY AT NIGHT, PASSAGE OF BLOODY-APPEARING URINE, PUFFINESS AROUND EYES, SWELLING OF HANDS AND FEET, ESPECIALLY IN CHILDREN, PAIN IN SMALL OF BACK JUST BELOW THE RIBS THAT IS NOT AGGRAVATED BY MOVEMENT, HIGH BLOOD PRESSURE
- PROTEINURIA (MICROALBUMINEMIA)
- UREMIA
- BONE PAIN, ALTERED HEIGHT OR LEAN BODY MASS
- UNBALANCED CALCIUM:PHOSPHORUS RATIOS
- ALTERED LIPID AND AMINO ACID LEVELS
- ABNORMAL BLOOD UREA NITROGEN (BUN):CREATININE RATIO
- PRESENCE OR HISTORY OF URINARY TRACT INFECTIONS
- FREQUENT WEIGHT SHIFTS
- LEG CRAMPS
- WEAKNESS, PALLOR, ANEMIA
- ITCHING AND DRY SKIN
- LOSS OF APPETITE
- DIFFICULTY SLEEPING
- SERUM CREATININE OVER 1.7 mg/dL FOR CHRONIC KIDNEY DISEASE
- PROTEIN-ENERGY MALNUTRITION OR WASTING

OVERVIEW OF RENAL NUTRITION

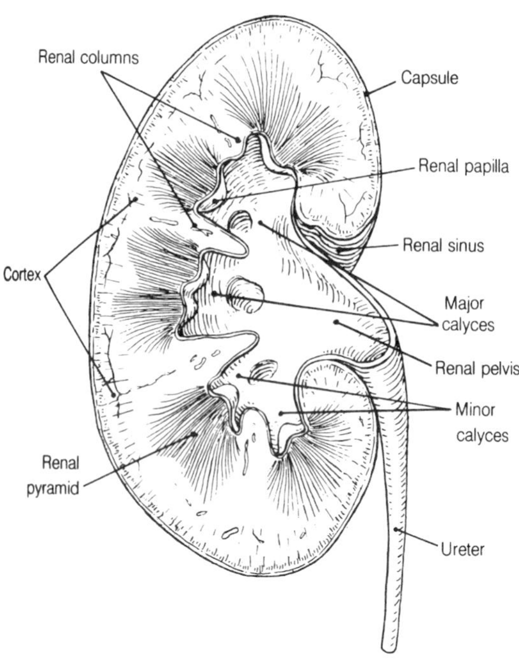

Figure 16–1 Anatomy of the Kidney. (Reprinted with permission from Hall-Craggs, ECB. *Anatomy as a Basis for Clinical Medicine.* 2nd Ed. Baltimore: Urban & Schwartzenberg, 1990.)

Subjective Global Assessment may be used for renal patients (National Kidney Foundation, 2000). Items used to assess nutritional status are weight change over the past 6 months, dietary intake and gastrointestinal (GI) symptoms, visual assessment of subcutaneous tissue, and muscle mass. Weight change is assessed by evaluating patient's weight during the past 6 months: loss of 10% of body weight over the past 6 months is severe, 5–10% is moderate, and less than 5% is mild; edema might obscure a greater amount of weight loss. Dietary intake is evaluated using a comparison of the patient's usual or recommended intakes to current intake. Duration and frequency of GI symptoms (e.g., nausea, vomiting, and diarrhea) are also assessed. The interviewer rates a 7-point scale with higher scores if patient has little or no weight loss, a better dietary intake, better appetite, and the absence of GI symptoms.

A registered dietitian with renal experience should be a central and integral part of the dietary management of both pediatric and adult patients (National Kidney Foundation, 2000). Registered dietitians are proficient in assessment and ongoing evaluation of patient's nutrition status and development of the nutrition plan of care and diet prescription.

All anthropometric indices (weight, height, and body mass index [BMI]), laboratory values, and dietary intakes deteriorate with worsening renal function in children with chronic renal insufficiency; disturbed nutritional intakes, bone biochemistry, and growth occurs early and suggest the need for collaboration between medical and dietetic intervention (Norman et al., 2000). Increased serum levels of inflammation may reduce nutrient intake and contribute to development of protein–energy malnutrition in dialysis patients (Mehrotra and Kopple, 2001).

Inflammation, with increased levels of specific cytokines (interleukin-6 and tumor necrosis factor alpha) and acute-phase proteins (C-reactive protein and serum amyloid A), has been found to be associated with vascular disease. The acute-phase response of inflammation causes loss of muscle mass and changes in plasma composition with decreases in serum albumin, prealbumin, and transferrin levels (Kaysen, 2001). Inflammation alters lipoprotein structure and function as well as endothelial structure and function to favor atherogenesis; it also increases atherogenic proteins in serum such as fibrinogen and lipoprotein. Because most dialysis patients have cardiovascular disease, a multifactorial approach is important.

In pediatrics, a registered dietitian skilled in the evaluation of growth as well as physical, developmental, educational, and social needs, will be needed. Assessing the child's nutritional status, developing the nutrition plan of care, providing education and counseling at the appropriate age level for patients, family, or caretakers, monitoring patient's nutritional status, evaluating adherence to nutrition prescription, assessing and monitoring adequacy of dialysis, and documentation of these services is all part of the job of the registered dietitian. Registered dietitians should manage the nutrition care and provide nutrition counseling for patients prior to starting dialysis and for those who have lost a kidney transplant and are returning to dialysis. http://www.kidney.org/professionals/doqi/guidelines/doqi_nut.html. Tables 16–1 to 16–3 give a brief background of the functionsof the kidneys and affects of renal activity.

TABLE 16–1 Human Kidney Functions

1. Waste removal
2. Erythropoietin secretion for red blood cell (RBC) production
3. Renin for blood pressure (BP) regulation
4. Vitamin D3 control for calcium (Ca):phosphorus (P) homeostasis
5. Control of potassium and phosphate
6. Acid-base balance (bicarbonate reabsorption and hydrogen ion secretion)
7. Carnitine synthesis to carry fatty acids from cytoplasm to mitochondria, for heart and skeletal muscle fuel. Note—lysine and methionine, vitamin C, iron, vitamin B6, and niacin are needed to produce carnitine.
8. Gluconeogenesis and glucose counterregulation (Gerich et al., 2001)

TABLE 16–2 Renal Hormonal Control

The kidney produces renin, which converts angiotensinogen to angiotensin I. Blood enzymes convert angiotensin I to angiotensin II, which then stimulates the adrenal gland to produce aldosterone. Increased sodium reabsorption results from aldosterone production. Blood pressure goes up as a result.

Antidiuretic hormone from the hypothalamus increases permeability of the distal and collecting tubules to increase water reabsorption.

The kidney accomplishes the final stage of conversion of vitamin D to its active form: 1,25-dihydroxy vitamin D, in the proximal tubule.

The kidney makes erythropoietin for RBC production. Erythropoietin deficiency is common in chronic renal anemia.

For More Information

- American Association of Kidney Patients
  http://www.aakp.org/
- American Foundation for Urologic Disease
  1128 N. Charles Street
  Baltimore, MD 21201
  1–800-242–2383
  http://www.afud.org
- American Kidney Fund
  6110 Executive Blvd., Suite 1010
  Rockville, MD 20852
  1–800-638–8299
  http://www.kidneyfund.org/

TABLE 16–3 Renal Notes

Body water = ⅔ extracellular water + ⅓ intracellular water

Renal functioning:	Decreased–glomerular filtration rate (GFR) decreases by 50%
	Insufficiency–GFR decreases by 75%
	Renal failure–GFR decreases by 85%
	End-stage renal diseases (ESRD) = GFR decreased by > 90%

BUN:creatinine ratio typically is 10:1 (creatinine doubles when renal function decreases by 50%)

Nitrogen (N) balance occurs via regulation of urea production rather than by urea hydrolysis (Young et al., 2000)

Chronic renal failure (GFR less than 20 mL/min)

Modification of protein and phosphorus intakes can slow progression of renal disease. Dietary phosphorus may be estimated using the formula (Boaz and Smetana, 1996): dietary phosphorus (mg) = 128 + 14 (protein intake in g).

- American Nephrology Nurses' Association
  http://anna.inurse.com/
- American Society of Pediatric Nephrology
  http://www.aspneph.com/
- European Dialysis and Transplant Association
  http://www.era-edta.org/
- Forum of End-Stage Renal Networks
  http://www.esrdnetworks.org/index.htm
- Health Sciences Library System—Kidney and Urologic Diseases
  http://www.hsls.pitt.edu/intres/internet_resources.html?page=16
- International Society of Nephrology
  http://www.isn-online.org/
- International Society for Peritoneal Dialysis
  http://www.ispd.org/
- Kidney Disease Outcomes Quality Initiative
  http://www.kidney.org/professionals/doqi/index.cfm
- Medicare Dialysis Sites
  http://www.medicare.gov/Health/Dialysis.asp
- National Kidney Foundation (NKF)
  30 East 33rd Street
  New York, NY 10016
  1–800-622–9010
  http://www.kidney.org/
  Cyber Nephrology: http://www.cybernephrology.org/
- NIH—National Kidney and Urologic Diseases Information Clearinghouse
  9000 Rockville Pike, Bldg. 31, Rm 8A52A
  Bethesda, MD 20852
  1–800-891–5390
  http://www.niddk.nih.gov
- Nephrology Calculator
  http://www.tinkershop.net/nephro.htm
- Nephrology News and Issues
  http://www.nephnews.com/
- Nephron Information Center
  http://www.nephron.com/
- Nephrology Links
  http://nephrologylinx.com/
- Nephro World
  http://www.nephroworld.com/
- Northwest Kidney Centers
  http://www.nwkidney.org/
- Renal Net—Kidney Information Clearinghouse
  http://www.renalnet.org/
- Renal Physicians Association
  http://www.renalmd.org/
- Renal World
  http://www.renalworld.com/
- U.S. Renal Data System
  http://www.usrds.org/
- World Kidney Fund
  http://www.worldkidneyfund.org/

INBORN ERRORS OF RENAL METABOLISM: VITAMIN-D-RESISTANT RICKETS, HARTNUP DISEASE

NUTRITIONAL ACUITY RANKING: LEVEL 3

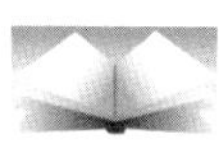

DEFINITIONS AND BACKGROUND

Vitamin D-resistant rickets is familial hypophosphatemia associated with decreased renal tubular reabsorption of phosphorous (P). Vitamin D is metabolized abnormally, and calcium absorption is decreased. Rickets or osteomalacia occurs. In poorly growing patients with X-linked hypophosphatemic rickets, growth hormone therapy combined with conventional treatment improves final height, phosphate retention, and radial bone mineral density (Baroncelli et al., 2001).

Hartnup disease is a rare familial condition characterized by hyperaminoaciduria. It results from the homozygous manifestation of a non-X-linked rare allele. The tryptophan-loading test is used to diagnose the disease. A red, scaly rash is seen on the face, neck, hands, and legs (symptoms resemble those of dietary pellagra). Emotional instability and delirium may exist in affected persons.

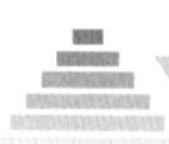

OBJECTIVES

- ▲ Correct malabsorption of vitamin D, calcium, and phosphorus in persons with **vitamin D-resistant rickets.**
- ▲ Correct behavioral side effects of persons with **Hartnup disease.** Ensure adequacy of protein.

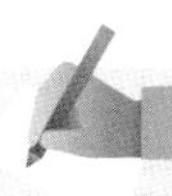

DIETARY AND NUTRITIONAL RECOMMENDATIONS

- **Vitamin D-resistant rickets.** Diet should include 4,800 international units (IU) of 1,25-dehydroxy-vitamin D3 plus oral phosphate in a quantity of 1.5–2 g phosphorus per day. Ensure diet provides adequate amounts of calcium. Be careful about mineral toxicities.
- **Hartnup disease.** Patient should be given oral nicotinamide therapy (40–200 mg/day) plus a high-protein diet or supplements. Oral neomycin should also be given.

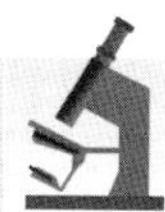

PROFILE

Clinical/History

Birth weight
Present weight
Length
Growth percentile
BMI
Blood pressure (BP)
Red, scaly rash
Rickets?

Lab Work

Blood urea nitrogen (BUN), creatine (creat)
Hemoglobin and hematocrit (H&H), Serum Fe
Cholesterol (chol), triglycerides (Trig)
Potassium (K+)
Glucose (gluc)
Ultrasound
Serum vitamin D
Albumin (Alb), prealbumin
Calcium (Ca++)
Phosphorus (P)
Tryptophan-loading test (Hartnup only)
Alkaline phosphatase (Alk phos)

Common Drugs Used and Potential Side Effects

- In vitamin D-resistant rickets, Ergocalciferol is a vitamin D analog that is used with phosphate supplements. After growth is completed, the drug is often reduced.
- Calcium replacements may be needed.
- Growth hormone therapy may be used; monitor for untoward side effects.

Herbs, Botanicals and Supplements

- Herbs and botanical supplements should not be used without discussing with physician.

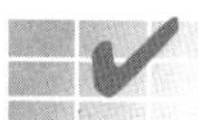

PATIENT EDUCATION

- ✓ Explain measures that are appropriate to specific condition.
- ✓ Encourage regular medical visits and nutritionist follow-up.

POLYCYSTIC KIDNEY DISEASE

NUTRITIONAL ACUITY RANKING: LEVEL 3

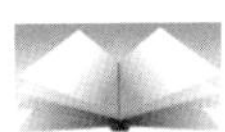

DEFINITIONS AND BACKGROUND

Polycystic kidney diseases (PKD) are disorders that causes multiple, fluid-filled, bilateral cysts in the kidneys and may also affect the liver, pancreas, colon, blood, and heart valves. Fluid-filled sacs or cysts of varying sizes that become larger as the disease progresses replace normal kidney tissue. PKD in its rare, autosomal dominant form affects 600,000 people in the United States at a rate of 1 in 400–1,000 persons; the autosomal recessive form occurs in 1 per 44,000 births; an acquired form occurs in patients on dialysis (http://www.cdc.gov/ncidod/EID/vol3no2/miller.htm) and often affects adults in midlife. Infants who are not treated may die before 1 month of age. The PKD1 gene accounts for 85% of autosomal dominant polycystic kidney disease (ADPKD), the most common human genetic disorder (Kleymenova et al., 2001). Children with autosomal recessive PKD experience high blood pressure, urinary tract infections, and frequent urination; their disease affects the liver, spleen, and pancreas, resulting in low blood-cell counts, varicose veins, and hemorrhoids. Because kidney function is crucial for early physical development, children with autosomal recessive PKD are usually smaller than average size.

PKD results from loss of function of either of two novel proteins, polycystin-1 or polycystin-2. Recent studies show that intracellular calcium signaling is important in kidney development, and defects in this signaling pathway are the basis of cyst formation in PKD (Somlo and Ehrlich, 2001).

Increased understanding of genetic and pathophysiologic mechanisms responsible for development of ADPKD, made possible by the advances of the last three decades, has laid the foundation for development of effective therapies (Qian et al., 2001). The concept that a polycystic kidney is a neoplasm in disguise is becoming increasingly accepted; therapies will benefit from information on cancer chemoprevention and chemosuppression.

Signs and symptoms include back or side pain, abnormally high blood pressure, progressive loss of kidney function, hematuria, vomiting, and chronic headaches. Most infants with autosomal recessive PKD also have unusual facial features (Potter's face) and failure to thrive. People with ADPKD can also experience urinary tract infections, liver and pancreatic cysts, abnormal heart valves, kidney stones, aneurysms in the brain, and diverticulosis. Proteinuria and microalbuminuria occur with a highly variable severity and are associated with progression of the autosomal form (Nakamura et al., 2001). Half of patients with PKD will require dialysis (http://www.niddk.nih.gov/health/kidney/pubs/polycyst/polycyst.htm). Laparoscopic surgery to remove the cysts may be beneficial for some patients. For others, transplantation is needed.

OBJECTIVES

- Prevent/treat chronic kidney disease.
- Minimize or alleviate nausea, vomiting, and anorexia.
- Bring hypertension under control where present.
- Correct or alleviate proteinuria or microalbuminemia.
- Manage dialysis when and if needed.
- Prepare for transplant, if planned.

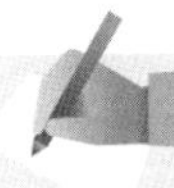

DIETARY AND NUTRITIONAL RECOMMENDATIONS

- Modify diet according to symptoms; sodium restriction may be beneficial for lowering blood pressure. Controlled protein intake (meeting recommended dietary allowance [RDA] for age) is recommended unless proteinuria is excessive, when lower levels are needed.
- Reduce or eliminate caffeine.

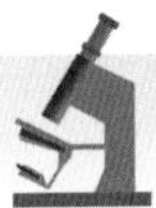

PROFILE

Clinical/History

Length or Height
Birth weight
Present weight
Growth percentile
BMI
Back or side pain
BP (very high)
Hematuria
Vomiting
Chronic headaches

Lab Work

BUN, Creat
H&H, Serum Fe, Percent Saturation
Serum ferritin
Mean cell volume (MCV)
Ultrasound
K+
Chol, Trig
Gluc
Serum vitamin D
Alb, pre-albumin
Proteinuria, micro-albuminemia
Ca++
Serum Phosphorus

Common Drugs Used and Potential Side Effects

- New drug therapy for PKD is an experimental drug called EKI-785.
- Angiotensin-converting enzyme (ACE) inhibitors are most frequently prescribed for hypertension; calcium channel blockers, diuretics, and beta-blockers may also be used. A common combined therapy is a diuretic plus an ACE inhibitor. Hypertensive ADPKD patients treated with diuretics may have a faster loss of renal function as compared with patients treated with ACE inhibitors, despite similar control (Ecder et al., 2001).
- Dilazep dihydrochloride, an antiplatelet drug, is effective in patients with immunoglobulin A nephropathy or diabetic nephropathy; it may be effective in reducing urinary albumin excretion in normotensive ADPKD patients with microalbuminuria (Nakamura et al., 2001).
- Antibiotics may be used to treat infections; monitor specific medicines for nutritional side effects.
- Analgesics may be useful for pain management.

Herbs, Botanicals and Supplements

- Herbs and botanical supplements should not be used without discussing with physician.

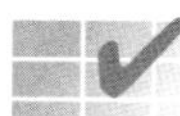

PATIENT EDUCATION

- ✓ Explain measures that are appropriate to specific condition.
- ✓ Encourage regular medical visits and nutritionist follow-up.

For More Information

- American Association of Kidney Patients
  100 South Ashley Drive, Suite 280
  Tampa, FL 33602
  1–800-749–2257
- National Kidney and Urologic Diseases Information Clearinghouse
  3 Information Way
  Bethesda, MD 20892-3580
  http://www.niddk.nih.gov/health/kidney/kidney.htm
- NIDDK
  http://www.niddk.nih.gov/health/kidney/pubs/polycyst/polycyst.htm
- Polycystic Kidney Disease Foundation
  4901 Main Street, Suite 200
  Kansas City, MO 64112
  1–800-753–2873
  http://www.pkdcure.org

GLOMERULONEPHRITIS, ACUTE

NUTRITIONAL ACUITY RANKING: LEVEL 3

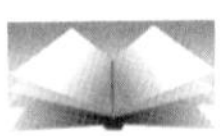

DEFINITIONS AND BACKGROUND

Inflammation in the glomeruli is called glomerulonephritis or simply nephritis. For example, after an antigen-antibody complex reaction, some complexes become trapped in the glomeruli. Edema, scarring, or inflamed glomeruli result. Untreated streptococcal infection can cause acute glomerulonephritis. Most conditions resolve after 3–12 months.

Uremia is the accumulation in the blood of waste substances ordinarily eliminated in the urine. This happens because the kidneys have lost their filtering ability as a result of temporary poisoning or severe kidney disease. Oliguria is a diminished amount of urine formation; anuria is a term that implies <400 cc/24 hours of urinary output.

Signs and symptoms of glomerulonephritis may include a decrease in urine volume, urine smell on breath and sweat, itching, vomiting, convulsions, rust-colored urine, and yellowish-brown skin discoloration. (See also acute renal failure.)

Additional processes that can damage the glomeruli and cause proteinuria include diabetes, hypertension, and other forms of kidney diseases.

Research shows that the level and type of proteinuria (whether the urinary proteins are only albumin or include other proteins) strongly determine the extent of damage and whether a patient is at risk for developing progressive kidney failure.

Proteinuria has also been shown to be associated with cardiovascular disease. Damaged blood vessels may lead to heart failure, stroke, or kidney failure.

OBJECTIVES

- ▲ Reduce elevated serum nitrogen levels from breakdown of endogenous or exogenous proteins.
- ▲ Reduce elevated blood pressure or edema.
- ▲ Spare protein for tissue repair.
- ▲ Improve renal functioning; prevent systemic complications.
- ▲ In children, avoid growth retardation over time.

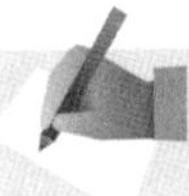

DIETARY AND NUTRITIONAL RECOMMENDATIONS

- For patients with oliguria, restrict fluid intake to 500–700 mL. Restrict protein intake when urinary output is <400 cc/24 hours or as physician deems necessary.
- For patients with uremia, diet should include high biologic value (HBV) proteins (eggs and milk); or essential amino acids (EAAs) 2–3 times normal should be included. Diet may be restricted to 0.6 g protein/kg; use at least 50% HBV proteins.
- If patient has edema or high blood pressure, restrict sodium intake to 2–3 g daily. In a child, 500–1,000 mg restriction may be needed.
- Use a high-calorie diet to spare protein, 35 kcal/kg (60% CHO, 30% fat.)
- When urinary output is reduced greatly, restrict phosphorus intakes as needed (e.g., low-phosphate diet of 5–10 mg/kg/day.) Potassium is often controlled by medications, but monitor values closely.
- Some patients may require dialysis to remove waste products.
- Vitamin D3, calcium, iron, and multivitamin intake should be increased when appropriate.
- Vegetarian diets and use of omega-3 fatty acids (Donadio et al., 1994) may be beneficial, especially for dyslipidemia in chronic kidney disease.

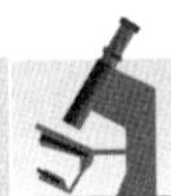

PROFILE

Clinical/History

Height
Weight
Edema-free adjusted body weight (aBWef)
Edema
BMI
BP
Temperature
Intake and output (I & O)
Oliguria or decrease in urine volume
Urine smell on breath and sweat
Itching
Vomiting
Convulsions
Rust-colored urine
Yellowish-brown skin discoloration

Lab Work

H&H, MCV
Serum Fe, total iron-binding capacity (TIBC), percent saturation
Serum ferritin
Glomerular filtration rate (GFR), creatine clearance (CrCl) levels
Renal x-rays
K+
Sodium (Na+)
Alb, prealbumin
Transferrin
BUN
Creat
White blood cell count (WBC)
Serum phosphorus
Specific gravity (decreased)
Aspartate aminotransaminase (AST)
Chol (increased)
Ca++
Serum copper (increased)

Common Drugs Used and Potential Side Effects

- When diuretics (such as Lasix) are used to reduce edema, watch for potassium wasting. Dehydration can elevate BUN; assess carefully.
- Antihypertensives have various effects; evaluate individually.

Herbs, Botanicals and Supplements

- Herbs and botanical supplements should not be used without discussing with physician.

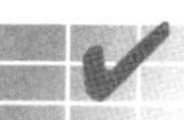

PATIENT EDUCATION

- ✔ Patients with ascites may become anorexic in the upright position. Position patient carefully for food intake.
- ✔ Fluid intake should be distributed carefully throughout patient's waking hours. Check for changes according to diarrhea, etc.
- ✔ Encourage frequent doctor or clinic visits to monitor renal functioning.
- ✔ A low-protein, low-phosphorus diet may be needed.

GLOMERULONEPHRITIS, CHRONIC

NUTRITIONAL ACUITY RANKING: LEVEL 3

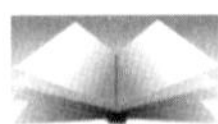

DEFINITIONS AND BACKGROUND

In chronic glomerulonephritis, repeated episodes of nephritis lead to loss of renal tissue and kidney function; glomeruli disappear and normal filtering is lost. Kidneys can no longer concentrate urine, and more urine is voided in an effort to rid the body of wastes. Protein and blood are lost in the urine. Blood pressure rises, causing vascular changes. Decreased proteinuria indicates an improved prognosis, whereas hypertension can delay improvement. Many diseases (including diabetes, hypertension, and other kidney diseases) can cause this inflammation, which leads to proteinuria. Chronic kidney disease (CKD) may be a result; also see chronic kidney disease entry.

Conservative treatment promotes protein restriction to correct metabolic and hormonal derangements. Many studies and the NKF support dietary protein restriction (0.6 g protein/kg body weight [BW]) for slowing the progression of renal disease in patients with or without diabetes (Pedrini et al., 1996).

Protein restriction is absolutely contraindicated in protein malnutrition, neoplasm, or infections. Protein restriction has its limitations: A renal dietitian is needed for appropriate teaching; commitment from the patient and family is needed; extra expense may be incurred for low-protein foods and amino acid analogs; growth and muscle mass may decline; and sufficient calorie intake is essential to prevent protein–calorie malnutrition (PCM).

OBJECTIVES

- Control hypertension and proteinuria.
- Correct metabolic abnormalities. Improve nutritional status and appetite.
- Reduce edema.
- Prevent further catabolism of protein to lower urea production and other protein waste products.
- Prevent complications, including growth failure, in children.

DIETARY AND NUTRITIONAL RECOMMENDATIONS

- Modify patient's diet according to disease progression; maintain sufficient levels of protein as long as kidneys can eliminate waste products of protein metabolism. As BUN rises to levels specified by age and identified by the physician as problematic, restrict protein intake to 0.6 g/kg. Control meat and milk intake, because they are high in both protein and phosphorus.
- Determine vitamins and nutrients provided by therapeutic diet and supplement to meet RDA, especially for calcium and B vitamins, which are easily lost in urine.
- Complete patient's energy requirements with carbohydrates and fat. For adults, 30–40 kcal/kg adjusted edema-free BW may be needed to use protein for tissue synthesis, etc.
- If lipids are elevated, fat and cholesterol may need to be restricted; monitor carefully.
- Restrict sodium intake for patients with edema or to control fluid retention. Carefully monitor sodium levels, because sodium depletion can occur during diuretic phase of chronic glomerulonephritis. Also check potassium and phosphorus levels.
- Children with uremia require vitamin D3 to promote growth and improve appetite; adults need to maintain bone health.
- Soy or vegetarian meals and use of omega-3 fatty acids (Donadio et al., 1994) may be beneficial.

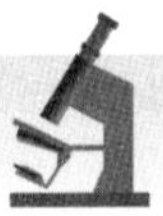

PROFILE

Clinical/History	Lab Work	
Height	Chol (often increased from proteinuria)	Proteinuria
Weight	Alb, prealbumin	Parathormone (PTH)
Edema-free adjusted by body weight (aBWef)	BUN	K+
Edema	Creat	Na+
Temperature	GFR, CrCl	Serum phosphorus
I & O	BMI	Serum Fe
BP (elevated)	WBC	TIBC, percent saturation, serum ferritin
	H&H	Renal x-rays
	Specific gravity (often decreased)	Kidney biopsy

Herbs, Botanicals and Supplements

- Herbs and botanical supplements should not be used without discussing with physician.

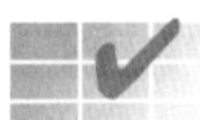

PATIENT EDUCATION

- ✔ Patient should not avoid drinking fluid to prevent nocturia.
- ✔ Fluid retention is better controlled by sodium restriction than by fluid restriction. Monitor patient carefully.
- ✔ Patients with edema are often thirsty despite fluid retention. Edema water is trapped and unavailable for body's use.
- ✔ Frequent doctor or clinic visits are recommended to evaluate renal functioning.
- ✔ Dietary protein restriction has its limitations—help from a renal dietitian is needed; commitment from patient and family is essential; extra expense is incurred for EAAs, keto-acid analogs (KAAs), and low-protein foods; growth and muscle mass may decline; calorie intake is essential to prevent PCM.
- ✔ Table 16–4 describes the findings of the Modified Diet in Renal Disease (MDRD) Study and its dietary guidance.

For More Information

- ✦ American Dietetic Association
  Pre-End Stage Renal Disease protocol
  www.eatright.org

TABLE 16–4 Modified Diet in Renal Disease (MDRD) Study

In the MDRD study, 840 adult patients with renal disease followed a low-protein (usually 0.6 for advanced disease) and low-phosphate diet (5–10 mg/kg/day). Keto and amino acid analogs were found to be useful (Gillis et al, 1995).

Evaluations of quality of life determined that among the usual-protein, low-protein, and very-low-protein groups, the very-low-protein diet was clearly the least palatable (Coyne et al, 1995). The imprecision of exchange lists is one factor causing difficulty in achieving target protein levels; one suggestion is to count grams of protein instead (MDRD Study Group, 1994).

Although 32 types of counseling strategies were employed, the most beneficial focused on psychosocial and behavioral approaches (Milas et al, 1995). Time spent by registered dietitians averaged from 183 to 116 minutes over a few to 25–36 months, respectively; more time was required for very-low-protein diets (Dolecek et al, 1995).

NEPHRITIS

NUTRITIONAL ACUITY RANKING: LEVEL 3

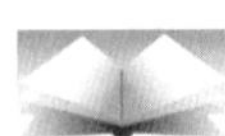

DEFINITIONS AND BACKGROUND

Nephritis, historically known as Bright's disease, is a kidney inflammation that results from a diffuse, progressive lesion affecting the renal parenchyma, interstitial tissue, and renal vascular system. The hereditary form is known as Alport Syndrome. The inflammation can become acute or chronic; it may result from scarlet fever, flu, or tonsillitis.

Nephritis may also reflect any altered kidney functioning. Fish oils may decrease loss of renal function by affecting eicosanoid and cytokine production, altering renal dynamics and decreasing inflammation (Donadio et al., 1994).

OBJECTIVES

- ▲ Reduce renal workload to allow healing.
- ▲ Improve or control excretion of waste products such as urea and sodium.
- ▲ Prevent edema resulting from sodium and fluid retention.
- ▲ Prevent uremia from nitrogen retention.
- ▲ Adjust electrolyte levels as needed (e.g., sodium, potassium, and chloride).
- ▲ Prevent systemic complications or net protein catabolism, as from poor intake.

DIETARY AND NUTRITIONAL RECOMMENDATIONS

- Determine fluid intake (measured output plus 500 mL insensible losses).
- Restrict sodium intake to 2–3 g if patient has hypertension or edema.
- In the case of renal failure, protein intake should be low (0.6 g/kg adjusted edema-free BW). Use 50% HBV proteins to ensure positive nitrogen balance.
- Check need for vitamin A, which may be low.
- Decrease phosphorus with a low-phosphate diet (5–10 mg/kg/day.)
- Provide adequate calories (35 kcal/kg BW).
- Use of fish oils may be beneficial to reduce inflammation.

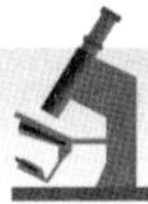

PROFILE

Clinical/History	Lab Work	
Height	BUN, Creat	AST
Weight	Chloride (Cl−)	Ca++
aBWef	GFR, CrCl	Proteinuria
Edema	Chol (may be increased)	H&H, serum Fe
BMI	Alb, prealbumin	TIBC, percent saturation, serum ferritin
I & O	Na+, K+	PTH
BP	RBP	Serum Cu (may be decreased)
Temperature	Phosphorus	

Herbs, Botanicals and Supplements

- ■ Herbs and botanical supplements should not be used without discussing with physician.

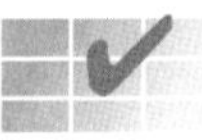

PATIENT EDUCATION

- ✔ Ensure dietary measures are appropriate for patient's current status.
- ✔ Consider discussing ways to include more fish oils in diet.

For More Information

- ✦ Hereditary Nephritis Foundation (Alport Syndrome)
  1390 W 6690 S, #202 H
  Murray, UT 84123
  (801) 262–5901
  http://www.cc.utah.edu/~cla6202/HNF.htm

NEPHROSCLEROSIS

NUTRITIONAL ACUITY RANKING: LEVEL 3

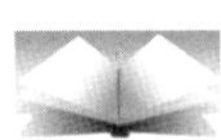

DEFINITIONS AND BACKGROUND

Hardening of the renal arteries, usually as a result of renal hypertension and generalized atherosclerotic heart disease, causes nephrosclerosis (historically known as arteriosclerotic Bright's disease). Albumin is lost in the urine, nitrogen waste products are retained, and retinal changes occur. Death may occur from circulatory failure or hypertension. Nephrosclerosis usually occurs in persons older than 35 years of age.

OBJECTIVES

- Reduce workload of circulatory system by decreasing excess weight, when present.
- Monitor abnormal protein status and nitrogen retention.
- Control hypertension.
- Prevent systemic complications.
- Control hyperglycemia, if patient has diabetes.
- Decrease elevated serum lipids.

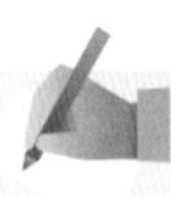

DIETARY AND NUTRITIONAL RECOMMENDATIONS

- If patient is obese, use a low-calorie diet.
- Protein intake should be normal, except during periods of nitrogen retention, when low protein (0.6 g/kg ideal body weight [IBW]) is useful.
- Diet should be low in cholesterol and saturated fats to lessen atherosclerotic heart disease. Linoleic acid seems to be important. Vegetarian diets, increased use of soy, folic acid, and omega-3 fatty acids should be considered.
- Monitor fluid intake according to patient's output. Intake should be adequate to eliminate wastes but controlled when retention occurs.
- Restrict sodium intake to reduce edema and hypertension.
- Control CHO intake with diabetes or hyperglycemia.

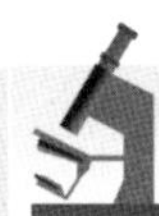

PROFILE

Clinical/History	Lab Work	
Height	H&H, serum Fe	Ca++, serum phosphorus
Weight	TIBC, percent saturation, serum ferritin	PTH
aBWef	Alb, prealbumin	Chol (increased)
Edema	Urinary albumin	AST
BMI	BUN, Creat	Trig
BP	GFR, CrCl	K+
I & O		Na+
Uremia		Gluc
		Urinary ketones

Herbs, Botanicals and Supplements

- Herbs and botanical supplements should not be used without discussing with physician.

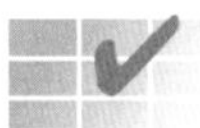

PATIENT EDUCATION

- Help patient control specific nutrients as needed (e.g., proteins, sodium, folic acid, lipids, fluid, etc.).
- Discuss shopping, meal preparation, and label reading.

NEPHROTIC SYNDROME

NUTRITIONAL ACUITY RANKING: LEVEL 3

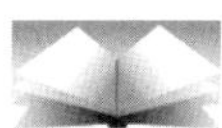

DEFINITIONS AND BACKGROUND

Not a disease in itself, nephrotic syndrome (also called nephrosis) causes massive proteinuria, with 3.5 g or more of protein lost within 24 hours. As much as 30 g could be lost as a result; albumin is especially affected. The common form of nephrotic syndrome in children is called "minimal change disease," and its cause is not known; prednisone may be prescribed.

Signs and symptoms of nephrotic syndrome include weight gain, hyperlipidemia, edema, chest pains, hypovitaminosis D, hypokalemia, and weakness. Adults who have nephrotic syndrome usually have some form of glomerulonephritis, with renal failure not far behind. Elevated low-density lipoprotein (LDL) cholesterol is also common from changes in lipoprotein production.

Dietary management centers on the problem of salt and water retention, protein depletion, hyperlipidemia, and loss of carrier proteins for vitamins and minerals (Devine and DiChiro, 1992). A very-high-protein diet will alter GFR; limit protein to decrease hyperfiltration. A low protein diet that provides adequate energy can maintain N balance in nephrotic syndrome. These patients have normal anabolic responses to dietary protein restriction (decreased amino acid oxidation) and feeding (increased protein synthesis and decreased degradation); proteinuria probably simulates conservation of dietary essential amino acids (Maroni, 1997).

In about 20% of children with nephrotic syndrome, kidney biopsy reveals scarring or deposits in the glomeruli. The two most common diseases that damage these filtering units are focal segmental glomerulosclerosis (FSGS) and membranoproliferative glomerulonephritis (MPGN). Rarely, a child may be born with a condition that causes nephrotic syndrome (congenital nephropathy).

OBJECTIVES

- Ensure efficient utilization of fed proteins, spared by use of adequate calories. Prevent muscle catabolism. If protein losses are severe, albumin infusion may be needed; this is rare.
- Reduce edema.
- Control sodium intake with otherwise uncontrolled hypertension (HPN).
- Monitor hypercholesterolemia, elevated triglycerides.
- Monitor patient for potassium deficits with certain diuretics.
- Replace any other nutrients, especially those at risk (calcium, vitamin D, etc.).
- Prevent or control renal failure.
- Correct anorexia.

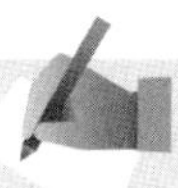

DIETARY AND NUTRITIONAL RECOMMENDATIONS

- Use a diet of modest protein restriction (0.8 g/kg in adults, with 50% HBV). Children should be given the RDA for their age because high protein levels may worsen proteinuria and will not improve serum albumin levels (Hogg et al., 2000).
- In the case of elevated levels of cholesterol and triglycerides, limit total fat and cholesterol; decrease intake of concentrated sugars and alcohol. Encourage use of linoleic acid and omega-3 fatty acids. A vegetarian, soy-based diet with amino acid replacements may also help to correct hyperlipoproteinemia (HLP) as well as loss of albumin (D'Amico et al., 1992).
- Carbohydrate intake should be high to spare protein for LBM. Increase fiber (25–35 g).
- Diet should provide 35 kcals/kg body weight daily.
- If patient has edema, sodium intake should be restricted to 2–3 g.
- Provide adequate sources of potassium, vitamin D, and calcium as tolerated. Replace zinc, vitamin C, folacin, and other nutrients. Monitor iron according to laboratory values.
- Fluid restrictions may be necessary if edema is refractory to diuretic therapy.
- Offer appetizing meals to increase intake.
- If required, use tube feedings (e.g., specialty renal products). Total parenteral nutrition (TPN) may also be beneficial.

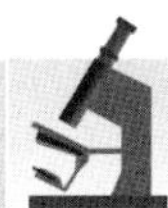

PROFILE

Clinical/History

Height
Weight (gains?)
aBWef
Edema
BMI
BP
I & O
Chest pains
Weakness

Lab Work

Alb, prealbumin
Proteinuria, uremia
Trig (increased)
Chol
H&H, serum Fe
TIBC, percent saturation, serum ferritin
Transferrin (increased)
Ceruloplasmin (decreased)
AST (increased)
Na+
K+ (hypokalemia?)
Serum phosphorus
Serum vitamin D
Hypovitaminosis D
Ca++
BUN, Creat
GFR, CrCl

Common Drugs Used and Potential Side Effects

- Diuretics. Thiazides such as Lasix deplete potassium. Others may spare or retain potassium (Aldactone, ACE inhibitors). Check need for dietary alterations.
- Corticosteroids such as Prednisone. Sodium restrictions may be needed. Potassium, nitrogen, or calcium losses may result. Muscle wasting or weight gain and other side effects are common.
- Cytotoxic agents may be used such as cyclophosphamide, chlorambucil, and cyclosporine. They are often used for a few months. Side effects include GI distress, nausea, and vomiting.
- Recent experience with ACE inhibitors (a type of blood pressure drug) indicates that these drugs help prevent protein from leaking into urine and keep kidneys from being damaged in children with nephrotic syndrome (NIDDK, 2001).

Herbs, Botanicals and Supplements

- Herbs and botanical supplements should not be used without discussing with physician.
- With cyclosporine, avoid use with Echinacea and St. John's wort because of counterproductive effects on drug.

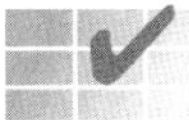

PATIENT EDUCATION

- ✓ Help patient plan appetizing meals. Sodium restriction is common.
- ✓ If patient has abdominal edema, careful positioning may increase comfort at mealtimes.
- ✓ Weight management plans will be needed if steroid use will be long-term.

PYELONEPHRITIS AND URINARY TRACT INFECTIONS

NUTRITIONAL ACUITY RANKING: LEVEL 3 (IF CHRONIC)

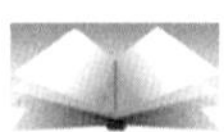

DEFINITIONS AND BACKGROUND

Bacterial invasion of the kidneys, pyelonephritis (the most common cause of urinary tract infection [UTI]) leads to fibrosis, scarring, and dilatation of the tubules, which impair renal function. *E. coli* most often causes upper UTIs; other organisms are found in complicated infections associated with diabetes mellitus, instrumentation, urinary stones, and immunosuppression (Roberts, 1999). With effective antibacterial therapy, the immune response by both T and B lymphocytes leads to antibodies that assist in bacterial eradication (Roberts, 1999).

Pyelonephritis does not require extensive medical nutrition therapy (Pachter, 1994). When patient is septic, hospitalization and treatment with parenteral antibiotics are needed. If patient does not improve rapidly, studies, including ultrasound and computed tomography (CT), are used to diagnose obstruction, abscess, or emphysematous pyelonephritis. Most of these complications are now rapidly treated percutaneously, with surgical therapy following as needed (Roberts, 1999).

Scarring of chronic pyelonephritis leads to loss of renal tissue and function; it sometimes progresses to end-stage renal disease. Hypertension is often present in chronic pyelonephritis.

Although not always a cause of UTIs, urinary incontinence requires attention. Check for vitamin B12 deficiency; decrease caffeine intake; and try bladder training (use of toilet every 2 hours). It also may be useful to maintain an adequate level of fluid intake to prevent onset of any UTIs.

Interstitial cystitis (painful bladder syndrome) causes an inflamed bladder wall and has no specific link to diet. But omission of alcohol, caffeine, citrus beverages, and tomatoes may give relief to some

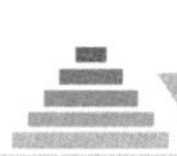

OBJECTIVES

- ▲ Preserve kidney function.
- ▲ Control blood pressure.
- ▲ Acidify urine to decrease additional bacterial growth.
- ▲ Force fluids unless contraindicated (Denman and Burton, 1992).

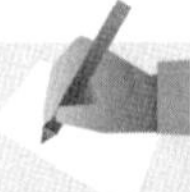

DIETARY AND NUTRITIONAL RECOMMENDATIONS

- Restrict excess sodium to control elevated blood pressure. However, some patients lose excessive amounts of sodium in their urine and must be monitored for depletion.
- Restrict protein intake if renal function is decreased. Otherwise, use sufficient amounts of HBV proteins, including foods such as meat, fish, poultry, eggs, and cheese.
- Restrict potassium when serum K+ is elevated. Check drugs first.
- Cranberries, plums, and prunes produce hippuric acid, which help to acidify urine. Corn, lentils, breads/starches, peanuts, and walnuts also tend to acidify urine. Cranberry juice contains hippuric acid and another substance that seems to prevent adherence of bacteria to urinary tract epithelial cells (Kontiokari et al., 2001; Pachter, 1994; Avorn, 1994). It is often suggested to consume 3 glasses daily of cranberry juice cocktail for this purpose. Although vitamin C is not necessarily effective in lowering urinary pH, sufficient levels of intake are needed to stimulate the anti-infective process.
- Avoid excess of caffeine for its diuretic effect. Stimulants such as caffeine rapidly leave bladder, a vulnerable site in which additional infections may begin.
- Vitamin A may be low; encourage improved intake, especially from carotenoids (Kavukcu et al., 1998).

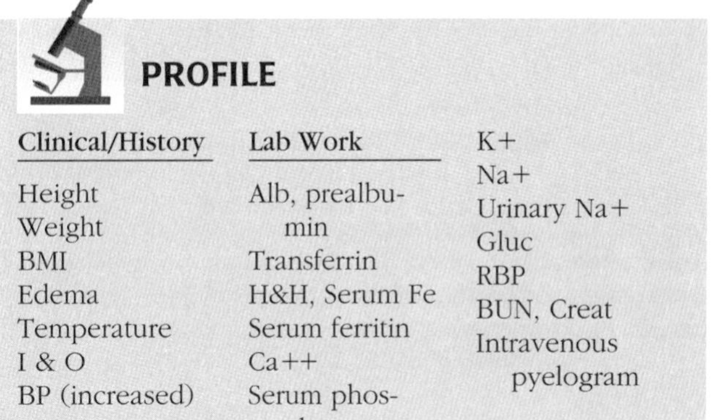

PROFILE

Clinical/History	Lab Work	
Height	Alb, prealbumin	K+
Weight	Transferrin	Na+
BMI	H&H, Serum Fe	Urinary Na+
Edema	Serum ferritin	Gluc
Temperature	Ca++	RBP
I & O	Serum phosphorus	BUN, Creat
BP (increased)		Intravenous pyelogram

Common Drugs Used and Potential Side Effects

- Urinary anti-infectives may be used. Ceftriaxone and gentamicin are cost-effective because only once-daily dosing is needed. With urinary anti-infectives, sufficient water and fluids should be ingested. Be careful with forced water diuresis, which impairs antibiotic effectiveness. Monitor responses to glucose changes in people with diabetes. Avoid use with alcohol.
- Sulfisoxazole (Gantrisin) can deplete folacin and vitamin K. Nausea and vomiting may also occur.
- Trimethoprim (Trimpex) and trimethoprim/sulfamethoxazole (Bactrim, Septra, Cotrim) may cause diarrhea, GI distress, and stomatitis. Use adequate fluid.
- Nitrofurantoin (Furadantin, Macrodantin) should be consumed with food or milk. An adequate protein diet

is needed. Nausea, vomiting, and anorexia are common. Diarrhea is less common.

- Quinolones include ofloxacin (Floxin), norfloxacin (Noroxin), ciprofloxacin (Cipro), and trovafloxin (Trovan). If Cipro (ciprofloxacin) is used, avoid taking with calcium supplements, milk, and yogurt; limit use of caffeine; monitor for nausea. If fluoroquinolone (Floxin, Maxaquin) is used, nausea is one side effect. Take separately from vitamin supplements.
- Penicillin products such as amoxicillin (Amoxil, Trimox, Wymox) and ampicillin may be used. If penicillin allergy exists, vancomycin may be used.

Herbs, Botanicals and Supplements

- Herbs and botanical supplements should not be used without discussing with physician. Blueberry, parsley, bearberry, yogurt, birch, and couch grass have been suggested for kidney and bladder infections, but no clinical trials have shown efficacy.

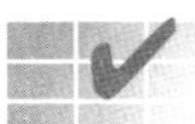

PATIENT EDUCATION

- ✔ Indicate which foods are palatable as sources of nutrients for dietary restrictions and for nutrients that tend to be low.
- ✔ Encourage appropriate fluid intake.
- ✔ Discuss acid ash diets as adjunct therapy only; medical therapy must be first.
- ✔ Limit caffeine and oral fluid intake at night, if needed.
- ✔ Showers, instead of baths, may be preventive.

For More Information

- Interstitial Cystitis Association (ICA)
  51 Monroe Street, Ste. 1402
  Washington, DC 20850
  1–800-435–7422
  www.ichelp.org
- National Bladder Foundation
  www.bladder.org

UROLITHIASIS/NEPHROLITHIASIS (KIDNEY STONES)

NUTRITIONAL ACUITY RANKING: LEVEL 2

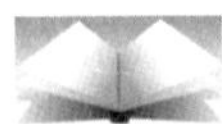

DEFINITIONS AND BACKGROUND

Kidney stones develop when salt and minerals in urine form crystals that coalesce and grow in size. Annually, 400,000 people are treated for this problem. In the South where there is a slightly higher prevalence, a history of hypertension, low use of calcium supplements, and low dietary intake of magnesium have been found among older women (Hall et al., 2001). Overall, major causes of renal stones are UTIs, dehydration, metabolic defects, cancer, immobilization, osteoporosis, and renal tubular acidosis (see Table 16–5).

High intake of dietary calcium seems to decrease risk of kidney stones; while supplemental calcium may increase risk. Regular calcium supplementation does not raise metabolites of calcium and oxalate in urine, and the proportion of oxalate to calcium is reduced; underlying mechanisms of changes seen in phosphate, calcium, and PTH and the observations on 1,25-(OH)2-cholecalciferol are not clear (Williams et al., 2001). Increased dietary calcium, in association with a reduction of the relative proportion absorbed, may be pertinent to the prevention of calcium oxalate rich stones. Timing of calcium intake in relation to oxalate intake and other factors in dairy products may also be related (Curhan et al., 1997).

Tea, coffee, caffeine, wine, and beer consumption may decrease risk; apple or grapefruit juices actually may aggravate risk (Curhan, 1996). Substituting milk for apple juice will not increase kidney stone risk in most normocalciuric adults who form calcium oxalate stones (Massey and Kynast-Gales, 1998). In addition, balanced diets containing moderate amounts of either beef or plant protein (legumes, seeds, nuts, and grains) are equally effective in reducing calcium oxalate kidney stone risk based on changes in urinary composition (Massey and Kynast-Gales, 2001).

Stones are formed by progressive deposition of crystalline material about an organic nidus; 10% of stones are organic (composed of cystine or uric acid) and 90% are inorganic (composed of calcium, magnesium, ammonium, oxalate, phosphate, or carbonate). Signs and symptoms include excruciating pain, nausea, vomiting, burning, and urinary frequency.

OBJECTIVES

- Determine predominant components and prevent recurrence in calculi-prone patients.
- Modify diet according to predominant component—there seldom is a single cause.
- To increase excretion of salts, dilute urine by increasing fluid volume to at least 2 L per 24 hours.

TABLE 16–5 Causes of and Predisposition to Renal Stones

1. Age—More common in middle age
2. Sex—Three times more common in males
3. Activity—Immobilization or excessive fluid losses from sweating
4. Climate—Hot climate and dehydration during summer months
5. Diminished water intake—During sleep, travel, illness, or from poor habits
6. Genetic disorders—Gout, primary hyperoxaluria
7. Metabolic disturbances—Bowel, endocrine, and renal problems that increase blood and urinary Ca^{++} and oxalate levels
8. Diet—Low intakes of calcium and fluid; high oxalates
9. Misuse of medications
10. Urinary tract infection or stagnation from blockage

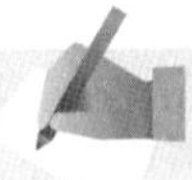

DIETARY AND NUTRITIONAL RECOMMENDATIONS

- Fluid intake should be high, as tolerated (2 quarts/day). Tea, coffee, wine, and beer are acceptable choices; apple or grapefruit juices should be limited (Curhan, 1996).
- Calcium oxalate stones. Calcium intake should be increased to more than 1,000 mg/day; good sources include skim milk, yogurt, broccoli, fortified orange juice, and ricotta or cheese. In patients' kidney stones and hypercalciuria, moderate protein intake decreases calcium excretion, mainly through a reduction in bone resorption and renal calcium loss, probably due to a decrease in exogenous acid load (Giannini et al., 1999). A diet reduced in oxalates is often needed, especially if patient hyperabsorbs oxalates (Juneja, 1992; Massey et al., 1993). Oxalates are found in spinach, strawberries, rhubarb, beets, nuts, chocolate, coffee, tea, cola, and wheat bran.
- Cystine stones. Use a diet low in cystine, methionine, and cysteine. Protein intake should be lessened but not severely restricted. Cystine stones usually are the result of a hereditary defect. Alkalize urine with agents like D-penicillamine.
- Uric acid stones. Resulting from purine metabolism, uric acid stones may require a reduction in foods that are high in purines (e.g., sardines, etc.). Uric acid stones may also result from gout, leukemia, cancer, etc. Alkalinize urine with citrate or bicarbonate.

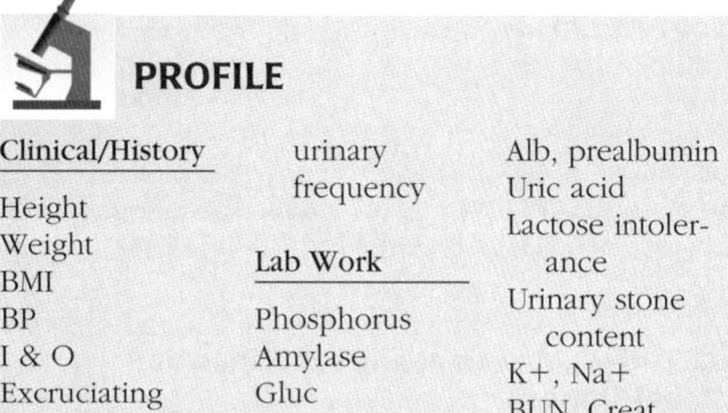

PROFILE

Clinical/History	Lab Work	
Height	Phosphorus	Alb, prealbumin
Weight	Amylase	Uric acid
BMI	Gluc	Lactose intolerance
BP	Urinary Ca++ (normal, 300–400 mg)	Urinary stone content
I & O	Ca++	K+, Na+
Excruciating pain		BUN, Creat
Nausea, vomiting		GFR, CrCl
Burning and urinary frequency		H&H, Serum Fe
		Serum oxalate levels

- Use of an acid ash or alkaline ash diet must be specifically determined by stone's composition. Acid ash is found in foods such as cranberries, plums, prunes, meat, and bread. Alkaline ash is found in foods such as milk, fruit, and vegetables. These diets are not well supported in the literature.

Common Drugs Used and Potential Side Effects

- For calcium oxalate or uric acid stones, allopurinol (Zyloprim) and probenecid usually are used instead of (or in conjunction with) a purine-restricted diet. Drink 10–12 glasses of fluid daily; avoid concomitant intake of vitamin C supplements. Maintain alkaline urine. Side effects include nausea, vomiting, diarrhea, and abdominal pain. Monitor renal and hepatic side effects.
- Thiazide diuretics sometimes are used to flush out the stone. Watch potassium levels; use replacements when needed. Control sodium intake; increase magnesium. Dry mouth or GI distress may occur.
- D-penicillamine requires B6 and zinc supplementation. Increase fluid intake with cystinuria. Take 1–2 hours before or after meals. Stomatitis, diarrhea, nausea, vomiting, and abdominal pain may occur.
- Pain medicine (Demerol, etc.) may be used. Dry mouth, constipation, nausea, or vomiting can occur.

Herbs, Botanicals and Supplements

- Herbs and botanical supplements should not be used without discussing with physician.

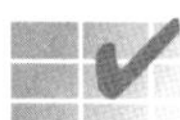

PATIENT EDUCATION

- ✓ Use dietary measures that are appropriate for condition and content of the stone. Discuss controversy about "ash" diets.
- ✓ Cranberry juice is a favorite beverage used to produce more acidic urine. Three glasses daily are recommended.
- ✓ Check calcium content of water supply. Distilled water may be required, because hard water contains more calcium.
- ✓ Vitamin B6 reduces production of oxalates by 50% and may help treatment (Curhan et al., 1999). Include good dietary sources daily.
- ✓ Increase fluid intake adequately.
- ✓ Vitamin C excess does not seem to affect oxalate stone formation even though oxalic acid is a by-product of vitamin C metabolism; routine restriction is unwarranted (Curhan et al., 1999).
- ✓ Use of cranberry concentrate tablets are marketed for prevention or treatment of UTIs but may not be beneficial for patients with a history of oxalate stones (Terris et al., 2001).

For More Information

- ✦ NIDDK
  http://www.niddk.nih.gov/health/kidney/pubs/stonadul/stonadul.htm
- ✦ American Foundation for Urologic Disease
  1128 North Charles Street
  Baltimore, MD 21201
  1-800-242-2383
  www.afud.org
- ✦ Oxalosis and Hyperoxaluria Foundation
  12 Pleasant Street
  Maynard, MA 01754
  1-888-712-2432

ACUTE RENAL FAILURE

NUTRITIONAL ACUITY RANKING: LEVEL 4

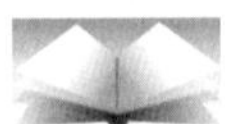

DEFINITIONS AND BACKGROUND

Acute renal failure (ARF) involves abrupt decline in renal function with waste retention. ARF occurs when the kidneys fail to function because of circulatory, glomerular, or tubular deficiency resulting from an abrupt cause: burns, severe crushing injuries, transfusions, antibiotics, nephrotoxicity, surgery or anesthesia, cardiac transplantation, shock, or sepsis. In children, the most common cause recently has been hemolytic uremic syndrome (HUS), caused by a specific strain of *Escherichia coli* bacteria with the need for transfusions, treatment of diarrhea, and dialysis. ARF is caused by diabetes in 43% of cases; hypertension in 23%; glomerulonephritis in 12%; polycystic kidney disease in 3%; and 18% from other causes. ARF occurs in about 5% of hospitalized patients, more often in surgical or trauma cases; frequently, this ARF is reversible.

The patient with ARF excretes less than 500 mL of urine daily; at least 600 mL is required to eliminate solute wastes. See Table 16–6. Signs and symptoms of ARF include anorexia, nausea, drowsiness, fatigue, itching, poor vision, headache, dyspnea, and weakness. Dialysis (daily or every other day) is necessary if other treatments fail, especially for hyperkalemia, pulmonary edema, uremia with malignant hypertension or seizures, heart failure, or pericarditis. African Americans, American Indians, and Hispanic Americans develop diabetes, nephropathy, and kidney failure at rates higher than average.

Scientists have described five stages in the progression to kidney failure in people with diabetes. Stages of progression to renal failure over several decades are indicated below (http://www.niddk.nih.gov/health/kidney/pubs/kdd/kdd.htm).

Stage I. The flow of blood through the kidneys, and therefore through the glomeruli, increases—this is called hyperfiltration—and kidneys are larger than normal. Some people remain in stage I indefinitely; others advance to stage II after many years.

Stage II. The rate of filtration remains elevated or at near-normal levels, and the glomeruli begin to show damage. Small amounts of albumin leak into urine—a condition known as microalbuminuria. In its earliest stages, microalbuminuria may not be detected on each evaluation. However, as the rate of albumin loss increases from 20–200 micrograms per minute, the finding of microalbuminuria becomes more constant. (Normal losses of albumin are less than 5 micrograms per minute.) A special test is required to detect microalbuminuria. People with type 1 and type 2 diabetes may remain in stage II for many years, especially if they have good control of their blood pressure and blood glucose levels.

Stage III. The loss of albumin and other proteins in the urine exceeds 200 micrograms per minute. It now can be detected during routine urine tests. Because such tests often involve dipping indicator strips into the urine, they are referred to as "dipstick methods." Stage III is sometimes referred to as "dipstick-positive proteinuria" (or "clinical albuminuria" or "overt diabetic nephropathy"). Some patients develop high blood pressure. The glomeruli suffer increased damage. The kidneys progressively lose the ability to filter waste, and blood levels of creatinine and urea-nitrogen rise. People with type 1 and type 2 diabetes may remain at stage III for many years.

Stage IV. This is referred to as "advanced clinical nephropathy." The GFR decreases to less than 75 mL per minute, large amounts of protein pass into the urine, and high blood pressure almost always occurs. Levels of creatinine and urea-nitrogen in the blood rise further.

Stage V. The final stage is kidney failure. The GFR drops to less than 10 mL per minute. Symptoms of kidney failure become apparent.

OBJECTIVES

- ▲ Correct underlying abnormality.
- ▲ Maintain homeostasis until kidneys resume adequate functioning.
- ▲ Maintain nitrogen, fluid, electrolyte, and mineral balances. Severe protein and amino acid restriction can slow recovery from ARF; histidine, arginine, tyrosine, cysteine, and serine are conditionally essential amino acids due to the inability to synthesize these in ARF (Rodriguez and Sandoval, 1997).
- ▲ Retard progression of renal failure.
- ▲ Prevent or correct uremia, hyperlipidemia, PCM, sepsis, and pulmonary complications.
- ▲ Lessen workload by reducing wastes (urea, uric acid, creatine, and electrolytes). Urea precursors include glutamine, alanine, and other ammonia nonessential amino acids (NAAs). Be aware of osmolarity of formulas.
- ▲ Preserve phospholipid pathways.
- ▲ Correct hyperglycemia from peripheral insulin resistance. Hemodialysis often improves this problem.
- ▲ Preserve LBM; control catabolism or weight loss. Twice weekly serum prealbumin measurements are valid assessments (Rodriguez and Sandoval, 1997).
- ▲ Prevent death.

TABLE 16–6 Phases of Acute Renal Failure

1. Anuric (14 days): Decreased output to less than 100 mL per day
2. Oliguric (8–14 days): Patient excretes 100–400 mL daily; abnormal fluid/electrolyte homeostasis occurs. Dialysis is needed to prevent permanent damage.
3. Diuretic (10 days): Patient gradually increases output of urine, up to several liters per day (400–4,000 mL). Fluid balance is critical.
4. Recovery (from 10 days to 3 months or up to 1 year): Patient gradually improves, although some loss of function may be permanent. ARF in acute care may be reversible, but mortality is still 50–75%. When toxic accumulation occurs, it may be fatal.

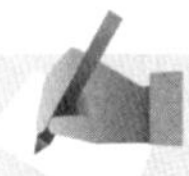

DIETARY AND NUTRITIONAL RECOMMENDATIONS

- Prevent catabolism. Ensure diet provides adequate calories (30–40 nonprotein kcals/kg BW). Controlyte, Polycose, fats, sugars, fruits, low-protein starches, and vegetables may be used. Use of fructose in ARF is controversial. If positive nitrogen balance does not result, try 35–45 kcals/kg.
- Restrict fluid intake to patient output plus 500 mL for insensible losses, etc. Err on the side of giving less rather than more. Patients may need more if excessive losses occur from diarrhea, vomiting, or surgical drains (Rodriguez and Sandoval, 1997).
- Diet should provide 0.6–0.8 g protein/kg BW at first, but that amount should increase to 1.2 g/kg BW as kidney function improves. In septic patients, higher levels of protein will be needed (see Table 16–7).
- Use at least 50% HBV proteins to provide proper ratio of EAAs to NAAs. Histidine and BCAAs also may be beneficial. Amin-Aid (American McGaw) is a mixture of amino acids and histidine without vitamins that can be used to give calories from CHOs, fats, and amino acids orally or with TF; other products are also available.
- If unable to eat, because gut function often declines in ARF, TPN or TF may be needed. Often, a diet with 50% CHO, 20% protein, and 30% fat is planned, with alternatives that are patient specific. While Nepro, Suplena, and other specific renal products are available for use with TF; monitor accordingly–there may be other standard or high stress products more appropriate for the patient. Glucose should be delivered at less than maximal oxidation rate of 5–7 mg/kg/minute to avoid increased carbon dioxide production (Rodriguez and Sandoval, 1997). Control use of lipids when there are elevated triglycerides.
- Always use TF if gut is intact. Where needed, TPN can help alleviate wasting or prolonged convalescence. Monitor glucose (hyperglycemia) and lipids (decreased triglyceride clearance).
- Control phosphorus with a low-phosphate diet (5–10 mg/kg/day), if needed.
- Supplement for calcium, folate, and vitamin B6; limit to 100 mg vitamin C to avoid excess oxalate deposition (Rodriguez and Sandoval, 1997). Add zinc, chromium, and vitamins K and A as needed but avoid excesses because of decreased renal excretion.
- If needed, restrict intake of potassium during anuric phase; monitor serum levels closely. During diuretic phase, too much potassium may be lost. Potassium-containing salt substitutes should only be used with a doctor's order or approval.
- Restrict sodium during anuric phase. During diuretic phase, excess sodium may be lost; liberalize with vomiting or diarrhea as well.
- Carnitine supplementation is not clearly supported in the literature.
- With hypertriglyceridemia or hyperlipidemia, use fewer simple sugars, more vegetarian meals (soy, etc.), and more omega-3 fatty acids.

TABLE 16–7 Controversies on Suggested Protein Intakes

The belief has been to use caution with protein intake–that protein excess leads to perfusion of remaining glomeruli and often to their destruction. The optimal nutritional regimen for patients with ARF may actually be high in protein and low in energy (Macias et al., 1996).

In one study of 40 patients, those with continuous venovenous hemofiltration showed no difference in protein catabolic rate between types of nutrition (oral, enteral nutrition [EN], PN); however, overall N balance was lower in those receiving nutritional support. When protein intake was low (less than 1 g/kg), high energy intakes reduced protein catabolism, but patients remained in negative N balance.

When protein intake is high enough to achieve N balance (1.5–1.8 g/kg), the protein catabolic rate is higher, but the increase is smaller when energy intake is low (25 kcal/kg daily).

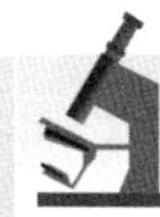

PROFILE

Clinical/History	Lab Work	
Height	BUN (over 30)	Mg++ (increased)
Weight	Creat	Alk phos
aBWef	Alb, pre-albumin	Transferrin
Edema	K+ (increased)	pH
BMI	Na+ (decreased)	Gluc (may be increased)
I & O	Urea	Azotemia
Temperature	Serum P (increased)	PT (to check need for vitamin K)
BP	GFR, CrCl	N balance
Oliguria (output 50–400 mL/day)	H&H, Serum Fe	Total lymphocyte count (TLC)
Anorexia, nausea	Ca++ (decreased)	Plasma carnitine (elevated from release from muscle and synthesis by liver)
Drowsiness, fatigue	Chol, Trig (increased)	
Itching	CO2 (decreased)	
Vision changes	Uric acid (increased)	
Headache, dyspnea	AST (increased)	
Weakness		

Common Drugs Used and Potential Side Effects

- Exchange amounts of protein may be released during tissue destruction, so patient has no capacity for urinary excretion during renal failure. Excessive sodium retention may occur, along with edema. Exchange resins (Kayexalate) may be used; take separately from calcium or antacids by several hours. Anorexia and constipation often result.

- Sorbitol may be given orally or by rectum to increase fluid and potassium loss through GI tract. Bloating, flatulence, or diarrhea can occur.
- Antacids should be monitored for mineral/electrolyte content (Maalox, Gelusil, Mylanta, etc.). Some types may be prohibited. Over-the-counter products should not be used at this time.
- Insulin may be needed with hyperglycemia or with TPN use. Watch for signs of hyperglycemia (blood glucose levels over 200 mg/dL should be addressed.) Hypergycemia must be avoided.

Herbs, Botanicals and Supplements

- Herbs and botanical supplements should not be used without discussing with physician.

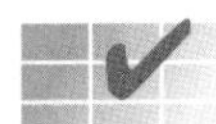

PATIENT EDUCATION

- ✔ Show patient how to monitor dietary intake of restricted nutrients and explain side effects of renal failure. Diet prescription should be followed carefully.
- ✔ Patient should monitor fluid status with daily weight measurement.
- ✔ Food labels should be read, and all foods should be measured carefully.

CHRONIC AND END-STAGE RENAL FAILURE

NUTRITIONAL ACUITY RANKING: LEVEL 4

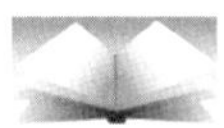

DEFINITIONS AND BACKGROUND

Chronic renal failure (CRF) is characterized by the inability of kidney function to return to normal after acute kidney failure or progressive renal decline from disease. CRF causes permanent reduction in function, eventually leading to end-stage renal disease (ESRD). **Azotemia** refers to excess urea and nitrogenous wastes in the bloodstream; this is a common finding.

There are between 2 and 13 million Americans with **chronic kidney disease (CKD)** and recent reports suggest that their treatment is currently suboptimal (Nissenson et al., 2001). **Pre-ESRD** care involves early detection of progressive renal disease, interventions to retard its progression, prevention of uremic complications, control of related conditions, adequate preparation for renal replacement therapy (RRT), and timely initiation of dialysis (Obrador et al., 1998). Mortality is remarkably high in the ESRD population; cardiovascular disease is the leading factor (Kaysen, 2001).

Protein–energy malnutrition (PEM) is common and is often present when dialysis therapy is initiated, indicating that deterioration in nutritional status often predates the onset of RRT. Biochemical and anthropometric indicators of PEM present at the initiation of dialysis are predictive of future morbidity and mortality risk (National Kidney Foundation, 2000). In patients with progressive CRF consuming uncontrolled diets, progressive declines in spontaneous protein and energy intake, serum proteins (e.g., serum albumin, transferrin), cholesterol lower than 150–180 mg/dL, total creatinine excretion, and anthropometric values are evident when the GFR falls below 50 mL/min and are particularly notable below a CrCl of about 25 mL/min (National Kidney Foundation, 2000). Early start of dialysis has been hypothesized to prevent deterioration of nutritional status and to lead to a better clinical outcome. The NKF Dialysis Outcomes Quality Initiative recommends that dialysis be started when renal Kt/V (urea) falls below 2.0/wk or the protein equivalent of total nitrogen appearance normalized to BW falls below 0.8 g/kg per day (Jansen et al., 2001).

Causes of CRF are varied, including diabetes, which alone causes many new cases each year. Pima Indians of Arizona have the world's highest incidence of type 2 diabetes mellitus (DM), and incidence of ESRD is 20 times higher in this group than the general United States population (Nelson et al., 1996). Both higher blood pressure and lower income are associated with a higher incidence of ESRD in both white and African-American men; disparities in BP and socioeconomic status relate to the excess risk of ESRD in black men compared with white men (Klag et al., 1997).

Other causes include hypoparathyroidism, recurrent acute or chronic glomerulonephritis, tubular disease, chronic hypercalcemia, chronic hyperkalemia, vascular diseases (ischemic disease, malignant hypertension, nephrosclerosis), pyelonephritis, renal calculi, renal neoplasms, collagen diseases such as systemic lupus erythematosus (SLE), amyloidosis, and analgesic abuse. Renal failure is three times more common in blacks than in whites, especially if hypertensive (Beto, 1995).

Signs and symptoms of CRF include severe headache, dyspnea, pitting edema of the hands and legs, failing vision, poor appetite, nausea and vomiting, abdominal pain, mouth ulcers, hiccups, bone and joint pain, fatigue, uremic convulsions, and pericarditis. In CKD, serum creatinine is > 1.7 mg/dL.

Mortality rises greatly with serum albumin levels below 3.5 g/dL. A low cholesterol level is another indicator of malnutrition in renal patients. Individuals undergoing dialysis who have a low-normal (less than approximately 150–180 mg/dL) nonfasting serum cholesterol have higher mortality than do those with higher cholesterol levels (National Kidney Foundation, 2000).

Patients with ESRD, who are receiving dialysis, tend to overestimate height to a greater extent than other populations, probably because of their high incidence of renal bone disease (Schnieder and Wilkens, 1997). TF may help infants and children overcome malnutrition and promote catch-up growth (Claris-Appiani et al., 1995).

Glutathione peroxidase helps prevent generation of free radicals and decreases risk of oxidative damage to tissues, including the kidney and its vascular supply. Poor selenium status is common in patients with CKD who adhere to low-protein diets because selenium is associated with protein (Smith and Temple, 1997). Poor selenium status exacerbates comorbid conditions such as congestive cardiomyopathy, skeletal myopathy, anemia, risk of cancer, and cardiac disease (CVD); therefore, it is important to correct poor selenium intake in renal patients.

Almost all patients with ESRD have elevated serum total homocysteine (tHcy) levels; use of a multivitamin supplement that contains 800 ug decreases these levels better than folic acid alone (Dierkes et al., 2001). Emerging research suggests some other vitamins such as pyridoxine, if provided in higher than normal amounts, may have an impact on reducing the risk of some aspects of renal cardiovascular disease (Makoff, 1999). It is, therefore, important to supplement some vitamins and use restraint in the supplementation of others. It is clear that renal failure patients, including predialysis, ESRD, and transplant patients need specialized supplementation to meet the requirements of renal disease management.

Better adherence to practices known to be of clinical benefit for patients with CKD not only will improve patient outcomes but also may reduce costs of care (Nissenson et al., 2001). A multidisciplinary effort is useful; billions are spent on ESRD services annually. Decreasing risks such as smoking, chronic anemia, and hypertension in renal patients may reduce death rates from cardiac heart disease (CHD). Early nutritional intervention may delay or prevent rapid progression of disease in some patients. The MDRD Study strongly suggests that control of protein and phosphorus help to delay progression of the disease (see Table 16–4).

OBJECTIVES

- ▲ Start working with high-risk patients (i.e., diabetics) when urine albumin/creatinine ratio is abnormal (>30). Start working with other patients when serum creatinine is greater than 1.5 mg/dl (women) or greater than 2.0 mg/dl (men) to limit further renal impairment and reduce kidney workload. Patients should see a team, including a renal dietitian.
- ▲ Normal postprandial repletion of amino acids is disrupted, possibly from metabolic acidosis (Garibotto et al., 1995). Control uremic symptoms and complications from accumulation of nitrogenous waste. Provide amino acids in proportion to minimal RDAs.
- ▲ Restore and maintain electrolyte balance; correct acidosis and anemias. The target hematocrit of 33% to less than 36% is desirable in most renal patients (Collins et al., 2000).
- ▲ Minimize tissue catabolism. Negative nitrogen balance is common.
- ▲ Maintain nutritional status, weight, appetite, and LBM.
- ▲ Postpone dialysis as long as possible.
- ▲ Maintain growth in children with adequate calories, vitamins, and minerals.
- ▲ Goal outcomes: blood pressure 125/75, nonsmoker, normal lipid profile, normal serum phosphorus, Hgb A1C <7, serum albumin 4.0, controlled C02 content, decreasing proteinuria, normal serum calcium, and EKG.
- ▲ Treat early problems related to kidney disease such as osteodystrophy, anemia.

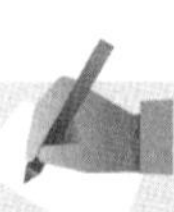

DIETARY AND NUTRITIONAL RECOMMENDATIONS

- Nondialyzed patients with advanced CRF (i.e., GFR <25 mL/min) should be prescribed a dietary energy intake of 35 kcal/kg/day for patients who are <60 years of age and 30 kcal/kg for patients >60 years of age (Kopple, 2001). CHO supplements may be needed; use fat additives if lipid levels are under control.
- For nondialyzed patients with CRF (GFR <25 mL/min), 0.60 g protein/kg/day should be prescribed; at least 50% should come from HBV sources (Kopple, 2001).
- Amino acid analogs (CHO skeleton of amino acids minus the amino group) may be used. EAAs can be given orally or by these keto-acid analogs (α-ketoisocaproate, etc.).
- If patient has edema, restrict sodium intake to 1–3 g of sodium. Restrict intake of phosphorus, if needed—low-phosphate diet (5–10 mg/kg/day.)
- Watch use of dietary potassium and salt substitutes if serum potassium levels are high. Liberalize with diarrhea or vomiting.
- Fluid intake should be equivalent to patient's output plus 500–1,000 mL for insensible losses. Monitor regularly.
- CHO intolerance is common. Fructose, galactose, and sorbitol are well tolerated.
- The typical renal failure diet is low in B vitamins; uremic factors affect folate and pyridoxine activities. In addition, retention of vitamin A or inappropriately high supplementation of vitamin C may cause toxicities, which exacerbate existing pathologies (Makoff, 1999). Provide extra vitamin B6, folic acid, and vitamin C, with RDA levels for other nutrients. Calcium (1,200–1,600 mg/day) also may be needed.
- With TPN, be careful not to use excesses of micronutrients because of reduced renal clearance. With TF, renal-specific products may be needed; monitor according to serum protein levels and other laboratory reports.

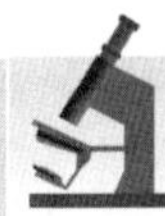

PROFILE

Clinical/History

- Height
- Weight
- aBWef
- Pitting edema, hands and legs
- BMI
- BP (increased)
- I & O
- Severe headache
- Dyspnea
- Failing vision
- Poor appetite, nausea and vomiting
- Abdominal pain
- Mouth ulcers, hiccups
- Bone and joint pain
- Fatigue
- Uremic convulsions
- Pericarditis

Lab Work

- Alb, prealbumin
- Transferrin
- Serum phosphorus (increased)
- BUN
- Creat
- GFR (below 10–15 mL/minute consider dialysis)
- Na+ (increased or decreased)
- K+ (increased)
- Ca++ (decreased)
- BUN:creatinine ratio (this ratio is altered by catabolic stress, low urine volume, and altered muscle mass)
- EKG
- Serum bicarbonate
- Uric acid (increased)
- Mg++ (increased)
- PTH
- Azotemia (excess urea and nitrogenous wastes)
- H&H, Serum Fe
- Serum ferritin, MCV, percent saturation
- pH
- CO2
- Cl−
- Chol, Trig
- Triceps skinfold (TSF), mid-arm circumference (MAC), mid-arm muscle circumference (MAMC)
- Renal biopsy
- DEXA scan

Common Drugs Used and Potential Side Effects

- For drugs to alleviate hypertension, monitor side effects.
- Phosphate binders such as calcium acetate or calcium carbonate to control serum phosphate levels. Nausea or vomiting may occur. Aluminum hydroxide is not used chronically because of accumulations in bone/brain tissue (National Institutes of Health, 1993). Calcium medications (gluconate, carbonate, or lactate) may increase calcium intake, which may be otherwise inadequate if milk is limited.

- In renal failure, patient is unable to convert vitamin D to its active form, and osteodystrophy can result from a lack of calcium use; ergocalciferol is a commonly used vitamin D analog. Extra water is needed to prevent constipation; monitor fluids carefully if urine output is decreased.
- Iron supplements may be needed to treat anemia. If recombinant human erythropoietin (r-HuEPO) is used, an iron supplement will be necessary (Sanders et al., 1994). Be careful not to overload with excesses and do not take supplements at the same time as calcium.
- In research, supplementation with histidine, an amino acid essential for renal patients, helps increase hemoglobin levels and promotes maintenance of a positive nitrogen balance.
- ACE inhibitors may be used to keep blood pressure under control; monitor specific side effects.
- Lipid-lowering medications may be used if cholesterol or triglyceride levels are high. Lipoprotein metabolism is often impaired in CKD and CRF.

Herbs, Botanicals and Supplements

- Herbs and botanical supplements should not be used without discussing with physician.

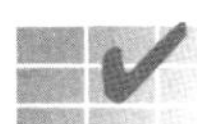

PATIENT EDUCATION

- ✔ Indicate which food sources must be restricted or used more frequently. Referral to a renal dietitian is suggested.
- ✔ Have patient consume appropriate amount of HBV proteins throughout the day.
- ✔ Taste changes may occur in patients with CKD—foods with sharp, distinct flavors may be needed. Lack of interest in red meats is common (Dobell et al., 1993).
- ✔ Low-protein wheat starch, hard candy, and jelly can be used.
- ✔ Discuss importance of dietary modification as an important element in therapy.
- ✔ Have patient weigh himself/herself daily.
- ✔ Reading food labels and measuring foods will be essential for control.
- ✔ Reading a restaurant menu, planning for box lunches, and dining away from home should be discussed.

For More Information

- ESRD Clinical Performance Measures (CPMs) Project http://www.hcfa.gov/quality/3m.htm
- NIDDK Patient Nutrition Guide http://www.niddk.nih.gov/health/kidney/pubs/kidney-failure/eat-right/eat-right.htm

HEMODIALYSIS

NUTRITIONAL ACUITY RANKING: LEVEL 4

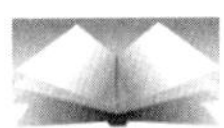

DEFINITIONS AND BACKGROUND

Hemodialysis is artificial filtering of blood by a machine, which is a catabolic process. Morbidity is largely related to physical fitness at the start of therapy. Among patients on hemodialysis, 33% have DM and 50% of deaths are related to cardiovascular disease (especially type IV HLP). Less protein is lost with hemodialysis than with peritoneal dialysis; nevertheless, amino acid losses still occur. The hemodialysis prognostic nutrition index (HD-PNI) can help identify patients who have a high risk of mortality; serum albumin and creatinine levels are used (Beto et al., 1999).

Chronic long-term dialysis can aggravate bone disease, anemia, and endocrine disorders and can lead to malnutrition if not monitored carefully. The NKF recommends strict criteria be used to diagnose malnutrition in patients maintained on dialysis: serum albumin lower than 3.4 g/dL, average body weight (ABW) lower than 90% ideal body weight (IBW), or documented protein intake lower than 0.8 g/kg. TF should be initiated for the small number who do not respond to medical, surgical, or psychiatric therapy, nutritional counseling, or food supplements (Kopple et al., 1996).

About 40% of patients undergoing maintenance dialysis suffer from varying degrees of PEM (Mehrotra and Kopple, 2001). Nutritional intervention can decrease malnutrition and mortality. Nutrient intake of patients receiving maintenance dialysis is also often inadequate, and evidence suggests toxins accumulate with renal failure that suppress appetite and contribute to nutritional decline once patients are on maintenance dialysis (Mehrota and Kopple, 2001). Adding organic nutrients (glucose, acetate) that supply energy to dialysis fluids may help treat malnutrition and body wasting in patients with CKD (Skutches and Sigler, 1997).

The Health Care Financing Administration's ESRD Core Indicators Project collects clinical information on prevalent adult patients receiving in-center hemodialysis (HD) care in the United States to assess quality of care (Frankenfield, 2000). This study has found that while hematocrit values, transferrin saturations, and iron prescription practices have improved over the last 5 years, significant opportunities to improve iron prescription practices still exist. Improvement of HD adequacy has been measured by baseline and annual urea reduction ratios (URRs) in representative samples of ESRD network patients; sustained improvement in HD care occurred after this ESRD Core Indicators Project was initiated (McClellan et al., 1999).

In HD patients, most with poor overall appetite may have good appetite for several specific foods, and increased intake of these foods may help to correct poor nutritional status; protein foods are often less desired (Ohri-Vachaspati et al., Correlates . . ., 1999). Decreased taste sensitivity has been shown to contribute to poor nutritional status in patients with renal disease, who have chronic uremia or are maintained using HD; salty, bitter, sucrose, and sour tastes all require a higher threshold (Middleton and Allman-Farinelli, 1999). This information may be helpful for developing palatable meals and dietary supplements for this population.

If TF is not tolerated, daily PN and intradialytic PN should be considered (Engel et al., 1995; Kopple et al., 1996). High-flux HD causes more amino acid losses than the conventional method (Hynote et al., 1995). Continuous venovenous hemodiafiltration (CVVHD) is less efficient than traditional HD; blood flows from dual-lumen central venous catheter and 1.5–2.0 g protein will be needed; this is used only in ARF.

Factors associated with inadequate protein nutrition in chronic HD are inadequate dialysis, inability to name any high-protein foods, need for help with shopping and cooking, poor appetite, and interdialytic fluid gain (Sehgal et al., 1998). Consistent use of EN supplements can improve nutritional status and serum albumin in HD patients (Beutler et al., 1997). There are sugar-free, lactose-free renal supplements available on the market.

In patients with renal disease treated with dialysis, diabetes comorbidity increases risk of vitamin B6 deficiency (Rock et al., 1997). Patients with diabetes who have dialysis are prone to hyperkalemia after meals, if insulin replacement is inadequate (Alton et al., 1993).

Pica (mostly ice but also starch, dirt, flour, and aspirin intake) has been found in patients who began chronic dialysis in a metropolitan area, especially in younger black patients and women (Ward and Kutner, 1999). Serum albumin levels tend to be low and serum phosphorus high; excessive interdialytic weight gains may also occur. Mean serum albumin levels tend to be lower in Asians on dialysis than in non-Asians; muscle and fat stores are more depleted; and population-specific anthropometric standards are scarce (Moretti et al., 2000).

An intensive program of dialysis and nutrition intervention can promote normal growth in children with ESRD maintained using HD (Tom et al., 1999). Children need adequate protein to encourage growth. Monitor potassium and phosphorus restrictions, because protein foods may be high in these nutrients. Fluid intake should be 20 mL/kg BW plus amounts equal to the previous day's output.

In HD patients who have moderate or severe malnutrition, energy supplements alone increase BW and body fat but do not improve nutritional status (Milano et al., 1998). Inadequate protein nutrition is independently associated with poor quality of life in HD patients. Poor physical and social function and high burden of kidney disease scores are found (Ohri-Vachaspati et al., Quality . . . 1999). The goals of the NKF Dialysis Outcomes Quality Initiative are to improve patient survival, reduce patient morbidity, increase efficiency of care, and improve quality of life (McCann, 1997).

Dyslipidemia is common in ESRD, and HD patients have increased cardiovascular morbidity and mortality. The high frequency of cardiovascular disease in dialysis patients may originate from disturbed CHO and lipid metabolism, oxidants and antioxidants, and the immuno-inflammatory system

(Schwedler et al., 2001). Chronic uremia is characterized by activation of an acute phase response and high serum levels of C-reactive protein (CRP), fibrinogen, and serum amyloid A can be found; CRP has been shown to predict cardiovascular and overall mortality in HD patients (Schwedler et al., 2001).

Treatment of secondary hyperparathyroidism (HPT) in patients with chronic renal disease has improved in recent years: skeletal pain, disabling fractures, tendon ruptures, and myriad other symptoms associated with HPT can now be avoided, and the quality of life of patients has improved (Yudd and Llach, 2000).

The role of the dietitian in caring for HD patients is further discussed in Table 16–8.

OBJECTIVES

- ▲ Compensate for protein losses. Replace lost amino acids, etc., without causing uremic symptoms.
- ▲ Spare protein adequately to allow for tissue repair and synthesis. Ensure energy and protein intakes are sufficient for growth in children.
- ▲ Modify electrolytes and fluid balance according to patient's tolerance.
- ▲ Prevent osteopenia, muscle weakness, cardiac arrhythmias, and hypertriglyceridemia.
- ▲ Provide follow-up for consistency of care in other settings or at home.
- ▲ Prevent or correct secondary HPT.

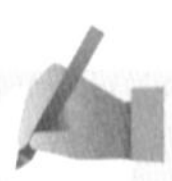

DIETARY AND NUTRITIONAL RECOMMENDATIONS

- Maintenance HD patients should be prescribed 1.2 g protein/kg/day; at least 50% should come from HBV sources (Kopple, 2001). Urea kinetic modeling may also be used to devise a protein prescription. National Renal diet suggests calculation of energy at 30–35 kcal/kg IBW. For patients who will not accept such a diet or are unable to maintain an adequate energy intake on that diet, a protein intake of up to 0.75 g protein/kg/day may be needed.
- Patients undergoing maintenance HD should be prescribed a dietary energy intake of 35 kcal/kg/day for patients who are <60 years of age and 30 kcal/kg for patients >60 years of age (Kopple, 2001). Try oral supplements before using other modes of feeding such as enteral or parenteral nutrition.
- For children, base initial protein intake on RDA for age plus an increment of 0.4 g/kg/day.
- Limit sodium intake unless there are large losses in dialysate or through vomiting or diarrhea. About 2–4 g of sodium is common and realistic.
- Check levels of potassium and phosphorus; modify diet accordingly. Dialysis removes very little phosphorus; low-phosphate diet (5–10 mg/kg/day) and limited dairy foods may be useful (American Dietetic Association, 1993). Potassium is often ordered as 40 mg/kg IBW.
- Fluid intake should be 500–1,000 mL plus the amount equal to the previous day's output or enough to permit a gain of 1–1.5 kg between treatments.
- Use vitamin supplementation to replace dialysate losses. Water-soluble vitamins are especially necessary but may not be needed daily. Vitamin B12 is not lost, for example. Folic acid (often need 1 mg), vitamin B6 (1.2–2.0 mg), vitamin C (50–100 mg), calcium (1,200–1,600 mg), and active vitamin D should be monitored and replaced at recommended levels. Be careful about zinc and vitamin A excesses. Carnitine may be supplemented, if needed. Use caution with parenteral solutions, especially for vitamins D and A. For children use RDA levels.
- Try oral supplements first. If TF is necessary, use an appropriate product to meet protein, kilocalorie, electrolyte, and volume needs. If low volume is needed, use a 1.5–2.0 kcal/mL product with small free-water flushes; a ratio of 150–200 nonprotein calories to nitrogen calories is suggested. Monitor electrolytes.
- Intradialytic parenteral nutrition (IDPN) helps malnourished patients on dialysis; try oral supplements first. IDPN improves serum albumin, BUN, total serum protein levels, and appetite in patients but may not be reimbursed (McQuiston et al., 1997).
- Fish oil supplementation may help reduce prostaglandin synthesis and may help improve hematocrit levels and symptoms of pruritus (Peck, 1997).

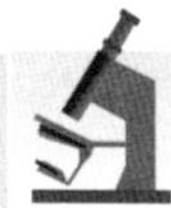

PROFILE

Clinical/History

Height
Weight
aBWef
Edema
BMI
BP
I & O
Temperature

Lab Work

Serum phosphorus
H&H, Serum Fe
Serum ferritin, percent saturation
BUN
Creat
GFR and CrCl (on HD, it will be below 10)
C-reactive protein
UUR or Kt/V
Gluc
Ca++
PTH
Uric acid
Alb, prealbumin
Transferrin
Parathyroid hormone
Na+
K+
Mg++
Urea
Serum B12, folacin (if MCV is increased)
Chol, Trig
N balance
TSF, MAC and MAMC in nonaccess arm
AST (decreased)
Serum bicarbonate (may be low)

Common Drugs Used and Potential Side Effects

- Control of hyperphosphatemia, maintenance of normocalcemia, and appropriate dosing of vitamin D analogues can prevent HPT in many cases. If severe HPT develops, many patients can still be controlled medically with correction of hyperphosphatemia and high doses of intravenous calcitriol. Phosphate binders may be used; those containing calcium (calcium acetate, calcium carbonate) may be prescribed and can cause nausea or vomiting. Aluminum products should be used for a short time period only. Long-term aluminum hydroxide (Alu-cap, Amphojel) may cause dementia, encephalopathy, or osteodystrophy (Committee on Nutrition, 1996). Sources of aluminum also include soda cans, drinking water, cooking utensils, and deodorant.
- Active vitamin D supplements may be prescribed; avoid long-term high doses.
- Carnitine is not clearly proven as essential; it is formed from lysine and methionine, requiring adequate vitamin C, niacin, iron, and B6. Red meat and dairy products are typical dietary sources. Some studies show improved exercise performance and fewer intradialytic muscle cramps; episodes of hypotension in patients undergoing hemodialysis occur when carnitine is given (Goral, 1998).
- Kayexalate may be needed to deplete excess serum potassium until serum levels return to normal. Anorexia, constipation, or diarrhea can occur. Take separately from calcium supplements or antacids.
- Excesses of vitamin–mineral supplements should be avoided. Supplements should be used to replace water-soluble vitamins in particular.
- Recombinant human erythropoietin (rHU-EPO) can be used to alleviate chronic anemia. Iron supplementation is usually needed when this is given.
- Cerivastatin, a new statin with powerful low-density lipoprotein–cholesterol (LDL-C) lowering capabilities, possesses some properties that may contribute to a reduction of coronary events in the patient with ESRD (Keane et al., 2001). Studies in this area have important implications for management of ESRD and HD patients.

Herbs, Botanicals and Supplements

- Herbs and botanical supplements should not be used without discussing with physician.

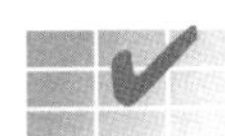

PATIENT EDUCATION

- ✓ Instruct patient to avoid use of carbonated beverages, which contain phosphates (colas). Increasing patient knowledge of hyperphosphatemia and its treatment may enhance dietary adherence to phosphorus restriction and use of phosphate binders; overall, patient understanding of hyperphosphatemia and its treatment is poor (Stamatakis et al., 1997).
- ✓ Provide information about dining away from home, home-delivered meals, etc.
- ✓ Discuss high-calorie, low-protein, mineral-controlled foods and supplements.
- ✓ Adequate care must be taken to ingest appropriate levels of protein and calories.
- ✓ Counsel patient regarding atherogenesis, if relevant.
- ✓ Discuss signs of uremia (nausea, vomiting, hiccups, fatigue, and weakness).
- ✓ Public Law 92–603 (July 1973) provides financial assistance via Medicaid to all persons covered by Social Security who have ESRD with dialysis.
- ✓ Avoidance of potassium-rich foods can create risk for low vitamin C intake. Vitamins C and B6 may be needed to maintain normal levels. Use of longer cooking times and extra water may help leach out excess potassium.
- ✓ Lack of interest in red meats, fish, poultry, eggs, sweets, and vegetables is common (Dobell et al., 1993). Work individually with patient to plan meals to ensure adequacy of protein intake.
- ✓ Trust and emotional support are essential.
- ✓ Energy and protein intakes increase when patients with ESRD participate in an exercise program during HD; appetites improve and protein intake is often 21 g greater in patients who exercise (Frey et al., 1999).
- ✓ Discuss maximum fluid gain (usually 3–5% of BW) between dialysis sessions. Noncompliance with fluid intake restrictions is common in patients with renal disease using HD and can lead to systemic and cardiac overload (Bushman, 1999). Teaching fluid management helps motivate patients to comply with their regimens; patients report that they feel better when their weight gains are within acceptable limits. (See Table 16–9.)

TABLE 16–8 Role of the Dietitian in Care of Hemodialysis Patients

The role of the dietitian is to support and maintain the nutritional status of dialysis patients. Anthropometry is performed at baseline and on a yearly basis. Close monitoring of nutritional status is completed by evaluating serum albumin and relevant biochemical data, appetite assessments, dietary energy and protein intakes, consumption of vitamins and minerals, and intake of oral supplemental foods, TF, and PN. Specified changes in serum albumin level or BW trigger action by the dietitian to prevent PCM.

The Hemodialysis (HEMO) Study is a randomized multicenter prospective clinical trial, supported by the National Institute of Diabetes, Digestive, and Kidney Diseases of the National Institutes of Health. The trial assesses effects of a standard versus higher dialysis dose and low versus high dialysis membrane flux on morbidity and mortality of chronic HD patients. This study exemplifies the important role of the dietitian in managing HD patients.

Data from Leung et al., 2001

TABLE 16–9 Fluid Equivalents

Equivalent Measures:
- 30 mL = 1 fluid oz = 2 tablespoons
- 240 mL = 8 fluid oz = 1 cup
- 2 cups = 1 lb fluid weight
- 2.2 lb = 1 kg fluid weight or 4 cups liquid

Sample Fluid Content:
- 1 whole popsicle = 90 mL
- 4 oz soup = 120 mL
- 6 oz juice = 180 mL
- 8 oz beverage = 240 mL
- 12 oz soda = 360 mL
- 16 oz milkshake = 480 mL

For More Information

- National Kidney Foundation–Nutrition Guidelines http://www.kidney.org/professionals/doqi/guidelines/doqi_nut.html

PERITONEAL DIALYSIS

NUTRITIONAL ACUITY RANKING: LEVEL 4

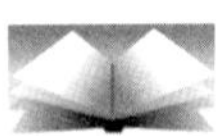

DEFINITIONS AND BACKGROUND

Peritoneal dialysis (PD) involves artificial filtering of the blood by a hyperosmolar solution (with osmosis to remove water and diffusion for glucose exchange/waste removal). Peritoneal renal dialysis removes metabolic wastes and excess fluid from the body but not so thoroughly that diet therapy is unnecessary. Considerable losses of protein and amino acids occur. Between PD treatments, the patient must return to a strict renal diet for CKD. Total calorie intake increases from glucose in dialysate in continuous ambulatory peritoneal dialysis (CAPD).

PD patients are more likely to have a primary diagnosis of glomerulonephritis, less likely to be of African-American heritage, and are younger than HD patients (Flanigan et al., 1998). PD may yield fewer growth problems in children than HD.

Types of PD include IPD (intermittent), CCPD (continuous cycling—used nearly 100% in children), and CAPD. In CAPD, there is fluid in the abdomen nearly 100% of the time; dialysis is performed four times daily; no partner is necessary. Electrolytes (potassium, phosphorus, sodium) need not be restricted as much; intake of proteins may be liberalized somewhat. With CAPD, extra glucose can increase weight and triglyceride levels. CHO absorption calculations should be individualized. One third of PD patients perform some form of automated peritoneal dialysis (APD) rather than CAPD (Flanigan, 1998). Intradialytic parenteral nutrition (IDPN) improves serum albumin, BUN, total serum protein levels, and appetite in patients (McQuiston et al., 1997).

The NKF Kidney Disease Outcomes Quality Initiative Clinical Practice Guidelines for Nutrition in CRF was published in the American Journal of Kidney Diseases and provides 27 clinical practice guidelines for adults and 10 clinical practice guidelines for children (Kopple, 2001). Among these is the recommendation that protein–energy nutritional status in these patients should be assessed by a panel of measures rather than by any single measure.

As with HD, the NKF recommends strict criteria be used to diagnose malnutrition in patients maintained on PD: serum albumin lower than 3.4 g/dL, ABW lower than 90% IBW, or documented protein intake lower than 0.8 g/kg. TF should be initiated for the small number of patients who do not respond to medical, surgical, or psychiatric therapy, nutritional counseling, or food supplements (Kopple et al., 1996). Whether high serum levels of CRP predict mortality in PD is not as clear as in HD, but there is a likely relationship, along with low serum albumin and low serum cholesterol levels (Fernandez-Reyes et al., 2000).

According to the USRDS, PD patients are hospitalized an average of 1.8 times per year (National Kidney Foundation, http://www.kidney.org/professionals/doqi/guidelines/doqiupd_vii.html). Chronic, long-term dialysis can aggravate bone problems, anemia, and endocrine disorders and can lead to malnutrition if not monitored carefully.

The Peritoneal Dialysis-Core Indicators Study (PD-CIS) retrospectively reviewed a random sample of PD patients from the United States ESRD program and found that 30% of the PD patients had a hematocrit below 30%; mean serum albumin for PD patients was 3.5 g/dL (Flanigan et al., 1998).

The NKF-Dialysis Outcomes Quality Initiative guidelines suggest that a target hematocrit of 33% to less than 36% is acceptable; fewer hospitalizations seem to occur within this range (Collins et al., 2000). The goals of the NKF-Dialysis Outcomes Quality Initiative are to improve patient survival, reduce patient morbidity, increase efficiency of care, and improve quality of life (McCann, 1997). If TF is not tolerated, daily PN and intradialytic PN should be considered.

OBJECTIVES

- Compensate for protein losses; 1–2 g protein may be lost per 2-L exchange.
- Ensure adequate sparing of protein for tissue repair and synthesis.
- Modify electrolytes and fluid balance according to patient's tolerance.
- Replace lost amino acids without causing uremic symptoms; 6–12 g of protein may be lost in dialysate.
- Prevent or correct anorexia, constipation, osteopenia, and growth delay.
- Alter calorie intake according to glucose absorption from the solution (e.g., 20 kcal/L of 1.5% solution; 60 kcal/L of 2.5% solution; 126 kcal/L of 4.5% solution).

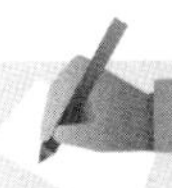

DIETARY AND NUTRITIONAL RECOMMENDATIONS

- Chronic PD patients should be prescribed 1.2–1.3 g protein/kg/day, at least 50% from HBV sources (Kopple, 2001). If there is peritonitis, 1.5 g/kg may be needed until infection subsides. For patients who will not accept such a diet or are unable to maintain an adequate energy intake on that diet, a protein intake of up to 0.75 g protein/kg/day may be needed.
- Children undergoing PD should be given RDA levels of protein, plus increments based on anticipated losses.
- Patients undergoing chronic PD should be prescribed a dietary energy intake of 35 kcal/kg/day for patients who are $<$60 years of age and 30 kcal/kg for patients $\geq$ 60 years of age (Kopple, 2001). At least one third of calories should come from CHOs (American Dietetic Association, 1993). In peritonitis, extra kilocalories may be needed until infection subsides.
- For children, follow RDA levels by age for energy and vitamins and minerals.

- Intake of sodium should be liberal, pending assessment of hydration, blood pressure, losses in dialysate, vomiting, and diarrhea. Usually, 2–4 g of sodium daily are used.
- Adjust phosphorus intake according to serum levels; low-phosphate diet (5–10 mg/kg/day) is commonly ordered.
- Fluid intake should be determined by patient's state of hydration—encourage or restrict according to intake and output. No more than 1 kg should be gained in 1 day. Fluid restriction is less common in PD.
- Supplement diet with multivitamins, especially vitamin B6 and folic acid. Monitor needs for calcium and vitamin D. Be careful about vitamin A; check serum levels. Monitor parenteral micronutrients carefully.
- If TF is needed, the formula indicated by protein, kilocalories, volume, and mineral needs of patient should be carefully chosen.

PROFILE

Clinical/History

Height
Weight
aBWef
Edema
BMI
BP
I & O
Temperature

Lab Work

Serum phosphorus (often increased)
H&H, Serum Fe
BUN
Creat
GFR, CrCl
UUR or Kt/V
Gluc
Ca++
PTH
Na+, K+
Uric acid
Alb, prealbumin
RBP
TSF, MAC, MAMC
Urea
Serum Folacin, B12 (only if MCV is elevated)
Chol, Trig
Mg++
AST (decreased)
Serum bicarbonate (may be low)

Common Drugs Used and Potential Side Effects

- Control of hyperphosphatemia, maintenance of normocalcemia, and appropriate dosing of vitamin D analogues can prevent secondary HPT. If severe HPT does occur, many patients can still be controlled with correction of hyperphosphatemia and high doses of intravenous calcitriol. Phosphate binders may be used; those containing calcium (calcium acetate, calcium carbonate) may be prescribed and can cause nausea or vomiting.
- Aluminum should be avoided in antacids, PN, albumin replacements, and dialysate, because it may cause encephalopathy and osteodystrophy (Committee on Nutrition, 1996). Aluminum products should be used for a short time period only. Long-term aluminum hydroxide (Alu-cap, Amphojel) may cause dementia, encephalopathy, or osteodystrophy (Committee on Nutrition, 1996). Sources of aluminum also include soda cans, drinking water, cooking utensils, and deodorant.
- Monitor any multivitamin–mineral supplementation for vitamins A and C, phosphorus, and magnesium. Avoid excesses.
- Lipid-lowering medications may be needed.

Herbs, Botanicals and Supplements

- Herbs and botanical supplements should not be used without discussing with physician.

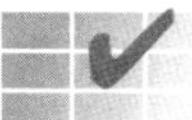

PATIENT EDUCATION

- Instruct patient to use salt substitutes carefully because of their potassium content.
- Have patient use milk sparingly if fluid and phosphorus restrictions are necessary. Fluid restrictions are not always needed with PD.
- Increasing patient knowledge of hyperphosphatemia and its treatment may enhance dietary adherence to phosphorus restriction and use of phosphate binders; overall, patient understanding of hyperphosphatemia and its treatment is poor (Stamatakis et al., 1997).
- Explain that vegetables may need to be leached before cooking to remove potassium, depending on serum K+ levels and need.
- Patient should learn how to recognize significant changes in dry weight (adjusted edema-free BW) or food intake. Discuss actions to be taken. Usually, 3–4 lb between IPD is allowed.

For More Information

- National Kidney Foundation–Nutrition Guidelines
  http://www.kidney.org/professionals/doqi/guidelines/nut_a02.html

RENAL TRANSPLANTATION

NUTRITIONAL ACUITY RANKING: LEVEL 4

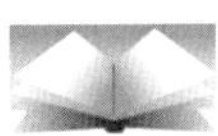

DEFINITIONS AND BACKGROUND

Renal transplantation is completed in ESRD when GFR drops to 10 mL/minute. Persons older than 60 years of age with poor health or history of cancer often cannot receive a transplant. Low-income patients with ESRD experience persistent financial barriers to transplantation that can be addressed with greater health benefits; but they also experience higher mortality that is caused by personal and/or environmental factors (Garg et al., 2001).

After a renal transplant, patient has a functioning donor kidney. High doses of glucocorticoid drugs are given to prevent rejection. The acute posttransplantation phase lasts up to 2 months; the chronic phase starts after 2 months. Complications of corticosteroid use include diabetes, osteoporosis, and hyperlipidemia. In the long term, cardiovascular morbidity remains the greatest risk for complications, followed by infections and malignancy (Matas, 1991).

Obesity decreases effectiveness of insulin receptors, increasing the tendency for glucose intolerance; weight control efforts are recommended. Early intensive dietary advice and follow-up helps control weight gain in the first year after renal transplantation (Patel, 1998).

Pediatric kidney transplantation has become an option for children with ESRD. Patient and graft survival rates, as well as long-term quality of life, have improved dramatically, a result of advances in surgical techniques, immunosuppression, and pre- and postoperative care (Papalois and Najarian, 2001). A child must reach a certain body surface area or weight (such as 20 kg) to receive a parent's kidney; siblings younger than 18 years of age generally are not allowed to donate a kidney.

OBJECTIVES

- Prevent infection and promote healing.
- Normalize diet to meet specific needs of patient and modify diet according to drug therapy to enhance outcome.
- Watch for abnormalities in calcium or phosphorus metabolism with hyperparathyroidism.
- Monitor for abnormal electrolyte levels (Na+, K+). Control BP carefully to prevent cardiac problems.
- Monitor CHO intolerance but make sure diet provides enough CHOs to spare proteins.
- Alleviate rejection episodes. Control infections, especially during acute phase. Support serum albumin levels to prevent additional infections.
- Force fluids unless contraindicated, as in retention. Match fluid output.
- Help patient adjust to a lifelong medical regimen during chronic phase. Improve survival rate by supporting immune response.
- Correct or manage complications that occur.
- Minimize weight gain.

DIETARY AND NUTRITIONAL RECOMMENDATIONS

- Progress from clear liquids to solids as quickly as possibly postoperatively. Monitor fluid status and adjust as needed.
- Daily intake of protein should be appropriate for RDAs (age, sex); 1.5 g/kg while on steroids may be recommended. Calories should be calculated as 30–35 kcal/kg or 1.3–1.5 BEE.
- Daily intake of sodium should be 2–4 g until drug regimen is reduced. Adjust potassium levels as needed.
- Daily intake of calcium should be 1–1.5 times the RDA to offset poor absorption. Children especially need adequate calcium for growth. Daily intake of phosphorus should be balanced with calcium intake.
- Supplement diet with vitamin D, magnesium, and thiamine as needed.
- Control CHO intake with hyperglycemia (50% total kilocalories) and limit concentrated sweets. Encourage complex CHOs.
- Plan fats at 30–35% of total kilocalories (encourage monounsaturated fats and omega-3 fatty acids). Low saturated fats and cholesterol may be needed. A low-fat regimen is recommended for prevention and treatment of hyperlipidemia.
- Reduce gastric irritants as necessary, if GI distress or reflux occurs.
- The special diet may be discontinued when drug therapy is reduced to maintenance levels. Encourage exercise and a weight control plan thereafter.

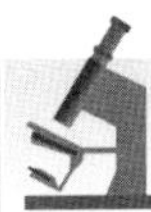

PROFILE

Clinical/History	Lab Work	
Height	Alb, prealbumin	WBC, TLC
Present weight	Ca++	Gluc
aBWef	Phosphorus	Chol, Trig
Edema	K+	N balance
BMI	Na+	GFR, CrCl
I & O	H&H, Serum Fe	Serum phosphorus
BP	BUN, Creat	AST, alanine aminotransferase (ALT)
Temperature	Mg++	Bilirubin
	TSF, MAC, MAMC	

Common Drugs Used and Potential Side Effects

Note—Patients are generally on 3–4 of the five drugs listed below.

- Corticosteroids (such as Prednisone, Solu-Cortef) are used for immunosuppression. Side effects include increased catabolism of proteins, negative nitrogen balance, hyperphagia, ulcers, decreased glucose tolerance, sodium retention, fluid retention, and impaired calcium absorption and osteoporosis. Cushing's syndrome, obesity, muscle-wasting, and increased gastric secretion may result. A higher protein intake and lower intake of simple CHOs may be needed.
- Cyclosporine does not retain sodium as much as corticosteroids. Nausea, vomiting, and diarrhea are common side effects. Hyperlipidemia, HPN, and hyperkalemia also may occur; decrease sodium and potassium as necessary. Elevated glucose and lipids may occur. The drug is also nephrotoxic; a controlled renal diet may be beneficial.
- Immunosuppressants such as Muromonab or Orthoclone (OKT3) and antithymocyte globulin (ATG) are less nephrotoxic than cyclosporine but can cause nausea, anorexia, diarrhea, and vomiting. Monitor carefully. Fever and stomatitis also may occur; alter diet as needed.
- Azathioprine (Imuran) may cause leukopenia, thrombocytopenia, oral and esophageal sores, macrocytic anemia, pancreatitis, vomiting, diarrhea, and other complex side effects. Folate supplementation and other dietary modifications (liquid or soft diet, use of oral supplements) may be needed. The drug works by lowering the number of T cells; it often is prescribed along with prednisone for conventional immunosuppression.
- Tacrolimus (Prograf, FK506) suppresses T-cell immunity; it is 100 times more potent than cyclosporine, thus requiring smaller doses. Side effects include GI distress, nausea, vomiting, hyperkalemia, and hyperglycemia.
- Even if serum Ca and P levels are in the normal range after kidney transplantation, calcium supplements may be needed to correct osteopenia.

Herbs, Botanicals and Supplements

- Herbs and botanical supplements should not be used without discussing with physician.
- With cyclosporine, avoid use with Echinacea and St. John's wort because of counterproductive effects on the drug.

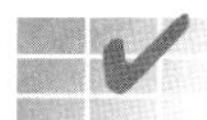

PATIENT EDUCATION

- ✓ Indicate which foods are sources of protein, calcium, and sodium in the diet.
- ✓ If patient does not drink milk, show how other sources of calcium may be used in diet. Calcium supplementation may be needed.
- ✓ Alcohol should be avoided unless permitted by doctor.
- ✓ Discuss control of hyperglycemia when appropriate.
- ✓ Patients should learn self-medication and when to seek medical attention.
- ✓ Discuss problems with long-term obesity and hypercholesterolemia.
- ✓ Encourage moderation in diet; promote adequate exercise.

For More Information

- American Council on Transplantation
  700 North Fairfax Street, Suite 505
  Alexandria, VA 22314
  (703) 836–4301

REFERENCES

Cited References

Alton M, et al. Glucose modulation of the disposal of an acute potassium load in patients with end-stage renal disease. *Am J Med*. 1993;94:475.

American Dietetic Association. Meeting the challenge of the renal diet. *J Am Diet Assoc*. 1993;93:637.

Avorn J, et al. Reduction of bacteriuria and pyuria after ingestion of cranberry juice. *JAMA*. 1994;271:751.

Baroncelli G, et al. Effect of growth hormone treatment on final height, phosphate metabolism, and bone mineral density in children with X-linked hypophosphatemic rickets. *Pediatr*. 2001;138:236.

Beto J, et al. Hemodialysis prognostic nutrition index as a predictor for morbidity and mortality in hemodialysis patients and its correlation to adequacy of dialysis. Council on Renal Nutrition National Research Question Collaborative Study Group. *J Ren Nutri*. 1999;9:2.

Beutler K, et al. Effect of oral supplementation on nutrition indicators in hemodialysis patients. *J Renal Nutri*. 1997;7:77.

Boaz M, Smetana S. Regression equation predicts dietary phosphorus intake from estimate of dietary protein intake. *J Am Diet Assoc*. 1996;96:1268.

Bushman M. Treating fluid noncompliance in the hemodialysis population using unit wide contests. *J Renal Nutri*. 1999;9:35.

Claris-Appiani A, et al. Catch-up growth in children with chronic renal failure treated with long-term enteral nutrition. *J Parenter Enteral Nutri*. 1995;19:175.

Collins A, et al. Hematocrit levels and associated medicare expenditures. *Am J Kidney Dis*. 2000;36:282.

Committee on Nutrition. Aluminum toxicity in infants and children. *Pediatrics*. 1996;97:413.

Curhan G. A prospective study of dietary and supplemental calcium and the risk of kidney stones in women. *Am J Epidemiol*. 1996; 143:515.

Curhan G, et al. Comparison of dietary calcium with supplemental calcium and other nutrients as factors affecting the risk for kidney stones in women. *Ann Int Med*. 1997;126:497.

Curhan G, et al. Intake of vitamins B6 and C and the risk of kidney stones in women. *J Am Soc Nephrol*. 1999;10:840.

D'Amico G, et al. Effect of vegetarian soy diet on hyperlipidemia in nephrotic syndrome. *Lancet*. 1992;339:1131.

Denman S, Burton J. Fluid intake and urinary tract infection in the elderly: questions and answers. *JAMA*. 1992;267:2245.

Devine W, DiChiro J. Current nutrition management of patients with renal disease. *Top Clin Nutri*. 1992;7:21.

Dierkes J, et al. Homocysteine lowering effect of different multivitamin preparations in patients with end-stage renal disease. *J Renal Nutri*. 2001;11:67.

Dobell E, et al. Food preferences and food habits of patients with chronic renal failure undergoing dialysis. *J Am Diet Assoc*. 1993; 93:1129.

Dolecek T, et al. Registered dietitian time requirements in the Modification of Diet in Renal Disease Study. *J Am Diet Assoc*. 1995; 95:1307.

Donadio J, et al. A controlled trial of fish oil in IgA nephropathy. *N Engl J Med*. 1994;331:1194.

Ecder T, et al. Diuretics versus angiotensin-converting enzyme inhibitors in autosomal dominant polycystic kidney disease. *Am J Nephrol*. 2001;21:98.

Engel B, et al. Strategies to identify and correct malnutrition in hemodialysis patients. *J Renal Nutri*. 1995;5:62.

Fernandez-Reyes M, et al. Nutritional status, comorbidity, and inflammation in hemodialysis. *Nephrologia*. 2000;20:540.

Flanigan M, et al. 1996 peritoneal dialysis—core indicators report. *Am J Kidney Dis*. 1998;32:E3.

Frankenfield D, et al. Anemia management of adult hemodialysis patients in the U.S. results: from the 1997 ESRD Core Indicators Project. *Kidney Int*. 2000;57:578.

Frey S, et al. Visceral protein status and caloric intake in exercising versus nonexercising individuals with end-stage renal disease. *J Renal Nutri*. 1999;9:71.

Garg P, et al. Income-based disparities in outcomes for patients with chronic kidney disease. *Semin Nephrol*. 2001;21:377.

Garibotto G, et al. Disposal of exogenous amino acids by muscle in patients with chronic renal failure. *Am J Clin Nutri*. 1995;62:136.

Gerich J, et al. Renal gluconeogenesis: its importance in human glucose homeostasis. *Diab care*. 2001;24:382.

Giannini S, et al. Acute effects of moderate dietary protein restriction in patients with idiopathic hypercalciuria and calcium nephrolithiasis. *Am J Clin Nutri*. 1999;69:267.

Goral S. Levocarnitine and muscle metabolism in patients with end-stage renal disease. *J Renal Nutri*. 1998;8:118.

Hall W, et al. Risk factors for kidney stones in older women in the southern United States. *Am J Med Sci*. 2001;322:12.

Hogg R, et al. Evaluation and management of proteinuria and nephrotic syndrome in children: recommendations from a pediatric nephrology panel established at the National Kidney Foundation Conference on Proteinuria, Albuminemia, Risk, Assessment, Detection, and Elimination (PARADE). *Pediatr*. 2000;105: 1242.

Hynote E, et al. Amino acid losses during hemodialysis: effects of high-solute flux and parenteral nutrition in acute renal failure. *J Parenter Enteral Nutri*. 1995;19:15.

Jansen M, et al. Renal function and nutritional status at the start of chronic dialysis treatment. *J Am Soc Nephrol*. 2001;12:157.

Juneja V. Idiopathic calcium oxalate lithiasis in a recurrent stone-forming patient. *J Renal Nutri*. 1992;2:165.

Kavukcu S, et al. Serum vitamin A and beta-carotene concentrations and renal scarring in urinary tract infections. *Arch Dis Child*. 1998;78:271.

Kaysen G. The microinflammatory state in uremia: causes and potential consequences. *J Am Soc Nephrol*. 2001;12:1549.

Keane W, et al. The CHORUS (Cerivastatin in Heart Outcomes in Renal Disease: Understanding Survival) protocol: a double-blind, placebo-controlled trial in patients with ESRD. *Am J Kidney Dis*. 2001;37:48S.

Klag M, et al. End-stage renal disease in African Americans and white men. *J Am Med Assoc*. 1997;277:1293.

Kleymenova E, et al. Tuberin-dependent membrane localization of polycystin-1: a functional link between polycystic kidney disease and the TSC2 tumor suppressor gene. *Mol Cell.* 2001;7:823.

Kontiokari T, et al. Randomized trial of cranberry-lingonberry juice and Lactobacillus GG drink for the prevention of urinary tract infections in women. *BMJ.* 2001;322:1571.

Kopple J. National kidney foundation K/DOQI clinical practice guidelines for nutrition in chronic renal failure. *Am J Kidney Dis.* 2001;37:66S.

Kopple J, et al. National Kidney Foundation position paper on proposed health care financing administration guidelines for reimbursement of enteral and parenteral nutrition. *J Renal Nutri.* 1996; 6:45.

Leung J, et al. The role of the dietitian in a multicenter clinical trial of dialysis therapy: The Hemodialysis (HEMO) Study. *J Ren Nutri.* 2001;11:101.

Macias W, et al. Impact of the nutritional regimen on protein catabolism and nitrogen balance in patients with acute renal failure. *J Parenter Enteral Nutri.* 1996;20:56.

Makoff R. Vitamin replacement therapy in renal failure patients. *Miner Electrolyte Metab.* 1999;25:349.

Maroni B. Mechanisms permitting nephrotic patients to achieve nitrogen equilibrium with a protein-restricted diet. *J Clin Invest.* 1997;99:2479.

Massey L, et al. Effect of dietary oxalate and calcium on urinary oxalate and risk of formation of calcium oxalate kidney stones. *J Am Diet Assoc.* 1993;93:901.

Massey L, Kynast-Gales S. Diets with either beef or plant proteins reduce risk of calcium oxalate precipitation in patients with a history of calcium kidney stones. *J Am Diet Assoc.* 2001;101:326.

Massey L, Kynast-Gales S. Substituting milk for apple juice does not increase kidney stone risk in most normocalciuric adults who form calcium oxalate stones. *J Am Diet Assoc.* 1998;98:303.

McCann L. National Kidney Foundation Dialysis Outcomes Quality Initiative. *J Renal Nutri.* 1997;7:39.

McClellan W, et al. Can dialysis therapy be improved? A report from the ESRD Core Indicators Project. *Am J Kidney Dis.* 1999;34: 1075.

McQuiston B, et al. Intradialytic parenteral nutrition efficacy: a retrospective study. *J Renal Nutri.* 1997;7:102.

MDRD Study Group. Reduction of dietary protein and phosphorus in the Modification of Diet in Renal Disease Feasibility Study. *J Am Diet Assoc.* 1994;94:986.

Mehrotra R, Kopple J. Nutritional management of maintenance dialysis patients: why aren't we doing better? *Annu Rev Nutri.* 2001; 21:343.

Middleton R, Allman-Farinelli M. Taste sensitivity is altered in patients with chronic renal failure receiving continuous ambulatory peritoneal dialysis. *J Nutri.* 1999;129:223S.

Milano M, et al. Energy supplementation in chronic hemodialysis patients with moderate and severe malnutrition. *J Renal Nutri.* 1998; 8:212.

Milas C, et al. Factors associated with adherence to the dietary protein intervention in the modification of diet in renal disease study. *J Am Diet Assoc.* 1995;95:1295.

Moretti H, et al. Prevalence of low albumin, suboptimal energy and muscle stores in Asian dialysis patients. *J Renal Nutri.* 2000;10:85.

Nakamura T, et al. Effect of dilazep dihydrochloride on urinary albumin excretion in patients with autosomal dominant polycystic kidney disease. *Nephron.* 2001;88:80.

National Institutes of Health. *Morbidity and mortality of renal dialysis: an NIH consensus statement.* Vol. 11, no. 1. Bethesda, MD: U.S. Department of Health and Human Services, 1993; 1–33.

National Kidney Foundation. Clinical practice guidelines for nutrition in chronic renal failure. K/DOQI, National Kidney Foundation. *Am J Kidney Dis.* 2000;35:1S. http://www.kidney.org/professionals/doqi/guidelines/doqi_nut.html

Nelson R, et al. Development and progression of renal disease in Pima Indians with noninsulin dependent diabetes mellitus. *N Engl J Med.* 1996;335:1636.

Nissenson A, et al. Opportunities for improving the care of patients with chronic renal insufficiency: current practice patterns. *J Am Soc Nephrol.* 2001;12:1713.

Nozaki J, et al. Homozygosity mapping to chromosome 5p15 of a gene responsible for Hartnup disorder. *Biochem Biophys Res Commun.* 2001;284:255.

Norman L, et al. Nutrition and growth in relation to severity of renal disease in children. *Pediatr Nephrol.* 2000;15:259.

Obrador G, et al. Pre-end-stage renal disease care in the United States: a state of disrepair. *J Am Soc Nephrol.* 1998;9:44S.

Ohri-Vachaspati P, et al. Correlates of poor appetite among hemodialysis patients. *J Renal Nutri.* 1999;9:182.

Ohri-Vachaspati P, et al. Quality of life implications of inadequate protein nutrition among hemodialysis patients. *J Renal Nutri.* 1999; 9:9.

Qian Q, et al. Treatment prospects for autosomal-dominant polycystic kidney disease. *Kidney Int.* 2001;59:2005.

Pachter L. Culture and clinical care: folk illness beliefs and behaviors and their implications for health care delivery. *JAMA.* 1994; 271:690.

Papalois V, Najarian J. Pediatric kidney transplantation: historic hallmarks and a personal perspective. *Pediatr Transplant.* 2001;5: 239.

Patel M. The effect of dietary intervention on weight gains after renal transplantation. *J Renal Nutri.* 1998;8:137.

Peck L. Essential fatty acid deficiency in renal failure: can supplements really help? *J Am Diet Assoc.* 1997;97:S150.

Pedrini M, et al. The effect of dietary protein restriction on the progression of diabetic and nondiabetic renal diseases: a meta-analysis. *Ann Intern Med.* 1996;124:627.

Rigalleau V, et al. Effects of low-protein diet on carbohydrate metabolism and energy expenditure. *J Renal Metab.* 1998;8:175.

Roberts J. Management of pyelonephritis and upper urinary tract infections. *Urol Clin North Am.* 1999;26:753.

Rock C, et al. Current prevalence of vitamin B6 deficiency in hemodialysis and peritoneal dialysis patients. *J Renal Nutri.* 1997; 7:10.

Rodriguez D, Sandoval W. Nutrition support in acute renal failure patients: current perspectives. *Support Line.* 1997;XIX:3.

Sanders H, et al. Nutritional implications of recombinant human erythropoietin therapy in renal disease. *J Am Diet Assoc.* 1994;94: 1023.

Schnieder R, Wilkens K. Actual and self-reported height in patients with end-stage renal disease. *J Renal Nutri.* 1997;7:83.

Schwedler S, et al. Inflammation and advanced glycation end products in uremia: simple coexistence, potentiation, or causal relationship? *Kidney Int.* 2001;59:32S.

Sehgal A, et al. Barriers to adequate protein nutrition among hemodialysis patients. *J Renal Nutri.* 1998;8:179.

Skutches C, Sigler M. Plasma glucose turnover and oxidation during hemodialysis: nutritional effect of dialysis fluid. *Am J Clin Nutri.* 1997;65:128.

Smith A, Temple K. Selenium metabolism and renal disease. *J Renal Nutri.* 1997;7:69.

Somlo S, Ehrlich B. Human disease: calcium signaling in polycystic kidney disease. *Curr Biol.* 2001;11:356.

Stamatakis M, et al. Factors influencing adherence in chronic dialysis patients with hyperphosphatemia. *J Renal Nutri.* 1997;7:144.

Terris M, et al. Dietary supplementation with cranberry concentrate tablets may increase the risk of nephrolithiasis. *Urology.* 2001; 57: 26.

Tom A, et al. Growth during maintenance hemodialysis: impact of enhanced nutrition and clearance. *J Pediatrics.* 1999;134:464.

Ward P, Kutner N. Reported pica behavior in a sample of incident dialysis patients. *J Renal Nutri.* 1999;9:14.

Williams C, et al. Why oral calcium supplements may reduce renal stone disease: report of a clinical pilot study. *J Clin Pathol.* 2001; 54:54.

Yudd M, Llach F. Current medical management of secondary hyperparathyroidism. *Am J Med Sci.* 2000;320:100.

Suggested Readings

Aparicio M, et al. Are supplemented low-protein diets nutritionally safe? *Am J Kidney Dis.* 2001;37:71S.

Boaz M, Smetana S. Regression equation predicts dietary phosphorus intake from estimate of dietary protein intake. *J Am Diet Assoc.* 1996;96:1268.

Brancati F, et al. Risk of end-stage renal disease in diabetes mellitus. *J Am Med Assoc.* 1997;278:2069.

Brunetti M, et al. Plasma sulfate concentration and hyperhomocystinemia in hemodialysis patients. *J Nephrol.* 2001;14:27.

Cappy C, Stine, et al. The effects of exercise during hemodialysis on physical performance and nutrition assessment. *J Renal Nutri.* 1999;9:63.

Cliffe M, et al. Can malnutrition in predialysis patients be prevented by dietetic intervention? *J Ren Nutri.* 2001;11:161.

Coburn J, Elangovan L. Prevention of metabolic bone disease in the pre-end-stage renal disease setting. *J Am Soc Nephrol.* 1998;9:71S.

Healy H, et al. Are metalloproteins and acute phase reactants associated with cardiovascular disease in end-stage renal failure? *Ann Clin Lab Sci.* 2000;30:295.

Heimburger O, et al. Hand-grip muscle strength, lean body mass, and plasma proteins as markers of nutritional status in patients with chronic renal failure close to start of dialysis therapy. *Am J Kidney Dis.* 2000;36:1213.

The HEMO Study Group. The Hemodialysis Pilot study: nutrition program and participant characteristics at baseline. *J Ren Nutri.* 1998;8:11.

Jones C, Newstead C, Will E, et al. Assessment of nutritional status in CAPD patients: serum albumin is not a useful measure. *Nephrol Dial Transplant.* 1997;12:1406.

Kaysen G, et al. Determinants of albumin concentration in hemodialysis patients. *Am J Kidney Dis.* 1997;29:658.

Landray M, et al. Epidemiological evaluation of known and suspected cardiovascular risk factors in chronic renal impairment. *Am J Kidney Dis.* 2001;38:537.

Lawson J, et al. Prevalence and prognostic significance of malnutrition in chronic renal insufficiency. *J Ren Nutri.* 2001;11:16.

Leon J, et al. Can a nutrition intervention improve albumin levels among hemodialysis patients? A pilot study. *J Ren Nutri.* 2001; 11:9.

Lorelli D, et al. The impact of pre-existing end-stage renal disease on survival in acutely injured trauma patients. *Am Surg.* 2001; 67:693.

Malatino L, et al. Hepatocyte growth factor predicts survival and relates to inflammation and intima media thickness in end-stage renal disease. *Am J Kidney Dis.* 2000;36:945.

Sezer S, et al. What happens after conversion of treatment to continuous ambulatory peritoneal dialysis from hemodialysis? *Adv Perit Dial.* 2000;16:177.

Sharma A. Reassessing hemodialysis adequacy in children: the case for more. *Pediatr Nephrol.* 2001;16:383.

Testa A, Plou A. Clinical determinants of interdialytic weight gain. *J Ren Nutri.* 2001;11:155.

Warady B, Hebert D, Sullivan E, et al. Renal transplantation, chronic dialysis, and chronic renal insufficiency in children and adolescents. The 1995 Annual Report of the North Am Pediatric Renal Transplant Cooperative Study. *Pediatr Nephrol.* 1997;11:49–64.

Whitson P, et al. Space flight and the risk of renal stones. *J Gravit Physiol.* 1999;6:87.

Wilkens K. Nutritional care and renal disease. In: Mahan K, Escott-Stump S, eds. *Krause's food, nutrition, and diet therapy.* 10th ed. Philadelphia: WB Saunders, 2000.

SECTION 17

ENTERAL AND PARENTERAL NUTRITION

CHIEF ASSESSMENT FACTORS

- INABILITY TO EAT ORALLY (MECHANICAL, GASTROINTESTINAL [GI], SURGICAL PROCEDURES)
- UNWILLINGNESS TO EAT (ANOREXIA NERVOSA, FEAR, ANXIETY, PSYCHOSIS)
- DISORDER OR DISEASE STATE :
  - GI OBSTRUCTION, CHRONIC DIARRHEA, CROHN'S DISEASE, SHORT-BOWEL SYNDROME, GI DISEASE FROM HIV INFECTION OR AIDS
  - PANCREATIC DISEASE
  - PULMONARY ASPIRATION OR PULMONARY COMPLICATIONS; VENTILATOR USE
  - CYSTIC FIBROSIS, FAILURE TO THRIVE, CHRONIC MALNUTRITION, VARIOUS CANCERS
  - SURGERY (PREOPERATIVE OR POSTOPERATIVE STATUS)
  - ORGAN TRANSPLANTATION
  - SEPSIS, TRAUMA, BURNS, AND OTHER EXCESSIVELY HIGH METABOLIC NEEDS
- THERAPIES SUCH AS RADIATION OR CHEMOTHERAPY, PAST OR CONCURRENT
- BENEFITS OF NUTRITIONAL INTERVENTION OUTWEIGH RISKS?
- AVAILABILITY OF APPROPRIATE LAB WORK
- ANTHROPOMETRIC MEASURES, SERIALLY
- OTHER PLANNED PROCEDURES AND IMPACT OF DELAYED NUTRITION SUPPORT

COMMENTS ABOUT ENTERAL AND PARENTERAL NUTRITION

The role of nutrition support has grown over the past few decades. Initially, total parenteral nutrition (TPN) was the ultimate standard of care. Then enteral nutrition (EN) was found to protect against translocation of intestinal bacteria, and gut function was also protected; TPN was considered to be a dangerous form of therapy (Jeejeebhoy, 2001). Critical review of the data does not show mucosal atrophy from use of TPN or increased bacterial translocation; overfeeding likely causes sepsis with TPN; and TPN is equally effective as an alternative to EN in patients at risk for malnutrition, who cannot be fed using the GI tract (Jeejeebhoy, 2001). Parenteral nutrition (PN) guidelines suggest that use of PN should be carefully managed (Fessler, 2001). Advances in technology have contributed to improved quality of life of patients under long-term home PN.

Many healthy elderly persons would not wish for tube feeding (TF) especially in the context of advanced disease or dementia. Despite this, the number of patients receiving gastrostomy TF continues to grow. Outcomes and ethical issues of TF must be considered; selection of appropriate patients is important. (American Dietetic Association, 2002) TF, when given in doses with too little water, can result in dehydration and "tube feeding syndrome" and should be carefully managed (Pardoe, 2001).

Full authorization to write diet and TF orders expedites patient-centered care and expands the dietitian's responsibilities beyond traditional dietetic practice. When dietitians are granted full authority to implement their nutritional recommendations, they write diet and TF orders on the physicians order sheets, change existing physician orders, and implement orders immediately, without a physician's co-signature (Wildish, 2001).

Fee schedules for payment of parenteral and enteral nutrition (PEN) items and services furnished under the prosthetic device benefit from the Social Security Act are under federal guidelines (Federal Register, 2001). Reasonable and prudent use of expensive products and supplies is expected.

Figure 17–1 provides a decision tree for interventions to treat malnutrition.

For More Information

- American Society for Parenteral and Enteral Nutrition (ASPEN)
  8630 Fenton Street, Suite 412
  Silver Spring, MD 20910
  http://clinnutr.org/

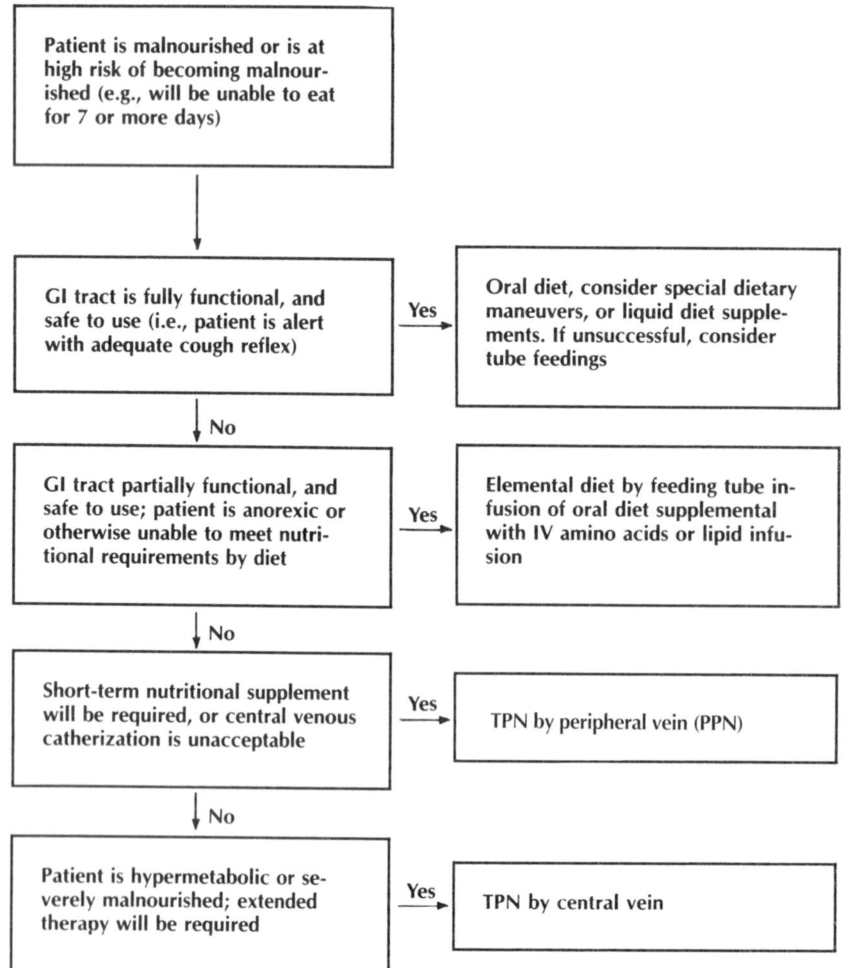

FIGURE 17–1 Decision tree for intervention in malnutrition. (Adapted with permission from Willard M. *Nutritional management for the practicing physician.* Reading, MA: Addison-Wesley, 1982;42.)

ENTERAL NUTRITION

NUTRITIONAL ACUITY RANKING: LEVEL 4 (HOME)

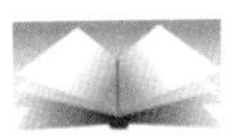

DEFINITIONS AND BACKGROUND

There are approximately 1,000 kcal available in the muscles, liver, and bloodstream as glucose or glycogen; daily replacement is crucial for brain and red blood cell survival. When oral feeding is not possible or is not safe, nutrients should be replaced by other means (see Table 17–1). Specialized nutrition support includes both EN and PN (American Dietetic Association, 1997). EN involves nutrition support via nasogastric tube, orogastric tube, gastrostomy, nasoduodenal or nasoenteric feeding, or jejunostomy for patients who are unable to consume adequate nutrients and fluid orally (see Fig. 17–2). Candidates must have a functioning GI tract for enteral feedings. PN is reserved for conditions in which EN is contraindicated, unsuccessful, or inadequate.

While EN, in its full definition, includes oral feeding, this chapter focuses on TF. EN is more economical than most parenteral feedings. EN yields better nutrient utilization by helping to maintain gut mucosal integrity. Trophic stimulation of the gut occurs with EN rather than PN.

EN has other advantages—IgA prevents absorption of enteric antigens; IgA increases with EN but not PN. Immunoenhancement from TF occurs when increased arginine, glutamine, long-chain polyunsaturated fatty acids (PUFAs), omega-3 fatty acids, and other related nutrients (vitamins A, C, and E and ribonucleic acids) have pharmacologic effects; decreased rates of complications by up to 75% can occur in surgical patients, and lengths of stay in the intensive care unit (ICU) are decreased by 20% (Alexander, 1993; Bower et al., 1995). Pneumonia, sepsis, and bacteremia are less common in patients who received enteral feedings supplemented with glutamine than those without (Houdijk et al., 1998; Wischmeyer et al., 2001).

Early enteral feeding is beneficial if patient is hemodynamically stable, depending on where the tube must be placed. Early intragastric EN is tolerated by many critically ill patients, including ventilated patients (Heyland et al., How well. . . 1999). An early postoperative feeding program can be cost-effective for patients undergoing bowel resection. The average variable direct cost savings per successful treatment patient was $1,531, which required an additional $108 of registered dietitian (RD) time; this protocol resulted in total cost savings of $4,450 per successful treatment (Hedberg et al., 1999).

Gastrostomy feeding may be helpful for young children to correct failure to thrive and other causes of malnutrition (Corwin et al., 1996). Minimal, hypocaloric feedings may be used with intravenous fluids or with PN after birth, especially in low-birth-weight infants, to stimulate GI tract motility and development (Berseth, 1995). Improved feeding tolerance and weight gains are noted, and there is less cholestasis, metabolic bone disease, and necrotizing enterocolitis (NEC) than in infants not given these feedings; optimal protein intake is 2.5–3.8 g/kg/day, with 100–110 kcal/kg/day (Turner-McKinley, 1996). Primary gastrostomy buttons have minimal complications and acceptable longevity; they are preferred devices of long-term enteral feeding in children (Ruangtrakool and Ong, 2000).

EN may be used in similar ways in other conditions as an adjunct to medical treatments. For example, in cancer patients who have undergone surgery, early EN with an enteral diet containing fish oil and medium-chain triglycerides (MCT)-structured lipid is well tolerated and improves physiological function (Swails et al., 1997). Total EN may not improve gut barrier function and may not provide any benefit over TPN in patients who undergo upper GI surgery (Reynolds et al., 1997). Nursing home residents with severe cognitive impair-

TABLE 17–1 Undesirable Practices Affecting the Nutritional Health of Hospital Patients*

Patients at risk for malnutrition have significantly higher length of stay, costs, and home health care needs despite the fact that most receive nutritional intervention while hospitalized (Chima et al., 1997).

1. Failure to record height and weight on admission; lack of weight curve tables
2. Rotation of staff at frequent intervals
3. Diffusion of responsibility for patient care
4. Prolonged use of glucose and saline intravenous feedings
5. Failure to observe or record patient food intake
6. Withholding meals because of diagnostic tests
7. Use of tube feedings of inadequate amount and uncertain composition, especially under unsanitary conditions
8. Ignorance of the composition of nutritional products (vitamins, etc.)
9. Failure to recognize altered needs as a result of injury, illness, trauma, sepsis, or surgery
10. Performance of surgery without ascertaining optimal nutritional status, and failure to replete stores after surgery
11. Failure to appreciate role of nutrition in prevention of and recovery from infection, especially with unwarranted reliance on antibiotics
12. Lack of communication between physician and dietitian
13. Delay of nutritional support until patient is in a state of advanced depletion, which may be irreversible
14. Limited availability of laboratory tests to assess nutritional status

*Adapted from Butterworth C. The skeleton in the hospital closet. *Nutrition Today.* 1974;March/April:8.

ment who receive TF do not survive longer than similar residents who are not tube fed (Mitchell et al., 1997).

Although TF is often started to prevent aspiration pneumonia from oral diet in stroke or demented patients, it can also increase risks according to neurogenic dysphagia studies. For most patients, a dedicated attempt to feed by hand is recommended (Finucane and Bunum, 1996). Because tube-fed patients in long-term acute-care facilities are routinely over- or underfed, only 25% receive their measured energy requirements (McClave et al., 1998). It is, therefore, important to carefully monitor how much feeding is actually given to a patient to determine if needs are being met.

Both underfeeding or overfeeding affect ventilatory status. It is, therefore, ideal to measure a patient's energy requirements using indirect calorimetry (IC) at least once. Uses of IC include assessing energy expenditure in patients who are critically ill, obese, or in whom estimation of requirements are difficult. It can also be used to assess effects induced by nutrition support on the cardiocirculatory and respiratory systems and to monitor the respiratory quotient (RQ) (Brand et al., 1997).

For obese patients, sepsis, wound infections, pneumonia, and other complications may be quite severe. Protein stores will be mobilized, and less protein is synthesized during critical illness. Actual body weight may be the best predictor of energy expenditure in healthy persons, but not in the critically ill. It is important not to overfeed. A hypocaloric, high-protein feeding may reduce hyperglycemia and promote nitrogen retention (Patino et al., 1999).

The definition of what constitutes gastric residual volumes as indicators of TF tolerance will vary. Volume of gastric residuals, which prompts holding or cessation of tube feedings vary from one facility to the next; one high volume should probably not prompt the clinician to stop TF but to monitor carefully and recheck frequently (Murphy and Bickford, 1999). Optimal patient positioning, use of prokinetic agents to improve gastric emptying, and careful abdominal examinations to evaluate for distention are important steps to consider.

For terminally ill individuals, consideration of a patient's advance directives or medical care guidelines must be part of the plan. When a patient's wishes are not known, TF is viewed as humane by a majority of internists (Hodges et al., 1994). When life-sustaining care includes nutrition and hydration, families and other surrogate decision makers sometimes reach different conclusions than when care consists of ventilators or other life support (Mayo, 1996). A multidisciplinary group can help with this important decision-making process.

Home nutrition support is the fastest growing segment of health care, usually for the management of short-bowel syndrome, bowel obstruction, chronic pancreatitis, enterocutaneous fistula, cancer, and severe dysphagia. Use of clinical practice guidelines or pathways may help practitioners to standardize nutrition support for patients (Wolfe and Mathiesen, 1997; Ireton-Jones et al., 1997). The American Dietetic Association recommends four or more medical nutrition therapy (MNT) visits for adults who are receiving EN (http://www.knowledgelinc.com/ada/mntguides/).

Cost Savings and Issues: MNT for patients who are tube fed saves thousands of dollars per case each year. Charts of home PEN (HPEN) patients were reviewed between 1991and 1996 and the annual cost of hospitalization related to HPEN ranged from $0–140,220 in PN patients and $0–39,204 in EN patients; solutions cost $55,193 for PN and $9,605 for EN (Reddy and Malone, 1998).

A multidisciplinary audit at 11 teaching hospitals assessed hidden costs related to EN (Silkroski et al., 1998). Each hospital delivered TF to an average of 38 patients daily using 13 different formulas over duration of 8 days. Problems involved feeding less than prescription, exceeding recommended hang time, and poor sanitation practices. Wastage of 18–62% of product was found at a cost of $26,846 annually per facility. Open and closed systems required 14 and 2 minutes of nursing staff time per patient per day, respectively; these sets cost $47,744 annually.

Patients receive an average of 52% of their goal for energy intake in the ICU primarily because prescriptions are incomplete or inadequate, EN delivery is frequently held for diagnostic tests and procedures, and the amount of formula is increased too slowly to reach the target amount; use of an EN protocol to address these issues is suggested (Spain et al., 1999). Providing a systematic approach for delivery of EN and PEN in the ICU results in quality improvement and cost savings (Schwartz, 1996).

TPN has been standard practice for children with cancer, who are unable to ingest adequate energy. In one study, 10 children with cancer and one with chemotherapy received home EN (HEN) therapy (over an average of 45 days). Tubes were well tolerated, and children experienced minimal complications despite neutropenia and thrombocytopenia. EN resulted in weight gain or maintenance in all but two children. Cost of HEN for all 11 children was $31,315 less than TPN costs (Ford and Pietcsh, 1999). Whenever possible, EN should be considered over TPN.

Nutrition support teams are associated with improved quality and cost-effective care. Teams are often able to decrease complications by 20–25%, decrease lengths of stay, and decrease readmission rates by approximately 43%—for every $1 spent on nutrition support teams, $4.20 is saved in health care costs (Hassell et al., 1994). Registered dietitians with special training and demonstrated competency in nutrition support are able to evaluate, write, or recommend TF or TPN orders (ASPEN, 2000). It is recommended dietitians pursue expanded clinical privileges for these practices, which are often institution-specific (Davis et al., 1995). Proper coding of malnutrition in medical records may also help improve reimbursement for MNT as provided by the qualified dietitian (Funk and Asyton, 1995).

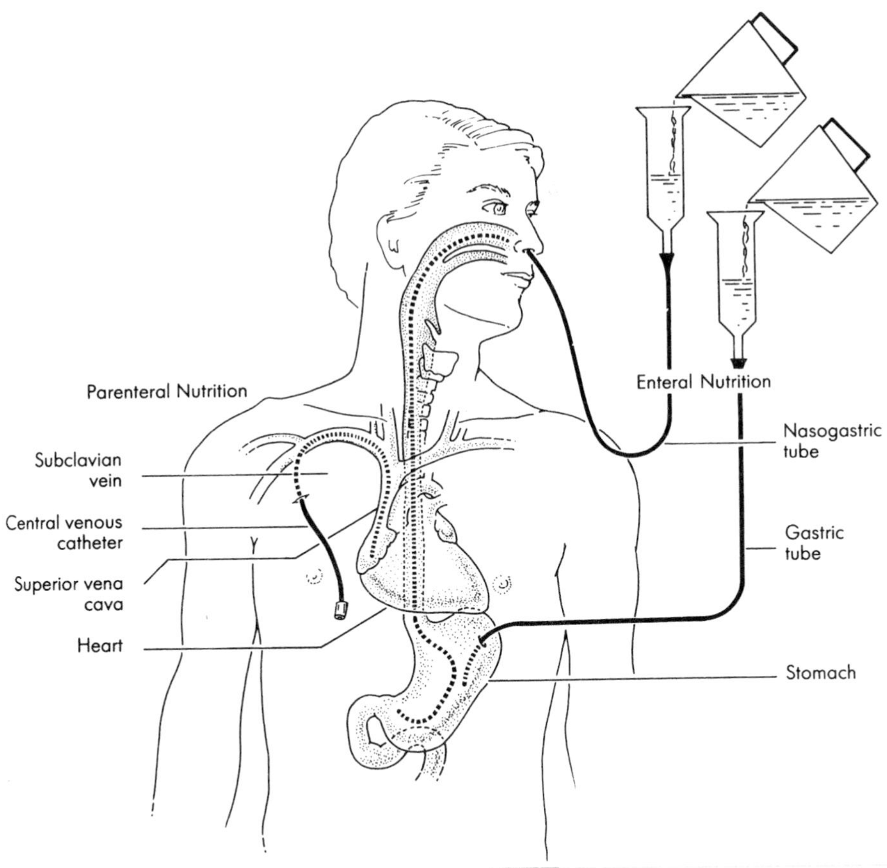

FIGURE 17–2 Enteral tube placement sites. (From Herbert V, Sharpe G. *Total nutrition: the only guide you'll ever need.* New York: St. Martin's Press, 1995.)

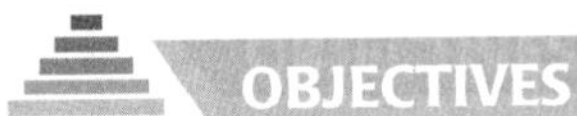

OBJECTIVES

- ▲ Meet 100% of recommended dietary allowances (RDAs) for vitamins and minerals. TF prescription is monitored for adequacy of proteins, carbohydrates (CHO), fat, vitamins, minerals, and water.
- ▲ Conduct a nutritionally focused physical exam including state of hydration, abdominal exam including possible GI intolerance, etc. Assess key factors: state of consciousness, general overall appearance, body composition, presence of respiratory distress, nausea, vomiting, abdominal distention, diarrhea, abdominal cramping, constipation, weight changes, hydration status, and abnormal laboratory values. Alter TF accordingly.
- ▲ Recommend or select feeding tube and site/location based on clinical condition, GI anatomy, and anticipated length of treatment.
- ▲ Formula selection includes type of feeding needed by individual and disorder, viscosity, and calories/mL. Elemental formulas should be limited to specific conditions in which digestion or absorption is impaired or in which polymeric diets have failed (Dietscher et al., 1998). See Table 17–2 for content selection.
- ▲ Monitor patient positioning. Head of bed should be elevated 60–90 degrees during feeding. One difficulty encountered in TF for critically ill patients is impaired gastric emptying: while the small bowel is ready, the stomach is not. A gastric feeding tube can be placed in a reverse Trendelenburg, right lateral decubitus position and 250 mg of erythromycin administered intravenously (Komenaka et al., 2000). For unconscious patient, turn to side to help with gastric emptying.
- ▲ Check residuals; if greater than 150 mL, hold feeding for 2 hours. Replace aspirate to reduce loss of electrolytes and gastric juices.
- ▲ For intermittent or bolus feedings, keep patient on his/her right side or keep head of bed elevated for 30 minutes after feeding to prevent aspiration. For patients at high risk for aspiration, who will be fed longer than 1 month, try a percutaneous gastrostomy (PEG) tube with continuous feeding. If aspiration persists, try a transjejunal tube with lower placement in the GI tract.
- ▲ Patient should be weighed on same scale at regular intervals. Patient should wear similar clothing.
- ▲ Adjust formula, as needed, for constipation, diarrhea, abdominal distention, and other signs of intolerance. Type, volume, and concentration may be altered.

TABLE 17–2 Sample Formulas

1. Blenderized–Homemade (watch for problems with avidin/biotin, Salmonella, nutrient density, viscosity)–Compleat
2. Polymeric 1 kcal/cc–Ensure, Osmolite, Isocal
3. Added fiber–Ensure with fiber, Boost/Fiber, Jevity, Impact with fiber, Replete with fiber
4. Calorically Dense–Ensure Plus, Boost Plus, Magnacal, Two Cal HN
5. High nitrogen–Ensure HN, Ensure Plus HN, Precision HN, Osmolite HN, Boost High Protein, Two Cal HN, Impact
6. Clear liquid–Citrotein, Nutrex, Ross SLD, Polycose, Controlyte
7. Critical care–Travasorb, Criticare HN, Impact
8. Predigested/elemental–Travasorb HN, Travasorb STD, Vivonex TEN
9. Disease-specific–Amin Aid, Hepatic Aid, Nutrihep, Nepro, Pulmocare, Stresstein, Suplena, TraumaCal, Traum-Aid, Travasorb Renal, Travasorb Hepatic, Advera for the immunocompromised
10. Peptide-based–Reabilan, Peptamen, Vital HN, Perative
11. Protein powder additives–Propac, Casec, ProMod

- Fiber-added formulas such as Ensure with fiber or Jevity may be appropriate with diarrhea or constipation, especially if formula will be used over time.
- Adding a few drops of blue food coloring to a formula (12 drops per liter) can help in distinguishing between normal lung aspirate and TF formula. Controversy exists regarding the practice of adding blue dye to feedings because of potential allergic reactions.
- For weight loss, 20 kcal/kg is recommended, 25 kcal/kg to maintain, 30 kcal/kg with mild stress factors, and 35–40 kcal/kg in moderate stress. Nitrogen needs will increase for burn or trauma patients, and the percentage of total kilocalories from protein should be increased in these cases.
- Maintenance levels of vitamins and minerals must be provided and monitored, especially if not given with chosen solution. Additional vitamins and minerals may be needed if volume of formula prescribed is not sufficient to meet RDAs.
- Ensure adequate free water is provided; usually 30 mL/kg in young adults with normal renal function. Determine percentage of free water in formula (70–85%) and subtract this amount from estimated needs; flushes may provide the difference. Monitor for congestive heart failure (CHF), renal, or liver failure, which may necessitate fluid restriction.
- Use feeding at safe temperatures: remove from refrigeration 10–15 minutes before feeding. Do not leave open or prepared feeding at room temperature for longer than 4 hours. Although it is possible to use homemade, blenderized feedings (Table 17–3), safe handling preparation techniques are especially important. Figure 17–3 describes critical control points in a Hazard Analysis Critical Control Points (HACCP) procedure for maintaining a clean TF product in a hospital setting. Figure 17–4 provides a quality assurance audit tool.

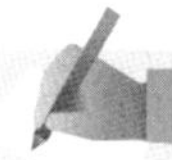

DIETARY AND NUTRITIONAL RECOMMENDATIONS

- Calculate kilocalories, protein, fluid, and nutrient needs according to age, sex, and medical status. Protein is generally 0.8–1.0 g/kg to maintain status, 1.25 for mild stress, 1.5 for moderate stress, and 1.75–2.0 for severe stress, trauma, or burns. The critically ill may need more calories and protein than other patients.
- Check patient's tolerance and side effects; alter formula content as appropriate.
- Sample new products to determine costs and convenience for HEN and institutional use.
- Estimate needs at 30–35 mL free H2O/kg body weight (BW) or 1 mL/kcal.
- Flush tubing with water (25–100 mL) every 3–6 hours for tube patency and before/after medications are given.
- In catabolic stress, glutamine-rich products such as Impact may be beneficial. In critical care, begin at slow rates, insert tube past pylorus if there is delayed gastric emptying. Feed with sensible energy goals such as 25 kcal/kg BW (Bell et al., 1994).
- With a gastrostomy tube, bolus or intermittent feeding is possible. For postpyloric or transpyloric placement, cyclic feedings may be better tolerated than continuous feedings.

TABLE 17–3 Homemade, Blenderized Tube Feeding (Shils/Bloch)

1. Wash hands and counters thoroughly before starting preparation.
2. Sanitize blender carefully before every use.
3. Blend together:
   10 g strained oatmeal
   50 g dextri-maltose
   50 g instant dry milk
   20 g strained liver
   568 g strained beef
   484 g strained green beans
   402 g strained applesauce
   85 mL vegetable oil
   200 mL orange juice
   300 mL whole milk
   500 mL water
4. Product yields: 1 kcal/mL (2,500 mL total volume; 1,312 mg calcium, 1,518 mg phosphorus, 24 mg iron, 7,582 international units (IU) vitamin A, 2.67 mg thiamine, 3.7 mg riboflavin, 27 mg niacin, 163 mg vitamin C, 2,550 mg sodium, 4,150 mg potassium.

Flow Process	*Hazard*	*Concern: CCP or CP*	*Control Criteria*	*Monitor Method: Procedure*	*Action Plan: Criteria Failure*
Purchase ↓	Contamination of enteral feeding products by chemical, microbiological or particulate matter; breakdown in quality control at point of production.	CP (CONTROL POINT)	• Purchase from approved, inspected and certified vendors.	• Monitor vendors for adherence to purchasing specifications. • Inspect delivery upon receipt. • Receive notification from vendors/FDA regarding quality control issues.	• Reject delivery not adhering to specifications without exception. • Follow food recall procedures to address quality control issues.
Receiving ↓	Contamination of enteral feeding products by chemical, microbiological or particulate matter through improper receiving methods.	CP	• Verify delivery based upon receiving criteria. • Immediately remove received enteral feeding products for appropriate storage.	• Monitor receiving process and vendor adherence to specifications for delivery. • Document vendor problems on Vendor Receiving Report.	• Coach/counsel employees in proper receiving techniques. • If necessary, revise receiving procedures according to HACCP guidelines.
Storage ↓	Contamination of enteral feeding products by chemical, microbiological or particulate matter due to improper storage and handling procedures.	CP	• Liquid protein module: verify adherence to temperature standards for freezer units prior to thawing and for refrigeration units during/after thawing. • MCT module and all other products: prevent from freezing and store at $< 86°$ F. Verify the correct temperature for dry storage areas. • Verify adherence to "first in first out" (FIFO), safety and sanitation standards in all storage areas. • Remove dented cans from circulation.	• Monitor temperatures in refrigeration/freezer units and dry storage areas. • Monitor product expiration dates. • Verify safety and sanitation process by conducting monthly Safety and Sanitation Inspections.	• Immediately remove enteral feeding products in affected refrigerator/freezer to a unit that is operating within standards; discard mixed or portioned product that has exceeded 2 hour limit of storage without temperature regulation. • Shut down and repair refrigerators/freezers unable to maintain temperature standards. • Remove products in affected dry storage areas to an area that meets temperature standard. • Return to vendor/discard products that have exceeded expiration date as noted by the manufacturer. • Return dented cans to vendor. • Coach/counsel employees in monitoring and action procedures.
Thaw ↓	Contamination of enteral feeding products due to inappropriate thawing and/or utilization of thawed item beyond specified time frame.	CCP (CRITICAL CONTROL POINT)	• Thaw liquid protein module and frozen Shakes completely using approved method of thawing under refrigeration only. Do not thaw at room temperature. • Label each unopened carton of liquid protein module with the date	• Monitor thawing temperature. *Do not use until completely thawed.* • Verify thawing schedule to enteral formula production schedule.	• Thaw fully if frozen and reject items of questionable quality. Discard thawed items that have exceeded expiration date. • Coach/counsel employees in proper thawing methods. • If necessary, revise thawing procedures according to HACCP guidelines.

(continued)

Figure 17–3 Critical Control Points in an HACCP Procedure for Tube Feedings

Flow Process	*Hazard*	*Concern: CCP or CP*	*Control Criteria*	*Monitor Method: Procedure*	*Action Plan: Criteria Failure*
↓			placed in the refrigerator for thawing. If unopened and unused after 5 days, the product is to be discarded. • Frozen shakes are labeled with an expiration date 12 days from transfer from freezer to thaw under refrigeration.		
Preparation ↓	Introduction of microbes, chemicals or particulates by process and/ or equipment cross contamination and/or employees.	CP	• Train employees in proper enteral feeding product handling techniques and sanitation. • Wash hands prior to preparing feedings or modular components. Prepare according to enteral formula recipe. • Use tap water for reconstituting Pediatric powders and Ceralyte. See Departmental HACCP Plan. *Note: Sterile water is used for the preparation and dilution of enteral feedings for neonates. For adult and pediatric feedings, distilled or sterile water is used upon specific order only.* • Clean and sanitize equipment and utensils prior to use. • Protect enteral feeding products from cross-contamination.	• Verify cleaning and sanitizing process. Observe that separation of enteral feeding products and raw or processed food items and cleaning compounds is maintained. • Verify adherence to enteral formula orders and recipes.	• Discard questionable enteral formula ingredients. • Reject ingredients not meeting acceptance criteria. Coach/counsel employees in proper enteral formula preparation methods. • If necessary, revise enteral formula preparation procedures according to HACCP guidelines.
Cold Holding ↓	Spores germinate and microorganisms multiply at temperatures above 40°F.	CCP	• Seal, label, and date (date opened) opened cartons of liquid protein module used. Store and hold under refrigeration at ≤40° F. Discard any open carton that has been unused after 48 hours of opening. • Seal, label, and date (date opened) opened bottles of MCT oil used. Store and hold in dry storage (do not refrigerate). Discard any open bottle that has been unused after 3 months of opening.	• Monitor refrigeration temperature and verify accuracy of temperature monitoring device. • Conduct daily inventory of prepared or open enteral feeding products to verify expiration and discard procedures.	• Monitor refrigeration temperature for ≤ 40°F. If temperature standards are not being met, immediately remove prepared or open enteral feeding products to refrigerator that maintains the required temperature. • Coach/counsel employees in enteral feeding product monitoring methods. • Discard formulas that have exceeded shelf life criteria.

(continued)

Flow Process	Hazard	Concern: CCP or CP	Control Criteria	Monitor Method: Procedure	Action Plan: Criteria Failure
↓			• Seal, label and date (date opened) opened cans of protein powder. Discard any opened can that has been unused after 1 month of opening. • Seal, label: formula, rate of administration, patient name, room # and date (date prepared) all reconstituted mixed enteral formula and portioned protein, fat or carbohydrate modules. • With the exception of unopened cans of enteral formula, MCT oil and powdered CHO module (which are stored at room temperature), store any mixed, reconstituted or portioned modules under refrigeration at ≤40°F until delivered to patient care units for administration. • Verify temperature accuracy of refrigeration monitor. • Inventory product to detect items at or near expiration.		
Delivery to Nursing Unit ↓	Surviving microorganisms can grow in inadequately maintained mixed enteral feeding products. Spores that survived can begin to grow during the inadequate temperature delivery process. Chemical and particulates cannot be destroyed.	CP	• After preparation, enteral feeding products will be stored on dinner meal service carts under refrigeration until delivered to nursing units according to delivery schedule.	• Monitor timeliness of delivery of enteral feeding products to nursing units.	• Discard mixed or portioned product that has exceeded 2 hour limit of storage without temperature regulation. • Coach/counsel employees in enteral feeding product delivery procedures. • If necessary, revise delivery procedures according to HACCP guidelines.
Cold Holding On Nursing Units ↓	Surviving microorganism can grow in inadequately maintained mixed or open enteral feeding products. Spores can survive and begin to	CCP	• Verify that all mixed enteral formulas, modular components and open containers of enteral feeding products are sealed, labeled as to contents, patient name, room # and dated. • Store and hold mixed	• Monitor refrigeration temperature and verify accuracy of temperature monitoring device. • Conduct daily inventory of prepared or open enteral feeding products to verify expiration and discard procedures.	• Monitor refrigeration temperature for ≤40°F. If temperature standards are not being met, immediately remove prepared or modular components to a refrigerator that maintains the required temperature.

(continued)

Flow Process	Hazard	Concern: CCP or CP	Control Criteria	Monitor Method: Procedure	Action Plan: Criteria Failure
↓	grow during the inadequate refrigeration holding process. Chemicals and particulates cannot be destroyed.		enteral feeding formulas and liquid protein module under refrigeration at ≤40°F in nourishment station refrigerators. • Verify temperature accuracy of refrigeration monitor. Inventory product to detect items at or near expiration. All mixed enteral formulas, opened containers of formula or containers of liquid protein module, MCT oil, CHO powder or protein powder are discarded 24 hours after the production date by Food & Nutrition staff. Opened cans of enteral formula are to be discarded by Nursing staff and are not to be stored in the refrigerator.		• Coach/counsel employees in enteral feeding product monitoring methods. • Discard formulas that have exceeded shelf life criteria.
Enteral Feeding Administration ↓	All enteral feeding products, at room temperature, can support microbial growth. Formula manipulation or using procedures that increase handling of formulas or administration systems increases the potential for contamination.	CCP	• Wash hands prior to handling feedings and administration systems. • Avoid touching any part of the container or administration system that will come in contact with the feeding. • Inspect seals and reservoirs for damage prior to utilization. • Assemble feeding systems on a clean, dry, disinfected surface. • Avoid adding medications directly to the feeding. If necessary, flush tube after administration with tap water. • Date/time each component of the system also indicating patient name and formula (on feeding bag). *Limit hang time of feeding to 4 hours.* • Empty feeding bags of product completely prior to pouring newly opened product into the bag.	• Monitor staff for adherence to proper enteral feeding administration techniques.	• Discard product that has exceeded limit for hang time. • Coach/Counsel staff on proper enteral formula administration procedures. • If necessary, revise enteral formula administration procedures according to HACCP guidelines.

(continued)

Flow Process	*Hazard*	*Concern: CCP or CP*	*Control Criteria*	*Monitor Method: Procedure*	*Action Plan: Criteria Failure*
↓			• Position container to prevent reflux of feeding up the feeding set. • Irrigate feeding tube with tap water (or as specified). • Change administration sets every 24 hours.		• Use administration sets with Y-ports and drip chambers and cap disconnected sets.
Sanitize (Ongoing process through various stages of the system)	Spread of microbes during the cleaning and sanitizing process. Introduction of microbes, chemicals or particulates by cross-contamination and/or employees.	CP	• Train employees in proper enteral feeding product handling techniques and sanitation. • Clean and sanitize surfaces, equipment, and utensils prior to use. • Protect products from contamination.	• Verify cleaning and sanitizing process. • Observe that separation of enteral feeding preparation and storage and sanitation processes is maintained.	• Re-clean and re-sanitize all preparation equipment. • Coach/counsel employees in proper sanitation procedures. • Discard enteral feeding products contaminated during sanitation process. • If necessary, revise sanitation procedures according to HACCP guidelines.

Quality Assessment & Improvement Program: HACCP Plan for Enteral Feeding Preparation & Administration

Completed by/Title:__________ Date: __________ Unit/Room#: __________

Patient Name: __________ Patient History Number: __________

Current Enteral Feeding Order: __________

Instructions: Review one patient on an enteral feeding. *For each "No" or "NA" explain in comments.

Direct Observation	*Yes*	*No**	*NA**	*Comments*
1. Enteral feeding product(s) received according to specification.				
2. Temperature standards for refrigeration and dry storage of enteral feeding product(s) met.				
3. Product usage according to FIFO; those exceeding expiration date returned/ 4. discarded.				
5. Liquid protein module and frozen shakes thawed under refrigeration; products labeled with date placed in refrigerator for thawing.				
6. Unopened and unused thawed liquid protein module discarded after 5 days; open cartons discarded after 48 hours.				
7. Unopened and unused thawed shakes discarded after 12 days.				
8. MCT oil, dry CHO powder and protein powder stored at room temperature; labeled with date opened. Opened and unused bottles/can discarded after 3/1 month(s).				
9. Employees wash hands prior to preparing enteral feedings or modular components.				
10. Cleaned and sanitized surface and equipment used to prepare enteral feedings or modular components.				
11. Enteral formula prepared according to recipe.				
12. Tap water used to reconstitute pediatric powdered formulas and Ceralyte; distilled or sterile water used in the preparation of enteral formulas upon specific order.				
13. Prepared enteral feedings kept separate from raw or processed food items and cleaning compounds.				
14. Reconstituted mixed enteral formulas and portioned protein, fat and carbohydrate modules sealed and labeled (formula, rate of administration, patient name and room number, date prepared).				

(continued)

Figure 17–4 Quality Assurance Audit Tool for Enteral Feeding Preparation and Administration

Direct Observation	*Yes*	*No**	*NA**	*Comments*
15. Temperature standard for refrigerated storage of reconstituted, mixed enteral formulas and portioned protein, fat and carbohydrate modules met.				
16. Inventory of reconstituted, mixed enteral formulas and portioned protein, fat and carbohydrate modules reveals none are past expiration date.				
17. Nursing staff wash hands prior to handling feedings and administration systems.				
18. Nursing staff avoid touching any part of the container or administration system that will come in contact with the feeding.				
19. Nursing staff assembles feeding system on a disinfected surface and inspects seals/reservoirs for damage.				
20. Medications are not added to feeding unless necessary. If added, tube is flushed with tap water (or as specified) after administration.				
21. Date/time each component of feeding system also feeding bag is labeled with patient name and formula.				
22. Hang time of feeding limited to 4 hours.				
23. Feeding bags completely emptied of product prior to pouring newly opened product into the bag.				
24. Disconnected sets are capped.				
25. Container is positioned to prevent reflux of feeding up set.				
26. Feeding tube is irrigated with tap water (or as specified).				
27. Administration sets changed every 24 hours.				

Additional Comments:____

- When patient is in transition back to oral diet or works during the day, night feeding may be used. It may be more energy-efficient than continuous feeding over 24 hours; nitrogen (N) balance may be poor unless calories are adequate. Oxygen consumption, N excretion, and urinary catecholamine levels are higher in continuous feeding over 24 hours (Campbell et al., 1990).
- See Table 17–4 for more considerations with enteral feeding and Table 17–5 for the role of the dietitian in nutrition support.

TABLE 17–4 Key Enteral Issues

FEEDING SITE SELECTION:

Consider any GI impairments or inability to absorb nutrients, vomiting, severe and persistent diarrhea, respiratory disease or skull surgery/fracture, or tendency to remove tubes by choice or inadvertently.

Nasogastric: Often used for temporary needs; tube placed into stomach from the nose.

Nasoenteric: For patients with impaired gastric emptying or in whom a gastric feeding is contraindicated

Nasojejunal: For patients at risk of pulmonary aspiration or with GI problems that preclude stomach placement such as mechanical problems or problems with gastric emptying or tolerance

Gastrostomy: Surgical incision or endoscopically placed PEG. PEG tubes allow long-term feeding. A low-profile device (button) can be used for long-term feedings or for improved body image.

Jejunostomy: Surgical incision into the jejunum to bypass inaccessible areas of the duodenum such as with short-bowel syndrome or obstructions from cancer, adhesions, stricture, or inflammatory disease. Percutaneous jejunostomy (PEJ) is a PEG with a transjejunal limb. A jejunostomy tube may cause some bowel necrosis; monitor carefully.

Gastrojejunostomy: Good for small bowel feeding when stomach must be decompressed (DeLegge et al., 1995).

CONTRAINDICATIONS FOR TUBE FEEDING

Impaired ability to digest or absorb nutrients (e.g., severe malabsorption disorders).

Severe and intractable diarrhea.

FORMULA SELECTION

Generic versus brand-name orders—It is generally more cost-effective to have an enteral formulary established, including multiple products, but one main brand of each category (standard/isotonic, isotonic with fiber, high nitrogen isotonic, elemental, high protein/high calorie for stress, critical care products, concentrated for patients with volume intolerance, malabsorption, specialty products for pulmonary or diabetes or immunocompromised or renal or hepatic patients). See also Table 17–1.

Substrates—CHO, protein, and fat (consider patient's ability to digest and absorb nutrients).

Elemental versus intact formulas—No superiority has been documented for elemental; if not sure of ability to digest fats, use MCTs (e.g., Osmolite or Isocal). Peptides and amino acids may be used for most patients.

Tolerance factors—Osmolality, calorie, and nutrient densities. In general, more free water is needed with a more concentrated formula.

FLUID NEEDS

Generally, 1 mL/kcal is recommended, unless patient needs fluid restriction; 30 mL/kg is most common for adults. Elderly individuals may require slight alterations, depending on organ function.

For CHF, renal failure (RF), or ascites: 20 mL/kg can also be used initially, progressing to 25 mL/kg as tolerated.

For patients with risk abnormal losses due to GI drainage, diarrhea, dehydration, and for those with other needs for extra water, 35–40 mL/kg may be used.

Children must receive adequate fluid, calculated by their body weight.

DELIVERY METHODS

Patient tolerance is key—Ability to meet needs without complications like nausea, vomiting, diarrhea, or glucosuria.

Bolus—Set amount given every 3–4 hours as a rapid syringe feeding; this closely resembles an oral diet for patients who are ambulatory or with long-term and well-established feedings.

Intermittent—Prescribed amount given every 3–4 hours by drip over 20–30 minutes.

Continuous—Controlled delivery of feeding over 24 hours. Less nausea and diarrhea are likely. Once stable, most patients may transfer to intermittent.

Cycled—Controlled delivery over 8–16 hours, allowing some rest periods for patient during 24 hours. Cyclic is well tolerated by older, malnourished, ambulatory patients (Hebuterne et al., 1995).

COMPLICATIONS

Evaluate for metabolic complications, e.g., low sodium, potassium, phosphate, and elevated glucose may occur. Patient may require sliding doses of insulin until hyperglycemia is resolved.

EN may have complications such as mechanical, metabolic, or GI effects.

Proper positioning greatly reduces risks of pulmonary aspiration. With mechanical ventilation, EN can be used with histamine-2 antagonists to facilitate gastric emptying, plus blue dye to detect aspiration, where permitted.

Small-bore tubes are associated with clogging. To prevent or correct mechanical clogging in small-bore tubes, flush regularly with water before and after all medications.

For GI concerns, check for residuals and hold feedings for amounts greater than 150 mL; stop for 4 hours and recheck. For diarrhea, check osmolality of feeding, rate, albumin level, and medications (e.g., sorbitol, magnesium).

Table 17–5 Role of a Nutrition Support Dietitian

Scope of Practice

The role of the nutrition support dietitian (NSD) has clearly emerged as a specialty practice. The goal of the NSD in this position, working in conjunction with other health care professionals, which include a pharmacist, nurse, and physician, is to support, restore, and maintain optimal nutritional health for individuals with potential or known alterations in nutritional status.

The NSD is a registered dietitian with clinical expertise or credentialing in nutrition support obtained through education, training, or experience in this field. The NSD assures optimal nutrition support through
(a) individualized nutrition screening and assessment;
(b) development of a MNT care plan and its implementation;
(c) monitoring and reassessment of an individual's response to the nutrition care delivered;
(d) development of a transitional feeding care plan or termination of a nutrition support care plan, as appropriate.

Other activities may include management of nutrition support services, including developing policies and procedures and supervising personnel and budgets; recommending and maintaining enteral and parenteral formularies; evaluating equipment for enteral feeding delivery; participating in nutrition support committees; and assuring optimal reimbursement for nutrition support activities.

The NSD should provide or assist with the education and training of patients, caregivers, and health care professionals concerning theories, principles, and practices of specialized nutrition support. Furthermore, the NSD may take an active role in research activities to include participation in or generation of research and outcomes studies, with evaluation, interpretation, and application of research results.

The NSD may practice in a variety of settings (e.g., acute and subacute facilities, ambulatory/outpatient clinics, long-term care facilities, home care) for all age groups and across all developmental stages along continuum of care. The NSD may not always work with a formal nutrition support service because the NSD practice may vary on the basis of the individual's position and practice environment, allowing the NSD to have independent, interdependent, and collaborative functions.

Sources: American Dietetic Association, 1998; Standards of Practice for Nutrition Support Dietitians, ASPEN (2000) at http://www.nutritioncare.org/profdev/standrds-diet.html; Fuhrman et al., 2001.

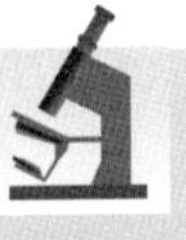

PROFILE

Clinical/History

Height
Weight
Body mass index (BMI)
Intake and output (I & O)
Diarrhea
Temperature
Nausea, vomiting

Lab Work

Albumin (Alb), prealbumin
Transferrin
Cholesterol (Chol), Triglycerides (Trig)
Calcium (Ca++), magnesium (Mg++)
Glucose (gluc)
Hemoglobin and hematocrit (H&H)
Sodium (Na+), potassium (K+)
Chloride (Cl−)
Chest x-ray
RQ (over 1.0 may indicate that caloric delivery is excessive)
Blood urea nitrogen (BUN), Creatine (creat)
Physical therapy (PT)
Serum insulin
Partial pressure of carbon dioxide (pCO2), partial pressure of oxygen (pO2)
Total lymphocyte count
Urine acetone
Phosphorus

Common Drugs Used and Potential Side Effects

- Combining prokinetic effects of erythromycin with proper patient positioning allows a rapid bedside transpyloric placement of feeding tubes (Komenaka et al., 2000).
- Drugs added to TF can greatly alter absorption of both the drugs themselves and the nutrients of the feeding. Monitor carefully for toxicity. Flush with 5–10 mL water after each medication is administered to prevent clogging.
- Metoclopramide (Reglan) has been used to prevent gastroenteritis (GE) reflux and aspiration in patients who are tube fed. Administration 10 minutes before tube insertion seems to increase success rate of tube passage. Gastric motility and relaxation of the pyloric sphincter are improved with this drug. However, chronic use may dislodge gastrostomy tubes; monitor closely.
- Antidiarrheal drugs (kaolin [Kaopectate], Lomotil) can be used to slow GI motility. Their use should not preclude a carefully planned fiber intake. Dry mouth is one common side effect.

- Antibiotics, H-2 antagonists, and sorbitol elixirs alter gut flora and can cause diarrhea because of their high osmolality.
- Dilantin should be administered separately from TF to prevent absorption problems. Tube feedings that are given continuously may need to be recalculated over 21 hours, for example, instead of 24 hours. Rate would have to be adjusted accordingly.

Herbs, Botanicals and Supplements

- Herbs and botanical supplements should not be used without discussing with physician.

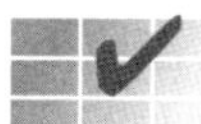

PATIENT EDUCATION

- ✔ Safe preparation of TF, used anywhere, is essential. Some ready-to-hang products may remain at room temperature for up to 36 hours; read product labels carefully.
- ✔ Patient/caretaker should be taught to review signs and symptoms of intolerance, how to manage simple problems, where to call for guidance, and when to call the physician.
- ✔ At least one follow-up phone call or home visit should be made to patients on HEN.
- ✔ If banana flakes are added to control diarrhea, monitor signs of hyperkalemia. Discuss problem with patient/caretaker.
- ✔ Patient should be allowed/encouraged to maintain social contacts at mealtime.
- ✔ When transitionally weaning young children to an oral diet, oral-motor, sensory, and developmental feeding problems may occur. Maintaining a positive relationship, checking for feeding readiness and oral stimulation, and developing a feeding plan should be attempted (Schauster and Dwyer, 1996).
- ✔ For elderly patients, weaning to oral diet, it is volume, rather than energy content, that limits voluntary food intake (Odlund et al., 1996). A careful assessment of total energy requirements and volume is needed.

For More Information

- ✦ American Dietetic Association
  Adult Enteral Nutrition protocol
  http://www.eatright.org

PARENTERAL NUTRITION

NUTRITIONAL ACUITY RANKING: LEVEL 4 (HOME)

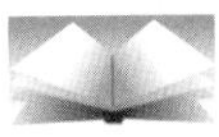

DEFINITIONS AND BACKGROUND

PN refers to intravenous feeding. It is an intravenous nutrient admixture given into the blood with a catheter placed in a vein; it contains protein, CHO, fat, vitamins, minerals, and other nutrients needed and is referred to as "total parenteral nutrition," "TPN," or "hyperalimentation" (http://www.clinnutr.org/). TPN lowers complication rates but does not influence overall mortality rate in surgical or critically ill patients (Heyland et al., 1998).

In all disease states, there is an association between presence of protein–energy malnutrition and poor clinical outcomes (American Gastroenterological Association, 2001). It is difficult to identify that PN makes a significant difference in patient outcomes and should not be automatically used in all surgical patients (Heyland et al., 2001). Quality of life and outcome measures are important indicators to monitor in patients who are critically ill. The following is a recommended list of generic measures: physical function (Katz's Activities of Daily Living Index, Karnofsky Index), mental function (Hospital Anxiety and Depression Scale, Profile of Mood State), measures of recovery (Glasgow Outcome Scale, return to work, return to home), and health-related quality of life (Sickness Impact Profile, Perceived Quality of Life Scale, (Black et al., 2001).

Critical review of the data (Jeejeebhoy, 2001) suggests that TPN does not cause mucosal atrophy or increase translocation of bacteria through the small intestine. Overfeeding, which is easy with TPN, can explain why in some cases TPN increases sepsis. Overall risks of TPN-induced complications have been exaggerated. When there is risk of malnutrition and EN is not tolerated, or there is gut failure, TPN is an equally effective and safe alternative (Jeejeebhoy, 2001).

PN may be most useful in patients undergoing surgery for esophageal or stomach cancers, in preoperative patients who are severely malnourished, and in patients with prolonged GI tract failure (American Gastroenterological Association, 2001). Indications are listed in Table 17–6. Placement sites are shown in Figure 17–5.

TABLE 17–6 Indications for TPN in Adults

General: Standard TPN is indicated for patients: (ASPEN, 1993)

1. Requiring long-term (over 10 days) supplemental nutrition because of the inability to receive daily energy, protein, or other nutrient requirements by oral or enteral tube feeding routes
2. Requiring total nutrition because of severe gut dysfunction or inability to tolerate enteral feedings

Specific: Standard TPN is routine for patients with: (ASPEN, 1993)

1. Dysfunction because of short-bowel syndrome, radiation enteritis, ischemic bowel, or malabsorption
2. Severely catabolic patients whose gut cannot be used within 5–7 days (such as closed head trauma, fractures, burns)
3. Disorders of the small bowel (inflammatory bowel disease [IBD], GI obstruction, inflammatory adhesions, severe diarrhea)
4. After bone-marrow transplantation
5. Cases with a high risk of aspiration
6. Severe acute necrotizing pancreatitis or other severe malnutrition when GI tract will not function for longer than 7–10 days
7. High-output enterocutaneous fistula (Meguid and Muscaritori, 1993)
8. AIDS or AIDS-related complex (ARC) with intractable diarrhea when enteral feeding is not successful
9. Hyperemesis gravidarum and for short intervals during pregnancy when oral intake is compromised, as with short bowel syndrome (SBS) and pancreatitis; the fetus can grow normally without metabolic or obstetric complications (Mamel et al., 1998)
10. After major surgery when enteral access cannot be established

Recommendations for Home Parenteral Nutrition in adult cancer patients (Schneider et al., 2001)

1. HPN may be offered to cancer patients with malnutrition or with inadequate/impossible oral intake
2. Patients need a multidisciplinary follow-up (oncologists, nutritionists, and pain specialists), and this follow-up will make treatment adaptations according to nutritional status possible; active participation of patients and/or their family is important
3. The benefit of HPN on the quality of life of terminally ill patients (vs. hydration) has not been clearly demonstrated. When life expectancy is below 3 months, and the Karnofsky index is below 50, the drawbacks of home artificial nutrition are more significant than the advantages; in this case, HPN is not recommended.
4. Prospective clinical trials are recommended to evaluate the impact of PN on quality of life in cancer patients.
5. Use of educational booklets that mention the telephone number of referring health care and what to do when a problem happens (e.g., fever on HPN) is recommended.

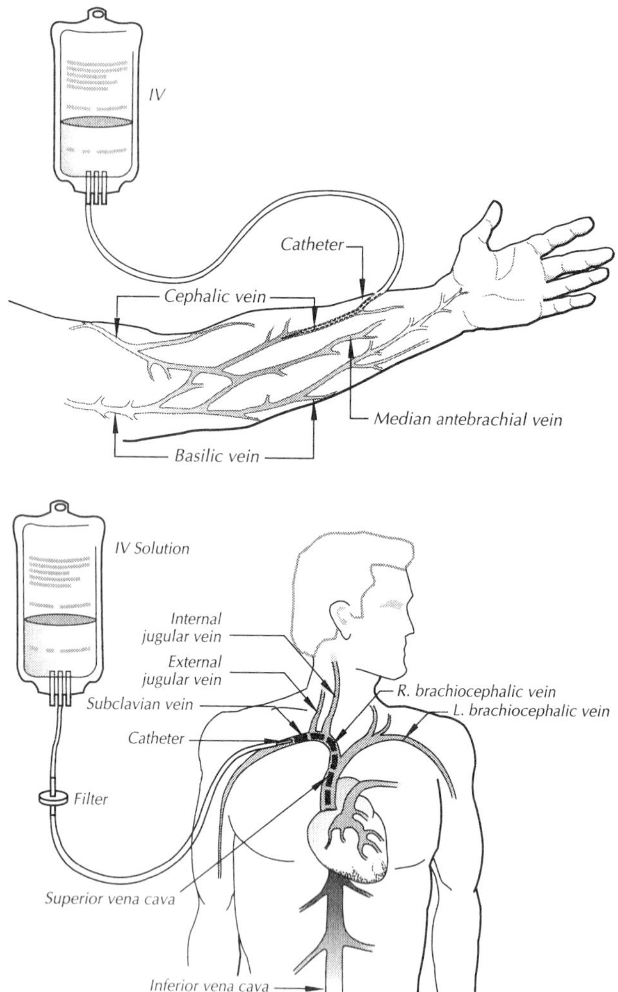

Figure 17–5 Parenteral Tube Placement Sites. From Zeman F, Niedart D. *Applications in medical and nutritional therapy*. Englewood Cliffs, NJ: Prentice-Hall, 1993.

In adults with SBS, small-bowel length is inversely related to risk of permanent intestinal failure; presence of the terminal ileum or colon is associated with increased survival rate and decreased likelihood of dependence on PN (Messing et al., 1999).

Central PN, partial PN, peripheral PN (PPN), and TPN are options for intravenous feeding (see Fig. 17–5). Indications for PPN include temporary losses of GI function (e.g., acute ileus) and occasions when short-term use is indicated such as after minor GI surgery. Adequate TPN/PPN support criteria include reaching a nutritional goal within 72 hours after initiation (Hester et al., 1996). PN may be given by continuous or cyclic infusion, altered according to patient tolerance.

Because a catheter is used, PN may indirectly contribute to increased infection rates in ICU via neutrophil suppression, serum microbial activity, early EN posttrauma results in better TLC count, N balance, less sepsis, pneumonia, and abdominal abscesses (Shronts, 1996). In most cases, gradual transition from PN to EN or oral nutrition is required; this prevents periods of inadequate nutrition where TPN might be discontinued before oral or enteral nutrition is adequate.

In general, PN is more expensive than EN and oral diets. Inappropriate initiation of PN, short-term use of PN, and metabolic complications associated with PN are less likely when patients receive management or consultation by multidisciplinary teams with expertise in nutrition and metabolic support (Trujillo et al., 1999). PN use that is not indicated or is preventable wastes over $500,000 per year, not including the cost of treating related complications. In a study in U.S. academic medical centers, 80% of hospitals and 41% of network partners reported using TPN formulas with excessive dextrose calories (Schloerb and Henning, 1998).

Specially trained registered dietitians may write TPN orders if granted clinical privileges by their institution or facility (Davis et al., 1995). Standardized practice guidelines should be used (Berger and Rosner, 1996). Use of clinical practice guidelines help practitioners administer nutrition support to patients (Wolfe and Mathiesen, 1997). The skills of specialists distinguish them from other practitioners; educators must realize the importance of specific PN training of adequate duration in didactic and clinical settings (Mueller et al., 1996). These skills include competency in fluid and electrolyte, acid-base monitoring, metabolic monitoring, and related areas.

To determine energy and nutrient requirements accurately, use of a programmed calculation may help to prevent administration of excessive glucose and energy in solutions. Practitioner enters basic anthropometric measures and a mean stress factor such as 20% greater than basal energy expenditure (BEE). Daily energy needs are calculated; one standard practice is to divide percentage of kilocalories from fat and CHO. A program is available at http://epen.kumc.edu (Schloerb, 2000).

Obese hospitalized patients who receive hypocaloric TPN, providing 2 g protein/kg ideal body weight (IBW) per day, can achieve N balance when compared with that of patients who received standard protein amounts in the TPN solution; weight change is not a problem (Choban et al., 1997; Patino et al., 1999).

PN may be performed safely at home with proper patient and family training and follow-up. Dependence on PN significantly impacts quality of life (Fish et al., 2000; DiMartini et al., 1998). Travel, sleep, exercise, and leisure activities are most often cited as being altered by HPN.

OBJECTIVES

- Maintain or replete lean body mass, avoiding or correcting malnutrition and its consequences.
- Assess calculations using height, weight, and age; or use indirect calorimetry. Determine appropriate patient requirements for calories, protein, vitamins, minerals, and fluid.

Some studies suggest use of hypocaloric feedings in obese patients to meet N balance, e.g., 50% resting energy expenditure (REE) plus adequate protein (Burge et al., Efficacy. . ., 1994). Fat and CHO make the balance of nonprotein calories after protein needs are estimated. During the flow phase of injury (days 3–15), 150–200 g dextrose per day and 1.5–2.0 g protein/kg IBW can limit negative N balance (Patino et al., 1999).

- Avoid substrate excesses and prevent refeeding syndrome (dextrose infusion followed by increased insulin release, causing shifts in phosphorus, K+, and magnesium).
- Maintain aseptic technique in all procedures for safe parenteral support. Lipid emulsions support rapid growth of most microorganisms and Center for Disease Control (CDC) suggests that lipid-containing PN solutions should be changed every 24 hours (Didier et al., 1998). For this reason, total nutrient admixtures (TNA) with all key nutrients in one bag have been discontinued in some institutions. All PN solutions regardless of lipid content should be used within 24 hours.
- Prevent or correct complications associated with PN (i.e., weight gain over 2 lb or 1 kg daily, indicating syndrome of inappropriate antidiuretic hormone [SIADH] or fluid overload, elevated glucose levels, cardiac arrhythmias, metabolic bone disease, etc.).
- Manage fluid requirements and monitor urinary and enteric outputs or extraneous losses. Avoid fluid overload, which actually may be more common than dehydration in these patients.
- Prevent essential fatty acid deficiency, which may occur when lipids are not administered (Abushufa et al., 1995); prevent excessive use of linoleic acid (Klein et al., 1991), which can cause inflammation and immunosuppression in patients with infection or sepsis.
- Formulate PN solutions according to patient conditions: for renal, review fluid and electrolytes, monitor essential amino acids (EAAs) in the solution. For hepatic, evaluate needs for fluid, electrolytes, and branched-chain amino acids (BCAAs). For pulmonary, increased lipids and decreased dextrose may be needed; the same is true for diabetes.
- IV solutions of calcium, phosphorus, and albumin may contain high aluminum levels (Davis et al., 1999). Risk of toxicity is greatest for infants and children with renal insufficiency who receive long-term PN.
- Transition back to enteral or oral intake when and if feasible.
- For HPN, allow patient to continue usual activity, employment, and a usual daily life.
- Monitor for long-term complications such as liver failure and metabolic bone disease. Parathyroid gland function may be abnormal in patients who receive long-term TPN; this may contribute to disturbed bone metabolism (Goodman et al., 2000).

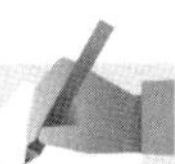

DIETARY AND NUTRITIONAL RECOMMENDATIONS

- Calculate needs for PN related to present enteral intake (calories, protein, fluid, vitamins, and minerals). Usually, 30–35 kcal/kg BW or IBW can be calculated, starting with 20–25 kcal/kg, or use the Harris-Benedict equation to determine BEE.
- Fat should be given daily as a calorie source. If tolerated, 4% total kilocalories should be given as fat to prevent essential fatty acid deficiency (EFAD); a 20% lipid emulsion yields 2 kcal/mL (Didier et al., 1998).
- Be careful not to overfeed because of risk of hyperglycemia, fatty liver, excessive CO2 production, etc. Maximum rate of glucose infusion should not exceed 5–6 mg/kg/minute, the rate of glucose oxidation or utilization.
- Provide weaning when patient is ready; use TF for interim nourishment as necessary. Progress to liquids and solids when patient is ready (e.g., bowel sounds, gag reflex, etc.). Infusion of PN nutrients may suppress appetite, prolonging PN use (Capell, 1996).
- Monitor phosphate needs from anabolism, malnutrition, etc. See Table 17–6.
- Glutamine infusion may be helpful in IBD or for stressed patients but not in hepatic encephalopathy. Glutamine-enriched PN has been associated with savings of $21,095 per patient when compared with standard solutions (MacBurney et al., 1994; Tremel et al., 1994). Short-chain fatty acids, soy, and fermentable fiber also may be needed to reduce TPN-induced bowel atrophy.
- Osmolality is important to monitor to prevent dehydration and other complications:
  D5W = osmolality of 252 mOsm per liter
  D10W = osmolality of 504 mOsm per liter
  D20W = osmolality of 1008 mOsm per liter
  D40W = osmolality of 2016 mOsm per liter
- Dextrose monohydrate in TPN yields 3.4 kcal/g, not 4 kcal/g. For unstable blood glucose, use fat at 10–20% of kilocalories, but avoid overfeeding and consider use of insulin.
- Intravenous vitamin A is only one-fourth to one-third available because it attaches to the plastic bags. Vitamin E is also a problem. Vitamin D is given as ergocalciferol in PN form; beware of excesses, because it may contribute to bone disease that is common in long-term TPN (Verhage et al., 1995). Vitamin K is generally only given weekly.
- Major mineral and micronutrient requirements in adult parenteral use are listed in Table 17–7. Water-soluble vitamins are needed daily; see Table 17–8. For mineral and electrolyte administration, see Table 17–9. Choline is important in metabolic pathways. Investigators are evaluating IV administration of choline for hepatic dysfunction from use of TPN (Shronts, 1997). This is not generally used in daily practice.
- For management of complications, see Table 17–10.

Table 17–7 Major Mineral and Micronutrient Requirements in Normal Adults

Nutrient	Recommended daily parenteral intake in normal adults
Major minerals	
Sodium	60–150 mEq
Potassium	40–100 mEq
Magnesium	8–24 mEq
Calcium	5–15 mEq
Phosphorus	10–30 mmol
Trace minerals	
Chromium	10–20 μg
Copper	0.3–1.2 mg
Iodine	70–140 μg
Iron	1–1.5 mg
Manganese	0.2–0.8 mg[a]
Molybdenum	19 μg
Selenium	20–80 μg
Zinc	2.5–4 mg
Fat-soluble vitamins	
A	3,300 IU
D	200 IU
E	10 IU
K	150 μg
Water-soluble vitamins	
Thiamine (B_1)	6 mg
Riboflavin (B_2)	3.6 mg
Pantothenic acid (B_5)	15 mg
Niacin (B_3)	40 mg
Pyridoxine (B_6)	6 mg
Biotin (B_7)	60 μg
Folic acid (B_9)	600 μg
Cobalamin (B_{12})	5 μg
Ascorbic acid (C)	200 mg

[a] Recent evidence suggests that manganese toxicity, manifesting as extrapyramidal manganese deposition and parkinsonian-like symptoms and/or chronic liver disease may develop with long-term PN. Many clinicians now limit manganese addition to PN solutions to <0.1 mg or eliminate it entirely.

Based on data from: American Gastroenterological Association. Medical position statement: parenteral nutrition. *Gastroenterology*. 2001;121:966.

Table 17–8 Daily Parenteral Multivitamin Requirements–(Derived from ASPEN Safe Practices, 1998)

Vitamin	*Adult Intake*	*Infants and Children under age 11*
Vitamin A	3,300 IU	2,300 IU
Vitamin D	200 IU	400 IU
Vitamin E	10 IU	7 IU
Vitamin K	2–4 mg **weekly**	200 μg
Ascorbic acid	100 mg	80 mg
Thiamine	3 mg	1.2 mg
Riboflavin	3.6 mg	1.4 mg
Niacin	40 mg	17 mg
Folic acid	400 μg	140 μg
Pantothenic acid	15 mg	5 mg
Vitamin B-6	4 mg	1 mg
Vitamin B-12	5 μg	1 μg
Biotin	60 μg	20 μg

Table 17-9 Daily Parenteral Electrolyte and Trace Element Requirements–(Derived from ASPEN Safe Practices, 1998. These values assume normal organ function.)

Electrolytes	Adult Intake	Term Neonates	Infants/Children	Teens
Acetate	As needed to maintain acid–base balance——————————————————>			
Calcium	10 mEq	3–4 mEq/kg	1–2.5 mEq/kg	10–20 mEq
Chloride	As needed	1–5 mEq/kg	2–5 mEq/kg	Individualize
Magnesium	10 mEq	0.3–0.5 mEq/kg	0.3–0.5 mEq/kg	10–30 mEq
Phosphorus/phosphate	30 mmol	1–2 mmol/kg	0.5–1 mmol/kg	10–40 mmol
Potassium	1–2 mEq/kg as needed	1–4 mEq/kg	2–3 mEq/kg	Individualize
Sodium	1–2 mEq/kg as needed	2–5 mEq/kg	2–6 mEq/kg	Individualize
Trace Element	**Adult Intake**	**Term Neonates**	**Under age 5**	**Age 5–18**
Chromium	10–15 μg	0.2 μg/kg	0.14–0.2 μg/kg	5–15 μg
Copper	0.3–0.5 mg	20 μg/kg	20 μg/kg	200–500 μg
Iodide	–	1 μg/kg	1 μg/kg	–
Manganese	60–100 μg	1 μg/kg	2–10 μg/kg	50–150 μg
Selenium	–	2–3 μg/kg	2–3 μg/kg	30–40 μg
Zinc	2.5–5 mg	300 μg/kg	100 μg/kg	2–5 mg

TABLE 17-10 Complications in Parenteral Nutrition

Pulmonary complications–Calculate needs and avoid overfeeding (minimal kilocalories may be best, e.g., 20–25 kcal/kg); CHO provision should not exceed 4–5 mg/kg/minute; avoid fluid excesses. Respiratory failure may occur in patients with limited pulmonary reserve. Prolonged mechanical ventilation can occur with carbon dioxide retention associated with overfeeding.

Lipid abnormalities–Decrease lipids if triglycerides are higher than 300 mg/dL; infuse over a longer time period; calculate that total kilocalories are not greater than 60% from lipids. Lipids over 2 g/kg/day can increase congestion of reticuloendothelial system and impair clearance of triglycerides.

Dehydration–Calculate needs as 30 mL/kg BW or as 1 mL/kcal given; alter as needed for diarrhea, medications used, ostomy, and losses from exudates such as burns or pressure ulcers. Include IV fluids from other non-PN sources.

Fluid overload–Calculate needs and decrease volume to meet needs; diuretics or dialysis may be needed; a higher concentration of dextrose or lipids may be needed if fluid restriction is required.

Hyperglycemia or blood glucose abnormalities–Reduce total grams of dextrose in the solution; add or increase insulin; consider use of lipids as partial substrate; advance feedings more slowly. Blood glucose over 220 mg/dL can cause hyperinsulinemia, increased intracellular transport of potassium and phosphate with hypokalemia, and hypophosphatemia as a result. Impaired phagocytosis and neutrophil clearance may also occur.

Hypoglycemia–Administer more dextrose; reduce or discontinue insulin use; gradually taper infusion rate during weaning.

Electrolyte abnormalities–Monitor fluid status, organ system function, and serum Na+, K+, P, Ca++, and Mg++ regularly. Determine relevant cause or mechanism. Physician will likely follow guidelines as follows:

- Hypernatremia: replace fluids with a more dilute TPN solution; decrease sodium.
- Hyponatremia: diuretic therapy with or without fluid restriction. Sometimes this occurs with fluid overload and total body water excess. Only occasionally, added sodium is required.
- Hyperkalemia: evaluate renal function; decrease K+ in solution and evaluate medications used; reduce exogenous supplements.
- Hypokalemia: increase K+ in solution and monitor K+-depleting diuretic use such as Lasix. Add additional K+ if needed.
- Hyperphosphatemia: evaluate renal function; decrease phosphate in solution and use phosphate binders if necessary.
- Hypophosphatemia: increase phosphate in solution and monitor for refeeding syndrome.
- Hypermagnesemia: decrease magnesium in solution.
- Hypomagnesemia: increase magnesium in solution and monitor refeeding. Consider if magnesium-wasting medications are being used. Additional Mg++ may be needed.
- Hypercalcemia: consider endocrine causes. Evaluate vitamin D, use isotonic saline, and add inorganic phosphate to solution until normal.
- Hypocalcemia: consider endocrine causes. Evaluate for hypoalbuminemia. Add additional calcium if needed.

Altered liver function–From excess energy may cause fatty infiltration and increased alkaline phosphatase. Occasionally, aspartate aminotransaminase (AST) and alanine aminotransferase (ALT) will be elevated as well. Hepatomegaly and cholestasis may also result at levels of 150% or more beyond total energy needs.

Renal function changes–Protein excesses over 2 g/kg daily can increase ureagenesis and decrease renal function or cause dehydration.

Catheter occlusion, venous thrombosis, phlebitis, sepsis–Contact physician or designated member of health care team for evaluation, diagnosis, and treatment of lines. For air embolism, place patient on his or her left side and lower head of bed (HOB) until resolved. Monitor for pneumothorax and ensure that trained staff handle catheters.

Adapted from: American Society for Enteral and Parenteral Nutrition. Guidelines for the use of parenteral and enteral nutrition in adult and pediatric patients. *J Parenter Enteral Nutri*. 2002; 17:1, Gottschlich M, et al. *Nutrition support dietetics curriculum*. 2nd ed. Silver Spring, MD: American Society for Enteral and Parenteral Nutrition, 1993.

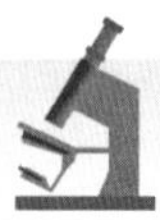

PROFILE

Clinical/History

- Height
- Weight (measure daily)
- BEE/REE
- BMI
- Serum Osm
- Blood pressure (BP)
- I & O
- Edema
- Skin turgor; physical signs of malnutrition

Lab Work

- Gluc (check daily or several times weekly once stable)
- Urinary glucose (check daily or several times weekly once stable)
- Alb; prealbumin (check weekly once stable)
- Retinol-binding protein (RBP)
- K+, Na+ (usually checked daily, then at least 3 times weekly once stable)
- BUN
- Creat (check weekly once stable)
- Alkaline phosphates (alk phos)
- Acetone
- Chol, Trig
- Transferrin
- PT or International Normalized Ratio (INR) (check weekly once stable)
- Chest x-ray
- Ca++, Mg++
- N balance
- Serum triglycerides (check weekly if receiving lipids)
- Serum phosphorus (check weekly once stable)
- Serum selenium
- Amylase, lipase
- Bilirubin
- Serum ammonia
- H&H, Serum Fe
- Serum folacin
- Serum B12
- AST, ALT
- White blood cell count (WBC), TLC
- pCO2, pO2

Common Drugs Used and Potential Side Effects

- Contact pharmacy for drugs that are stable and compatible with PN solutions or nutrient additives. Often, H-2 blockers, steroids, and insulin may be added to PN solutions.
- TPN does not reduce toxicity associated with chemotherapy.
- The nurse often administers Vitamin K subcutaneously once a week.

Herbs, Botanicals and Supplements

- Herbs and botanical supplements should not be added to any intravenous feedings.

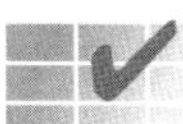

PATIENT EDUCATION

- ✓ Discuss with patient/caretakers the goals of the PN, especially if home TPN will be used. Discuss aseptic technique, I & O records, TPN pump use, medications, additives, and complications.
- ✓ Teach transition processes when and if patient is ready. Assistance from a registered dietitian is recommended (Sousa, 1994; American Dietetic Association, 1994). Nausea and vomiting may occur; eating some type of concentrated CHO during transition is helpful (Nichol et al., 1995). Transition may be possible from TPN to TF if patient tolerates one-third to one-half of kilocalorie needs by that route. To wean from TPN to oral diet, start with sips of clear liquids and advance, if tolerated, to full liquids by the second day; use lactose-free liquids at first. When intake is greater than 500 kcal orally, reduce TPN by 50%. When patient is consuming two-thirds to three-fourths of estimated needs orally, discontinue TPN by tapering (first hour by 50%, second hour by 75%, and third hour 100%).
- ✓ Home TPN (HPN) requires aseptic technique and meticulous catheter care. Infection control measures should be discussed, because catheter-related bloodstream infections are the most critical complication. Change bag, tubing, and cassette every 24 hours or as recommended by home care agency. Long-term consequences should be discussed (such as trace element deficiencies and metabolic problems).
- ✓ Solutions must be prepared under sterile conditions.
- ✓ Discuss problems: when to call the doctor, when to call the dietitian, and when to call the pharmacist or nurse.
- ✓ Discuss psychosocial issues related to adaptation to PN, oral deprivation, and lifestyle changes.
- ✓ Quality of life tends to decline with long-term TPN use. Encourage patient to participate in favorite activities as much as possible.
- ✓ Promote positive communications and collaboration among members of the health care team.

REFERENCES

Cited References

Abushufa R, et al. Essential fatty acid status in patients on long-term home parenteral nutrition. *J Parenter Enteral Nutri*. 1995;19:286.

Alexander J. Immunoenhancement via enteral nutrition. *Arch Surg*. 1993;128:1242.

American Dietetic Association. Position of the American Dietetic Association. Ethical and legal issues in nutrition, hydration, and feeding. *J Am Diet Assoc*. 2002;102:716.

American Dietetic Association. Position of the American Dietetic Association. Nutrition monitoring of the home parenteral and enteral patient. *J Am Diet Assoc*. 1994;94:664.

American Dietetic Association. Position of the American Dietetic Association. The role of registered dietitians in enteral and parenteral nutrition support. *J Am Diet Assoc*. 1997;97:302.

American Dietetic Association. Standards of professional practice for dietetics professionals. *J Am Diet Assoc*. 1998;98:83.

American Gastroenterological Association. Medical position statement: parenteral nutrition. *Gastroenterology*. 2001;121:966.

American Society for Enteral and Parenteral Nutrition. Guidelines for the use of parenteral and enteral nutrition in adult and pediatric patients. *J Parenter Enteral Nutri*. 2002;26(Suppl 1):18.

American Society for Enteral and Parenteral Nutrition. Safe practices. *J Parenter Enter Nutri*. 1998;22:49.

Bell S, et al. Experience with enteral nutrition in a hospital population of acutely ill patients. *J Am Diet Assoc*. 1994;94:414.

Berger J, Rosner F. Ethics of practice guidelines. *Arch Intern Med*. 1996;156:2051.

Berseth C. Minimal enteral feedings. *Clin Perinatol*. 1995;22:195.

Black N, et al. Review of outcome measures used in adult critical care. *Crit Care Med*. 2001;29:2119.

Bower R, et al. Early enteral administration of a formula (Impact) supplemented with arginine, nucleotides, and fish oil in intensive care unit patients: results of a multicenter, prospective, randomized clinical trial. *Crit Care Med*. 1995;23:436.

Brandi L, et al. Indirect calorimetry in critically ill patients: clinical applications and practical advice. *Nutrition*. 1997;13:349.

Burge J, et al. Copper decreases ascorbic acid stability in total parenteral nutrition solutions. *J Am Diet Assoc*. 1994;94:777.

Burge J, et al. Efficacy of hypocaloric total parenteral nutrition in hospitalized obese patients: a prospective, double-blind randomized trial. *J Parenter Enteral Nutri*. 1994;18:203.

Campbell I, et al. Comparison of the metabolic effects of continuous postoperative enteral feeding and feeding at night only. *Am J Clin Nutri*. 1990;52:1107.

Capell B. Parenterally infused nutrients may suppress appetite. *Support Line*. 1996;XVIII:10.

Chima C, et al. Relationship of nutritional status to length of stay, hospital costs, and discharge status of patients hospitalized in the medicine service. *J Am Diet Assoc*. 1997;97:975.

Choban P, et al. Hypo-energetic nutrition support in hospitalized obese patients: a simplified method for clinical application. *Am J Clin Nutri*. 1997;66:546.

Corwin D, et al. Weight and length increases in children after gastrostomy placement. *J Am Diet Assoc*. 1996;96:874.

Davis A, et al. Advancing clinical privileges for nutrition support practitioners: the dietitian as a model. *Nutr Clin Pract*. 1995;10:98.

Davis A, et al. Aluminum: a problem trace metal in nutrition support. *Nutr Clin Pract*. 1999;14:227.

DeLegge M, et al. Percutaneous endoscopic gastrojejunostomy: a dual center safety and efficacy trial. *J Parenter Enteral Nutri*. 1995; 19:239.

Didier M, et al. Total nutrient admixtures appear safer than lipid emulsion alone as regards microbial contamination. *J Parenter Enteral Nutr*. 1998;22:291.

Dietscher J, et al. Nutritional response of patients in an intensive care unit to an elemental formula vs. a standard enteral formula. *J Am Diet Assoc*. 1998;98:335.

DiMartini A, et al. Quality of life after small intestine transplantation and among home parenteral nutrition patients. *Parenter Enter Nutr*. 1998;22:357.

Federal Register. Medicare program; replacement of reasonable charge methodology by fee schedules for parenteral and enteral nutrients, equipment, and supplies. Final rule. *Fed Regist*. 2001;66:45173.

Fessler T. Appropriateness of adult parenteral nutrition use in a large hospital. *Nutr in Clin Practice*. 2001;16:153.

Finucane T, Bunum J. Use of tube feeding to prevent aspiration pneumonia. *Lancet*. 1996;348:1421.

Fish J, et al. Recent developments in home total parenteral nutrition. *Gastroenterology*. 2000;2:327–330.

Ford C, Pietcsh J. Home enteral tube feeding in children after chemotherapy or bone marrow transplantation. *Nutr Clin Pract*. 1999;14:19.

Fuhrman M, et al. The American Society for Parenteral and Enteral Nutrition (A.S.P.E.N.) Standards of Practice for nutrition support dietitians. *J Am Diet Assoc*. 2001;101:825.

Funk K, Asyton C. Improving malnutrition documentation enhances reimbursement. *J Am Diet Assoc*. 1995;95:468.

Goodman W, et al. Altered diurnal regulation of blood ionized calcium and serum parathyroid hormone concentrations during parenteral nutrition. *Am J Clin Nutri*. 2000;71:560.

Hassell J, et al. Nutrition support team management of enterally fed patients in a community hospital is cost-effective. *J Am Diet Assoc*. 1994;94:993.

Hebuterne X, et al. Acute renutrition by cyclic enteral nutrition in elderly and younger patients. *JAMA*. 1995;273:638.

Hedberg A, et al. Economic implications of an early postoperative enteral feeding protocol. *J Am Diet Assoc*. 1999;99:802.

Heyland D, et al. How well do critically ill patients tolerate early, intragastric enteral feeding? Results of a prospective, multicenter trial. *Nutr Clin Pract*. 1999;14:23.

Heyland D, et al. Total parenteral nutrition in the critically ill patient: a meta-analysis. *JAMA*. 1998;280:2013.

Heyland D, et al. Total parenteral nutrition in the surgical patient: a meta-analysis. *Can J Surg*. 2001;44:102.

Hodges M, et al. Tube feeding: internists' attitudes regarding ethical obligations. *Arch Intern Med*. 1994;154:1013.

Houdijk A, et al. Randomized trial of glutamine-enriched enteral nutrition on infectious morbidity in patients with multiple trauma. *Lancet*. 1998;352:772.

Ireton-Jones C, et al. Clinical pathways in home nutrition support. *J Am Diet Assoc.* 1997;97:1003.

Jeejeebhoy K. Enteral and parenteral nutrition: evidence-based approach. *Proc Nutr Soc.* 2001;60:399.

Jeejeebhoy K. Total parenteral nutrition: potion or poison? *Am J Clin Nutri.* 2001;74:160.

Klein S, et al. Lipolytic response to metabolic stress in critically ill patients. *Crit Care Med.* 1991;19:776.

Komenaka I, et al. Erythromycin and position facilitated placement of postpyloric feeding tubes in burned patients. *Dig Surg.* 2000; 17:578.

MacBurney M, et al. A cost-evaluation of glutamine-supplemented parenteral nutrition in adult bone marrow transplant patients. *J Am Diet Assoc.* 1994;94:1263.

Mamel J, et al. Total parenteral nutrition during pregnancy in a patient requiring long-term nutrition support. *Nutr Clin Pract.* 1998; 13:123.

Mayo T. Forgoing artificial nutrition and hydration: legal and ethical considerations. *Nutr Clin Pract.* 1996;11:254.

McClave S, et al. Are patients fed appropriately according to their caloric requirements? *J Parenter Enter Nutri.* 1998;22:375.

Meguid M, Muscaritoli M. Current uses of total parenteral nutrition. *Am Fam Physician.* 1993;47:383.

Messing B, et al. Long-term survival and parenteral nutrition dependence in adult patients with the short bowel syndrome. *Gastroenterol.* 1999;117:1043.

Mitchell S, et al. The risk factors and impact on survival of feeding tube placement in nursing home residents with severe cognitive impairment. *Arch Int Med.* 1997;157:327.

Mueller C, et al. Order writing for parenteral nutrition by registered dietitians. *J Am Diet Assoc.* 1996;96:764.

Murphy L, Bickford V. Gastric residuals in tube feeding: how much is too much? *Nutr Clin Pract.* 1999;14:304.

Nichol J, et al. The prevalence of nausea and vomiting in pediatric patients receiving home parenteral nutrition. *Nutr Clin Pract.* 1995;10:189.

Odlund A, et al. Energy-enriched hospital food to improve energy intake in elderly patients. *J Parenter Enter Nutri.* 1996;20:93.

Olree K, Skipper A. The role of nutrition support dietitians as viewed by chief clinical and nutrition support dietitians: implications for training. *J Am Diet Assoc.* 1997;97:1255.

Pardoe E. Tube feeding syndrome revisited. *Nutr in Clinical Practice.* 2001;16:144.

Patino J, et al. Hypocaloric support in the critically ill. *World J Surg.* 1999;23:553.

Reddy P, Malone M. Cost and outcome analysis of home parenteral and enteral nutrition. *JPEN.* 1998;22:302.

Reynolds J, et al. Does the role of feeding modify gut barrier function and clinical outcome in patients after major upper gastrointestinal surgery? *J Parenter Enter Nutri.* 1997;21:196.

Ruangtrakool R, Ong T. Primary gastrostomy button: a means of long-term enteral feeding in children. *J Med Assoc Thai.* 2000; 83:151.

Schauster H, Dwyer J. Transition from tube feedings to feedings by mouth in children: preventing eating dysfunction. *J Am Diet Assoc.* 1996;96:277.

Schloerb P. Electronic parenteral and enteral nutrition. *J Parenter Enter Nutri.* 2000;24:23.

Schloerb P, Henning J. Patterns and problems of adult total parenteral nutrition use in U.S. academic medical centers. *Arch Surg.* 1998;133:7.

Schwartz D. Enhanced enteral and parenteral nutrition practice and outcomes in an intensive care unit with a hospital-wide performance improvement process. *J Am Diet Assoc.* 1996;96:484.

Shronts E. Enteral versus parenteral nutrition: a clinical review. *Support Line.* 1996;XVIII:10.

Shronts E. Essential nature of choline with implications for total parenteral nutrition. *J Am Diet Assoc.* 1997;97:639.

Silkroski M, et al. Tube feeding audit reveals hidden costs and risks of current practice. *Nutr in Clin Pract.* 1998;13:283.

Sousa A. Benefits of dietitian home visits. *J Am Diet Assoc.* 1994;94: 1149.

Schneider S, et al. Standards, options, and recommendations for home parenteral or enteral nutrition in adult cancer patients. *Bull Cancer.* 2001;288:605.

Spain D, et al. Infusion protocol improves delivery of enteral tube feeding in the critical care unit. *J Parenter Enter Nutri.* 1999;23: 288.

Swails W, et al. Effect of a fish oil structured lipid-based diet on prostaglandin release from mononuclear cells in cancer patients after surgery. *J Parenter Enter Nutri.* 1997;21:266.

Tremel H, et al. Glutamine dipeptide-supplemented parenteral nutrition maintains intestinal function in the critically ill. *Gastroenterology.* 1994;107:1595.

Trujillo E, et al. Metabolic and monetary costs of avoidable parenteral nutrition use. *J Parenter and Enteral Nutri.* 1999;23:109.

Turner-McKinley L. Dilemmas in feeding extremely low-birth-weight infants. *Support Line.* 1996;XVIII:1.

Verhage A, et al. Increase in lumbar spine bone mineral content in patients on long-term parenteral nutrition without vitamin D supplementation. *J Parenter Enteral Nutri.* 1995;19:431.

Wildish D. Medical directive: authorizing dietitians to write diet and tube-feeding orders. *Can J Diet Pract Res.* 2001;62:204.

Wischmeyer P, et al. Glutamine administration reduces Gram-negative bacteremia in severely burned patients: a prospective, randomized, double-blind trial versus isonitrogenous control. *Crit Care Med.* 2001;29:2075.

Wolfe B, Mathiesen K. Clinical practice guidelines in nutrition support: can they be based on randomized clinical trials? *J Parenter Enter Nutri.* 1997;21:1.

Suggested Readings

Allred C, et al. Malnutrition and clinical outcomes: the case for medical nutrition therapy. *J Am Diet Assoc.* 1996;96:361.

Ahronheim J, et al. State practice variations in the use of tube feeding for nursing home residents with severe cognitive impairment. *J Am Geriatr Soc.* 2001;49:148.

Bloch A, Mueller C. Methods of nutritional support. In: Mahan K, Escott-Stump S, eds. *Krause's food, nutrition, and diet therapy.* 10th ed. Philadelphia: WB Saunders, 2000.

Borum M, et al. The effect of nutritional supplementation on survival in seriously ill hospitalized adults: an evaluation of the SUPPORT data. Study to Understand Prognoses and Preferences for Outcomes and Risks of Treatments. *J Am Geriatr Soc.* 2000;48:33S.

Burck R. Feeding, withdrawing, and withholding: ethical perspectives. *Nutr Clin Pract.* 1996;11:243.

Dorner B, et al. To "feed or not to feed" dilemma. *J Am Diet Assoc.* 1997;97: S172.

Fernandex-Alvarex J, et al. Management of spontaneous congenital chylothorax: oral medium-chain triglycerides versus total parenteral nutrition. *Am J Perinatol.* 1999;16:415.

Grave-Fisher G, Opper F. An interdisciplinary nutrition support team improves quality of care in a teaching hospital. *J Am Diet Assoc.* 1996;96:176.

Gura K. National Advisory Groups' total parenteral nutrition (TPN) guidelines: why they are needed and causes for concern. *Nutr in Clin Pract.* 1999;14:318.

Hester D, et al. Evaluation of the appropriate use of parenteral nutrition in an acute care setting. *J Am Diet Assoc.* 1996;96: 602.

Jeppesen P, et al. Essential fatty acid deficiency in patients receiving home parenteral nutrition. *Am J Clin Nutri.* 1998;68:126.

JCAHO Board of Directors. *Comprehensive Accreditation Manual for Hospitals.* Oakbrook Terrace, IL: JCAHO, 2001. http://www.jcaho.org/standards_frm.html

Kayser-Jones J, et al. A prospective study of the use of liquid oral dietary supplements in nursing homes. *J Am Geriatr Soc.* 1998; 46:1378.

Lykins T, Clark. Nutrition support clinical pathways. *Nutr Clin Pract.* 1996;11:16.

Matarese L. Indirect calorimetry: technical aspects. *J Am Diet Assoc.* 1997;97:S154.

Metheny N, et al. pH concentrations of pepsin and trypsin in feeding tube aspirates as predictors of tube placement. *J Parenter Enter Nutri.* 1997;21:279.

Schanler R, et al. Feeding strategies for premature infants: randomized trial of gastrointestinal priming and tube-feeding method. *Pediatrics.* 1999;103:434.

Skipper A, et al. Knowing brand names affects patient preferences for enteral supplements. *J Am Diet Assoc.* 1999;99:91.

Storm H, Lin P. Forms of carbohydrate in enteral nutrition formulas. *Support Line.* 1996;XVIII:7.

Verhage A, et al. Neurologic symptoms due to possible chromium deficiency in long-term parenteral nutrition that closely mimic metronidazole-induced syndromes. *J Parenter Enter Nutri.* 1996;20:123.

APPENDIX A

Nutritional Review

CARBOHYDRATES AND FIBER

Carbohydrates are essential for life. The brain and central nervous system require a continuously available glucose supply. When it is necessary, lean body mass is metabolized to provide glucose for these tissues. Generally, 90% of carbohydrates are absorbed from a mixed diet. Replacement of dietary carbohydrates with protein may decrease risk of ischemic heart disease in women; caution is suggested because protein intakes are usually associated with higher saturated fatty acids (SFA) and cholesterol intake (Hu et al., 1999).

Sugar replacers are sugar-free sweeteners; they are carbohydrates (usually sugar alcohols) but not sugars (McNutt, 2000). Unlike calorie-free intense sweeteners such as saccharin and aspartame, they are used in the same amount as sugars. Sugar replacers have the same bulk and volume. Sugar replacers are usually labeled as "sugar free" or "no sugar added." These products include: mannitol, erythritol, isomalt, lactitol, maltitol, xylitol, sorbitol, and hydrogenated starch hydrolysate.

Both soluble and insoluble fiber play an important role in maintenance of health. Except in a few therapeutic situations, fiber should be obtained from food sources. Between 20 and 35 g/day is recommended (American Dietetic Association, 1997). All dietary fibers, regardless of type, are readily fermented by microflora of the small intestines, producing short chain fatty acids (acetate, propionate, and butyrate). Insoluble fibers (bran, cereal, vegetables) increase fecal volume (bulk) and decrease colonic transit time by virtue of their ability to increase water-holding capacity. They have no effect on serum cholesterol but are useful in reducing appendicitis, constipation, diverticulosis, and perhaps colon cancer; however, mineral depletion may occur with excess use. Soluble fibers (fruit, barley, oat bran, legumes) decrease serum cholesterol by decreasing the enterohepatic recycling of bile acids resulting in increased use of cholesterol for bile synthesis, which in turn alters enzyme activities related to cholesterol synthesis, stabilizes blood glucose levels, and helps maintain mineral nutriture. They have little effect on fecal bulk or transit time. An overview of carbohydrate and fiber classifications is listed in Table A-1.

FATS, LIPIDS, AND FATTY ACID REVIEW

The usual American diet contains 35–40% fat kilocalories; a better goal is 30% daily. Fats are carriers for fat-soluble vitamins and essential fatty acids (EFAs). However, when fat intake is decreased to 25% of energy, it is possible to achieve overall improved macronutrient intake without sacrificing micronutrient intakes (Swinburn et al., 1999).

Fat is essential for cell membranes, serves as an insulating agent for organ padding, and is a rich source of calories. Generally, 95% of fat from the diet is absorbed. One to two percent of calories should be available as linoleic acid, which prevents EFA deficiency. At risk for EFA deficiency are people with low body fat stores, very malnourished persons, and premature low birth weight (LBW) infants.

Lipase is needed for long-chain triglycerides (TG with long-chain fatty acids [LCFA]) and medium-chain triglycerides (TG with medium-chain fatty acids [MCFA]) to metabolize into free fatty acids (FFAs). Most fat emulsions contain LCT and can compromise immune function, elevate serum lipids, impair alveolar diffusion capacity, or decrease reticular endothelial system. MCFAs produced from MCTs are transported to the liver via the portal vein, therefore, not requiring micelle or chylomicron formation; they are now being investigated for intravenous fat use.

Polyunsaturated fatty acid (PUFA) status of elderly women may be more fragile and more dependent on exogenous supply of long-chain PUFAs than that of younger women (Babin et al., 1999). Older women have much lower levels of linoleic acid in their TG and cholesterol levels than younger women.

Trans-fatty acids are made by hydrogenation of vegetable oils to form more solid products (i.e., margarine). The process increases the amount of saturation and converts natural cis-double bonds to trans-double bonds. The ADA supports a new food label including the amount of trans fat in a serving of a food (Stahl, 2000).

Sphingolipids have a common feature—a sphingoid base backbone such as d-erythro-sphinosine. These lipids include ceramides, sphingomyelins, cerebrosides, gangliosides, and sulfatides; sphingolipids in plants, fungi, and yeasts include mainly cerebrosides and phosphoinositides (Vesper et al., 1999). Dairy products, eggs, and soybeans contain the most in our diet; fruit has a tiny bit. They are not essential nutrients but are hydrolyzed throughout the gastrointestinal (GI) tract to regulate growth, differentiation, apoptosis, and other cellular functions. They inhibit colon carcinogenesis, reduce low-density lipoprotein (LDL) levels, and increase high-density lipoprotein (HDL) levels. Dietary constituents such as cholesterol, fatty acids, and mycotoxins alter their metabolism. Figure A-1 shows how fat in the body changes over a lifetime. Table A-2 describes typical sources of fatty acids in the American diet.

TABLE A-1 Carbohydrate and Fiber Classifications

Type		Food Sources
Monosaccharides		
Glucose		Corn syrup, honey, fruits, vegetables
Fructose		High fructose corn syrup, honey, fruits, vegetables
Galactose		Milk sugar (as a part of lactose)
Mannose		Of little nutritional value; found in poorly digested fruit structures
Disaccharides		
Glucose + Fructose = Sucrose		Table sugar, cane or beet sugars, maple sugar, some natural fruits and vegetables
Glucose + Galactose = Lactose		Milk, cream, whey
Glucose + Glucose = Maltose		Malt sugar, sprouting grains, partially digested starch
Oligosaccharides		
Galactose + Glucose + Fructose = Raffinose		Beans and other legumes
Lactose + Galactose + Glucose + Fructose = Stachyose		Beans and other legumes
Polysaccharides–digestible		
Starch (amylose and amylopectin)		Modified food starch, potatoes, beans, breads, pasta, rice, other starchy products such as tapioca
Glycogen		Muscle storage form of glucose
Polysaccharides–indigestible (fiber)		
Insoluble Fibers	–Cellulose	Soybean hulls, fruit membranes, legumes, carrots, other vegetables
	–Lignin (noncarbohydrate)	Wheat straw, alfalfa stems, tannins, cottonseed hulls
	–Cutin (noncarbohydrate)	Apple or tomato peels, seeds in berries, peanut or almond skins, onion skins
	–Insoluble hemicelluloses	Corn hulls, wheat and corn brans; brown rice
Soluble Fibers	–Pectin	Citrus pulp, apple pulp, sugar beet pulp, banana, cabbage and Brassica foods, legumes (such as kidney beans), alfalfa leaves, sunflower heads
	–Soluble hemicelluloses	Soy fiber concentrate, barley hulls
	–Gums and mucilages	Oats, gum arabic, guar gum from legumes, psyllium from plantains, xanthan from prickly ash trees

Adapted from Wardlaw G. *Perspectives in nutrition*. 4th ed. New York: McGraw-Hill, 1999.

OTHER FATTY ACID ISSUES AND SUBSTANCES

Carnitine

When carnitine is in short supply, production of ATP slows down or halts altogether. Deficiency in heart or skeletal muscle reduces muscle efficiency. In renal failure, carnitine may actually be a useful additive to the diet to improve fatty acid metabolism. Carnitine does not enhance athletic performance and is not a "fat burner."

Function: Carnitine transports fatty acids into mitochondria, where they undergo beta-oxidation.

Sources: Carnitine is normally produced in the liver from essential amino acids lysine and methionine.

Myo-Inositol

Myo-inositol has been distributed as a "vitamin," but there is no current evidence that dietary intake is necessary for good health.

Functions: Inositol phosphates liberated from glycerophosphatides acts as secondary messenger in the release of intracellular of calcium, which in turn causes activation of certain

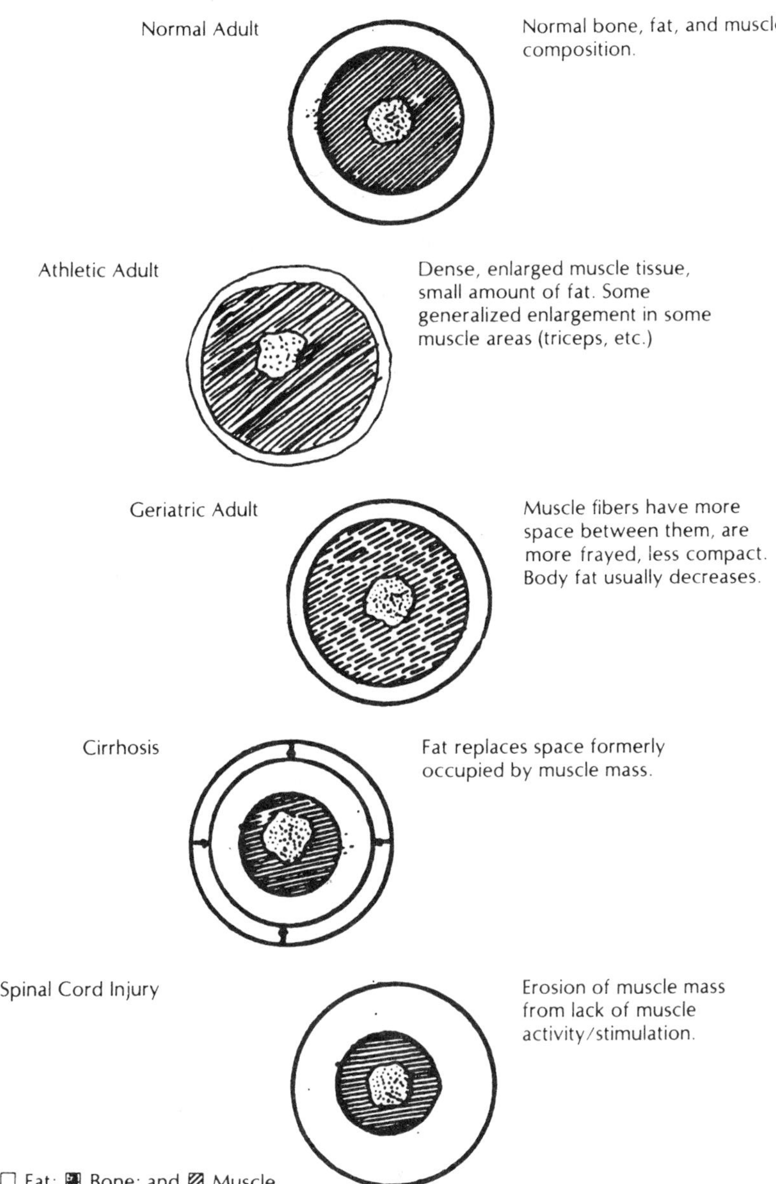

FIGURE A–1 Changes in muscle mass, bone, and body fat in different life stages or disease conditions. (From Brown W, et al. The distribution of body fat in relation to habitual activity. *Ann Hum Biol.* 1977;4:537.)

cellular enzymes and produces hormonal responses; possible role in diabetes mellitus or in renal failure.

Sources: Found as phytic acid in plants and as phospholipid in animals.

PROTEINS AND AMINO ACIDS

Amino acids and proteins are the building blocks of life. All growth and repair functions of the body require utilization and availability of amino acids in the proper proportion and amounts. The main protein source in the American diet is animal protein: Beef contributes 18% of protein, poultry 14%, milk 9%, bread 7%, cheese 6%, seafood 4%, eggs 3%, fresh pork 3%, ham 3% , and pasta 2% according to the 1989–1991 Continuing Survey of Food Intake by Individuals (Smit et al., 1999). Average Total Protein Needs = Infants: 1,700 mg/kg body weight (40% essential); Children: 700 mg/kg body weight (36% essential); Adults: 425 mg/kg body weight (19% essential). Table A-3 indicates which amino acids are essential and those that can be made by the body (nonessential).

To produce the nonessential amino acids from dietary intake of the essentials, it is recommended that the limited amino acids be consumed within a 24-hour period of each other. Protein synthesis requires all amino acids; an insufficient amount of any one may impede or slow formation of

TABLE A-2 Fats and Fatty Acids

Class	Fatty Acid Component	Key Food Sources; other comments
Fatty Acids		
Omega-3-family	Alpha-Linolenic acid (polyunsaturated)—an essential fatty acid	Vegetable oils (soybean, canola, or rapeseed) and nuts
	Eicosapentaenoic acida (EPA)* (polyunsaturated)	Fish, especially salmon, mackerel, eel, tuna, and herring
	Docosahexanoic acid (DHA) (polyunsaturated)	Fish (same as EPA)
Omega-6-family	Linoleic acid—(polyunsaturated) an essential fatty acid	Vegetable oils (safflower, sunflower, corn, soybean, peanut)
	Conjugated linoleic acid (CLA)—group of isomers produced by rumen bacteria and are naturally rich in milk fat; CLA may inhibit atherosclerosis, increase bone formation, reduce inflammatory joint disease, and reduce body fat accumulation (Scimeca and Miller, 2000)	
	Arachidonic acid* (polyunsaturated) metabolic essential fatty acid	Animal tissues (very low—there is no good dietary source of arachidonic acid)
Omega-9	Oleic acid (monounsaturated)	Vegetable oils and lipids
Acyl-glycerols	made of glycerol esterified to fatty acids	
Triglycerides (triacylglycerols) [TAG]	Glycerol with 3 esterified fatty acids	Fats and oils
Mono and diglycerides	Glycerol with 1 or 2 esterified fatty acids	Additive in low fat foods
Phospholipids		
Glycerophosphatides	Glycerol with 2 fatty acids and a nitrogen base	Egg yolks, liver, wheat germ, peanuts (lecithin)
Sphingophosphatides	Sphingosine with 1esterified fatty acid (a ceramide)	Found in myelin of nerve tissue (low in food supply)
Glycolipids		
Cerebrosides, gangliosides	A ceramide linked to a monosaccharide or an oligosaccharide	Found in nerve and brain tissue (low in food supply)
Sterols		
Cholesterol	Steroid nucleus (synthesized from acetyl CoA) often with 1 esterified fatty acid (i.e., cholesterol steroid hormones, bile acids, and salts)	Liver, heart, and other organ meats
Fat-soluble vitamins		
A,D, E, and K	Lipid soluble, some esterified with 1 fatty acid	Various food sources

*EPA and arachidonic acids are transformed into eicosanoids for prostaglandin, leukotriene, thromboxane, and prostacyclin synthesis. Prostaglandins are used in many diverse hormone-like compounds. Thromboxanes are vasoconstrictors (platelets); leukotrienes are for chemotaxis (leukocytes); prostacyclins are vasodilators (blood

TABLE A-3 Amino Acid Classification

ESSENTIAL AMINO ACIDS: Must be consumed from diet	CONDITIONAL AMINO ACIDS: These amino acids are generally nonessential except in illness, stress	NONESSENTIAL AMINO ACIDS: Generally made by the body if adequate nitrogen is available
Histidine (aromatic)	Arginine (basic)	Alanine (neutral)
Isoleucine (neutral)	Cysteine (sulfur)	Asparagine (acidic)
Leucine (neutral)	Glutamine (acidic)	Aspartic acid (acidic)
Lysine (basic)	Tyrosine (aromatic)	Glutamic acid (acidic)
Methionine (sulfur)		Glycine (neutral)
Phenylalanine (aromatic)		Ornithinine (basic)
Threonine (neutral)		Proline (cyclic)
Tryptophan (aromatic)		Serine (neutral)
Valine (neutral)		

Source: Shils M, et al. *Modern nutrition in health and disease.* 9th ed. Baltimore: Williams & Wilkins, 1999.

the polypeptide chain. For valine, leucine, and isoleucine, the requirement of each is increased by excess of the other branched-chain amino acids (BCAAs).

Protein requirement is inversely related to calories when the latter are deficient. Generally, more than 90% of protein is absorbed from the diet. Older women who eat 80% of their total daily protein at their noon meal have greater whole-body protein retention than do women whose protein is distributed throughout the day (Arnal, 1999). Dietary protein utilization is affected by other macronutrients eaten at the same time; therefore, it is important to determine protein quality under standard conditions (Gaudichon et al., 1999). Foods of high biologic value (HBV) contain approximately 40% EAAs. See Table A-4 for biologic value of proteins.

Protein absorption is delayed in those who ingested milk fat or sucrose with protein compared with those who ingested protein alone. The net protein utilization of milk protein is greater when the protein is ingested with sucrose versus alone or with milk fat. Albumin synthesis is lower in men consuming a diet high in vegetable protein compared to animal protein but can be increased by consuming high-quality protein (Caso et al., 2000). EAAs from oral or parenteral sources are considered to be utilized similarly.

Common **nitrogen** end-products from amino acid degradation include aspartate, glutamate, ornithine, tyrosine, taurine, and ammonia. Common **carbon** end-products include pyruvate, oxaloacetate, ketones, succinate, alpha-ketoglutarate, ketobutyrate, and carbon dioxide. Proteins are made from amino acids—histamine is a product of histidine; carnitine is a product of lysine; creatine and choline are made from methionine; neurotransmitters are made from tryptophan or tyrosine; purines and pyrimidines are made from glutamine; creatine and hemoglobin are made from glycine; glutathione is made from cysteine; ethanolamine and choline come from serine.

MINERALS

Minerals are inorganic compounds, containing no carbon structures. There are 22 essential minerals known to be needed from the diet. Macrominerals (needed in large amounts) include calcium, phosphorus, magnesium, potassium, sodium, chloride, and sulfur. Trace minerals include iron, copper, selenium, fluoride, iodine, chromium, zinc, manganese, molybdenum, cobalt, and others. Table A-5 describes adverse effects of excesses.

MACROMINERALS

Minerals that are needed at levels of 100 mg daily or more are known as macrominerals. Estimated intakes of 12 different minerals have been studied and reported by Hunt and Meacham (2001); where available, these data are included in the following mineral descriptions.

TABLE A-4 Chemical Score and Net Protein Utilization of Common Foods

Protein	*Biologic Value (Chemical Score)*	*Net Protein Utilization (in Rats)*
Whole egg	100	94
Human milk	100	87
Cow's milk	95	82
Soya bean	74	65
Sesame	50	54
Groundnut	65	47
Cottonseed	81	59
Maize (corn)	49	52
Millet	63	44
Rice, polished	67	59
Wheat, whole	53	48

Biologic value of food proteins: 100% is ideal. Adapted from Joint FAO/WHO Ad Hoc Expert Committee. Energy and protein requirements. WHO technical report #522, Geneva, World Health Organization, 1973; 67.

TABLE A-5 Adverse and Toxic Effects of Excessive Intakes of Mineral Nutrients

Nutrient	*Excessive Acute Oral or Enteral Intake*	*Excessively Elevated Circulating Concentration*	*Excessive Tissue/Total-Body Accumulation*
Calcium	Bitter taste	Lethargy Somnolence Coma Anorexia Constipation Subcutaneous fat necrosis	Hypercalcemia
Chromium	For chromates: Nausea and vomiting For chromic salts: None known	Increased insulin sensitivity and hypoglycemia (theoretical)	None known
Copper	Nausea Vomiting GI hemorrhage	Hemolytic anemia Jaundice	Chronic hepatic cirrhosis Acute hepatic necrosis Jaundice
Iron	Nausea Vomiting Metallic taste Discolored (black) stools	Increased susceptibility to gram-negative septicemias Dizziness Peripheral vascular collapse Anaphylaxis (to iron dextrans)	Hemosiderosis Splenomegaly Negative chromium balance Increased susceptibility to intracellular infections Hemochromatosis (genetic predisposition or iron overloading)
Magnesium	Laxative effect Diarrhea	Transient hypocalcemia Respiratory paralysis Cardiac arrest	None known
Manganese	None known	None known	Schizophrenia-like psychotic disorder Parkinson's disease-like neurologic disorder
Molybdenum	None known	None known	Hypercupruria Genu valgum (in India)
Nickel	Allergic reactions (dermatitis or rash)	Allergic reactions (dermatitis or rash)	None known
Phosphorus	Hypocalcemia (with possible resultant tetany)	None known	None known
Selenium	None known	Peripheral vascular collapse	Weakened fingernails and toenails Dental enamel defects Hair loss Dermatitis Generalized tremor Garlic odor of breath
Silicon	Gritty taste	None known	None known
Zinc	Nausea Vomiting Metallic taste Epigastric distress Gastric erosion	Sweating Dizziness Tachycardia	T cell dysfunction Phagocytic dysfunction Elevated LDL/HDL ratio in serum lipid pattern

Calcium

Calcium absorption is dependent upon the calcium needs of the body, foods eaten, and the amount of calcium in foods eaten. Vitamin D, whether from diet or exposure to the ultraviolet light of the sun, increases calcium absorption. Calcium absorption tends to decrease with increased age for both men and women. According to recent USDA surveys, average calcium intakes for women and younger men are below their recommended dietary allowance (RDA). The average calcium intake by women 20–29 years of age was about 778 mg per day, and the intake by women 30–50 years of age was about 719 mg; average calcium intake by men 20–29 years of age was 1,075 mg. New RDA for calcium is 1,000 mg for most adults; 1,300 for teenagers; 1,200 mg for those over age 50.

Roles: For strong bones and teeth, nerve irritability, muscle contraction, heart rhythm, blood coagulation, enzymes, osmotic pressure, intercellular cement, maintenance of cell membranes, and permeability helps protect against high blood pressure.

About 60% is bound to protein, mostly albumin. About 30–60% absorption occurs with intakes of 400–1,000 mg.

Sources: In 1990, ¾ of the calcium in our diet came from dairy products. Milk and cheese products remain the primary source of calcium for Americans (Hunt and Meacham, 2001). Foods that contain small amounts of calcium but are not considered good sources can contribute significant amounts of calcium to an individual's diet if these foods are eaten often or in large amounts—oysters, dried fruit, green leafy vegetables, salmon and sardines with bones, molasses, and tofu. Some foods, such as orange juice, bread, and ready-to-eat cereals, are not normally good sources of calcium but may have had calcium added. Most instant-prepared cereals are fortified with calcium; check labels on the carton or package for the percentage of the U.S. RDA. Phytates and excessive protein or zinc decrease absorption. Calcium-fortified soy milk does not provide as much calcium as cow's milk, and the calcium from soy milk is absorbed only 75% as efficient as from cow's milk (Heaney et al., 2000). Chinese vegetables that contain high oxalate levels may not provide good calcium bioavailability (Weaver et al., 1997). Calcium is lost in cooking some foods even under the best conditions. To retain calcium, cook foods in a minimal amount of water and for the shortest possible time.

Calcium Substitutes for Milk:

1 cup plain nonfat yogurt = 452 mg
3 oz sardines, canned, with bones = 372 mg
1 cup fruited low fat yogurt = 345 mg
1 cup almonds = 332 mg
1 cup Brazil nuts = 260 mg
1 cup frozen yogurt = 240 mg
1 cup oysters = 226 mg
1 cup rhubarb = 174 mg
3 oz salmon, canned, with bones = 167 mg
1 cup pork and beans = 138 mg
1 cup spinach, cooked = 138 mg
1 T blackstrap molasses = 137 mg
1 cup tofu = 130 mg
1 cup dates = 130 mg
1 cup peanuts = 107 mg
1 cup cranberry sauce = 104 mg
1 cup dried apricots = 100 mg
½ cup turnip greens = 99 mg
½ cup kale, cooked = 90 mg
1 cup broccoli, cooked = 72 mg

Signs of Deficiency: Hypocalcemia, tetany, paresthesia, hyperirritability, muscle cramps, convulsions, and stunting in growth. Premenstrual syndrome (PMS) is associated with a calcium deficiency, and calcium supplements often alleviate the symptoms of PMS (Schrezenmeir and Miller, 2000).

Signs of Excess: Hypercalcemia, loss of intestinal tone, kidney failure, and psychosis. Recommending excessive calcium use in the general, unsupervised public may not be advisable; this mineral has antagonistic effects on vitamin D and boron that cannot be overlooked (Mertz, 1994).

Chloride

Chloride constitutes about 3% of total mineral content in the body. It is the main extracellular ion, along with sodium. No RDA or upper limit (UL) levels have been established.

Roles: Digestion (HCl in stomach), acid-base balance, O2/CO2 exchange in red blood cells (RBCs), and fluid balance.

Sources: Table salt, salt substitutes containing potassium chloride, processed foods made with table salt, sauerkraut, snack chips, and green olives.

Signs of Deficiency: Hypochlorhydria and disturbed acid-base-balance.

Signs of Excess: Disturbed acid-base balance.

Magnesium

Magnesium is a mineral needed by every cell of the body; half of the stores are found inside cells of body tissues and organs, and half are combined with calcium and phosphorus in bone. Only 1% of magnesium in the body is found in blood. The body works hard to keep blood levels of magnesium constant. Results of two national surveys indicated that the diets of most adult men and women do not provide the recommended amounts of magnesium. Adults age 70 and over eat less magnesium than younger adults, and non-Hispanic black subjects consume less magnesium than either non-Hispanic white or Hispanic subjects. In spite of poor intakes, magnesium deficiency is rarely seen in the United States in adults. RDA varies by age but is typically 420 mg for men and 320 mg for women. UL for supplemental magnesium for adolescents and adults is 350 mg daily.

Roles: Magnesium is needed for more than 300 biochemical reactions in the body. It helps maintain normal muscle contraction, nerve transmission and function, heart rhythm, energy metabolism and protein synthesis, enzyme activation (ADP, ATP), glucose utilization, prevention of atherosclerosis, bone matrix and growth, and normal Na+/K+ pump. Maintaining an adequate magnesium intake is a positive lifestyle modification for preventing and managing high blood pressure. Magnesium deficiency can cause metabolic changes that may contribute to heart attacks and strokes; population surveys have associated higher blood levels of magnesium with lower risk of coronary heart disease. Magnesium deficiency may also be a risk factor for postmenopausal osteoporosis. Elevated blood glucose levels increase the loss of magnesium in the urine, which in turn lowers blood levels of magnesium; this explains why low blood levels of magnesium (hypomagnesemia) are seen in poorly controlled type 1 and type 2 diabetes.

Sources: Green vegetables such as spinach provide magnesium, because the center of the chlorophyll molecule contains magnesium. Nuts, seeds, and some whole grains (wheat germ, bran) are also good sources of magnesium. Although magnesium is present in many foods, it usually occurs in small amounts. As with most nutrients, daily needs for magnesium cannot be met from a single food. Eating a wide variety of foods, including five servings of fruits and vegetables daily and plenty of whole grains, helps to ensure an adequate intake. Other sources include avocado, pumpkin seeds, cocoa, chocolate, soybeans, dried beans, peas, beet greens and other green leafy vegetables, meats, seafood, milk, tofu, and chili. Intake from a meal may be 45–55% absorbed. Beware of excess phytates. In the United States, milk and cheese contribute to the diets of infants and toddlers, as well as adolescents; beverages such as instant coffee are often contributors of magnesium to the diets of adults and seniors (Hunt and Meacham, 2001).

Water can provide magnesium, but the amount varies according to the water supply. "Hard" water contains more magnesium than "soft" water. Dietary surveys do not estimate magnesium intake from water, which may lead to underestimating total magnesium intake and its variability.

Signs of Deficiency: Hypomagnesemia. Poor growth, confusion, disorientation, loss of appetite, depression, tetany with muscle contractions and cramps, tingling, numbness, abnormal heart rhythms, coronary spasm, abnormal nerve function with seizures or convulsions, hyperirritability, and even death. When magnesium deficiency does occur, it is usually due to excessive loss of magnesium in urine from diabetes, antibiotics, diuretics, or excessive alcohol use, GI system disorders that cause a loss of magnesium or limit magnesium absorption, or chronically low intake of magnesium. Chronic or excessive vomiting, diarrhea, and fat malabsorption may also result in magnesium depletion.

Signs of Excess: Hypermagnesemia. Mental status changes, nausea, diarrhea, appetite loss, muscle weakness, difficulty breathing or respiratory failure, extremely low blood pressure, and irregular heartbeat. High doses of magnesium supplements, which may be added to laxatives, can promote diarrhea. Magnesium toxicity is more often associated with kidney failure, when the kidney loses the ability to remove excess magnesium. Very large doses of laxatives also have been associated with magnesium toxicity, even with normal kidney function. The elderly are at risk of magnesium toxicity, because kidney function declines with age, and they are more likely to take magnesium-containing laxatives and antacids.

Phosphorus

Phosphorus is second only to calcium in quantity in the human body. About 80% is in the skeleton and teeth as calcium phosphate; 20% is in extracellular fluid and cells. About 10% is bound to protein. RDA for adult men and women is 700 mg/day. UL for adults varies from 3–4 g/day.

Roles: Energy metabolism (ADP, ATP); fat, amino acid, and carbohydrate (CHO) metabolism, calcium (Ca^{++}) regulation, vitamin utilization, bones and teeth, osmotic pressure, DNA coding, buffer salts, fatty acid transport, oxygen transport and release, leukocyte phagocytosis, and microbial resistance.

Sources: Protein-rich foods such as meat, poultry, fish, egg yolks, dried beans and nuts, whole grains, enriched breads and cereals, milk, cheese, and dairy products. Also found in peas, corn, chocolate, and seeds. Excessive intake of soft drinks increases phosphorus intake, often causing an unbalanced intake of calcium. About 70% of oral intake is absorbed. In the United States, milk and cheese products contribute the main sources of phosphorus for infants, toddlers, and adolescents; meat/poultry/fish products contribute more to the diets of adults and seniors (Hunt and Meacham, 2001).

Signs of Deficiency: Hypophosphatemia, neuromuscular and hematologic changes, rickets, osteomalacia, and renal changes. Deficiency is rare but may occur in those persons who take phosphate binders, total parenteral nutrition (TPN) without phosphate, and prematurity.

Signs of Excess: Hyperphosphatemia, especially problematic in renal failure. Nutritional secondary hyperparathyroidism may occur, with fragile bones and fractures.

Potassium

Potassium constitutes about 5% of total mineral content in the body. It is the main intracellular ion. No specific RDA exists.

Roles: Nerve conduction, muscle contraction, glycolysis, glycogen formation, protein synthesis and utilization, acid-base balance, cellular enzyme functioning, and water balance.

Sources: Fruits and vegetables (see below), dried beans and peas, whole grains, and whole and skim milk. In the United States, milk and cheese products contribute the main sources of potassium for infants, toddlers, and adolescents; meat/poultry/fish products contribute more to the diets of adults and seniors, with vegetables a secondary source (Hunt and Meacham, 2001).

Each food listed contains > 500 mg K+ per serving:

1 t cream of tartar (on cereal, etc.)
1 cup prune or tomato juice
1 ¼ cup orange or citrus juice
1 medium banana (1 small banana, 400 mg)
7–8 dates or 4 figs
7 large prunes or 1/2 cup dark raisins
6 fresh apricots
1 ½ cups milk (any kind)
½ cantaloupe
1 cup broccoli
¾ cup winter squash
1 large white or sweet potato
½ avocado (600 mg)
2 T molasses
½ cup nuts
¾ cup dry beans, cooked
½ t salt substitute (most brands)

Signs of Deficiency: Hypokalemia. Muscle weakness, cardiac arrhythmia, paralysis, bone fragility, decreased growth, weight loss, and even death.

Signs of Excess: Hyperkalemia. Paralysis, muscular weakness, arrhythmias and heart disturbances, and even death.

Sodium

Sodium constitutes about 2% of total mineral content in the body. It is the main extracellular ion, along with chloride. No specific RDA exists.

Roles: Nerve stimulation, muscle contraction, acid-base balance, regulation of blood pressure, and glucose transport into cells. Sodium is the major extracellular fluid cation.

Sources: Milk, cheese, eggs, meat, fish, poultry, beets, carrots, celery, spinach, chard, seasoned salts, baking powder and soda, table salt (NaCl), many drugs and preservatives, some drinking water, and salt added to processed foods.

More than 95% from a mixed diet is absorbed. In the United States, infants receive the greatest amount of sodium from milk and cheese products; grain products are the primary source for all other age groups, and meat/poultry/fish are secondary sources for adults and seniors (Hunt and Meacham, 2001).

Signs of Deficiency: Hyponatremia, water intoxication, anorexia, nausea, muscle atrophy, poor growth, weight loss, confusion, coma, and even death.

Signs of Excess: Hypernatremia. Confusion, coma. High blood pressure and calcium excretion from bones may result. Heart failure and edema may also result from excesses.

Sulfur

Sulfur exists as part of the amino acids, methionine, cystine, and cysteine and as part of the antioxidant glutathione peroxidase and other organic molecules. No specific RDA exists.

Roles: Amino acids (methionine, cystine, cysteine), thiamin molecule, coenzyme A, biotin and pantothenic acid, connective tissue metabolism, penicillin, sulfa drugs, insulin molecule, heparin, and keratin of skin, hair, and nails.

Sources: Meat, poultry, fish, eggs, dried beans and legumes, Brassica family vegetables (broccoli, cabbage, etc.), and wheat germ.

Signs of Deficiency: Not specific but likely to occur with hypoalbuminemia.

Signs of Excess: Uncommon because excess is excreted in the urine as sulfate, usually in combination with calcium. This may result in hypercalciuria (often after a high protein meal).

TRACE MINERALS

Elements that are found in minute amounts in body tissues and are specific to the function of certain enzymes. They are typically not found in free ionic state but are bound to other proteins.

Copper

Copper has recently received attention as an antioxidant, especially in coronary heart disease. Copper and ascorbic acid supplements may be provided on alternate days if supplementation or TPN use is prolonged, because the two nutrients counteract each other's absorption (Burge et al., 1994). Concentrations of copper are highest in the liver, brain, heart, and kidney; skeletal muscle also contains a large percentage because of total mass (Anderson, 2000). About 90% of copper is bound as ceruloplasmin and is transported to other tissues, mainly by albumin. New RDA is 900 mcg daily for men and women. UL was set at 10 mg/day.

Roles: Skeletal development, immunity, formation of red blood cells and leukopoiesis, phospholipid synthesis, electron transport, pigmentation, aortic elasticity, connective tissue formation, and central nervous system (CNS) and myelin sheath structure.

Sources: Liver, kidney, shellfish such as oysters, nuts, dried beans and legumes, cocoa, eggs, prunes, and potatoes. Note: Milk is low in copper. Daily intake of copper in the United States is 2–5 mg; however, many persons have a lower intake than this because fresh foods are low in copper. Meat/poultry/fish are primary sources in the United States for all age groups except infants, for whom infants' foods are the primary source of copper (Hunt and Meacham, 2001). Approximately 30–60% of oral intake is absorbed. Absorption is enhanced by acid and decreased by calcium. Approximately 94% of copper is tightly bound to ceruloplasmin.

Signs of Deficiency: Hypochromic anemia, cardiomyopathy, aortic aneurysms, elevated cholesterol levels, neutropenia, skeletal abnormalities and osteoporosis, decreased skin and hair pigmentation, Menke's disease or kinky-hair syndrome, dermatitis, anorexia, diarrhea, and reduced immune responses. Deficiency is rare in adults, except with celiac sprue, protein-losing enteropathies, and nephrotic syndrome. Requirement is increased by excessive zinc intake.

Signs of Excess: Rare, but liver cirrhosis, biliary cirrhosis, and other liver disorders (including Wilson's disease) may contribute to the retention of copper. Abnormalities in red blood cell formation, copper deposits in the brain, and liver damage occur. Excesses may decrease vitamin A absorption.

Fluoride

Fluoride is found in nearly all drinking waters and soils. The American Dietetic Association affirms that fluoride is an important element for all mineralized tissues and that appropriate consumption aids bone and tooth (American Dietetic Association, 2000). RDA is 3 mg/day for men and women. UL is set at 10 mg/day.

Roles: Calcium uptake, some role in prevention of calcified aortas, resistance to dental caries, collapsed vertebrae, and osteoporosis, formation of hydroxyapatite, and enamel growth.

Sources: Fluoridated water, tea, seafood and marine fish with bones, infant foods to which bone meal has been added, and 80–90% of oral intake is absorbed.

Signs of Deficiency: Dental caries, calcification of aorta, and anemia. Possibly bone thinning and osteoporosis.

Signs of Excess: Bony outgrowths at the spine. Tooth mottling, pitting, and discoloration (fluorosis) at doses of greater than 2–3 ppm in the drinking water. Use of water with an excessively high natural fluoride level may be associated with increased risk of hip fracture in women but not in men (Kurttio et al., 1999). Excess can result in neurologic problems; this feature is valuable in rat poison, for example.

Iron

Iron deficiency anemia is the most common nutrient deficiency in the world. Anemias are still relatively common in toddlers, teenage girls, and women of childbearing age (Looker et al., 1997). Functional iron is found in hemoglobin, myoglobin, and enzymes. Storage iron is found in ferritin, hemosiderin, and transferrin. Iron is conserved and reused at a rate of 90% daily; the rest is excreted, mainly in bile. Dietary iron must be consumed to meet the 10% gap to prevent deficiency. New RDA is 8 mg for men and postmenopausal women and 18 mg for premenopausal women. Pregnant women need 27 mg per day. UL for iron is 45 mg daily.

Roles: Responsible for carrying oxygen to cells through hemoglobin and myoglobin, skeletal muscle functioning, cognitive functioning, leukocyte functions and T-cell immunity, cellular enzymes, and cytochrome content for normal cellular respiration.

Sources: Heme sources—lean meat (such as liver), seafood (clams, oysters), and poultry and egg yolk. Nonheme sources—dried beans and peas, dried fruits such as dried apricots, dark molasses, cocoa, baking chocolate, green leafy vegetables (leaf lettuce, spinach), outer layer of grains, potatoes (especially if eaten frequently), and whole grain and fortified breads and cereals. Sulfur amino acids and vitamin C increase iron absorption. Excessive calcium intake, oxalic, tannic, and phytic acids can reduce absorption; e.g., decreasing calcium intake at lunch and dinner increases iron absorption in healthy women (Gleerup et al., 1995).

Serum iron is largely bound to transferrin. Distribution is under control of interleukin-1. About 5–15% is absorbed as ferrous iron; 15–25% of oral intake of heme iron is absorbed (meat, fish, poultry); 2–20% of oral intake of nonheme iron is absorbed (legumes, grains, and fruit). In the United States, grain products provide the highest amount of dietary iron for all age groups except infants, for whom infant foods are the best source (Hunt and Meacham, 2001).

Signs of Deficiency: Hypochromic anemia, fatigue and weakness, pallor, dyspnea, decreased resistance to infection, koilonychia, spoon-shaped nails, impaired learning ability, headache, tachycardia, glossitis, cheilosis, and dysphagia. Deficiency is defined as having an abnormal value for two of three laboratory tests of iron status (erythrocyte protoporphyrin, transferrin saturation, or serum ferritin); iron deficiency anemia is defined as iron deficiency plus low hemoglobin (Looker et al., 1997).

Signs of Excess: Iron deposits, liver damage (cirrhosis), diabetes mellitus, and skin pigmentation. GI distress (Trumbo, 2001). Hereditary or secondary hemochromatosis. Transfusion overload is rare but may be found in persons with sickle cell anemia or thalassemia major. Excess may occur from taking iron supplements daily or from multiple sources.

Zinc

Zinc is so ubiquitous in cellular metabolism that even minor impairment in supply is likely to have multiple biologic and clinical effects. Zinc deficiency causes a reduction in antibody responses and cell-mediated responses of the immune system. Zinc absorption is affected by level of zinc in the diet and any interfering substances, such as phytates, calcium, cadmium, folic acid, excessive fiber, and copper. Albumin is the major plasma carrier. New RDA is 11 mg for men, 8 mg for women. UL 40 mg.

Roles: ACTH-stimulated steroidogenesis in adrenals and sexual maturation, fatty acid, CHO, protein and nucleic acid metabolism, CO2 transport, amino acid breakdown from peptides, oxidation of vitamin A, reproduction, growth, enzymes (such as alcohol dehydrogenase, alkaline phosphatase, lactic acid dehydrogenase), wound healing, catalyst for hydrogenation, immunity, night vision, alcohol detoxification in the liver, heme synthesis, taste and smell acuity, synthesis of glutathione, and collagen precursors. Zinc status may influence serum leptin levels possibly via effects on production of interleukin-2 and tumor necrosis factor; serum leptin levels decrease during zinc restriction and increase during supplementation (Mantzoros et al., 1998).

Zinc supplementation has been shown to be effective in reducing morbidity and mortality from diarrhea, malaria, HIV infection, sickle cell anemia, renal disease, and GI disorders by preventing the immune system response from being diminished (Fraker et al., 2000). Zinc gluconate lozenges do not always alleviate cold symptoms in children and adolescents; more nausea, bad taste, mouth, tongue, or throat discomfort, and diarrhea may occur (Macknin et al., 1998).

Sources: Seafood (especially oysters), poultry, meat (red meat such as beef and liver especially), eggs, milk, peanuts, oatmeal, whole corn, whole grains (whole wheat or rye bread), wheat germ, and yeast. The average American diet contains 10–15 mg daily. Meat/poultry/fish are the primary sources of zinc for all age groups of Americans except infants, for whom infant foods provide the richest source (Hunt and Meacham, 2001). Zinc is distributed in the body with proteins such as albumin, transferrin, ceruloplasmin, and gamma globulin. Animal sources are better utilized; vegetarian diets must be monitored for zinc deficiency. Phytates, excess copper, and fiber can decrease absorption by forming complexes. Calcium and phosphate salts also decrease absorption; 10–40% from meals is absorbed in the duodenum and the jejunum. Vitamin D can increase bioavailability.

Signs of Deficiency: Dermatitis and skin lesions, hypoglycemia, growth failure and hypogonadism, mild anemia, decreased taste acuity, alopecia, diarrhea, apathy, depression, and impaired wound healing. Zinc deficiency has a significant impact on development and on immune function; premature infants and children are at greatest risk (Costello and Grumstrup-Scott, 2000). In children with zinc deficiency, severe growth depression is seen. Strict vegetarians, preschoolers who do not eat meat, adolescent females, and those on a chronically high phytate diet may also be at risk, especially if other disease states are present.

Signs of Excess: Low levels of serum copper and lowered HDL cholesterol may result. Excessive zinc intake is probably self-limiting because of GI distress that occurs. Zinc toxicity can occur in renal dialysis if not carefully monitored.

ULTRA-TRACE MINERALS

Boron

Boron can be found in the brain and the bone; it is also found in the spleen and thyroid. It is found in foods such as sodium borate; it is absorbed at a rate of 90%. No RDA has been set, but a UL of 20 mg was established.

Roles: Mineral metabolism in animals and man. Cell membrane functioning. It may function in a role similar to estrogen in bone metabolism and strengthening (Anderson, 2000).

Sources: Drinking water, wine, cider and beer, noncitrus fruits, leafy vegetables, nuts, and legumes. Note: Protein foods and grains are low in boron. In the United States, infant foods provide the most for infants; fruits and fruit juices provide the most for toddlers; milk and cheese foods provide the most in adolescent diets; and beverages provide the most for adults and seniors (Hunt and Meacham, 2001).

Signs of Deficiency: None known at this time.

Signs of Excess: Reproductive and developmental effects (Trumbo, 2001).

Chromium

Chromium is closely related to insulin action. Absorption ranges from 0.5 to 2%. Chromium needs transferrin for distribution. No specific RDA exists.

Roles: Insulin molecule (part of glucose tolerance factor [GTF]), some inhibition of vascular disorders from aortic plaque, fatty acid, triglyceride and cholesterol metabolism, normal glucose metabolism, nucleic acid stability, regulation of gene expression, and peripheral nerve functioning.

Sources: Oysters, liver, potatoes, eggs, vegetable oil, brewer's yeast, whole grains and bran, shortening, nuts, and peanuts. Dairy products, fruits, and vegetables are low in chromium. Phytates and oxalates can decrease absorption.

Signs of Deficiency: Glucose intolerance, increased FFA levels, low respiratory quotient, peripheral neuropathy, impaired fertility and growth, and perhaps elevated cholesterol and triglycerides. Deficiency may be found in severe malnutrition, in diabetes, or in elderly patients with cardiovascular disease.

Signs of Excess: None known.

Cobalt

Most cobalt appears in the body with vitamin B12 stores in the liver (Anderson, 2000). Cobalt may share intestinal transport with iron and is increased in patients with low iron intake iron stores. No specific RDA exists.

Roles: Treatment of some anemias, part of structure of cobalamin in vitamin B12, role in immunity, and healthy nerves and red blood cells.

Sources: Seafood (oysters, clams), meats (such as liver), poultry, some grains, and cereals. Note: Cow's milk is very low. More than 50% of dietary cobalt is absorbed.

Signs of Deficiency: Weakness, anemia, and emaciation. Usually in conjunction with vitamin B12 deficiency and low intake of protein foods. Lack of intrinsic factor, gastrectomy, or malabsorption syndromes may also cause deficiency.

Signs of Excess: Polycythemia, bone marrow hyperplasia, reticulocytosis, and increased blood volume may result.

Iodine

With the iodization of salt, iodine deficiency has been almost eliminated in the United States and Western nations. Millions of people are at risk in other nations. The thyroid gland maintains 75% of the body's iodine; the rest is throughout the body, as in the gastric mucosa and blood. Iodide content of vegetables varies by the content of the local soil. Absorption is 50–100% from the gut. New RDA is 150 μg/day for both men and women. UL is 1.1 mg daily.

Roles: Energy metabolism, proper thyroid functioning, normal growth and reproduction, prevention of goiter, and regulation of cellular metabolism and temperature. Iodine is found with T3 and T4 distribution.

Sources: Iodized salt, seaweed, seafood (clams, oysters, sardines, lobster, and saltwater fish). Less good sources may include cream (in milk), eggs, drinking water in various areas, plant leaves (broccoli, spinach, turnip greens), cranberries, and legumes. Iodized salt should be encouraged for pregnant women. Goitrogens in cabbage, turnips, rapeseeds, peanuts, cassava, and soybeans may block uptake of iodine by body cells; heating and cooking inactivate them.

Signs of Deficiency: Enlarged thyroid gland and related goiter and hypothyroidism. Cretinism, deaf-mutism, abnormal fetal growth, and brain development.

Signs of Excess: Excess may depress thyroid activity or can lead to elevated TSH levels (Trumbo, 2001), hyperthyroidism, high levels of thyroid hormone, and possibly a hyperthyroidism goiter.

Manganese

Manganese affects reproductive capacity, pancreatic function, and carbohydrate metabolism. Less than 5% is absorbed from diet. It is transported bound to a macroglobulin, transferrin, or transmanganin. Human milk tends to be low in manganese levels. An adequate intake (AI) level has been set at 2.3 mg for men and 1.8 mg for women. The UL has been established at 11 mg.

Roles: Polysaccharide and fatty acid metabolism, enzyme activation, tendon and skeletal development, possible role in hypertension, fertility and reproduction (role with squalene as a precursor of cholesterol and sex hormones), melanin and dopamine production, energy and glucose production, and possible roles in blood and ear labyrinth formation.

Sources: Tea, coffee, whole grains, wheat germ and bran, blueberries, peas, beans and dried legumes, nuts, spinach, and cocoa powder. Sources of manganese are plant foods, not animal foods. In the United States, infant foods provide the highest amount of manganese for infants; grain products are primary sources for all other age groups and beverages, fruits, vegetables, desserts, and mixed dishes are secondary sources (Hunt and Meacham, 2001).

Signs of Deficiency: Nausea, vomiting, transient dermatitis, color changes in hair, hypocholesterolemia, growth retardation, weight loss, and slow growth of hair and beard. In animals, sterility and striking skeletal abnormalities occur. Beware of excess calcium, phosphorus, iron, or magnesium supplementation. Manganese, cobalt, and iron complete for pathways.

Signs of Excess: This rarely occurs in those who mine manganese for a living. Excesses accumulate in the liver and CNS; neurologic side effects like those in Parkinson's disease occur.

Molybdenum

Molybdenum is important mostly for its role in xanthine oxidase. About 40–100% of intake is absorbed from the duodenum in protein-bound form. It is readily absorbed from the stomach and small intestine and excreted in the urine. New RDA is 45 μg for both men and women. The UL was set at 2 mg.

Roles: Flavoproteins, copper antagonist, component of sulfite oxidase, aldehyde oxidase and xanthine oxidase, iron storage, energy metabolism, and degradation of cysteine and methionine through sulfite oxidase.

Sources: Legumes, whole grain breads and cereals, dark green leafy vegetables, milk and dairy products, and organ meats. Milk and cheese products provide the most molybdenum for infants, toddlers, and adolescents; grain products provide the most for adults and seniors (Hunt and Meacham, 2001).

Signs of Deficiency: Tachycardia, tachypnea, visual and mental changes, headache, nausea, and vomiting. This has been seen in patients with long-term TPN that is deficient in molybdenum.

Signs of Excess: Impaired reproduction and growth and gout-like syndrome can occur. Excess is rare, because it is usually just excreted in the urine.

Selenium

Cellular and plasma glutathione are the functional parameters for measuring selenium status. Selenium intake in the U.S. is generally very good; deficiency is not seen here. More than 50% dietary intake is absorbed (average range, 35–85%). It is transported protein-bound to albumin from the duodenum. A new RDA level for selenium was set at 55 μg/day for both men and women to achieve the best antioxidant levels; UL were also set at 400 μg.

Roles: Protein biosynthesis, spares vitamin E, cell wall protection as an antioxidant (glutathione peroxidase), protein matrix of teeth, protection against mercury toxicity, some role in fertility, liver function, heart muscle function, and growth.

Selenium functions within mammals primarily as selenoproteins, which contain selenium as selenocysteine. Glutathione catalyzes the reduction of peroxides that can cause cellular damage.

Eleven selenoproteins have been identified: cellular or classical glutathione peroxidase, plasma glutathione peroxidase (extracellular), phospholipid hydroperoxide glutathione peroxidase, GI glutathione peroxidase, iodothyronine deiodinase, selenoproteins P and W, thioredoxin reductase, and selenophosphate synthetase (Holben and Smith, 1999).

Sources: Seafood and fish, chicken, egg yolks, meats (especially kidney, liver), whole grain breads and cereals, wheat germ, foods grown in selenium-rich soil, including garlic, dairy products, Brazil nuts, and onions. Dietary selenium is found with protein in animal tissue. Muscle meats, organ meats, and seafood are dependable sources of selenium. Grains and seeds have variable amounts dependent on the soil. Dietary intake of selenium alters retention of selenium; the human body retains and distributes selenium from broccoli and inorganic salts differently (Finley, 1999).

Signs of Deficiency: Muscle weakness and pain, carcinogenesis, and cardiomyopathy. Keshan disease is a selenium deficiency that occurs in China where soil levels are quite low; cardiomyopathy is the main symptom. Kashin-Beck disease is common in preadolescents and adolescents; it is caused by a virus and has effects similar to osteoarthritis with stiffness and swelling of the elbows, knees, and ankles.

Signs of Excess: Symptoms of toxicity have only been reported in China with selenosis (skin and nail changes, decaying of teeth, neurologic abnormalities).

LESS STUDIED ULTRA-TRACE MINERALS

Aluminum, Arsenic, Cadmium, Lead, Lithium, and Tin

Not much is known about roles, functions, or purpose in the human body. For all age groups, grain products (mainly cornbread, pancakes, biscuits, muffins, and yellow cake) provide the highest amount of aluminum in the diet; beverages contribute secondarily (Hunt and Meacham, 2001).

Nickel

No RDA has been set, but UL was established at 1 mg per day, because decreased body weight can occur with excess as noted in animal studies (Trumbo, 2001).

Suspected Roles: Growth, reproduction, iron and zinc metabolism, hematopoiesis, DNA and RNA, and enzyme activation.

Sources: Grains and vegetables. Note: Less than 10% is absorbed. It is transported by serum albumin.

Silicon

No RDA or UL have been established.

Suspected Roles: Normal bone growth and calcification, normal collagen and connective tissue formation (especially in the presence of Ca++), and development of atherosclerosis with decreased silicon in aorta is experimental.

Sources: Most foods—only minute amounts are needed. Grains and beer are good sources.

Vanadium

No RDA has been set, but UL was established at 1.8 mg per day, because renal lesions have been noted in animal studies (Trumbo, 2001).

Suspected Roles: Possible roles in growth, lipid metabolism, and reproduction. Early trials with vanadium indicate that there may be a role in treatment of diabetes mellitus (DM); it has the ability to mimic insulin and lower blood pressure (BP) and glucose levels (Verma et al., 1998).

Sources: Leafy green vegetables and cereal grains.

VITAMINS

Vitamins were named as such "vital amines" in 1912, because they seemed to be important to life. Once it was known that they contain few amine groups, the "e" was dropped. There are 13 known vitamins (four fat-soluble and nine water-soluble). They are organic compounds, containing carbon structures. Research indicates that oxidative stress may form the biological basis for a number of medical conditions such as tissue injury after trauma, cardiovascular disease, and cancer (Rock et al., 1996). Regular use of multivitamin supplements with minerals may reduce risk of fetal death associated with maternal cigarette smoking (Wu et al., 1998).

The best nutritional strategy for promoting optimal health and reducing the risk of chronic disease is to obtain adequate nutrients from a wide variety of foods; supplementation is appropriate when well-accepted, peer-reviewed, scientific evidence shows safety and effectiveness (American Dietetic Association, 1996). A potential role for vitamin C, vitamin E, and the carotenoids in modifying risks has stimulated intense research efforts. Eating more fruits and vegetables rather than taking supplements is currently the recommendation for most individuals.

FAT-SOLUBLE VITAMINS

Vitamin A (Retinol, Retinal, Retinoic Acid)

Vitamin A is best known for its role in vision and skin integrity. Its provitamins include beta-carotene and cryptoxanthin. From 7–65% of vitamin A from the diet is absorbed. Dietary retinyl esters are hydrolyzed in the intestine by the pancreatic enzyme, pancreatic triglyceride lipase (PTL), and intestinal brush border enzyme, phospholipase B (Harrison and Hussain, 2001). Once in the cell, retinol is complexed with cellular retinol-binding protein type 2 (CRBP2), a substrate for reesterification of the retinol by the enzyme lecithin:retinol acyltransferase (LRAT); retinol not bound is esterified by acyl-CoA acyltransferase (Harrison and Hussain, 2001). Retinol-binding protein (RBP) is used to evaluate transport. Retinyl esters are incorporated into chylomicrons.

Stress can increase excretion; zinc or protein deficiency can decrease transport. Dietary vitamin A is transported via chylomicrons; 90% of vitamin A is stored in the liver. New RDA is 900 μg for men, 700 μg for women. UL is 3,000 μg/day.

Functions: Vision (especially night), gene regulation, growth, prevention of early miscarriage, immunity against infection (e.g., measles), corticosterones, weight gain, proper bone, tooth, and nerve development, membrane functions, and epithelial tissue integrity in lungs and trachea especially. Vitamin A supplementation is used to treat some forms of cancer and the degenerative eye disease retinitis pigmentosa.

Sources: Fish liver oils, egg yolk, animal livers, dairy products, butter and fortified margarine, and cream.

Signs of Deficiency: Xerophthalmia, night blindness, follicular hyperkeratosis or thickening of skin around hair follicles, drying of the whites of the eyes, eventual blindness, spots on the whites of the eyes, risk of infections, and death.

Vulnerable Populations: Anorexia nervosa, burns, biliary obstruction, cancer, cirrhosis, celiac disease, cystic fibrosis, drug use (cholestyramine, mineral oil, neomycin), hookworm, hepatitis of infectious origin, giardiasis, kwashiorkor, malaria, measles, pancreatic disease, pneumonia, pregnancy, prematurity, rheumatic fever, tropical sprue, and zinc deficiency.

Signs of Excess: Headache, peeling of skin, enlarged spleen and kidneys, bone thickening and joint pain, drying of the mucous membranes, and liver damage. Vitamin A is known for its teratogenic affects; if pregnant women are using a supplement, they should consider taking it in the form of beta-carotene (Voyles et al., 2000). Caution should be given to supplement use in women of childbearing age, because many women don't know they are pregnant in the earliest stages; supplements with retinol should be avoided during the first trimester, if vitamin A deficiency is not present. Long-term supplementation with retinol (7576 RE or 25,000 IU daily) may have adverse effects on blood lipid levels and alkaline phosphatase (alk phos) levels (Cartmel et al., 1999).

Carotenoids: There are more than 500 natural carotenoids. Two beta-carotene molecules are equivalent to one molecule of vitamin A. Beta-carotene is found in deep yellow, orange, or dark green fruits and vegetables such as carrots, mixed vegetables, vegetable soup, cantaloupe, spinach, broccoli, sweet potatoes, collards, peaches, apricots, and papaya.

The bioavailability of carotenoids from vegetables is low, and the fat required for adequate absorption is low (van het Hof et al., 2000). Between 9 and 17% of dietary carotenes are absorbed. A decline in lutein intake (leafy green vegetables) in all age groups has occurred, especially among white women, while lycopene intake has increased among men (Nebeling et al., 1997). Carotenoids may have a role in prevention of some types of cancer through enhancement of immune response, inhibition of mutagenesis, and protection against oxidative damage to cells (Vandenlangenberg et al., 1996). In addition, α-carotenes, β-cryptoxanthin, lutein plus zeaxanthin, and lycopenes may contribute to these important functions. Persons at risk for developing lung cancer, i.e., current smokers and workers exposed to asbestos, should be discouraged from taking beta-carotene supplements; the CARET study was stopped 21 months early because of substantial evidence of harm (Omenn et al., 1996). With new RDA levels, no recommendations were made for beta-carotene, because there is not enough evidence for an RDA.

Signs of Excess: Hypercarotenodermia (yellowing of skin with clear whites of eyes).

Vitamin D (Ergocalciferol or D2, Cholecalciferol or D3)

The main function of vitamin D is bone metabolism and calcium homeostasis. Vitamin D is actually a prohormone rather than just a vitamin (DeLuca, 1993). Total body–sun exposure provides equivalent of 250 μg (10,000 I.U.) vitamin D daily, suggesting that this is a physiological limit. Bile salts are required for absorption; 90% of dietary intake is absorbed. There is decreased production with aging. Active metabolite = 1,25-dihydroxyvitamin D3. Transport occurs via chylomicrons to the liver. New RDA is 200 IU for most people, 400 IU for people age 51–70. UL is 50 μg/day for adults.

Functions: Utilization of calcium and phosphorus, volume and acidity of gastric secretions, growth of soft tissues, bone calcification, growth and repair, tooth formation, effects on parathormone (PTH), and renal/intestinal phosphate absorption. The RDA for vitamin D may prevent osteomalacia in adults who are not exposed to sunlight, but higher vitamin D intakes are needed to help prevent osteoporosis and secondary hyperparathyroidism (Vieth, 1999). Supplemental vitamin D may also help prevent some cancers, osteoarthritis progression, multiple sclerosis (MS), and hypertension.

Sources: Cod liver oil, sunshine, eggs (one yolk = 27 IU), liver, salmon, sardines, fish roe, tuna (3 ½ oz = 200–300 IU), herring (3 ½ oz = 330 IU), vitamin-D-fortified milk (8 oz = 100 IU), fortified margarine, and irradiated yeast. Brief and casual exposure to sunlight equals approximately 200 IU of vitamin D (Haddad, 1992).

Signs of Deficiency: Bowed legs, rickets in children, and osteomalacia in adults. Hypovitaminosis D is related to lowered vitamin D intake, less exposure to ultraviolet light, anticonvulsant use, renal dialysis, nephrotic syndrome, hypertension (HPN), DM, winter season, high PTH and alk phos levels, and lower levels of ionized calcium and albumin (Thomas et al., 1998). Hypovitaminosis D is common in general medical inpatients, including those with vitamin D intakes exceeding the RDA amount without apparent risk factors for deficiency.

Vulnerable Populations: Biliary obstruction, celiac disease, cystic fibrosis, DM, drug use (bile salt binders, glucocorticoids, phenobarbital, primidone, mineral oil), end-organ failure, Fanconi's disease, hepatic disease, HPN, primary hypophosphatemia, hypoparathyroidism, inflammatory bowel disease, intestinal malabsorption, lack of exposure to sunlight, lymphatic obstruction, nephrotic syndrome, pancreatitis, parathyroid surgery, postmenopausal status, prematurity, renal disease and dialysis, small bowel resection, and tropical sprue.

Signs of Excess: Poor appetite, nausea, vomiting, increased urination, weakness, thirst, itchy skin, kidney failure, calcium deposits throughout the body, and nervousness. Use of oral contraceptives (OCAs) is associated with increased levels of vitamin D (Harris and Dawson-Hughes, 1998).

Vitamin E (α-Tocopherol, gamma-Tocopherol)

The main function of vitamin E is as a membrane antioxidant. Tocotrienols plus other forms affect cholesterol metabolism, carotid arteries, and immunity against cancer. Natural form is d-alpha-tocopherol (need 22 IU); dl-alpha-tocopherol is synthetic and less effective (need 33 IU). The new RDA is 15 mg for adults. UL is 1,000 mg.

Functions: Antioxidant along with vitamin C and selenium, anticoagulant and vitamin K antagonist, intracellular respiration, hemopoietic agent, roles in muscular, vascular, reproductive, and CNS systems, some role in reproduction, neutralizes free radicals, protects against cataracts, may relieve discomforts of rheumatoid arthritis, protects against effects of the sun, smog, and lung disease, may protect against Alzheimer's disease, and cellular membrane integrity. Vitamin E is a protective factor in the prevention of coronary disease mortality, especially among the elderly (Kritchevsky et al., 1995; Losonczy et al., 1996). High dose (1,800 IU) vitamin E supplements may help reduce risk of retinopathy or nephropathy in patients with type 1 diabetes; retinal blood flow is significantly increased (Bursell et al., 1999).

RDA for Vitamin E levels are now 15 mg for both men and women (equal to 22 IU of natural source vitamin E or 33 IU of synthetic sources) (Monsen, 2000). *ULs were also set for vitamin E—1 g/day.*

Sources: Salad oils (safflower and sunflower oils), margarine, grain products, seeds and nuts, green leafy vegetables (spinach, asparagus, broccoli, turnip greens), avocado, dried prunes, and wheat germ. Note: Normal requirements increase with use of PUFAs. Normal needs are 15 mg daily, but with PUFAs, normal requirements double daily. Overall, 20–40% is absorbed with meals. Bile and pancreatic secretions are needed. Very low-density lipoproteins (VLDL) and LDL carry it to tissues. Gamma-tocopherol is more common in the United States food supply (as in soybean oil); it is less useful to the body.

Signs of Deficiency: Rupture of red blood cells, nerve damage, impaired bone mineralization, impaired vitamin A storage, and prolonged blood coagulation. Vitamin E is one of the least toxic vitamins, but at high doses it can antagonize the utilization of other fat-soluble vitamins.

Vulnerable Populations: Alzheimer's disease, arthritis, biliary cirrhosis, bronchopulmonary dysplasia, cardiovascular diseases, cystic fibrosis, drug use (cholestyramine, clofibrate, oral contraceptives, triiodothyronine), high intake of PUFA in diet, malabsorption syndromes, malnutrition, musculoskeletal disorders, pancreatic diseases, pregnancy, prematurity, pulmonary diseases, and steatorrhea.

Signs of Excess: Excessive intake does not seem to cause hypervitaminosis but has caused isolated cases of dermatitis, fatigue, pruritus ani, acne, vasodilation, hypoglycemia, GI symptoms, increased requirement for vitamin K and impaired coagulation, and muscle damage.

Vitamin K (Phylloquinone K-1, Menaquinone K-2, Menadione K-3)

First isolated from alfalfa, vitamin K is also known as phylloquinone in green plants and as menaquinone in bacterial synthesis. It is important for normal blood clotting and calcium metabolism. The new RDA is 120 μg for men and 90 μg for women. No UL was established.

Functions: Antihemorrhagic factor, normal blood coagulation, calcium metabolism, and bone mineralization. Low vitamin K intakes are associated with an increased incidence of hip fractures (Booth et al., 2000).

Sources: Plant foods are better sources of vitamin K, including kale, Brussels sprouts, spinach, cauliflower, and cabbage, lettuce (eaten in large amounts), fish, liver, meat, eggs, cereal, and some fruits. Note: Because men hemorrhage more often than women, it may be necessary to review vitamin K intake by males. Intestinal bacteria make about 50% of the bodily requirement. A sterile gut or malabsorption can create deficiency. Vitamin K absorption is optimal with bile and pancreatic juice; 10–70% of dietary intake is usually absorbed. Beware: Vitamin E excesses can reduce absorption. Warfarin (Coumadin) blocks regeneration of active, reduced vitamin K, thus prolonging clotting time (monitored through prothrombin time [PT] or International Normalized Ratio (INR,) where 2–3 is desired.).

Signs of Deficiency: Bleeding and hypoprothrombinemia. Vitamin K deficiency is rare but can be found in lipid malabsorption, chronic antibiotic therapy, and liver disease. Giving an injection of vitamin K upon birth prevents hemorrhagic disease of the newborn.

Vulnerable Populations: Calcium disorders, drug use (anticoagulants, cholestyramine, mineral oil, neomycin, and other antibiotics), hepatic biliary obstruction, hepatocellular disease, malabsorption syndromes, postmenopausal women at risk for hip fractures, prematurity, and small bowel disorders.

Signs of Excess: Prolonged bleeding time. Menadione can be toxic if given in excessive does; severe jaundice in infants or hemolytic anemia may result.

WATER-SOLUBLE VITAMINS

Thiamin (Vitamin B1)

Known as the "morale" vitamin, thiamin is beneficial for nerve and heart function and for CHO metabolism. Thiamin is mainly a coenzyme for decarboxylations of 2-keto acids and transketolations (Combs, 2000). High CHO intakes, pregnancy, lactation, increased basal metabolic rate (BMR), and antibiotic use will increase needs. As calorie intake from protein and fat increases, thiamin requirement decreases. The extent of absorption varies widely. Thiamin hydrochloride is the common supplemental form. RDA is 1.2 mg/day for men and 1.1 mg for women. No UL was established.

Functions: Prevents beriberi; role in cell respiration, RNA and DNA formation, protein catabolism, growth, appetite, normal muscle tone in cardiac and digestive tissues, neurologic functioning, CHO metabolism as coenzyme in energy-producing Krebs' cycle, and thiamin pyrophosphate (TPP) at pyruvic acid step. Magnesium, manganese, riboflavin, and vitamin B6 are synergists. Acetylcholine synthesis requires thiamin.

Sources: Pork, yeast, dried legumes, organ and lean meats, whole grains such as oats and whole wheat, nuts, cornmeal, brown rice, enriched flours and breads/cereals, dried milk, wheat germ, dried egg yolk or whole egg, green peas, and seeds. Note: Two slices of bread or one slice of bread and one serving of cereal will provide 15% of the daily RDA. Some nutrients are thiamin-sparing; others destroy the nutrient. Thiamin is spared by fat, protein, sorbitol, and vitamin C; antagonists include raw fish, tea, coffee, blueberries, and red cabbage. Avoid cooking with excessive water and alkaline products such as baking soda; thiamin is lost readily.

Signs of Deficiency: Anorexia, calf muscle weakness, weight loss, and cardiac and neurologic signs (mental confusion, muscular wasting, edema in wet beriberi, peripheral neuropathy, tachycardia). In dry beriberi, energy deprivation and inactivity are causes. Wernicke's encephalopathy is due to thiamin deficiency and often associated with malnutrition and alcoholism. TPN without multi-vitamin (MVI) use can lead to symptoms of Wernicke's encephalopathy; problems disappear within a few days after intravenous thiamin use (Hahn et al., 1998).

Vulnerable Populations: Alcoholism, cancers, cardiomyopathies, CHO (high intakes), celiac disease, children with congenital heart disease before and after surgery (Shamir, 2000), congestive heart failure, fever, high parenteral glucose loading, lactation and pregnancy, tropical sprue, and thyrotoxicosis.

Signs of Excess: Respiratory failure and death with large doses (1,000 times nutritional needs). With 100 times the normal dose, headache, convulsions, muscular weakness, cardiac arrhythmia, and allergic reactions have been noted.

Riboflavin (Vitamin B2)

Riboflavin is important in CHO metabolism and maintenance of healthy mucous membranes. It is the main coenzyme in redox reactions of fatty acids and the tri-carboxylic acid (TCA) cycle (Combs, 2000). RDA is 1.3 mg/day for men, 1.1 for women. No UL was established.

Functions: Cell respiration, oxidation reduction, conversion of tryptophan to niacin, component of retinal pigment, involvement in all metabolisms (especially fat), purine degradation, adrenocortical function, coenzyme in electron transport as flavin adenine dinucleotide (FAD)/flavin mononucleotide (FMN), healthy mucous membranes, skin and eyes, growth, and proper functioning of niacin and pyridoxine.

Sources: Milk, cheese, egg whites, legumes, peanuts, fish, poultry, meats, yeast, broccoli, spinach, asparagus, and fortified grains. Note: Body size, BMR, growth, activity excesses, and fat metabolism affect daily requirements. Beware of excesses of niacin and methylxanthines. Light destroys riboflavin; buy milk in opaque cartons. As protein intake increases, the need for riboflavin decreases. Riboflavin is spared by dextrins and starch and is found in greater amounts in protein foods. Cheilosis gives a magenta-colored tongue.

Signs of Deficiency: Photophobia, lacrimation, itchy and burning eyes or lips, mouth, and tongue. Fissures and scaling of lips, angular stomatitis, dermatitis, greasy nasolabial folds, purple, swollen tongue, and peripheral neuropathy. Riboflavin deficiency is most commonly found in developing countries like India and can lead to deficiency of B6 and B2 and impairment of psychomotor function. Riboflavin metabolism is affected by certain diseases, infections, drugs, and hormones (Lakshmi, 1998).

Vulnerable Populations: Alcoholism, cancers, chronic infections, drug use (broad-spectrum antibiotics, chloramphenicol), gastrectomy, and low oral intake during childhood, pregnancy, or lactation.

Signs of Excess: There is no known toxicity.

Niacin (Nicotinic Acid—NA, Nicotinamide—Nam)

Niacin serves as coenzyme for several dehydrogenases (Combs, 2000). Niacin requirements are related to protein and calorie intake. RDA is 16 mg/day for men, 14 for women. UL was established at 35 mg for men and women.

Functions: Prevention of pellagra (along with other B-complex vitamins), needed to treat tuberculosis (TB) with isoniazid (INH), part of nicotinamide adenine dinucleotide (NAD) in metabolism, use of CHO, protein, and fat in energy metabolism, growth, conversion of vitamin A to retinol, and metabolism of fatty acids, serum cholesterol, and triglycerides. Nicotinic acid is often used as a vasodilator; nicotinamide is less vasodilating.

Sources: Yeast, organ meats, meat, poultry, salt water fish, nuts and legumes, coffee and tea, dairy products, potatoes, and enriched breads and cereals. Sixty mg of tryptophan is equivalent to 1 mg of niacin. Diet supplies 31% of niacin intake as tryptophan. Milk and eggs are good sources of tryptophan but not niacin.

Signs of Deficiency: Muscular weakness, inflammation of the tongue, anorexia, abnormal intestinal function and indigestion, skin eruptions, abnormal brain functioning. Severe deficiency leads to pellagra; one sign of pellagra is Casal's collar, a rough, red dermatitis; others include diarrhea, dementia, or even death (also called the three D's of pellagra). Pellagra is commonly seen in undernourished areas of Africa. A 3-year prospective study found that pellagra patients had a low incidence of HIV infection compared to the general population (Pitche et al., 1999).

Vulnerable Populations: Alcoholism, cancers, chronic diarrhea, cirrhosis, DM, and TB.

Signs of Excess: Histamine release, causing flushing of skin (when using 1–2 g of nicotinic acid daily in an effort to lower cholesterol levels). Megadoses should be avoided.

Vitamin B6 (Pyridoxol, Pyridoxal, Pyridoxamine)

Vitamin B6 is primarily known for its role in AA metabolism (Combs, 2000). RDA is 1.3–1.7 mg/day for men and 1.3–1.5 mg for women. UL was established at 100 mg/day for adult men and women.

Functions: Protein metabolism, coenzymes (-ases), conversion of tryptophan to niacin, fat metabolism (changing linoleic to arachidonic acid), CHO metabolism, synthesis of folic acid (with possible role in homocysteine metabolism and atherosclerosis), glandular and endocrine functions, nerve and brain energy, antibodies, may work against dental caries in the pregnant (PG) patient, role in dopamine and serotonin metabolism, glycogen phosphorylase, healthy red blood cells, and immunity.

Sources: Muscle and organ meats, poultry, fish, tuna, and salmon, whole grain cereals (such as oatmeal), walnuts, legumes (garbanzo beans), soybeans and peanuts, potatoes, yeast, bananas, corn, cabbage, yams, raisins and prunes, watermelon, avocado, and eggs. Note: enteric bacteria can make Vitamin B6 in healthy persons. About 96% of dietary vitamin B6 is absorbed. Infants need three times as much vitamin B6 as adults. Needs increase with increased protein intake, decrease with fatty acids, or decrease with other B-complex vitamins. High protein intakes may deplete vitamin B6 levels.

Signs of Deficiency: Convulsions in infants, anemias, and skin disorders. Weakness, sleeplessness, peripheral neuropathies, cheilosis, stomatitis, and impaired immunity (Combs, 2000). The vitamin is widely distributed throughout the diet; deficiency is rare, except in alcoholics, individuals taking isoniazid without B6 supplementation, or women taking oral contraceptives.

Vulnerable Populations: Alcoholism, drug use (cycloserine, dilantin, hydralazine, isoniazid, oral contraceptives, penicillamine), elderly status, pregnancy, and TB with INH treatment and no vitamin replacement.

Signs of Excess: Sensory neuropathy with gait changes and peripheral sensation and muscle incoordination.

Vitamin B12 (Cobalamin, Cyanocobalamin)

Vitamin B12 is known for its role as a coenzyme in metabolism of propionate, amino acids, and single carbon fragments (Combs, 2000). It is known as a growth stimulator and is informally called "extrinsic factor." Many people over age 50 lose the ability to absorb B12 from foods and should consider using more fortified foods. New RDA is 2.4 μg for adults. No UL was established.

Functions: Coenzymes, blood cell formation, nucleoproteins and genetic material, nutrient metabolism, growth, nerve tissue, thyroid functions, metabolism, transmethylation, myelin formation, and possible role in homocysteine metabolism and control of atherosclerosis.

Sources: Liver, kidney, muscle meats, eggs, cheese, milk, shellfish, and fish. Fermented foods such as soy sauce, tempeh, miso, and fortified foods such as soy milk. Vitamin B12 is not found in plant foods; monitor use of meat-free vegetarian diets. For best absorption, riboflavin, niacin, magnesium, and vitamin B6 are needed.

Signs of Deficiency: Pernicious anemia, poor vision, and some psychiatric disturbances. Monitor persons after total gastrectomy for megaloblastic anemia, when intrinsic factor is not available. Moderate intake of animal products does not restore normal vitamin B12 status in persons who had inadequate intake of B12 during childhood because of macrobiotic diets (Van Dusseldorp et al., 1999).

Vulnerable Populations: Adolescents with poor diets, disorders of gastric mucosa, gastrectomy, genetic defects (apoenzymes, absence of transcobalamin II, absence of ileal receptors), intestinal infections, malabsorption due to ileal resection or disease, prolonged daily intake of megadoses of folic acid, and strict vegetarians.

Signs of Excess: No toxicity is known.

Folic Acid (Folic Acid, Polyglutamyl Folacins)

Folic acid works primarily as a coenzyme in single-carbon metabolism (Combs, 2000). Folic acid can be made in the intestines with help from biotin, protein, and vitamin C. Only 25–50% of dietary folacin is bioavailable. Fortification of more commonly eaten foods has been implemented to provide adequate folic acid for vulnerable populations, especially for current knowledge about cardiovascular disease and neural tube defects (Oakley, 1998). New RDA is 400 μg for adults. UL is 1,000 μg/day.

Synthetic folic acid increases blood folate levels more effectively than food sources of folate, especially among women with a history of neural tube defects (Neuhouser, 1998). The new Dietary Reference Intakes (DRIs) express folate in "folate equivalents," which account for the difference between natural sources and more bioavailable supplemental sources. Dietary folate equivalents from fortified foods provide 1.7 times the micrograms of added folic acid; use of this term is recommended for planning and evaluating people's intake (West Suitor and Bailey, 2000).

Pteroylglutamic acid is the pharmacologic form. About 90% of circulating folacin is bound to albumin. Some drugs interfere with utilization such as sulfasalazine (Azulfidine), phenytoin (Dilantin), and methotrexate.

Functions: Prevents megaloblastic and macrocytic anemias, needed for growth, hemoglobin, amino acid metabolism, prevents excessive buildup of homocysteine in the body, which may be a precursor of atherosclerosis, and reduces the incidence of neural tube defects by 45% in women who receive 400 μg/day (Swain and St. Clair, 1997). Its protective role against cervical and colon cancer is being studied. The positive risk of breast cancer and alcohol intake may be weakened by adequate intake of folate such as 600 vs. 150–299 μg/day (Zhang et al., 1999). Elevations in homocysteine levels are found in persons with cardiovascular disease; there is some biologic plausibility but currently no proof that folate supplements may prevent heart disease, stroke, and peripheral artery disease (Swain and St Clair, 1997).

Folate is required for many one-carbon reactions involved in synthesis of phospholipids, DNA, proteins, and neurotransmitters. Metabolism of folate and choline is interdependent; choline is used as a methyl donor (to convert homocysteine to methionine) when folate intake is low. Synthesis of phosphatidylcholine is insufficient to maintain choline status when intakes of folate and choline are low; therefore, over 250 mg choline is required by adults daily when folate levels are low (Jacob et al., 1999).

Sources: Foods with highest folate content include: liver, cold cereals (not bran), pinto and navy beans (cooked), asparagus, raw spinach, romaine lettuce, broccoli, instant breakfast, bran and granola cereals, and avocados. Major contributors also include brewer's yeast, oranges, and orange juice (Hine, 1996). Other good sources include nuts, whole grains, kidney, bananas, lima beans, grapefruits and their juice, beets, wheat germ, and fortified breads and cereals.

Signs of Deficiency: Decrease in total number of cells (pancytopenia) and large red blood cells with a macrocytic or megaloblastic anemia. Neural tube defects in newborns may result. Deficiency is common, especially during pregnancy, with oral contraceptive use, in malabsorption syndromes, or in alcoholics, teens, or elderly individuals.

Vulnerable Populations: Alcoholism, cancers, drug use (aspirin, cycloserine, dilantin, methotrexate, oral contraceptives, primidone, pyrimethamine), hematologic diseases (pernicious anemia, sickle cell anemia, thalassemia), vitamin B12 deficiency, malabsorption syndromes, and pregnancy.

Signs of Excess: Epileptic seizures seen in rats (Combs, 2000). May cause zinc deficiency by forming nonabsorbable complexes in gut.

Pantothenic Acid

Pantothenic acid is a coenzyme in fatty acid metabolism (Combs, 2000). Pantothenic acid is digested "from everywhere;" it does not have reported requirements (Bender, 1999). <u>RDA for adult men and women is 5 mg/day. UL is not established.</u>

Functions: Coenzyme A, metabolism, synthesis of cholesterol and fatty acids, adrenal gland activity, acetyl transfer, antibodies, normal serum glucose, electrolyte control and hydration, prevents premature graying in some animals, heme synthesis, choline to acetylcholine, and healthy red blood cells.

Sources: Liver, organ meats, egg yolks, legumes, peanuts, yeast, salmon, mushrooms, broccoli, kale, avocado, whole grains, lean muscle meats, poultry, milk, yeast, and molasses. Needs increased by one-third in pregnancy and lactation; 50% is bioavailable from diet.

Signs of Deficiency: Deficiency is rare, but patient's complaint may include burning feet syndrome, vomiting, paresthesias, and leg cramps. People at risk for deficiency include persons with chronic ulcerative colitis.

Vulnerable Populations: Alcoholism, elderly women, liver disease, pregnancy.

Signs of Excess: Mild GI distress and diarrhea.

Biotin

Biotin is a coenzyme for carboxylations (Combs, 2000). <u>RDA is 30 μg/day for adult men and women. UL was not established.</u>

Functions: Coenzyme in CO2 fixation, deamination, decarboxylation, synthesis of fatty acids, CHO metabolism, oxidative phosphorylation, leucine catabolism, and carboxylation of pyruvic acid to oxaloacetate.

Sources: Liver, kidney, milk, egg yolk, yeast, nuts, legumes, chocolate, fish, and soy flour. Note: Synthesized by intestinal bacteria. Biotin is called the "antiraw egg white" factor because raw egg white decreases biotin availability with avidin. Be wary of extended antibiotic use or prolonged unsupplemented TPN use. Probably, 50% of dietary biotin is absorbed from the small intestine.

Signs of Deficiency: Inflammation of the skin and lips. Biotin-binding protein avidin can cause problems if raw eggs whites are consumed. Biotin deficiency leads to impaired glucose tolerance (Bender, 1999). Other symptoms include dermatitis, alopecia, paralysis, depression, nausea, hepatic steatosis, hypercholesterolemia, and glossitis.

Vulnerable Populations: Excessive intake of raw egg whites (avidin), genetic conditions (beta-methyl-crotonyglycinuria, propionic l-acidemia), and inadequate parenteral provision with long-term use.

Signs of Excess: There are no known toxic effects.

Choline

Choline is a methyl-rich compound (almost considered to be a B-vitamin) that is required for phospholipid synthesis and neurotransmitter function. Internal synthesis of phosphatidylcholine is insufficient to maintain choline status when intakes of folate and choline are low; choline is used as a methyl donor (to convert homocysteine to methionine) when folate intake is low; more than 250 mg choline is required by adults daily in these instances (Jacob et al., 1999). <u>RDA is set</u>

at 550 mg/day for adult men, 425 mg/day for adult women. UL level has been set at 3.5 g/day.

Functions: Methyl donor, lipotrophic agent, some role in muscle control and in short-term memory with the neurotransmitter acetylcholine, component of sphingomyelin, emulsifier in bile, and component of pulmonary surfactant (CO2/O2 exchange). It helps the body absorb and use fats, especially for cell membranes.

Sources: Eggs and high protein animal products such as liver, dairy foods, soybeans, peanuts, cauliflower, lettuce, and chocolate. Lecithin is one form of choline precursor, as is phosphatidylcholine. Liver can synthesize/resynthesize. Average daily intake is 400–900 mg. High fat intake accelerates deficiency.

Signs of Deficiency: Insufficient phospholipid synthesis and neurotransmitter function would be expected.

Signs of Excess: None known at this time.

Vitamin C (Ascorbic Acid, Dehydroascorbic Acid)

Vitamin C is a reductant in hydroxylations in biosynthesis of collagen and carnitine and in metabolism of drugs and steroids (Combs, 2000). Vitamin C is needed via an exogenous source by all humans and is found in fruits and vegetables. Men who do not smoke may want to take 90–100 mg daily to minimize their risk of chronic disease (Carr and Frei, 1999). About 90% of dietary intake is absorbed. New RDA for vitamin C for women is 75 mg for men, 90 mg to reach saturation levels (Monsen, 2000). ULs were also set for vitamin C at 2,000 mg/day.

Concentration of vitamin C in plasma and other body fluids does not increase in proportion to increasing daily doses of vitamin C and tends to approach an upper limit; there is no pharmacokinetic justification for use of megadoses of vitamin C over 200 mg/day (Blanchard et al., 1997). Bioavailability is complete at 200 mg vitamin C as a single dose; at single doses of 500 mg and higher, bioavailability declines and absorbed amounts are excreted (Levine et al., 1996).

Functions: Hydroxylation (lysine and proline) in collagen formation and wound healing, norepinephrine metabolism, tryptophan to serotonin transformation, folic acid metabolism, antioxidant as a scavenger of superoxide radicals and to protect vitamins A and E, changing ferric iron to ferrous iron, prevention of infection, intracellular respiration, tyrosine metabolism, intercellular structures of bone, teeth, and cartilage, prevention of scurvy, believed to defer aging with collagen turnover process, reducing agent, elevation of HDL cholesterol in the elderly, and lowering of serum cholesterol. Serum ascorbic acid level influences cholesterol homeostasis in women (Simon and Hudes, 1998).

Dietary antioxidants, including vitamins C and E, may protect against atherosclerotic disease, especially in individuals older than 55 years of age (Kritchevsky et al., 1995). Vitamin C supplements may be protective against cognitive impairment (Paleologos et al., 1998). High serum levels of ascorbic acid are independently inversely associated with blood lead levels; if this relationship is causal, intake of vitamin C may have public health implications (Simon and Hudes, 1999). Individuals with diabetes tend to have a significantly lower mean plasma level of vitamin C (Johnston and Thompson, 1998).

Sources: Citrus fruits, strawberries, collard greens, Brussels sprouts, broccoli, red and green peppers, tomatoes, cantaloupe, currants, gooseberries, liver, plant leaves (e.g., broccoli), and baked potato. Note: No more than 1 g/day is stored in liver tissue. Body reserves may be up to 1,500 mg, or a 30- to 40-day supply. An excretion of 50% is normal. Men are found to have lower serum levels than women. Smoking decreases serum levels; increasing the intake of vitamin C is recommended for smokers. Increased intake removes greater amounts of nicotine. Avoid high levels of pectin, iron, copper, and zinc from the diet.

Signs of Deficiency: The first symptom of deficiency is fatigue; treatment with vitamin C results in quick recovery and alleviation of symptoms. Scurvy reveals swollen, bleeding gums, eventual tooth loss, lethargy, fatigue, poor wound healing, edema, hemorrhages, weak bones or cartilage and connective tissues, rheumatic pains in the legs, muscular atrophy, skin lesions, and psychological changes including depression and hypochondria.

Vulnerable Populations: Achlorhydria, alcoholism, Alzheimer's disease, burns, cancers, chronic diarrhea, DM, elevated cholesterol, infants whose mothers consumed over 400 mg daily during pregnancy, nephrosis, pregnancy, severe trauma, surgical wounds, and TB.

Signs of Excess: GI distress and diarrhea. Excesses do not produce a hypervitaminosis but have been linked to oxalate kidney stones or gout in susceptible persons. In addition, excesses may aggravate high serum ferritin levels in 30% of African Americans and 12% of non-African Americans; they may also harm persons with hereditary hemolytic anemias (Herbert, 1995).

RECOMMENDED DIETARY ALLOWANCES AND DIETARY REFERENCE INTAKES

The Dietary Reference Intakes (DRIs) are nutrient-based reference values for use in planning and assessing diets and for other purposes. They replace the RDAs that have been published since 1941 by the National Academy of Sciences. The Standing Committee on the Scientific Evaluation of Dietary Reference Intakes of the Food and Nutrition Board, Institute of Medicine (IOM), and National Academies of Sciences determined them, with help from Health Canada. The IOM is a private, nonprofit organization that provides health policy advice under a congressional charter granted to the National Academy of Sciences.

Each of the ten editions of the RDAs was a single report. The DRI values comprise seven reports. The first one, published in August 1997, covers nutrients related to bone health (calcium, phosphorus, magnesium, vitamin D, and fluoride). Ultimately, the DRI's will be a three-level system that offers guidelines for minimum, optimum, and maximum nutrient intakes; Estimated Average Requirements, Recommended Dietary Allowances and Upper Levels. The National Academies recently released the fourth in a series of reports presenting the dietary reference values for nutrient intake by Americans and Canadians (Trumbo et al, 2001.) The final document regarding macronutrients was not available at the time of printing. To find the new data, access the search at the Institute of Medicine site (http://wwwsearch.nationalacademies.org/)

EARs will be the mean amounts of nutrients required to prevent nutrient deficiency. This means that half of the population will need more, and half will need less. EARs will be further defined by specific age/gender categories allowing for more accurate guidelines for all ages of the population.

RDAs: After computing the EARs for each age/gender category and its standard deviation, the Food and Nutrition Board (FNB) then establishes RDAs to meet the nutrient requirements of each specified category.

ULs are defined as the upper limit of intake known or predicted to be safe for each age/gender category. Amounts taken above this level could cause toxicity and adverse physiologic and psychologic effects.

TABLE A-6 Recommended Dietary Allowances[a] Revised 1989 (Abridged) Designed for the Maintenance of Good Nutrition of Practically All Healthy People in the United States[1]

Category	Age (years) or condition	Weight[b] (kg)	Weight[b] (lb)	Height[b] (cm)	Height[b] (in)	Protein (g)
Infants	0.0–0.5	6	13	60	24	13
	0.5–1.0	9	20	71	28	14
Children	1–3	13	29	90	35	16
	4–6	20	44	112	44	24
	7–10	28	62	132	52	28
Males	11–14	45	99	157	62	45
	15–18	66	145	176	69	59
	19–24	72	160	177	70	58
	25–50	79	174	176	70	63
	51 +	77	170	173	68	63
Females	11–14	46	101	157	62	46
	15–18	55	120	163	64	44
	19–24	58	128	164	65	46
	25–50	63	138	163	64	50
	51 +	65	143	160	63	50
Pregnant						60
Lactating	1st 6 months					65
	2nd 6 months					62

[a]The allowances, expressed as average daily intakes over time, are intended to provide for individual variations among most normal persons as they live in the United States under usual environmental stresses. Diets should be based on a variety of common foods in order to provide other nutrients for which human requirements have been less well defined.

[b]Weights and heights of Reference Adults are actual medians for the US population of the designated age, as reported by NHANES II. The median weights and heights of those under 19 years of age were taken from Hamill et al (1979). The use of these figures does not imply that the height-to-weight ratios are ideal.

TABLE A-7 Dietary Reference Intakes: Recommended Intakes for Individuals, Vitamins Food and Nutrition Board, The Institute of Medicine, National Academies

Life Stage Group	Vitamin A (μg/d)[a]	Vitamin C (mg/d)	Vitamin D (μg/d)[b,c]	Vitamin E (mg/d)[d]	Vitamin K (μg/d)	Thiamin (mg/d)	Riboflavin (mg/d)	Niacin (mg/d)[e]	Vitamin B_6 (mg/d)	Folate (μg/d)[f]	Vitamin B_{12} (μg/d)	Pantothenic Acid (mg/d)	Biotin (μg/d)	Choline[g] (mg/d)
Infants														
0–6 mo	400*	40*	5*	4*	2.0*	0.2*	0.3*	2*	0.1*	65*	0.4*	1.7*	5*	125*
7–12 mo	500*	50*	5*	5*	2.5*	0.3*	0.4*	4*	0.3*	80*	0.5*	1.8*	6*	150*
Children														
1–3 y	**300**	**15**	5*	**6**	30*	**0.5**	**0.5**	**6**	**0.5**	**150**	0.9	2*	8*	200*
4–8 y	**400**	**25**	5*	**7**	55*	**0.6**	**0.6**	**8**	**0.6**	**200**	1.2	3*	12*	250*
Males														
9–13 y	**600**	**45**	5*	**11**	60*	**0.9**	**0.9**	**12**	**1.0**	**300**	1.8	4*	20*	375*
14–18 y	**900**	**75**	5*	**15**	75*	**1.2**	**1.3**	**16**	**1.3**	**400**	2.4	5*	25*	550*
19–30 y	**900**	**90**	5*	**15**	120*	**1.2**	**1.3**	**16**	**1.3**	**400**	2.4	5*	30*	550*
31–50 y	**900**	**90**	5*	**15**	120*	**1.2**	**1.3**	**16**	**1.3**	**400**	2.4	5*	30*	550*
51–70 y	**900**	**90**	10*	**15**	120*	**1.2**	**1.3**	**16**	**1.7**	**400**	2.4[h]	5*	30*	550*
>70 y	**900**	**90**	15*	**15**	120*	**1.2**	**1.3**	**16**	**1.7**	**400**	2.4[h]	5*	30*	550*
Females														
9–13 y	**600**	**45**	5*	**11**	60*	**0.9**	**0.9**	**12**	**1.0**	**300**	1.8	4*	20*	375*
14–18 y	**700**	**65**	5*	**15**	75*	**1.0**	**1.0**	**14**	**1.2**	**400**[i]	2.4	5*	25*	400*
19–30 y	**700**	**75**	5*	**15**	90*	**1.1**	**1.1**	**14**	**1.3**	**400**[i]	2.4	5*	30*	425*
31–50 y	**700**	**75**	5*	**15**	90*	**1.1**	**1.1**	**14**	**1.3**	**400**[i]	2.4	5*	30*	425*
51–70 y	**700**	**75**	10*	**15**	90*	**1.1**	**1.1**	**14**	**1.5**	**400**	2.4[h]	5*	30*	425*
>70 y	**700**	**75**	15*	**15**	90*	**1.1**	**1.1**	**14**	**1.5**	**400**	2.4[h]	5*	30*	425*
Pregnancy														
≤18 y	**750**	**80**	5*	**15**	75*	**1.4**	**1.4**	**18**	**1.9**	**600**[j]	2.6	6*	30*	450*
10–30 y	**770**	**85**	5*	**15**	90*	**1.4**	**1.4**	**18**	**1.9**	**600**[j]	2.6	6*	30*	450*
31–50 y	**770**	**85**	5*	**15**	90*	**1.4**	**1.4**	**18**	**1.9**	**600**[j]	2.6	6*	30*	450*
Lactation														
≤18 y	**1,200**	**115**	5*	**19**	75*	**1.4**	**1.6**	**17**	**2.0**	**500**	2.8	7*	35*	550*
19–30 y	**1,300**	**120**	5*	**19**	90*	**1.4**	**1.6**	**17**	**2.0**	**500**	2.8	7*	35*	550*
31–50 y	**1,300**	**120**	5*	**19**	90*	**1.4**	**1.6**	**17**	**2.0**	**500**	2.8	7*	35*	550*

NOTE: This table (taken from the DRI reports, see www.nap.edu) presents Recommended Dietary Allowances (RDAs) in **bold type** and Adequate Intakes (AIs) in ordinary type followed by an asterisk (*). RDAs and AIs may both be used as goals for individual intake. RDAs are set to meet the needs of almost all (97 to 98 percent) individuals in a group. For healthy breastfed infants, the AI is the mean intake. The AI for other life stage and gender groups is believed to cover needs of all individuals in the group, but lack of data or uncertainty in the data prevent being able to specify with confidence the percentage of individuals covered by this intake.

[a]As retinol activity equivalents (RAEs). 1 RAE = 1 μg retinol, 12 μg β-carotene, 24 μg α-carotene, or 24 μg β-cryptoxanthin in foods. To calculate RAEs from REs of provitamin A carotenoids in foods, divide the REs by 2. For preformed vitamin A in foods or supplements and for provitamin A carotenoids in supplements, 1 RE = 1 RAE.

[b]Cholecalciferol. 1 μg cholecalciferol = 40 IU vitamin D.

[c]In the absence of adequate exposure to sunlight.

[d]As α-tocopherol. α-Tocopherol includes RRR-α-tocopherol, the only form of α-tocopherol that occurs naturally in foods, and the 2R-stereoisometric forms of α-tocopherol (RRR-, RSR-, RRS-, and RSS-α-tocopherol) that occur in fortified foods and supplements. It does not include the 2S-stereoisometric forms of α-tocopherol (SRR-, SSR-, SRS-, and SSS-α-tocopherol), also found in fortified foods and supplements.

[e]As niacin equivalents (NE). 1 mg of niacin = 60 mg of tryptophan; 0–6 months = preformed niacin (not NE).

[f]As dietary folate equivalents (DFE). 1 DFE = 1 μg food folate = 0.6 μg of folic acid from fortified food or as a supplement consumed with food = 0.5 μg of a supplement taken on an empty stomach.

[g]Although AIs have been set for choline, there are few data to assess whether a dietary supply of choline is needed at all stages of the life style, and it may be that the choline requirement can be met by endogenous synthesis at some of these stages.

[h]Because 10 of 30 percent of older people may malabsorb food-bound B_{12}, it is advisable for those older than 50 years to meet their RDA mainly by consuming foods fortified with B_{12} or a supplement containing B_{12}.

[i]In view of evidence linking folate intake with neural tube defects in the fetus, it is recommended that all women capable of becoming pregnant consume 400 μg from supplements or fortified foods in addition to intake of food folate from a varied diet.

[j]It is assumed that women will continue consuming 400 μg from supplements or fortified food until their pregnancy is confirmed and they enter prenatal care, which ordinarily occurs after the end of the periconceptional period—the critical time for formation of the neural tube.

TABLE A-8 Dietary Reference Intakes (DRIs): Tolerable Upper Intake Levels (UL[a]), Vitamins Food and Nutrition Board, The Institute of Medicine, National Academies

Life Stage Group	Vitamin A (μg/d)[b]	Vitamin C (mg/d)	Vitamin D (μg/d)	Vitamin E (mg/d)[c,d]	Vitamin K	Thiamin	Riboflavin	Niacin (mg/d)[d]	Vitamin B_6 (mg/d)	Folate (μg/d)[d]	Vitamin B_{12}	Pantothenic Acid	Biotin	Choline (g/d)	Carot-enoids[e]
Infants															
0–6 mo	600	ND[f]	25	ND	ND	ND	ND	ND	ND	ND	ND	ND	ND	ND	ND
7–2 mo	600	ND	25	ND	ND	ND	ND	ND	ND	ND	ND	ND	ND	ND	ND
Children															
1–3 y	600	400	50	200	ND	ND	ND	10	30	300	ND	ND	ND	1.0	ND
4–8 y	900	650	50	300	ND	ND	ND	15	40	400	ND	ND	ND	1.0	ND
Males, Females															
9–13 y	1,700	1,200	50	600	ND	ND	ND	20	60	600	ND	ND	ND	2.0	ND
14–18 y	2,800	1,800	50	800	ND	ND	ND	30	80	800	ND	ND	ND	3.0	ND
19–70 y	3,000	2,000	50	1,000	ND	ND	ND	35	100	1,000	ND	ND	ND	3.5	ND
>70 y	3,000	2,000	50	1,000	ND	ND	ND	35	100	1,000	ND	ND	ND	3.5	ND
Pregnancy															
≤18 y	2,800	1,800	50	800	ND	ND	ND	30	80	800	ND	ND	ND	3.0	ND
19–50 y	3,000	2,000	50	1,000	ND	ND	ND	35	100	1,000	ND	ND	ND	3.5	ND
Lactation															
≤18 y	2,800	1,800	50	800	ND	ND	ND	30	80	800	ND	ND	ND	3.0	ND
19–50 y	3,000	2,000	50	1,000	ND	ND	ND	35	100	1,000	ND	ND	ND	3.5	ND

[a]UL = The maximum level of daily nutrient intake that is likely to pose no risk of adverse effects. Unless otherwise specified, the UL represents total intake from food, water, and supplements. Due to lack of suitable data, ULs could not be established for vitamin K, thiamin, riboflavin, vitamin B_{12}, pantothenic acid, biotin, or carotenoids. In the absence of ULs, extra caution may be warranted in consuming levels above recommended intakes.

[b]as preformed vitamin A only.

[c]As α-tocopherol; applies to any form of supplemental α-tocopherol.

[d]The ULs for vitamin E, niacin, and folate apply to synthetic forms obtained from supplements, fortified foods, or a combination of the two.

[e]β-Carotene supplements are advised only to serve as a provitamin A source for individuals at risk of vitamin A deficiency.

[f]ND = Not determinable due to lack of data of adverse effects in this age group and concern with regard to lack of ability to handle excess amounts. Source of intake should be from food only to prevent high levels of intake.

SOURCES: Dietary Reference Intakes for Calcium, Phosphorus, Magnesium, Vitamin D, and Fluoride (1997); Dietary Reference Intakes for Thiamin, Riboflavin, Niacin, Vitamin B_6, Folate, Vitamin B_{12}, Pantothenic Acid, Biotin, and Choline (1998); Dietary Reference Intakes for Vitamin C, Vitamin E, Selenium, and Carotenoids (2000); and Dietary Reference Intakes for Vitamin A, Vitamin K, Arsenic, Boron, Chromium, Copper, Iodine, Iron, Manganese, Molybdenum, Nickel, Silicon, Vanadium, and Zinc (2001). These reports may be accessed via www.nap.edu.

TABLE A-9 Dietary Reference Intakes: Recommended Intakes for Individuals, Elements Food and Nutrition Board, The Institute of Medicine, National Academies

Life Stage Group	*Calcium (mg/d)*	*Chromium (µg/d)*	*Copper (µg/d)*	*Fluoride (mg/d)*	*Iodine (µg/d)*	*Iron (mg/d)*	*Magnesium (mg/d)*	*Manganese (mg/d)*	*Molybdenum (µg/d)*	*Phosphorus (mg/d)*	*Selenium (µg/d)*	*Zinc (mg/d)*
Infants												
0–6 mo	210*	0.2*	200*	0.01*	110*	0.27*	30*	0.003*	2*	100*	15*	2*
7–12 mo	270*	5.5*	220*	0.5*	130*	**11**	75*	0.6*	3*	275*	20*	**3**
Children												
1–3 y	500*	11*	**340**	0.7*	**90**	**7**	**80**	1.2*	**17**	**460**	**20**	**3**
4–8 y	800*	15*	**440**	1*	**90**	**10**	**130**	1.5*	**22**	**500**	**30**	**5**
Males												
9–13 y	1,300*	25*	**700**	2*	**120**	**8**	**240**	1.9*	**34**	**1,250**	**40**	**8**
14–18 y	1,300*	35*	**890**	3*	**150**	**11**	**410**	2.2*	**43**	**1,250**	**55**	**11**
19–30 y	1,000*	35*	**900**	4*	**150**	**8**	**400**	2.3*	**45**	**700**	**55**	**11**
31–50 y	1,000*	35*	**900**	4*	**150**	**8**	**420**	2.3*	**45**	**700**	**55**	**11**
51–70 y	1,200*	30*	**900**	4*	**150**	**8**	**420**	2.3*	**45**	**700**	**55**	**11**
>70 y	1,200*	30*	**900**	4*	**150**	**8**	**420**	2.3*	**45**	**700**	**55**	**11**
Females												
9–13 y	1,300*	21*	**700**	2*	**120**	**8**	**240**	1.6*	**34**	**1,250**	**40**	**8**
14–18 y	1,300*	24*	**890**	3*	**150**	**15**	**360**	1.6*	**43**	**1,250**	**55**	**9**
19–30 y	1,000*	25*	**900**	3*	**150**	**18**	**310**	1.8*	**45**	**700**	**55**	**8**
31–50 y	1,000*	25*	**900**	3*	**150**	**18**	**320**	1.8*	**45**	**700**	**55**	**8**
51–70 y	1,200*	20*	**900**	3*	**150**	**8**	**320**	1.8*	**45**	**700**	**55**	**8**
>70 y	1,200*	20*	**900**	3*	**150**	**8**	**320**	1.8*	**45**	**700**	**55**	**8**
Pregnancy												
≤18 y	1,300*	29*	**1,000**	3*	**220**	**27**	**400**	2.0*	**50**	**1,250**	**60**	**13**
10–30 y	1,000*	30*	**1,000**	3*	**220**	**27**	**350**	2.0*	**50**	**700**	**60**	**11**
31–50 y	1,000*	30*	**1,000**	3*	**220**	**27**	**360**	2.0*	**50**	**700**	**60**	**11**
Lactation												
≤18 y	1,300*	44*	**1,300**	3*	**290**	**10**	**360**	2.6*	**50**	**1,250**	**70**	**14**
19–30 y	1,000*	45*	**1,300**	3*	**290**	**9**	**310**	2.6*	**50**	**700**	**70**	**12**
31–50 y	1,000*	45*	**1,300**	3*	**290**	**9**	**320**	2.6*	**50**	**700**	**70**	**12**

NOTE: This table presents Recommended Dietary Allowances (RDAs) in **bold type** and Adequate Intakes (AIs) in ordinary type followed by an asterisk (*). RDAs and AIs may both be used as goals for individual intake. RDAs are set to meet the needs of almost all (97 to 98 percent) individuals in a group. For healthy breastfed infants, the AI is the mean intake. The AI for other life stage and gender groups is believed to cover needs of all individuals in the group, but lack of data or uncertainty in the data prevent being able to specify with confidence the percentage of individuals covered by this intake.

SOURCES: Dietary Reference Intakes for Calcium, Phosphorus, Magnesium, Vitamin D, and Fluoride (1997); Dietary Reference Intakes for Thiamin, Riboflavin, Niacin, Vitamin B_6, Folate, Vitamin B_{12}, Pantothenic Acid, Biotin, and Choline (1998); Dietary Reference Intakes for Vitamin C, Vitamin E, Selenium, and Carotenoids (2000); and Dietary Reference Intakes for Vitamin A, Vitamin K, Arsenic, Boron, Chromium, Copper, Iodine, Iron, Mangenese, Molybdenum, Nickel, Silicon, Vanadium, and Zinc (2001). These reports may be accessed via www.nap.edu.

TABLE A-10 Dietary Reference Intakes (DRIs): Tolerable Upper Intake Levels (UL[a]), Elements Food and Nutrition Board, The Institute of Medicine, National Academies

Life Stage Group	Arsenic[b]	Boron (mg/d)	Calcium (g/d)	Chromium	Copper (μg/d)	Fluoride (mg/d)	Iodine (μg/d)	Iron (mg/d)	Magnesium (mg/d)[c]	Manganese (mg/d)	Molybdenum (μg/d)	Nickel (mg/d)	Phosphorus (g/d)	Selenium (μg/d)	Silicon[d]	Vanadium (mg/d)[e]	Zinc (mg/d)
Infants																	
0–6 mo	ND[f]	ND	ND	ND	ND	0.7	ND	40	ND	ND	ND	ND	ND	45	ND	ND	4
7–12 mo	ND	ND	ND	ND	ND	0.9	ND	40	ND	ND	ND	ND	ND	60	ND	ND	5
Children																	
1–3 y	ND	3	2.5	ND	1,000	1.3	200	40	65	2	300	0.2	3	90	ND	ND	7
4–8 y	ND	6	2.5	ND	3,000	2.2	300	40	110	3	600	0.3	3	150	ND	ND	12
Males, Females																	
9–13 y	ND	11	2.5	ND	5,000	10	600	40	350	6	1,100	0.6	4	280	ND	ND	23
14–18 y	ND	17	2.5	ND	8,000	10	900	45	350	9	1,700	1.0	4	400	ND	ND	34
19–70 y	ND	20	2.5	ND	10,000	10	1,100	45	350	11	2,000	1.0	4	400	ND	1.8	40
>70 y	ND	20	2.5	ND	10,000	10	1,100	45	350	11	2,000	1.0	3	400	ND	1.8	40
Pregnancy																	
≤18 y	ND	17	2.5	ND	8,000	10	900	45	350	9	1,700	1.0	3.5	400	ND	ND	34
19–50 y	ND	20	2.5	ND	10,000	10	1,100	45	350	11	2,000	1.0	3.5	400	ND	ND	40
Lactation																	
≤18 y	ND	17	2.5	ND	8,000	10	900	45	350	9	1,700	1.0	4	400	ND	ND	34
19–50 y	ND	20	2.5	ND	10,000	10	1,100	45	350	11	2,000	1.0	4	400	ND	ND	40

[a]UL = The maximum level of daily nutrient intake that is likely to pose no risk of adverse effects. Unless otherwise specified, the UL represents total intake from food, water, and supplements. Due to lack of suitable data, ULs could not be established for arsenic, chromium, and silicon. In the absence of ULs, extra caution may be warranted in consuming levels above recommended intakes.

[b]Although the UL was not determined for arsenic, there is no justification for adding arsenic to food or supplements.

[c]The ULs for magnesium represent intake from a pharmacological agent only and do not include intake from food and water.

[d]Although silicon has not been shown to cause adverse effects in humans, there is no justification for adding silicon to supplements.

[e]Although vanadium in food has not been shown to cause adverse effects in humans, there is no justification for adding vanadium to food and vanadium supplements should be used with caution. The UL is based on adverse effects in laboratory animals and these data could be used to set a UL for adults but no children and adolescents.

[f]ND = Not determinable due to lack of data of adverse effects in this age group and concern with regard to lack of ability to handle excess amounts. Source of intake should be from food only to prevent high levels of intake.

SOURCES: Dietary Reference Intakes for Calcium, Phosphorus, Magnesium, Vitamin D, and Fluoride (1997); Dietary Reference Intakes for Thiamin, Riboflavin, Niacin, Vitamin B_6, Folate, Vitamin B_{12}, Pantothenic Acid, Biotin, and Choline (1998); Dietary Reference Intakes for Vitamin C, Vitamin E, Selenium, and Carotenoids (2000); and Dietary Reference Intakes for Vitamin A, Vitamin K, Arsenic, Boron, Chromium, Copper, Iodine, Iron, Manganese, Molybdenum, Nickel, Silicon, Vanadium, and Zinc (2001). These reports may be accessed via www.nap.edu.

REFERENCES

Cited References

American Dietetic Association. Position of The American Dietetic Association: the impact of fluoride on health. *J Am Diet Assoc.* 2000; 100:1208.

American Dietetic Association. Position of The American Dietetic Association: health implications of dietary fiber. *J Am Diet Assoc.* 1997;97:1157.

American Dietetic Association. Position of the American Dietetic Association: vitamin and mineral supplementation. *J Am Diet Assoc.* 1996;96:73.

Arnal M, et al. Protein pulse feeding improves protein retention in elderly women. *Am J Clin Nutri.* 1999;69:1202.

Anderson J. Minerals. In: Mahan L, Escott-Stump S. *Krause's food, nutrition, and diet therapy.* 10th ed. Philadelphia: WB Saunders, 2000.

Babin F, et al. Differences between polyunsaturated fatty acid status of noninstitutionalized elderly women and younger controls: a bioconversion defect can be suspected. *Euro J Clin Nutri.* 1999; 53:591.

Baumgartner T. Trace elements in clinical nutrition. *Nutr Clin Pract.* 1993;8:251.

Bender D. Optimum nutrition: thiamin, biotin, and pantothenate. *Proc Nutr Soc.* 1999;58:427.

Blanchard J, et al. Pharmacokinetic perspectives on megadoses of ascorbic acid (review). *Am J Clin Nutri.* 1997;66:1165.

Booth S, et al. Dietary vitamin K intakes are associated with hip fracture but not with bone mineral density in elderly men and women. *Am J Clin Nutri.* 2000;71:1201.

Burge J, et al. Copper decreases ascorbic acid stability in total parenteral nutrition solutions. *J Am Diet Assoc.* 1994;94:777.

Bursell S, et al. High-dose vitamin E supplementation normalizes retinal blood flow and creatinine clearance in patients with type 1 diabetes. *Diab Care.* 1999;22:1245.

Carr A, Frei B. Toward a new recommended dietary allowance for vitamin C based on antioxidant and health effects in humans. *Am J Clin Nutri.* 1999;69:1086.

Caso G, et al. Albumin synthesis is diminished in men consuming a predominantly vegetarian diet. *J Nutri.* 2000;130:528.

Combs G. Vitamins. In: Mahan L, Escott-Stump S. *Krause's food, nutrition, and diet therapy.* 10th ed. Philadelphia: WB Saunders, 2000.

Costello R, Grumstrup-Scott J. Zinc: What role might supplements play? *J Am Diet Assoc.* 2000;100:371.

DeLuca H. Vitamin D: 1993. *Nutrition Today.* 1993;28:6.

Finley J. The retention and distribution by healthy young men of stable isotopes of selenium consumed as selenite, selenate, or hydropenically-grown broccoli are dependent on the isotopic form. *J Nutri.* 1999;129:865.

Fraker P, et al. The dynamic link between the integrity of the immune system and zinc status. *J Nutri.* 2000;130:1399S.

Gaudichon C, et al. Net postprandial utilization of 15-N-labeled milk protein nitrogen is influenced by diet composition in humans. *J Nutri.* 1999;129:890.

Gleerup A, et al. Iron absorption from the whole diet: comparison of the effect of two different distributions of daily calcium intake. *Am J Clin Nutri.* 1995;61:97.

Haddad J. Vitamin D: solar rays, the Milky Way, or both? *N Engl J Med.* 1992;326:1213.

Hahn J, et al. Wernicke encephalopathy and beriberi during total parenteral nutrition attributable to multivitamin infusion shortage. *Pediatrics.* 1998;101:E10.

Harris S, Dawson-Hughes B. The association of oral contraceptive use with plasma 25-hydroxyvitamin D levels. *J Am Col Nutri.* 1998; 17:282.

Harrison E, Hussain M. Mechanisms involved in the intestinal digestion and absorption of dietary vitamin A. *J Nutri.* 2001;131:1405.

Heaney R, et al. Bioavailability of the calcium in fortified soy imitation milk, with some observations on method. *Am J Clin Nutri.* 2000;71:1166.

Herbert V. Vitamin C supplements and disease—counterpoint (editorial). *J Am Col Nutri.* 1995;14:112.

Hine R. What practitioners need to know about folic acid. *J Am Diet Assoc.* 1996;96:451.

Holben D, Smith A. The diverse role of selenium with selenoproteins: a review. *J Am Diet Assoc.* 1999;99:836.

Hu F, et al. Dietary protein and risk of ischemic heart disease in women. *Am J Clin Nutri.* 1999;70:221.

Hunt C, Meacham S. Aluminum, boron, calcium, copper, iron, magnesium, manganese, molybdenum, phosphorus, potassium, sodium and zinc: concentrations in common Western foods and estimated daily intakes by infants, toddlers, and male and female adolescents, adults, and seniors in the United States. *J Am Diet Assoc.* 2001;101: 1058.

Jacob R, et al. Folate nutriture alters choline status of women and men fed low choline diets. *J Nutri.* 1999;129:712.

Johnston C, Thompson L. Vitamin C status of an outpatient population. *J Am Col Nutri.* 1998;17:366.

Kritchevsky S, et al. Dietary antioxidants and carotid artery wall thickness: the ARIC study. *Circulation.* 1995;92:2142.

Kurttio P, et al. Exposure to natural well water and hip fracture: a cohort analysis in Finland. *Am J Epid.* 1999;150:817.

Kutsky R. *Handbook of vitamins, minerals, and hormones.* 2nd ed. New York: Von Nostrand Reinhold Company, 1981.

Lakshmi A. Riboflavin metabolism—relevance to human nutrition. *Indian J Med Res.* 1998;108:182.

Levine M, et al. Vitamin C pharmacokinetics in healthy volunteers: evidence for a recommended dietary allowance. *Proc Natl Acad Sci.* 1996;93:3704.

Looker A, et al. Prevalence of iron deficiency in the United States. *JAMA.* 1997;277:973.

Losonczy K, et al. Vitamin E and vitamin C supplement use and risk of all-cause and coronary heart disease mortality in older persons: the Established Populations for Epidemiologic Studies of the Elderly. *Am J Clin Nutri.* 1996;64:190.

Macknin M, et al. Zinc gluconate lozenges for treating the common cold in children: a randomized controlled trial. *J Am Med Assoc.* 1998;279:1962.

Mantzoros C, et al. Zinc may regulate serum leptin concentrations in humans. *J Am Col Nutri.* 1998;17:270.

McNutt K. What clients should know about sugar replacers. *J Am Diet Assoc.* 2000;100:466.

Mertz, W. A balanced approach to nutrition for health. The need for biologically essential minerals and vitamins. *J Am Diet Assoc.* 1994; 94:1259.

Monsen E. Dietary Reference Intakes for antioxidant nutrients: vitamin C, vitamin E, selenium, and carotenoids. *J Am Diet Assoc.* 2000; 100:637.

Monsen E. New dietary reference intakes proposed to replace the recommended dietary allowances. *J Am Diet Assoc.* 1996;96: 754.

Nebeling L, et al. Changes in carotenoid intake in the United States: the 1987 and 1992 National Health Interview Surveys. *J Am Diet Assoc.* 1997;97:991.

Neuhouser M, et al. Absorption of dietary and supplemental folate in women with prior pregnancies with neural tube defects and controls. *J Am Col Nutri.* 1998;17:625.

Oakley G. Eat right and take a multivitamin (editorial). *N Engl J Med.* 1998;338:1060.

Omenn G, et al. Risk factors for lung cancer and for intervention effects in CARET, the beta-carotene, and retinol efficacy trial. *J Nat'l Cancer Inst.* 1996;88:1550.

Paleologos M, et al. Cohort study of vitamin C intake and cognitive impairment. *Am J Epid.* 1998;148:164.

Pitche P, et al. Prevalence of HIV infection in patients with pellagra and pellagra-like erythemas. *Med Trop.* 1999;59:365.

Pugliese M, et al. Nutritional rickets in suburbia. *J Am Col Nutri.* 1998;17:637.

Rock C, et al. Update on the biological characteristics of the antioxidant micronutrients: vitamin C, vitamin E, and the carotenoids. *J Am Diet Assoc.* 1996;96:693.

Schrezenmeir J, Miller G. Calcium. *J Am Col Nutri.* 2000;19:83S.

Scimeca J, Miller G. Health benefits of conjugated linoleic acid. Proceedings of a symposium held October 2, 1999, at the 40th Annual Meeting of the American College of Nutrition in Washington, DC. *J Am Col Nutri.* 2000;19:469S.

Shamir R. Thiamine deficiency in children with congenital heart disease before and after corrective surgery. *J Parenter Enteral Nutri.* 2000;24:154.

Simon J, Hudes E. Relation of serum ascorbic acid to blood lead levels. *J Am Med Assoc.* 1999;281:2289.

Simon J, Hudes E. Relation of serum ascorbic acid to serum lipids and lipoproteins in U.S. adults. *J Am Col Nutri.* 1998;17:250.

Smit E, et al. Estimates of animal and plant protein intake in U.S. adults: results from the Third National Health and Nutrition Examination Survey 1988–1991. *J Am Diet Assoc.* 1999;99:813.

Stahl P. What's new at the FDA: informing consumers about trans fat labeling. *JAMA.* 2000;100:1133.

Swain R, St. Clair L. The role of folic acid in deficiency states and prevention of disease. *J Fam Practice.* 1997;44:138.

Swinburn B, et al. Effects of reduced-fat diets consumed ad libitum on intake of nutrients, particularly antioxidant vitamins. *J Am Diet Assoc.* 1999;99:1400.

Teasley-Strausburg K, et al. Trace mineral solutions. In: Teasley-Strausburg K, ed. *Nutrition support handbook: a compendium of produce with guidelines for usage.* Cincinnati: Harvey Whitney Books, 1992; 117.

Thomas M, et al. Hypovitaminosis D in medical patients. *N Engl J Med.* 1998;338:777.

Trumbo P, et al. Dietary Reference Intakes: vitamin A, vitamin K, arsenic, boron, chromium, copper, iodine, iron, manganese, molybdenum, nickel, silicon, vanadium, and zinc. *J Am Diet Assoc.* 2001;101:294.

Van Dusseldorp M, et al. Risk of persistent cobalamin deficiency in adolescents fed a macrobiotic diet in early life. *Am J Clin Nutri.* 1999;69:664.

Vandenlangenberg G, et al. Influence of using different sources of carotenoid data in epidemiologic studies. *J Am Diet Assoc.* 1996; 96:1271.

van het Hof K, et al. Dietary factors that affect the bioavailability of carotenoids. *J Nutri.* 2000;130:503.

Verma A, et al. Nutritional factors that can favorably influence the glucose/insulin system: vanadium. *J Am Col Nutri.* 1998;17:11.

Vesper H, et al. Sphingolipids in food and the emerging importance of sphingolipids to nutrition (review). *J Nutri.* 1999;129:1239.

Vieth R. Vitamin D supplementation, 25-hydroxyvitamin D concentrations, and safety (review). *Am J Clin Nutri.* 1999;69:842.

Voyles L, et al. High levels of retinol intake during the first trimester of pregnancy result from use of over-the-counter vitamin/mineral supplements. *J Am Diet Assoc.* 2000;100:1068.

Weaver C, et al. Calcium bioavailability from high oxalate vegetables: Chinese vegetables, sweet potatoes, and rhubarb. *J Food Sci.* 1997; 62:524.

West Suitor C, Bailey L. Dietary folate equivalents: interpretation and results. *J Am Diet Assoc.* 2000;100:88.

Wu T, et al. Maternal cigarette smoking, regular use of multivitamin/mineral supplements and risk of fetal death: the 1988 National Maternal and Infant Health Survey. *Am J Epid.* 1998;148:215.

Zhang S, et al. A prospective study of folate intake and the risk of breast cancer. *J Am Med Assoc.* 1999;281:1632.

Suggested Readings

Anderson J, Garner S. *Calcium and phosphorus in health and disease.* Boca Raton: CRC Press, 1996.

Andersen L, et al. Evaluation of a food frequency questionnaire with weighed records, fatty acids, and alpha-tocopherol in adipose tissue and serum. *Am J Epid.* 1999;150:75.

Anderson J. Minerals. In: Mahan K, Escott-Stump S, eds. *Krause's food, nutrition, and diet therapy.* 10th ed. Philadelphia: WB Saunders, 2000.

Berdanier C. *Advanced nutrition: macronutrients.* Boca Raton: CRC Press, 1995.

Booth S, et al. Assessment of phylloquinone and dihydrophylloquinone dietary intakes among a nationally representative sample of U.S. consumers using 14-day food diaries. *J Am Diet Assoc.* 1999; 99:1072.

Brighenti F, et al. Effect of consumption of a ready-to-eat breakfast cereal containing inulin on the intestinal milieu and blood lipids in healthy male volunteers. *Euro J Clin Nutri.* 1999;53:726.

Brouwer I, et al. Dietary folate from vegetables and citrus fruits decreases plasma homocysteine concentrations in humans in a dietary controlled trial. *J Nutri.* 1999;129:1135.

Campbell N. How safe are folic acid supplements? *Arch Int Med.* 1996;156:1638.

Cartmel B, et al. Effects of long-term intake of retinol on selected clinical and laboratory indexes. *Am J Clin Nutri.* 1999;69:937.

Castenmiller J, et al. The food matrix of spinach is a limiting factor in determining the availability of beta-carotene and to a lesser extent of lutein in humans. *J Nutri.* 1999;129:349.

Crouse J, et al. A randomized trial comparing the effect of casein with that of soy protein containing varying amounts of isoflavones on plasma concentrations of lipids and lipoproteins. *Arch Int Med.* 1999;159:2070.

Cynober L. *Amino acid metabolism and therapy in health and nutritional disease.* Boca Raton: CRC Press, 1995.

Devaraj S, et al. The effects of alpha tocopherol supplementation on monocyte function. *J Clin Invest.* 1996;98:756.

Flynn M, et al. Lipoprotein response to a National Cholesterol Education Program step II diet with and without energy restriction. *Metabolism: Clin and Exprimental.* 1999;48:822.

Ford E, Bowman B. Serum and red blood cell folate concentrations, race, and education: findings from the Third National Health and Nutrition Examination Survey. *Am J Clin Nutri.* 1999;69:476.

Gausseres N, et al. Whole-body turnover in humans fed a soy protein-rich vegetable diet. *Euro J Clin Nutri.* 1997;51:308.

Gregory J, et al. Urinary excretion of folate by nonpregnant women following a single oral dose of folic acid is a functional index of folate nutritional status. *J Nutri.* 1998;128:1907.

Guttormsen A, et al. Determinants and vitamin responsiveness of intermediate hyperhomocystinemia (> 40 umol/liter): The Hordaland Homocysteine Study. *J Clin Invest.* 1996;98:2174.

Haken V. Interactions between drugs and nutrients. In: Mahan K, Escott-Stump S, eds. *Krause's food, nutrition, and diet therapy.* 9th ed. Philadelphia: WB Saunders, 1996.

Hallikainen M, Uusitupa M. Effects of 2 low-fat stanol ester-containing margarines on serum cholesterol concentrations as part of a low-fat diet in hypercholesterolemic subjects. *Am J Clin Nutri.* 1999;69:403.

Hemila H, et al. Vitamin C and other compounds in vitamin C rich food in relation to risk of tuberculosis in male smokers. *Am J Epid.* 1999;150:632.

Herbert V, Sharpe G. *Total nutrition: the only guide you'll ever need.* New York: St. Martin's Press, 1995.

Hirschmann J, Raugi G. Adult scurvy. *J Am Acad Dermatol.* 1999;41:895.

Huang C, et al. The bioavailability of beta-carotene in stir- or deep-fried vegetables in men determined by measuring the serum response to a single ingestion. *J Nutri.* 2000;130:534–540.

Innis S, et al. Variability in the trans fatty acid content of foods within a food category: implications for estimation of dietary trans fatty acid intakes. *J Am Col Nutri.* 1999;18:255.

Jacques P, et al. The effect of folic acid fortification on plasma folate and total homocysteine concentrations. *N Engl J Med.* 1999;340:1449.

Jenkinson A, et al. Dietary intakes of polyunsaturated fatty acids and indices of oxidative stress in human volunteers. *Euro J Clin Nutri.* 1999;53:523.

Kelly P, et al. Unmetabolized folic acid in serum: acute studies in subjects consuming fortified food and supplements. *Am J Clin Nutri.* 1997;65:1790.

Kleemola P, et al. The effect of breakfast cereal on diet and serum cholesterol: a randomized trial in North Karelia, Finland. *Euro J Clin Nutri.* 1999;53:716.

Krinsky N, Sies H. Antioxidant vitamins and beta-carotene in disease prevention. *Am J Clin Nutri.* 1995;62:1299S.

Kritchevsky S, et al. Dietary antioxidants and carotid artery wall thickness: The ARIC Study. *Circulation.* 1995;92:2142.

LeFur C, et al. Influence of mental stress and circadian cycle on postprandial ischemia. *Am J Clin Nutri.* 1999;70:213.

Lewis C, et al. Estimated folate intakes: data updated to reflect food fortification, increased bioavailability, and dietary supplement use. *Am J Clin Nutri.* 1999;70:198.

Lichtenstein A, et al. Effects of different forms of dietary hydrogenated fats on serum lipoprotein cholesterol levels. *N Engl J Med.* 1999;340:1933.

Losonczy K, et al. Vitamin E and vitamin C supplement use and risk of all-cause and coronary heart disease mortality in older persons: the Established Populations for Epidemiologic Studies of the Elderly. *Am J Clin Nutri.* 1996;64:190.

Louheranta A, et al. A high-trans fatty acid diet and insulin sensitivity in young healthy women. *Metabolism: Clin and Experimental.* 1999;48:870.

Lykkesfeldt J, et al. Ascorbate is depleted by smoking and repleted by moderate supplementation: a study in male smokers and nonsmokers with matched dietary antioxidant intakes. *Am J Clin Nutri.* 2000;71:530.

Lyle B, et al. Supplement users differ from nonusers in demographic, lifestyle, dietary and health characteristics. *J Nutri.* 1998;128:2355.

Mares-Perlman J, et al. Zinc intake and sources in the U.S. adult population: 1976–1980. *J Am Col Nutri.* 1995;14:349.

Martin A, et al. Effect of fruits, vegetables, or vitamin E—rich diet on vitamins E and C distribution in peripheral and brain tissues: implications for brain functions. *J Gerontol A Biol Sci Med Sci.* 2000;55: B144.

Miwa K, et al. Vitamin E deficiency in variant angina. *Circulation.* 1996;94:14.

Monsen E. New dietary reference intakes proposed to replace the recommended dietary allowances. *J Am Diet Assoc.* 1996;96:754.

Omenn G. An assessment of the scientific basis for attempting to define the Dietary Reference Intake for beta-carotene. *J Am Diet Assoc.* 1998;98:1406.

Perry H, et al. Longitudinal changes in serum 25-hydroxy-vitamin D in older people. *Metabolism: Clin and Experimental.* 1999;48:1028.

Rock C, et al. Bioavailability of beta-carotene is lower in raw than in processed carrots and spinach in women. *J Nutri.* 1998;128:913.

Ramakrishna T. Vitamins and brain development. *Physiol Res.* 1999;48:175–187.

Rock C. Dietary reference intakes, antioxidants, and beta-carotene. *J Am Diet Assoc.* 1998;98:1410.

Ruxton C, et al. Guidelines for sugar consumption in Europe: Is a quantitative approach justified? *Euro J Clin Nutri.* 1999;53:503.

Schwartz J. Role of polyunsaturated fatty acids in lung disease. *Am J Clin Nutri.* 2000;71:393S.

Spiller G. *Handbook of lipids in human nutrition.* Boca Raton: CRC Press, 1996.

Strauss R. Comparison of serum concentrations of a-tocopherol and beta-carotene in a cross-sectional sample of obese and nonobese children (NHANES III). *J Pediatr.* 1999;134:172.

Stuerenburg H. CSF copper concentrations, blood-brain barrier function, and ceruloplasmin synthesis during the treatment of Wilson's disease. *J Neural Transm.* 2000;107:321.

Takamatsu S, et al. Effects on health of dietary supplementation with 100 mg d-alpha-tocopherol acetate, daily for 6 years. *J Int Med Research.* 1995;23:342.

Thorpe J, et al. Prior protein intake may affect phenylalanine kinetics measured in healthy adult volunteers consuming 1 g protein/kg/d. *J Nutri.* 1999;129:343.

Utinger R. The need for more vitamin D (editorial). *N Engl J Med.* 1998;338:828.

Vandenlangenberg G, et al. Influence of using different sources of carotenoid data in epidemiologic studies. *J Am Diet Assoc.* 1996;96:1271.

Van Asselt D, et al. Free and protein-bound cobalamin absorption in healthy middle-aged and older subjects. *J Am Geriatr Soc.* 1996;44:949.

van den Heuvel E, et al. Oligofructose stimulates calcium absorption in adolescents. *Am J Clin Nutri.* 1999;69:544.

Welch G, Loscalzo J. Homocysteine and atherosclerosis. *N Engl J Med.* 1998;338:1042.

Whitmyre S. Water, electrolytes, and acid-base balance. In: Mahan K, Escott-Stump S, eds. *Krause's food, nutrition, and diet therapy.* 10th ed. Philadelphia: WB Saunders, 2000.

Will J, et al. Serum vitamin C concentrations and diabetes: findings from the third National Health and Nutrition Examination Survey. *Am J Clin Nutri.* 1999;70:49.

Wolever T, et al. Day-to-day consistency in amount and source of carbohydrate intake associated with improved blood glucose control in type 1 diabetes. *J Am Col Nutri.* 1999;18:242.

Yates A, et al. Dietary reference intakes: the new basis for recommendations for calcium and related nutrients, B vitamins and choline. *J Am Diet Assoc.* 1998;98:699.

APPENDIX B

Dietetic Process, Forms, and Counseling Tips

INTRODUCTION

The American Dietetic Association maintains responsibility for education, practice standards, and credentialing of dietetic professionals. Practice and job analyses are conducted to determine current trends as well as future goals. Standards from the Joint Commission on Accreditation of Healthcare Organizations (JCAHO) set the expectation that quality care will lead to positive outcomes. Leadership and continuous performance improvement are two areas that are considered to be critical for maintaining quality services (Escott-Stump et al., 2000). JCAHO will support chronic-disease management programs where services are provided at a lower cost across the continuum of care. Other important trends and issues include the following:

1. Dietitians and technicians work in a variety of settings but are concentrated in acute care, long-term care, and the community (Bryk and Soto, 1999). Because they possess a wide scope of knowledge in nutrition and management, dietetics professionals are also in an ideal position to advance to foodservice management jobs (Stonebrook, 1999). They may also seek positions in home health care; of the 7.5 million new jobs created in the U.S. during the first half of the 1990s, home care positions were among the top 10 (Campbell, 1999).
2. Dietetics professionals perform a variety of tasks including clinical services, food services, nutrition information, and public health functions. Levels of responsibility tend to increase with years of experience. Dietetics educators and practitioners need to consider cross-training to meet future demands of practice (Gates and Sandoval, 1998). Learning should be continuous, supportive, stimulating and empowering, lifelong, understanding, confidence-building, and creative (Duyff, 1999).
3. Most dietitians work in settings that are supportive of interdisciplinary teamwork. Dietitians are comfortable in their work and want more responsibility, but some are uncomfortable with change. They must position their nutrition services as being vital to cost-effective, high-quality care; augment their skills in consultation, training, nutrition support, and outcomes research; and strengthen collaborative ties with key home health care professionals (Schiller et al., 1998). In the future, dietitians will need to be more proactive, take on new skills, acquire more knowledge, readily market their services, take risks, and work to overcome traditional stereotypes (Dahlke et al., 2000).
4. Employer and practitioner surveys suggest expansion of responsibilities to include more physical assessment, certification to perform cardiopulmonary resuscitation, assessment of need for adaptive feeding equipment, leading work site wellness, teaching exercise education, and provision of home care services. Order-writing privileges by dietitians allow orders for tube feeding (TF) and total parenteral nutrition (TPN) orders to be implemented quickly and effectively (Moreland et al., 2002; Myers et al., 2002).
5. Dietetic professionals will need to be cross-trained, versatile, flexible, creative, and proactive (Balch, 1996). Consultation is an area in which the profession is likely to excel. Up-skilling has become a major trend in health care; it has implications for the profession's scope of practice, licensure, malpractice liability considerations (Visocan, 1998), and other standards for care.
6. Patients who are moderately or severely malnourished have higher health care costs than those who remain well nourished (Abron, Braunschweig, 1999). Medical nutrition therapy (MNT) has the potential to pay for itself with savings in utilization for other services (Sheils et al., 1999). If MNT had been covered in 1998, by 2004 approximately $2.3 billion would have been saved through reduced hospital spending through Medicare part A (Johnson, 1999).
7. Changes in hospital foodservice operation are expected in several areas—71% will serve fewer meals to in-patients, 73% will employ less staff, 70% will have smaller expense budgets, and 61% will generate more revenue (Silverman et al., 2000). Foodservice managers who desire to improve patient satisfaction should focus attention on meeting or exceeding patient expectations for food and service quality (Lau and Gregoire, 1998).
8. Cost-effectiveness analysis is a great tool to use in a clinical setting to prove the worth of certain services for prevention and treatment of chronic diseases (Naglak et al., 1998). Nutrition therapists can use this information to negotiate a disease-state management contract with companies (Israel and McCabe, 1999).
9. Clinical nutrition managers are in a position of opportunity in the health care arena. They have power and leadership roles and can increase power and influence through support from other managers, acquisition of resources, identification of opportunities, and use of available information (Mislevy et al., 2000).
10. Nutrition education is an essential component of the

curricula for the majority of health care professionals with nutrition principles, identification of nutrition risk factors, and timely referral to a qualified dietetics professional as the main focus (American Dietetic Association, Position . . .1998). In a survey of clinical nutrition training programs for physicians, 13 programs focused primarily on adult nutrition, seven on pediatrics, 12 taught nutrition as the sole focus, eight were within gastroenterology, and two within endocrinology; most programs included training in research (Heimburger et al., 1998). Dietitians should actively seek involvement in these programs when possible.

11. Two tiers of nutrition services exist: basic nutrition education where advice may be provided by most health care professionals; the second tier is "an intensive approach to the management of chronic disease and requires significantly more training in food and nutrition science than is commonly provided by the curriculum of other health professionals. It requires a broad knowledge base to translate complex diet prescriptions into meaningful individualized dietary modifications for the lay person" (Fox, 2000). Registered dietitians are currently the single identifiable group of health care professionals with standardized education, clinical training, continuing education, and national credentialing requirements necessary to be directly reimbursed as a provider of nutrition therapy.

12. Routine contact, communication, and interaction between physicians and dietitians are vital if physicians are to recognize dietitians' responsibilities and competencies and to collaborate with them when providing MNT to patients (Boyhtari and Cardinal, 1997).

13. Medicare coverage of diabetes, renal, enteral, and parenteral nutrition in acute care should continue at current level with a multidisciplinary approach (Fox, 2000). MNT and lifestyle counseling are also integral components where pharmacotherapy is indicated (American Dietetic Association, 1999).

14. Strong management and leadership skills are needed in moving nutrition into the next era of health care; nutritionists must manage their own competence as well as that of others who report to them (Dodds and Polhamus, 1999).

15. Demonstration of effectiveness is essential, especially in this era of evidence-based medicine and accountability (Barr et al., 2001). Health-related quality of life (HRQL) is a patient-related concept that can be measured as part of outcomes evaluation. Beyond biochemical and physical improvements, a "quality of life assessment" is an important step in determining if the best outcomes have been achieved (see Figure B-1). Biologic factors, symptoms, functional status, health perceptions, and quality of life function along a continuum (Wilson and Cleary, 1995). A nutrition quality of life instrument is now available.

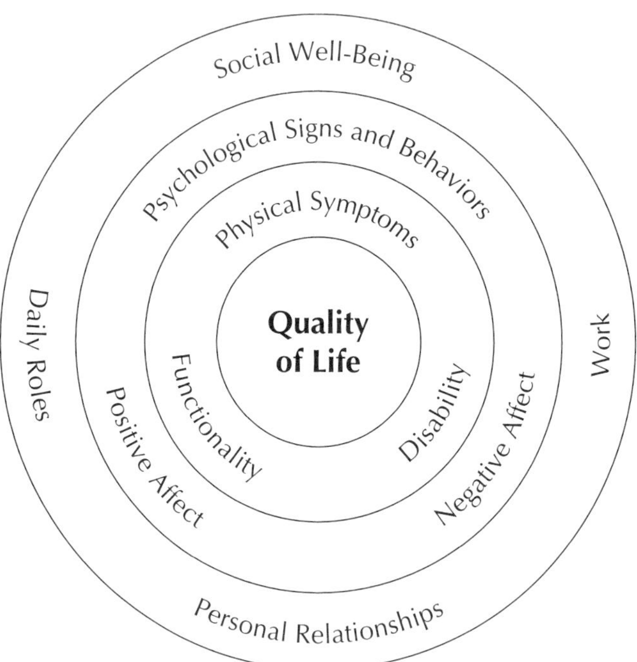

Figure B-1 Quality of life assessments should include a review of subjective perceptions and objective measurements of health status (based on Testa and Simonson, 1996).

THE DIETETIC PROCESS AND ROLE OF THE REGISTERED DIETITIAN ON THE HEALTH TEAM

Disease management is an approach to patient care that emphasizes coordinated, comprehensive care along the continuum of disease and across health care delivery systems. Evidence-based medicine is an approach to practice and teaching that integrates pathophysiological rationale, diagnosis, etiology, prognosis with valid and current clinical research evidence (Meakins, 2002.) Multidisciplinary teams are ideally suited to develop, lead, and implement evidence-based disease management programs, because they play an essential role in the preventive, diagnostic, and therapeutic decisions for patients throughout the course of their disease. (Ellrodt et al., 1997). Figures B-2A and B-2B provide suggested nutritional care processes and flow chart.

THE SPECIFIC ROLE OF THE DIETITIAN INCLUDES:

Nutritional Risk Screening

1. JCAHO now requires a home care provider to screen for moderate to high nutritional risk for all home care patients (Campbell, 1999) and institutionalized patients. A trained professional can then identify nutritional risk factors and prioritize the level of dietitian involvement.

2. The need to screen patients earlier than within the first 24 hours after admission has resulted in use of more preadmission screenings. Critical pathways should be developed first; patients are called at home prior to admission, leading to greater patient satisfaction and better screening outcomes (Baird Schwartz and Gudzin, 2000).

3. Screening factors should be developed for the specific setting and type of population typically seen (Council on Practice Quality Management Committee, 1994). Cultural sensitivity is crucial in this process. Identify priority patients from nutritional screening in Table B-1. Assign screenings as low risk (level 1), moderate risk (level 2), and high risk (level 3). See Appendix D for nutritional acuity rankings for different diagnoses.

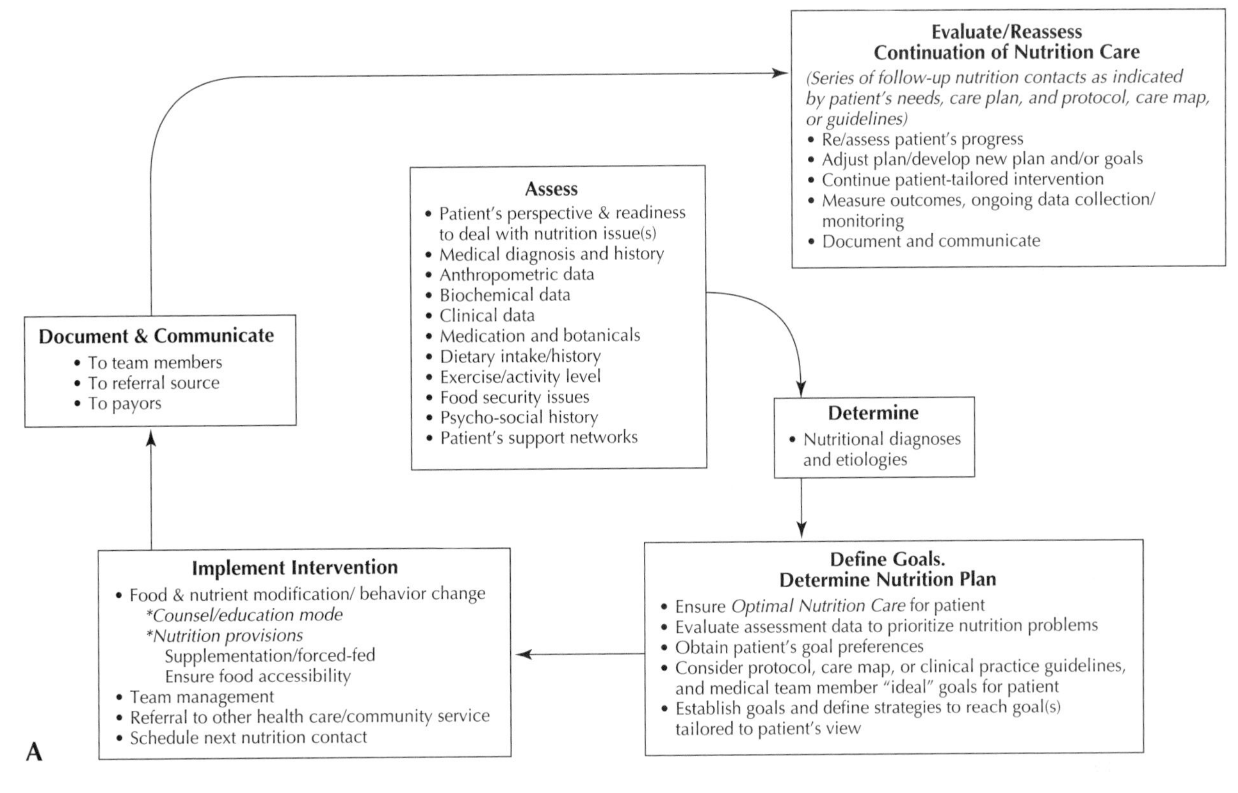

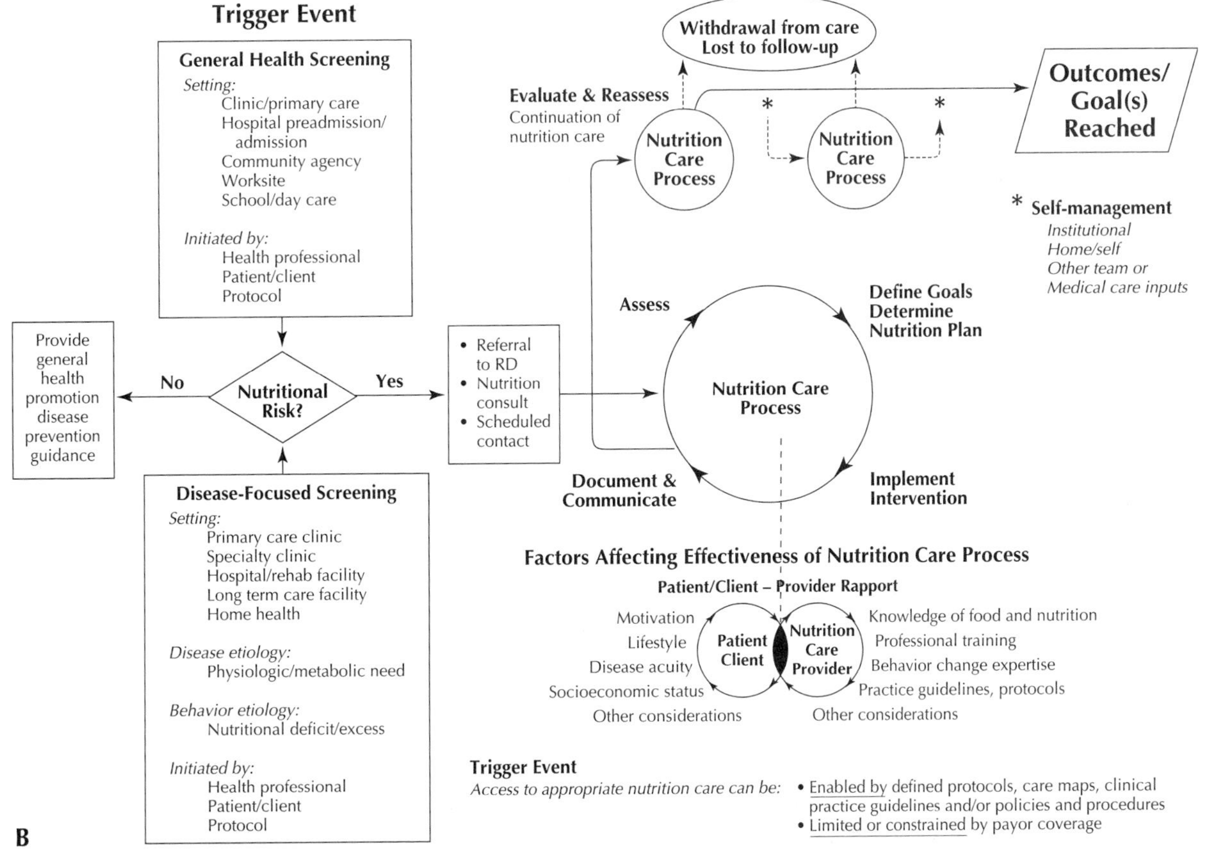

Figure B-2 (A and B) Suggested Nutritional Care Process (Adapted from Splett and Myers, 2001), used with permission.

TABLE B-1 Identifying Priority Patients from Nutrition Screening

1. Admitting diagnosis: 1 POINT EACH

AIDS-HIV
Alcohol and/or drug abuse
Bowel obstruction
Cachexia/failure to thrive
Cancer/leukemia
Cerebrovascular accident (CVA)
Chronic obstructive pulmonary disease (COPD)
Cirrhosis
Congestive heart failure (CHF)
Coronary artery disease (CAD)
Crohn's disease
CVA or subdural hematoma, recent
Dehydration
Diabetes (uncontrolled or new onset)
Dysphagia
Eating disorders
Gastrointestinal bleeding
Hepatic encephalopathy
Hepatitis
Hypertension
Inflammatory bowel disease
Malabsorption
Malnutrition
Multiple sclerosis
Nephrotic syndrome
Neutropenia
Obesity
Pancreatitis
Parkinson's disease
Peritonitis
Pressure ulcer, stages 2–4 or multiple sites
Renal failure, with or without dialysis
Sepsis
Tuberculosis

2. Other factors: 1 POINT EACH

Albumin < 3.0 g/dl
Cancer and surgical patients who are underweight, have swallowing problems, or mouth sores
Clear liquid diets, partial parenteral nutrition (PPN), or nil per os (NPO, nothing by mouth) greater than 5 days
Complex modified diets
Intensive care unit (ICU) patients
Patients older than 75 years
Tube feeding, new or complex

Nutritional Priority Score: high risk (4+ points)___ moderate risk (2–3 points)____ low risk (0–1 point)____

Assessment

The nutritional status of patients can affect the integrity of external or other body tissues; in high-risk patients, the tissues can manifest specific nutrient-based lesions (Kight et al., 1999). JCAHO requires physical examination for manifestations of nutrient deficiency or excess. Factors required for a thorough nutritional assessment include the following: clinical assessment (physical examination, dietary intake), anthropometric assessment (weight for height, midarm muscle circumference, skinfold thickness), hematological assessment (hemoglobin, red cell morphology, ferritin, other stores), biochemical assessment (albumin, transferrin, creatinine-height index, zinc, other parameters; see Figure B-2. immune status (delayed cutaneous hypersensitivity, total lymphocyte count [TLC], T cells), and miscellany (hand grip strength, darkness adaptation, taste acuity). For a simplified assessment, use the Subjective Global Assessment (Figure B-3). See Table B-2, then see Figure B-4 for a grid to determine levels of malnutrition using some of these data)

Steps for assessment:

1. Read medical history, review laboratory data and medications, and conduct physical assessment for nutritional problems.
2. Establish a medical database and key nutritional problem list.
3. Qualified nutrition professionals should be prepared to conduct nutrition physical exams (Kight et al., 1999) or review physical examination as conducted by physician. Interpret or identify nutritional deficiency. Make a nutritional diagnosis such as "nutrient imbalance, code #D7.003" (Kight, 1994). See Figure B-3.
4. Prioritize level of care for patient. See Table B-1.
5. Identify patient's level of readiness for changes that are required.
6. Take a home-based diet history or record a typical daily intake (3- to 7-day records are more accurate when available). See Figure B-5 for a Nutrition History Form and Figure B-6 for a Food Intake Record format.
7. For a <u>Food Diary</u>, have patient list everything he/she eats or drinks during a 24-hour period, recording the amount of each food, time food was consumed, method of preparation and ingredients, related activities or symptoms, with whom, and emotional atmosphere at the time. Have patient record no more than one 24-hour period per form.
8. Determine calorie and protein requirements. Protein and energy requirements are listed in Tables B-3 to B-4.
9. Select appropriate diet and feeding mode.
10. Complete nutritional assessment forms—see Figures B-7 and B-9. Forms will change for an out-patient setting.

TABLE B-2 Sample Laboratory Values

Each facility has its own values according to laboratory procedures. The following ranges are estimated and sample values (other units are in parentheses).

Normal Serum Values

Coagulation Tests:
- Bleeding time = 1–3 minutes Ivy; 2–4 minutes Duke
- Coagulation time = 6–10 minutes
- Erythrocyte sedimentation rates = 0–10 mm/hour (males); 0–15 mm/hour (females)
- International Normalized Ratio (INR) = 2–3
- Prothrombin time = 11–16 seconds control; 70–110% of control value

Amylase = 60–180 Somogyi units/dL
Bicarbonate = 22–28 mEq/L (22–28 mmol/L)
Bilirubin, total = 0.15–1.0 mg/dL
Calcium = 9–11 mg/dL (2.3–2.8 mmol/L)
Carotene = 48–200 mg/dL
Ceruloplasmin = 27–37 mg/dL
Chloride = 95–105 mEq/L (95–105 mmol/L)
Copper = 70–155 mg/dL
Creatine phosphokinase (CPK) = 0–145 units/L
Creatinine = 0.7–1.4 mg/dL
Glycohemoglobin = 5.5–8.5%; also called "hemoglobin A, C"
Glucose, fasting = 70–110 mg/dL (3.9–6.1 mmol/L)
Lactic acid dehydrogenase (LDH) = 200–680 units/mL
Lipase = less than 1.5 units
Lipids: total serum = 450–850 mg/dL
- Cholesterol = 120–210 mg/dL; 20–30% high-density lipoprotein (HDL), 60–70% low-density lipoprotein (LDL)
- Triglycerides = less than 160 mg/dL (less than 2.09 mmol/L)
- Total fatty acids = 190–240 mg/dL

Phospholipids = 60–350 mg/dL
Lymphocytes = over 1,500/mm3
Magnesium = 1.8–3 mg/dL (0.8–1.2 mmol/L)
Nitrogen balance = goal of 1–4 g/24 hours UUN
Nitrogen, nonprotein, serum = 15–35 mg/dL
Osmolality, serum = 280–295 mOsm/L (280–295 mmol/kg)
Oxygen as partial pressure of oxygen (pO2) = 80–100 mm Hg
Partial pressure of carbon dioxide (pCO2) = 35–45 mm Hg
pH, arterial, plasma = 7.36–7.44
Phenylalanine, serum = less than 3 mg/dL
Phosphatase, serum:
- acid = 0.5–2 Bodansky units
- alkaline = 2–4.5 Bodansky units (30–135 units/L)

Phosphate, inorganic, serum 2.5–5 mg/dL (0.8–1.6 mmol/L)
Phosphorus = 2.5–4 mg/dL
Potassium, serum = 3.5–5.5 mEq/L (3.5–5 mmol/L)
Proteins, serum: total = 6–8 g/dL
- Albumin = 3.5–5 g/dL (35–50 g/L); usually 40% of total proteins
- C-reactive protein (CRP) = 0; is elevated with inflammation
- Globulin = 1.5–3 g/dL
- Prealbumin (transthyretin) = 16–35 mg/dL
- Retinol-binding protein = 2.6–7.6 mg/dL
- Transferrin = 170–370 mg/dL (1.7–3.7 g/L)

Respiratory quotient (RQ) = from carbohydrate (CHO) 1, from mixed diet 0.85, from protein 0.8, from fat 0.7
Sodium, serum = 136–145 mEq/L (135–145 mmol/L)
Sulfates, serum, inorganic = 0.5–1.5 mg/dL
Transaminases (liver, muscle, brain): aspartate aminotransaminase (AST) (SGOT) = 5–40 units/mL
alanine aminotransferase (ALT) (SGPT) = 5–35 units/mL
Blood urea nitrogen (BUN) = 8–18 mg/dL (3–6.5 mmol/L)
Uric acid = 4.0–9.0 mg/dL
Vitamin A = 125–150 IU/dL or 20–80 mg/dL
Vitamin B6 = 3.6–18.0 mg/L
Vitamin B12 = 200–900 mg/L
Vitamin C = 0.6–2 mg/dL
Zinc = 0.75–1.4 mg/mL or up to 79 mg/dL

(continued)

TABLE B-2 Sample Laboratory Values (*Continued*)

Blood Cell Values
Erythrocyte count = 4.5–6.2 million/mm3 (males); 4.2–5.4 million/mm3 (females)
Ferritin = 20–300 mg/mL (males); 20–120 mg/mL = (females)
Folate = 2–20 mg/mL
Iron = 75–175 mg/dL (males); 65–165 mg/dL (females)
Iron-binding capacity, total = 240–450 mg/dL (18–59% saturation)
Hematocrit = 40–54% (males); 37–47% (females)
Hemoglobin = 14–17 g/dL (males); 12–15 g/dL (females)
Mean cell volume (MCV) = 80–94 cu/microns
Mean cell hemoglobin (MCH) = 26–32 picograms
Mean cell hemoglobin concentration = 32–36%
White blood cells = 4.8–11.8 thousand/mm^3
Lymphocytes = 24–44% total white blood cell count (WBC)
TLC = % lymphocytes × WBC/100; normal = 12,000/mm3; deficient = <900/mm3

Normal Urine Values
Acetone = 0
Aldosterone = 6–16 mg/24 hours
Ammonia = 20–70 mEq/L
Amylase = 260–950 Somogyi units/24 hours
Calcium, normal diet = less than 250 mg/24 hours
Creatine = less than 100 mg/24 hours (higher in pregnancy/children)
Creatinine = 15–25 mg/kg body weight (BW) in 24 hours
Estrogens = 4–25 mg/24 hours (males); 4–60 mg/24 hours (females), higher in pregnancy
Hemoglobin, myoglobin = 0
5-hydroxyindoleacetic acid (5-HIAA) = 0
Osmolality = 300–800 mOsm/kg
Oxalate = 20–60 mg/24 hours
pH = 4.6–8 with average of 6 (diet-dependent)
Protein = less than 30 mg/24 hours (0 qualitative)
Specific gravity = 1.003–1.030
Sugar = 0
Urea nitrogen = 2–20 g/24 hours (450–700 mmol/day)
Vanillylmandelic acid (VMA) = 1.8–8.4 mg/24 hours

Stool Values
Fat = less than 7 g/24 hours in a 3-day period
Nitrogen = less than 2.5 g per day

Specific Lab Tests and Panels (Veldee, 1995)
Renal Values:
Glomerular filtration rate (GFR) = 110–150 mL/minute (males); 105–132 mL/minute (females)
Urea clearance = 40–65 mL/minute standard; 60–100 mL/minute maximum
Thyroid Values:
T3 (concentration) = 50–210 mg/dL serum
T4 (concentration) = 4.8–13.2 mg/dL serum
Thyroid-stimulating hormone (TSH) = less than or equal to 0.2 micro-unit/L
Radioactive iodine uptake = 9–19% in 1 hour; 10–50%/24 hours
Protein-bound iodine = 3.6–8.8 mg/dL

Nutrition Screen Panel: For preliminary assessment early in stay of parameters such as albumin, prealbumin/transthyretin, ascorbic acid, carotene, zinc, zinc protophyrin/heme ratio, and cholesterol.

Geriatric Screen Panel: To identify nutrient deficiencies common in elderly individuals—all nutrition screening data plus vitamins B12, B6, and D.

Nutrition Monitoring Panel: For acute care, TPN, and tube-fed patients, once weekly—albumin, prealbumin/transthyretin, C-reactive protein, ascorbic acid, zinc, and zinc protophyrin/heme ratio; others as needed.

Nutrition Wound Healing Panel: For weekly monitoring of patients with significant wounds—includes albumin, prealbumin/transthyretin, C-reactive protein, ascorbic acid, zinc, and retinol.

Home Parenteral Nutrition Panel: Used 1–2 times annually at routine clinic visits—albumin, prealbumin/transthyretin, zinc, copper, zinc protophyrin/heme ratio, ionized calcium, phosphate, magnesium, ascorbic acid, triglycerides, AST, alkaline phosphatase.

Figure B-3 **SUBJECTIVE GLOBAL ASSESSMENT (SGA)**

Select appropriate categories with a check mark. Numerical values are assigned and used for scoring. Patient may self-report the sections 1–4; medical or nutritional staff will complete numbers 5, 6, and the SGA score.

1-Weight

Weight ________ Height ___feet and ___inches

Overall loss in past 6 months: Amt.= #_____lbs; % loss = _____ (20%+ 4 pts; 10–19.9% 3 pts; 6–9.9% 2 pts; 2–5.9% 1 pt; 0–1.9% 0 pts)

Overall loss in past 1 month: Amt.= #_____lbs; % loss = _____ (10%+ 4 pts; 5–5.9.9% 3 pts; 3–4.9% 2 pts; 2–2.9% 1pt; 0–1.9% 0 pts)

Change in past 2 weeks:_____increased (0) _____no change (0) _____ decreased (1).

2-Food Intake (over past month)

_____No change recently (0)

_____Change: more than usual (0)___ less than usual (1) _____

Now taking: normal food but less than normal (1)___ little solid food (2) ___ only liquids (3)___ only nutritional supplements (3)___ very little of anything (4)___ only tube feedings or nutrition by vein___

Supplement: (circle) nil, vitamin, minerals, # _____frequency/week.

3-Symptoms (longer than 2 weeks)

_____no problems eating (0) _____nausea (1) _____vomiting (3) _____diarrhea (3)

_____anorexia/no appetite (3) _____constipation (1) _____mouth sores (2) _____dry mouth (1)

_____pain (3)—(where_____________)

_____ things taste funny or have no taste (1) ____smells bother (1)

_____other (1):________________________(depression, financial worries, dental problems, etc.)

4-Functional capacity (activity over the past month)

_____normal with no limitations (0) _____not usual, but up and about with normal activity (1)

_____not feeling up to most things, but in bed less than half the day (2)

_____able to do little activity and spend most of the day in bed or chair (3)

_____seldom out of bed

****

5-Disease and its relation to nutritional requirements

Primary diagnosis (specify)______________________________ Stage_______________

Cancer (1), AIDS (1), Pulmonary or cardiac cachexia (1), Pressure ulcers/wound/fistula (1), Trauma (1), Age Greater than 65 years (1)

Metabolic demand (stress): _____no stress—no stress, fever, steroids (0)

_____low stress—temp 99–101° less than 72 hours, low-dose steroids (1)

_____moderate stress—moderate stress, temp 101–102° about 72 hours, moderate steroid use (2)

_____high stress—high-stress factors, temp over 102° over 72 hours, over 30 mg prednisone equivalents per day (3)

6-Physical (for each trait specify: 0 = normal, 1+ = mild, 2+ = moderate, 3+ =severe)

_____Loss of subcutaneous fat (triceps, chest)

_____Muscle wasting (quadriceps, deltoids)

_____Ankle edema

_____Sacral edema

_____Ascites

_____Mucosal lesions

_____Cutaneous lesions

_____ Hair change

SGA rating (select one):

A_____Well nourished (no weight loss or recent nonfluid gain; no intake deficit or recent improvement noted; no symptoms of nutritional impact; no functional deficits or recent improvement noted; no physical deficit or improvements shown recently)

B_____Moderately (or suspected of being) malnourished (5% weight loss in 1 month or 10% in 6 months; definite decreased intake; presence of nutritional impact symptoms; moderate functional deficit or recent deterioration; evidence of mild to moderate loss of subcutaneous fat and/or muscle mass and/or muscle tone on palpation)

C_____Severely malnourished (over 5% weight loss in 1 month or over 10% weight loss in 6 months; severe deficits in intake; presence of nutritional impact symptoms; severe functional deficit or recent functional deterioration; obvious signs of malnutrition such as severe loss of subcutaneous tissues or possible edema)

Derived from: Detsky A, et al. Subjective global nutritional assessment. *J Parenter Enteral Nutri.* 1987;11:8; and Dr. Faith Ottery, 1998 (Ottery and Associates, 215–351–4050).

		Weight as a percentage of calculated optimum body weight			
		<60%	60% to 75%	76% to 90%	>90%
Serum albumin level (g/dL)	<2.5	Severe PEM	Severe PEM	Moderate malnutrition	Protein malnutrition (kwashiorkor)
	2.5–3.0	Severe PEM	Moderate malnutrition	Moderate malnutrition	Protein malnutrition (kwashiorkor)
	3.1–3.5	Moderate malnutrition	Moderate malnutrition	Mild malnutrition	Mild malnutrition
	>3.5	Energy malnutrition (marasmus)	Energy malnutrition (marasmus)	Mild malnutrition	No malnutrition present

Figure B-4 Criteria grid for determining malnutrition diagnosis. (Adapted from Funk K, Ayton C. Improving malnutrition documentation enhances reimbursement. *J Am Diet Assoc.* 1995;95:468.)

Plan

1. Establish a nutritional care plan to give directional stimulus to treatment efforts. Include evaluation of previous nutritional practices, knowledge of diet and of normal nutrition, and need for further instructions.

2. Formulate objectives with patient and physician. Contact family when appropriate.

3. Determine goals (i.e., maintenance, anabolism, etc.). Consider quality of life factors as relevant to patient (see Fig. B-1).

4. The care plan is developed in cooperation with other disciplines (Escott-Stump, 1997). Consider nutritional problems and determine course of action for the following:

Treat: Procedures and dietary adjustment to meet goals, including oral, enteral nutrition (EN), or parenteral nutrition (PN) modes. Consider underlying malnutrition, medications, chronic or acute illnesses, and patient goals.

Diagnose: Request more data—food diary, laboratory or other available tests, nutrient or calorie intake analyses, and possibly a home visit.

Educate: Explain relationship of diet to disorder and disease, plus patient's/client's role in management. Use a client-centered approach. Explain diet—dietary principles, ways to change and improve habits, written materials, sample menus, and meal patterns. Use plate method as a simple method to teach meal planning; plate serves as a pie chart that shows proportions of the plate that should be covered by different foods (Camelon, 1998). Use nutrition counseling skills, converting theory into practice and science into art (Snetselaar, 1997). The goal is to promote desirable outcomes by promoting healthful behavior and involving patient and family in care decisions (Escott-Stump et al., 2000).

5. Document on appropriate forms. Figures B-8 and B-9 provide sample care plan, cardex, and assessment forms that are available for use in hospitals or nursing homes. Figure B-10 provides a physical assessment tool to track changes, often in an extended care facility.

6. Attend care plan meetings. Figure B-11 describes a master plan of care used in an extended care facility.

Implementation

1. Carry out plans: this may include use of established care maps or clinical pathways.

2. Participate in medical rounds. Consult and advise physician about necessary referrals, adaptive feeding equipment, special wishes or needs of patient, etc. Maintain medical team communication by making rounds or actively participating in conferences.

3. Complete anthropometric measurements.

4. Evaluate food–drug interactions; counsel accordingly.

5. Coordinate transitional feedings.

6. Monitor food intake, nitrogen balance, and laboratory values.

7. Advise and provide MNT as needed.

8. When permitted, write and edit diet/nutritional orders.

9. Conduct group classes and outpatient conferences when needed. Use appropriate audiovisual aids and teaching tools. Teach using principles of adult education, lifestyle change management, and stages; see Table B-5. For education, dietitians have a responsibility as intervention specialists to provide health behavior counseling and to promote specific medical and lifestyle changes (Insull, 1992).

Figure B-5 NUTRITION HISTORY FORM

NAME ______________________________ DATE ___________

OCCUPATION ______________________________

HEIGHT _____′ _____″
PRESENT WEIGHT _______

To be completed by dietitian
GOAL WEIGHT _____ BMI ____

1. How would you generally describe your eating habits? Good Fair Poor
2. Has your appetite changed recently? Yes No
3. How many times a day do you eat? ______________
4. How long does it usually take to complete a meal?______________
5. When you chew your food, do you______ take your time? ______ chew a few times, then swallow?
6. Do you use a straw to drink beverages? Yes No
7. Do you chew gum? Yes No How often? ______
8. Number of carbonated beverages daily ____________
9. Number of caffeine beverages daily (coffee, regular colas, and tea)
   _____ cups of coffee (regular)
   _____ cans of cola (regular, diet, Mellow Yellow ®, Mountain Dew®)
   _____ cups of tea (regular)
10. Do you have dentures? Yes No If so, do you wear them at mealtime? Yes No
11. Do you have any problems chewing? Yes No
12. Do you take any vitamin/mineral supplements? ______________________________
13. List any foods that you do **NOT** tolerate: ______________________________
14. Are you now or have you ever followed any special diet?______________
    If so, what type of diet?______________________________
15. How often do you eat out? ________times a week. What types of restaurants?______________

Source: The American Dietetic Association. *MNT Across the Continuum*. 2nd ed. Chicago, IL:1998. Used with permission.

10. Write meaningful nutrition notes: physicians prefer a goal-oriented, concise note format more than three to one over other outcome-focused documentation (Klein et al., 1997).

Evaluation

Monitor patient's nutritional progress: portion control, ingredient control, meal quality, and delivery system (oral, tube feeding, parenteral nutrition). Evaluate according to evidence-based practice guides such as *Medical Nutrition Therapy Across the Continuum,* MNTACC (Myers et al., 2001; American Dietetic Association, 1996).

1. Evaluate care plan and outcomes; determine which goals, if any, have been met. Monitor efficacy of therapy and nutritional interventions.
2. Evaluate using comparisons with JCAHO, state, and other federal and local regulations; they also should include comparisons with professional standards of care established by diagnosis or disease state, as available from the American Dietetic Association and other accrediting agencies.
3. Audit nutritional care—when feasible, give a follow-up call to patient after discharge or conduct a home visit. See Table B-6 for sample patient education outcomes.
4. Document evaluation with progress notes. See Table B-7.
5. Figure B-12 shows how a concept map can be used to teach dietetic students how to think critically and how to evaluate clinical care (Roberts, 1995).
6. To effectively monitor quality of care, clinicians must monitor their own work or that of their peers via care audits; see Figure B-13 for an example format.
7. Test knowledge of patient/client and family members.
8. Determine changes that have occurred—weight, dietary behavior, laboratory data.

Reassessment

1. Monitor and evaluate nutritional status of patient to determine any new steps that should be completed to allow patient to succeed in nutritional goals (as inpatient, outpatient, or in the home).
2. Identify necessary changes in care (nutrient or fluid needs, mode of intake).
3. Implement needed changes.
4. Compare outcomes with care maps, clinical pathways, or other resources used. Figure B-14 provides a sample care map format, into which specific facility information can be written. Figure B-15 is a sample critical pathway for a general patient admission.
5. Document on Nutrition Progress Notes page (See sample in Figure B-16.).

Figure B-6 FOOD INTAKE RECORD

Please indicate which foods you eat.

	Less than once a week	Not daily but at least once a week	Daily
Milk, yogurt			
Cheese			
Red meat			
Poultry			
Fish			
Eggs			
Mixed dishes			
Dried beans, legumes			
Peanut butter			
Nuts			
Breads, cereal			
Potatoes, pasta, rice			
Fruits, juices			
Vegetables			
Margarine, butter			
Cooking oil			
Sour cream, salad dressing			
Ice cream			
Cookies, cake, pie			
Candy			
Soft drink			
Coffee			
Tea, iced tea			
Alcohol			

Describe your usual daily eating pattern (include amount eaten).

Time	Meal	Food/method of preparation	Amount eaten	Calculations (for RD)
	Breakfast			
	Snack			
	Lunch			
	Dinner			
	Snack			

Source: The American Dietetic Association. *MNT Across the Continuum*. 2nd ed. Chicago, IL:1998. Used with permission.

TABLE B-3 Common Calculations Related to Protein and Energy Expenditure

For Healthy Persons—Calculations of Energy (Derived from Shils et al., 1999).

	Sedentary	Moderate	Active
Overweight	20–25 kcal/kg	30 kcal/kg	35 kcal/kg
Normal weight	30 kcal/kg	35 kcal/kg	40 kcal/kg
Underweight	30 kcal/kg	40 kcal/kg	45–50 kcal/kg

For Hospitalized Patients—Using estimates are based on body mass index (BMI) (Note: Feeding programs should support a patient being within 10–15 lb of desirable weight range (such as BMI). Adapted from: American Gastroenterological Association, 2001.

BMI (kg/ m^2)	Energy required (kcals/kg/day)
<15	35–40
15–19	30–35
20–29	20–25
>30	15–20

SEVERITY OF WEIGHT CHANGES

Determination of Weight Changes: unplanned weight loss can affect morbidity and mortality:
%Weight change = {usual weight − actual weight/usual weight} × 100%

more than 2% in 1 week
more than 5% in 1 month
more than 7.5% in 3 months
more than 20% in unlimited period of time
more than 40% usually incompatible with life

Use of Healthy Body Weight (HBW): less strict than "ideal" body weight (IBW).

Calorie Estimations from Nutrients:

Carbohydrate 4 kcal/g oral diet or 3.4 kcals/g (hydrated dextrose in TPN)
Protein 4 kcal/g
Fat 9 kcal/g
Alcohol 7 kcal/g

Basal metabolic rate = energy expenditure at rest; kilocalories required to maintain minimal physiological functioning (i.e., heart beating, breathing, etc.). Factors affecting basal metabolic rate and calorie include:

1. Age. Infants need more kilocalories per square meter of body surface than any other age groups. Basal metabolic rate (BMR) declines after maturity.
2. Body Size. Total BMR relates to body size; large persons require more kilocalories for basal and activity levels.
3. Body Composition. Lean tissue is more active than fatty tissue. An obese person generally has more total lean body mass as well as adipose tissue, therefore has a higher metabolic rate than a lean person.
4. Climate. A damp or hot climate decreases BMR, and a cold climate increases BMR. Changes are slight.
5. Hormones. Thyroxine increases BMR; sex hormones and adrenalin alter BMR mildly; low zinc intake may lower BMR.
6. Fever. BMR increases by 7% for each degree above normal, F.; 10% for each degree C.
7. Growth. BMR increases during anabolic stages (pregnancy, childhood, teen years, and anabolic stages of wound healing).

(continued)

TABLE B-3 Common Calculations Related to Protein and Energy Expenditure (*Continued*)

Various methods are used to determine BMR and calorie needs for sick individuals. Several of the most common methods include the following calculations:

METHOD A: Standard Calculations (Harris Benedict Equation)

Harris & Benedict (1919) practiced calorimetry to evaluate basal energy expenditure (BEE) (energy to fuel basic life functions at rest in a thermally neutral environment, 10 or more hours after eating). The study was performed on healthy, ambulatory persons and may overestimate by 7–24% in sick or elderly persons. Total Energy Expenditure (TEE) = BEE × Activity and Injury Factors. Note: For some conditions, BEE has been overestimated when actual resting energy expenditure (REE) is measured by indirect calorimetry. In other cases, BEE has underestimated patient needs.

Calculate basal needs: Harris-Benedict Equation:

Men BEE (kcal) = [66 + 13.7 × weight (kg) + 5 × height (cm) − 6.8 × age (years)].

Women BEE (kcal) = [655 + 9.6 × weight (kg) + 1.7 × height (cm) − 4.7 × age (years)]

Add activity factor: normal BMR x 1.25 for weight maintenance. For weight gain, use maintenance energy + 1,000 kcals (Shils, 1999)

Add stress factors (Shils et al., 1999):

- Mild starvation = .85–1.00 × BEE
- Postoperative recovery without complications = 1.0–1.05 × BEE
- Cancer =1.1–1.45 × BEE
- Peritonitis = 1.05–1.25 × BEE
- Severe infection or multiple trauma = 1.3–1.55 × BEE
- Pressure ulcers or long-bone fracture = 1.25–1.30 × BEE
- Burns (over 40% body surface area) = 2 × BEE

METHOD B: Critical Care Assessments

Indirect Calorimetry: Calculation of energy expenditure by measuring gas exchange (VO2 and VCO2 represent intracellular metabolism).

It is helpful for patients in the ICU. For REE, use a metabolic cart.

REE includes specific dynamic action for digestion and absorption (slightly above BEE) and is considered relatively equivalent in clinical context. BEE and REE are estimations. REE can be from normal to below normal in mild starvation such as that which occurs in the hospital setting.

It may be useful to defer weight repletion until a patient's critical episode subsides; keep in mind that needs generally normalize again in 20–50 days.

Prevent overfeeding, which can cause fluid overload, increased CO2 production, and hepatic aberrations. Use Ireton Jones calculation.

Newer studies using indirect calorimetry have found that the energy needs of critically ill or injured adults are not as high as previously thought.

TABLE B-4 Protein Needs/Degree of Illness

- 6.25 g of dietary protein = 1 g of nitrogen; therefore, estimated nitrogen requirements × 6.25 = estimated protein needs in grams.
- Normal nitrogen needs = 1 g N/300 kcal. Illness nitrogen needs = 1 g N/120–180 kcal.
- Note: If energy is not provided in adequate amounts, protein tissues become a substrate.
- Amino acids (AAs) = 1 g/kg 3 4 kcal = AA calories (in TF or TPN).
- Nonprotein Calories (NPC) = total kilocalories less AA kilocalories; NPC kilocalories for a patient are often based on 40% fat, 60% CHO.

Method 1 (protein)	**Increments of Increased Protein Requirements**
No illness	100% basal needs
Mild illness	130% basal needs
Moderate illness	160% basal needs
Severe illness	200% basal needs
Method 2 (kcals and protein)	Kcals and Protein Requirements
Mild stress	35 kcal/kg + 1 g protein/kg
Moderate stress	45 kcal/kg + 1.5 g protein/kg

Recommended Daily Protein Intake *

Clinical condition	*Protein requirement (g/kg IBW per day)*[a]
Normal	0.8
Metabolic stress (illness/injury)	1.0–1.5
Acute renal failure (undialyzed)	0.8–1.0
Hemodialysis	1.2–1.4
Peritoneal dialysis	1.3–1.5

IBW, ideal body weight.

* Adapted from The American Gastroenterological Association, 2001.

[a] Additional protein intake may be needed to compensate for excess protein loss in specific patient populations such as those with burn injury, open wounds, and protein-losing enteropathy or nephropathy. Lower protein intake may be necessary in patients with chronic renal insufficiency not treated by dialysis and certain patients with hepatic encephalopathy.

Figure B-7 INITIAL NUTRITION ASSESSMENT (Adult)

NAME:____ **DATE:**________ **RECORD#:**_____________________________

DOB:__________ **Age:**___ **GENDER:** Male___Female___
REFERRING PHYSICIAN:__________________

DIAGNOSES:
PROBLEMS: 1) 2) 3) 4)

Vision Problems: **Hearing Problems:** **Ambulation Problems:**
Occupation: **Hours of Work:** **Stress Level:**
Household Members' Ages /Health:
Ethnic Background:
Country of Origin: **Years in U.S.:** **Years in School:** **Language:** **Needs Interpreter:**

Family Hx: **CAD/Athero:** **HTN:** **High Chol:** **DM:** **CVA:** **CA:** Site **Other:**
Medical Hx: Onset of Disease: ______________ (mo/yr) Type of Treatment:
Previous MNT Yes No If yes, when: _________ where: ___________________________________
Diet Order_______________________________________**Nourishments**______________________
Relevant Labs: **Gluc** **BUN** **Creat** **Chol** **TG** **Ca++** **Phos** **Na++** **K+** **Alb** **Hgb/Hct**
I & O______**Other:**____
Medications/Interactions____
____
Laxatives: ________________ **Diuretics:**___________________**Insulin:**_____________________________
Vitamins/Minerals___________________________**Herbs/Botanicals**_________________________________

Weight History:
Height: Current Weight: Usual Weight: Wt Changes over __________mo/yr
Highest Weight: Lowest Weight: Desired Weight/Why_________________________________
Attempts at Wt Changes:
Activity: Type: Duration/Frequency:
Food Allergies:
Food Aversions:

Appetite: good/fair/poor **Difficulty chewing/swallowing** **Nausea/vomiting/constipation/diarrhea**
Food Purchase/Prep:
Religious, Ethnic, Economic: **Food Assist:**
Psychosocial Factors: **Smokes:** **ppd**

Readiness to Learn:

Nutritional Status: ___**Mild protein–calorie malnutrition (weight loss under 5%, albumin 3.2 or higher)**
___**Nutritional marasmus (alb over 3.2 g/dl, weight loss over 10%)**
___**Kwashiorkor (alb below 3.2 g/dl; weight loss under 10%)**
___**Mixed PCM (malnutrition with hypoalbuminemia and weight loss 25% or more)**

Dietary Intake Analysis: Meal/Snack Times:_____________________

Kcal_______ CHO____g(___%) Pro______g(___%) Fat_______g (___%) Sat Fat ______ Chol_____mg
Na_____g K____g Ca____mg Fe____mg Folate____mg Mg______mg B6____mg vit E_____IU Fiber_____g
ETOH_____ Caffeine_____mg H_2O_______cc Findings:_________________________________
ASSESSED NEEDS: Protein ___ g/Kg/day =____ Kcals____ kcals/Kg/day=____ Fluids:____cc/Kg/day=_____

Dietitian:____________________________**Date of Review:**________**Follow-Up Date:**_______

Adapted from: The American Dietetic Association. *MNT Across the Continuum*. 2nd ed. Chicago, IL:1998.

TECHNICIAN CARE PLAN CARD — NURSING HOME

ADDRESSOGRAPH

DIAGNOSES/MEDICAL HISTORY			At 90 Days	At 180 Days	At 270 Days	REASSESSMENT: 1 YEAR
RESIDENT STATUS	ADMISSION DATA		COMMENT/DATE			
Alertness	Normal	Impaired				
Ability to feed self	Normal	Impaired	Assist/total			
Chewing	Normal	Impaired	Dentures/missing teeth			
Swallowing	Normal	Impaired	Speech therapy			
Taste	Normal	Impaired				
Vision	Normal	Impaired	Glasses/blind			
Hearing	Normal	Impaired	HOH			
Communication Skills	Normal	Impaired				
Mental abilities	Normal	Impaired				
Bowel function	Normal	Impaired	Incontinent			
Bladder function	Normal	Impaired	Incontinent – force fluids			
Ambulation/mobility	Normal	Impaired	Assist/wheelchair			
Appetite (% intake)	Normal	Impaired				
Skin integrity	Normal	Impaired	P. ulcer Stage I II III IV			
WEIGHT STATUS	Male/Female	Ht	Adm. wt.			
Est. protein needs	NL 1g/kg	Other:				
IBW range:	Normal	Below 75%	Est. kcal needs:			
Usual wt:	WNL	Above 120%	Goal:			
Weight changes	None	Loss/gain	Past 3 mos:			
Fluid needs	NL 30 mL/kg	Impaired	Fluid needs:			
SIGNED/DATE	N/A	N/A				

LABS/DATE/CONCERN	RELEVANT MEDS.
FBS	Insulin:
Alb/Prealbumin Total Protein	Corticosteroids:
BUN Creatinine	Diuretics:
Lytes: Na+ K+	Laxatives:
H & H Fe B12	Vitamins/minerals:
Lipids: TG Chol	Other:
Other:	

DISLIKES:

LIKES:

PREVIOUS DIETS:

RELIGION: C P J Other:

FOOD ALLERGIES:

SUPPLEMENTS (Item/When)

BEVERAGE PREFERENCES:
B L D

EXCHANGES	B	L	D	HS	C	P	F
Milk							
Veg.							
Fruits							
Breads							
Meats							
Fats							
TOTAL							

Special Alert
Blind
Other:

MENUS:
Weekly--Self-Select ____Family ____
House: Standard ____Special ____

Meal Location: Room
DINING ROOM: Table #

NAME ______________ Room ______ Diet Order ______________ MENUS MEAL LOCATION

Figure B-8 Sample technician care plan card–nursing home.

HOSPITAL **NUTRITION HISTORY AND CARE PLAN FORM**

ADDRESSOGRAPH	NO.	MEDICAL DIAGNOSES/CLINICAL PROBLEMS

INIT.	RESPONSIBLE DIETITIAN	INIT.	UNIT TECHNICIAN	INIT.	OTHER STAFF MEMBERS

CL. PROB. NO.	EXPECTED PATIENT OUTCOMES	NUTRITION INTERVENTIONS	INIT./ DATE	EVALUATION	INIT./ DATE
		DIET INSTRUCTIONS:			

LABS	DATE	DATE	DATE	DATE	DATE
BS					
Sodium					
Potassium					
Chloride					
HGB					
HCT					

Albumin					
BUN					
Creat.					
T. Pro.					
Chol.					
Trig.					
Amylase					

Phos.					
Ht.					
Wt.					
% IBW/HBW					
Other					

DRUGS	INTERACTION

HOSPITAL NUTRITION HISTORY AND CARE PLAN

SUBJECTIVE:

Date interviewed ________
Home diet ____________ Compliance G F P
Present Appetite G F P Home Appetite G F P
Recent surgery, illness or stress ____________
Meals/day ________ Snacks ________
Meals eaten home ______ Away ______ Where ______
Recent weight □'s Y N ___#
Bowel habits: Normal Constipated Diarrhetic
Dental: Chewing Swallowing
Dentures: Y N Partials
Physical limitations: ____________
Lifestyle: ____________

	B	L	D	10	PM	HS
Meat						
Bread						
Veg.						
Fruit						
Fat						
Milk W 2% S						

NOURISHMENTS:
AM
PM
HS

MEAL PATTERN/FOOD HABITS

FOOD GROUPS	DAY	WK.	USUAL EATING PATTERN
Cheese			
Meat/poultry			
Eggs			
Veg.			
Starch veg.			
Fruits			
Starch			
Fats			
Dessert			
Sugar/candy			
Alcohol			
Beverage			
Meals out			

DIET HISTORY

1. Who shops
2. Who cooks
3. No. in household
4. No. eating together
5. Meal eaten where
6. Occupation
7. Activity level
8. Exercise
How often
9. Religious influence
10. Cultural influence
11. Sodium intake— Table
Cooking
Salty foods
12. Dietetic products
13. Supplements/vitamins

Previous Hx:

ALLERGIES:	INTOLERANCES:
Other:	

Figure B-9 Sample nutritional assessment form—hospital. (Adapted with permission from Food and Nutrition Services Department, Aliquippa Hospital, Aliquippa, PA.)

Figure B-10 Sample Nutrition Physical Assessment tool.

Body System	Normal	Abnormal	Severe	Considerations
Weight for age	At ideal BMI, or normal for age	Thin Overweight/obese	Emaciated Morbid obesity	Recent illness? Poor eating habits?
Hair	Firmly attached Normal distribution Lustrous, shiny	Thin Sparse Dull, dry	Depigmented Easily pluckable Brittle, very dry Corkscrew hairs	Chemotherapy? Chemical treatments? Protein or biotin deficits? Vitamin C deficiency?
Eyes	Bright, clear Pink conjunctiva	Sunken, dull Pale, dry conjunctiva Poor vision Photophobia	Xerosis Keratomalacia Night blindness	Vitamins A or zinc deficiencies? Riboflavin deficiency for conjunctival inflammation?
Lips	Good color, moist	Swollen, red Dry, cracked	Fissured Bleeding	Riboflavin, pyridoxine, niacin deficiencies?
Gums	Pink, firm	Sore, spongy Red, swollen	Bleed easily	Vitamin C deficiency?
Tongue	Pink Papillae present	Purple or magenta White or gray coating Smooth, slick	Beefy red Burning Fissured	Riboflavin, pyridoxine, folic acid, niacin, vitamin B12 or iron deficiencies?
Teeth	Clean, intact All present	Dentures in good repair Missing, loose or chipped teeth Loss of tooth enamel	Edentulous Poorly fitted or loose dentures Rampant caries	Poor dietary habits? Calcium deficiency?
Neck	No swelling	Small nodule	Goiter	Iodine excess or deficiency?
Skin	Smooth, slightly moist Good color	Pale Dry, scaly Nasolabial seborrhea Bruises easily Hyperpigmented Pressure ulcer stage 1 Impaired wound healing	Pellagrous dermatitis Pressure ulcers stage 2–4	Iron deficiency? Vitamins A, C, or zinc deficiency? Essential fatty acid or protein deficiency? Niacin excess?
Bloodstream	Normal lab values	Anemia, mild	Anemia, hemolytic or microcytic/hypochromic, or megaloblastic Prolonged clotting time	Vitamin E, iron, copper, folate, vitamin B12 deficiencies? Vitamin K deficiency?
Heart	Strong, regular heartbeat	Arrhythmias Palpitations	High output failure Cardiomegaly	Potassium excess or deficits? Thiamin or selenium deficiency?
Lungs	Adequate breathing	Respiratory muscle weakness	Respiratory failure Pneumonia	Protein, phosphorus deficiencies?
Legs	Well developed Firm muscles No joint/bone pain	Calf tenderness Flaccid muscles Aches	Edema Bowed legs or rickets Bone or joint pain	Protein deficiency? Vitamin D, calcium, Vitamin A or C deficiencies?
Abdomen	No swelling or pain	Mildly edematous Diarrhea	Hepatomegaly Ascites	Protein or fat deficiencies? Niacin or zinc deficiencies?
Hands and nails	Normal, smooth	Brittle, thin nails Atrophied fine muscles	Spoon-shaped nails Transverse depigmentation	Iron deficiency? Protein deficiency?
Musculoskeletal	Normal muscular and bone development	Calf muscle tenderness Wasted appearance Muscle pain Decreased grip strength	Paralysis Osteoporosis Bone fractures	Thiamin, protein, vitamin C deficiencies?
Neurologic	Normal reflexes No developmental delay	CVA Limited reflexes Irritability Mild disorientation	Convulsions Comatose Seizures Dementia Peripheral neuropathy	Thiamin, vitamins B6 or B12, folate, niacin, iodine, phosphorus, calcium or magnesium deficiencies?
General appearance	Normal development of muscles, fat	Loss of subcutaneous fat	Severe emaciation with sunken or hollow cheeks	Calorie or fluid deficits?

Evaluations: Nutrition status—Normal______Abnormal because of____________________________
Recommendations/Goals:____
Dietitian's Signature:________________ Date:__________

Adapted from: Halsted C, et al. Preoperative nutritional assessment. In Quigley E, Sorrell M eds. *The gastrointestinal surgical patient: preoperative and postoperative care*. Baltimore: Williams & Wilkins, 1994; 27–49; Shils M, et al. *Modern nutrition in health and disease*. 9th ed. Baltimore: Williams & Wilkins, 1999; 886.

DIETARY MASTER PLAN OF CARE — EXTENDED CARE FACILITY

Problem	Plan of Action	Goal
1. Needs assistance at mealtime	1. Nursing will cut meat, open milk, arrange food. Dietary should mark meal cards with appropriate color to indicate feeding assistance needed.	1. Adequate intake of basic foods. Adequate fluid and calorie intake. Meet energy and nutrient needs of patient.
2. Cannot self-feed	2. Spoon feeding by Nursing will be needed.	2. Adequate intake of basic foods so that fluid, calorie, protein, and nutrient needs are met.
3. Cannot swallow (dysphagia)	3. Tube feeding will be administered by Nursing. Progress as tolerated to thick pureed diet.	3. Tube feeding should be calculated to provide adequate calories, protein, and nutrients to meet needs of patient. Adequate fluid intake.
4. Blind	4. Tray arranged by Nursing. May require bowls from Dietary if patient wishes to feed self.	4. Adequate intake of basic foods so that fluid, calorie, protein, and nutrient needs are met.
5. No teeth or poorly fitting dentures or difficulty in chewing	5. Modify food consistency (moisture) or texture (chopping, mincing) to meet patient needs. Either mechanical soft diet or pureed foods. Be aware of weight losses.	5. Adequate intake of basic foods in altered form to ensure that calories, fluid, protein, and nutrient needs are met. Progress from pureed when possible.
6. Poor appetite or refuses to eat or poor calorie intake	6. Offer encouragement at mealtimes. Assist if needed. Spoon feed if necessary. If severe, may tube feed. Offer preferred foods and/or provide nutritional supplement between meals (by Nursing). Suggest occupational therapy group feeding ("lunch bunch"). Identify causation, treatments.	6. Increase intake of calories, protein, fluids, and other nutrients to meet needs. Correct anorexia, weight loss.
7. Fluid retention (edema)	7. Control sodium content of diet. Offer diet as ordered by physician. (May be "no added salt," 2–3 g sodium diet, or other restriction.) Check/monitor albumin, I & O.	7. Lessen edema. Prevent further complications. Control sodium intake through diet. Correct protein malnutrition, if evident.
8. Will not complete meals	8. Encourage self-help. If patient falls asleep, remind patient to finish meals.	8. Monitor feeding process to ensure adequate intake of fluid, protein, calories and other nutrients.
9. Dietary inadequacy	9. Encourage foods from all four basic food groups. (If patient refuses citrus fruits, vitamin C may be lacking. If milk, calcium is at risk. If meats, protein may be lacking. If vegetables, vitamins and fiber may be low.) Encourage dessert last.	9. Monitor dietary intake to improve intake of food groups so that nutrients are no longer lacking. Evaluate and maintain calorie levels.
10. Buying foods from snack machines while on modified diet	10. Ask nursing to watch patient so that snacks are not brought in by family or purchased by patient. Discuss problem with the patient to explain role of the diet in treatment plan.	10. Reduce cheating on diet. Increase adherence to diet.
11. Elevate blood sugar or uncontrolled diabetes	11. Control intake of carbohydrates, sweets. Follow calorie-controlled diet as ordered by doctor. Offer substitutes when diet is not consumed.	11. Adhere to diabetic diet. Adequate intake of protein, calories, fluid, and nutrients. Limit side effects of diabetes.
12. Constipation	12. Add fiber and fluid unless contraindicated. Crushed bran can be added to hot cereal for pureed diets. Milk or prune juice may also be helpful if tolerated. Add activity if feasible. If TF, use fiber—added product.	12. Alleviate constipation. Prevent obstruction.
13. Pressure ulcer	13. Add extra protein and calories to meals and snacks. Add a supplement or tube feed if necessary. Extra vit. C and zinc.	13. Heal ulcer. Prevent further skin breakdown.
14. Significant weight loss, especially rapid	14. Add snacks or supplements between meals. Use nutrient-dense foods at mealtime. Weigh regularly (once weekly) with same clothing.	14. Promote return to healthy/ideal body weight. Prevent morbidity/mortality.

Figure B-11 Dietary master plan of care—extended care facility.

TABLE B-5 Patient Education and Counseling Tips

Chief Assessment Factors

1. Socioeconomic factors.
2. Cultural, religious beliefs and background.
3. Age and sex of patient and significant others (SOs).
4. Birth order of patient and family involvement.
5. Occupation.
6. Medical status and medical history.
7. Marital status; number and ages of children.
8. Cognitive status; educational level.
9. Readiness to learn and staging: precontemplation, contemplation, preparation, action, or maintenance (Baldwin and Falciglia, 1995).
10. Emotional status (stress, acceptance of illness, chronic disease, or condition).
11. Instructor's ability to teach; awareness and use of teaching/learning principles and adult learner theories.

Principles of Learning

1. The recipient must value information.
2. Pace should be adequate for learner (i.e., small steps).
3. Environment should be conducive to learning (e.g., free of distractions and stress), and patient should be ready to learn (e.g., free of pain).
4. Information must be meaningful, relevant, and organized. Material should be logical in sequence.
5. Counselor must be truly interested in sharing the information.
6. Adequate follow-up should be available for reinforcement of facts and principles.
7. For adult learners, information that is useful in the present is more meaningful than facts learned for the "future." Adults tend to prefer problem-solving information (e.g., survival skills) over learning facts alone.

Principles of Teaching

1. Counselor must first listen to patient. Involve patient in setting mutual objectives.
2. Small segments of information should be presented in understandable language in small, manageable "sound bites."
3. An organized plan should be used to teach. Clear objectives should be established, with timelines and short- and long-term outcomes.
4. Feedback should be used with each step. Be prepared to receive evaluation (peer review) from patient; improve as needed.
5. Good eye contact should be maintained with patient. Be aware, however, that direct or prolonged eye contact would be seen as rude or threatening by some cultures. Know your client.
6. Appropriate teaching tools or audiovisual aids should be used as appropriate. Using a 6th–8th grade reading level is suggested with easy layout, visual appeal, and illustrations.
7. Questions must be allowed for clarification.
8. Praise and positive reinforcement should be offered to learner. Carl Rogers emphasizes use of "unconditional positive regard" for all persons.

Counseling Tips

1. Knowledge does not automatically ensure compliance. Behavioral change takes time and encouragement.
2. Trial and error will be common for patient in learning new behaviors.
3. Increase in self-esteem comes with improvement in behavior.
4. Counselor should appropriately foster independence.
5. Empathy is an important part of humanistic care.
6. Counselor serves as an "intervention specialist" (Insull, 1992). The therapeutic nature of patient–clinician relationship draws from its capacity to meet the needs of both parties. The term "connexional" has been used to describe the powerful experience shared: an immediacy of awareness of patient's situation, a sense of being part of the larger whole, and a lingering feeling of joy, peacefulness, and awe (Matthews et al., 1993).
7. The "patient centered" approach to counseling is effective. Steps include assessing stage of change and motivation level of client, assessing past experiences with dietary changes, assessing anticipated challenges, identifying challenges and obstacles, identifying coping strategies and skills, setting goals, identifying steps needed for follow-up, and anticipating lapses and relapses (Rosal et al., 2001).
8. Goal setting as a strategy for behavioral change requires that the patient recognize the need for change, establish a goal, monitor goal-related activity, and use self-reward for goal attainment (Weber Cullen et al., 2001).

(continued)

TABLE B-5 Patient Education and Counseling Tips (*Continued*)

Counseling for End-of-Life or Hospice Patients (adapted from Lattanzi-Licht M and Gallagher-Allred C presentation at Food and Nutrition Conference and Exhibition, October 23, 2001):

1. Attempt to reduce fears related to eating.
2. Recognize stages of terminal illness: fear of abandonment, finding a natural and realistic approach, building bridges, and ownership of the experience.
3. Pain management is most important for quality of life.
4. Respect individual's cultural beliefs and needs.
5. Identify a patient advocate who will address concerns as care progresses.
6. Help maintain self-esteem and dignity.
7. Comfort foods can be important to patient satisfaction; identify and address these needs on a meal-to-meal basis.
8. Look for hidden messages from patient; communicate with other health care team members.

TABLE B-6 Sample Outcome Audits–Patient Education

This patient education audit identifies the ability of the patient to demonstrate or verbalize how he or she will or has changed behaviors after nutritional instructions.

Any Patient

1. Patient is able to identify the basic food pyramid and can select his or her menu accurately according to desired amounts.
2. Patient is able to explain importance of his or her diet to his or her health.
3. Patient is able to plan 1 day's menus and snacks from his/her dietary pattern.
4. Patient is able to incorporate economic/ethnic food choices into his/her prescribed diet.
5. Patient has been following diet at home for period of time. Patient is able to describe elements of this diet with accuracy.
6. Patient expresses recognition of need to lose/gain weight.
7. Patient is allergic to foods, as documented by tests, observation, family, etc.
8. Patient likes/refuses to eat specific foods and/or beverages.

Liquid Diets

1. Patient is able to progress to solid foods at this time.
2. Patient is able to tolerate only clear/full liquids at this time.
3. Patient is able to name high-protein liquids that can be consumed on this diet.

Protein-Altered Diets

1. Patient can identify foods that contain protein of high biologic value.
2. Patient can name foods to include/omit in diet to increase/decrease protein content of meals and snacks.

Mineral Diets (Iron, Potassium, Calcium, etc.)

1. Patient is able to name foods that are high/low in mineral.
2. Patient is able to accurately select menu choices for days that include/exclude foods that are high in mineral.
3. Patient is able to plan menus for home that are high/low in mineral.

Vegetarian Diet

1. Patient is able to identify correctly two or more complementary protein foods.
2. Patient is able to plan menus that provide adequate protein and vitamin B12, zinc, etc. for age and sex.

Tube Feeding

1. Patient does/does not tolerate specific tube feeding as ordered.
2. Patient will receive calories in product used, with flush of ___mL every ___hours.
3. Patient or significant other is able to prepare tube feeding as ordered for use at home (when home feedings are ordered).

Bland

1. Patient is able to identify foods to avoid on bland diet.
2. Patient is able to explain rationale for excluding caffeine-containing beverages or foods, black pepper, alcohol.

(*continued*)

TABLE B-6 Sample Outcome Audits—Patient Education (*Continued*)

Postgastrectomy or Dumping Syndrome (for any reason)

1. Patient is able to verbalize effects of diet on dumping syndrome.
2. Patient is able to explain guidelines to be followed to prevent dumping syndrome, e.g., beverages are served 30 minutes before or after meals; concentrated sweets omitted or severely limited.

High Fiber

1. Patient is able to verbalize foods that can be used to increase fiber in his or her diet, to desired level of ___g daily.
2. Patient is able to explain role of fiber in his or her particular disorder.
3. Patient is able to describe purpose of adequate fluids in dietary regimen and is able to consume ___ mL daily.

Low Fat

1. Patient is able to name foods that he or she must omit for the low-fat diet.
2. Patient is able to explain role of fat in his or her condition.
3. Patient is able to note grams of fat from a given food label.

Cardiac Care

1. Patient is able to name three beverages that are high in caffeine.
2. Patient is able to describe modifications in his or her diet that will be needed to prevent further coronary complications: saturated versus unsaturated fats, sodium and potassium, fiber, etc., and use of the DASH diet.
3. Patient is able to categorize correctly into the proper food pyramid lists.
4. Patient is able to plan menus for home use that include appropriate modifications.
5. Patient is able to name snack foods that can be included in dietary plan.

Low Cholesterol

1. Patient is able to describe simple definitions for cholesterol, saturated, polyunsaturated, and monounsaturated fats.
2. Patient is able to identify foods that have high cholesterol content.
3. Patient is able to name vegetable oils that may be used in diet.
4. Patient is able to describe three cooking methods that are acceptable for dietary regimen.
5. Patient is able to name foods that are good sources of monounsaturated fats.

Hyperlipidemia Diets

1. Patient is able to explain principal restrictions for his/her diet regarding calories, carbohydrate, fat, alcohol, and cholesterol.
2. Patient is able to plan days of menus within dietary restrictions.
3. Patient is able to discuss role of soluble fiber.

Hypoglycemia Diet

1. Patient is able to verbalize reasons for eating frequently.
2. Patient is able to describe reactions that can occur when concentrated carbohydrates are eaten or with omission of meals.
3. Patient is able to describe role of protein and fats in diet.
4. Patient is able to name sources of concentrated carbohydrate that are portable.

Diabetic Diets

1. Patient is able to explain relationship of diet to complications of diabetes.
2. Patient is able to name foods that contain CHO.
3. Patient is able to categorize into the correct food pyramid lists.
4. Patient is able to verbalize a simple definition of diabetes.
5. Patient is able to describe role of medications with food intake.
6. Patient is able to explain rationale for following a prudent diet to prevent complications (heart disease, etc.).
7. Patient is able to explain how proper spacing of meals affects his/her disorder.
8. Patient is able to describe symptoms of ketoacidosis and insulin shock and can name foods to take or avoid for each condition.
9. After looking at several food labels, patient is able to point out ingredients that mean "sugar" or carbohydrate.
10. Patient is able to describe techniques for managing special events (travel, parties, restaurants, holiday meals, etc.).

(*continued*)

TABLE B-6 Sample Outcome Audits–Patient Education (*Continued*)

Reducing Diets

1. Patient is able to verbalize his or her primary motivation for losing weight and has identified his or her current level of readiness for change in behaviors.
2. Patient is able to describe his or her realistic goal for weight loss–either short-term or long-term, including a timetable.
3. Patient is able to list foods that are low in calories and may be eaten as snacks.
4. Patient is able to categorize foods into the proper food pyramid categories.
5. Patient is able to demonstrate proper technique for recording food intake at home.
6. Patient has demonstrated weight loss over a certain time frame.

Sodium Restrictions

1. Patient is able to name foods that are naturally high in sodium.
2. Patient is able to name foods that have been processed or prepared with excesses of sodium.
3. Patient is able to explain difference between "salt" and "sodium" in foods.
4. Patient is able to list seasonings that can be used at home, in place of salt and salt-containing seasonings.
5. Patient is able to plan menus for home that will be low in sodium.
6. Patient is able to identify salt substitutes that he or she can use for his or her condition.
7. Patient is able to discuss how other nutrients (e.g., potassium, calcium, magnesium) play a role in the specific condition.

Gliadin-Free/Gluten-Restricted Diet

1. Patient is able to examine food labels and to name ingredients that must be avoided.
2. Patient is able to list products that must be avoided in diet.
3. Patient is able to plan menus that can be used at home.
4. Patient is able to adapt recipes for use at home.

Lactose Intolerance

1. Patient is able to name foods or beverages that must be avoided.
2. Patient is able to plan menus that are nutritionally complete for calcium but are lactose-restricted.
3. Patient demonstrates awareness that he or she can tolerate up to __ mL of lactose per day at this time.
4. Patient is able to discuss difference between lactose intolerance and milk allergy.

Renal Diets

1. Patient is able to describe restrictions that are needed in regard to protein, sodium, potassium, fluid, calories, and phosphorus.
2. Patient is able to plan menus that are balanced for the restricted nutrients.
3. Patient is able to name "free" foods that he or she can eat as desired.
4. Patient is able to discuss how foods, nutrients, and prescribed medications may interact.

TABLE B-7 Documentation: Charting Notes

Using the "SOAP" (or other designated) method of charting will permit the dietitian to communicate his or her role in the health care team. There are now many methods of chart documentation; the primary concern is that the accepted method is used and that assessment findings/actions are communicated concisely and accurately. The following guidelines may be used to develop effective notes:

SOAP Format:

S–Subjective information regarding current status as reported by patient or others (e.g., nausea, difficulty with chewing and swallowing, notable food habits that affect dietary treatment, comments about usual food intake elsewhere). Enclosing them in quotation marks may indicate actual comments from patient.

O–Objective and measurable data from the medical record of patient's weight, height, ideal weight, laboratory data, diet orders, drug orders, etc. or from documented medical notes and records. Known and observed eating habits and facts are part of these data.

A–Assessment of patient's "S" and "O" by dietitian. For example, dietitian may respond to patient's statements about eating excessive amounts of sweets and elevated blood glucose levels by writing that "Dietary intake exceeds the order for the restricted calorie diet." The assessment should make the "P" (Plans) section a natural consequence for activity.

P–Plans and recommended follow-up:

Treatment. Alterations in diet; changes in consistency of diet; supplemental feedings; prosthetic feeding aid; change in feeding modality.
Diagnosis. Request for more diagnostic tests; completion of an actual food diary for several days.
Education. Diet classes; personalized instructions to patients and significant others.

(continued)

TABLE B-7 Documentation: Charting Notes (*Continued*)

Progress Notes

Patient Progress: Dietary intake (calorie counts, gross nutrient inadequacies); problems with eating or feeding; food acceptance or rejection due to dislikes, allergies, intolerances, poor appetite, environmental factors, cultural factors, food quality; understanding of modified diet instructions being presented. If a patient refuses treatment or care, he or she must be informed of the consequences; all speech/learning/comprehension deficits should be considered, and progress notes should support refusal as a right of the patient (Robinson, 1996).

Specific Dietary Information: Unusual diet patterns; composition of calculated diets; significant nutrient deficiencies in diets as ordered, comments about multiple nutrient restrictions that are difficult or unacceptable to the patient; precautions in the use of the diet; composition of tube feeding when not specifically ordered; suggestions for change in a diet order with given rationale; nourishments and supplements as part of the diet regimen; explanation or interpretation of an unusual diet prescription.

Information Related to Diet Instructions: Record of initial instructions and patient responses; patient progress in accepting and understanding diet; ability to follow a diet order; suggested referrals to outside agencies or programs; appointments made to outpatient nutrition counseling services.

Nutrition History: Comments about diet obtained from patient, including an interpretation of such observations.

Follow-Up: Outcomes of nutritional services. Suggested changes. Referral to other services, agencies, and food programs. Contact with physician or other health care provider. Contact with reimbursement companies or managed-care organizations.

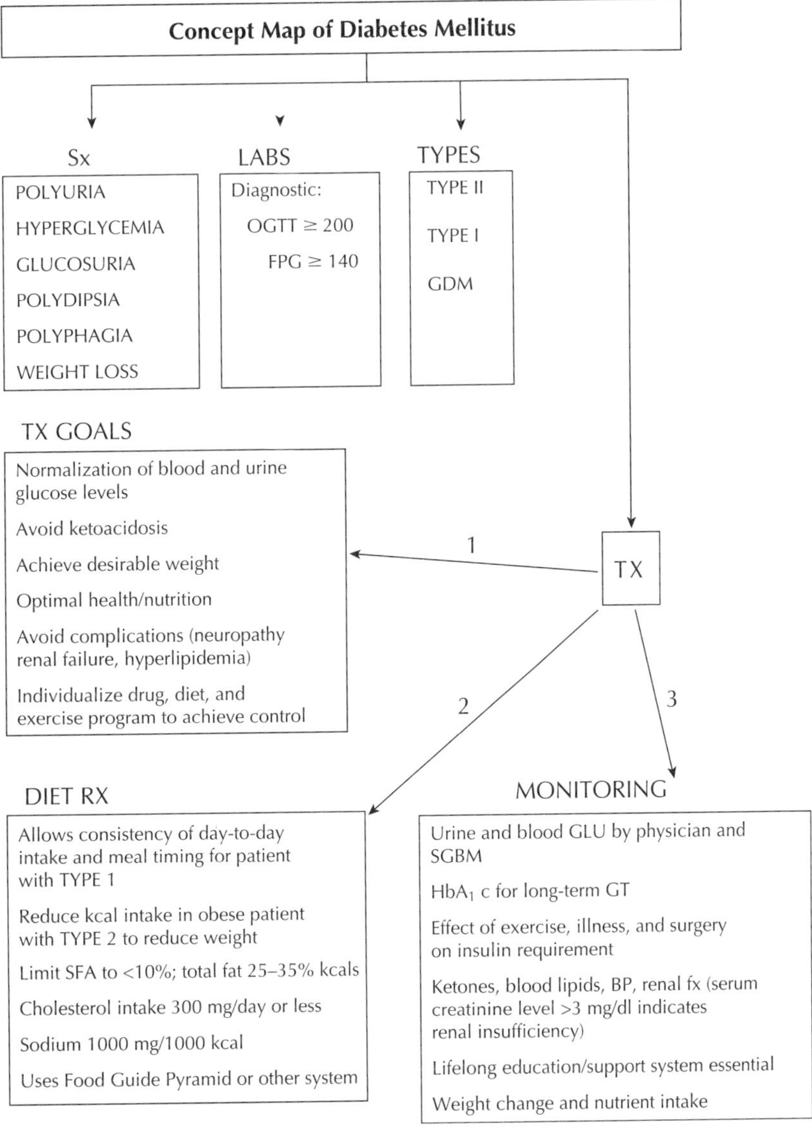

Figure B-12 Concept map of diabetes mellitus (Roberts, 1995).

Figure B-13 Nutritional Care Audit

Medical Unit______________**Responsible Dietitian** ______________________**Date of Audit**________

Nutrition Screening

- Patient screened within 24 hours of admission; assessment date is recorded.
- All available screening data are recorded in screening.
- Screening risk score is documented.

Patient Assessment

- Patient assessment is performed on the date designated from screening.
- Nutritional assessment complete for anthropometric, biochemical, clinical, and dietary evaluations.
- Patient nutrition status and recommendations are validated in medical record and dietary cardex.
- All pertinent information is on the assessment form.
- Recommendations outlined in the assessment are valid and appropriate for patient or medical condition.

Follow-up/Monitoring

- Pertinent nutrition issues are addressed in the follow-up process.
- All important information (for other dietitians to follow) from the follow-up is noted on the patient cardex card.
- Progress and/or problem resolution is noted on the interdisciplinary care plan (as applicable).
- Discharge planning is addressed.

Patient Education

- Patient education is addressed in a timely fashion.
- Education is appropriate to patient's condition, age, abilities, etc.
- Education and expected compliance is documented.
- Relevant information from patient's education session is documented.

Nutrient or Calorie Count

- Count is initiated when appropriate for patient situation.
- Count information is charted daily for duration indicated.
- Count information is clearly noted in designated site.

Food Allergies

- RD visits patient for whom severe food allergies are noted on admission.
- RD charts in the medical record within 24 hours of admission, validating awareness of known food allergies by the Nutrition Department.
- RD corrects chart or computer entry when an allergy is an intolerance.
- RD investigates questionable information when dealing with food allergies.

Communication

- Important information from all above processes/services are on the care plan, cardex, chart, or other designated site.
- RD communicates appropriate information through diet techs, kitchen staff, and other team members.
- The computer, phone, notes, fax, and other communication methods have been used to effectively communicate pertinent information.

Interdisciplinary Care Planning

- All relevant nutrition-related problems are entered on patient interdisciplinary care plan.
- Clear goals are included on care plan.
- Initiation of care planning process is noted on patient cardex card.

Adapted by: Cynthia Brylinsky, MS, RD, 2001.

Care Map = who, what, and when
Guidelines of Care = how

Care Map for (Disease) ______________________

Care Map	Day 1	Day 2	Day 3	Day 4	Day 5
Consults					
Lab Tests					
Diagnostic Treatments					
Treatments/Assessments					
Medications					
Diet					
Activity					
Teaching					
Psychosocial					
Discharge Planning					
Other					

Figure B-14 Care map format.

Discharge Planning

Involvement with discharge planning and overseeing reimbursement for nutrition support are important roles for dietitians in home care services (Foltz, Arensberg, and Schiller, 1996).

1. Discharge plans should include current diet prescription, supplemental feedings, TF and TPN details, food allergies and intolerances, problems with chewing and swallowing or nausea and vomiting, diarrhea, pressure ulcers, other nutritional needs, weight, height, usual BW, recent weight changes, summary of interventions and counseling, name of dietitian, and phone number for contact (Escott-Stump, 1996). Determination of BMI is also important. See Table B-8.

2. Determine needs for home care—tube feeding, TPN, and/or oral feeding.

3. Educate patient, family, or caretakers.

4. Refer to other agencies when appropriate. See Table B-9 for selected information sites. Table B-10 lists dietetic practice groups of The American Dietetic Association; these are often excellent resources and contacts.

5. Document services; submit copy to agency, physician, or other healthcare professional. If records are computerized, submit as per standard operating procedure.

6. Manage and evaluate resources, plans, and outcomes. A multidisciplinary case-management approach is best.

7. Serve as patient advocate with reimbursement agencies and care facilities. Communicate, communicate, communicate!

TABLE B-8 Discharge Planning Summary

Wt____Ht______ UBW_______ BMI_____ Recent weight changes__________ Goal Wt________________
Current diet prescription_______________________________Supplemental feedings____________________
TF and TPN details ____
Food allergies and intolerances____
Problems with chewing and swallowing or N & V, diarrhea___________________________________
Pressure ulcers, other nutritional needs____
Summary of interventions and counseling____
Name of dietitian and phone number for contact ____________________________________

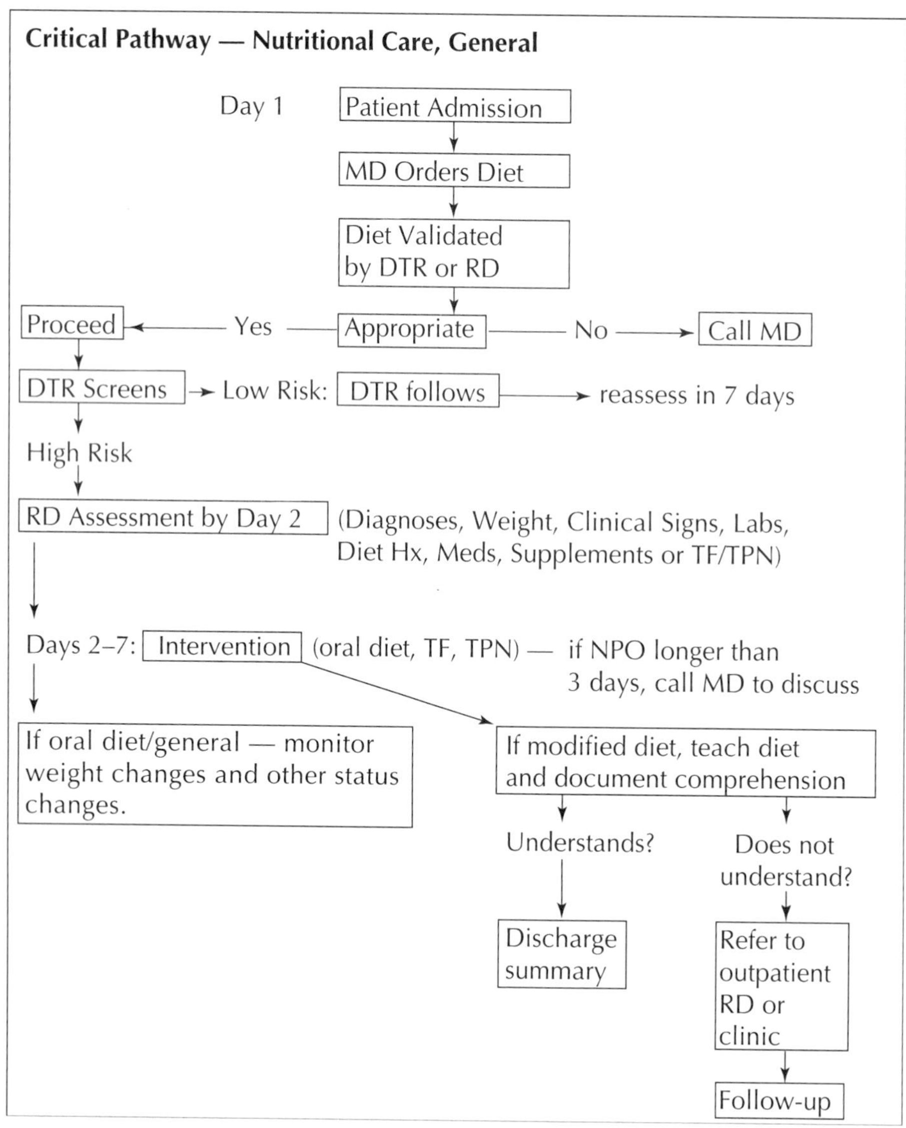

Figure B-15 **Sample critical pathway–nutritional care, general.**

Figure B-16 NUTRITION PROGRESS NOTES:

Patient:______________________________ ID #______________________

Ht: __________ Wt: __________ IBW: __________ Usual Wt: __________

Current diet/nutrition support order: ______________________________

Estimated needs: ______________ kcal per Kg ______________g protein per Kg

NUTRITIONAL DIAGNOSIS OR PROBLEM LIST:

1. Increased/alteration in nutrition needs r/t: ______________________________
2. Decreased/inadequate nutrient intake r/t: ______________________________
3. Alteration in biochemistries: ______________________________
4. Alteration in knowledge regarding therapeutic diet/food-drug interaction: ______________________________
5. Other: ______________________________

INTERVENTION

___None required. Follow-up per nutrition protocol.

___Food preferences obtained to optimize intake/patient satisfaction.

___Supplements/nourishments ordered,______________________.

___Patient educated regarding______________________.

___Preferred method of learning discussed: visual___auditory___reading___hands-on___.

___Outpatient Nutrition Clinic recommended; Referral completed on date__________.

___Monitor: _____ basic metabolic panel; _____ albumin/prealbumin; _____ glucose q __ hours; _____ lytes daily/weekly; _____ liver panel/triglycerides weekly; _____ weight daily/biweekly/weekly; other______________________

RECOMMENDATIONS

Recommended actions:

____

____

____

EVALUATION/GOALS

____Nutrient intake currently adequate/inadequate,______________________________

____Comprehension of education: good/fair/poor, r/t______________________________

____Expected adherence to education: good/fair/poor, r/t ______________________________

____Other:______________________________

CODING FOR REIMBURSEMENT:________DRG__________ICD Code_____MNT Code

DIETITIAN'S SIGNATURE:______________________DATE:__________

TABLE B-9 Selected Associations, Clearinghouse, and Information Centers

Food & Nutrition Associations:

AMERICAN INSTITUTE OF NUTRITION
9650 Rockville Pike
Bethesda, MD 20814-3990
(301) 530-7050

AMERICAN SOCIETY OF CLINICAL NUTRITION
9650 Rockville Pike
Bethesda, MD 20814-3998
(301) 530-7110

CULINARY INSTITUTE OF AMERICA
433 Albany Post Road
Hyde Park, NY 12538
(914) 452-9600

INSTITUTE OF FOOD TECHNOLOGISTS
221 North LaSalle Street, Suite 300
Chicago, IL 60601
(312) 782-8424

INTERNATIONAL ASSOCIATION OF CULINARY PROFESSIONALS
304 West Liberty Street, Suite 201
Louisville, KY 40202
(502) 581-9786

SOCIETY FOR NUTRITION EDUCATION
2001 Killebrew Drive, Suite 340
Minneapolis, MN 55425-1882
(612) 854-0035

THE AMERICAN DIETETIC ASSOCIATION
216 W. Jackson Boulevard
Chicago, IL 60606
(312) 899-0040 / (800) 366-1655

Health/Medical Organizations

ALCOHOL:

NATIONAL CLEARINGHOUSE FOR ALCOHOL INFORMATION
PO Box 2345
Rockville, MD 20852
(301) 468-2600

ALLERGY AND ASTHMA:

AMERICAN ACADEMY OF ALLERGY ASTHMA AND IMMUNOLOGY
611 East Wells Street
Milwaukee, WI 53202
(414) 272-6071 / (800) 822-2762

FOOD ALLERGY NETWORK
10400 Eaton Place, Suite 107
Fairfax, VA 22030-2208
(703) 691-3179

ARTHRITIS:

ARTHRITIS FOUNDATION
1330 West Peachtree Street
Atlanta, GA 30309
(404) 872-7100 / (800) 283-7800

ARTHRITIS INFORMATION CLEARINGHOUSE
PO Box 9782
Arlington, VA 22209
(703) 558-4999

CANCER:

AMERICAN CANCER SOCIETY
1599 Clifton Road, NE
Atlanta, GA 30329-4251
(404) 329-7920 / (800) ACS-2345

AMERICAN INSTITUTE FOR CANCER RESEARCH
1759 R Street, NW
Washington, DC 20009
(202) 328-7744 / (800) 843-8114

CANCER INFORMATION CLEARINGHOUSE
National Cancer Institute, Office of Cancer Communications
9000 Rockville Pike, Building 31, Room 10A18
Bethesda, MD 20205
(301) 496-5583 or (800) 4-CANCER

CARDIOLOGY:

AMERICAN HEART ASSOCIATION
7272 Greenville Avenue
Dallas, TX 75231
(214) 373-6300 / (800) 242-8721

CONSUMER INFORMATION:

CONSUMER INFORMATION CENTER
Room G-142, 18th and F Streets NW
Washington, DC 20405

DIABETES:

NATIONAL DIABETES INFORMATION CLEARINGHOUSE (NDIC)
1 Information Way
Bethesda, MD 20892-3560
(301) 654-3327

DIGESTIVE DISEASES:

NATIONAL DIGESTIVE DISEASE INFORMATION CLEARINGHOUSE (NDDIC)
2 Information Way
Bethesda, MD 20892-3570
(301) 654-3810

NUTRITION AND FOOD:

FOOD AND NUTRITION INFORMATION CENTER
National Agricultural Library Building, Room 304
10301 Baltimore Boulevard
Beltsville, MD 20705
(301) 344-3719

FOOD AND WATER SAFETY:

MEAT AND POULTRY HOTLINE
U.S. Department of Agriculture: (800) 535-4555

SEAFOOD SAFETY
American Seafood Institute: (800) EAT-FISH

WATER SAFETY
Safe Drinking Water Hotline: (800) 426-4791

HANDICAPS/DISABILITIES:

CLEARINGHOUSE ON THE HANDICAPPED
400 Maryland Avenue SW, 3119 Switzer Building
Washington, DC 20202
(202) 245-0080

(continued)

TABLE B-9 Selected Associations, Clearinghouse, and Information Centers (*Continued*)

HEALTH FRAUD:
NATIONAL COUNCIL AGAINST HEALTH FRAUD RESOURCE CENTER
300 East Pink Hill Road
Independence, MO 64057
(816) 228-4595

HEALTH INFORMATION:
CENTER FOR HEALTH PROMOTION AND EDUCATION
Centers for Disease Control
1600 Clifton Road, Building 1, SSB-249
Atlanta, GA 30333
(404) 329-3492

CLEARINGHOUSE ON HEALTH INDEXES
National Center for Health Statistics
Division of Epidemiology and Health Promotion
3700 East-West Highway, Room 2-27
Hyattsville, MD 20782

NATIONAL HEALTH INFORMATION CLEARINGHOUSE
PO Box 1133
Washington, DC 20013-1133
(207) 429-9091/(800) 336-4797

HIGH BLOOD PRESSURE:
HIGH BLOOD PRESSURE INFORMATION CENTER
120-80 National Institutes of Health
Bethesda, MD 20205
(703) 558-4880

MEDICAL ASSOCIATIONS:
AMERICAN ACADEMY OF FAMILY PHYSICIANS
8880 Ward Parkway
Kansas City, MO 64114-2797
(816) 333-9700

AMERICAN MEDICAL ASSOCIATION
515 North State Street
Chicago, IL 60610
(312) 464–5000

NATIONAL ACADEMY OF SCIENCES
Institute of Medicine, Food & Nutrition Board
2101 Constitution Avenue, NW
Washington, DC 20418
(202) 334-2587

MEDICATIONS:
FOOD AND DRUG ADMINISTRATION (FDA)
Office of Consumer Affairs, Public Inquiries
5600 Fishers Lane (HFE-88)
Rockville, MD 20857
(301) 443-3170

MENTAL HEALTH:
NATIONAL CLEARINGHOUSE FOR MENTAL HEALTH INFORMATION
Public Inquiries Section
5600 Fishers Lane, Room 15C-05
Rockville, MD 20857
(301) 443-4513

PEDIATRICS:
AMERICAN ACADEMY OF PEDIATRICS
141 Northwest Point Boulevard
Elk Grove Village, IL 60007-1098
(847) 228-5005

MARCH OF DIMES BIRTH DEFECTS FOUNDATION
1275 Mamaroneck Avenue
White Plains, NY 10605
(914) 428-7100

NATIONAL ASSOCIATION OF PEDIATRIC NURSE ASSOCIATES AND PRACTITONERS
1101 Kings Highway, N., Suite 206
Cherry Hill, NJ 08034-1931
(609) 667-1773

REHABILITATION:
NATIONAL REHABILITATION INFORMATION CENTER
4407 Eighth Street NE
Washington, DC 20017-2299
(202) 635-5822

SMOKING:
OFFICE ON SMOKING AND HEALTH
Technical Information Center
5600 Fishers Lane, Park Building, Room 116
Rockville, MD 20857
(301) 443-1690

SPORTS:
AMERICAN COLLEGE OF SPORTS MEDICINE
Box 1440
Indianapolis, IN 46206-1440
(317) 637-9200

PRESIDENT'S COUNCIL ON PHYSICAL FITNESS AND SPORTS
701 Pennsylvania Avenue, NW, Suite 250
Washington, DC 20004
(202) 272-3421

WOMEN'S HEALTH:
ASSOCIATION OF WOMEN'S HEALTH, OBSTETRIC AND NEONATAL NURSES
700 14th Street, NW, Suite 600
Washington, DC 20005
(202) 662-1608

NATIONAL CENTER FOR HEALTH EDUCATION IN MATERNAL AND CHILD HEALTH
2000 15th Street, North, Suite 701
Arlington, VA 22201
(703) 524-7802

NATIONAL CLEARINGHOUSE FOR FAMILY PLANNING INFORMATION
PO Box 2225
Rockville, MD 20852
(301) 881-9400

Food Industry Organizations & Associations
AMERICAN BAKERS ASSOCIATION
1350 I Street, NW, Suite 1290
Washington, DC 20005
(202) 789-0300

AMERICAN FROZEN FOOD INSTITUTE
2000 Corporate Ridge, Suite 1000
McLean, VA 22102
(703) 821-0770

AMERICAN MEAT INSTITUTE
P.O. Box 3556
Washington, DC 20007
(703) 841-2400

(*continued*)

TABLE B-9 Selected Associations, Clearinghouse, and Information Centers (*Continued*)

CALORIE CONTROL COUNCIL
1101 15th Street, NW, Suite 202
Washington, DC 20005
(202) 785-3232

CHOCOLATE MANUFACTURERS ASSOCIATION
7900 Westpart Drive, Suite A-320
McLean, VA 22102
(703) 790-5011

EGG NUTRITION CENTER
1819 H Street, NW, Suite 520
Washington, DC 20006
(202) 833-8850

FOOD MARKETING INSTITUTE
800 Connecticut Avenue, NW, Suite 400
Washington, DC 20006
(202) 452-8444

GROCERY MANUFACTURERS OF AMERICA
1010 Wisconsin Avenue, NW, Suite 900
Washington, DC 20007
(202) 337-9400

INSTITUTE OF SHORTENING AND EDIBLE OILS, INC.
1750 New York Avenue, N.W.
Washington, DC 20006
(202) 783-7960

INTERNATIONAL APPLE INSTITUTE
6707 Old Dominion Drive, Suite 320
McLean, VA 22101
(703) 442-8850

INTERNATIONAL DAIRY FOODS ASSOCIATION
1250 H Street, NW, Suite 900
Washington, DC 20005
(202) 737-4332

NATIONAL ASSOCIATION OF MARGARINE MANUFACTURERS
1101 15th Street, NW, Suite 202
Washington, DC 20005
(202) 785-3232

NATIONAL CATTLEMEN'S BEEF ASSOCIATION
1301 Pennsylvania Avenue, NW, Suite 300
Washington, DC 20004
(202) 347-0288

NATIONAL CONFECTIONERS ASSOCIATION
7900 Westpark Drive, Suite A-320
McLean, VA 22102
(703) 821-0770

NATIONAL DAIRY COUNCIL
10255 West Higgins Road, Suite 900
Rosemont, IL 60018-5616
(847) 803-2000

NATIONAL FISHERIES INSTITUTE
1901 North Fort Myer Drive, Suite 400
Arlington, VA 22209
(703) 524-8880

NATIONAL FOOD PROCESSORS ASSOCIATION
1401 New York Avenue, NW, Suite 400
Washington, DC 20005
(202) 639-5900

NATIONAL MILK PRODUCERS FEDERATION
1840 Wilson Boulevard, Suite 400
Arlington, VA 22201
(703) 243-6111

NATIONAL PASTA ASSOCIATION
2101 Wilson Boulevard, Suite 920
Arlington, VA 22201
(703) 528-6507

NATIONAL PEANUT COUNCIL
1500 King Street, Suite 301
Alexandria, VA 22314
(703) 838-9500

NATIONAL PORK BOARD
122 C Street, NW, Suite 875
Washington, DC 20001
(202) 347-3600

NATIONAL RESTAURANT ASSOCIATION
1200 17th Street, NW
Washington, DC 20036-3097
(202) 331-5900

NATIONAL TURKEY FEDERATION
1225 New York Avenue, NW, Suite 400
Washington, DC 20005
(202) 898-0100

PRODUCE MARKETING ASSOCIATION
1500 Casho Mill Road
P.O. Box 6036
Newark, DE 19714-6036
(302) 738-7100

SALT INSTITUTE
700 N. Fairfax Street
Suite 600
Alexandria, VA 22314-2040
(703) 549-4648

SNACK FOOD ASSOCIATION
1711 King Street, Suite 1
Alexandria, VA 22314
Phone: (703) 836-4500

THE SUGAR ASSOCIATION, INC.
1101 15th Street, NW, Suite 600
Washington, DC 20005
(202) 785-1122

UNITED FRESH FRUIT & VEGETABLE ASSOCIATION
727 N. Washington Street
Alexandria, VA 22314
(703) 836-3410

WHEAT FOODS COUNCIL
5500 South Quebec Street, Suite 111
Englewood, CA 80111
(303) 694-5828

TABLE B-10 American Dietetic Association Practice Groups

Clinical
- Diabetes Care and Education
- Dietitians in General Clinical Practice
- Dietitians in Nutrition Support
- Dietetics in Physical Medicine and Rehabilitation
- Nutrition in HIV/AIDS
- Oncology Nutrition
- Pediatric Nutrition
- Perinatal Nutrition
- Renal Dietitians
- Weight Management

Community
- Complementary Care
- Dietitians in Developmental & Psychiatric Disorders
- Food and Culinary Professionals
- Gerontological Nutritionists
- Hunger, Malnutrition, and Environmental Nutrition
- Public Health Nutrition
- Vegetarian Nutrition

Consultation and Business
- Consultant Dietitians in Health Care Facilities
- Dietitians in Business and Communications
- Nutrition Entrepreneurs
- Sports and Cardiovascular Nutritionists

Education and Research
- Dietetic Educators of Practitioners
- Nutrition Education of Health Professionals
- Nutrition Education for the Public
- Research

Management
- Clinical Nutrition Management
- Dietetic Technicians in Practice
- Management in Food and Nutrition Systems
- School Nutrition Services

For more information or to contact a practice group, write to the following address:
The American Dietetic Association
216 West Jackson Boulevard
Chicago, IL 60606-6995
1-800-877-1600

RATIONALE FOR DIAGNOSTIC-RELATED GROUP TABLES (TABLE B-11)

In the United States, medical costs have soared higher than other expenses in cost-of-living evaluations. To curb excessive growth in medical charges, diagnostic-related groups (DRGs) were established by the federal government as reasonable costs per diagnosis, recognizing regional differences as well as differences in size of facilities. It is good practice for hospitals to admit and discharge patients expediently and to provide excellent care, especially to receive payment for the services rendered.

Malnourished patients have longer lengths of stay, higher costs, and more deaths. One goal of health care includes assurance that patient will have a satisfactory or improved status during hospitalization and that rapid discharge to home, other rehabilitative or skilled nursing center, or other site will occur within a reasonable time frame. Payment methods to hospitals and other facilities are often related to DRGs. If a patient lingers in the facility longer than a typical DRG suggests, this becomes an "outlier," and expenses will exceed payments to the facility in many cases. It is best to standardize care and to "manage" care to keep expenses in line while providing the best level of care.

Authors have described the effect of DRGs on hospital malnutrition and vice versa. In some institutions, it is possible to obtain more money per case when malnutrition is listed as a comorbidity factor or a complication. In one study of coding for malnutrition, additional reimbursement of $12,326 was possible by coding with the additional International Classification of Diagnoses, 9th edition (ICD-9) codes (Funk and Ayton, 1995).

Managed care organizations (MCOs) tend to estimate and reimburse for specific services at a given rate. The trend to "cost-justify" all services through managed care will continue. Reimbursement of services by a registered dietitian is a cost-effective way to control health care costs in many diagnoses. Dietitians must market their skills to companies by emphasizing how they can reduce costs and improve outcomes (Hahn, 1996).

Because nutritional status affects immunity, wound healing, and other factors related to medical care, a sample population was selected to create Table B-11. Lengths of stay for uncomplicated procedures vary and, therefore, are not listed. Actual DRG codes are assigned by the institution and scrutinized by the government. For more information, contact the medical records, admitting, or fiscal departments of local hospitals for more specific local or regional information.

TABLE B-11 Sample DRGs and ICD-9 Codes

This chart was created to serve as a guide for planning nutritional care according to ICD-9 codes and to designate typical DRGs that are assigned. It is essential to designate the appropriate codes to ensure that nutritional conditions such as protein–calorie malnutrition (PCM) are listed for comorbidity and complications and to obtain reimbursement (see Table B-12).

CONDITION AND ICD-9 INTERNATIONAL CODE	*DRG CODE EXAMPLE*	*Section of this Book*
Pregnancy (650)	#373	One
Infertility (628.9)	#369	
Dental difficulties/oral disorders:	#185	Two
Edentulism (525.1)		
Broken or wired jaw (802.2)		
Mouth ulcers (528.9)		
Tongue disorders (529.9)		
Periodontal disease (523.9)	#185	
Skin disorders:	#284	
Acne (706.1)	#284	
Psoriasis (696.1)	#283	
Chronic urticaria (708.9)	#284	
Infantile eczema (692.9)	#284	
Acrodermatitis enteropathica (686.8)	#278	
Dermatitis herpetiformis (692.9)	#284	
Pressure ulcer (707.0)	#271	
Vitamin deficiencies:	#297	
Xerophthalmia (264.7)	#47	
Cheilosis (266.0)	#297	
Scurvy (267)	#297	
Food allergy/allergic reactions	#447	
Asthma (493)	#97	
Food poisoning (005.9)	#183	
Ménière's syndrome	#73	
Biliary atresia (751.61)	#208	Three
Cerebral palsy (343.9)	#35	
Cleft palate (749)	#52 surgical #74 medical	
Congenital heart disease	#137	
Cystic fibrosis (277)	#298	
Cystinosis (270)	#299	
Down's syndrome (758)	#429	
Failure to thrive (783.4)	#298	
Inborn errors of CHO metabolism	#299	
Hirschsprung's disease (751.3)	#190	
Homocystinuria (270.4)	#299	
Low-birth-weight infant (765.1)	#385	
Maple syrup urine disease (270.3)	#299	
Necrotizing enterocolitis	#184	
Phenylketonuria (270.1)	#299	
Prader-Willi syndrome (759.8)	#385	
Tyrosinemia (270.4)	#299	
Wilson's disease (275.1)	#299	
Alzheimer's disease (331.0)	#429	Four
Amyotrophic lateral sclerosis (335.20)	#12	
Anorexia nervosa (307.1)	#428	
Coma (780.0)	#27	
Depression (311)	#426	
Epilepsy (345.9)	#25	
Huntington's chorea (333.4)	#12	
Multiple sclerosis (340)	#13	
Myasthenia gravis (358)	#12	
Neurological trauma/spinal cord injury (952.9)	#9	
Parkinson's disease (332)	#12	
Psychosis	#430	

(*continued*)

TABLE B-11 Sample DRGs and ICD-9 Codes (*Continued*)

CONDITION AND ICD-9 INTERNATIONAL CODE	*DRG CODE EXAMPLE*	*Section of this Book*
Bronchial asthma	#96	Five
Acute respiratory failure (799.1)	#87	
Pneumonia/bronchitis	#90	
Chronic obstructive pulmonary disease (496)	#88	
Cor pulmonale (416.9)	#145	
Pulmonary embolus (415.1)	#78	
Tuberculosis (011.9)	#80	
Atherosclerosis, ischemic heart disease (414)	#132	Six
Cerebrovascular disease (436)	#131	
Congestive failure or shock (428)	#127	
Heart valve disorder	#136	
Hyperlipoproteinemias (272.4)	#299	
Hypertension (401.9)	#134	
Myocardial infarction (410.9)	#121	
Peripheral vascular disease (443.9)	#130	
Achalasia (530.3)	#183	Seven
Heartburn/esophagitis (553.3)	#183	
Dyspepsia (536.8)	#183	
Gastric retention (536.8)	#183	
Gastritis/gastroenteritis (535.5)	#183	
Pernicious vomiting (536.2)	#183	
Peptic ulcer/complications (533.9)	#176	
Gastrectomy or vagotomy (43.89)	#155	
Diarrhea (558.9)	#183	
Dysentery (009.0)	#183	
Malabsorption syndrome (579.9)	#183	
Gluten-induced enteropathy (579.0)	#183	
Tropical sprue (579.1)	#183	
Lactose malabsorption (271.3)	#183	
Constipation (564)	#183	
Irritable colon (564.1)	#183	
Diverticular diseases (562.11)	#183	
Enteritis or Crohn's disease (555.9)	#179	
Intestinal fistula (569.81)	#189	
Ileitis (558.9)	#183	
Ulcerative colitis/ileostomy (556)	#149	
Ileostomy, permanent (46.23)	#149	
Colostomy (46.10)	#149	
Anal procedures (e.g., hemorrhoidectomy) (49.46)	#157	
Intestinal lipodystrophy (Whipple's disease)	#188	Eight
Pancreatitis (577.0)	#204	
Pancreatic insufficiency (577.8)	#204	
Zollinger-Ellison syndrome (251.5)	#176	
Cholecystitis (574.0)	#208	
Cholecystectomy (574.0)	#195	
Jaundice (782.4)	#464	
Hepatitis (573.3)	#206	
Biliary cirrhosis (571.6)	#207	
Alcoholic liver disease (571.3)	#202	
Alcohol dependence (305)	#436	
Ascites (789.5)	#464	
Hepatic cirrhosis (571.5)	#202	
Liver transplant	#191	
Hepatic encephalopathy and/or coma (572.2)	#206	
Insulin-dependent diabetes mellitus (250.01)	#295	Nine
Noninsulin-dependent diabetes mellitus (250.00)	#294	
Gestational diabetes (648.8)	#372	

(*continued*)

TABLE B-11 Sample DRGs and ICD-9 Codes (*Continued*)

CONDITION AND ICD-9 INTERNATIONAL CODE	*DRG CODE EXAMPLE*	*Section of this Book*
Ketoacidosis and/or coma (250.11)	#294	Nine (*Continued*)
Hypoglycemia (251.2)	#297	
Hyperinsulinism (251.1)	#301	
Addison's disease (255.4)	#301	
Hyperthyroidism (242.9)	#301	
Hypothyroidism (244.9)	#301	
Goiter (240.9)	#301	
Diabetes insipidus (253.5)	#301	
Gout (274.9)	#245	
Cushing's syndrome (255.0)	#301	
Parathyroid disorders (252)	#301	
Altered calcium metabolism (275.4)	#297	
Pregnancy-induced hypertension (642.4)	#372	
Obesity (278.0)	#297	Ten
Underweight or general debility (269.9)	#297	
Kwashiorkor, severe PCM (260)	#297	
Nutritional marasmus (261)	#297	
Other severe PCM/nutritional edema (262)	#297	
Malnutrition, moderate degree (263)	#297	
Malnutrition, mild degree (263.1)	#297	
Malnutrition, other PCM (263.8)	#297	
Muscular dystrophy (359.1)	#256	Eleven
Osteoarthritis (715.9)	#245	
Osteomalacia (268.2)	#245	
Osteoporosis (733)	#245	
Rheumatoid arthritis (714)	#242	
Scleroderma	#241	
Systemic lupus erythematosus (710)	#241	
Nutritional anemias (281)	#395	Twelve
Iron-deficiency anemia (280.9)	#395	
Sickle-cell anemia (282.6)	#395	
Brain tumor	#10	Thirteen
Cancer (e.g., leukemia 209.9 or lymphoma 202.8)	#403	
Radiotherapy	#409	
Chemotherapy	#410	
Electrolyte imbalances (K+, Ca++, Mg++, Na+ 275–6)	#297	Fourteen
Amputation (84.17)	#114	
Appendectomy/complications (47)	#164	
Bowel surgery	#148	
Jejunoileal bypass (45.91)	#288	
Gastric bypass or stapling (44.31)	#288	
Craniotomy	#1	
Retinal cataract surgery	#36	
Hysterectomy, abdominal (68.4)	#353	
Coronary bypass/cardiac catheterization (36.10)	#106	
Total hip arthroplasty (81.59)	#209	
Tonsillectomy/adenoidectomy (28.3)	#57–58	
Acquired immune deficiency syndrome	#423	Fifteen
Bacterial endocarditis (421)	#126	
Burns (949)	#457	
Fever, unknown origin (780.6)	#419	
Fracture, hip (821)	#210 surgical #236 medical	
Infectious mononucleosis (075)	#421	
Poliomyelitis (045.9)	#20	

(*continued*)

TABLE B-11 Sample DRGs and ICD-9 Codes (*Continued*)

CONDITION AND ICD-9 INTERNATIONAL CODE	*DRG CODE EXAMPLE*	*Section of this Book*
Rheumatic fever (390)	#241	Fifteen (*Continued*)
Typhoid fever (002)	#423	
Glomerulonephritis, acute (580.9)	#332	Sixteen
Glomerulonephritis, chronic (582.9)	#332	
Nephritis (583.9)	#332	
Nephrosclerosis (403.9)	#332	
Nephrotic syndrome (581.9)	#326	
Pyelonephritis, chronic (590.0)	#320	
Urolithiasis (592.9)	#323	
Renal failure, acute (584.9)	#316	
Renal failure, chronic (585)	#316	
Renal dialysis: hemodialysis (39.95)	#317	
Renal dialysis: peritoneal (54.98)	#317	
Postrenal transplantation (55.69)	#302	
Vitamin D-resistant rickets (275.3)	#299	
Hartnup disease (270)	#299	

TABLE B-12 Codes For Nutrition Reimbursement for Registered Dietitians

The American Dietetic Association announced three new current procedural codes (CPT) for MNT. The codes have been released by the Health Care Financing Administration (HCFA) and included in American Medical Association's *Current Procedural Terminology CPT 2001* book, page 300.

MNT, provided by a registered dietitian, is a service that involves a comprehensive assessment of a patient's overall nutritional status, medical data, and diet history, followed by intervention to prescribe a personalized course of treatment. Registered dietitians are specialized practitioners with academic and professional training in nutrition and are credentialed through the national credentialing agency, the Commission on Dietetic Registration.

97802 **Medical nutrition therapy: initial assessment and intervention, individual face-to-face with patient, each 15 minutes**

97803 **Reassessment and intervention, individual face-to-face with patient, each 15 minutes**

97804 **Medical nutrition therapy assessment and/or intervention performed by a physician, see Evaluation and Management or Preventive Medicine service codes**

http://www.eatright.org/gov/mntannounce.html

REFERENCES

Cited References

Abron, Braunschweig C. Creating a clinical registry: prospects, problems, and preliminary results. *J Am Diet Assoc.* 1999;99:467.

American Dietetic Association. *Medical nutrition therapy across the continuum.* Chicago: American Dietetic Association, 1996.

American Dietetic Association. Medical nutrition therapy and pharmacotherapy. *J Am Diet Assoc.* 1999;99:227.

American Dietetic Association. Position of The American Dietetic Association: nutrition education for health care professionals. *J Am Diet Assoc.* 1998;98:343.

American Gastroenterological Association. Medical Position Statement: parenteral nutrition. *Gastroenterology.* 2001;121:966.

Baird, Schwartz D, Gudzin D. Preadmission nutrition screening: expanding hospital-based nutrition services by implementing earlier nutrition interventions. *J Am Diet Assoc.* 2000;100:81.

Balch G. Employers' perceptions of the roles of dietetics practitioners: challenges to survive and opportunities to thrive. *J Am Diet Assoc.* 1996;96:1301.

Baldwin T, Falciglia D. Application of cognitive behavioral theories to dietary change in clients. *J Am Diet Assoc.* 1995;95:1315.

Barr J, et al. Case problem: quality of life outcomes assessment–How can you use it in Medical Nutrition Therapy? *J Am Diet Assoc.* 2001; 101:1064.

Boyhtari M, Cardinal B. The role of clinical dietitians as perceived by dietitians and physicians. *J Am Diet Assoc.* 1997;97:851.

Bryk JA, Soto TK. Membership database of the American Dietetic Association. *J Am Diet Assoc.* 1999;99:102.

Camelon K. The Plate Model: a visual method of teaching meal planning. *J Am Diet Assoc.* 1998;98:10.

Campbell S. Practice report of The American Dietetic Association: home care—an emerging practice area for dietetics. *J Am Diet Assoc.* 1999;99:1453.

Council on Practice Quality Management Committee. ADA's definitions for nutrition screening and nutrition assessment. *J Am Diet Assoc.* 1994;94:838.

Dahlke R, et al. Focus groups as predictors of dieitians' roles on interdisciplinary teams. *J Am Diet Assoc.* 2000;100:455.

Detsky A, et al. Subjective global nutritional assessment. *J Parenter Enteral Nutri.* 1987;11:8.

Dodds J, Polhamus B. Self-perceived competence of advanced public health nutritionists in the United States. *J Am Diet Assoc.* 1999; 99:808.

Duyff R. The value of lifelong learning: key element in professional career development. *J Am Diet Assoc.* 1999;99:538.

Ellrodt G, et al. Evidence-based disease management. *J Am Med Assoc.* 1997;278:1687.

Escott-Stump S. Continuity of nutrition care. *Hospital Food & Nutrition Focus.* 1996;13:7.

Escott-Stump S, et al. Joint Commission on Accreditation of Healthcare Institutions: friend or foe? *J Am Diet Assoc.* 2000;100:839.

Escott-Stump S. Managing nutrition services. In: Jackson R, ed. *Nutrition and food services for integrated health care: a handbook for leaders.* Gaithersburg, MD: Aspen Publishers, 1997; 149.

Foltz, Arensberg M, Schiller R. Dietitians in home care: a survey of current practice. *J Am Diet Assoc.* 1996;96:347.

Fox T. Institute of Medicine urges Medicare coverage of medical nutrition therapy. *J Am Diet Assoc.* 2000;100:166.

Funk K, Ayton C. Improving malnutrition documentation enhances reimbursement. *J Am Diet Assoc.* 1995;95:468.

Gates G, Sandoval W. Teaching multiskilling in dietetics education. *J Am Diet Assoc.* 1998;98:278.

Hahn N. Home is where the jobs are. *J Am Diet Assoc.* 1996;96:334.

Harris J, Benedict F. *A biometric study of basal metabolism in man.* Publication no. 279. Washington, DC: Carnegie Institute of Washington, 1919.

Heimburger D, et al. Survey of clinical nutrition training programs for physicians. *Am J Clin Nutri.* 1998;68:1174.

Insull W. Dietitians as intervention specialists: a continuing challenge for the 1990s. *J Am Diet Assoc.* 1992;92:551.

Israel D, McCabe M. Using disease-state management as the key to promoting employer sponsorship of medical nutrition therapy. *J Am Diet Assoc.* 1999;99:583.

Johnson R. The Lewin Group study—What does it tell us and why does it matter? *J Am Diet Assoc.* 1999;99:426.

Kight M, et al. Conducting physical examination rounds for manifestations of nutrient deficiency or excess: an essential component of JCAHO assessment performance. *Nutrition in Clinical Practice.* 1999;14:93.

Kight M. *Dietetic-specific nutritional diagnostic codes.* Tucson, AZ: Biodietetic Associates, 1994.

Klein C, et al. Physicians prefer goal-oriented note format more than three to one over other outcome-focused documentation. *J Am Diet Assoc.* 1997;97:1306.

Lau C, Gregoire M. Quality ratings of a hospital foodservice department by inpatients and post-discharge patients. *J Am Diet Assoc.* 1998;98:1303.

Matthews D, et al. Making "connexions:" enhancing the therapeutic potential of patient-clinician relationships. *Ann Intern Med.* 1993; 118:973.

Meakins JL. Innovation in surgery: the rules of evidence. *Am J Surg.* 2002;183:399.

Mislevy J, et al. Clinical nutrition managers have access to sources of empowerment. *J Am Diet Assoc.* 2000;100:1038.

Moreland K, et al. Development of implementation of the Clinical Privileges for Dietitian Nutrition Order Writing program at a long-term acute care hospital. *J Am Diet Assoc.* 2002;102:72.

Myers E, et al. Clinical Privileges: missing piece of the puzzle for clinical standards that elevate responsibilities and salaries for registered dietitians? *J Am Diet Assoc.* 2002;102:123.

Myers E, et al. Evidence-based practice guides vs. protocols: what's the difference? *J Am Diet Assoc.* 2001;101:1085.

Naglak M, et al. What to consider when conducting a cost-effectiveness analysis in a clinical setting. *J Am Diet Assoc.* 1998;98:10.

Roberts C, et al. Concept mapping: an effective instructional strategy for diet therapy. *J Am Diet Assoc.* 1995;95:908.

Robinson G. Applying the 1996 JCAHO nutrition care standards in a long-term care setting. *J Am Diet Assoc.* 1996;96:400.

Rosal M, et al. Facilitating dietary change: the patient-centered counseling model. *J Am Diet Assoc*. 2001;101:332.

Schiller M, et al. Administrators' perceptions of nutrition services in home health care agencies. *J Am Diet Assoc*. 1998;98:56.

Sheils J, et al. The estimated costs and savings of medical nutrition therapy: the Medicare population. *J Am Diet Assoc*. 1999;99: 428.

Shils M, et al, eds. *Modern nutrition in health and disease*. Baltimore: Williams & Wilkins, 1999.

Silverman D. *Laboratory values for assessing and monitoring nutritional status*. Columbus, OH: Ross Laboratories, 1994.

Silverman M, et al. Current and future practices in hospital foodservice. *J Am Diet Assoc*. 2000;100:76.

Snetselaar L. *Nutrition counseling skills for medical nutrition therapy*. Gaithersburg, MD: Aspen Publishers, 1997.

Splett P, Myers E. A proposed model for effective nutrition care. *J Am Diet Assoc*. 2001;101:361.

Testa M, Simonson D. Current concepts: assessment of quality-of-life outcomes. *N Engl J Med*. 1996;334:13.

Veldee M. Judicious and efficient utilization of laboratory nutrition tests. *Support Line*. 1995;XVII:9.

Weber, Cullen K, et al. Using goal setting as a strategy for dietary behavior change. *J Am Diet Assoc*. 2001;101:562.

Wilson I, Cleary P. Linking clinical variables with health-related quality of life: a conceptual model of patient outcomes. *JAMA*. 1995; 273:59.

Suggested Readings

American Dietetic Association. Standards of Professional Practice for Dietetics Professionals. *J Am Diet Assoc*. 1998;98:83.

Arena J, Walters P. Do you know what a dietetic technician can do? A focus on clinical technicians and their expanded roles and responsibilities. *J Am Diet Assoc*. 1997;97: S139.

Berger J, Rosner F. The ethics of practice guidelines. *Arch Int Med*. 1996;156:2051.

Betkoski D, Ometer L. Documenting your future: how to write a business plan. *J Am Diet Assoc*. 2000;100:293.

Biesemeier C. Case manager/registered dietitian partnerships: teaming up to achieve positive patient outcomes. *J Care Mgt*. 1997; 3:72.

Biesemeier C, Chima C. Computerized patient record: are we prepared for our future practice? *J Am Diet Assoc*. 1997;97:1099.

Dodd J. Look before you leap—but do leap. *J Am Diet Assoc*. 1999; 99:422.

Dwyer J. Scientific underpinnings for the profession: dietitians in research. *J Am Diet Assoc*. 1997;97:593.

Eck L, et al. A model for making outcomes research standard practice in clinical dietetics. *J Am Diet Assoc*. 1998;98:451.

Evans-Stoner N. Nutrition assessment: a practical approach. *Nursing Clin N America*. 1997;32:637.

Glanz K, et al. Why Americans eat what they do: taste, nutrition, cost, convenience, and weight control concerns as influences on food consumption. *J Am Diet Assoc*. 1998;98:10.

Hammond K. Physical assessment: a nutritional perspective. *Nursing Clin N America*. 1997;32:779.

Harris-Davis E, Haughton B. Model for multicultural nutrition counseling competencies. *JAMA*. 2000;100:1178.

Keys A, et al. *The biology of human starvation, vol. 1*. Minneapolis: University of Minnesota Press, 1950, pp. 184–208.

Lacey K, Cross N. A problem-based nutrition care model that is diagnostic driven and allows for monitoring and managing outcomes. *J Am Diet Assoc*. 2002;102:578.

Laramee S. Nutrition services in managed care: new paradigms for dietitians. *J Am Diet Assoc*. 1996;96:336.

Miller M, Kinsel K. Patient-focused care and its implications for nutrition practice. *J Am Diet Assoc*. 1998;98:177.

Olendzki B, et al. Nutrient Intake Report: a coordination of patient dietary assessment between physicians and registered dietitians. *J Am Diet Assoc*. 1998;98:10.

Physicians' desk reference for drug therapy. Oradell, NJ: Medical Economics Company, current edition.

Porter C, Matel J. Are we making decisions based on evidence? *J Am Diet Assoc*. 1998;98:404.

Rhoades P, et al. An objective method of assessing the clinical abilities of dietetics interns. *J Am Diet Assoc*. 1998;98:7.

Roberts C, et al. Concept mapping: an effective instructional strategy for diet therapy. *J Am Diet Assoc*. 1995;95:908.

Sandrick K. Is nutritional diagnosing a critical step in the nutrition care process? *J Am Diet Assoc*. 2002;102:427.

Simmons M, Vaughan L. Patient nutrition acuity as a predictor of the time required to perform medical nutrition therapy. *J Am Diet Assoc*. 1999;99:167.

Stein K. Diet office redesign to enhance satisfaction and reduce costs. *J Am Diet Assoc*. 2000;100:512.

Stein K. Foodservice in correctional facilities. *J Am Diet Assoc*. 2000; 100:508.

Stonebrook A. Education and certification influence the nutrition and management knowledge of long-term care foodservice managers. *J Am Diet Assoc*. 1999;99:553.

Swails W, et al. A proposed revision of current ICD-9-CM malnutrition code definitions. *J Am Diet Assoc*. 1996;96:370.

Trissler R. From aspartame to Xenical: a look at the FDA review process. *J Am Diet Assoc*. 1999;99:797.

Visocan B. Up-skilling and dietetics professionals. *J Am Diet Assoc*. 1998;98:9.

Wallach J. *Interpretation of diagnostic tests*. 6th ed. Boston: Little, Brown & Co., 1996.

Westbrook N. Applying the 1995 JCAHO standards to dietetic practice in home care. *J Am Diet Assoc*. 1996;96:404.

Witte S, et al. Standards of practice criteria for clinical nutrition managers. *J Am Diet Assoc*. 1997;97:673.

Zeman F, Ney D. *Applications in medical nutrition therapy*. 2nd ed. Englewood Cliffs, NJ: Prentice-Hall, 1996.

Multiple-Condition Case Studies

PRACTICE CASE STUDIES AND CONCEPT MAPS

Using the concept map formats, write a summary for each of the patients in the following case studies. Add as many details as needed to make the case complete. The concept map should help to identify key areas and visualize the cases more clearly. The concept map for the sample case below follows after the case. The concept maps for all other chapter case studies appear in order at the end of Appendix C.

Sample Case: Chronic Diarrhea 0 Weight Loss in Elderly Women

Marian J. has entered the acute-care facility where you work as a clinical dietitian. She is a 79-year-old white female who has been widowed and living alone for the past 7 years. Her only son lives near her and visits her in the hospital each evening. From a review of her medical record, it is noted that she has been admitted for chronic diarrhea and weight loss of 10 lb (she currently weighs 145 lb). She has osteoarthritis in her wrists and ankles, hypertension with a current reading of 170/100, and history of a cerebrovascular accident (CVA) 5 years ago with minimal residual deficits. She is relatively sedentary because of her osteoarthritis. Marian previously was prescribed a low-sodium diet and was given a diet instruction sheet at the doctor's office. She has her own teeth, which are in good condition. Recently, she has complained to her son of being more "sad" than usual. What nutritional plan and actions should be developed?

Primary concern:

diarrhea with resulting weight loss of 10 lb

Secondary concerns:

osteoarthritis, which makes it difficult to eat and to walk quickly
hypertension, which is regulated by medications
history of CVA
mild depression of recent onset

Additional information and data are needed for a thorough assessment:

1. Diarrhea entry (pp. 293)—determine cause; discuss any history of food allergy and intolerances, recent use of antibiotics, medication history. Marian cannot identify anything unusual in her diet recently and has not taken antibiotics. Check laboratory values.
2. Weight loss—identify cause (from diarrhea, inadequate intake from recent depression, etc.). Obtain a thorough weight history (before this weight loss, Marian's height was 5 feet, 2 inches and weight 155 lb; she was overweight by 35 to 45 lb all of her married life).
3. Osteoarthritis (pp. 467)—evaluate weight history and use of medications (she takes Trilisate during periods of flare).
4. Hypertension (pp. 249)—Marian did not take her prescribed diuretics on a regular basis before her stroke; since that time, she does take them faithfully. Her excess weight probably contributed to the hypertension. The current reading of 170/100 is "high normal" for her while on medication; it usually runs 145/95.
5. History of cerebrovascular accident (pp. 236)—Marian indicates that the most problematic concern she has is some recent depression, which prevents her from eating a full meal as usual. Her medication to control hypertension is all that has been used until now.

Prescribed Medications:

Trilisate for osteoarthritis
Bumex for hypertension

Self-Prescribed Medications:
Mineral oil for ("for regularity")

Diet History: Usual Intake at Home

Breakfast (7:30 AM)
Corn flakes/whole milk and 2 t sugar
Black coffee

Lunch (11:30 AM)
Peanut butter/jelly sandwich
1 cup canned tomato soup
¾ cup canned pears

Snack (3:00 PM)
½ cup sherbet
Black coffee

Dinner (6:00 PM)
Chicken or beef/gravy
Buttered noodles
½ cup green beans
1 cup whole milk

Allergies, Food Likes, and Dislikes:

Does not eat pork and dislikes fish intensely

Other Information:

The doctor has prescribed Kaopectate for the diarrhea and it seems to be effective. He also ordered a general/2 g sodium diet. Marian is not eating well in the facility and seems depressed.

Sample Care Plan:

1. Objectives:

Short-Term—Resolve diarrhea and increase overall fiber from diet. Request that the doctor consider changing the diet to high fiber/no salt added so that Marian's appetite can improve with more seasoned foods. Diarrhea and weight loss have been attributed to the use of Trilisate; the doctor has changed her medication to Lodine, with less likelihood of causing any anorexia or diarrhea. Yogurt or acidophilus milk may be used to recolonize flora in the intestinal tract.

Extra fluids are essential during this time. Check electrolyte status until diarrhea resolves. Monitor weights to see if rehydration helps Marian to recover a few of the lost pounds.

The doctor has ordered an antidepressant temporarily; depression is common after a CVA. An antidepressant may help Marian recover her appetite.

Discuss with Marian the effects of mineral oil on fat-soluble vitamin absorption and how it may also contribute to some diarrhea. Advise her that the high-fiber diet she has been given will help normalize bowel function.

When her appetite returns, some suggested alterations in her dietary pattern may include: use of a high-fiber cereal at breakfast; use of more fresh fruits each day (especially oranges, bananas, and apples for potassium, pectin fiber, and low sodium content); use of skim milk instead of whole milk with at least 3 cups daily, if tolerated; addition of a salad or some raw vegetables with lunch or dinner to enhance vitamin and mineral content of her diet, as well as fiber.

For her blood pressure, it may be recommended that she try some of the lower sodium/lower fat soups that are now available on the market. Easy-to-prepare foods are now available from the grocery store at reasonable prices so that she can readily plan her meals and maintain her independence.

2. Follow-Up Session:

Approximately 2 weeks after returning home, Marian sees you in the Ambulatory Nutrition Clinic for a follow-up visit. She feels much better and has regained 3 lb that were lost from the diarrhea, which has resolved.

Long-Term Objectives—Discuss with Marian how to maintain weight after diarrhea has resolved. To help her mobility and reduce stress on the joints, additional weight gain should not be the plan. For her goal weight of 140 lb (minimal planned weight loss), a plan of 1,500–1,600 calories would be shared, using simplified exchange lists that also are low in added salt.

Her son brings her dinner meals approximately three times weekly. He also has made contact with the local Meals on Wheels program to enroll his mother at your suggestion. They provide a hot meal that generally is lower in sodium and fat upon request.

Although her activity level is not significantly improved, she does try to participate in daily exercises for strengthening and stretching. This has improved her range of motion and energy level. She sees the physical therapist each week for some resistance training exercises that she can follow at home. Her spirits also have improved, and her doctor has discontinued the antidepressant medication.

Marian no longer uses mineral oil as a laxative and has faithfully adopted high-fiber foods into her daily pattern. She indicates that your advice about fiber foods has not been as difficult as she expected. She is now including 3–4 fruits and vegetables daily, with the long-range goal of "5 a day." This is beneficial not only for her hypertension and for normal bowel function but also to protect against future cerebrovascular accidents as far as possible.

Marian agrees to call you if she has other questions or concerns about her diet. The high-fiber diet remains the emphasis, with consideration also to lower sodium foods but not so low that she loses her appetite. She and her son are pleased with your interventions; you plan to stay in contact once every 6 months by telephone. A concept map of this case follows on page 781. A blank format is at the end of the chapter.

PRACTICE CASE STUDIES

Section 1 Case Study: Normal Life-Cycle Conditions

Josie is a 15-year-old white teen who is pregnant. She has a history of disordered eating and was hospitalized for this problem approximately 2 years ago. Her weight before the pregnancy was 95 lb and she was 5 feet 1 inch in height. She is now 24 weeks pregnant and weighs 102 lb. Her serum albumin level is 3.4 g/dL; blood glucose is 110 mg/100 mL. There is no other blood work available at this time. You are her outpatient dietitian and are now scheduled to see her twice a month until she delivers.

What assessment data do you ask for? What are essential aspects to include in her care plan? What counseling tips will you consider as you talk with her, considering both the pregnancy and the history of disordered eating?

See Concept Map for Section 1 Case Study at the end of Appendix C.

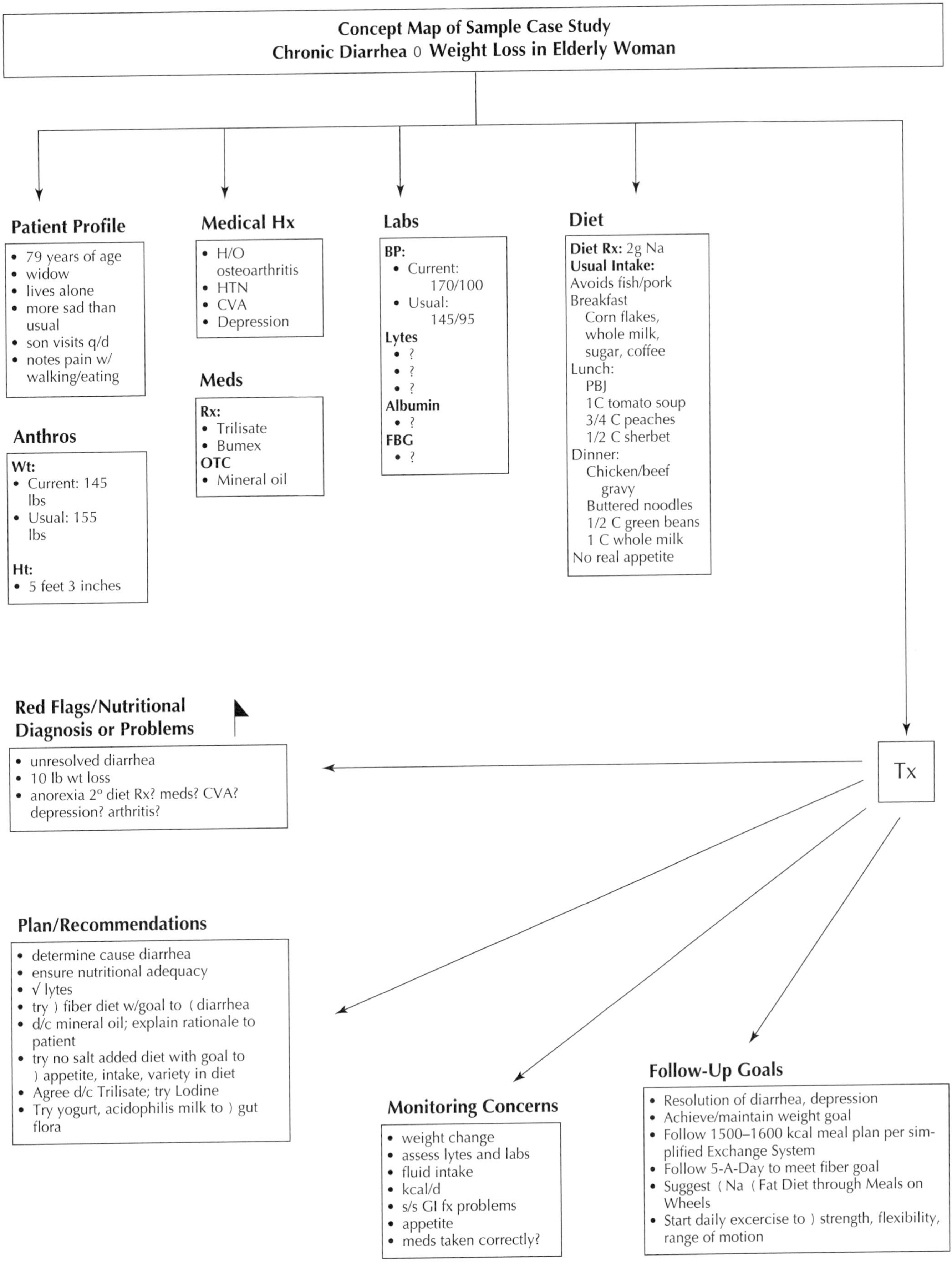
Concept Map of Sample Case Study
Chronic Diarrhea 0 Weight Loss in Elderly Woman
Patient Profile
• 79 years of age
• widow
• lives alone
• more sad than usual
• son visits q/d
• notes pain w/ walking/eating
Anthros
Wt:
• Current: 145 lbs
• Usual: 155 lbs
Ht:
• 5 feet 3 inches
Medical Hx
• H/O osteoarthritis
• HTN
• CVA
• Depression
Meds
Rx:
• Trilisate
• Bumex
OTC
• Mineral oil
Labs
BP:
• Current: 170/100
• Usual: 145/95
Lytes
• ?
• ?
• ?
Albumin
• ?
FBG
• ?
Diet
Diet Rx: 2g Na
Usual Intake:
Avoids fish/pork
Breakfast
Corn flakes, whole milk, sugar, coffee
Lunch:
PBJ
1C tomato soup
3/4 C peaches
1/2 C sherbet
Dinner:
Chicken/beef gravy
Buttered noodles
1/2 C green beans
1 C whole milk
No real appetite
Red Flags/Nutritional Diagnosis or Problems
• unresolved diarrhea
• 10 lb wt loss
• anorexia 2° diet Rx? meds? CVA? depression? arthritis?
Tx
Plan/Recommendations
• determine cause diarrhea
• ensure nutritional adequacy
• √ lytes
• try) fiber diet w/goal to (diarrhea
• d/c mineral oil; explain rationale to patient
• try no salt added diet with goal to) appetite, intake, variety in diet
• Agree d/c Trilisate; try Lodine
• Try yogurt, acidophilis milk to) gut flora
Monitoring Concerns
• weight change
• assess lytes and labs
• fluid intake
• kcal/d
• s/s GI fx problems
• appetite
• meds taken correctly?
Follow-Up Goals
• Resolution of diarrhea, depression
• Achieve/maintain weight goal
• Follow 1500–1600 kcal meal plan per simplified Exchange System
• Follow 5-A-Day to meet fiber goal
• Suggest (Na (Fat Diet through Meals on Wheels
• Start daily excercise to) strength, flexibility, range of motion

Section 2 Case Study: Dietary Practices and Miscellaneous Conditions

Nathan is a 24-year-old black male who presents at your nutrition office with gastrointestinal (GI) distress, recent acute gastroenteritis, and low albumin and serum electrolytes. His doctor has diagnosed food allergies, including wheat and egg allergies. He is also lactose intolerant. He has brought a 7-day food diary for you to review.

What additional assessment data do you need? What nutritional care plan will you develop? How will you follow up his care and nutritional status? What guidance will you offer in regard to label reading, dining in restaurants, packing a lunch for work, and holiday meals?

See Concept Map for Section 2 Case Study at the end of Appendix C.

Section 3 Case Study: Special Pediatric Conditions

Kyle is a 6-month-old white male with cerebral palsy and failure to thrive. He is below the 5th percentile on the growth charts for height and weight. His mother is 20 years old, and the father is absent. Kyle and his mother have been referred to your services by the pediatrician to conquer the failure to thrive. Kyle has a low hemoglobin and hematocrit (H&H), low blood glucose level, and low blood urea nitrogen (BUN)/creatinine. You find that Kyle's mother started cow's milk at 6 weeks because it was "supposed to be good for him." She has not introduced any cereal, fruits, vegetables, or meats into his diet; she feeds him 4 oz of milk four times daily. Kyle requires use of a special nipple because he cannot close his lips completely around a bottle.

What additional assessment data do you need? What nutritional care plan factors should be considered? Design a nutritional care plan and establish goals for Kyle's recovery and growth.

See Concept Map for Section 3 Case Study at the end of Appendix C.

Section 4 Case Study: Neurologic and Psychiatric Conditions

Stanley is a 42-year-old male with a history of schizophrenia and tardive dyskinesia. He has taken many types of antipsychotics during the previous 20 years. He has lived in a nursing home since suffering a mild stroke. He is paralyzed on the right side and has mild dysphagia. You are assigned to his floor in the Veterans Administration Medical Center. Stanley's medical record indicates that he has a blood pressure that averages 150/95, blood glucose levels of 135 mg/100 mL, H&H slightly below normal, and other normal laboratory values.

What additional nutritional information do you need? For Stanley's current status, the doctor has ordered a mechanical soft diet, but you note some coughing with meals. Should you ask for a speech therapy consult? What other nutritional care plan factors will you need to know? What are some common medications that cause tardive dyskinesia? What are some risks noted for stroke patients who must also take antipsychotics?

See Concept Map for Section 4 Case Study at the end of Appendix C.

Section 5 Case Study: Pulmonary Disorders

Marissa is a 28-year-old black female with cystic fibrosis, which was diagnosed when she was 12 years old. She now has extensive problems with chronic pneumonia and bouts of atelectasis. She takes three or four antibiotics to prevent additional pulmonary infections. Recently, elevated blood sugar levels have been noted on doctor's visits. Although a diagnosis of diabetes has not been made, Marissa has been advised to see you in the outpatient clinic to discuss management of diabetes and cystic fibrosis. She is 5 feet 8 inches in height and weighs 125 lb.

What additional factors do you need to complete her nutritional assessment? What care plan factors must be addressed? Because shopping is a tedious prospect for Marissa, what suggestions do you have to simplify the shopping and meal preparation process for her? She lives alone. Develop recipe adaptations to her favorite meal of barbecued chicken with fried potatoes and greens, with sweet potato pie for dessert.

See Concept Map for Section 5 Case Study at the end of Appendix C.

Section 6 Case Study: Cardiovascular Disorders

Sonny is a youthful 72-year-old man with arteriosclerosis and a recent valve replacement surgery. He has come to see you in your clinic office upon referral by his physician. He has experienced a 10-lb weight loss since his surgical procedure and has lost his appetite. He wants to return to his usual practice of walking 5 miles per day but does not have the energy to do so. His lab work reveals a low H&H, normal glucose, albumin level of 3.2 g/dL, serum cholesterol of 275 g/dL, and high homocysteine level with low serum folate.

What suggestions do you have for Sonny's dietary regimen? Design a dietary plan that includes his favorite foods of scrambled eggs and bacon. What shopping tips do you have for him? Sonny has been taking a supplement from a local Chinese market, containing several herbs that you are not familiar with. Who should you contact to find out more about the content of these supplements? Should you talk with his doctor about this practice? Sonny wants you to advise him about incremental increases in his activity program. Should you offer advice on this subject?

See Concept Map for Section 6 Case Study at the end of Appendix C.

Section 7 Case Study: Gastrointestinal Disorders

Naomi is a 52-year-old white woman who is married and has two grown children. Recently, her daughter called you to make an appointment regarding Naomi's GI complaints. She has suffered for 10 years with Crohn's disease and has recently been diagnosed with acute pancreatitis. She is unable to consume solid foods with liquids at the same meal; she has nausea after meals and cannot sleep if she has eaten too close to bedtime. Naomi also has high blood pressure and a family history of cardiovascular disease. She is 5 feet 3 inches and weighs 172 lb. Her lab work is not available because she is from another state. She takes Lasix for her blood pressure and prednisone for the inflammatory bowel disease.

What nutritional assessment data should you seek? What types of nutritional guidance would you offer to Naomi regarding: nausea, liquid and solid food consumption, foods to limit for lowering blood pressure and reducing cardiovascular risks, foods to assist with some weight loss, other nutritional issues related to inflammatory bowel disease and pancreatitis? What side effects do her medications have? What suggestions can you offer?

See Concept Map for Section 7 Case Study at the end of Appendix C.

Section 8 Case Study: Pancreatic, Hepatic, and Biliary Disorders

William is a 65-year-old American Indian male with liver failure and recent encephalopathy. His current blood work reveals a low H&H, albumin of 2.5 mg/dL, glucose of 160 mg/100 mL, elevated serum ammonia levels, and BUN and creatinine that are slightly elevated. William's doctor advises you that he probably has early renal failure. His height is 6 feet 2 inches and his weight is 220 lb. He takes ferrous sulfate, Glynase, and lactulose.

What other information should you seek to develop a nutritional care plan? What dietary advice may be useful to William? If William is allowed to go home from the hospital, what type of diet should be prescribed for use at home? What medication side effects are likely?

See Concept Map for Section 8 Case Study at the end of Appendix C.

Section 9 Case Study: Endocrine Disorders

Tyler is a 60-year-old white male with a recent diagnosis of hyperthyroidism; he has long-term diabetes. His doctor referred him to you and indicates that he has lost approximately 25 lb in a 6-month period. He is taking Tapazole and Humulin insulin. From a diet history, you find that Tyler consumes approximately 2,500 kcal and 50 g of protein each day. He does not consume excessive amounts of carbohydrate, and his blood glucose levels tend to be easily controlled by the insulin. His laboratory work indicates a low H&H, slightly low BUN and creatinine, and normal glucose.

What type of nutritional care plan would you design? Because Tyler enjoys dining in restaurants, especially Italian and Mexican, what types of foods would you recommend for him? Tyler travels a lot on business and skips breakfast regularly. What suggestions do you have for him while he is "on the road?"

See Concept Map for Section 9 Case Study at the end of Appendix C.

Section 10 Case Study: Weight Control and Malnutrition

Sarai is a 32-year-old Native American who has been referred by her doctor to your weight control clinic. Her height is 5 feet 1 inch, and her weight is 182 lb. She has a history of diabetes controlled by diet, gallstones, and knee replacement surgery. Sarai is willing to work with you at this time on a nutritional plan that allows her to lose 1–1.5 lb weekly over the next 6 months. She needs to join a support group because her family does not think she needs any weight loss; she is "just fine as she is." Her laboratory work is normal at this time for all factors other than a slightly low H&H.

What types of questions would you ask regarding her dietary habits? Sarai works in a factory where she must stand all day on her feet. She gets hungry and takes frequent breaks. What suggestions do you have for Sarai's snack breaks? With her knee replacement, Sarai is not able to walk great distances without pain. What type of referral might be useful for her to inquire about reasonable exercises?

See Concept Map for Section 10 Case Study at the end of Appendix C.

Section 11 Case Study: Musculoskeletal, Arthritic, and Collagen Disorders

Suzanne is a 50-year-old white female with a diagnosis of lupus and multiple allergies, including milk allergy. She has come to see you in the outpatient clinic of the hospital where you work. She has no available lab work but tells you that she tends to fatigue easily and to have a lot of GI distress. Recently, she has had chronic mild diarrhea after meals. Her height is 5 feet 6 inches and she weighs 120 lb.

What additional information should you request from her physician? What type of nutritional care plan might you begin to design for Suzanne? What types of foods are tolerable for diarrhea? List several suggestions. Is there a special diet for lupus? Suzanne has copies of four diets that she uses in sequence to try to cure her disease. What advice would you offer to her about these diets?

See Concept Map for Section 11 Case Study at the end of Appendix C.

Section 12 Case Study: Anemias and Blood Disorders

Lenora is a 14-year-old black female who has sickle-cell anemia. She eats well but has no energy for her after-school sports activities. She takes a multivitamin supplement twice a week. She currently is using nighttime tube feedings from 8 pm to 8 am. Lenora weighs 120 lb and is 5'8"; she recently lost 12 lb after a bout of influenza and tends to lose weight easily.

What nutritional parameters do you need to assess her nutritional status further? What suggestions do you have for Lenora to include more fruits, vegetables, and nutrients needed for added vitamins B6, A, E, and folic acid? What suggestions do you have for Lenora to be able to participate in sports more regularly?

See Concept Map for Section 12 Case Study at the end of Appendix C.

Section 13 Case Study: Cancer

Ed is a 68-year-old retired farmer. He recently has been diagnosed with throat cancer and severe anemia. He is unable to swallow thin liquids and uses thickened beverages for most of his meals. His height is 5 feet 10 inches, and his weight is 160 lb. He has had radiation therapy to his throat and will have another few months of this treatment. His prognosis is poor, and he wants advice on how to make meals more appealing. He has significant anorexia and mouth sores.

What nutritional assessment factors should you seek? What type of nutritional care plan would be useful for Ed? Plan a high-calorie, high-protein diet that uses thickened liquids and soft foods that he can tolerate. What other suggestions would you offer?

See Concept Map for Section 13 Case Study at the end of Appendix C.

Section 14 Case Study: Surgical Disorders

Matt is a white 12-year-old boy who has recently undergone surgery for a fractured femur. He has a history of asthma, takes theophylline, and uses inhalers. He is a "chocolate fiend" and is unwilling to give up his chocolate bars two times daily. He eats poorly and skips all fruits and vegetables. His surgical wound is not healing well, and his doctor has not prescribed any vitamin–mineral supplements. When Matt goes home, he will eventually return to school, where he likes to play hockey.

What nutritional parameters do you need to assess his nutritional status further? What side effects are common from asthma medications? What suggestions do you have for Matt to include more fruits, vegetables, and nutrients needed for wound healing? How can you use Matt's desire to play hockey as a reinforcer for improving his diet and ensuring a faster recovery? What negotiation skills will you need?

See Concept Map for Section 14 Case Study at the end of Appendix C.

Section 15 Case Study: Hypermetabolic, Infectious, Traumatic, and Febrile Conditions

Marcus is a 35-year-old black male who has been diagnosed as HIV-positive. He has made an appointment to see you in the outpatient nutrition clinic because he wants advice on how to stay healthy. His height is 6 feet 4 inches, and his weight is 240 lb. Currently, his total lymphocyte count (TLC) is low, as is his H&H. He has an albumin level of 3.6 mg/dL and other normal laboratory values. He has begun taking AZT and two experimental medications, under doctor's supervision.

What factors should you monitor for Marcus? What side effects might he experience on AZT? What are some common long-term problems associated with being HIV-positive? If Marcus wants to try supplemental foods and beverages, which might you recommend and why? What tips can you offer to provide symptom relief for problems such as diarrhea?

See Concept Map for Section 15 Case Study at the end of Appendix C.

Section 16 Case Study: Renal Disorders

Aaron is a 75-year-old white male in your skilled nursing facility. He has chronic renal failure and is blind. He uses adaptive feeding equipment and receives dialysis three times weekly. Recently, his renal dietitian has called you to note that his albumin level has dropped to 2.4 gm/dL; his phosphorus levels are high and serum K+ is elevated slightly. Because of his osteoarthritis, Aaron takes a lot of pain medication. He wears dentures and follows a mechanical soft diet.

What nutritional information should you address first? What tips are useful for Aaron to maintain his self-feeding ability despite his blindness? What guidance will you offer regarding his nutritional care plan?

See Concept Map for Section 16 Case Study at the end of Appendix C.

Section 17 Case Study: Enteral and Parenteral Nutrition

Sophie is an 80-year-old Jewish grandmother of six. She lives with her daughter, who provides gastrostomy tube feeding without problems for Sophie at home. Sophie has had problems with elevated lipid levels recently, and her doctor is concerned. You have been called as the home-care dietitian to make a visit and to discuss Sophie's needs. Her height is 4 feet 11 inches and her weight is 140 lb; her serum cholesterol is 250 mg/dL. Her tube feeding runs 70 mL/hour of standard product, yielding 1 kcal/mL.

What is she currently receiving in calories? How would you suggest making adjustments for her elevated lipid levels? At Sophie's age, would you support the daughter's request to aggressively treat the hypercholesterolemia with medications? Because Sophie is nonambulatory, what other suggestions do you have for her nutritional care plan?

See Concept Map for Section 17 Case Study at the end of Appendix C.

CONCEPT MAPS FOR PRACTICE CASE STUDIES

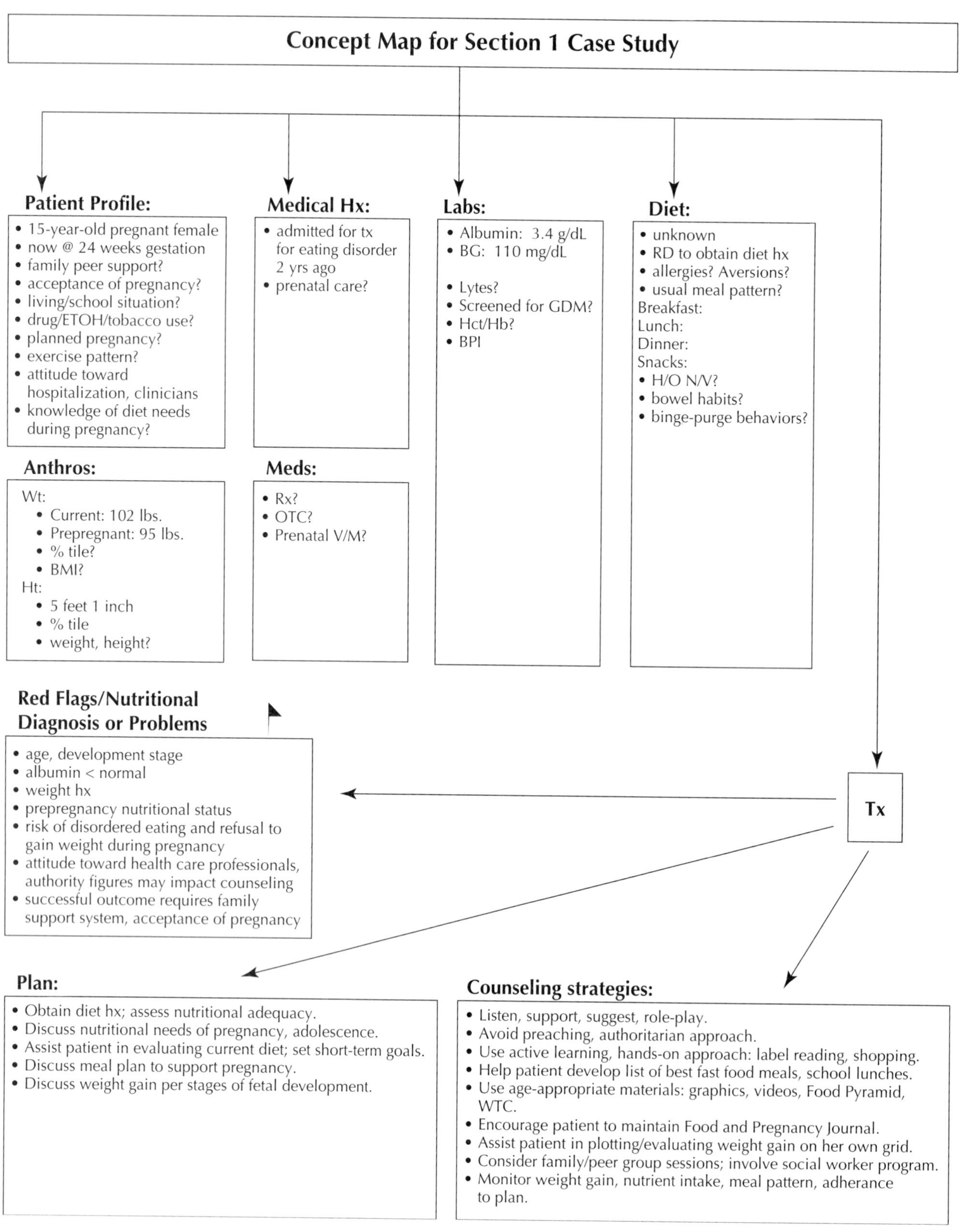

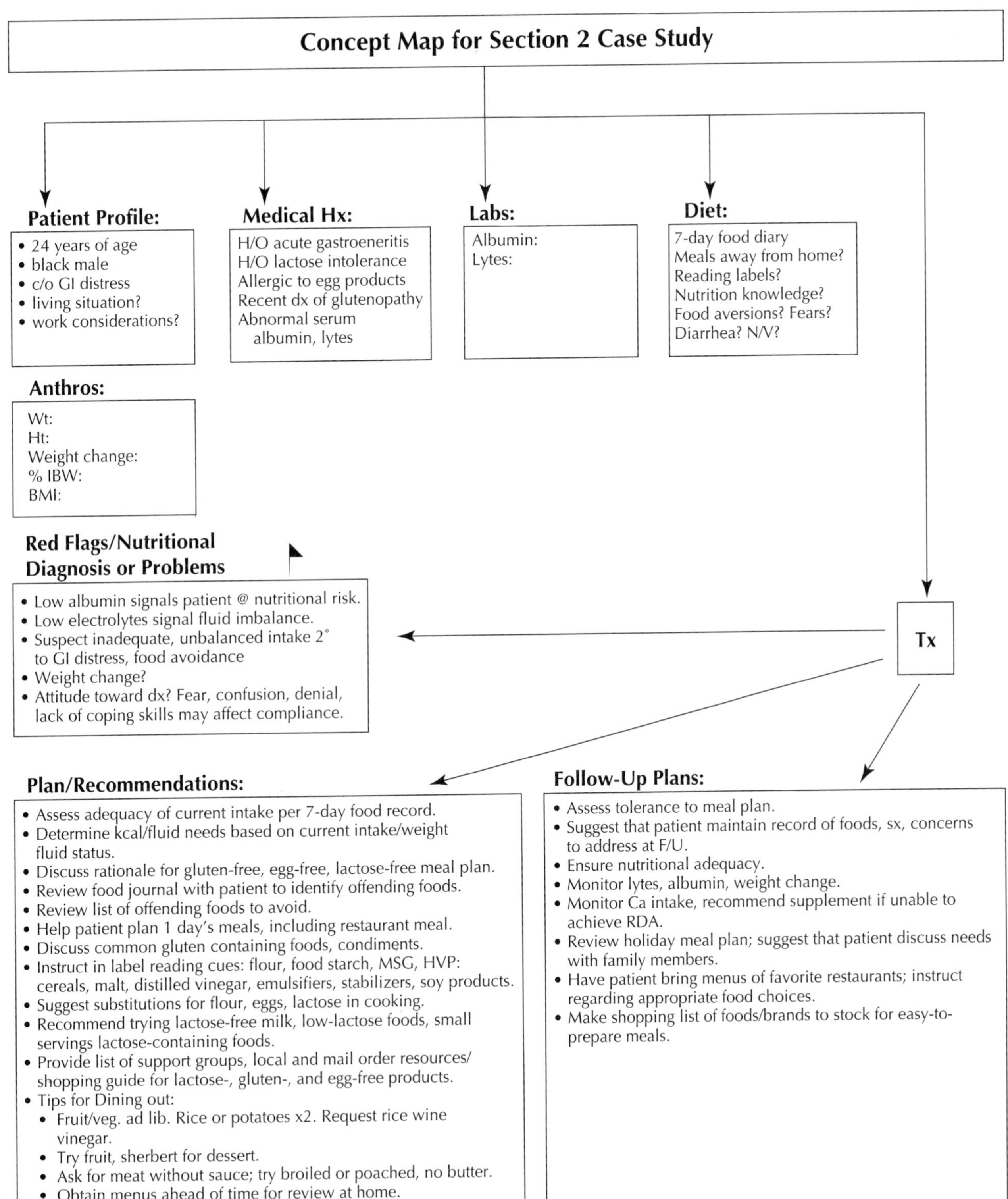
Concept Map for Section 2 Case Study
Patient Profile:
• 24 years of age
• black male
• c/o GI distress
• living situation?
• work considerations?
Medical Hx:
H/O acute gastroenteritis
H/O lactose intolerance
Allergic to egg products
Recent dx of glutenopathy
Abnormal serum albumin, lytes
Labs:
Albumin:
Lytes:
Diet:
7-day food diary
Meals away from home?
Reading labels?
Nutrition knowledge?
Food aversions? Fears?
Diarrhea? N/V?
Anthros:
Wt:
Ht:
Weight change:
% IBW:
BMI:
Red Flags/Nutritional Diagnosis or Problems
• Low albumin signals patient @ nutritional risk.
• Low electrolytes signal fluid imbalance.
• Suspect inadequate, unbalanced intake 2° to GI distress, food avoidance
• Weight change?
• Attitude toward dx? Fear, confusion, denial, lack of coping skills may affect compliance.
Tx
Plan/Recommendations:
• Assess adequacy of current intake per 7-day food record.
• Determine kcal/fluid needs based on current intake/weight fluid status.
• Discuss rationale for gluten-free, egg-free, lactose-free meal plan.
• Review food journal with patient to identify offending foods.
• Review list of offending foods to avoid.
• Help patient plan 1 day's meals, including restaurant meal.
• Discuss common gluten containing foods, condiments.
• Instruct in label reading cues: flour, food starch, MSG, HVP: cereals, malt, distilled vinegar, emulsifiers, stabilizers, soy products.
• Suggest substitutions for flour, eggs, lactose in cooking.
• Recommend trying lactose-free milk, low-lactose foods, small servings lactose-containing foods.
• Provide list of support groups, local and mail order resources/ shopping guide for lactose-, gluten-, and egg-free products.
• Tips for Dining out:
• Fruit/veg. ad lib. Rice or potatoes x2. Request rice wine vinegar.
• Try fruit, sherbert for dessert.
• Ask for meat without sauce; try broiled or poached, no butter.
• Obtain menus ahead of time for review at home.
Follow-Up Plans:
• Assess tolerance to meal plan.
• Suggest that patient maintain record of foods, sx, concerns to address at F/U.
• Ensure nutritional adequacy.
• Monitor lytes, albumin, weight change.
• Monitor Ca intake, recommend supplement if unable to achieve RDA.
• Review holiday meal plan; suggest that patient discuss needs with family members.
• Have patient bring menus of favorite restaurants; instruct regarding appropriate food choices.
• Make shopping list of foods/brands to stock for easy-to-prepare meals.

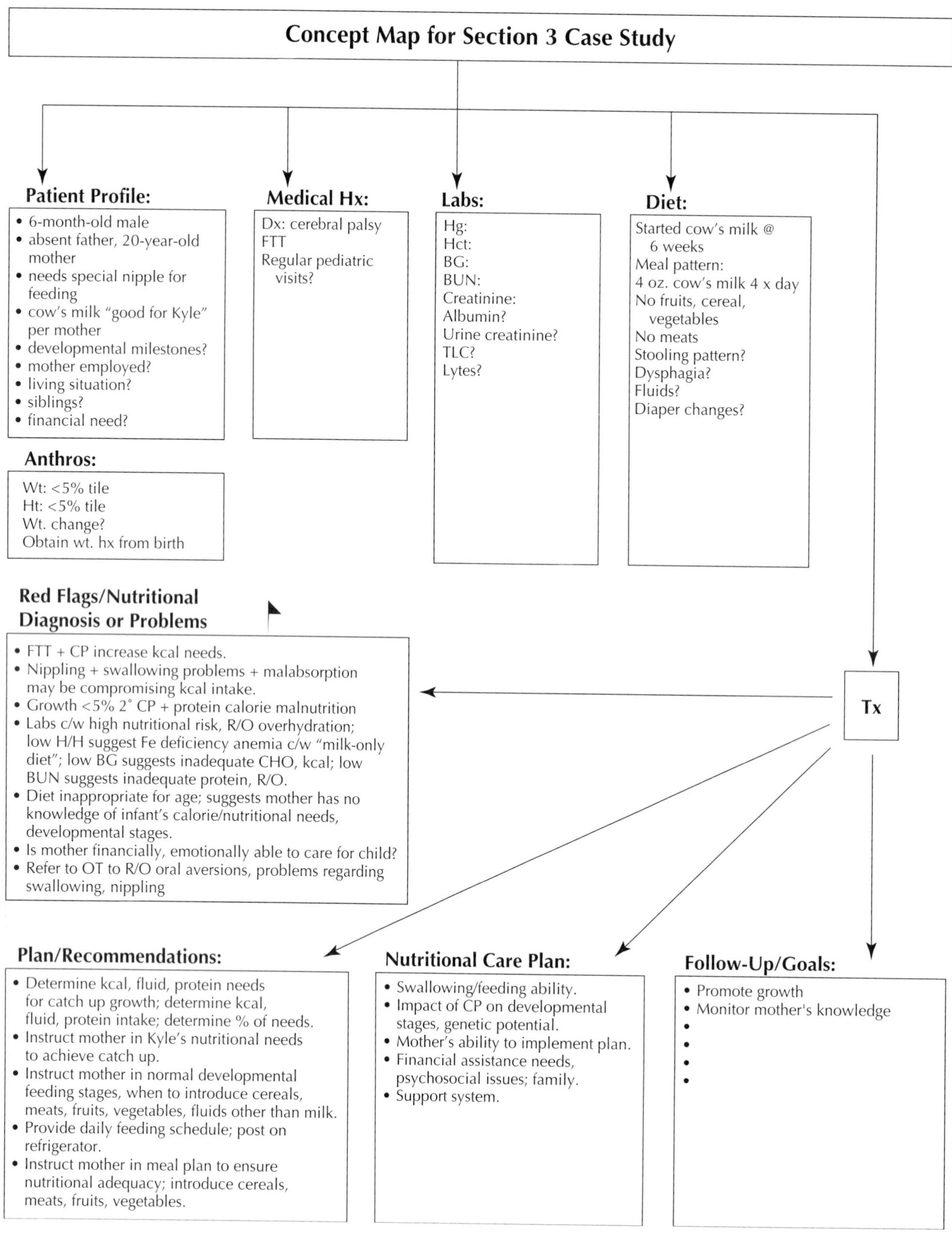
Concept Map for Section 3 Case Study
Patient Profile:
• 6-month-old male
• absent father, 20-year-old mother
• needs special nipple for feeding
• cow's milk "good for Kyle" per mother
• developmental milestones?
• mother employed?
• living situation?
• siblings?
• financial need?
Medical Hx:
Dx: cerebral palsy
FTT
Regular pediatric visits?
Labs:
Hg:
Hct:
BG:
BUN:
Creatinine:
Albumin?
Urine creatinine?
TLC?
Lytes?
Diet:
Started cow's milk @ 6 weeks
Meal pattern:
4 oz. cow's milk 4 x day
No fruits, cereal, vegetables
No meats
Stooling pattern?
Dysphagia?
Fluids?
Diaper changes?
Anthros:
Wt: <5% tile
Ht: <5% tile
Wt. change?
Obtain wt. hx from birth
Red Flags/Nutritional Diagnosis or Problems
• FTT + CP increase kcal needs.
• Nippling + swallowing problems + malabsorption may be compromising kcal intake.
• Growth <5% 2° CP + protein calorie malnutrition
• Labs c/w high nutritional risk, R/O overhydration; low H/H suggest Fe deficiency anemia c/w "milk-only diet"; low BG suggests inadequate CHO, kcal; low BUN suggests inadequate protein, R/O.
• Diet inappropriate for age; suggests mother has no knowledge of infant's calorie/nutritional needs, developmental stages.
• Is mother financially, emotionally able to care for child?
• Refer to OT to R/O oral aversions, problems regarding swallowing, nippling
Tx
Plan/Recommendations:
• Determine kcal, fluid, protein needs for catch up growth; determine kcal, fluid, protein intake; determine % of needs.
• Instruct mother in Kyle's nutritional needs to achieve catch up.
• Instruct mother in normal developmental feeding stages, when to introduce cereals, meats, fruits, vegetables, fluids other than milk.
• Provide daily feeding schedule; post on refrigerator.
• Instruct mother in meal plan to ensure nutritional adequacy; introduce cereals, meats, fruits, vegetables.
Nutritional Care Plan:
• Swallowing/feeding ability.
• Impact of CP on developmental stages, genetic potential.
• Mother's ability to implement plan.
• Financial assistance needs, psychosocial issues; family.
• Support system.
Follow-Up/Goals:
• Promote growth
• Monitor mother's knowledge

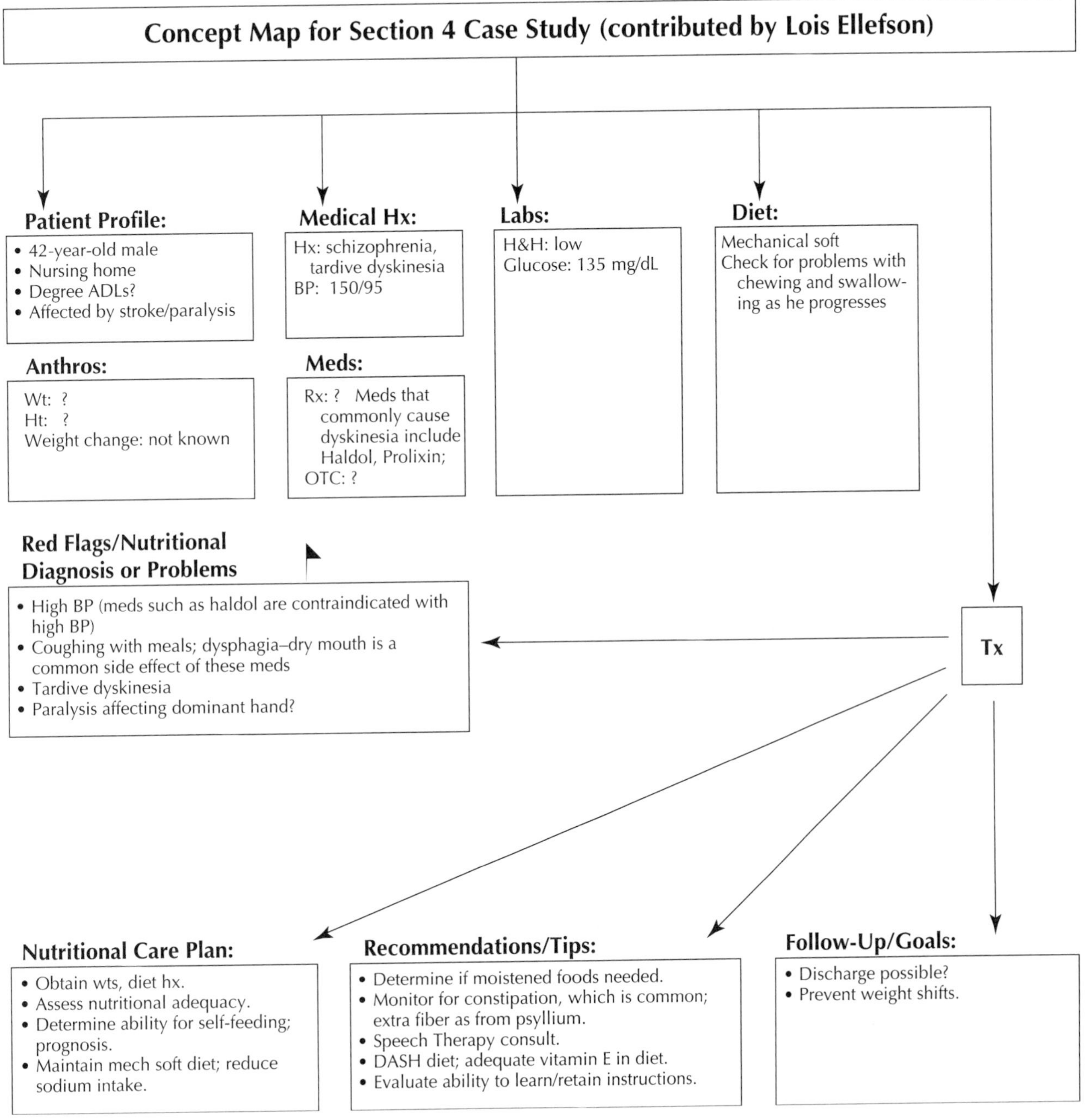
Concept Map for Section 4 Case Study (contributed by Lois Ellefson)
Patient Profile:
• 42-year-old male
• Nursing home
• Degree ADLs?
• Affected by stroke/paralysis
Medical Hx:
Hx: schizophrenia, tardive dyskinesia
BP: 150/95
Labs:
H&H: low
Glucose: 135 mg/dL
Diet:
Mechanical soft
Check for problems with chewing and swallowing as he progresses
Anthros:
Wt: ?
Ht: ?
Weight change: not known
Meds:
Rx: ? Meds that commonly cause dyskinesia include Haldol, Prolixin;
OTC: ?
Red Flags/Nutritional Diagnosis or Problems
• High BP (meds such as haldol are contraindicated with high BP)
• Coughing with meals; dysphagia–dry mouth is a common side effect of these meds
• Tardive dyskinesia
• Paralysis affecting dominant hand?
Tx
Nutritional Care Plan:
• Obtain wts, diet hx.
• Assess nutritional adequacy.
• Determine ability for self-feeding; prognosis.
• Maintain mech soft diet; reduce sodium intake.
Recommendations/Tips:
• Determine if moistened foods needed.
• Monitor for constipation, which is common; extra fiber as from psyllium.
• Speech Therapy consult.
• DASH diet; adequate vitamin E in diet.
• Evaluate ability to learn/retain instructions.
Follow-Up/Goals:
• Discharge possible?
• Prevent weight shifts.

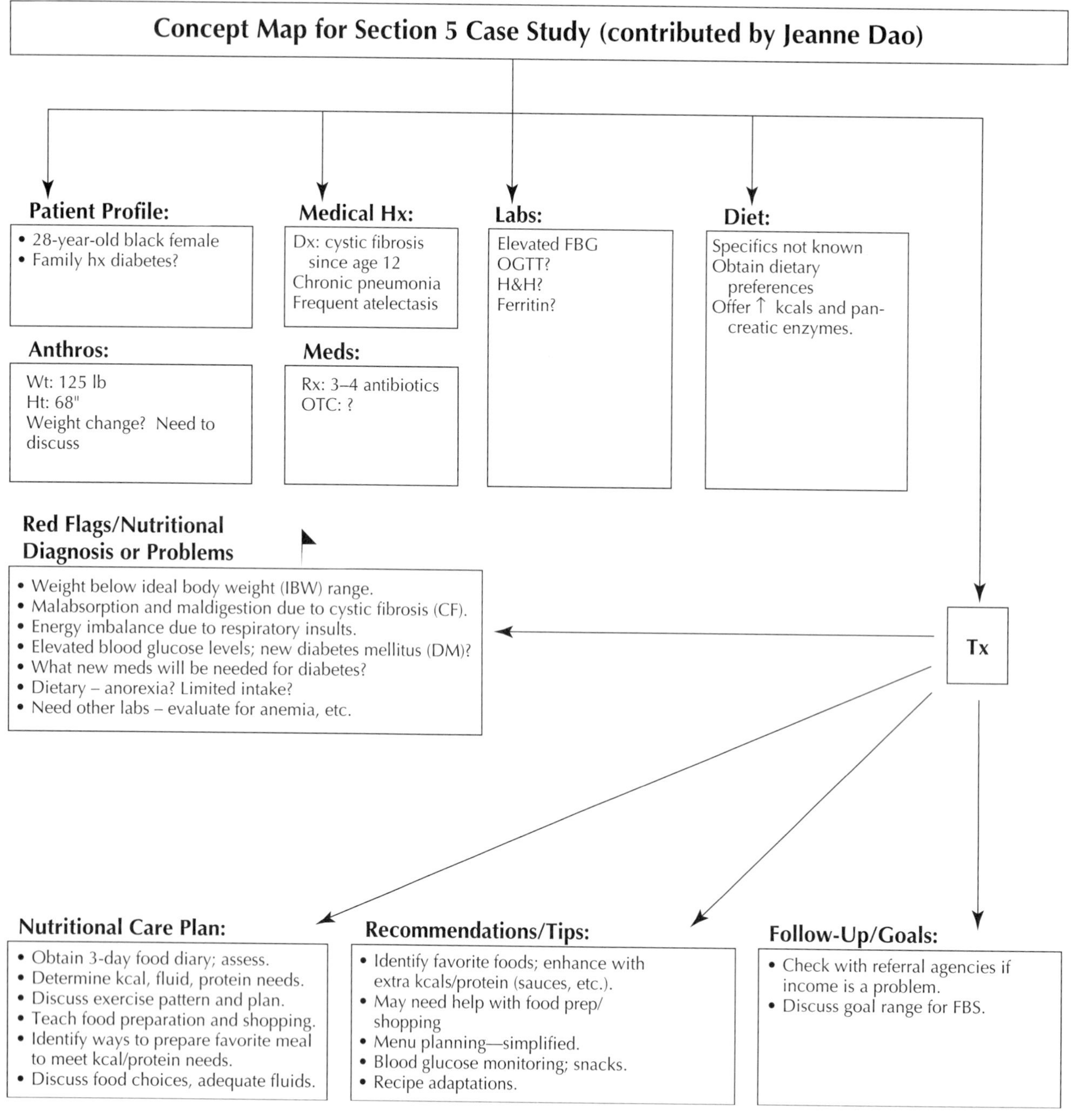
Concept Map for Section 5 Case Study (contributed by Jeanne Dao)
Patient Profile:
• 28-year-old black female
• Family hx diabetes?
Medical Hx:
Dx: cystic fibrosis since age 12
Chronic pneumonia
Frequent atelectasis
Labs:
Elevated FBG
OGTT?
H&H?
Ferritin?
Diet:
Specifics not known
Obtain dietary preferences
Offer ↑ kcals and pancreatic enzymes.
Anthros:
Wt: 125 lb
Ht: 68"
Weight change? Need to discuss
Meds:
Rx: 3–4 antibiotics
OTC: ?
Red Flags/Nutritional Diagnosis or Problems
• Weight below ideal body weight (IBW) range.
• Malabsorption and maldigestion due to cystic fibrosis (CF).
• Energy imbalance due to respiratory insults.
• Elevated blood glucose levels; new diabetes mellitus (DM)?
• What new meds will be needed for diabetes?
• Dietary – anorexia? Limited intake?
• Need other labs – evaluate for anemia, etc.
Tx
Nutritional Care Plan:
• Obtain 3-day food diary; assess.
• Determine kcal, fluid, protein needs.
• Discuss exercise pattern and plan.
• Teach food preparation and shopping.
• Identify ways to prepare favorite meal to meet kcal/protein needs.
• Discuss food choices, adequate fluids.
Recommendations/Tips:
• Identify favorite foods; enhance with extra kcals/protein (sauces, etc.).
• May need help with food prep/ shopping
• Menu planning—simplified.
• Blood glucose monitoring; snacks.
• Recipe adaptations.
Follow-Up/Goals:
• Check with referral agencies if income is a problem.
• Discuss goal range for FBS.

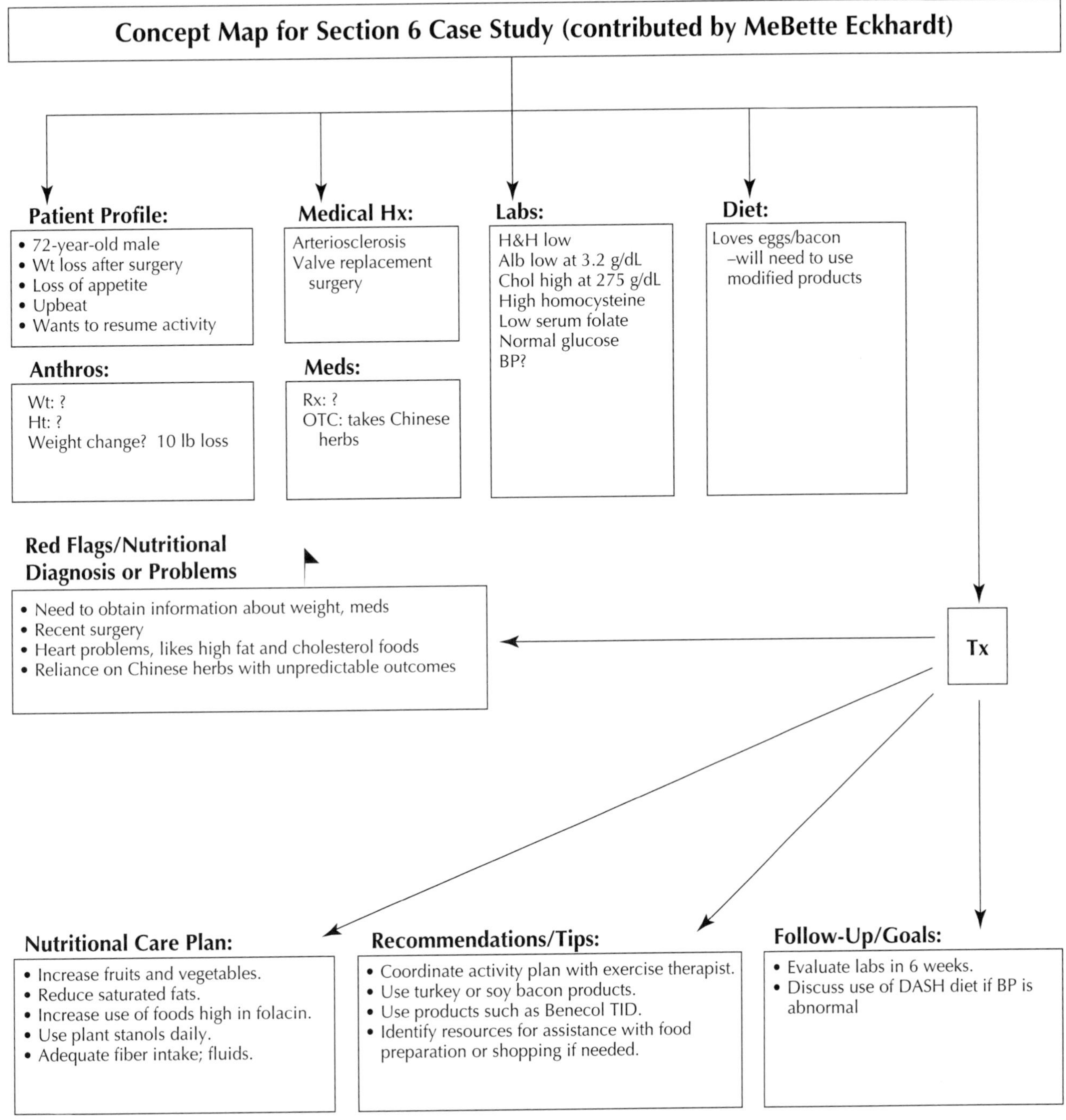
Concept Map for Section 6 Case Study (contributed by MeBette Eckhardt)
Patient Profile:
• 72-year-old male
• Wt loss after surgery
• Loss of appetite
• Upbeat
• Wants to resume activity
Medical Hx:
Arteriosclerosis
Valve replacement surgery
Labs:
H&H low
Alb low at 3.2 g/dL
Chol high at 275 g/dL
High homocysteine
Low serum folate
Normal glucose
BP?
Diet:
Loves eggs/bacon
–will need to use modified products
Anthros:
Wt: ?
Ht: ?
Weight change? 10 lb loss
Meds:
Rx: ?
OTC: takes Chinese herbs
Red Flags/Nutritional Diagnosis or Problems
• Need to obtain information about weight, meds
• Recent surgery
• Heart problems, likes high fat and cholesterol foods
• Reliance on Chinese herbs with unpredictable outcomes
Tx
Nutritional Care Plan:
• Increase fruits and vegetables.
• Reduce saturated fats.
• Increase use of foods high in folacin.
• Use plant stanols daily.
• Adequate fiber intake; fluids.
Recommendations/Tips:
• Coordinate activity plan with exercise therapist.
• Use turkey or soy bacon products.
• Use products such as Benecol TID.
• Identify resources for assistance with food preparation or shopping if needed.
Follow-Up/Goals:
• Evaluate labs in 6 weeks.
• Discuss use of DASH diet if BP is abnormal

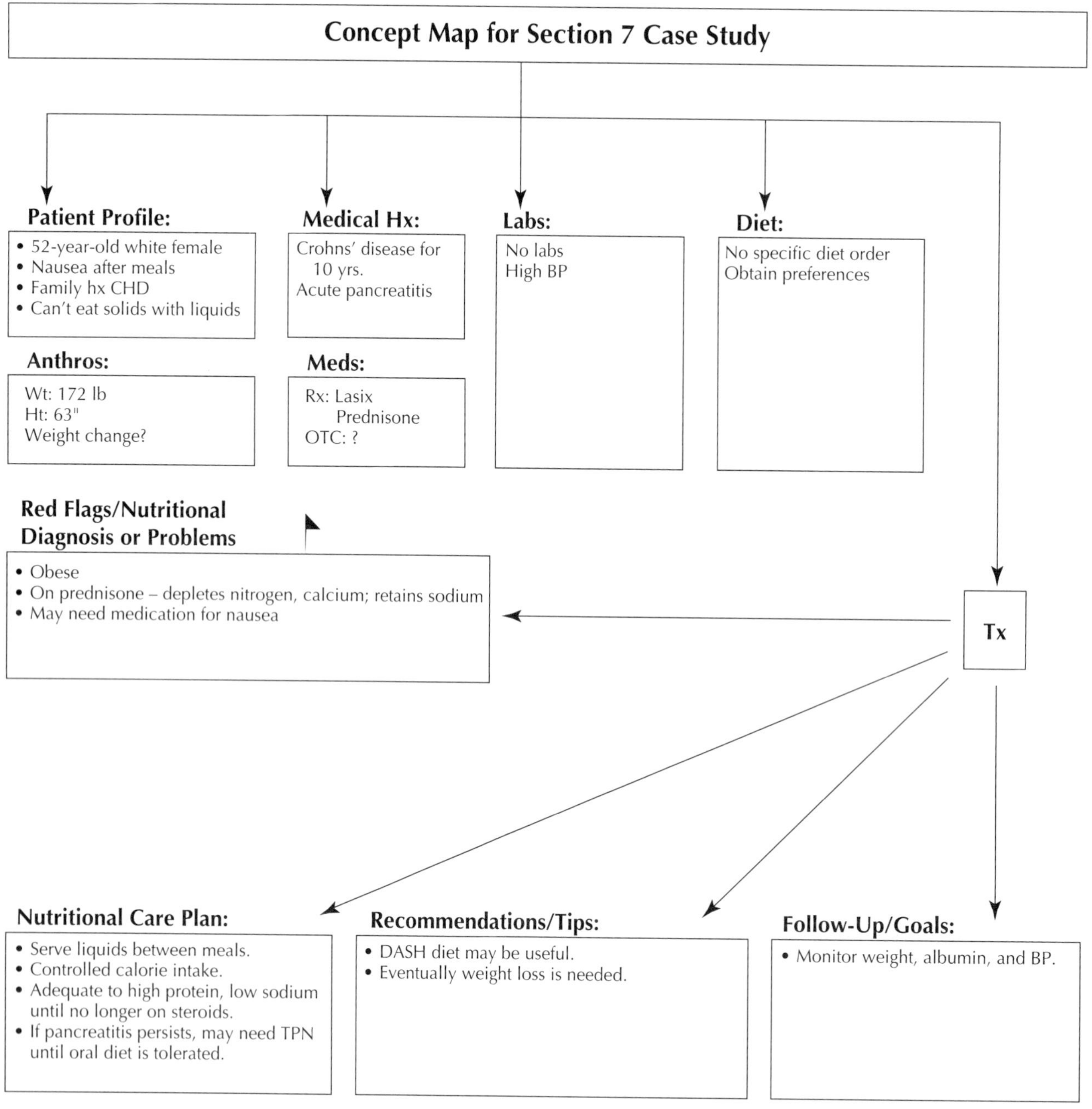
Concept Map for Section 7 Case Study
Patient Profile:
• 52-year-old white female
• Nausea after meals
• Family hx CHD
• Can't eat solids with liquids
Medical Hx:
Crohns' disease for 10 yrs.
Acute pancreatitis
Labs:
No labs
High BP
Diet:
No specific diet order
Obtain preferences
Anthros:
Wt: 172 lb
Ht: 63"
Weight change?
Meds:
Rx: Lasix
Prednisone
OTC: ?
Red Flags/Nutritional Diagnosis or Problems
• Obese
• On prednisone – depletes nitrogen, calcium; retains sodium
• May need medication for nausea
Tx
Nutritional Care Plan:
• Serve liquids between meals.
• Controlled calorie intake.
• Adequate to high protein, low sodium until no longer on steroids.
• If pancreatitis persists, may need TPN until oral diet is tolerated.
Recommendations/Tips:
• DASH diet may be useful.
• Eventually weight loss is needed.
Follow-Up/Goals:
• Monitor weight, albumin, and BP.

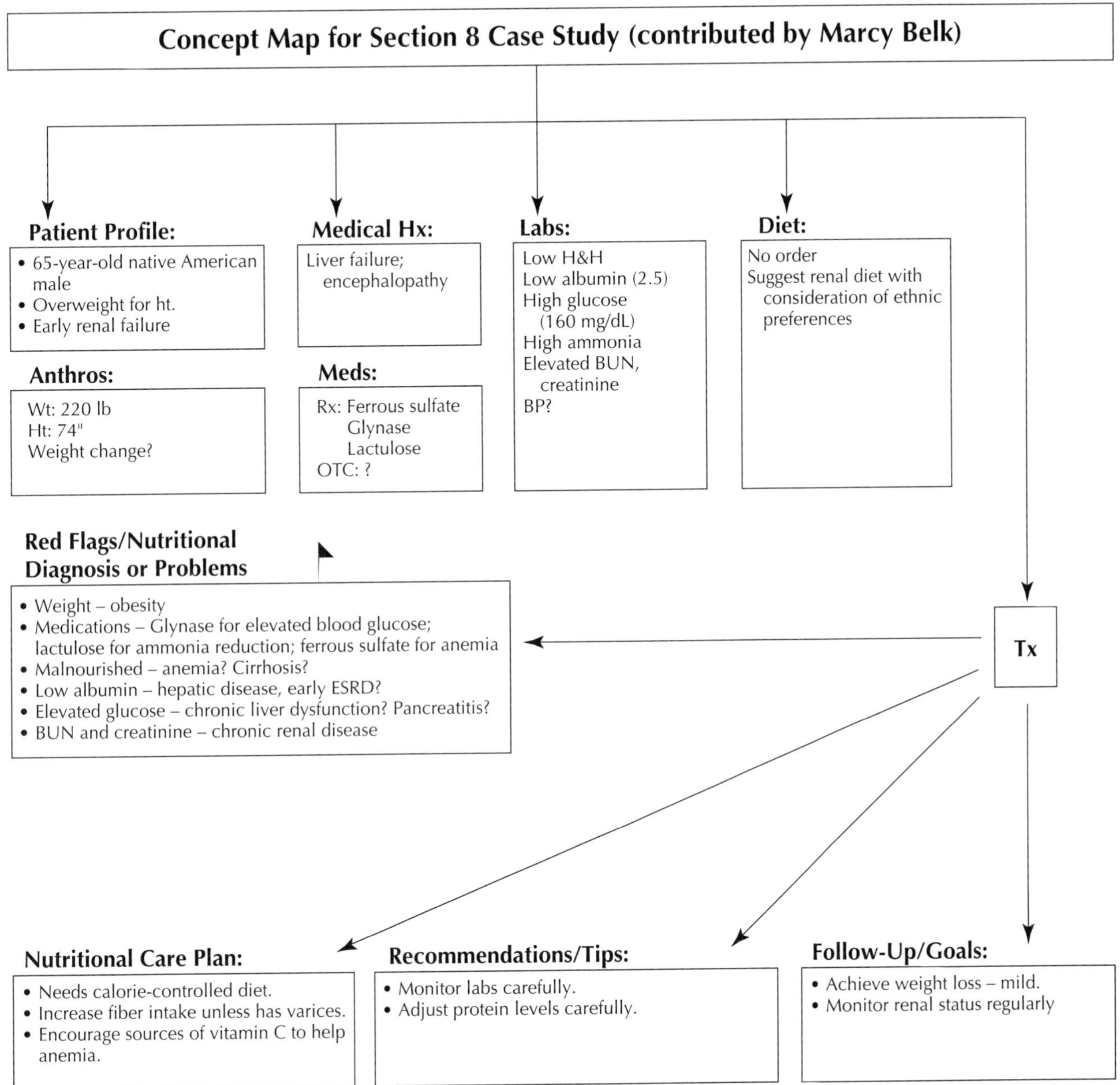
Concept Map for Section 8 Case Study (contributed by Marcy Belk)
Patient Profile:
• 65-year-old native American male
• Overweight for ht.
• Early renal failure
Medical Hx:
Liver failure; encephalopathy
Labs:
Low H&H
Low albumin (2.5)
High glucose (160 mg/dL)
High ammonia
Elevated BUN, creatinine
BP?
Diet:
No order
Suggest renal diet with consideration of ethnic preferences
Anthros:
Wt: 220 lb
Ht: 74"
Weight change?
Meds:
Rx: Ferrous sulfate
Glynase
Lactulose
OTC: ?
Red Flags/Nutritional Diagnosis or Problems
• Weight – obesity
• Medications – Glynase for elevated blood glucose; lactulose for ammonia reduction; ferrous sulfate for anemia
• Malnourished – anemia? Cirrhosis?
• Low albumin – hepatic disease, early ESRD?
• Elevated glucose – chronic liver dysfunction? Pancreatitis?
• BUN and creatinine – chronic renal disease
Tx
Nutritional Care Plan:
• Needs calorie-controlled diet.
• Increase fiber intake unless has varices.
• Encourage sources of vitamin C to help anemia.
Recommendations/Tips:
• Monitor labs carefully.
• Adjust protein levels carefully.
Follow-Up/Goals:
• Achieve weight loss – mild.
• Monitor renal status regularly

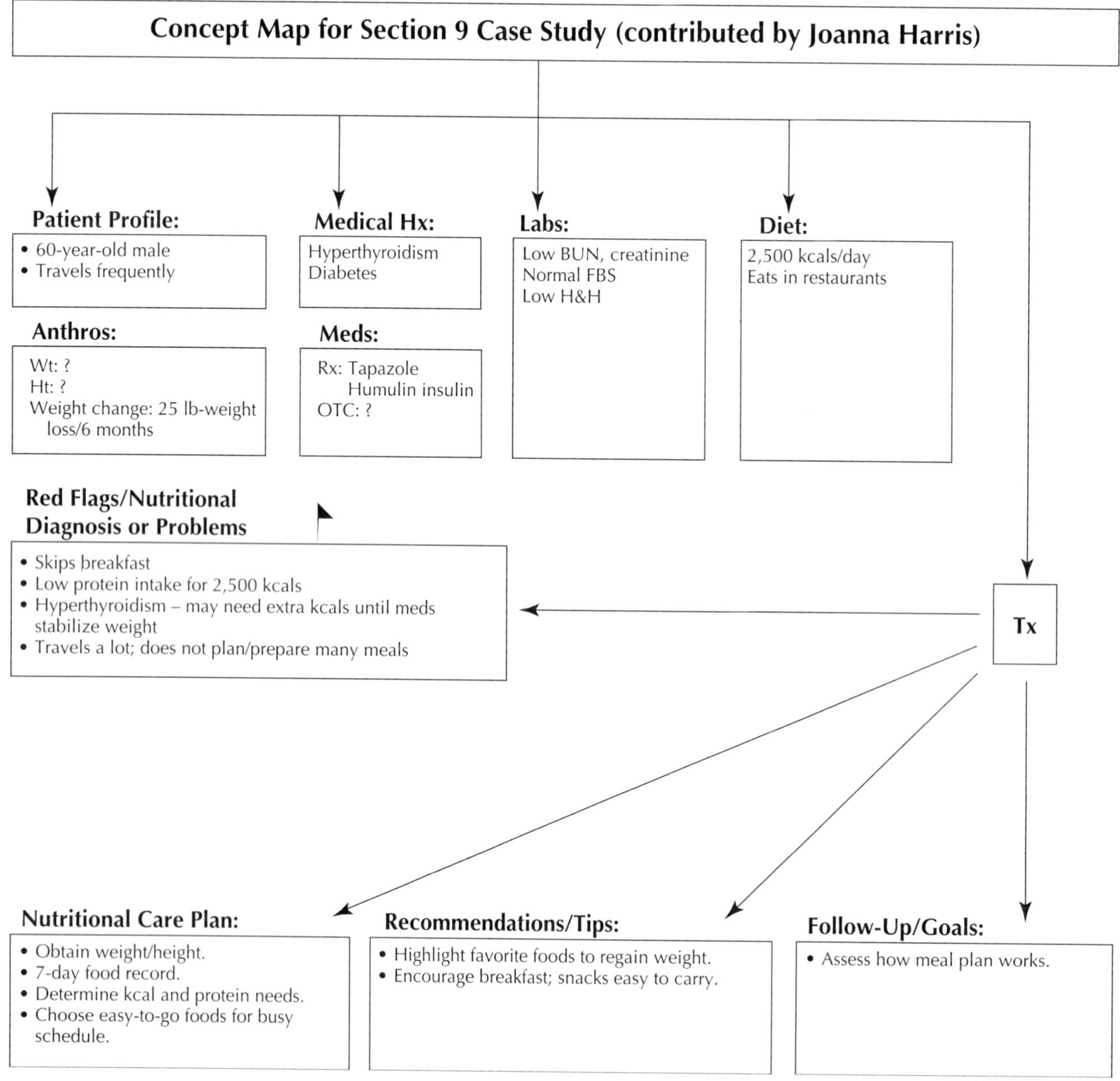
Concept Map for Section 9 Case Study (contributed by Joanna Harris)
Patient Profile:
• 60-year-old male
• Travels frequently
Medical Hx:
Hyperthyroidism
Diabetes
Labs:
Low BUN, creatinine
Normal FBS
Low H&H
Diet:
2,500 kcals/day
Eats in restaurants
Anthros:
Wt: ?
Ht: ?
Weight change: 25 lb-weight loss/6 months
Meds:
Rx: Tapazole
Humulin insulin
OTC: ?
Red Flags/Nutritional Diagnosis or Problems
• Skips breakfast
• Low protein intake for 2,500 kcals
• Hyperthyroidism – may need extra kcals until meds stabilize weight
• Travels a lot; does not plan/prepare many meals
Tx
Nutritional Care Plan:
• Obtain weight/height.
• 7-day food record.
• Determine kcal and protein needs.
• Choose easy-to-go foods for busy schedule.
Recommendations/Tips:
• Highlight favorite foods to regain weight.
• Encourage breakfast; snacks easy to carry.
Follow-Up/Goals:
• Assess how meal plan works.

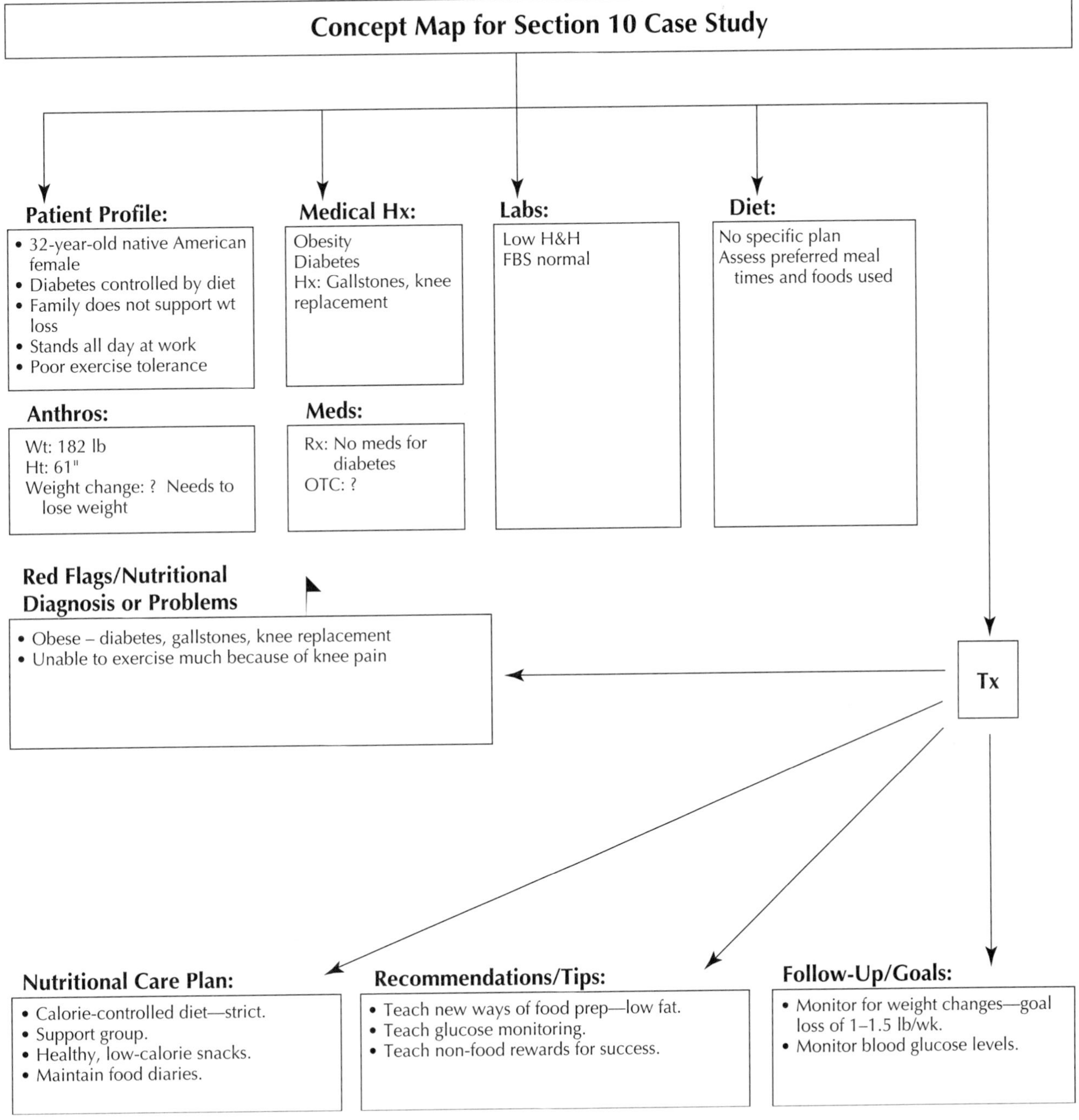
Concept Map for Section 10 Case Study
Patient Profile:
• 32-year-old native American female
• Diabetes controlled by diet
• Family does not support wt loss
• Stands all day at work
• Poor exercise tolerance
Medical Hx:
Obesity
Diabetes
Hx: Gallstones, knee replacement
Labs:
Low H&H
FBS normal
Diet:
No specific plan
Assess preferred meal times and foods used
Anthros:
Wt: 182 lb
Ht: 61"
Weight change: ? Needs to lose weight
Meds:
Rx: No meds for diabetes
OTC: ?
Red Flags/Nutritional Diagnosis or Problems
• Obese – diabetes, gallstones, knee replacement
• Unable to exercise much because of knee pain
Tx
Nutritional Care Plan:
• Calorie-controlled diet—strict.
• Support group.
• Healthy, low-calorie snacks.
• Maintain food diaries.
Recommendations/Tips:
• Teach new ways of food prep—low fat.
• Teach glucose monitoring.
• Teach non-food rewards for success.
Follow-Up/Goals:
• Monitor for weight changes—goal loss of 1–1.5 lb/wk.
• Monitor blood glucose levels.

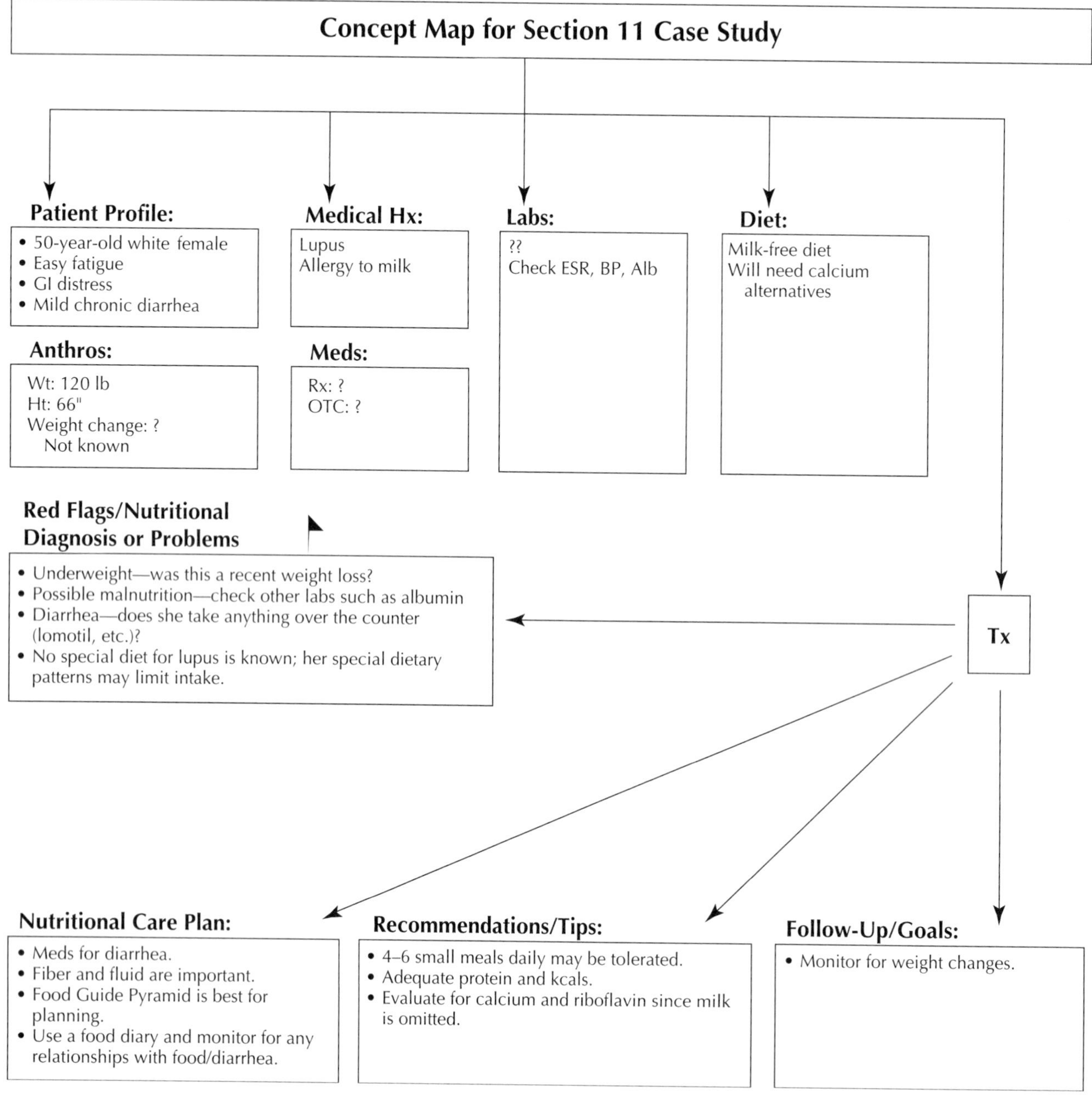
Concept Map for Section 11 Case Study
Patient Profile:
• 50-year-old white female
• Easy fatigue
• GI distress
• Mild chronic diarrhea
Medical Hx:
Lupus
Allergy to milk
Labs:
??
Check ESR, BP, Alb
Diet:
Milk-free diet
Will need calcium alternatives
Anthros:
Wt: 120 lb
Ht: 66"
Weight change: ? Not known
Meds:
Rx: ?
OTC: ?
Red Flags/Nutritional Diagnosis or Problems
• Underweight—was this a recent weight loss?
• Possible malnutrition—check other labs such as albumin
• Diarrhea—does she take anything over the counter (lomotil, etc.)?
• No special diet for lupus is known; her special dietary patterns may limit intake.
Tx
Nutritional Care Plan:
• Meds for diarrhea.
• Fiber and fluid are important.
• Food Guide Pyramid is best for planning.
• Use a food diary and monitor for any relationships with food/diarrhea.
Recommendations/Tips:
• 4–6 small meals daily may be tolerated.
• Adequate protein and kcals.
• Evaluate for calcium and riboflavin since milk is omitted.
Follow-Up/Goals:
• Monitor for weight changes.

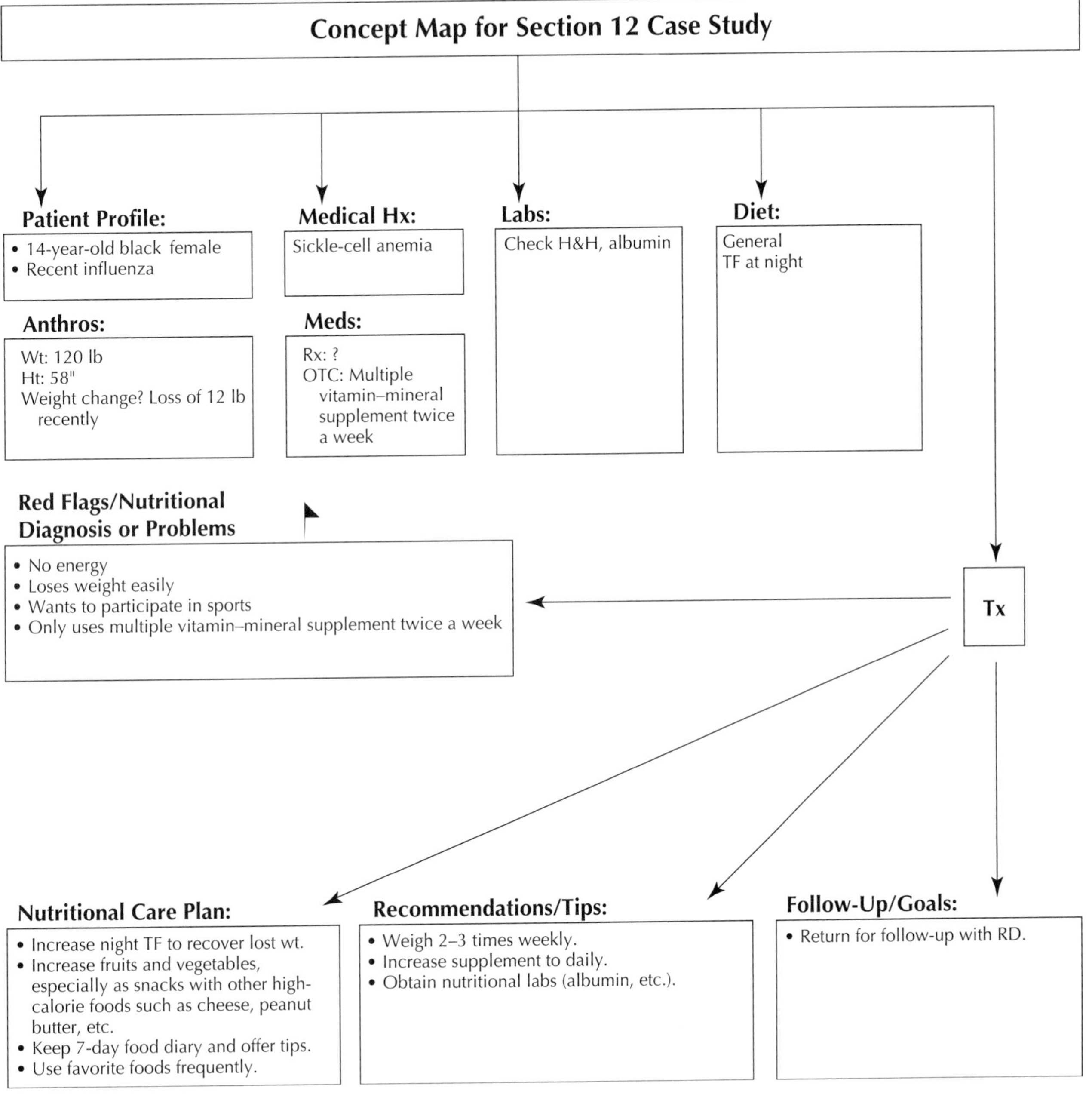
Concept Map for Section 12 Case Study
Patient Profile:
• 14-year-old black female
• Recent influenza
Medical Hx:
Sickle-cell anemia
Labs:
Check H&H, albumin
Diet:
General
TF at night
Anthros:
Wt: 120 lb
Ht: 58"
Weight change? Loss of 12 lb recently
Meds:
Rx: ?
OTC: Multiple vitamin–mineral supplement twice a week
Red Flags/Nutritional Diagnosis or Problems
• No energy
• Loses weight easily
• Wants to participate in sports
• Only uses multiple vitamin–mineral supplement twice a week
Tx
Nutritional Care Plan:
• Increase night TF to recover lost wt.
• Increase fruits and vegetables, especially as snacks with other high-calorie foods such as cheese, peanut butter, etc.
• Keep 7-day food diary and offer tips.
• Use favorite foods frequently.
Recommendations/Tips:
• Weigh 2–3 times weekly.
• Increase supplement to daily.
• Obtain nutritional labs (albumin, etc.).
Follow-Up/Goals:
• Return for follow-up with RD.

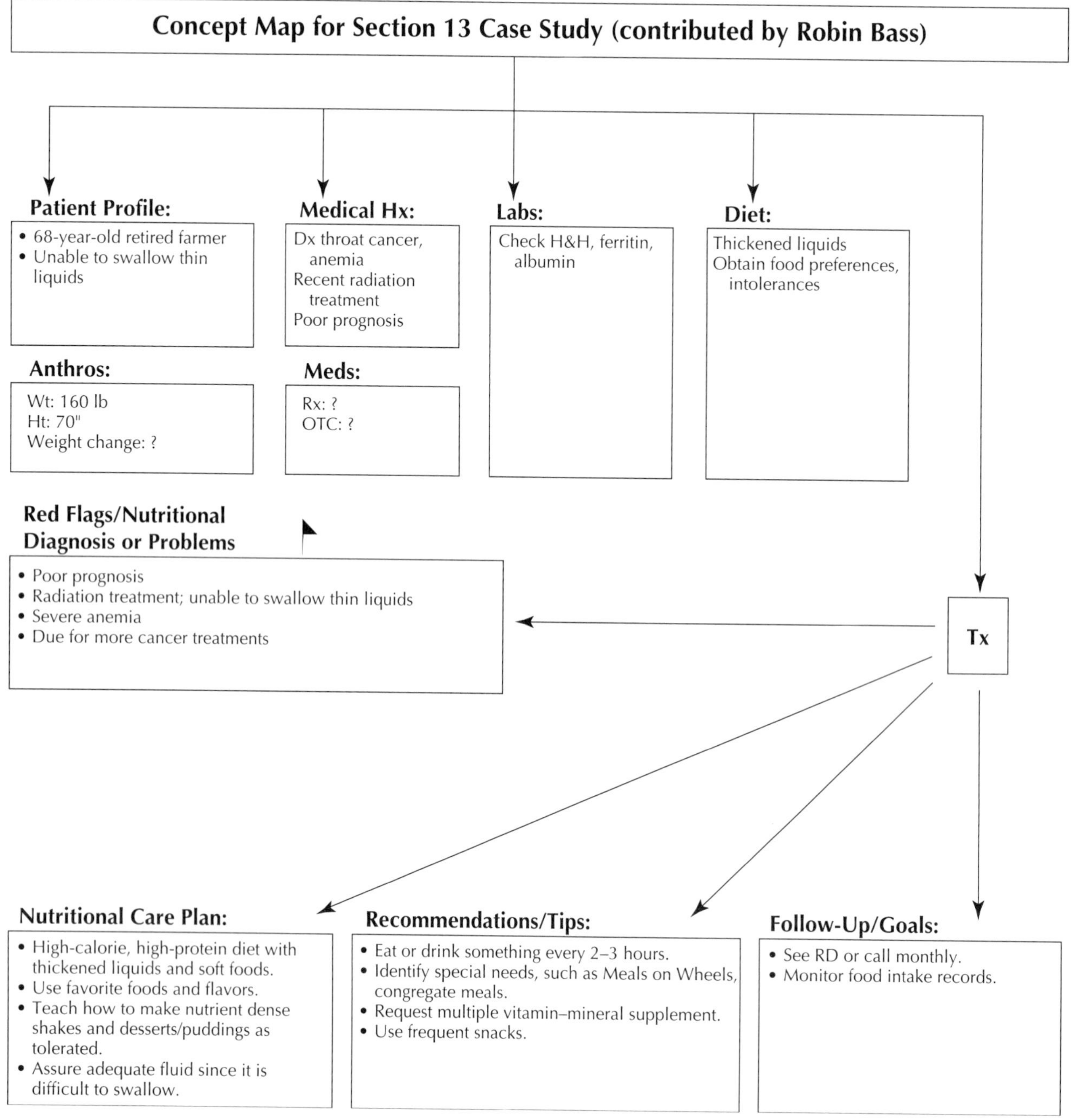
Concept Map for Section 13 Case Study (contributed by Robin Bass)
Patient Profile:
• 68-year-old retired farmer
• Unable to swallow thin liquids
Medical Hx:
Dx throat cancer, anemia
Recent radiation treatment
Poor prognosis
Labs:
Check H&H, ferritin, albumin
Diet:
Thickened liquids
Obtain food preferences, intolerances
Anthros:
Wt: 160 lb
Ht: 70"
Weight change: ?
Meds:
Rx: ?
OTC: ?
Red Flags/Nutritional Diagnosis or Problems
• Poor prognosis
• Radiation treatment; unable to swallow thin liquids
• Severe anemia
• Due for more cancer treatments
Tx
Nutritional Care Plan:
• High-calorie, high-protein diet with thickened liquids and soft foods.
• Use favorite foods and flavors.
• Teach how to make nutrient dense shakes and desserts/puddings as tolerated.
• Assure adequate fluid since it is difficult to swallow.
Recommendations/Tips:
• Eat or drink something every 2–3 hours.
• Identify special needs, such as Meals on Wheels, congregate meals.
• Request multiple vitamin–mineral supplement.
• Use frequent snacks.
Follow-Up/Goals:
• See RD or call monthly.
• Monitor food intake records.

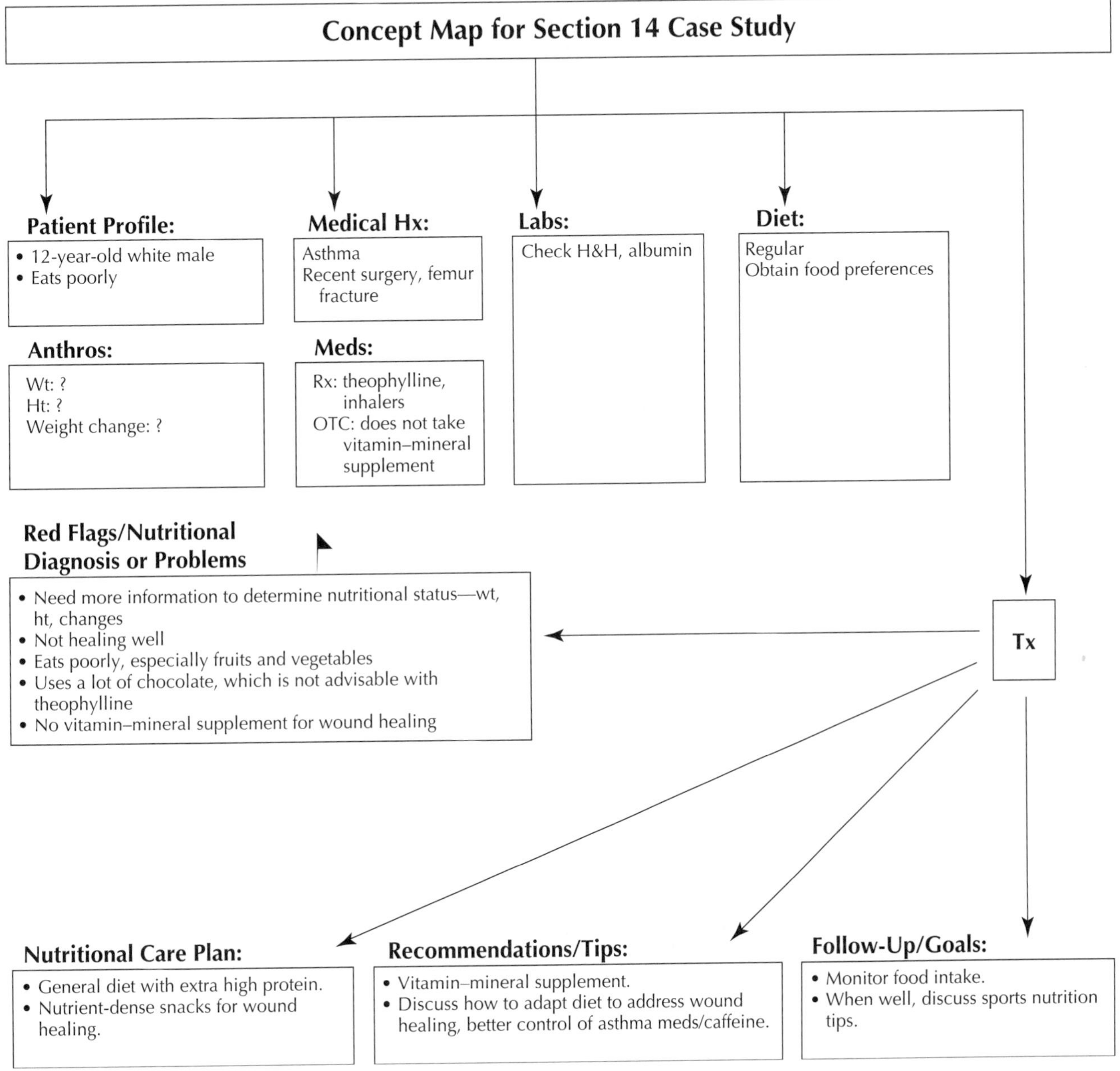

Concept Map for Section 14 Case Study
Patient Profile:
• 12-year-old white male
• Eats poorly
Medical Hx:
Asthma
Recent surgery, femur fracture
Labs:
Check H&H, albumin
Diet:
Regular
Obtain food preferences
Anthros:
Wt: ?
Ht: ?
Weight change: ?
Meds:
Rx: theophylline, inhalers
OTC: does not take vitamin–mineral supplement
Red Flags/Nutritional Diagnosis or Problems
• Need more information to determine nutritional status—wt, ht, changes
• Not healing well
• Eats poorly, especially fruits and vegetables
• Uses a lot of chocolate, which is not advisable with theophylline
• No vitamin–mineral supplement for wound healing
Tx
Nutritional Care Plan:
• General diet with extra high protein.
• Nutrient-dense snacks for wound healing.
Recommendations/Tips:
• Vitamin–mineral supplement.
• Discuss how to adapt diet to address wound healing, better control of asthma meds/caffeine.
Follow-Up/Goals:
• Monitor food intake.
• When well, discuss sports nutrition tips.

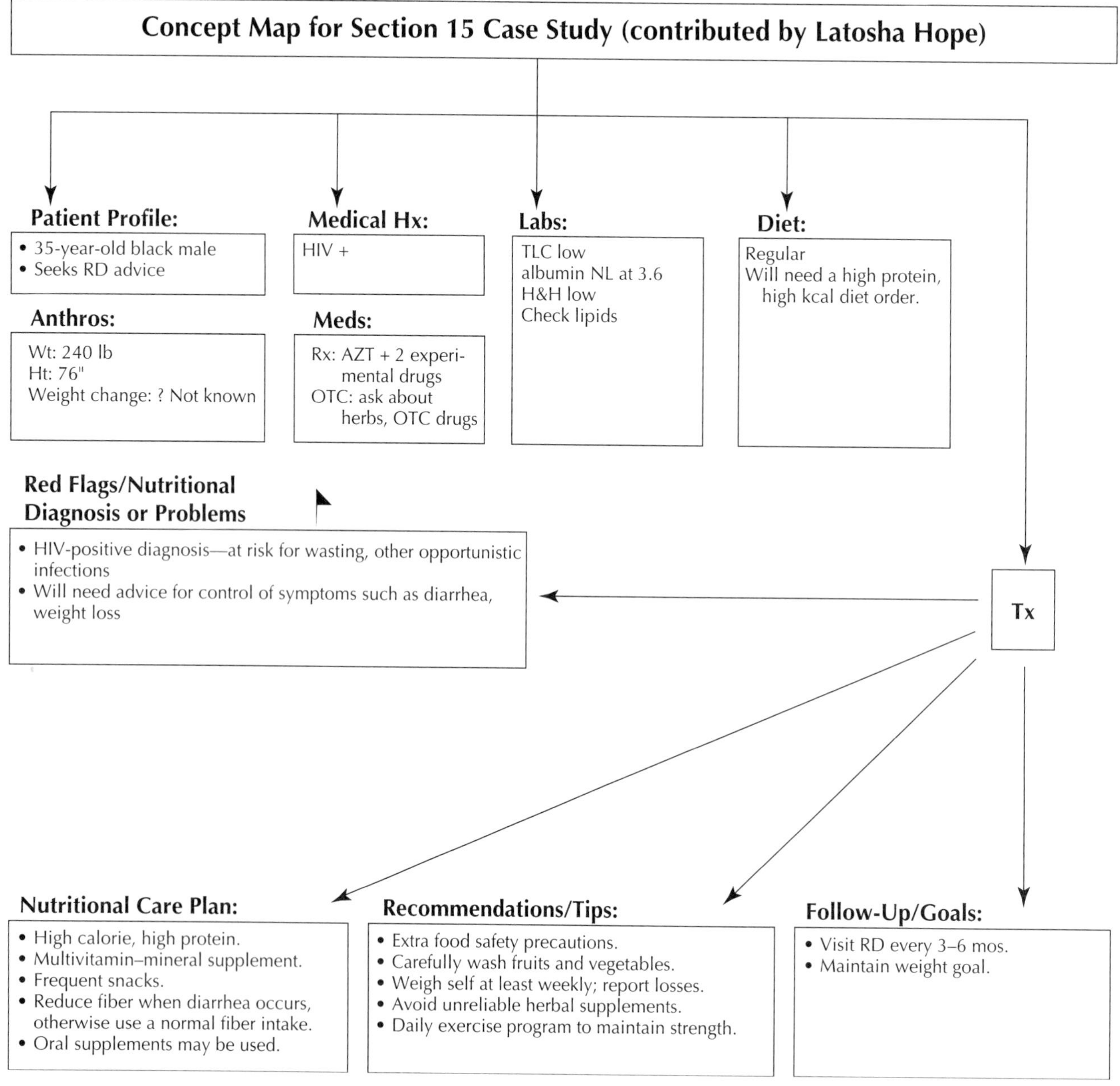

Concept Map for Section 15 Case Study (contributed by Latosha Hope)
Patient Profile:
• 35-year-old black male
• Seeks RD advice
Medical Hx:
HIV +
Labs:
TLC low
albumin NL at 3.6
H&H low
Check lipids
Diet:
Regular
Will need a high protein, high kcal diet order.
Anthros:
Wt: 240 lb
Ht: 76"
Weight change: ? Not known
Meds:
Rx: AZT + 2 experimental drugs
OTC: ask about herbs, OTC drugs
Red Flags/Nutritional Diagnosis or Problems
• HIV-positive diagnosis—at risk for wasting, other opportunistic infections
• Will need advice for control of symptoms such as diarrhea, weight loss
Tx
Nutritional Care Plan:
• High calorie, high protein.
• Multivitamin–mineral supplement.
• Frequent snacks.
• Reduce fiber when diarrhea occurs, otherwise use a normal fiber intake.
• Oral supplements may be used.
Recommendations/Tips:
• Extra food safety precautions.
• Carefully wash fruits and vegetables.
• Weigh self at least weekly; report losses.
• Avoid unreliable herbal supplements.
• Daily exercise program to maintain strength.
Follow-Up/Goals:
• Visit RD every 3–6 mos.
• Maintain weight goal.

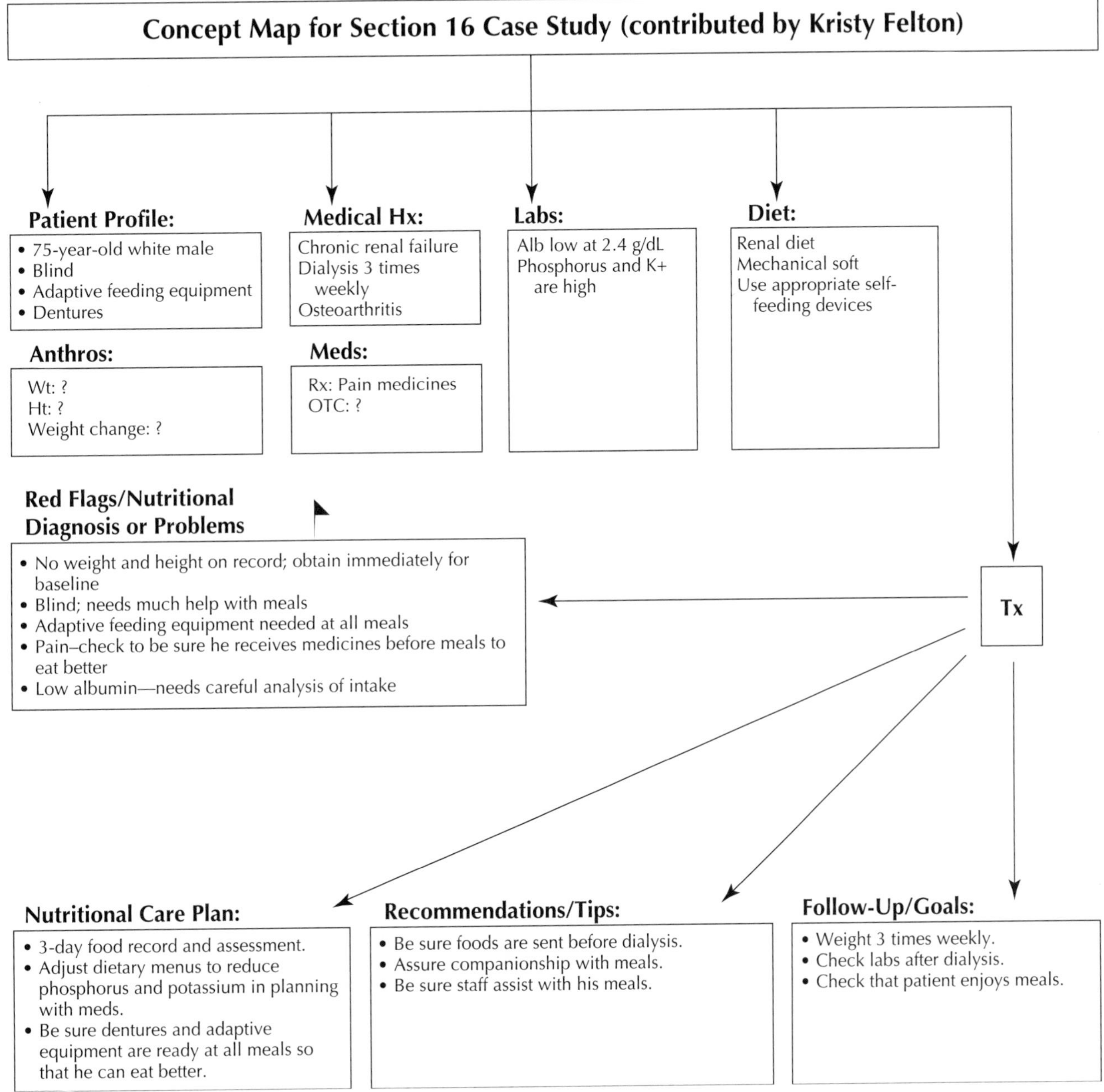
Concept Map for Section 16 Case Study (contributed by Kristy Felton)
Patient Profile:
• 75-year-old white male
• Blind
• Adaptive feeding equipment
• Dentures
Medical Hx:
Chronic renal failure
Dialysis 3 times weekly
Osteoarthritis
Labs:
Alb low at 2.4 g/dL
Phosphorus and K+ are high
Diet:
Renal diet
Mechanical soft
Use appropriate self-feeding devices
Anthros:
Wt: ?
Ht: ?
Weight change: ?
Meds:
Rx: Pain medicines
OTC: ?
Red Flags/Nutritional Diagnosis or Problems
• No weight and height on record; obtain immediately for baseline
• Blind; needs much help with meals
• Adaptive feeding equipment needed at all meals
• Pain–check to be sure he receives medicines before meals to eat better
• Low albumin—needs careful analysis of intake
Tx
Nutritional Care Plan:
• 3-day food record and assessment.
• Adjust dietary menus to reduce phosphorus and potassium in planning with meds.
• Be sure dentures and adaptive equipment are ready at all meals so that he can eat better.
Recommendations/Tips:
• Be sure foods are sent before dialysis.
• Assure companionship with meals.
• Be sure staff assist with his meals.
Follow-Up/Goals:
• Weight 3 times weekly.
• Check labs after dialysis.
• Check that patient enjoys meals.

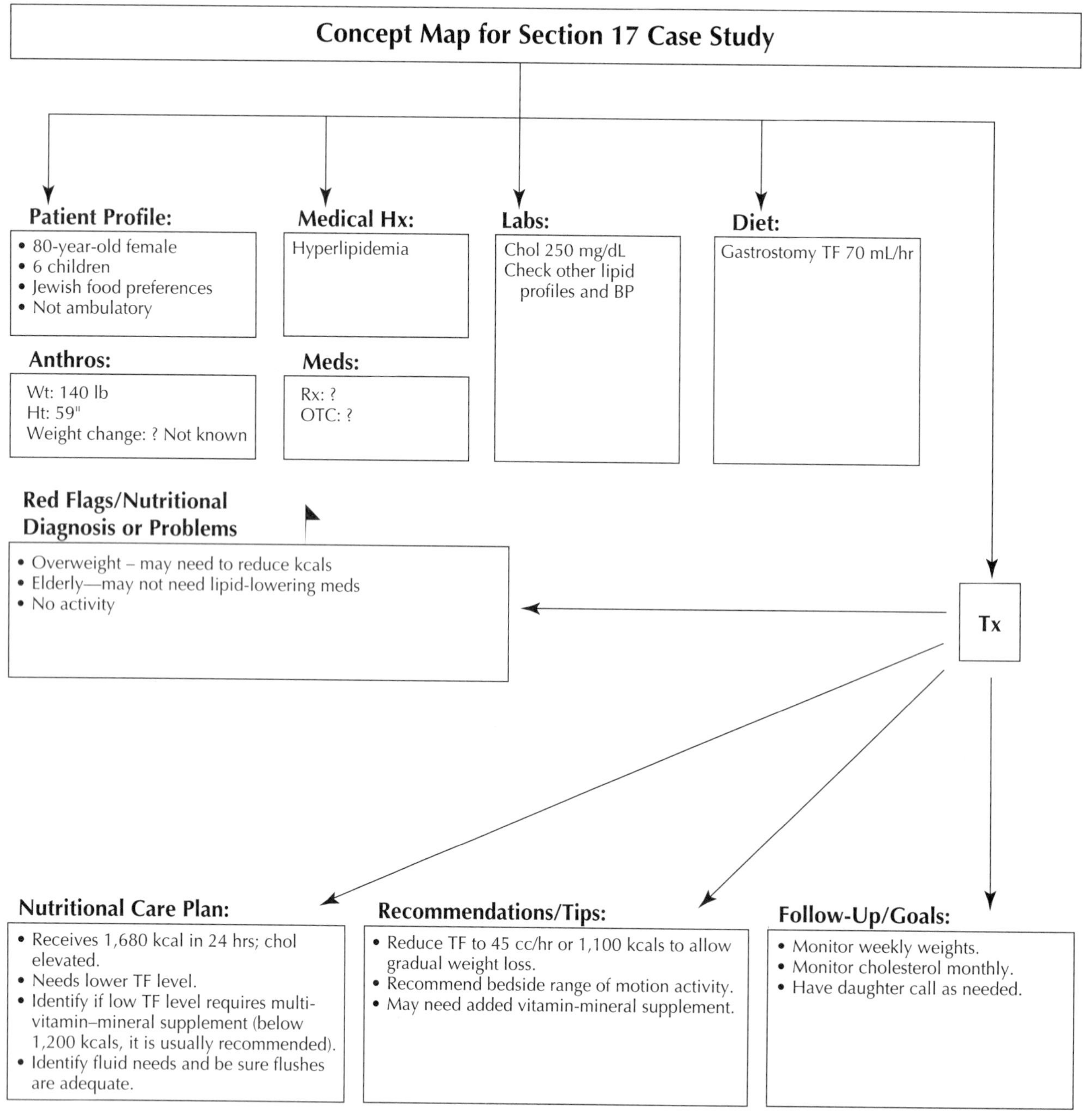
Concept Map for Section 17 Case Study
Patient Profile:
• 80-year-old female
• 6 children
• Jewish food preferences
• Not ambulatory
Medical Hx:
Hyperlipidemia
Labs:
Chol 250 mg/dL
Check other lipid profiles and BP
Diet:
Gastrostomy TF 70 mL/hr
Anthros:
Wt: 140 lb
Ht: 59"
Weight change: ? Not known
Meds:
Rx: ?
OTC: ?
Red Flags/Nutritional Diagnosis or Problems
• Overweight – may need to reduce kcals
• Elderly—may not need lipid-lowering meds
• No activity
Tx
Nutritional Care Plan:
• Receives 1,680 kcal in 24 hrs; chol elevated.
• Needs lower TF level.
• Identify if low TF level requires multi-vitamin–mineral supplement (below 1,200 kcals, it is usually recommended).
• Identify fluid needs and be sure flushes are adequate.
Recommendations/Tips:
• Reduce TF to 45 cc/hr or 1,100 kcals to allow gradual weight loss.
• Recommend bedside range of motion activity.
• May need added vitamin-mineral supplement.
Follow-Up/Goals:
• Monitor weekly weights.
• Monitor cholesterol monthly.
• Have daughter call as needed.

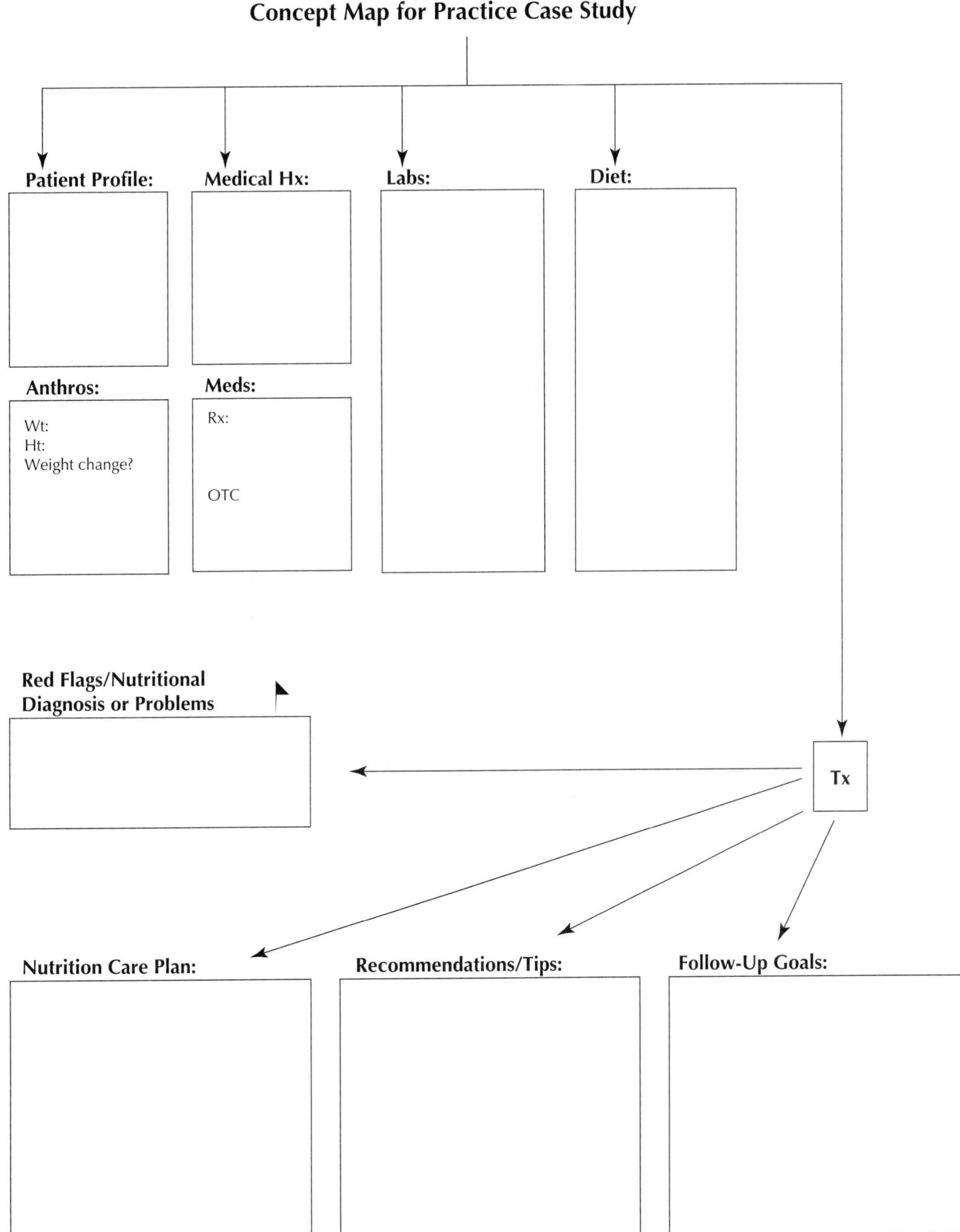

(Concept map examples and the concept map template were contributed by Candyce M. Roberts, MS, RD.)

A P P E N D I X

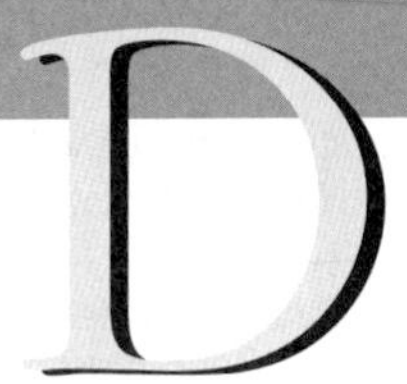

Nutritional Acuity Ranking for Dietitian Services

More than 75 dietitians, clinical nutrition managers, and specialists were surveyed regarding this ranking; the results are tabulated below. Consensus levels are indicated by each diagnosis/condition in this text. 51 surveys were tabulated, with rankings 1–4 considering:

- TIME SPENT (average): for assessment, planning, monitoring, counseling, follow-up contacts
- DEPTH OF KNOWLEDGE/EXPERIENCE SUGGESTED FOR A DIETITIAN TO PROVIDE ADEQUATE CARE.

For this study, facility size or setting was not evaluated. Patients were considered in the continuum of care—regardless of setting. Where mostly "unable to rank," the next highest level of consensus was chosen for this text.

Acuity Rating for Dietitian Service by Diagnosis/Condition	*Level 1: Minimal*	*Level 2: Moderate*	*Level 3: High*	*Level 4: Extensive*	*Unable to Rank*	*Comments: Total Returned*
Life Cycle:						
Pregnancy, uncomplicated	31	17	0	0	3	51
Pregnancy with complications	0	15	29	4	3	51
Infant, normal admission 0–6 mos.	23	18	2	1	7	51
Infant, normal admission 6–12 mos.	24	14	3	0	10	51
Child, normal admission 1–6 yrs.	29	15	0	0	7	51
Child, normal admission, 7–12 yrs.	29	15	0	0	7	51
Adolescent, normal admission	32	12	1	0	6	51
Athlete, sports nutrition advisement	4	25	11	0	11	51
Dietary Practices/Miscellany:						
Cultural food pattern, adaptation/ advisement	15	30	4	0	2	51
Vegetarian, advisement on planning	7	35	9	0	0	51
Kosher dietary patterns, advisement	21	26	2	0	2	51
Dental difficulties	17	29	5	0	0	51
Oral disorders (periodontal disease, etc.)	20	25	4	0	2	51
Temporomandibular joint dysfunction	19	18	5	0	9	51
Skin disorders, such as acne or allergies	36	12	1	0	2	51
Pressure ulcer, stage 1 or 2	2	30	14	0	5	51
Pressure ulcer, stage 3 or 4	0	10	24	15	2	51
Vitamin deficiency counseling	1	27	17	4	2	51
Food allergy, simple	17	26	6	1	1	51
Food allergy, multiple	0	20	24	6	1	51
Chinese restaurant syndrome	15	23	3	0	10	51
Food poisoning, preventive counseling	26	16	1	0	8	51
Food poisoning, corrective therapy	9	27	6	1	8	51
Migraine headache	15	23	4	2	7	51
Ménière's syndrome	18	14	4	1	14	51

(continued)

Acuity Rating for Dietitian Service by Diagnosis/Condition	*Level 1: Minimal*	*Level 2: Moderate*	*Level 3: High*	*Level 4: Extensive*	*Unable to Rank*	*Comments: Total Returned*
Pediatric Disorders:						
Adrenoleukodystrophy	0	1	8	12	30	51
Biliary atresia	0	2	16	17	16	51
Cerebral palsy	0	9	23	10	9	51
Cleft palate	0	11	19	12	9	51
Congenital heart disease	1	17	12	13	8	51
Cystic fibrosis	0	0	19	20	12	51
Cystinosis (Fanconi's syndrome)	0	1	14	8	28	51
Down's syndrome	2	23	10	7	9	51
Failure to thrive, pediatric	0	0	11	33	7	51
Fetal alcohol syndrome	2	4	14	14	17	51
Inborn errors of CHO metabolism	0	0	6	37	8	51
Hirschsprung's disease (megacolon)	1	4	8	19	19	51
Homocystinuria	0	0	5	40	6	51
Large-for-gestational-age infant	5	17	14	2	13	51
Low-birth-weight infant	3	9	17	14	8	51
Myelomeningocele	2	13	8	10	18	51
Maple syrup urine disease	0	0	3	37	11	51
Necrotizing enterocolitis	0	0	9	35	7	51
Childhood obesity counseling	0	8	26	10	7	51
Phenylketonuria	0	1	8	36	6	51
Prader-Willi syndrome	0	1	21	19	10	51
Rickets, nutritional	0	10	21	8	12	51
Spina bifida	0	11	14	12	14	51
Tyrosinemia	0	0	12	25	14	51
Wilson's disease	0	4	17	14	16	51
Neuropsychiatric Disorders:						
Alzheimer's disease or other dementias	8	25	9	6	3	51
Amyotrophic lateral sclerosis	0	14	20	6	11	51
Anorexia nervosa	0	2	15	24	10	51
Bulimia	1	2	17	28	3	51
Cerebral aneurysm	6	22	14	4	5	51
Coma	1	11	23	10	6	51
Depression, mild	25	15	8	0	3	51
Depression with numerous meds	6	29	11	3	2	51
Epilepsy or seizure disorders	17	16	10	5	3	51
Guillain-Barré syndrome	3	10	21	10	7	51
Huntington's chorea	1	14	16	3	17	51
Multiple sclerosis	1	22	18	5	5	51
Myasthenia gravis	3	18	19	3	8	51
Neurological trauma, spinal cord	0	9	24	15	3	51
Parkinson's disease	4	28	15	4	0	51
Psychosis	17	21	8	2	3	51
Substance abuse and withdrawal/ rehabilitation	11	24	12	1	3	51
Tardive dyskinesia	10	8	5	1	27	51
Trigeminal neuralgia	13	9	8	0	21	51
Pulmonary:						
Bronchial asthma	28	14	6	0	3	51
Respiratory distress syndrome, any age	5	24	15	6	1	51
Acute respiratory failure	2	7	27	10	5	51
Bronchiectasis	14	14	3	1	19	51
Bronchitis, acute	28	16	2	0	5	51
Bronchial pneumonia	14	29	4	0	4	51
Chronic obstructive pulmonary diseases	1	22	22	4	2	51
Chylothorax	3	5	18	11	14	51

(continued)

Acuity Rating for Dietitian Service by Diagnosis/Condition	*Level 1: Minimal*	*Level 2: Moderate*	*Level 3: High*	*Level 4: Extensive*	*Unable to Rank*	*Comments: Total Returned*
Cor pulmonale	2	15	8	4	22	51
Pulmonary embolus	14	22	7	3	5	51
Pulmonary tuberculosis	10	19	12	3	7	51
Sarcoidosis	5	16	11	2	17	51
Thoracic empyema	8	10	6	2	25	51
Transplantation, lung	0	0	8	30	13	51
Transplantation, heart-lung	0	0	7	31	13	51
Cardiovascular Disorders:						
Angina pectoris	18	20	4	2	7	51
Arteritis, temporal or giant cell	15	15	2	1	18	51
Atherosclerosis, coronary heart disease	0	21	22	5	3	51
Cardiac tamponade	12	10	8	1	20	51
Cardiac transplantation	0	0	12	32	7	51
Cerebrovascular accident (stroke)	1	13	21	12	4	51
Congestive heart failure	1	23	18	7	2	51
Cardiac cachexia	0	3	34	14	0	51
Heart valve diseases	11	19	18	3	0	51
Hyperlipidemia	0	15	31	5	0	51
Hypertension	3	32	11	3	2	51
Myocardial infarction, acute	3	24	17	3	4	51
Pericarditis	8	21	11	5	6	51
Peripheral vascular disease	7	25	13	3	3	51
Thrombophlebitis	19	18	6	2	6	51
Gastrointestinal Disorders:						
Esophageal stricture or spasm	2	19	24	3	3	51
Achalasia	4	17	15	1	14	51
Esophageal trauma	0	13	28	9	1	51
Esophageal varices	1	15	28	4	3	51
Heartburn, hiatal hernia, esophagitis	15	27	5	2	2	51
Dyspepsia or indigestion	22	25	2	0	2	51
Gastric retention	4	20	24	1	2	51
Gastritis or gastroenteritis	10	27	10	2	2	51
Hypertrophic gastritis (Ménétrièr's disease)	4	11	15	1	20	51
Pernicious vomiting, one week +	0	9	30	12	0	51
Peptic ulcer	10	31	7	1	2	51
Gastrectomy and/or vagotomy	0	6	31	12	2	51
Diarrhea (acute enteritis)	5	25	16	3	2	51
Dysentery or traveler's diarrhea	18	21	8	1	3	51
Fat malabsorption syndrome	0	1	30	19	1	51
Celiac disease (gluten-enteropathy)	0	1	23	26	1	51
Tropical sprue	0	1	22	22	6	51
Lactose malabsorption or maldigestion	3	29	10	8	1	51
Constipation	28	21	1	0	1	51
Megacolon, acquired	1	19	11	6	14	51
Irritable colon/spastic colitis	5	24	16	5	1	51
Diverticular diseases	3	32	12	2	2	51
Peritonitis	4	20	18	6	3	51
Carcinoid syndrome	1	15	13	7	15	51
Crohn's disease (regional enteritis)	0	1	23	26	1	51
Intestinal fistula	0	1	21	27	2	51
Ulcerative colitis	0	2	20	27	2	51
Ileostomy	1	7	30	12	1	51
Colostomy	3	13	24	10	1	51
Intestinal lipodystrophy (Whipple's disease)	0	2	16	17	16	51
Intestinal lymphangiectasia	0	3	13	9	26	51
Short-bowel syndrome	0	0	17	33	1	51
Hemorrhoids, hemorrhoidectomy	36	14	0	0	1	51

(continued)

Acuity Rating for Dietitian Service by Diagnosis/Condition	*Level 1: Minimal*	*Level 2: Moderate*	*Level 3: High*	*Level 4: Extensive*	*Unable to Rank*	*Comments: Total Returned*
Hepatic/Biliary/Pancreatic Disorders:						
Jaundice	19	19	7	2	4	51
Hepatitis	3	23	17	6	2	51
Alcoholic liver disease	0	4	36	5	6	51
Ascites	1	7	36	5	2	51
Hepatic cirrhosis	0	0	33	15	3	51
Portacaval shunt for portal hypertension	3	12	18	11	7	51
Liver transplantation	0	0	5	35	11	51
Hepatic encephalopathy, failure or coma	0	0	8	41	2	51
Pancreatitis, acute	0	8	25	16	2	51
Pancreatitis, chronic	0	9	32	9	1	51
Pancreatic insufficiency	1	8	25	17	0	51
Zollinger-Ellison syndrome	1	4	22	8	16	51
Gallbladder disease, surgical or nonsurgical	14	27	6	3	1	51
Biliary cirrhosis	2	6	26	12	5	51
Cholestatic liver disease	0	9	25	12	5	51
Endocrine Disorders:						
Insulin-dependent diabetes mellitus	0	2	28	17	4	51
Non-insulin-dependent diabetes mellitus	0	13	25	12	1	51
Diabetic gastroparesis	0	8	25	7	4	44
Diabetic ketoacidosis or coma	0	4	24	22	1	51
Hyperosmolar hyperglycemic nonketotic coma	0	9	15	19	1	44
Hypoglycemia	0	22	23	6	0	51
Hyperinsulinism	2	14	21	12	2	51
Adrenocortical insufficiency, chronic	3	16	18	6	8	51
Addison's disease	5	15	10	6	15	51
Acromegaly	6	20	3	2	20	51
Hyperaldosteronism	5	18	8	3	17	51
Hypopituitarism	9	19	7	2	14	51
Pheochromocytoma	6	16	5	3	21	51
Hyperthyroidism	7	29	5	3	7	51
Hypothyroidism	8	28	7	2	6	51
Diabetes insipidus	6	17	17	2	9	51
Syndrome of inappropriate ADH (SIADH)	3	17	20	2	9	51
Cushing's syndrome	3	21	16	1	10	51
Parathyroid disorders (altered calcium)	4	10	24	13	0	51
Gestational diabetes	0	5	22	20	4	51
Pregnancy-induced hypertension	3	16	21	6	5	51
Weight Control & PCM:						
Obesity, nonsurgical counseling	3	20	13	15	0	51
Underweight or general debility	2	20	16	12	1	51
Protein-calorie malnutrition: kwashiorkor	0	2	21	27	1	51
Protein-calorie malnutrition: marasmus	0	2	20	28	1	51
Rheumatic & Musculoskeletal Disorders:						
Ankylosing spondilitis	12	7	6	0	26	51
Immobilization, extended	5	26	13	2	5	51
Gout	23	20	8	0	0	51
Muscular dystrophy	7	21	14	1	8	51
Osteoarthritis (degenerative joint disease)	20	21	3	0	7	51
Osteomyelitis, acute	12	24	2	1	12	51
Osteomalacia	7	26	11	1	6	51
Osteoporosis	3	35	8	1	4	51
Paget's disease (osteitis deformans)	8	16	5	2	20	51
Polyarteritis nodosa	9	14	4	0	24	51
Rheumatoid arthritis	19	20	6	1	5	51
Ruptured intervertebral disc	25	11	6	1	8	51

(continued)

Acuity Rating for Dietitian Service by Diagnosis/Condition	*Level 1: Minimal*	*Level 2: Moderate*	*Level 3: High*	*Level 4: Extensive*	*Unable to Rank*	*Comments: Total Returned*
Scleroderma (systemic sclerosis)	8	12	14	4	13	51
Systemic lupus erythematosa	8	14	18	5	6	51
Anemias/Related Blood Disorders:						
Aplastic anemia	6	24	11	4	6	51
Anemia, iron deficiency	7	35	7	2	0	51
Anemia, nutritional (folic acid, copper, etc.)	0	23	21	4	3	51
Anemia, pernicious or vitamin B12	0	26	19	3	3	51
Anemia from parasitic infestation	14	20	7	2	8	51
Anemia, sideroblastic	7	20	7	3	14	51
Hemochromatosus (iron overloading)	4	23	16	3	5	51
Hemorrhage, acute or chronic	14	24	5	2	6	51
Sickle cell anemia	12	21	10	3	5	51
Polycythemia vera (Osler's disease)	12	10	3	1	25	51
Thrombocytic purpura	15	11	1	3	21	51
Thalassemia (Cooley's anemia)	8	16	4	1	22	51
Cancers:						
Cancer (general or unlisted types)	1	18	22	8	2	51
Leukemia, acute	1	10	23	13	4	51
Leukemia, chronic	1	12	27	9	2	51
Bone marrow transplantation	1	1	1	39	9	51
Brain tumor	3	13	21	11	3	51
Breast cancer	3	23	22	3	0	51
Bronchial carcinoma (lung cancer)	0	8	31	9	3	51
Choriocarcinoma	1	11	23	5	11	51
Esophageal cancer	0	0	24	25	2	51
Gastric carcinoma	0	0	25	24	2	51
Hepatic carcinoma	0	3	23	24	1	51
Intestinal carcinoma	0	1	24	24	2	51
Lymphoma, Hodgkin's disease	3	10	25	8	5	51
Lymphoma, non-Hodgkin's	4	13	23	6	5	51
Myeloma (simple or multiple)	4	14	27	1	5	51
Oral cancer	0	4	24	21	2	51
Osteosarcoma	4	10	24	8	5	51
Pancreatic carcinoma	0	2	22	23	4	51
Prostate cancer	10	22	13	1	5	51
Radiation colitis or enteritis	0	4	24	19	4	51
Wilm's tumor (embryoma of kidney)	1	5	9	7	29	51
Surgical Conditions:						
Surgery, general	18	25	4	1	3	51
Hyponatremia	11	23	15	1	1	51
Hypernatremia	11	23	15	1	1	51
Hypokalemia	8	24	17	1	1	51
Hyperkalemia	5	23	19	2	2	51
Hypocalcemia	8	21	18	1	3	51
Hypercalcemia	7	23	18	1	2	51
Hypomagnesemia	8	22	17	2	2	51
Hypermagnesemia	6	27	13	3	2	51
Phosphate imbalances	6	21	19	3	2	51
Amputation, one or more limbs	7	20	18	1	5	51
Appendectomy	38	7	2	0	4	51
Bowel surgery	0	14	29	7	1	51
Jejunoileal bypass surgery	0	3	24	16	8	51
Gastric bypass or stapling	1	2	29	16	3	51
Cesarean delivery	39	6	2	0	4	51
Cataract surgery	43	4	0	0	4	51
Hysterectomy, abdominal	40	7	0	0	4	51
Pelvic exenteration	23	7	12	1	8	51

(continued)

Acuity Rating for Dietitian Service by Diagnosis/Condition	*Level 1: Minimal*	*Level 2: Moderate*	*Level 3: High*	*Level 4: Extensive*	*Unable to Rank*	*Comments: Total Returned*
Open heart surgery	0	16	19	14	2	51
Pancreatic surgery	3	5	25	16	2	51
Parathyroidectomy	16	15	13	4	3	51
Spinal surgery	14	22	9	1	5	51
Total hip arthroplasty	11	26	7	2	5	51
Tonsillectomy and adenoidectomy	40	7	1	0	3	51
Trauma, Stress, Infections:						
AIDS and HIV infection	0	7	20	24	0	51
Ascariasis	9	2	7	1	32	51
Bacterial endocarditis	8	8	12	4	19	51
Burns and minor thermal injury	4	13	22	9	3	51
Burns and major thermal injury	0	0	5	39	7	51
Candidiasis	9	27	11	0	4	51
Encephalitis or Reye's syndrome	4	20	14	1	12	51
Chronic fatigue syndrome	15	22	4	1	9	51
Fever, greater than 102°	12	22	12	3	2	51
Fracture, hip	9	29	9	2	2	51
Fracture, long-bone	15	23	10	1	2	51
Herpes simplex I and II	29	15	2	0	5	51
Herpes zoster (shingles)	29	14	3	1	4	51
Infection, general	22	22	4	0	3	51
Infectious mononucleosis	30	14	3	1	3	51
Influenza (flu, respiratory)	29	11	3	0	8	51
Meningitis	14	17	7	0	13	51
Multiple organ dysfunction	0	0	9	37	5	51
Pelvic inflammatory disease	28	13	3	0	7	51
Poliomyelitis	21	17	5	0	8	51
Rheumatic fever	20	17	4	1	9	51
Sepsis or septicemia	5	11	21	12	2	51
Toxic shock syndrome	18	16	4	5	8	51
Trauma	2	8	20	17	4	51
Trichinosis	12	20	5	2	12	51
Typhoid fever	13	17	4	2	15	51
Renal Disorders:						
Inborn errors—Vitamin-D-resistant rickets	1	2	22	16	10	51
Hartnup disease	2	4	10	7	28	51
Polycystic kidney disease	5	7	13	13	13	51
Glomerulonephritis, acute	3	6	28	11	3	51
Glomerulonephritis, chronic	2	3	28	13	5	51
Nephritis (Bright's disease)	3	8	21	9	10	51
Nephrosclerosis	3	7	20	7	14	51
Nephrotic syndrome	2	5	27	14	3	51
Pyelonephritis	7	11	21	5	7	51
Urolithiasis (renal stones)	7	24	12	0	8	51
Renal failure, acute	1	1	18	29	2	51
Renal failure, chronic	0	1	21	28	1	51
Hemodialysis	0	1	18	30	2	51
Peritoneal renal dialysis	0	0	17	29	5	51
Renal transplantation	0	0	13	33	5	51
Enteral/Parenteral Nutrition:						
Home tube feeding	0	1	19	23	8	51
Home total parenteral nutrition	0	0	9	34	8	51
*TOTALS:	2,147	3,973	4,040	2,489	1,966	14,615 Total rankings

*Summary: Most diagnoses were level 3 (28%) or level 2 (27%), totaling 55%. Of the remaining conditions, 17% were ranked at level 4 and 15% at level 1; 13% of respondents found that they could not rank certain disorders because of unfamiliarity. Overall, 72% of all conditions warrant the services of a Registered Dietitian at moderate, high, or extensive levels of involvement.

APPENDIX 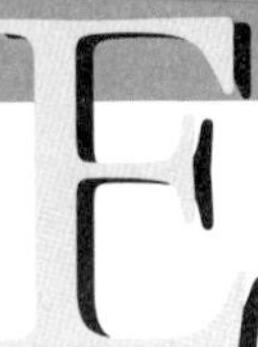

Complementary Nutrition—Herbals and Botanicals

The philosophy that food can be health promoting beyond its nutritional value has gained acceptance within the public arena and among the scientific community as foods are linked to disease prevention and treatments (American Dietetic Association, 1995). Herbal supplement use is going up while supporting evidence for these herbs is going down (Shah and Grant, 2000). Dietitians are uniquely qualified to translate sound scientific evidence into practical applications. Dietitians consider themselves knowledgeable about use of functional foods and nutrient supplements, but only 10% feel confident about the roles of herbs in prevention and treatment of illnesses (Lee et al., 2000).

Functional foods are foods that provide health benefits beyond basic nutrition and are adjunctive to a balanced diet. Fish provides fish oils; fermented dairy products have probiotics; and beef has conjugated linoleic acid. Many plants contain biologically active chemicals known as phytochemicals. Phenolic phytochemicals are the largest group of phytochemicals, the most important groups being flavonoids, phenolic acids, and polyphenols. Phenolics are biologically active compounds that may possess some disease-prevention properties (King and Young, 1999). Oats provide beta-glucan, soy provides isoflavones, flaxseed provides lignins and α-linolenic acid, garlic provides organosulfur compounds, broccoli and cruciferous vegetables provide isothiocyanates and indoles, citrus fruits provide liminis, cranberry provides polymeric compounds, tea provides cachectin, and wine provides phenolics (Hasler et al., 1998).

Increasing numbers of patients use herbal medicines but do not tell their health care providers. Consumers are testing many new products, some more effective than others. There are 29,000 different dietary supplements available to consumers, and an average of 1,000 new products are added yearly according to the Food and Drug Administration (FDA) (Stein, 2000). Practitioners who refer their patients to a medical herbalist should assess for specific skills, educational background, national qualifications, experience, hours of supervised clinical practice, professionalism, association memberships, and willingness to communicate openly with the referring practitioner (Libster, 1999). It is also important to find out whether he/she sells particular brands of herbal products and bases clinical decisions on information provided by the manufacturer.

Nutrition therapy is an integral part of many complementary therapies for cancer, arthritis, chronic back pain, human immunodeficiency virus (HIV), gastrointestinal (GI) problems, and eating disorders (Hamilton, 1998). Chinese herbal formulations may reduce some symptoms of patients with irritable bowel syndrome (IBS) (Bensoussan, 1998). Red-yeast rice is the fermented product of rice on which red yeast has been grown; it has been a dietary staple in Asian countries and helps to lower total cholesterol levels (Heber et al., 1999). Rice-bran oil contains tocotrienols, powerful antioxidants that belong to the vitamin E family and protect against cardiac heart disease (CHD) and some forms of cancer (McCaskill and Zhang, 1999).

Echinacea seems to be an effective treatment for upper respiratory tract infections (UTIs), if taken when the symptoms first appear. Fresh garlic has been found to help lower cholesterol. Ginkgo may help improve cognitive function in patients with Alzheimer's disease. Ginseng may also help with cognitive function, but more research is needed. Saw Palmetto helps those with benign prostatic hyperplasia. St John's Wort helps with depression, while Valerian may provide relief for people with insomnia.

DHEA expanded the definition of dietary supplements, while distinguishing them from drugs or food additives. Nonvitamin nonmineral (NVNM) supplements are classified inconsistently, and information on prevalence of use is limited (Radimer, 2000). Reported use in the NHANES III survey was highest for garlic and lecithin. Use of NVNM supplements increased greatly as a result of the passage of the DHEA (Hankin, 2000). Because the DHEA does not mandate substantiation of products' efficacy, there may be risks with their consumption. Clients do not understand that these are drugs and may interact with one another or with foods. Legally, they are dietary supplements, but they are drugs as far as their actions in the body. Medicinal herbs should actually be viewed as experimental drugs. Although FDA regulates additives and drugs, premarket review of dietary supplements is minimal; research is needed in this area (Hankin, 2000). Figure E-1 shows a form that can be used to solicit appropriate assessment information from a patient or client.

Adverse reactions are discovered postmarketing through case studies versus clinical trials for pharmaceuticals. Gingko biloba may cause GI problems, headaches, allergic skin reactions, or bleeding disorders. Ma huang can cause stroke or dangerous increases in blood pressure (BP). St John's wort

Final Report—March 2002

Most CAM modalities have not yet been scientifically studied and found to be safe and effective. The fact that many Americans are using CAM modalities should not be confused with the fact that most of these modalities remain unproven by high-quality clinical studies. The White House Commission on Complementary and Alternative Medicine Policy believes that conventional and CAM systems of health and healing should be held to the same rigorous standards of good science, as stated in its final report of March 2002. More funding for research is needed to determine the possible benefits and limitations of a variety of CAM modalities. Well-designed scientific research and demonstration projects can help to determine which CAM modalities and approaches are clinically effective and cost-effective. With information from these studies, the public can make informed, intelligent decisions about their own health and well-being and the appropriate use of CAM interventions.

The Commission endorsed the following 10 guiding principles to shape the process of making recommendations:

1. A wholeness orientation in health care delivery. Health involves all aspects of life—mind, body, spirit, and environment—and high-quality health care must support care of the whole person.
2. Evidence of safety and efficacy. The Commission is committed to promoting the use of science and appropriate scientific methods to help identify safe and effective CAM services and products and to generate evidence that will protect and promote the public health.
3. The healing capacity of the person. People have a remarkable capacity for recovery and self-healing, and a major focus of health care is to support and promote this capacity.
4. Respect for individuality. Each person is unique and has the right to health care that is appropriately responsive to him or her, respecting preferences and preserving dignity.
5. The right to choose treatment. Each person has the right to choose freely among safe and effective care or approaches, as well as among qualified practitioners who are accountable for their claims and actions and responsive to the person's needs.
6. An emphasis on health promotion and self-care. Good health care emphasizes self-care and early intervention for maintaining and promoting health.
7. Partnerships as essential to integrated health care. Good health care requires teamwork among patients, health care practitioners (conventional and CAM), and researchers committed to creating optimal healing environments and to respecting the diversity of all health care traditions.
8. Education as a fundamental health care service. Education about prevention, healthy lifestyles, and the power of self-healing should be made an integral part of the curricula of all health care professionals and should be made available to the public of all ages.
9. Dissemination of comprehensive and timely information. The quality of health care can be enhanced by promoting efforts that thoroughly and thoughtfully examine the evidence on which CAM systems, practices, and products are based and make this evidence widely, rapidly, and easily available.
10. Integral public involvement. The input of informed consumers and other members of the public must be incorporated in setting priorities for health care and health care research and in reaching policy decisions, including those related to CAM, within the public and private sectors.

From the Executive Summary (http://www.whccamp.hhs.gov/es.html.)

can reduce the effectiveness of prescription drugs and may inhibit iron absorption. Nonsteroidal anti-inflammatory agents may negate the usefulness of feverfew in treatment of migraines (Miller, 1998). Feverfew, garlic, gingko, and ginseng may alter bleeding time and should not be used with warfarin. Kyushin, licorice, plantain, uzara root, hawthorn, and ginseng may interfere with digoxin action (Miller, 1998). Evening primrose oil and borage should not be used with anticonvulsants, because they lower the seizure threshold. Immunostimulants (Echinacea) should not be used with immunosuppressants (corticosteroids and cyclosporine). Tannic acids are present in saw palmetto. Kelp ingested as a source of iodine may interfere with thyroid replacement therapies. Licorice can offset the pharmacologic effect of spironolactone. Karela and ginseng can affect blood glucose levels and should not be used by patients with diabetes mellitus (DM). Ginseng may also add to the effects of estrogens or corticosteroids and can elevate BP. Table E-1 provides a more complete list of potential interactions between botanicals and drugs.

Figure E-1 **Herbal, Botanical and Dietary Supplement Intake Form**

Your health care professional needs the following information about your usual supplement and dietary habits to develop a personal plan for you. Please complete all sections completely and accurately.

NAME ______________________ AGE __________ DATE __________

1. What kind of supplements do you use? (Check all that apply)

___ None
___ Multivitamin/mineral supplement
___ Herbal or botanical supplement
___ Amino acid or protein supplement
___ Fiber supplement
___ Other (see question 14 checklist at end of this form)

2. How long have you used this supplement(s)?

___ 1 month or less
___ 3 months
___ 6 months
___ 1 year
___ more than one year (specify) ______________________

3. How long do you plan to use this supplement(s)?

___ Indefinitely
___ 1 year
___ 6 months
___ 3 months
___ 1 month or less

4. What are your primary reason(s) for taking this supplement(s)?

___ For its preventive effect against disease/medical condition
___ To help treat a disease/medical condition
___ General wellness
___ Energy
___ Weight loss
___ Pregnancy/lactation
___ Other (specify)

If used to *treat* specific medical condition: What are your medical symptoms?
____

5. How long have you had these symptoms/medical condition?

___ 1 week or less
___ 1 month
___ 3 months
___ 6 months
___ 1 year
___ More than 1 year (specify)

6. Have symptoms improved since you started taking this supplement?

___ Yes (explain how)______________________________
___ No

7. Are you currently taking or have recently taken any over-the-counter or prescription medications, including oral contraceptives?

___ Yes (specify)
___ No

8. Do you have any additional illnesses or medical conditions?

___ Yes (specify)______________________________
___ No

9. Are you pregnant or breastfeeding?
___ Yes
___ No

10. Do you drink alcohol?
___ Yes
___ No

If yes, how often?
___ Rarely
___ Occasionally
___ Often
___ Never

If yes, how much at one sitting?
___ 1 glass
___ 2 glasses
___ 3 glasses or more

11. Do you smoke?
___ Yes
___ No

If yes, how often and how much?
___ 1–5 cigarettes, cigars, pipes per day
___ 1 pack per day
___ 2 packs per day
___ More than 2 packs per day

12. Are you allergic to any medications, foods, plants, or flowers?
___ Yes (specify) ____________________
___ No

13. Are you on a self- or medically-prescribed eating plan/diet?
___ Yes (specify) ____________________
___ No

14. What specific supplement(s) do you take, amount you take, and how often do you take it?

	Amount/Dose	Number of Doses (per day or week)
Aloe	________	________
Amino acid(s)	________	________
Black cohosh	________	________
Bee pollen	________	________
Calcium	________	________
Cat's claw	________	________
Chondroitin	________	________
Chromium	________	________
Coenzyme Q10	________	________
Creatine	________	________
"Andro"/DHEA	________	________
Dong quai	________	________
Echinacea	________	________
Evening primrose oil	________	________
Feverfew	________	________
Fiber	________	________
Fish oil/DHA	________	________
Folic acid	________	________
Garlic	________	________
Ginger	________	________
Ginkgo biloba	________	________
Ginseng	________	________

Goldenseal	____________	______________________________
Grapeseed extract	____________	______________________________
Iron	____________	______________________________
Kava	____________	______________________________
Ma huang/ephedra	____________	______________________________
Milk thistle	____________	______________________________
Multiple vitamin/mineral	____________	______________________________
Peppermint	____________	______________________________
Pyruvate	____________	______________________________
St John's wort	____________	______________________________
Saw palmetto	____________	______________________________
SAM-e	____________	______________________________
Valerian	____________	______________________________
Vitamin B complex	____________	______________________________
Vitamin C	____________	______________________________
Vitamin D	____________	______________________________
Vitamin E	____________	______________________________
Other	____________	______________________________

Sources: American Dietetic Association. *Sports nutrition: a guide for the professional working with active people*. Chicago, IL: American Dietetic Association, 2000; and The American Dietetic Association. Special report from the Joint Working Group on Dietary Supplements, 2000. Used with permission.

TABLE E-1 Potential Drug Interactions Between Dietary Supplements/Botanicals and Prescription Drugs

Dietary Supplement/ Botanical	*Primary Uses or Actions*	*Potential Drug Interactions*	*Potential Outcome(s) of Drug Interaction*	*Recommended Action(s)*
Belladonna (leaf and root)	Anticholinergic, sedative, respiratory antispasmodic	Additive anticholinergic effects with drugs such as tricyclic antidepressants, some antihistamines, phenothiazines, and quinidine (22)[a]	Symptoms of excessive anticholinergic activity (eg, sedation, dry mouth, difficult urination) may occur.	Caution. Use low dosage of belladonna and titrate to effectiveness, monitoring side effects.
Chasteberry	Premenstrual syndrome (PMS), menopausal symptoms, dysmenorrhea	Hormone replacement therapy, oral contraceptives (23)	Herb use with hormones could potentiate or antagonize effects; results depend on dose of herb.	Use combinations cautiously and under medical supervision. Use lowest effective dose of herb.
Chromium	Trace element involved in glycemic control. Used in weight loss, diabetes, and dyslipidemia	Insulin, hypoglycemic agents	Chromium may potentiate effects of insulin and hypoglycemics, causing hypoglycemia (theoretical) (24).	Monitor blood glucose levels and adjust doses of insulin or hypoglycemics as needed.
Coenzyme Q-10 (Ubiquinone, Co-Q10)	Immunostimulant, cardiovascular diseases, periodontal disease	"Statins" (eg, lovastatin, cerivastatin, pravastatin, simvastatin, atorvastatin, fluvastatin), gemfibrozil, tricyclic antidepressants (eg, amitriptyline, nortriptyline, desipramine), glyburide	Statins, gemfibrozil, tricyclic antidepressants, and glyburide decrease endogenous levels of CoQ-10 (25–27).	The significance of drug-induced decreases in endogenous CoQ-10 levels is uncertain. Supplementation with CoQ-10 or increases in the current CoQ-10 dosage are potential options to offset this effect.

(continued)

TABLE E-1 Potential Drug Interactions Between Dietary Supplements/Botanicals and Prescription Drugs (*Continued*)

Dietary Supplement/ Botanical	*Primary Uses or Actions*	*Potential Drug Interactions*	*Potential Outcome(s) of Drug Interaction*	*Recommended Action(s)*
Coenzyme Q-10 (cont.)		Warfarin	Decreased warfarin effects. CoQ-10 may act similarly to vitamin K (28).	Monitor INR values and adjust warfarin dose as necessary.
Danshen	Circulatory disorders, cardiovascular ischemic disease	Antiplatelet drugs; ticlopidine, clopidogrel, aspirin	Additive effect, increased risks of bleeding and/or bruising (29).	Caution advised. Monitor for excessive bleeding and bruising.
		Warfarin	Additive anticoagulant effects (reflected in INR values), with increased bleeding risks (18,19,30).	Best to avoid combination. If used, monitor INR closely and adjust warfarin dosage.
Dong quai	"Woman's tonic": PMS, menopausal symptoms, menstrual cramps	Warfarin, aspirin, clopidogrel, ticlopidine	Dong quai contains "coumadin-like" substances and may potentiate anticoagulants and platelet-altering drugs (31,32).	Avoid in patients using anticoagulants or antiplatelet drugs. More information is needed.
Echinacea	Antiviral, immunostimulant	Warfarin	Additive effect with warfarin (may increase INR) (33.34).	Avoid use with warfarin.
		Immunosuppressants	Antagonistic effects (theoretical) (35).	Avoid combinations.
Ephedra or Ma huang (contains ephedrine and derivative alkaloids)	Central nervous system (CNS) stimulant, respiratory stimulant, bronchodilator, anorexiant	Digoxin, halothane (anesthetic)	Combination can cause arrhythmias (22,29).	Avoid combinations.
		Hypoglycemic agents	Increased blood glucose (23).	Caution: Monitor blood glucose.
		Monoamine oxidase inhibitor (MAOI) antidepressants	Increased blood pressure and heart rate (29).	Avoid combination.
		Antihypertensives	Antagonistic effects (6,29).	Avoid combination.
		Oxytocin	Can cause severe hypertension (22).	Avoid combination.
		Theophylline and caffeine	Increased CNS stimulation and possible increase in heart rate and blood pressure (6,23).	Caution advised. If combinations are used, initiate with low doses of herb.
		Dexamethasone (steroid)	Increased metabolism of dexamethasone may diminish effects of steroid. Treatment failure is possible (23).	Avoid combination.
Feverfew	Migraine headache, inflammatory conditions, menstrual irregularities	Warfarin, antiplatelet drugs (eg, clopidogrel, ticlopidine, aspirin)	Decreased platelet aggregation (via cyclo-oxygenase and phospholipase A2 inhibition) by herb may cause increased bleeding or bruising risks (11, 20,34).	Avoid use with warfarin. Use caution in combination with antiplatelet drugs.

(*continued*)

TABLE E-1 Potential Drug Interactions Between Dietary Supplements/Botanicals and Prescription Drugs (*Continued*)

Dietary Supplement/ Botanical	*Primary Uses or Actions*	*Potential Drug Interactions*	*Potential Outcome(s) of Drug Interaction*	*Recommended Action(s)*
Feverfew (cont.)		Nonsteroidal anti-inflammatory drugs (NSAIDs) (eg, ibuprofen, indomethacin, diclofenac, celecoxib)	Decreases herb's anti-inflammatory action (29).	If using feverfew for anti-inflammatory purposes, do not combine with NSAIDs.
Garlic	Antimicrobial, immunostimulant, cardiovascular diseases, dyslipidemia therapy	Warfarin	Increased risks of bleeding, with possible elevations in INR values (10,29, 35–37).	More information is needed, but caution with warfarin therapy is recommended. Monitor INR and symptoms of bleeding.
		Antiplatelet agents (eg, clopidogrel, ticlopidine, aspirin)	Increased risks of bleeding or bruising (10,29,35,36).	Caution: Use only with physician supervision.
		Hypoglycemic agents (insulin and oral hypoglycemics)	Garlic may increase insulin levels with need to decrease hypoglycemic agent dosages (29,35).	Monitor glucose levels with initiating therapy in those who have diabetes.
Ginger	Antinauseant (eg, motion sickness), anti-inflammatory	Warfarin, antiplatelet drugs (eg, clopidogrel, ticlopidine, aspirin) (26,27,29)	Decreased platelet aggregation (via thromboxane inhibition) may increase risk of bleeding (10).	Avoid use with drugs that affect bleeding and platelet function.
		Antihypertensive drugs	May cause unpredictable blood pressure responses (increase or decrease) (35).	Caution: Monitor and adjust doses according to response.
		Hypoglycemic drugs	Additive effects may decrease blood glucose (22,35).	Monitor blood glucose and adjust doses of herb or drugs as necessary.
Ginkgo biloba	Circulatory disorders (eg, impotence, Alzheimer's disease, intermittent claudication)	Warfarin, antiplatelet drugs (eg, clopidogrel, ticlopidine, aspirin)	Ginkgo inhibits platelet aggregation and may increase bleeding risks with these drugs (10,11, 23,29,34). INR values may be increased.	Avoid combinations with warfarin and antiplatelet drugs. More information is needed, but cases of spontaneous bleeding have been reported (38,39).
Ginseng (especially Panax or Asian ginseng)	Stress adaptation, performance, digestive aid, impotence. Multiple active ingredients that can vary with type.	Warfarin	Can increase or decrease effects or warfarin. Unpredictable action, but most reports have shown a decrease in INRs (10,11,20,29).	Avoid use with warfarin.
		Antiplatelet drugs (eg, clopidogrel, ticlopidine, aspirin)	Possible additive or antagonist effects on platelet function (10,11,29).	Caution with drugs that affect bleeding and platelet function.
		Insulin, oral hypoglycemics MAOI antidepressants	Fluctuations in blood glucose (10). Potentiates action of MAOIs. Cases of headache, insomnia, tremors, irritability, visual hallucination reported (10,11).	Use cautiously (unpredictable). Avoid combinations.

(*continued*)

TABLE E-1 Potential Drug Interactions Between Dietary Supplements/Botanicals and Prescription Drugs (*Continued*)

Dietary Supplement/ Botanical	*Primary Uses or Actions*	*Potential Drug Interactions*	*Potential Outcome(s) of Drug Interaction*	*Recommended Action(s)*
Ginseng (cont.)		CNS stimulants, caffeine, hormones, steroids, antipsychotics	Can exaggerate responses to all of these medications (eg, CNS stimulation, increased blood pressure and heart rate) (29).	Use cautiously and only with supervision. Effects can vary.
Grapefruit juice		Alprazolam, buspirone, cisapride, cyclosporine, diazepam, isradipine, felodipine, nicardipine, nifedipine, nisoldipine, lovastatin, atorvastatin, tacrolimus (Note: This is not a complete listing)	Decreases drug metabolism in the gut (via P450-CYP3A4 inhibition), resulting in increases in response to many "susceptible" medications. Potentially dangerous interactions! (7,40,41).	Severity and consequence of interaction depends on several factors. Consult pharmacist regarding specific interactions. One glass of juice can have effects lasting up to 24 hours.
Hawthorn	Numerous cardiovascular actions, including vasodilatory, inotropic, antiarrhythmic effects	Digoxin, angiotensin-converting enzyme (ACE) inhibitors (eg, lisinopril); most cardiovascular medications can be affected	Hawthorn has potent cardiac effects and can potentiate the effects of most cardiovascular medications (10,29, 35,42).	Use only under close medical supervision. Decreasing dosages of other cardiovascular medications may be necessary if hawthorn is added to therapy, especially digoxin. Hawthorn can take up to 2 weeks for onset of effects.
Indian snakeroot	Mild essential hypertension, mental illness	Digoxin	Arrhythmias (especially bradycardia) and angina (6).	Avoid. Reactions can be severe.
		Barbiturates (e.g., phenobarbital)	Increased sedation (22).	Use combination cautiously.
		Levodopa (plain)	Decreased levodopa effectiveness with increased extrapyramidal symptoms (6,22).	Avoid with levodopa, but safe to use with levodopa/ carbidopa.
		Sympathomimetics (eg, albuterol, pseudoephedrine)	Increases in blood pressure (6).	Caution. Use low doses of herb and titrate slowly to effect.
		Antihypertensives, diuretics (eg, furosemide, hydrochlorothiazide, torsemide)	Increased effect of both drugs and herb (eg, decreased blood pressure) (6).	Caution: Monitor blood pressure and adjust doses.
		MAOI antidepressants (eg, phenelzine, tranylcypromine)	CNS excitation and increased blood pressure.	Avoid combination. Separate herb from drugs by 3 to 4 days.
		Beta-blockers (eg, metoprolol, atenolol, propranolol, bisoprolol)	Enhanced beta blockade, with decreased heart rate and blood pressure (6).	Avoid combination.
		Neuroleptics (eg, tranquilizers)	Increased effects of both herb and drugs (22).	Caution advised.
Kava Kava	Anxiolytic, euphoric	CNS stimulants	Possible antagonistic effects. Results are unpredictable (29).	Avoid combinations (theoretical).

(continued)

TABLE E-1 Potential Drug Interactions Between Dietary Supplements/Botanicals and Prescription Drugs (*Continued*)

Dietary Supplement/ Botanical	*Primary Uses or Actions*	*Potential Drug Interactions*	*Potential Outcome(s) of Drug Interaction*	*Recommended Action(s)*
Kava Kava (cont.)		CNS depressants (eg, alcohol, barbiturates, anxiolytics)	Additive CNS depressant effects (10,22,29).	Use only under close medical supervision.
		Benzodiazepines (eg, alprazolam, diazepam, lorazepam, triazolam)	Severe CNS effects. Cases of comatose states have been reported (22,29,43).	Avoid. Dangerous combination.
L-tryptophan (5-HTP or 5-hydroxy-tryptophan) (precursor to serotonin)	Insomnia, depression, enhanced athletic performance	MAOI antidepressants	Can exacerbate conditions of psychosis or hypomania (25).	Need more information.
		SSRI antidepressants	"Serotonin syndrome" is possible (44).	Avoid most combinations.
		Serotonin receptor antagonists (eg, cyproheptadine, methysergide)	Antagonistic interaction. Decreased effects of L-tryptophan (theoretical).	Avoid combinations.
Licorice root	Gastric or duodenal ulcers, antibacterial-anti-inflammatory, expectorant.	Digoxin	Potentiates digoxin toxicity through potassium loss (22,29).	Monitor potassium level and replace as necessary.
		Steroids (especially hydrocortisone)	May potentiate effects of steroids (23,29).	Avoid combination.
		Progesterone, estrogens	Licorice may have estrogenic or antiestrogenic effects (35).	Use cautiously.
		Antihypertensive medications	Increased sodium and water retention may offset effects of drugs and increase blood pressure (11,45).	Avoid combinations.
		Thiazide and loop diuretics (eg, furosemide, hydrochlorothiazide)	Offsets of diuretics by increasing sodium and water retention. Potentiates risks of hypokalemia (11,45).	Avoid combinations.
		Spironolactone (diuretic)	Spironolactone especially antagonized (10).	Avoid combinations
Melatonin	Sleep cycle adjuster (eg, "jet lag"), sleeping aid, immunostimulant	CNS depressants (eg, alcohol, benzodiazepines, barbiturates)	Possible additive CNS depression (theoretical).	Use cautiously. Use of low doses of melatonin is recommended.
		Immunosuppressants, corticosteroids	Antagonistic effects (46).	Avoid combinations.
Niacin (nicotinic acid, nicotinamide, vitamin B3)	Lipid-lowering agent (at higher doses), vertigo, peripheral vascular disorders	"Statins" (eg, lovastatin, cerivastatin, pravastatin, simvastatin, atorvastatin, fluvastatin) (cholesterol-lowering agents)	Increased risks of myopathy (severe reaction is possible) (6,25).	Combination should only be used under medical supervision.

(*continued*)

TABLE E-1 Potential Drug Interactions Between Dietary Supplements/Botanicals and Prescription Drugs (*Continued*)

Dietary Supplement/ Botanical	*Primary Uses or Actions*	*Potential Drug Interactions*	*Potential Outcome(s) of Drug Interaction*	*Recommended Action(s)*
Niacin (cont.)		Antidiabetic medications	May interfere with glucose control (6).	Monitor glucose levels and adjust doses as necessary.
		Carbamazepine	Increased carbamazepine levels (25).	Caution: Use only under physician supervision. Monitor carbamazepine levels.
Omega-3-fatty acids (fish oil fatty acids)	Cardiovascular diseases, immune disorders, antioxidant	Warfarin, antiplatelet drugs (eg, aspirin, clopidogrel, ticlopidine)	Increased bleeding and bruising risks. Blocks cyclo-oxygenase and decreases platelet adhesion, with increases in bleeding time (46,47).	Use cautiously. Monitor for unusual bleeding and bruising.
St. John's wort	Antidepressant, anxiolytic	SSRIs (eg, fluoxetine, paroxetine, sertraline, citalopram), MAOI antidepressants (eg, phenelzine)	Little data available on simultaneous use of these drugs with St. John's wort. Theoretically, they could compete for the same receptors or be additive in their effects (9,10,11,29,48).	St. John's wort should only be used under medical supervision. All other medications should be reviewed to minimize potential interactions.
		SSRIs (eg, fluoxetine, paroxetine, sertraline, citalopram)	Risk of inducing a "serotonin syndrome" with symptoms such as confusion, agitation, tremors, seizures (48,49).	St. John's wort should only be used under medical supervision. All other medications should be reviewed to minimize potential interactions.
		Cyclosporine	Decrease in cyclosporine blood levels. Loss of therapeutic effect, with possible transplant rejection (12).	Avoiding combination is recommended. Monitor cyclosporine levels with concurrent use.
		Digoxin	Decreased digoxin levels (13).	Use caution; if combined, monitor digoxin levels and adjust dose accordingly.
		Oral contraceptives	Increased rate of hormone metabolism. Cases of breakthrough and irregular menstrual bleeding. Decreased effectiveness of oral contraceptive therapy is possible (14).	More information needed on this interaction, but caution is advised. Report unusual symptoms to physician.
		Protease inhibitors (HIV drugs) (eg, indinavir, ritonavir, nelfinavir, amprenavir, saquinavir)	Decreased blood levels of these drugs, which may cause treatment failure or drug resistance (15,16).	Avoid combinations.
		Non-nucleoside reverse transcriptase inhibitors (HIV drugs) (eg, nevirapine, delavirdine, efavirenz)	Decreased blood levels of these drugs, which may cause treatment failure or drug resistance (15,16).	No data to confirm at this time. Suspected interaction because herb affects protease inhibitors. Avoid until more is known.

(*continued*)

TABLE E-1 Potential Drug Interactions Between Dietary Supplements/Botanicals and Prescription Drugs (*Continued*)

Dietary Supplement/ Botanical	*Primary Uses or Actions*	*Potential Drug Interactions*	*Potential Outcome(s) of Drug Interaction*	*Recommended Action(s)*
St. John's wort (cont.)		Theophylline	Possible decrease in theophylline blood levels (50).	Only one case report at this time. Caution advised. Monitor theophylline levels if the herb is added to drug regimen.
		Warfarin	Increased warfarin metabolism, with resulting decreased in INR values (secondary to induction of P450-CYP2C9 isozymes) (14).	Risk/benefit must be assessed. If herb added to or removed from warfarin therapy, INR should be monitored until stabilized values are assured.
		Calcium channel blockers (eg, amlodipine, diltiazem, felodipine, isradipine, nicardipine, nifedipine, verapamil)	Possible decreases in calcium channel blocker levels, resulting in increased blood pressure and heart rate and anginal symptoms (17).	Theoretical interaction. No cases yet reported. Monitor blood pressure and heart rate if herb added to therapy.
Saw palmetto	Benign prostatic hypertrophy	Finasteride	Herb and drug may have similar mechanism of action, so additive or antagonistic effects are possible.	Current practice is to avoid until more information is available.
		Testosterone	Herb has antiandrogenic effects (10).	Need more information.
		Oral contraceptives and hormone replacement therapy	Herb has antiestrogenic effects (10,35).	Weight risks versus benefit.
Valerian	Antianxiety, sleep aid	Benzodiazepines (eg, diazepam, glurazepam, lorazepam, alprazolam, temazepam, triazolam), sedatives, CNS depressants	No conclusive reports have shown interactions, but common sense suggests additive potentials with these medications (11, 23,29).	Use caution when combining any medications that cause drowsiness or affect mental functioning, including alcohol. Use low doses of herb initially and titrate to desired response.
		Barbiturates (eg, phenobarbital)	Additive effects could cause excessive sedation (10,11, 23,29).	
		Alcohol	Inconclusive reports with alcohol, but could be additive risk of sedation (10,11,35).	
Vitamin B-6 or pyridoxine	Vitamin associated with neural function	Phenobarbital, phenytoin	Chronic, high-dose pyridoxine consumption may lower blood levels of these two medications. In cases of epilepsy treatment, seizure control could be compromised (6).	If pyridoxine is added to either drug regimen, keep vitamin at lowest effective dose. Monitor therapy with serum drug levels.

(continued)

TABLE E-1 Potential Drug Interactions Between Dietary Supplements/Botanicals and Prescription Drugs (*Continued*)

Dietary Supplement/ Botanical	*Primary Uses or Actions*	*Potential Drug Interactions*	*Potential Outcome(s) of Drug Interaction*	*Recommended Action(s)*
Vitamin E	Many actions	Warfarin	Vitamin E may increase the bleeding risks of patients on warfarin. INR values can be elevated, possibly due to interference with production of vitamin K-dependent clotting factors (5,6,25).	Avoid doses >400 IU/day. If unusual bruising or bleeding occurs, lower dose. Increases in INR and bleeding time are possible.
Yohimbe (plant) Yohimbine (drug)	Erectile dysfunction, hypertension, alpha-2-blocker activity	Tricyclic antidepressants (eg, amitriptyline, nortriptyline)	Can cause fluctuations in blood pressure (23,29).	Avoid combinations.
		MAOI antidepressants (eg, phenelzine)	Herb has mild MAOI activity; additive effects are possible (9,29).	Caution. Best to avoid, monitor for side effects if used.
		Antianxiety medications	May counteract benefits of anxiolytics.	Avoid if possible.
		Stimulants, appetite suppressants, decongestants	Additive stimulant effects. MAOI interaction is possible (eg, increased blood pressure) (29).	Avoid combinations.
		Antihypertensives	Antagonistic effects. Yohimbe can increase blood pressure (29).	Best avoided. If used, monitor blood pressure closely.
		Clonidine	Antagonism of clonidine can precipitate hypertensive crisis or withdrawal symptoms (depending on clonidine usage) (23).	Avoid combination.
		Phenothiazines (eg, prochlorperazine, promethazine, perphenazine)	Increased alpha-2 antagonism (23).	Combination is contraindicated.
Zinc	Immunostimulant, viral illness, enhances athletic performance, diabetes, male fertility	Immunosuppressants	Antagonistic effects (theoretical).	Avoid combination.
		Fluoroquinolones (eg, levofloxacin, ofloxacin, ciprofloxacin) and tetracycline	Zinc can bind these antibiotics in the gut and prevent absorption, resulting in possible treatment failure (29).	Separate administration of zinc from these antibiotics by at least 4 hours.

[a]Sources provided in reference list at end of chapter.

AGENCIES FOR UPDATES AND RESOURCES ON HERBALS, BOTANICALS, DIETARY SUPPLEMENTS

American Botanical Council
P.O. Box 144345, Austin, TX 78714-4345, (512) 926-4900, Fax: (512) 926-2345
Web site: http://www.herbalgram.org

American Cancer Society
Complementary & Alternative Methods / Dietary and Herbal Remedies
Web site: http://www.cancer.org/alt_therapy/nav_dietary.html

American Council on Science and Health
1995 Broadway, Second Floor , New York, NY 10023-5860. (212) 362 7044, Fax: (212) 362-4919
Web site: http://www.acsh.org/

American Dietetic Association
216 West Jackson Boulevard, Suite 800, Chicago, IL 60606-6995
Consumer Nutrition Hotline: (800) 366-1655
Web site: http://www.eatright.org/; http://www.eatright.org/nuresources.html

American Heart Association
Position on Vitamin and Mineral Supplements
Web site: http://www.americanheart.org/Heart_and_Stroke_A_Z_Guide/vitamin.html

American Herbal Products Association
8484 Georgia Ave., Suite 370, Silver Spring, MD 20910. (301) 588-1171, Fax: 301-588-1174
Web site: http://www.ahpa.org/

American Medical Association (AMA)
Vitamins and Minerals
Web site: http://www.ama-assn.org/insight/gen_hlth/vitamins/vitamins.htm

American Nutraceutical Association
Web site: http://www.americanutra.com/association.html

Center for Science in the Public Interest (CSPI)
Nutrition Action Health Letter
1875 Connecticut Avenue, N.W., Suite 300, Washington, D.C. 20009. (202)332-9110, Fax: 202/265-4954
Customer Service Office E-mail: circ@cspinet.org

Consumer Lab.com
Web site: http://www.consumerlab.com/index.html

Ergogenic Aids/Athletic Supplements
Web Site: http://www.geocities.com/HotSprings/Spa/9971/index.html

Federal Trade Commission (FTC)
600 Pennsylvania Avenue, N.W., Washington, D.C. 20580. (202)326-2222
Consumer Response Center: Toll-Free (877)FTC-HELP (382-4357)
Web site: http://www.ftc.gov/ftc/who.htm
Alternative Medicines Web site: http://www.ftc.gov/bcp/conline/pubs/health/whocares/altmeds.htm

U. S. Food and Drug Administration
Center for Food Safety and Applied Nutrition (CFSAN)
200 C Street SW, Washington, DC 20204
Food Information Line: 1-800-FDA-4010
To report a problem or illness caused by a dietary supplement, FDA at 1-800-FDA-1088
Dietary Supplements
Web site: http://vm.cfsan.fda.gov/~dms/supplmnt.html
Special Nutritionals Adverse Event Monitoring System (A searchable database from the FDA)
Web site: http://www.fda.gov/medwatch/how.htm

Food and Nutrition Information Center (FNIC)
National Agricultural Library, Room 304, 10301 Baltimore Avenue, Beltsville, MD 20705-2351.
(301)504-5719, FAX:(301)504-6409
Web site: http://www.nal.usda.gov/fnic/etext/000015.html

Health Care Reality Check
The Georgia Council Against Health Fraud, Inc.
Web site: http://www.hcrc.org/

Herb Research Foundation
1007 Pearl St., Suite 200 Boulder, CO 80302. (800) 748-2617, Outside the USA, (303) 449-2265.
Web site: http://www.herbs.org/

HerbMed Alternative Medicine Foundation, Inc.
Web site: http://www.amfoundation.org/herbmed.htm

Intelihealth
Vitamin and Nutrition Resource Center
Web site: http://www.intelihealth.com/IH/ihtIH/WSIHW000/325/325.html

Institute of Food Technologists
The Society for Food Science and Technology
221 N. LaSalle St., 300, Chicago, IL 60601-1291. (312) 783-8424
Web site: http://www.ift.org/

Journal of Performance Enhancement
Guide to Dietary Supplements
Web site: http://members.tripod.com/mprevost/Supplement_guide_frame.htm

Mayo Health Oasis Clinic
Web site: http://www.mayohealth.org/

MEDLINE Plus Health Information, National Library of Medicine
Vitamin and Mineral Supplements
Web site: http://www.nlm.nih.gov/medlineplus/vitaminandmineralsupplements.html

National Academy of Sciences, Institute of Medicine, Food, and Nutrition Board
Institute of Medicine
2101 Constitution Ave., NW, Washington, D.C. 20418
Web site: http://www4.nas.edu/IOM/IOMHome.nsf/Pages/Food+and+Nutrition+Board

National Council for Reliable Health Information (NCRHI)
P.O. Box 1276, Loma Linda, CA 92354. (909) 824-4690, Fax (909) 824-4838
Web site: http://www.ncrhi.org/

The National Institutes of Health (NIH), National Center for Complementary and Alternative Medicine (NCCAM)
P.O. Box 8218, Silver Spring, MD 20907-8218. (301) 589-5367, Toll Free: (888)644-6226, TTY/TDY: (888)644-6226, Fax: (301)495-4957
Web site: http://altmed.od.nih.gov/

NCCAM's CAM Citation Index (CCI) consists of approximately 180,000 bibliographic citations dated from 1963–1999. The CAM citations were extracted from the National Library of Medicine's MEDLINE database.
Web site: http://nccam.nih.gov/nccam/databases.html

NCCAM Clearinghouse
Web site: http://nccam.nih.gov/nccam/fcp/clearinghouse/index.html

The National Institutes of Health (NIH), National Institute of Mental Health
NIMH Public Inquiries
6001 Executive Blvd., Rm. 8184, MSC 9663, Bethesda, MD 20892-9663. (301) 443-4513, Fax: (301) 443-4279
Web site: http://www.nimh.nih.gov/

The National Institutes of Health, Office of Dietary Supplements
Building 31, Room 1B25, 31 Center Drive, MSC 2086, Bethesda, MD 20892-2086.
(301) 435-2920, Fax: (301) 480-1845
Web site: http://odp.od.nih.gov/ods/about/about.html
Facts about Dietary Supplements: Web site: http://www.cc.nih.gov/ccc/supplements/intro.html

RxList.com
Herbal Monographs and Frequently Asked Questions on Herbs from RxList.com
Web site: http://www.rxlist.com/alternative.htm#herbal_mon

USDA-Iowa State Database of the Isoflavone Content of Foods
Web site: http://www.nal.usda.gov/fnic/foodcomp/Data/isoflav/isoflav.html

U.S. Pharmacopeia
(800) 822-8772
Web site: http://www.usp.org/

U.S. Soy Foods Directory
Indiana Soybean Board
Web site: http://www.soyfoods.com/

Vegetarian Nutrition Dietetic Practice Group
Web site: http://www.andrews.edu/nufs/vndpg.html

The VERIS Research Information Service
Web site: http://www.veris-online.org/default.htm

REFERENCES

Cited references

American Dietetic Association. Position of the American Dietetic Association: phytochemicals and functional foods. *J Am Diet Assoc.* 1995;95:496.

Bensoussan A, et al. Treatment of irritable bowel syndrome with Chinese herbal medicine: a randomized controlled trial. *JAMA.* 1998; 280:1585.

Hamilton K. An overview of herbal and nutritional integrative medicine: a registered dietitian's perspective. *Support Line.* 1998;XX:5.

Hankin J. Keeping up with the increasing popularity of nonvitamin, nonmineral supplements. *J Am Diet Assoc.* 2000;100:419.

Heber D, et al. Cholesterol-lowering effects of a proprietary Chinese red-yeast-rice dietary supplement. *Am J Clin Nutri.* 1999;69:231.

King A, Young G. Characteristics and occurrence of phenolic phytochemicals. *J Am Diet Assoc.* 1999;99:21.

Lee Y, et al. The knowledge, attitudes, and practices of dietitians licensed in Oregon regarding functional foods, nutrient supplements, and herbs as complementary medicine. *J Am Diet Assoc.* 2000;100:543.

Libster M. Guidelines for selecting a medical herbalist for consultation and referral: consulting a medical herbalist. *J Alt and Complementary Medicine.* 1999;5:457.

McCaskill D, Zhang F. Use of rice bran oil in foods. *Food Technology.* 1999;53:50.

Miller L. Herbal medicinals: selected clinical considerations focusing on known or potential drug–herb interactions. *Arch Int Med.* 1998;158:2200.

Radimer K, et al. Nonvitamin, nonmineral dietary supplements: issues and findings from NHANES III. *J Am Diet Assoc.* 2000;100: 447.

Sarubin A. *A health professional's guide to popular dietary supplements.* Chicago, IL: The American Dietetic Association, 2000.

Shah P, Grant K. An overview of common herbal supplements. *Support Line.* 2000;22:3.

Stein K. Herbal supplements or prescription drugs: a risky combination? *J Am Diet Assoc.* 2000;100:412.

White House Commission on Complementary and Alternative Medicine Policy. Executive Summary (http://www.whccamp.hhs.gov)

References for Table E-1

1. Richman A, Witkowski J. Herbs by the numbers. *Whole Foods Magazine.* 1997;10:20.
2. Johnston B. One third of the nation's adults use herbal remedies. *HerbalGram.* 1997;40:49.
3. Eisenberg D. Trends in alternative medicine use in the United States: 1990–1997. *JAMA.* 1998;280:1569.
4. Eisenberg D, Kessler R, Foster C, et al. Unconventional medicine in the United States: prevalence, costs, and patterns of use. *N Engl J Med.* 1993;328:246–252.
5. Hansten P. Drug interactions. In: Yound L, ed. *Applied therapeutics.* 6th ed. Vancouver, WA: Applied Therapeutics, Inc, 1995.
6. American Society of Health-System Pharmacists. *AHFS drug information.* Bethesda, MD: ASHP, Inc, 1998.
7. Bailey D, Arnold J, Spence J. Grapefruit juice and drugs: how significant is the interaction? *Clin Pharmacokin.* 1994;26:91.
8. Brevoort P. The U.S. botanical market: an overview. *HerbalGram.* 1996;36:49.
9. American Herbal Products Associations. *Botanical safety handbook.* Boca Raton, FL: CRC Press, 1997.
10. Miller L. Herbal medicinals: selected clinical considerations focusing on known or potential drug-herb interactions. *Arch Intern Med.* 1998;158:2200.
11. Klepser T, Klepser M. Unsafe and potentially safe herbal therapies. *Am J Health-Syst Pharm.* 1999;56:125.
12. Ruschitzka F, Meier P, Turina M. Acute heart transplant rejection due to St. John's wort. *Lancet.* 2000;355:548.
13. Johne A, Brockmoller J, Bauer S. Pharmacokinetic interaction of digoxin with an herbal extract from St. John's wort (*Hypericum perforatum*). *Clin Pharmacol Ther.* 1999;66:338.
14. Yue Q, Berquist C, Gerden B. Safety of St. John's wort (*Hypericum perforatum*). *Lancet.* 2000;355:575.
15. Lumpkin M, Alpert S. *Risk of drug interactions with St. John's wort and indinavir and other drugs.* Washington, DC: FDA CDER Public Health Advisory, 2000. URL: www.fda.gov/cder/drug/advisory/stjwort.htm
16. Piscitelli S, Burstein A, Chaitt D, et al. Indinavir concentrations and St. John's wort. *Lancet.* 2000;355:547.
17. Pharmacist's Letter/Prescriber's Letter Therapeutic Research Faculty. *Natural medicines comprehensive database.* 1st ed. Stockton, CA: Therapeutic Research Faculty, 2000.
18. Yu C, Chan J, Sanderson J. Chinese herbs and warfarin potentiation by danshen. *J Intern Med.* 1997;241:337.
19. Eisenberg D. Trends in alternative medicine use in the United States: 1990–1997. *JAMA.* 1998;280:1569.
20. Eisenberg D, Kessler R, Foster C, et al. Unconventional medicine in the United States: prevalence, costs, and patterns of use. *N Engl J Med.* 1993;328:246.
21. Hansten P. Drug interactions. In: Yound L, ed. *Applied therapeutics.* 6th ed. Vancouver, WA: Applied Therapeutics, Inc, 1995.
22. American Society of Health-System Pharmacists. *AHFS drug information.* Bethesda, MD: ASHP, Inc, 1998.
23. Bailey D, Arnold J, Spence J. Grapefruit juice and drugs: how significant is the interaction? *Clin Pharmacokin.* 1994;26:91.
24. Brevoort P. The U.S. botanical market: an overview. *HerbalGram.* 1996;36:49.
25. American Herbal Products Associations. *Botanical safety handbook.* Boca Raton, FL: CRC Press, 1997.
26. Miller L. Herbal medicinals: selected clinical considerations focusing on known or potential drug–herb interactions. *Arch Intern Med.* 1998;158:2200.
27. Klepser T, Klepser M. Unsafe and potentially safe herbal therapies. *Am J Health-Syst Pharm.* 1999;56:125.
28. Ruschitzka F, Meier P, Turina M. Acute heart transplant rejection due to St. John's wort. *Lancet.* 2000;355:548.
29. Johne A, Brockmoller J, Bauer S. Pharmacokinetic interaction of

digoxin with an herbal extract from St. John's wort (*Hypericum perforatum*). *Clin Pharmacol Ther*. 1999;66:338.

30. Yue Q, Berquist C, Gerden B. Safety of St. John's wort *(Hypericum perforatum)*. *Lancet*. 2000;355:575.
31. Lumpkin M, Alpert S. *Risk of drug interactions with St. John's wort and indinavir and other drugs*. Washington, DC: FDA CDER Public Health Advisory, 2000. URL: www.fda.gov/cder/drug/advisory/stjwort.htm
32. Piscitelli S, Burstein A, Chaitt D, et al. Indinavir concentrations and St. John's wort. *Lancet*. 2000;355:547.
33. Pharmacist's Letter/Prescriber's Letter Therapeutic Research Faculty. *Natural medicines comprehensive database*. 1st ed. Stockton, CA: Therapeutic Research Faculty, 2000.
34. Yu C, Chan J, Sanderson J. Chinese herbs and warfarin potentiation by danshen. *J Intern Med*. 1997;241:337.
35. Chan K, Lo A, Woo K. The effects of danshen (Salvia miltiorrhiza) on warfarin pharmacodynamics and pharmacokinetics of warfarin enantiomers in rats. *J Pharm Pharmacol*. 1995;47:402.
36. Janetzky K, Morreale A. Probable interaction between warfarin and ginseng. *Am J Health-Syst Pharm*. 1997;54:692.
37. Herbal roulette. *Consumer Reports*. 1995;60:698.
38. The German Commission E. *The complete german E monographs: therapeutic guide to herbal medicines*. 1st ed. Boston, MA: American Botanical Council, 1998.
39. Brinker F. *Herb contraindications and drug interactions*. 2nd ed. Sandy, OR: Eclectic Medical Publications, 1998.
40. Mertz W. Interaction of chromium with insulin: a process report. *Nutr Rev*. 1998;56:174.
41. *MICROMEDEX Healthcare Series*. Vol. 101. Englewood, CO: MICROMEDEX Inc, 1999.
42. Aberg F, Appelkvist E, Broijersen A, et al. Gemfibrozil-induced decrease in serum ubiquinone and alpha- and gamma-tocopherol levels in men with combined hyperlipidemia. *Eur J Clin Invest*. 1998;28:235.
43. Folkers K, Langsjoen P, Willis R, et al. Lovastatin decreases coenzyme Q levels in humans. *Proc Natl Acad Sci (USA)*. 1990;87:8931.
44. Spigset O. Reduced effect of warfarin caused by ubidecarenone. *Lancet*. 1994;334:1372.
45. *Facts and comparisons. the review of natural products*. St. Louis, MO: Wolters Kluwer Company, loose-leaf version (updated quarterly). 1998.
46. Tam L. Warfarin interactions with Chinese traditional medicines: danshen and methyl salicylate medicated oil. *Aust NZ J Med*. 1995;25:258.
47. Lo A, Chan K, Yeung J, et al. Dangqui *(Angelica sinensis)* affects the pharmacodynamics but not the pharmacokinetics of warfarin in rabbits. *Eur J Drug Metab Pharmacokinet*. 1995;20:55.
48. Liu J, Xu S, Yao X, et al. Angelol-type coumarins from Angelica pubescence F. biserrata and their inhibitory effect on platelet aggregation. *Phytochemistry*. 1995;39:1099.
49. Winslow L. Herbs as medicines. *Arch Intern Med*. 1998;158:2192.
50. de Lemos M, Sunderji R. Herbal interactions with warfarin. *Vancouver Hospital & Health Sciences Centre Drug and Therapeutics Newsletter*. May, 1999. Available at http://www.vhpharmsci.com/document/article21.htm. Accessed March 16, 2000.
51. Newall C, Anderson L, Philpson J. *Herbal medicine: a guide for healthcare professionals*. London, UK: The Pharmaceutical Press, 1996.
52. Robbers J, Speedie M, Tyler V. *Pharmacognosy and pharmacobiotechnology*. Baltimore, MD: Williams & Wilkins, 1996.
53. Sunter WH. Warfarin and garlic. *Pharm J*. 1991;246:722.
54. Matthews M Jr. Association of ginkgo biloba with intracerebral hemorrhage. *Neurology*. 1998;50:1993.
55. Rowin J, Lewis S. Spontaneous bilateral subdural hematosis associated with chronic ginkgo biloba ingestion have also occurred. *Neurology*. 1996;46:1775.
56. Fuhr U. Drug interactions with grapefruit juice: extent, probable mechanism and clinical relevance. *Drug Safety*. 1998;18:251.
57. Ameer B, Weintraub R. Drug interactions with grapefruit juice. *Clin Pharmacokinet*. 1997;33:103.
58. Upton R, ed. *Hawthorn leaf with flower: quality control, analytical and therapeutic monograph*. Santa Cruz, CA: American Herbal Pharmacopoeia, 1999; 1–29.
59. Almeida J, Grinsley E. Coma from a health food store: interaction between kava and alprazolam. *Ann Intern Med*. 1996;125:940.
60. Messiha F. Fluoxetine: adverse effects and drug interactions. *J Toxicol; Clin Toxicol*. 1993;31:603.
61. Holt G. *Food & possible interactions with drugs: revised and expanded edition*. Chicago, IL: Precept Press, 1998.
62. *Nonherbal dietary supplements. Pharmacist's letter continuing education booklet*. 1998;98:1–51.
63. Martindale W. *Martindale: the extra pharmacopoeia*. Taunton, MA: Pharmaceutical Press, 1999.
64. Gordon J. SSRIs and St. John's wort: possible toxicity? *Am Fam Physician*. 1998;57:950.
65. Mills K. Serotonin syndrome: a clinical update. *Crit Care Clin*. 1997;13:763.
66. Nebel A, Schneider B, Baker R. Potential metabolic interaction between St. John's wort and theophylline. *Ann Pharmacother*. 1999;33:502.

Suggested Resources

American Botanical Council. *The complete German commission E monographs: therapeutic guide to herbal medicines*. Boston, MA: Integrative Medicine Communications, 1998.

American Dietetic Association / Hudnall M. *Vitamins, minerals, and dietary supplements*. New York: John Wiley & Sons, 1999. Web site: http://www.eatright.org/.

American Dietetic Association/American Pharmaceutical Association Special Report. *Health care professional's guide to evaluating dietary supplements*. From the Joint Working Group on Dietary Supplements, 2000. Web site: http://www.eatright.org/.

American Herbal Products Association. *Botanical safety handbook*. Boca Raton, FL: CRC Press, 1997.

Brinker F. *Herb contraindications and drug interactions*. Sandy, OR: Eclectic Medical Publications, 1998.

Cohen MH, Eisenberg DM. Potential physician malpractice liability associated with complementary and integrative medical therapies. Ann Intern Med 2002;136:596.

Helmsfield S, et al. Garcinia cambogia (hydroxycitric acid) as a potential antiobesity agent: a randomized controlled trial. *JAMA*. 1998; 280:1610.

Michalczyk D. Complementary/alternative medicine: another path to MNT coverage? *J Am Diet Assoc*. 2000;100:632.

PDR for herbal medicine: physician's desk reference for herbal medicines. Montvale, NJ: Medical Economics Company, 1998. Web site: http://www.emery-pratt.com/PromoMed/pdrherbal.htm (ordering information); http://www.pdr.net/ for electronic edition.

Pierce A. *American pharmaceutical practical guide to natural medicines*. New York: The Stonesong Press, Inc., 1999.

Pszczola D. Addressing functional problems in fortified foods. *Food Technology*. 1998;52:38.

Robbers J, Tyler V. *Tyler's herbs of choice: the therapeutic use of phytomedicinals*. Binghamton, NY: Haworth Herbal Press, 1999.

Sinclair S. Migraine headaches: nutritional, botanical, and other alternative approaches. *Altern Med Rev*. 1999;4:86.

Tyler V. *The honest herbal: a sensible guide to the use of herbs and related remedies*. 4th edition. New York: Pharmaceutical Products Press, 1999.

United States General Accounting Office. Report to Congressional Committees Food Safety. *Improvements needed in overseeing the safety of dietary supplements and "functional foods."* Washington, DC: Government Printing Office, 2000.

Winslow L, Roll D. Herbs as medicines. *Arch Int Med*. 1998;158:2192.

Winter H. *Vitamins, herbs, minerals, & supplements: the complete guide*. Tucson, AZ: Fisher Books, 1998.

INDEX

Note: Page numbers followed by f indicate figures; those followed by t indicate tables.

G

T